APPLIED
Biopharmaceutics & Pharmacokinetics

fourth edition

Notice

APPLIED Biopharmaceutics & Pharmacokinetics

fourth edition

Leon Shargel, PhD
Vice President and Technical Director
National Association of Pharmaceutical Manufacturers
Ronkonkoma, New York

Adjunct Associate Professor
School of Pharmacy
University of Maryland
Baltimore, Maryland

Andrew Yu, PhD
Associate Professor of Pharmaceutics
Albany College of Pharmacy
Albany, New York*

*Present affiliation
HFD-520 CDER, FDA, Rockville, MD.
(The contents of this book reflect the personal views of the authors and not that of the FDA.)

McGraw-Hill
Medical Publishing Division

New York St. Louis San Francisco Auckland Bogotá Caracas Lisbon London
Madrid Mexico City Milan Montreal New Delhi San Juan
Singapore Sydney Tokyo Toronto

Applied Biopharmaceutics & Pharmacokinetics, Fourth Edition

3 4 5 6 7 8 9 0 HPC/HPC 0 9 8 7 6 5 4 3 2 1 0

ISBN: 0-8385-0278-4

Library of Congress Cataloging-in-Publication Data

Shargel, Leon, 1941–
Applied biopharmaceutics and pharmacokinetics / Leon Shargel, Andrew Yu. —4th ed.
p. cm.
Includes bibliographical references and index.
ISBN 0-8385-0278-4 (case : alk. paper)
1. Biopharmaceutics. 2. Pharmacokinetics. I. Yu, Andrew B. C., 1945– . II. Title
[DNLM: 1. Biopharmaceutics. 2. Pharmacokinetics. QV 38 S531a 1999]
RM301.4.S52 1999
615′.7—dc21
DNLM/DLC
for Library of Congress 98-49079

Editor-in-Chief: Cheryl L. Mehalik
Production Service: York Production Services
Art Coordinator: Eve Siegel
Cover Design: Aimee Nordin
Illustrator: Wendy Beth Jackelow

CONTENTS

15. MULTIPLE-DOSAGE REGIMENS / 419

16. NONLINEAR PHARMACOKINETICS / 449

17. APPLICATION OF PHARMACOKINETICS IN CLINICAL SITUATIONS / 475

PREFACE TO THE 4TH EDITION

For this edition, we have included the theme of active learning and outcome-based objectives. Moreover, we have continued to integrate basic pharmaceutical sciences with clinical pharmacy practice. As with our previous editions, we have emphasized the understanding of the basic concepts in biopharmaceutics and pharmacokinetics and the application of these concepts to drug therapy.

Basic biopharmaceutic and pharmacokinetic principles are supplemented, whenever possible, with situation analysis questions designed to engage students to learn not just "the basic facts and equations" but to "analyze and integrate" these principles into patient care and drug consultation situations. Although drug therapy is not the primary goal of this text, a greater clinical focus has been included in the chapters, and over 50 new drugs entries are cited in this new edition. New developments and changes in biopharmaceutics, bioavailability, population pharmacokinetics, pharmacodynamics, metabolism, and drug delivery are presented. This new edition may be used as a textbook for an integrated course in biopharmaceutics and pharmacokinetics or as the textbook for each course taught separately.

Encouraging active learning in biopharmaceutics and pharmacokinetics requires the creation of a text with minimum mathematical skills and illustrative problem solving examples. In this edition, we revised our learning objectives and added several new features:

Learning Problems

These elements assist in learning basic biopharmaceutic and pharmacokinetic concepts including computation skills by problem solving. Peer discussions are encouraged. The learning objectives include understanding basic kinetic concepts, applying equations, and doing dose calculations. Solutions with annotated comments are provided at the end of the book.

Practice Focus

Advanced skills are examined here that are necessary beyond the basics in applying biopharmaceutic and pharmacokinetic knowledge to drug therapy. Some of the situations considered include: how basic pharmacokinetics can be applied to drug-specific situations when some key information is missing; what pharmacokinetic parameters and assumptions are necessary for proper drug therapy; how valid are the data and the pharmacokinetic assumptions; and how practitioners deal with problems of missing information in clinical practice. The practical focus shows how drug therapy can be optimized using basic biopharmaceutics and pharmacokinetic principles.

FAQ for Each Chapter

These sections are designed to clarify frequently asked questions on biopharmaceutic and pharmacokinetic concepts and their applications often encountered by students during self-learning or didactic lectures. From our experience, an alternative approach may make sense for some readers and give fresh insight to others.

Application of Pharmacokinetics to Drug Therapy

The application of pharmacokinetics to drug therapy using pharmacokinetic models is more fully discussed using an integrated approach. Basic pharmacokinetic models are compared with other approaches including physiological models, population pharmacokinetics, statistical moment, clinical pharmacokinetics, and therapeutic drug monitoring.

The success of this textbook is due to the valuable comments from readers, including colleagues; faculty; and students, and academic reviewers who include:

Joseph S. Adir, Ph.D.
Professor and Assistant Dean
Howard University,
College of Pharmacy
Washington, DC

Kim Hancock, Ph.D.
Assistant Professor of
Pharmaceuticals
Ferris State University,
College of Pharmacy

M. Delwar Hussain
Assistant Professor of
Pharmaceutics
University of Wyoming,
School of Pharmacy

Srikumaran Melethil, Ph.D.
Professor of Pharmaceutics & Medicine
University of Missouri-Kansas City

Gail Palmgren, Pharm.D.
Clinical Assistant Professor
Auburn University,
School of Pharmacy

We welcome and appreciate their comments and have incorporated many of their suggestions into this edition. We are grateful to the many students, especially J. Lee and R. Asher, for their contributions.

Leon Shargel
Andrew B.C. Yu

1

REVIEW OF MATHEMATICAL FUNDAMENTALS

The mathematics presented here are for review purposes only. For a more complete discussion of fundamental principles, a suitable textbook in mathematics should be consulted.

ESTIMATION AND THE USE OF CALCULATORS AND COMPUTERS

Most of the mathematics needed for pharmacokinetics and other calculations presented in this book may be performed with pencil, graph paper, and logical thought processes. A scientific calculator with logarithmic and exponential functions will make the calculations less tedious. Special computer softwares (see Appendix B) are available for disease state calculations in clinical pharmacokinetics.

Whenever a calculation affecting drug dose is made, one should mentally approximate whether the answer is correct given the set of information. For example, for a given problem, consider whether the number in the answer has the correct magnitude and units; eg, if the correct answer should be between 100 mg and 200 mg, then answers such as 12.5 mg or 1250 mg would have to be wrong.

The units for the answer to a problem should be carefully checked; eg, if the expected answer is a concentration unit, then mg/L or μg/mL are acceptable; and units such as liters or mg/hr are definitely wrong. Wrong units may be caused by an incorrect substitution or by the selection of an incorrect formula. In pharmacokinetic calculation, the answer is only correct if both the number and the units are correct.

Approximation

Approximation is a useful process for checking whether the answer to a given set of calculations is probably correct. Approximation can be performed with pencil and paper and sometimes with a pencil, graph paper, and ruler. The procedure is especially useful in a busy environment when answers must be checked quickly.

To estimate a series of computations, round the numbers and write the numbers using scientific notation. Then perform the series of calculations, remembering the laws of exponents. For example, estimate the answer to the following problem:

$$\frac{58 \times 489}{2114 \times 0.04} \approx \frac{6 \times 10 \times 5 \times 10^2}{2 \times 10^3 \times 4 \times 10^{-2}} \approx \frac{30 \times 10^3}{8 \times 10} \approx 400$$

The precise answer to the above calculation is 335.4. Notice, the approximated answer should be somewhat less than 400, since $30 \div 8$ is between 3 and 4.

For some pharmacokinetic problems, data, such as time versus drug concentration, may be placed on either regular or semilog graph paper. The approximated answer to the problem may be obtained by inspection of the line that is fitted to all the data points. Graphical methods for solving pharmacokinetic problems are given in the latter half of this chapter.

Calculators

A scientific handheld calculator is essential for calculations. Most scientific calculators have exponential and logarithmic functions which are frequently used in pharmacokinetics. Additional functions such as mean, standard deviation, and linear regression analysis are used to determine the half-life of drugs. Statistical parameters, such as correlation coefficient, are used to determine how well the model agrees with the observed data.

Exponents and Logarithms

Exponents

In the expression,

$$N = b^x \tag{1.1}$$

x is the exponent, b is the base, and N represents the number when b is raised to the xth power, ie, b^x. For example,

$$1000 = 10^3$$

whereby 3 is the exponent, 10 is the base, and 10^3 is the third power of the base, 10. The numeric value, N in equation 1.1, is 1000. In this example, it can be reversely stated that the log of N to the base 10 is 3. Thus, taking the log of the number N has the effect of "compressing" the number; some numbers are easier to handle when "compressed" or transformed to base 10. Transformation simplifies many mathematical operations.

Laws of Exponents	Example
$a^x \cdot a^y = a^{x+y}$	$10^2 \cdot 10^3 = 10^5$
$(a^x)^y = a^{xy}$	$(10^2)^3 = 10^6$
$\frac{a^x}{a^y} = a^{x-y}$	$\frac{10^2}{10^4} = 10^{-2}$
$\frac{1}{a^x} = a^{-x}$	$\frac{1}{10^2} = 10^{-2}$
$\sqrt[y]{a} = a^{1/y}$	$\sqrt[3]{a} = a^{1/3}$

Logarithms

The logarithm of a positive number N to a given base b is the exponent (or the power) x to which the base must be raised to equal the number N. Therefore, if

$$N = b^x \tag{1.2}$$

then

$$\log_b N = x \tag{1.3}$$

For example, with common logarithms (log), or logarithms using base 10,

$$100 = 10^2$$
$$\log 100 = 2$$

The number 100 is considered the *antilogarithm* of 2.

Natural logarithms (ln) use the base e, whose value is 2.718282. To relate natural logarithms to common logarithms, the following equation is used:

$$2.303 \log N = \ln N \tag{1.4}$$

Exponential Expression	**Logarithmic Statement**
$10^3 = 1000$	$\log 1000 = 3$
$10^2 = 100$	$\log 100 = 2$
$10^1 = 10$	$\log 10 = 1$
$10^0 = 1$	$\log 1 = 0$
$10^{-1} = 0.1$	$\log 0.1 = -1$
$10^{-2} = 0.01$	$\log 0.01 = -2$
$10^{-3} = 0.001$	$\log 0.001 = -3$

Laws of Logarithms

$$\log ab = \log a + \log b$$

$$\log \frac{a}{b} = \log a - \log b$$

$$\log a^x = x \log a$$

$$-\log \frac{a}{b} = + \log \left(\frac{b}{a}\right)$$

Of special interest is the following relationship:

$$\ln e^{-x} = -x \tag{1.5}$$

Equation 1.5 can be compared with the following example:

$$\log 10^{-2} = -2$$

A logarithm does not have units. A logarithm is dimensionless and is considered a real number. The logarithm of 1 is zero; the logarithm of a number less than 1 is a negative number, and the logarithm of a number greater than 1 is a positive number.

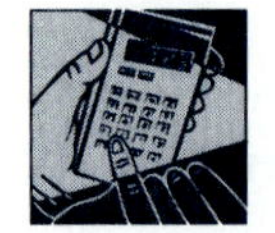

PRACTICE PROBLEMS

Many calculators and computers have logarithmic and exponential functions. The following problems review methods for calculations involving logarithmic or exponential functions using a calculator. Earlier editions of this text demonstrate the use of logarithmic and exponential tables to perform these problems. Before starting any new calculations, be sure to clear the calculator of any previous numbers.

1. Find the log of 35.

Solution
Enter the number 35 into your calculator.
Press the LOG function key.
Answer = 1.5441
(For some calculators, the LOG function key is pressed first, followed by the number; the answer is obtained by pressing the = key).
Notice that the correct answer for log 35 is the same as calculating the exponent of 10, which will equal 35 as shown below.

$35 = 10^{1.5441}$

Estimation—Since the number 35 is between 10 and 100 (ie, 10^1 and 10^2), then the log of 35 must be between 1.0 and 2.0.

2. Find the log of 0.028
Estimation—Since the number 0.028 is between 10^{-1} and 10^{-2}, then the log of 0.028 must be between −1.0 and −2.0.

Solution
Use the same procedure above.
Enter the number 0.028 into your calculator.
Press the LOG function key.
Answer = −1.553

3. Find the antilog of 0.028.
The process for finding an antilog is the reverse of finding a log. The antilog is the number that corresponds to the logarithm, such that the antilog for 3 (in base 10) is 1000 (or 10^3). This problem is the inverse of Practice Problem 2, above. In this case, the calculation determines what the number is when 10 is raised to 0.028 (ie, $10^{0.028}$).

Solution
The following methods may be used, depending upon the type of calculator being used.

Method 1
If your calculator has a function key marked 10^x then do the following:
Enter 0.028.
Press 10^x.
Answer = 1.0666

Method 2
Some calculators assume that the user knows that 10^x is the *inverse* of log x. For this calculation:
Enter 0.028.
Press the key marked INV.
Then press key marked LOG.
Answer = 1.0666

4. Evaluate $e^{-1.3}$

Solution
The following methods may be used, depending upon the type of calculator being used.

Method 1
If your calculator has a function key marked e^x, then do the following:
Enter 1.3.
Change the sign to minus by pressing the key marked ±.
Press e^x.
Answer = 0.2725

Method 2
Some calculators assume that the user knows that e^x is the *inverse* of ln x. For this calculation:
Enter 1.3.
Change the sign to minus by pressing the key marked ±.
Press the key marked INV.
Then press key marked LN.
Answer = 0.2725
Thus, $e^{-1.3} = 0.2725$

5. Find the value of k in the following expression:

$$25 = 50e^{-4k}$$

Solution

$$e^{-4k} = \frac{25}{50} = 0.50$$

Take the natural logarithm, ln for both sides of the equation:

$$\ln e^{-4k} = \ln 0.50$$

From Equation 1.5, $\ln e^{-x} = -x$. Therefore, $\ln e^{-4k} = -4k$ and $\ln 0.50 = -0.693$ (Calculator: Enter 0.5, then press LN function key.)

$$-4k = -0.693$$
$$k = -0.693/-4 = 0.173$$

6. A very common problem in pharmacokinetics is to evaluate an expression such as

$$C_p = C_p^0 e^{-kt}$$

For example, find the value of C_p in the following equation when $t = 2$:

$$C_p = 35e^{-0.15t}$$

Solution

Using a calculator:
Enter 0.15
Press ± key = −0.15
Multiply by 2 = −0.30
Press e^x function key = 0.7408
Multiply by 35 = 25.93

$$C_p = 35e^{-0.15t} = 35(0.7408) = 25.93$$

Because $e^{-x} = 1/e^x$, as the value for x becomes larger, then the value for e^{-x} becomes smaller.

Spreadsheets for Performing Calculations

Spreadsheet software, such as LOTUS 123, QUATRO PRO and EXCEL, is available on many personal computers, including both the MAC and IBM compatible PCs. These spreadsheets are composed of a grid as shown in Figure B-2 of Appendix B. Detailed spreadsheet operation examples are found in Appendix B.

CALCULUS

Since pharmacokinetics considers drugs in the body to be in a dynamic state, calculus is an important mathematic tool for analyzing drug movement quantitatively. Differential equations are used to relate the concentrations of drugs in various body organs over time. Integrated equations are frequently used to model the cumulative therapeutic or toxic responses of drugs in the body.

Differential Calculus

Differential calculus is a branch of calculus that involves finding the rate at which a variable quantity is changing. For example, a specific amount of drug X is placed in a beaker of water to dissolve. The rate at which the drug dissolves is determined by the rate of drug diffusing away from the surface of the solid drug and is expressed by the *Noyes Whitney equation*:

$$\text{Dissolution rate} = \frac{dX}{dt} = \frac{DA}{l}(C_1 - C_2)$$

where d = denotes a very small change; X = drug X; t = time; D = diffusion coefficient; A = effective surface area of drug; l = length of diffusion layer; C_1 = surface concentration of drug in the diffusion layer; and C_2 = concentration of drug in the bulk solution.

The derivative dX/dt may be interpreted as a change in X (or a derivative of X) with respect to a change in t.

In pharmacokinetics, the amount of drug in the body is a variable quantity (dependent variable), and time is considered to be an independent variable. Thus, we consider the amount of drug to vary with respect to time.

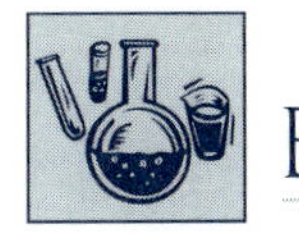

EXAMPLE

The concentration C of a drug changes as a function of time t:

$$C = f(t) \tag{1.6}$$

Consider the following data:

Time (hr)	Plasma Concentration of Drug C (μg/mL)
0	12
1	10
2	8
3	6
4	4
5	2

The concentration of drug C in the plasma is declining by 2 μg/mL for each hour of time. The rate of change in the concentration of the drug with respect to time (ie, derivative of C) may be expressed as:

$$\frac{dC}{dt} = 2\mu\text{g/mL/hr}$$

Here, $f(t)$ is a mathematical equation that describes how C changes, expressed as

$$C = 12 - 2t \tag{1.7}$$

Integral Calculus

Integration is the reverse of differentiation and is considered as the summation of $= f(x) \cdot dx$; the integral sign $\int$ implies summation. For example, given the function $y = ax$, plotted in Figure 1-1, the integration would be $\int ax \cdot dx$. Figure 1-2 is a graph of the function $y = Ae^{-x}$, commonly observed after an intravenous bolus drug injection. The integration process is actually a summing up of the small individual pieces under the graph. When x is specified and is given boundaries from a to b, then the expression becomes a definite integral, ie, summing up of the area from $x = a$ to $x = b$.

A *definite* integral of a mathematical function is the sum of individual areas under the graph of that function. There are several reasonably accurate numerical methods for approximating an area. These methods can be programmed into a computer for rapid calculation. The *trapezoidal rule* is a numerical method frequently used in pharmacokinetics to calculate the area under the plasma–drug concentration versus time curve, called area under the curve (AUC). For example, Figure 1-2 contains a curve depicting the elimination of a drug from the plasma after a

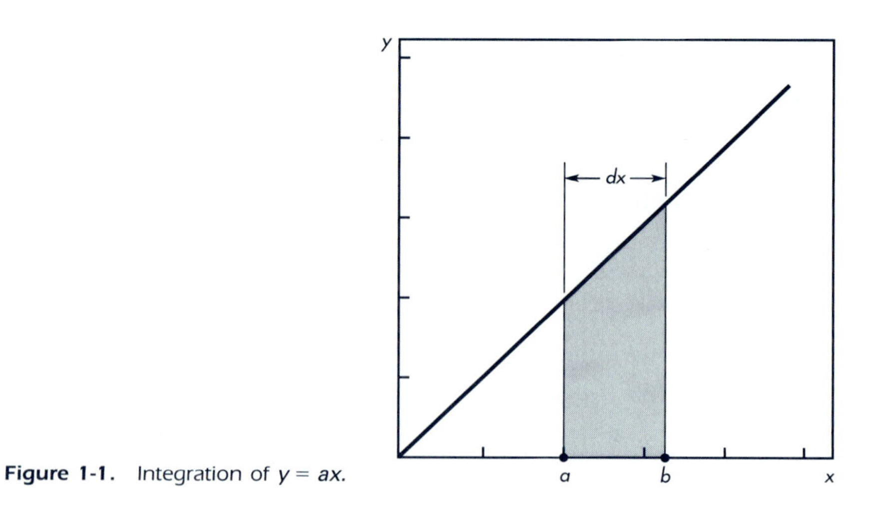

Figure 1-1. Integration of $y = ax$.

single intravenous injection. The drug plasma levels and the corresponding time intervals plotted in Figure 1-2 are as follows:

Time (hr)	Plasma Drug Level μg/mL
0.5	38.9
1.0	30.3
2.0	18.4
3.0	11.1
4.0	6.77
5.0	4.10

The area between time intervals is the area of a trapezoid and can be calculated with the following formula:

$$[\mathrm{AUC}]_{t_{n-1}}^{t_n} = \frac{C_{n-1} + C_n}{2}(t_n - t_{n-1}) \quad \textbf{(1.8)}$$

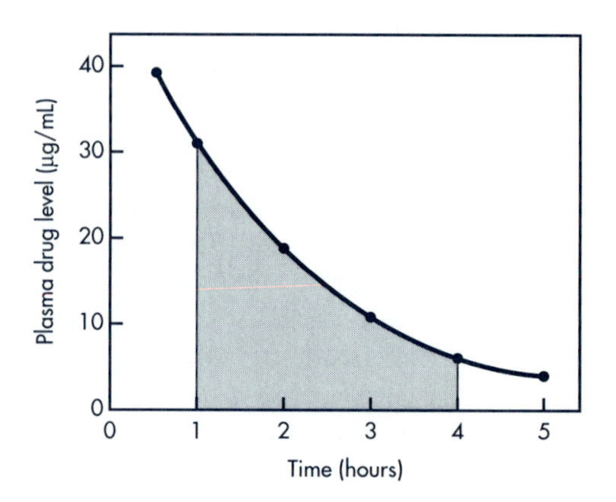

Figure 1-2. Graph of the elimination of drug from the plasma after a single IV injection.

where [AUC] = area under the curve, t_n = time of observation of drug concentration C_n, and t_{n-1} = time of prior observation of drug concentration corresponding to C_{n-1}.

To obtain the AUC from 1 to 4 hours in Figure 1-2, each portion of this area must be summed. The AUC between 1 and 2 hours is calculated by proper substitution into Equation 1.8:

$$[\mathrm{AUC}]_{t1}^{t2} = \frac{30.3 + 18.4}{2}(2 - 1) = 24.35\ \mu\mathrm{g\ hr/mL}$$

Similarly, the AUC between 2 and 3 hours is calculated as 14.75 μg hr/mL, and the AUC between 3 and 4 hours is calculated as 8.94 μg hr/mL. The total AUC between 1 and 4 hours is obtained by adding the three smaller AUC values together.

$$\begin{aligned}[\mathrm{AUC}]_{t1}^{t4} &= [\mathrm{AUC}]_{t1}^{t2} + [\mathrm{AUC}]_{t2}^{t3} + [\mathrm{AUC}]_{t3}^{t4} \\ &= 24.35 + 14.75 + 8.94 \\ &= 48.04\ \mu\mathrm{g\ hr/mL}\end{aligned}$$

The total area under the plasma drug level versus time curve (Fig. 1-2) is obtained by summation of each individual area between two consecutive time intervals using the trapezoidal rule. The value on the y axis when time equals zero is estimated by back extrapolation of the data points using a log linear plot (ie, log y versus x).

This numerical method of obtaining the AUC is fairly accurate if sufficient data points are available. As the number of data points increases, the trapezoidal method of approximating the area becomes more accurate.

The trapezoidal rule assumes a linear or straight-line function between data points. If the data points are spaced widely, then the normal curvature of the line will cause a greater error in the area estimate.

At times, the area under the plasma level time curve is extrapolated to $t = \infty$. In this case the residual area $[\mathrm{AUC}]_{tn}^{t\infty}$ is calculated as follows:

$$[\mathrm{AUC}]_{tn}^{t\infty} = \frac{C_{pn}}{k} \tag{1.9}$$

where C_{pn} = last observed plasma concentration at t_n and k = slope obtained from the terminal portion of the curve.

The trapezoidal rule written in its full form to calculate the AUC from $t = 0$ to $t = \infty$ is as follows:

$$[\mathrm{AUC}]_0^{\infty} = \sum [\mathrm{AUC}]_{tn-1}^{tn} + \frac{C_{pn}}{k}$$

GRAPHS

The construction of a curve or straight line by plotting observed or experimental data on a graph is an important method of visualizing relationships between variables. By general custom, the values of the independent variable (x) are placed on the horizontal line in a plane, or on the abscissa (x axis), whereas the values of the dependent variable are placed on the vertical line in the plane, or on the ordinate (y axis), as demonstrated in Figure 1-3. The values are usually arranged so that they

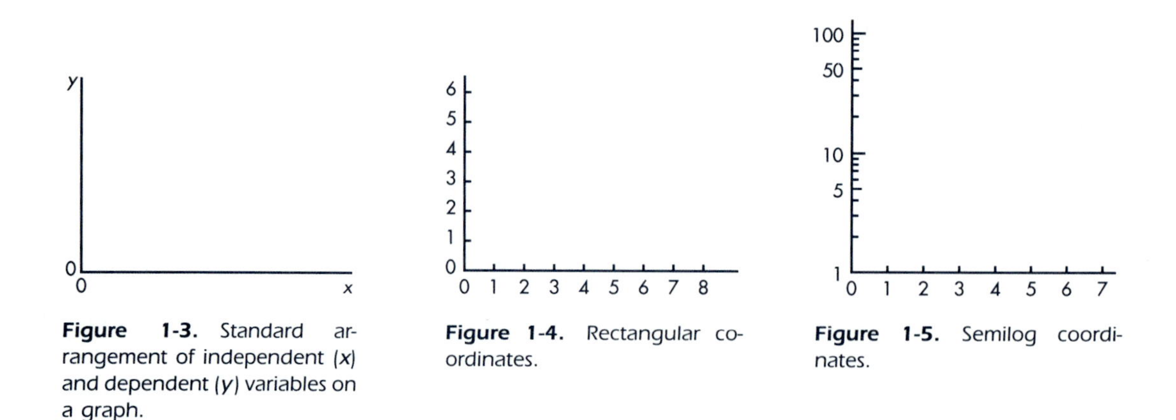

Figure 1-3. Standard arrangement of independent (x) and dependent (y) variables on a graph.

Figure 1-4. Rectangular coordinates.

Figure 1-5. Semilog coordinates.

increase from left to right and from bottom to top. The values may be spaced arbitrarily along each axis to optimize any observable relationships between the two variables.

In pharmacokinetics, time is the independent variable and is plotted on the abscissa (x axis), whereas drug concentration is the dependent variable and is plotted on the ordinate (y axis).

Two types of graph paper are usually used in pharmacokinetics. These are Cartesian or rectangular coordinate graph paper (Fig. 1-4) and semilog graph paper (Fig. 1-5).

Semilog paper is available with one, two, three, or more cycles per sheet, each cycle representing a 10-fold increase in the numbers, or a single $\log_{10}$ unit. This paper allows placement of the data at logarithmic intervals so that the numbers need not be converted to their corresponding log values prior to plotting on the graph.

Curve Fitting

Fitting a curve to the points on a graph implies that there is some sort of relationship between the variables x and y, such as dose of drug versus pharmacologic effect (eg, lowering of blood pressure). Moreover, the relationship is not confined to isolated points but is a continuous function of x and y. In many cases, a hypothesis is made concerning the relationship between the variables x and y. Then, an empirical equation is formed that best describes the hypothesis. This empirical equation must satisfactorily fit the experimental or observed data.

Physiological variables are not always linearly related. However, the data may be arranged or transformed to express the relationship between the variables as a straight line. Straight lines are very useful for accurately predicting values for which there are no experimental observations. The general equation of a straight line is

$$y = mx + b \tag{1.10}$$

where m = slope and b = y intercept. Equation 1.10 could yield any one of the graphs shown in Figure 1-6, depending on the value of m. The absolute magnitude of m gives some idea of the steepness of the curve. For example, as the value of m approaches 0, the line becomes more horizontal. As the absolute value of m be-

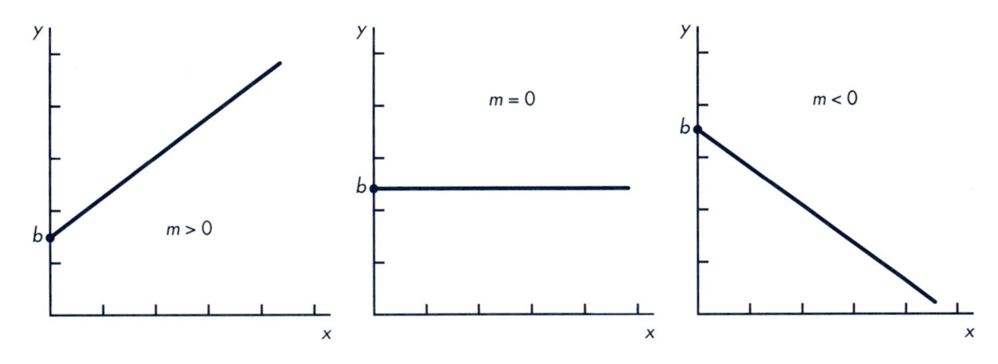

Figure 1-6. Graphic demonstration of variations in slope (m).

comes larger, the line slopes further upward or downward, depending on whether m is positive or negative, respectively. For example, the equation

$$y = -15x + 7$$

would indicate a slope of -15 and a y intercept at $+7$. The negative sign indicates that the curve is sloping downward from left to right.

Determination of the Slope

Slope of a Straight Line on a Rectangular Coordinate Graph

The value of the slope may be determined from any two points on the curve (Fig. 1-7). The slope of the curve is equal to $\Delta y/\Delta x$, as shown in the following equation:

$$\text{Slope} = \frac{y_2 - y_1}{x_2 - x_1} \qquad \textbf{(1.11)}$$

The slope of the line plotted in Figure 1-7 would be

$$m = \frac{2 - 3}{3 - 1} = \frac{-1}{2}$$

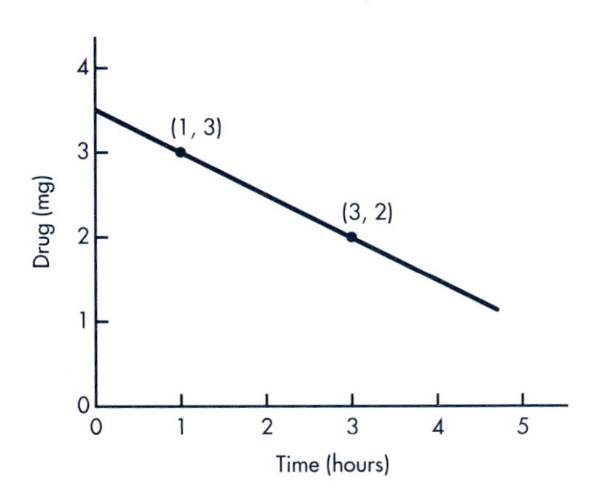

Figure 1-7. Graphic representation of a line with a slope value of $m = -1/2$.

Because the y intercept is equal to 3.5, the equation for the curve by substitution into Equation 1.10 would be

$$y = -\frac{1}{2}x + 3.5$$

Slope of a Straight Line on a Semilog Graph

When using semilog paper, the y values are plotted on a logarithmic scale without performing actual logarithmic conversions, whereas the corresponding x values are plotted on a linear scale. Therefore, to determine the slope of a straight line on semilog paper graph, the y values must be converted to logarithms, as shown in the following equation:

$$\text{Slope} = 2 \cdot 3\,\frac{(\log y_2 - \log y_1)}{x_2 - x_1} = \frac{\ln y_2 - \ln y_1}{x_2 - x_1} \qquad \textbf{(1.12)}$$

The slope value is often used to calculate k, a constant that determines the rate of drug decline:

$$k = 2.3 \text{ slope}$$

Least-Squares Method

Very often an empirical equation is calculated to show the relationship between two variables. Experimentally, data may be obtained that suggest a linear relationship between an independent variable x and a dependent variable y. The straight line that characterizes the relationship between the two variables is called a *regression line.* In many cases, the experimental data may have some error and therefore show a certain amount of scatter or deviations from linearity. The *least-squares method* is a useful procedure for obtaining the line of best fit through a set of data points by minimizing the deviation between the experimental and the theoretical line. In using this method, it is often assumed, out of simplicity, that there is a linear relationship between the variables. If a linear line deviates substantially from the data, it may suggest the need for a nonlinear regression model, although several variables (multiple linear regression) may be involved. Nonlinear regression models are complex mathematical procedures that are best performed with a computer program (see Appendix B).

When the equation of a linear model is examined, the dependent variables can be expressed as the sum of products of the independent *variables* and *parameters.* In nonlinear models, at least one of the parameters appears as other than a coefficient.

For example,

Linear model: $y = ax$, $y = ax + bx + cx^2$, $y = ax + bx_1 + cx^2$,
Nonlinear model: $y = ax/(b + cx)$, $y = 10e^{-3x}$
(a, b, and c are parameters and x and x_1 are variables)

The second nonlinear example as written is nonlinear, but may be transformed to a linear equation by taking the natural log on both sides.

$$\ln y = -3x$$

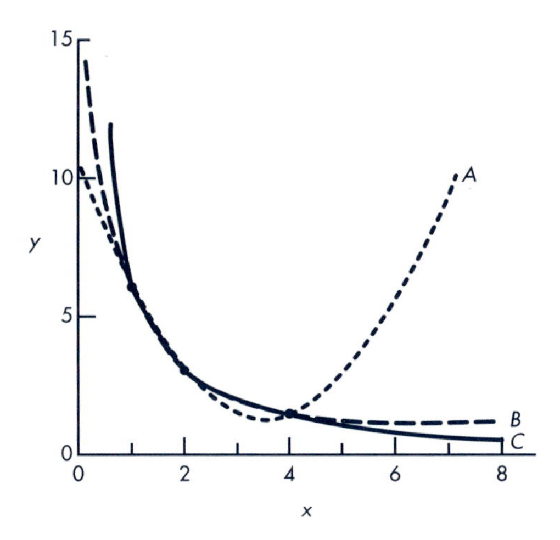

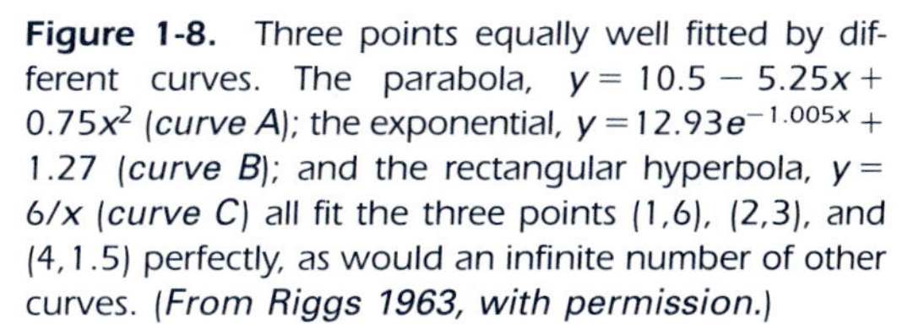
Figure 1-8. Three points equally well fitted by different curves. The parabola, $y = 10.5 - 5.25x + 0.75x^2$ (*curve A*); the exponential, $y = 12.93e^{-1.005x} + 1.27$ (*curve B*); and the rectangular hyperbola, $y = 6/x$ (*curve C*) all fit the three points (1,6), (2,3), and (4,1.5) perfectly, as would an infinite number of other curves. (*From Riggs 1963, with permission.*)

Problems of Fitting Points to a Graph

When x and y data points are plotted on a graph, a relationship between the x and y variables is sought. Linear relationships are useful for predicting values for the dependent variable y, given values for the independent variable x.

The linear regression calculation using the least-squares method is used for calculation of a straight line through a given set of points. However, it is important to realize that, when using this method, one has already assumed that the data points are related linearly. Indeed, for three points, this linear relationship may not always be true. As shown in Figure 1-8, Riggs (1963) calculated three different curves which accurately fit the data. Generally, one should consider the *law of parsimony*, which broadly means "keep it simple"; that is, if a choice between two hypotheses is available, choose the more simple relationship.

If a linear relationship exists between the x and y variables, one must be careful as to the estimated value for the dependent variable y, assuming a value for the independent variable x. *Interpolation*, which means filling the gap between the observed data on a graph, is usually safe and assumes that the trend between the observed data points is consistent and predictable. In contrast, the process of *extrapolation* means predicting new data beyond the observed data, and assumes that the same trend obtained between two data points will extend in either direction beyond the last observed data points. The use of extrapolation may be erroneous if the regression line no longer follows the same trend beyond the measured points.

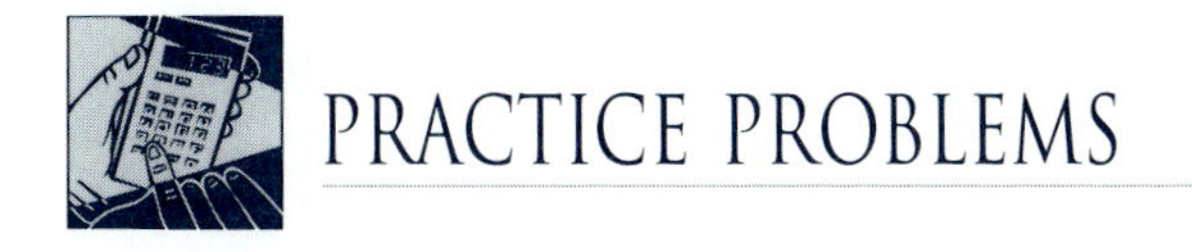

PRACTICE PROBLEMS

1. Plot the following data and obtain the equation for the line that best fits the data by (a) using a ruler and (b) using the method of least squares.

x (mg)	y (hr)	x (mg)	y (hr)
1	3.1	5	15.3
2	6.0	6	17.9
3	8.7	7	22.0
4	12.9	8	23.0

Solution

a. Ruler

Place a ruler on a straight edge over the data points and draw the best line that can be observed. Take any two points and determine the slope by the slope formula given in Equation 1.11 and the y intercept. This method can give a reasonably quick approximation if there is very little scatter in the data.

b. Least-Squares Method

In the least-squares method the slope m and the y intercept b (Eq. 1.13) are calculated so that the average sum of the deviations squared is minimized. The deviation, d, is defined by

$$b + mx - y = d \tag{1.13}$$

If there are no deviations from linearity, then $d = 0$ and the exact form of Equation 1.13 is as follows:

$$b + mx - y = 0$$

To find the slope, m, and the intercept, y, the following equations are used:

$$m = \frac{\sum (x) \sum (y) - n \sum (xy)}{[\sum (x)]^2 - n \sum (x^2)} \tag{1.14}$$

where n = number of data points.

$$b = \frac{\sum (x) \sum (y) - n \sum (x^2) \sum y}{[\sum (x)]^2 - n \sum (x^2)} \tag{1.15}$$

where $\sum$ is the sum of n data points.

Using the data above, tabulate values for x, y, x^2, and xy as shown below:

x	y	x^2	xy
1	3.1	1	3.1
2	6.0	4	12.0
3	8.7	9	26.1
4	12.9	16	51.6
5	15.3	25	76.5
6	17.9	36	107.4
7	22.0	49	154.0
8	23.0	64	184.0
—	—	—	—
$\sum x = 36$	$\sum y = 108.9$	$\sum x^2 = 204$	$\sum xy = 614.7$

Now substitute the values into Equations 1.14 and 1.15.

$$b = \frac{(36)(614.7) - (204)(108.9)}{(36)^2 - (8)(204)} = 0.257 \text{ mg}$$

$$m = \frac{(36)(108.9) - (8)(614.7)}{(36)^2 - (8)(204)} = 2.97 \text{ mg/hr}$$

Therefore, the linear equation that best fits the data is

$$y = 2.97x + 0.257$$

Although an equation for a straight line is obtained by the least-squares procedure, the reliability of the values should be ascertained. A *correlation coefficient*, r is a useful statistical term which indicates the relationship of the x, y data to a straight line. For a perfect linear relationship between x and y, $r = +1$ if the slope is ascending and -1 if the slope is descending. If $r = 0$, then no linear relationship between x and y exists. Usually, $r \geq 0.95$ demonstrates good evidence or a strong correlation that there is a linear relationship between x and y.

2. Determination of Slope Can Be Carried Out Using the Calculator. Many calculators have a statistical linear regression program to determine the slope of the regression line and the coefficient of correlation. The calculator must be cleared and the statistical routine initiated. For regular linear regression, the data may be entered directly in pairs as follows:

a. Linear Regression

Enter Time	Enter Concentration
0	0
2	20
4	40

In this case, the slope should be 10 if linear regression is performed correctly, and the process is zero order. This slope value should be close to the slope determined by graphical method on regular graph paper.

b. Log Linear Regression

In this case, the data below is not a linear relationship but can be transformed (take the log of concentration) to make the data linear. Use the same linear regression program above, except, each time after concentration is entered, press LOG as shown below:

Enter Time	Enter Concentration	Key Stroke
0	10	LOG
2	5	LOG
4	2.5	LOG

The slope obtained should approximate the value determined by graphical method on the semilog paper. The slope value is -0.151.

If the LN key above is pressed each time instead of LOG in all the steps above, the slope would be -0.346, or equal to $-k$, the elimination constant. This is a shortcut method sometimes used to determine k of a first-order process. The regression involves regressing ln concentration versus time directly, ie, $\ln C$ versus t, since $\ln C = -kt + \text{Intercept}$, the slope m is $-k$ (see later section of this chapter).

UNITS IN PHARMACOKINETICS

For an equation to be valid, the units or dimensions must be constant on both sides of the equation. In pharmacokinetics many different units are used, as listed in Table 1.1. For an accurate equation, both the integers and the units must balance. For example, a common expression for total body clearance is:

$$Cl_T = kV_D \tag{1.16}$$

After insertion of the proper units for each term in the above equation from Table 1.1,

$$\frac{\text{mL}}{\text{hr}} = \frac{1}{\text{hr}}\,\text{mL}$$

Thus, the above equation is valid as shown by the equality mL/hr = mL/hr.

An important rule in using equations with different units is that the units may be added, subtracted, divided, or multiplied as long as the final units are consistent and valid. When in doubt, check the equation by inserting the proper units. For example,

$$\text{AUC} = \frac{FD_0}{kV_D} = \text{concentration} \times \text{time} \tag{1.17}$$

$$\frac{\mu\text{g}}{\text{mL}}\,\text{hr} = \frac{1\ \text{mg}}{\text{hr}^{-1}\ \text{liter}} = \mu\text{g hr/mL}$$

Certain terms have no units. These terms include logarithms and ratios. Percent may have no units and is mathematically expressed as a decimal between 0 and 1

TABLE 1.1 Common Units Used in Pharmacokinetics

PARAMETER	SYMBOL	UNIT	EXAMPLE
Rate	$\frac{dD}{dt}$	$\frac{\text{Mass}}{\text{Time}}$	mg/hr
	$\frac{dc}{dt}$	$\frac{\text{Concentration}}{\text{Time}}$	μg/mL hr
Zero-order rate constant	k_0	$\frac{\text{Concentration}}{\text{Time}}$	μg/mL hr
		$\frac{\text{Mass}}{\text{Time}}$	mg/hr
First-order rate constant	k	$\frac{1}{\text{Time}}$	1/hr or hr^{-1}
Drug dose	D_0	Mass	mg
Concentration	C	$\frac{\text{Mass}}{\text{Volume}}$	μg/mL
Plasma drug concentration	C_p	$\frac{\text{Drug}}{\text{Volume}}$	μg/mL
Volume	V	Volume	mL or L
Area under the curve	AUC	Concentration × time	μg hr/mL
Fraction of drug absorbed	F	No units	0 to 1
Clearance	Cl	$\frac{\text{Volume}}{\text{Time}}$	mL/hr
Half-life	$t_{1/2}$	Time	hr

or as 0 to 100%, respectively. On occasion, percent may indicate mass/volume, volume/volume, or mass/mass. Table 1.1 lists common pharmacokinetic parameters with their symbols and units.

A constant is often inserted in an equation to quantitate the relationship of the dependent variable to the independent variable. For example, *Fick's Law of Diffusion* relates the rate of drug diffusion dQ/dt to the change in drug concentration C, the surface area of the membrane A, and the thickness of the membrane h. In order to make this relationship an equation, a diffusion constant D is inserted:

$$\frac{dQ}{dt} = \frac{DA}{h} \times \Delta C \qquad \textbf{(1.18)}$$

To obtain the proper units for D, the units for each of the other terms must be inserted:

$$\frac{\text{mg}}{\text{hr}} = \frac{D(\text{cm}^2)}{\text{cm}} \times \frac{\text{mg}}{\text{cm}^3}$$

$$D = \text{cm}^2/\text{hr}$$

The diffusion constant D must have the units of area/time or cm^2/hr if the rate of diffusion is in mg/hr.

Graphs should always have the axes (abscissa and ordinate) properly labeled with units. For example, in Figure 1-7 the amount of drug on the ordinate (y axis) is given in milligrams and the time on the abscissa (x axis) is given in hours. The equation that best fits the points on this curve is the equation for a straight line, or $y = mx + b$. Because the slope $m = \Delta y/\Delta x$, then the units for the slope should be milligrams per hour. Similarly, the units for the y intercept b should be the same units as those for y, namely, milligrams.

MEASUREMENT AND THE USE OF SIGNIFICANT FIGURES

Every measurement is performed within a certain degree of accuracy, which is limited by the instrument used for the measurement. For example, the weight of freight on a truck may be accurately measured to the nearest 0.5 kg, whereas the mass of drug in a tablet may be measured to 0.001 g (1 mg). Measuring the weight of freight on a truck to the nearest mg is not necessary and would require a very costly balance or scale to detect a change in a mg quantity.

Significant figures are the number of accurate digits in a measurement. If a balance measures the mass of a drug to the nearest mg, measurements containing digits representing less than a mg are inaccurate. For example, in reading the weight or mass of a drug of 123.8 mg from this balance, the 0.8 mg is only approximate; the number is therefore rounded to 124 mg and reported as the observed mass.

For practical calculation purposes, all figures may be used until the final number (answer) is obtained. However, the answer should retain only the number of significant figures made in the least accurate initial measurement.

UNITS FOR EXPRESSING BLOOD CONCENTRATIONS

Various units have been used in pharmacology, toxicology, and the clinical laboratory to express drug concentrations in blood, plasma, or serum. Drug concentrations or drug levels should be expressed as mass/volume. The expressions mcg/mL, μg/mL, and mg/L are equivalent and are commonly reported in the literature. Drug concentrations may also be reported as mg% or mg/dL, both of which indicate milligrams of drug per 100 mL (deciliter). Two older expressions for drug concentration occasionally used in veterinary medicine are the terms ppm and ppb, which indicate the number of parts of drug per million parts of blood (ppm) or per billion parts of blood (ppb). One ppm is equivalent to 1.0 μg/mL. The accurate interconversion of units is often necessary to prevent confusion and misinterpretation.

STATISTICS

All measurements have some degree of error. An *error* is the difference between the true or absolute value and the observed value. Errors in measurement may be determinate (constant) or indeterminate (random, accidental). Determinate errors may be minimized in analytical procedures by using properly calibrated instrumentation, standardized chemicals, and appropriate blanks and control samples. Indeterminate errors are random and occur due to chance. For practical purposes, several measurements of a given sample are usually performed, and the result averaged. The mean ± SD is often reported. SD or standard deviation (see Appendix A) is a statistical way of expressing the spread between the individual measurements from the mean. A small SD relative to the mean value is indicative of good consistency and reproducibility of the measurements. A large SD indicates poor consistency and data fluctuations. Frequently, the variability of the measurements may be expressed as RSD or relative standard deviation, which is calculated by the SD divided by the mean of the data. RSD allows variability to be expressed on a percent basis and is useful in comparing the variability of two sets of measurements when the means are different.

In measurements involving a single subject or sample, only measuring error is involved. On the other hand, when two or more samples or subjects in a group are measured, there is usually variation due to individual differences. For example, the weight of each student in a class is likely different from the others due to individual physical differences such as height and sex. Therefore, in determining the weight of a group of students, we deal with variations due to biologic differences as well as weighing errors. A major error in group measurement is *sampling error*, an error due to nonuniform sampling. Sampling is essential because the measurement of all members in the group is not practical.

We use statistics to obtain a valid interpretation of the experimental data. Statistics is the logical use of mathematics, which includes (1) experimental design, (2) collection of data, (3) analysis of data, (4) interpretation of data, and (5) hypothesis testing. A more complete discussion of statistics is found in Appendix A.

TABLE 1.2 Dosing Unit Based on Body Weight or Body Surface Area[a]

METHOD	ORAL DRUG UNIT	INFUSION UNIT	REMARKS
General	mg	mg/hr	BW not used
BW	mg/kg	mg/kg/hr	Known BW
BSA	mg/1.73 m^2	mg/1.73 m^2/hr	Estimated BSA

[a]BW, body weight; BSA, body surface area

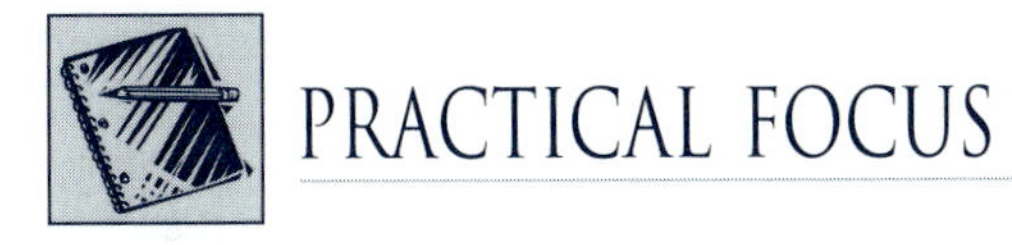

PRACTICAL FOCUS

In pharmacokinetics and therapeutics, plasma or tissue samples are often monitored to determine if a prescribed dose needs to be adjusted. Comparisons of literature data from several medical centers are often made. The pharmacist should to be familiar with all units involving dosing and be able to make conversions. Some physicians prescribe a drug dose based on body weight while others prefer the body surface area method. Significant differences in plasma drug concentrations may result if the dose is based on a different method. Drug concentrations may also be different if a dose is injected rapidly versus infused over a period of time. Table 1.2 lists some of the common methods of dosing.

Most potent drugs are dosed precisely for the individual patient and the body weight of the patient should be known. For example, theophylline is dosed at 5 mg/kg. Since the body weight (BW) of individuals may vary with age, sex, disease, and nutritional states, an individualized dose based on body weight would more accurately reflect the appropriate therapy needed for the patient. For drugs with a narrow therapeutic index and potential for side effects, dosing based on body surface is common. During chemotherapy with antitumor drugs, many drugs are dosed according to the body surface area (BSA) of the patient. The body surface area may be determined from the weight of the patient using the empirical equation:

$$BSA = \left(\frac{BW}{70\ \text{kg}}\right)^{0.73} \times 1.73\ \text{m}^2$$

where BSA = body surface area in square meters, and BW = body weight in kilograms. Some common units and conversions used in pharmacokinetics and toxicology are listed in Table 1.3.

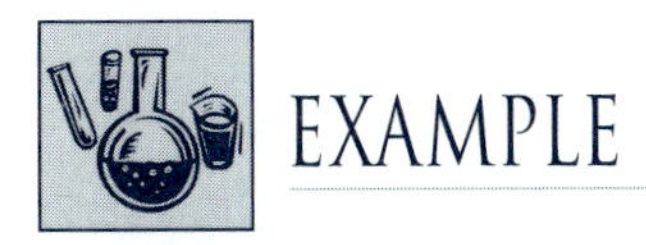

EXAMPLE

The rate of ethanol elimination in four alcoholics undergoing detoxification was reported to be 17 to 33 mg/dL/hr (Jones, 1992). (1) What is the rate of elimination in μg/mL/hr? (2) The peak blood concentration in one subject (SP) is 90 μg/dL, what is his peak blood concentration in μg/mL? (3) Which category would

TABLE 1.3 Pharmacokinetic Units and Conversions

UNITS IN VOLUME	VOLUME (BASED ON BODY WEIGHT)
mL	mL/kg
dL	dL/kg
L	L/kg
CONCENTRATION	**WEIGHT CONVERSION**
gm/L	1 kg = 1000 g
mg/L	1 gm = 1000 mg
mg/dL	1 mg = 1000 μg
mg/mL	1 μg = 1000 ng
ng/mL	1 ng = 1000 pg
pg/mL	
Examples of Concentration Conversion Used in Toxicology and Therapeutics	
1 mg% = 1 mg/dL	
1 mg/L = 1 μg/mL	
1 μg/L = 1 ng/mL	
1 ng/L = 1 pg/mL	

SP belong to according to the following classification for blood alcohol (where values are in mg %)?

a. >0.55 mg %—fatal
b. 0.50–0.55 mg %—dead drunk
c. 0.10–0.50 mg %—illegal
d. 0.05–0.10 mg %—questionable
e. <0.05 mg %—safe

Solution

1. 17 μg/dL/hr = 17000 μg/100 mL/hr = 170 μg/mL/hr
   33 μg/dL/hr = 33000 μg/100 mL/hr = 330 μg/mL/hr
2. 90 mg/dL = 90 μg/100 mL = 0.9 μg/mL
3. 90 mg/dL = 0.090 mg/dL = 0.090 mg %
   Subject SP is questionable.

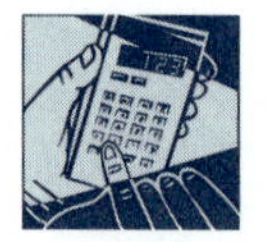

PRACTICE PROBLEM

The volume of distribution of theophylline is *0.7 L/kg*. In most patients, the optimal benefits of theophylline therapy are seen at serum concentration of >10 mg/L, setting a plasma drug concentration of *5 mg/L* lower therapeutic limit may result in reduced clinical efficacy (Eder and Bryan, 1996). (1) What is the volume of distribution of a 20-year-old male patient weighing 70 kg? (2) What is the total dose for the patient if he is dosed at 5 mg/kg?

Solution

(1) (5 mg/L is an alternative way to express 5 μg/mL)
Volume of the patient = 0.7 L/kg × 70 kg = 49 L

(2) Dose of the patient = 5 mg/kg × 70 kg = 350 mg

RATES AND ORDERS OF REACTIONS

Rate

The rate of a chemical reaction of process is the velocity with which the reaction occurs. Consider the following chemical reaction:

drug $A \rightarrow$ drug B

If the amount of drug A is decreasing with respect to time (that is, the reaction is going in a forward direction), then the rate of this reaction can be expressed as follows:

$$-dA/dt$$

Since the amount of drug B is increasing with respect to time, the rate of the reaction can also be expressed as:

$$+dB/dt$$

Usually only the parent (or pharmacologically active) drug is measured experimentally. The metabolites of the drug or the products of the decomposition of the drug may not be known or may be very difficult to quantitate. The rate of a reaction is determined experimentally by measuring the disappearance of drug A at given time intervals.

Rate Constant

The order of a reaction refers to the way in which the concentration of drug or reactants influences the rate of a chemical reaction or process.

Zero-Order Reactions

If the amount of drug A is decreasing at a constant time interval t, then the rate of disappearance of drug A is expressed as

$$\frac{dA}{dt} = -k_0 \qquad \textbf{(1.19)}$$

The term k_0 is the zero-order rate constant and is expressed in units of mass/time (eg, mg/min). Integration of Equation 1.19 yields the following expression:

$$A = -k_0 t + A_0 \qquad \textbf{(1.20)}$$

where A_0 is the amount of drug at $t = 0$. Based on this expression (Eq. 1.20), a graph of A versus t would yield a straight line (Fig. 1-9). The y intercept would be equal to A_0, and the slope of the line would be equal to k_0.

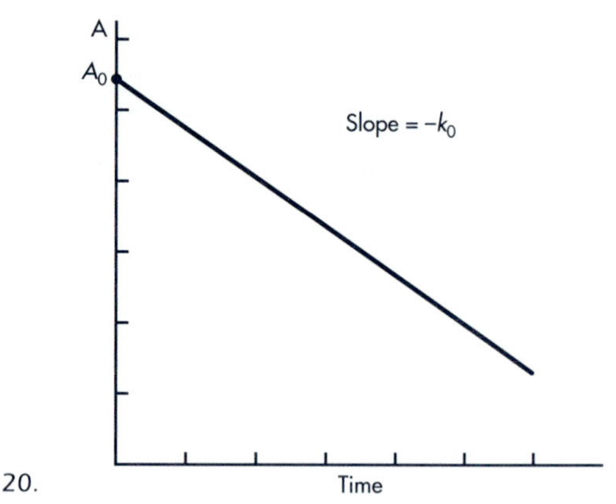

Figure 1-9. Graph of Equation 1.20.

Equation 1.20 may be expressed in terms of drug concentration which can be measured directly.

$$C = -k_0 t + C_0 \qquad \textbf{(1.21)}$$

C_0 is the drug concentration at time 0, C is the drug concentration at time t, k_0 is the zero-order decomposition constant.

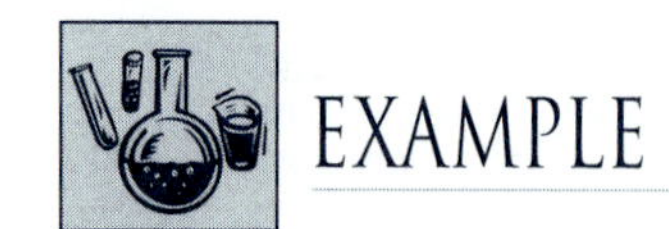

EXAMPLE

A pharmacist weighs exactly 10 g of a drug and dissolves it in 100 mL of water. The solution is kept at room temperature, and samples are removed periodically and assayed for the drug. The pharmacist obtains the following data:

Drug Concentration (mg/mL)	Time (hr)
100	0
95	2
90	4
85	6
80	8
75	10
70	12

From these data, a graph constructed by plotting the concentration of drug versus time will yield a straight line. Therefore, the rate of decline in drug concentration is of zero order.

The zero-order rate constant k_0 may be obtained from the slope of the line or by proper substitution into Equation 1.21.

If

C_0 = concentration of 100 mg/mL at $t = 0$

and

$$C = \text{concentration of 90 mg/mL at } t = 4 \text{ hr}$$

then

$$90 = -k_0(4) + 100$$

and

$$k_0 = 2.5 \text{ mg/mL hr}$$

Careful examination of the data will also show that the concentration of drug declines 5 mg/mL for each 2-hour interval. Therefore, the zero-order rate constant may be obtained by dividing 5 mg/mL by 2 hours:

$$k_0 = \frac{5 \text{ mg/mL}}{2 \text{ hr}} = 2.5 \text{ mg/mL hr}$$

First-Order Reactions

If the amount of drug A is decreasing at a rate that is proportional to the amount of drug A remaining, then the rate of disappearance of drug A is expressed as

$$\frac{dA}{dt} = -kA \qquad (1.22)$$

where k is the first-order rate constant and is expressed in units of time^{-1} (eg, hr^{-1}). Integration of Equation 1.21 yields the following expression:

$$\ln A = -kt + \ln A_0 \qquad (1.23)$$

Equation 1.23 may also be expressed as

$$A = A_0 e^{-kt} \qquad (1.24)$$

Because ln = 2.3 log, Equation 1.23 becomes

$$\log A = \frac{-kt}{2.3} + \log A_0 \qquad (1.25)$$

When drug decomposition involves a solution, starting with initial concentration C_0, it is often convenient to express the rate of change in drug decomposition, dC/dt in terms of drug concentration, C, rather than amount because drug concentration is assayed. Hence,

$$\frac{dC}{dt} = -kC \qquad (1.26)$$

$$\ln C = kt + \ln C_0 \qquad (1.27)$$

Equation 1.27 may be expressed as

$$C = C_0 e^{-kt} \qquad (1.28)$$

Because ln = 2.3 log, Equation 1.27 becomes

$$\log C = \frac{-kt}{2.3} + \log C_0 \qquad (1.29)$$

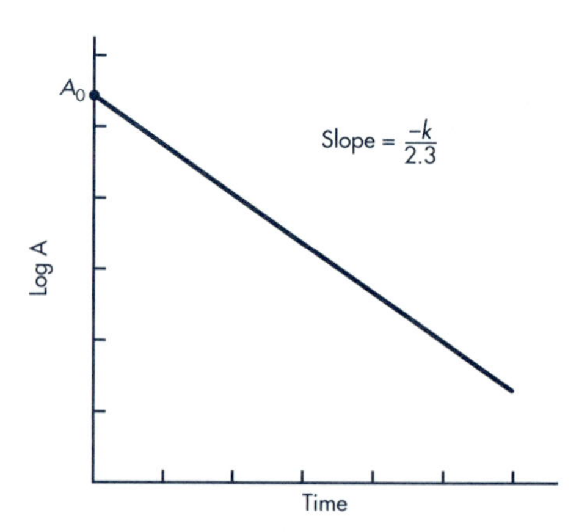

Figure 1-10. Graph of Equation 1.25.

According to Equation 1.25, a graph of log A versus t would yield a straight line (Fig. 1-9), the y intercept would be log A_0, and the slope of the line would be equal to $-k/2.3$ (Fig. 1-10). Similarly, a graph of log C versus t would yield a straight line according to Equation 1.29. The y intercept would be log C_0, and the slope of the line would be equal to $-k/2.3$. For convenience, C versus t may be plotted on semilog paper without the need to convert C to log C. An example is shown in Figure 1-11.

Half-Life

Half-life ($t_{1/2}$) expresses the period of time required for the amount or concentration of a drug to decrease by one half.

First-Order Half-Life

The $t_{1/2}$ for a first-order reaction may be found by means of the following equation:

$$t_{1/2} = 0.693/k \qquad \textbf{(1.30)}$$

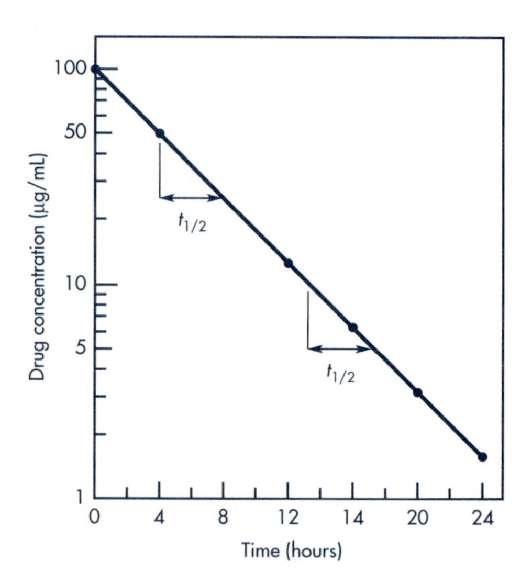

Figure 1-11. This graph demonstrates the constancy of the $t_{1/2}$ in a first-order reaction.

It is apparent from this equation that for a first-order reaction, $t_{1/2}$ is a constant. No matter what the initial amount or concentration of drug is, the time required for the amount to decrease by one half is a constant (Fig. 1-11).

Zero-Order Half-Life

In contrast to the first-order $t_{1/2}$, the $t_{1/2}$ for a zero-order process is not constant. The zero-order $t_{1/2}$ is proportional to the initial amount or concentration of the drug and is inversely proportional to the zero-order rate constant k_0:

$$t_{1/2} = \frac{0.5\ A_0}{k_0} \qquad \textbf{(1.31)}$$

Because the $t_{1/2}$ changes as drug concentrations decline, the zero-order $t_{1/2}$ has little practical value.

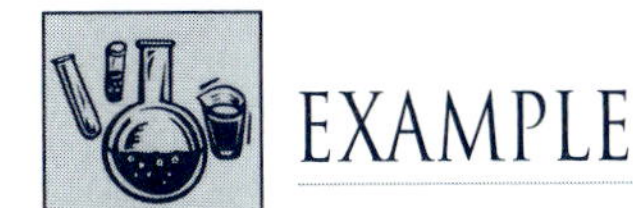

EXAMPLE

A pharmacist dissolves exactly 10 g of a drug into 100 mL of water. The solution is kept at room temperature, and samples are removed periodically and assayed for the drug. The pharmacist obtains the following data:

Drug Concentration (mg/mL)	Time (hr)	Log Drug Concentration
100.0	0	2.00
50.0	4	1.70
25.0	8	1.40
12.5	12	1.10
6.25	16	0.80
3.13	20	0.50
1.56	24	0.20

With these data, a graph constructed by plotting the logarithm of the drug concentrations versus time will yield a straight line on rectangular coordinates. More conveniently, the drug concentration values can be plotted directly at a logarithmic axis on semilog paper against time, and a straight line will be obtained (Fig. 1-11). The relationship of time versus drug concentration in Figure 1-11 indicates a first-order reaction.

The $t_{1/2}$ for a first-order process is constant and may be obtained from any two points on the graph that show a 50% decline in drug concentration. In this example, the $t_{1/2}$ is 4 hr. The first-order rate constant may be found by (1) obtaining the product of 2.3 times the slope or (2) by dividing 0.693 by the $t_{1/2}$, as follows:

$$\text{Slope} = -\frac{k}{2.3} = \frac{\log y_2 - \log y_1}{x_2 - x_1}$$

$$-k = \frac{2.3(\log 50 - \log 100)}{4 - 0} \qquad k = 0.173\ \text{hr}^{-1}$$

$$k = \frac{0.693}{t_{1/2}}$$

$$k = \frac{0.693}{4} = 0.173\ \text{hr}^{-1}$$

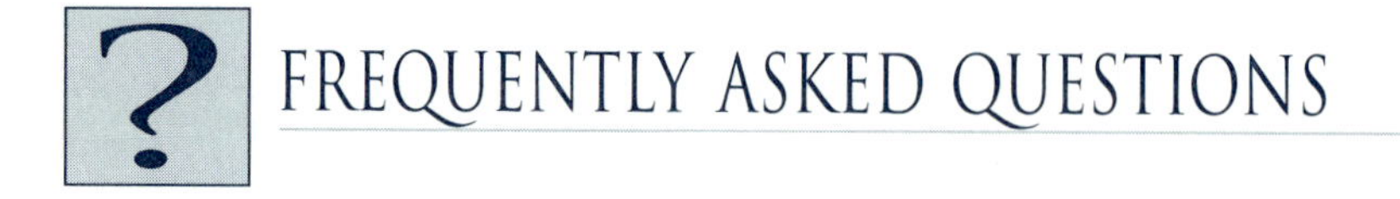

FREQUENTLY ASKED QUESTIONS

1. How do I know my graph is plotted on the semilog paper?

2. I plotted the plasma drug concentration versus time data on semilog paper, and got a slope with an incorrect k. Why?

3. I performed linear regression t versus $\ln C_p$. How do I determine the C_p^0 from the intercept?

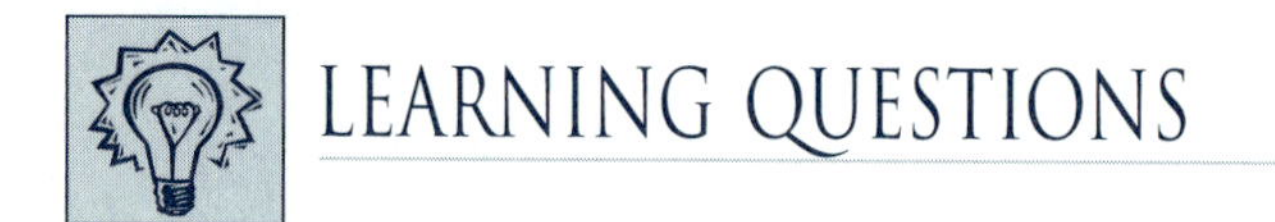

LEARNING QUESTIONS

1. Plot the following data on both semilog graph paper and standard rectangular coordinates.

Time (min)	Drug A (mg)
10	96
20	89
40	73
60	57
90	34
120	10
130	2.5

a. Does the decrease in the amount of drug A appear to be a zero-order or first-order process?

b. What is the rate constant k?

c. What is the half-life $t_{1/2}$?

d. Does the amount of drug A extrapolate to zero on the x axis?

e. What is the equation for the line produced on the graph?

2. Plot the following data on both semilog graph paper and standard rectangular coordinates.

Time (min)	Drug A (mg)
4	70
10	58
20	42

30	31
60	12
90	4.5
120	1.7

Answer Questions **a, b, c, d,** and **e** set forth in the preceding problem.

3. A pharmacist dissolved a few milligrams of a new antibiotic drug into exactly 100 mL of distilled water and placed the solution in a refrigerator (5°C). At various time intervals, the pharmacist removed a 10-mL aliquot from the solution and measured the amount of drug contained in each aliquot. The following data were obtained.

Time (hr)	Antibiotic (μg/mL)
0.5	84.5
1.0	81.2
2.0	74.5
4.0	61.0
6.0	48.0
8.0	35.0
12.0	8.7

a. Is the decomposition of this antibiotic a first-order or zero-order process?
b. What is the rate of decomposition of this antibiotic?
c. How many milligrams of antibiotics were in the original solution prepared by the pharmacist?
d. Give the equation for the line that best fits the experimental data.

4. A solution of a drug was freshly prepared at a concentration of 300 mg/mL. After 30 days at 25°C, the drug concentration in the solution was 75 mg/mL.
a. Assuming first-order kinetics, when will the drug decline to one half of the original concentration?
b. Assuming zero-order kinetics, when will the drug decline to one half of the original concentration?

5. How many half-lives ($t_{1/2}$) would it take for 99.9% of any initial concentration of a drug to decompose? Assume first-order kinetics.

6. If the half-life for decomposition of a drug is 12 hours, how long will it take for 125 mg of the drug to decompose 30%? Assume first-order kinetics and constant temperature.

7. Exactly 300 milligrams of a drug is dissolved into an unknown volume of distilled water. After complete dissolution of the drug, 1.0-mL samples were removed and assayed for the drug. The following results were obtained:

Time (hr)	Concentration (mg/mL)
0.5	0.45
2.0	0.3

Assuming zero-order decomposition of the drug, what was the original volume of water in which the drug was dissolved?

8. For most drugs, the overall rate of drug elimination is proportional to the amount of drug remaining in the body. What does this imply about the kinetic order of drug elimination?

9. A single cell is placed into a culture tube containing nutrient agar. If the number of cells doubles every 2 minutes and the culture tube is completely filled in 8 hours, how long does it take for the culture tube to be only half full of cells?

10. The volume of distribution of warfarin is 9.8 ± 4.2 L. Assuming normal distribution, this would mean that 95% of the subjects would have a volume of distribution ranging from ____ L to ____ L.

11. Which of the following functions has the steepest declining slope? (t is the independent variable and y is the dependent variable.)
a. $y = 2\ e^{-3t}$
b. $y = 3\ e^{-2t}$
c. $y = 2\ e^{t}$

12. Which of the following equations predicts y increasing as t increases? (t is a positive number.)
a. $y = 2\ e^{-3t}$
b. $y = 3\ e^{-2t}$
c. $y = 2\ e^{t}$

13. Which of the following would result in an error message when you take the log of x using the calculator?
a. $x = 2.5$
b. $x = 0.024$
c. $x = 10^{-2}$
d. $x = -0.2$

14. Which of the following equation(s) would have the greatest value at t equal to zero assuming t is not negative.
a. e^{-3t}
b. $3\ e^{-2t}$
c. $2/e^{t}$

REFERENCES

Riggs DS: *The Mathematical Approach to Physiological Problems.* Baltimore, Williams & Wilkins, 1963, p 51

BIBLIOGRAPHY

Bolton S: *Pharmaceutical Statistics.* New York, Marcel Dekker, 1984

Eder AF, Bryan WA: Theophylline: Recent consensus and current controversy. *Am Assoc Clin Chem* TDX/Tox, **17:** Jan, p1051, 1996

Jones AW: Disappearance rate of ethanol from the blood of human subjects: Implications in forensic toxicology. *J Forensic Sci* May, 104–118, 1992

Randolph LK, Cuminera JL: Statistics. In Gennaro AR (ed), *Remington's Pharmaceutical Sciences,* 17th ed. Easton, Mack, 1985, pp 104–139

Thomas GB: *Calculus and Analytic Geometry.* Reading, MA, Addison-Wesley, 1960

2

INTRODUCTION TO BIOPHARMACEUTICS AND PHARMACOKINETICS

BIOPHARMACEUTICS

Biopharmaceutics considers the interrelationship of the physicochemical properties of the drug, the dosage form in which the drug is given, and the route of administration on the rate and extent of systemic drug absorption. Thus, biopharmaceutics involves factors that influence the (1) protection of the activity of the drug within the drug product, (2) the release of the drug from a drug product, (3) the rate of dissolution of the drug at the absorption site, and (4) the systemic absorption of the drug. Figure 2-1 is a general scheme describing this dynamic relationship.

The study of biopharmaceutics is based on fundamental scientific principles and experimental methodology. These methods must be able to assess the impact of the physical and chemical properties of the drug, drug stability and large scale production of the drug and drug product on the biological performance of the drug. Moreover, biopharmaceutics considers the requirements of the drug and dosage form in a physiological environment and the drug's intended therapeutic use and route of administration.

Studies in biopharmaceutics use both *in-vitro* and *in-vivo* methods. *In-vitro* methods are procedures employing test apparatus and equipment without involving laboratory animals or humans. *In-vivo* methods are more complex studies involving human subjects or laboratory animals. Some of these methods will be discussed in Chapter 5. Historically, pharmacologists evaluated the relative systemic drug availability *in vivo* after giving a drug product to an animal or human and then comparing specific pharmacologic, clinical, or possible toxic responses. For example, a drug such as isoproterenol causes an increase in heart rate when given intravenously but has no observable effect on the heart when given orally at the same dose level. Therefore, systemic drug availability may differ according to the route

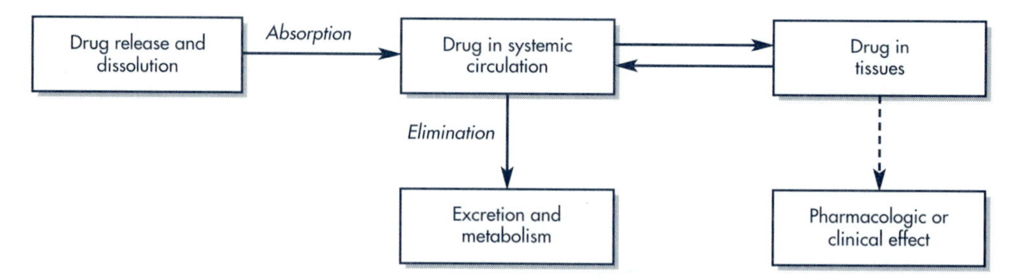

Figure 2-1. Scheme demonstrating the dynamic relationship between the drug, the drug product, and the pharmacologic effect.

of administration. In addition, the bioavailability (a measure of systemic availability of a drug) may differ from one drug product to another containing the same drug. This difference in drug bioavailability may be manifested by observing the difference in the therapeutic effectiveness of the drug products.

PHARMACOKINETICS

Pharmacokinetics involves the kinetics of drug absorption, distribution, and elimination (ie, excretion and metabolism). The description of drug distribution and elimination is often termed *drug disposition.* The study of pharmacokinetics involves both experimental and theoretical approaches. The experimental aspect of pharmacokinetics involves the development of biological sampling techniques, analytical methods for the measurement of drugs and metabolites, and procedures that facilitate data collection and manipulation. The theoretical aspect of pharmacokinetics involves the development of pharmacokinetic models that predict drug disposition after drug administration. The application of statistics is an integral part of pharmacokinetic studies. Statistical methods are used for pharmacokinetic parameter estimation and data interpretation. Statistical methods are applied to pharmacokinetic models to determine data error and structural model deviations. Mathematics and computer techniques form the theoretical basis of many pharmacokinetic methods. Classical pharmacokinetics is a study of theoretical models focusing mostly on model development and parameterization.

CLINICAL PHARMACOKINETICS

Clinical pharmacokinetics is the application of pharmacokinetic methods in drug therapy. Clinical pharmacokinetics involves a multidisciplinary approach to individually optimized dosing strategies based on the patient's disease state and patient-specific considerations. The study of clinical pharmacokinetics of drugs in disease states requires input from medical and pharmaceutical research. Table 2.1 is a list of 10 age-adjusted rates of death from 10 leading causes of death in the USA, 1993. The influence of many diseases on drug disposition is not adequately studied. Age, gender, genetic, and ethnic differences can also result in pharmacokinetic differences that may affect the outcome of drug therapy. The study of pharmacokinetic differences of drugs in various population groups is termed *population*

TABLE 2.1 Ratio of Age-Adjusted Death Rates, by Male/Female Ratio from the 10 Leading Causes of Death in the USA, 1993

DISEASE	RANK	MALE:FEMALE
Disease of heart	1	1.9
Malignant neoplasms	2	1.5
Cerebrovascular diseases	3	1.2
Chronic obstructive pulmonary diseases	4	1.6
Accidents and others*	5	2.6
Pneumonia and influenza	6	1.6
Diabetes mellitus	7	1.2
HIV infections	8	6.3
Suicide	9	4.4
Homicide and legal intervention	10	3.8

*Death due to adverse effects suffered as defined by CDC.

Source: CDC-MMWR (Morbidity and Mortality Weekly Report), March 1, 45:8, 1996.

pharmacokinetics (Sheiner and Ludden, 1992). Another important aspect of pharmacokinetics is *therapeutic drug monitoring* (TDM). When drugs with narrow therapeutic indices are used in patients, it is necessary to monitor plasma drug concentrations closely by taking periodic blood samples. The pharmacokinetic and drug analysis services necessary for safe drug monitoring are generally provided by the *clinical pharmacokinetic service* (CPKS). Some drugs frequently monitored are the aminoglycosides and anticonvulsants. Other drugs closely monitored are those used in cancer chemotherapy in order to minimize adverse side effects (Rodman and Evans, 1991).

PHARMACODYNAMICS

Pharmacodynamics refers to the relationship between the drug concentration at the site of action (receptor) and pharmacologic response, including biochemical and physiologic effects that influence the interaction of drug with the receptor. The interaction of a drug molecule with a receptor causes the initiation of a sequence of molecular events resulting in a pharmacologic or toxic response. Pharmacokinetic-pharmacodynamic models are constructed to relate plasma drug level to drug concentration in the site of action and establish the intensity and time course of the drug. Pharmacodynamics and pharmacokinetic-pharmacodynamic models are discussed more fully in Chapter 19.

TOXICOKINETICS AND CLINICAL TOXICOLOGY

Toxicokinetics is the application of pharmacokinetic principles to the design, conduct and interpretation of drug safety evaluation studies (Leal et al, 1993) and used in validating dose related exposure in animals. Toxicokinetic data aids in the interpretation of toxicologic findings in animals and extrapolation of the resulting data to humans. Toxicokinetic studies are performed in animals during preclinical drug development and may continue after the drug has been tested in clinical trials.

Clinical toxicology is the study of adverse effects of drugs and toxic substances (poisons) in the body. The pharmacokinetics of a drug in an over-medicated (intoxicated) patient may be very different from the pharmacokinetics of the same drug given in therapeutic doses. At very high doses, the drug concentration in the body may saturate enzymes involved in the absorption, biotransformation, or active renal secretion mechanisms thereby changing the pharmacokinetics from *linear* to *nonlinear* pharmacokinetics. Nonlinear pharmacokinetics is discussed in Chapter 16. Drugs frequently involved in toxicity cases include acetaminophen, salicylates, morphine and the tricylic antidepressants (TCA). Many of these drugs can be assayed conveniently by fluorescence immunoassay (FIA) kits.

MEASUREMENT OF DRUG CONCENTRATIONS

Sensitive, accurate, and precise analytical methods are available for the direct measurement of drugs in biologic samples, such as milk, saliva, plasma, and urine. Measurements of drug concentrations in these biological samples are generally validated so that accurate information is generated for pharmacokinetic and clinical monitoring. In general, chromatographic methods are more discriminating since chromatography separates the drug from other related materials that may cause assay interference.

Sampling of Biologic Specimens

Only a few biologic specimens may be obtained safely from the patient to gain information as to the drug concentration in the body. *Invasive* methods include sampling blood, spinal fluid, synovial fluid, tissue biopsy, or any biologic material that requires parenteral or surgical intervention in the patient. In contrast, *noninvasive* methods include sampling of urine, saliva, feces, expired air, or any biologic material that can be obtained without parenteral or surgical intervention. The measurement of drug concentration in each of these biologic materials yields different information.

Drug Concentrations in Blood, Plasma, or Serum

Measurement of drug concentration (levels) in the blood, serum, or plasma is the most direct approach to assessing the pharmacokinetics of the drug in the body. *Whole blood* contains the cellular elements including red blood cells, white blood cells, platelets, and various other proteins, such as albumin and globulins. In general, serum or plasma is used for drug measurement. To obtain *serum,* whole blood is allowed to clot and the serum is collected from the supernatant after centrifugation. *Plasma* is obtained from the supernatant of centrifuged whole blood to which an anticoagulant, such as heparin, has been added. Therefore, the protein content of serum and plasma is not the same. Plasma perfuses all the tissues of the body including the cellular elements in the blood. Assuming that a drug in the plasma is in dynamic equilibrium with the tissues, then changes in the drug concentration in plasma will reflect changes in tissue drug concentrations.

Plasma Level–Time Curve

The plasma level–time curve is generated by measuring the drug concentration in plasma samples taken at various time intervals after a drug product is administered.

The concentration of drug in each plasma sample is plotted on rectangular coordinate graph paper against the corresponding time at which the plasma sample was removed. As the drug reaches the general (systemic) circulation, plasma drug concentrations will rise up to a maximum. Usually absorption of a drug is more rapid than elimination. As the drug is being absorbed into the systemic circulation, the drug is distributed to all the tissues in the body and is also simultaneously being eliminated. Elimination of a drug can proceed by excretion or biotransformation or a combination of both.

The relationship of the drug level–time curve and various pharmacologic parameters for the drug is shown in Figure 2-2. MEC and MTC represent the *minimum effective concentration* and *minimum toxic concentration* of drug, respectively. For some drugs, such as those acting on the autonomic nervous system, it is useful to know the concentration of drug that will just barely produce a pharmacologic effect (ie, MEC). Assuming the drug concentration in the plasma is in equilibrium with the tissues, the MEC reflects the minimum concentration of drug needed at the receptors to produce the desired pharmacologic effect. Similarly, the MTC represents the drug concentration needed to just barely produce a toxic effect. The *onset time* corresponds to the time required for the drug to reach the MEC. The *intensity* of the pharmacologic effect is proportional to the number of drug receptors occupied, which is reflected in the observation that higher plasma drug concentrations produce a greater pharmacologic response, up to a maximum. The *duration* of drug action is the difference between the onset time and the time for the drug to decline back to the MEC.

In contrast, the pharmacokineticist can also describe the plasma level–time curve in terms of such pharmacokinetic terms as peak plasma level, time for peak plasma level, and area under the curve, or AUC (Fig. 2-3). The time of peak plasma level is the time of maximum drug concentration in the plasma and is a rough marker of average rate of drug absorption. The peak plasma level or maximum drug con-

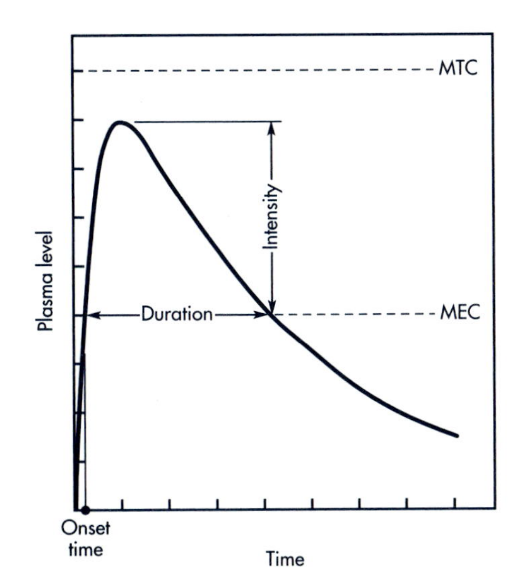

Figure 2-2. Generalized plasma level–time curve after oral administration of a drug.

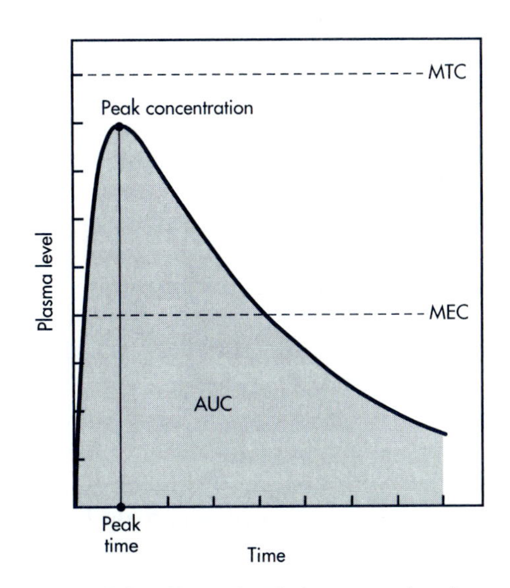

Figure 2-3. Plasma level–time curve showing peak time and concentration. The shaded portion represents the AUC (area under the curve).

centration is related to the dose, the rate constant for absorption, and elimination constant of the drug. The AUC is related to the amount of drug absorbed systemically. These and other pharmacokinetic parameters are discussed in succeeding chapters.

Drug Concentrations in Tissues

Tissue biopsies are occasionally removed for diagnostic purposes such as the verification of a malignancy. Usually, only a small sample of tissue is removed, making drug concentration measurement difficult. Drug concentrations in tissue biopsies may not reflect drug concentration in other tissues nor drug concentration in the tissue from which the biopsy material was removed. For example, if the tissue biopsy was for the diagnosis of a tumor within the tissue, the blood flow to the tumor cells may not be the same as the blood flow to other cells in this tissue. In fact, for many tissues, blood flow to one part of the tissues need not be the same as the blood flow to another part of the same tissue. The measurement of the drug concentration in tissue biopsy material may be used to ascertain if the drug reached the tissues and obtained the proper concentration within the tissue.

Drug Concentrations in Urine and Feces

Measurement of drug in *urine* is an indirect method to ascertain the bioavailability of a drug. The rate and extent of drug excreted in the urine reflects the rate and extent of systemic drug absorption. The use of urinary drug excretion measurements to establish various pharmacokinetic parameters is discussed in Chapter 10.

Measurement of drug in *feces* may reflect drug that has not been absorbed after an oral dose or may reflect drug that has been expelled by biliary secretion after systemic absorption. Fecal drug excretion is often performed in mass balance studies in which the investigator attempts to account for the entire dose given to the patient. For a mass balance study, both urine and feces are collected and their drug content measured. For certain solid oral dosage forms that do not dissolve in the gastrointestinal tract but slowly leach out drug, fecal collection is performed to recover the dosage form. The undissolved dosage form is then assayed for residual drug.

Drug Concentrations in Saliva

Saliva drug concentrations have been reviewed for many drugs for therapeutic drug monitoring (Pippenger and Massoud, 1984). Because only free drug diffuses into the saliva, saliva drug levels tend to approximate free drug rather than total plasma drug concentration. The saliva/plasma drug concentration ratio is less than 1 for many drugs. The saliva/plasma drug concentration ratio is mostly influenced by the pKa of the drug and pH of the saliva. Weak acid drugs and weak base drugs with pKa significantly different than pH 7.4 (plasma pH) generally have better correlation to plasma drug levels. The saliva drug concentrations taken after equilibrium with the plasma drug concentration generally provide more stable indication of drug levels in the body. The use of salivary drug concentrations as a therapeutic indicator should be used with caution and preferably used as a secondary indicator.

Forensic Drug Measurements

Forensic science is the application of science to personal injury, murder, and other legal proceedings. Drug measurements in tissues obtained at autopsy or in other bodily fluids such as saliva, urine, and blood may be useful if the person has taken an overdose of a legal medication, has been poisoned, or has been using drugs of abuse such as opiates (eg, heroin), cocaine or marijuana. The appearance of social drugs in blood, urine, and saliva drug analysis show short-term drug abuse. These drugs may be eliminated rapidly, making it more difficult to prove that the subject has been using drugs of abuse. The analysis for drugs of abuse in hair samples by very sensitive assay methods, such as gas chromatography coupled with mass spectrometry, provides information regarding past drug exposure. A recent study (Cone et al, 1993) showed that the hair samples from subjects who were known drug abusers contained cocaine and 6-acetylmorphine, a metabolite of heroine (diacetylmorphine).

Significance of Measuring Plasma Drug Concentrations

The intensity of the pharmacologic or toxic effect of a drug is often related to the concentration of the drug at the receptor site, usually located in the tissue cells. Because most of the tissue cells are richly perfused with tissue fluids or plasma, checking the plasma drug level is a responsive method of monitoring the course of therapy.

Clinically, individual variations in the pharmacokinetics of drugs are quite common. Monitoring the concentration of drugs in the blood or plasma ascertains that the calculated dose actually delivers the plasma level required for therapeutic effect. With some drugs, receptor sensitivity in individuals varies so that monitoring of plasma levels is needed to distinguish the patient who is receiving too much of a drug from the patient who is supersensitive to the drug. Moreover, the patient's physiologic functions may be affected by disease, nutrition, environment, concurrent drug therapy, and other factors. Pharmacokinetic models allow more accurate interpretation of the relationship between plasma drug levels and pharmacologic response. In the absence of pharmacokinetic information, plasma drug levels are relatively useless in dosage adjustment. For example, suppose a single blood sample from a patient was assayed and found to contain 10 μg/mL. According to the literature, the maximum safe concentration of this drug is 15 μg/mL. In order to apply this information properly, it is important to know when the blood sample was drawn, what dose of the drug was given, and the route of administration. If the proper information is available, the use of pharmacokinetic equations and models may describe the blood level–time curve accurately.

Monitoring of plasma drug concentrations allows for the adjustment of the drug dosage in order to individualize and optimize therapeutic drug regimens. In the presence of alteration in physiologic functions due to disease, monitoring plasma drug concentrations may provide a guide to the progress of the diseased state and enable the investigator to modify the drug dosage accordingly. Clinically, sound medical judgment and observation are most important. Therapeutic decisions should not be based solely on plasma drug concentrations.

In many cases, the pharmacodynamic response to the drug may be more important to measure than just the plasma drug concentration. For example, the electrophysiology of the heart including an electrocardiogram (ECG) is important to assess in patients medicated with cardiotonic drugs such as digoxin. For an anticoagulant drug, such as dicumarol, prothrombin clotting time may indicate whether proper dosage was achieved. Most diabetic patients taking insulin will monitor their own blood or urine glucose levels.

For drugs that act irreversibly at the receptor site, plasma drug concentrations may not accurately predict pharmacodynamic response. Drugs used in cancer chemotherapy often interfere with nucleic acid or protein biosynthesis to destroy tumor cells. For these drugs, the plasma drug concentration does not relate directly to the pharmacodynamic response. In this case, other pathophysiologic parameters and side effects are monitored in the patient to prevent adverse toxicity.

BASIC PHARMACOKINETICS AND PHARMACOKINETIC MODELS

Basic pharmacokinetics involves the quantitative study of various kinetic processes of drug disposition in the body. The biological nature of drug distribution and disposition is complex, and drug events often happen simultaneously. Basic pharmacokinetics requires (1) a thorough knowledge of anatomy and physiology and (2) an understanding of the concepts and limitations of mathematical models.

Drugs are in a dynamic state within the body. A *model* is a *hypothesis* using mathematical terms to concisely describe quantitative relationships. Simplifying assumptions are made to describe a complex biologic system concerning the movement of drugs. Various mathematical models can be devised to simulate the rate processes of drug absorption, distribution, and elimination. These mathematical models make possible the development of equations to describe drug concentrations in the body as a function of time.

The predictive capability of a model lies in the proper selection and development of mathematical function(s) that parameterize the essential factors governing the kinetic process. The key parameters in a process is commonly estimated by fitting the model to the experimental data known as *variables*. A pharmacokinetic function relates an *independent* variable to a *dependent* variable. For example, a model may predict the drug concentration in the liver 1 hour after an oral administration of a 20 mg dose. The independent variable is time and the dependent variable is the drug concentration in the liver. Based on a set of time versus drug concentration data, a model equation is derived to predict the liver drug concentration with respect to time. The drug concentration depends on the time after the administration of the dose.

A model may be *empirically* or *physiologically* based. The model that simply interpolates the data and allows an empirical formula to estimate drug level over time is justified when limited information is available. Empirical models are practical but not very useful in explaining the mechanism of the actual process by which the drug is absorbed, distributed and eliminated in the body.

Physiologically based models also have limitations. Using the example above and apart from the necessity to sample tissue and monitor blood flow to the liver *in vivo*, the investigator needs to understand the following questions. What does liver drug concentration mean? Should the drug concentration in the blood within the tissue be determined and subtracted from the drug in the liver tissue? What type of cell is representative of the liver if a selective biopsy liver tissue sample can be collected without contamination from its surroundings? Indeed, depending on the spatial location of the liver tissue from the hepatic blood vessels, tissue drug concentrations can differ. Moreover, changes in the liver blood perfusion will alter the tissue drug concentration. If the heterogeneous liver tissue is homogenized and assayed, the homogenized tissue only represents a hypothetical concentration that matches no real liver tissue. Most generated pharmacokinetic information depends on the method of tissue sampling, timing of the sample, drug analysis, and the predictive model selected. The need to approximate the real system (assuming uniformity within a given space or region) with a model is necessary and rational. Assumptions are inherent in all pharmacokinetic models even when a physiologic model is considered. A detailed physiologic model is more difficult but can reveal organ-specific or suborgan-regional information. In general, most pharmacokinetic models assume that the plasma drug concentration reflects drug concentrations globally within the body. Based on knowledge of the physiologic and biochemical composition of the body organs, the drug concentration in the liver may be estimated by knowing the liver extraction ratio for the drug.

A great number of models have been developed to estimate regional and global information about drug disposition in the body. Some physiologic pharmacokinetic models are discussed in Chapter 20. Pharmacokinetic processes are discussed in separate chapters under the topics of drug absorption, drug distribution, drug elimination, and pharmacokinetic drug interactions involving one or all the above processes. Theoretically, an unlimited number of models may be constructed to describe the kinetic processes of drug absorption, distribution, and elimination in the body depending on the degree of detailed information considered. Practical considerations have limited the growth of new pharmacokinetic models.

For example, assume a drug is given by intravenous injection and that the drug rapidly dissolves (distributes) in the body fluids. A pharmacokinetic model that describes this situation is a tank containing a volume of fluid that is rapidly equilibrated with the drug. In the human body, a fraction of the drug would be continually eliminated as a function of time (Fig. 2-4). The concentration of the drug in the tank after a given dose is governed by two parameters: (1) the fluid volume of the tank that will dilute the drug, and (2) the elimination rate of drug per unit of time. In pharmacokinetics, these parameters are assumed to be constants. If a known set of drug concentrations in the tank is determined at various time intervals, then the volume of fluid in the tank and the rate of drug elimination can be estimated.

Because drug concentrations is dependent on time, the two variables in this example, drug concentration and time, are called *dependent* and *independent* variables, respectively. In practice, pharmacokinetic parameters are determined experimentally from a set of drug concentrations collected over various times known as *data*. The number of parameters needed to describe the model depends on the complexity of the process and on the route of drug administration. In general, as the number of parameters that need to be evaluated increases, accurate estimation of these parameters becomes increasingly more difficult. With complex pharmacokinetic models, computer programs are used to facilitate parameter estimation.

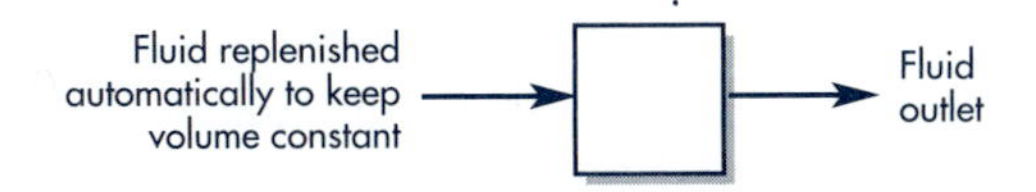

Figure 2-4. Tank with a constant volume of fluid equilibrated with drug. The volume of the fluid is 1.0 L. The fluid outlet is 10 mL/min. The fraction of drug removed per unit of time is 10/1000, or 0.01 min^{-1}.

However, for the parameters to be valid, the number of data points should always exceed the number of parameters in the model.

Pharmacokinetic models are used to:

1. Predict plasma, tissue, and urine drug levels with any dosage regimen.
2. Calculate the optimum dosage regimen for each patient individually.
3. Estimate the possible accumulation of drugs and/or metabolites.
4. Correlate drug concentrations with pharmacologic or toxicologic activity.
5. Evaluate differences in the rate or extent of availability between formulations (bioequivalence).
6. Describe how changes in physiology or disease affect the absorption, distribution, or elimination of the drug.
7. Explain drug interactions.

Because a model is based on a hypothesis and simplifying assumptions, a certain degree of caution is necessary when relying totally on the pharmacokinetic model to predict drug action. For some drugs, plasma drug concentrations are not useful in predicting drug activity. For other drugs, disease state and compensatory response from the body may modify the response of a drug. If a simple model does not fit accurately all the experimental observations, a new, more elaborate model may be proposed and subsequently tested. Since limited data are generally available in most clinical situations, pharmacokinetic data should be interpreted along with clinical observations rather than replacing sound judgment by the clinician. Development of pharmacometric, statistical models may help to improve prediction of drug levels among patients in the population (Sheiner and Beal, 1982; Mallet et al, 1988). However, it will be some time before these methods become generally accepted.

Compartment Models

The body can be represented as a series, or systems, of compartments that communicate reversibly with each other. A compartment is not a real physiologic or anatomic region but is considered as a tissue or group of tissues that have similar blood flow and drug affinity. Within each compartment, the drug is considered to be uniformly distributed. Mixing of the drug within a compartment is rapid and homogeneous and is considered to be "*well stirred*," so that the drug concentration represents an average concentration, and each drug molecule has an equal probability of leaving the compartment. Compartment models are based on linear assumptions using linear differential equations.

Conceptually, drugs move dynamically in and out of compartments. Rate constants are used to represent the overall rate processes of drug entry into and exit from the compartment. The model is an open system since drug can be eliminated from the system.

A compartmental model provides a simple way of grouping all the tissues into one or more compartments where drugs move to and from the central or plasma compartment. At any time, the amount of drug in the body is simply the sum of drug present in the central compartment plus the drug present in the tissue compartment. Although the tissue compartment does not represent a specific tissue, the mass balance accounts for the drug present in all the tissues. Knowing the parameters of the two-compartment model, one can estimate the amount of drug left in the body and the amount of drug eliminated from the body at any time. The compartmental models are particularly useful when there is little information known about the tissues.

If the tissue drug concentrations and binding are known, physiologic pharmacokinetic models, which are based on actual tissues and blood flow, describe the data more realistically. Physiologic pharmacokinetic models are frequently used in describing drug distribution in animals, because tissue samples are easily available for assay. On the other hand, tissue samples are often not available for human subjects, and approximations are often made in applying physiologic models to humans. Compartmental models form the basis of physiologic and other advanced models. Unlike physiological models, parameters, such as half-life, are kinetically determined from the data. In contrast, most physiological models assume an average set of blood flow for individual subjects, a major disadvantage in trying to predict individualized dosing.

Mammillary Model

The mammillary model is the most common compartment model used in pharmacokinetics. The model consists of one or more peripheral compartments connected to a central compartment. The central compartment is assigned to represent plasma and highly perfused tissues which rapidly equilibrate with drug. The mammillary model is a strongly connected system since one can estimate the amount of drug in any compartment of the system after drug is introduced into a given compartment. When an intravenous dose of drug is given, the drug enters directly into the central compartment. Elimination of drug occurs from the central compartment since the organs involved in drug elimination, primarily kidney and liver, are well-perfused tissues.

Several types of compartment models are described in Figure 2-5. The pharmacokinetic rate constants are represented by the letter k. Compartment 1 represents the plasma or central compartment, and compartment 2 represents the tissue

MODEL 1. One-compartment open model, IV injection.

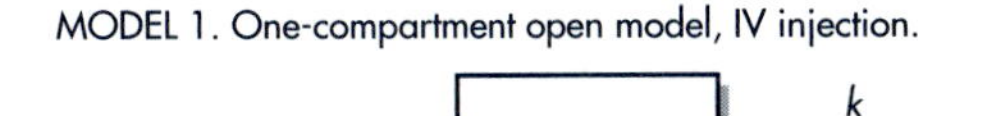

MODEL 2. One-compartment open model with first-order absorption.

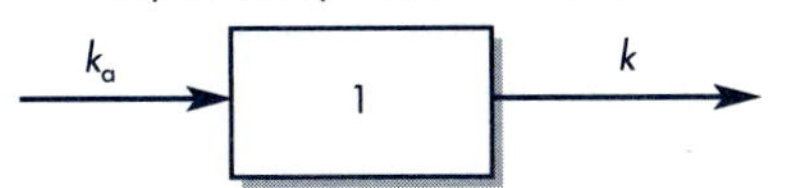

MODEL 3. Two-compartment open model, IV injection.

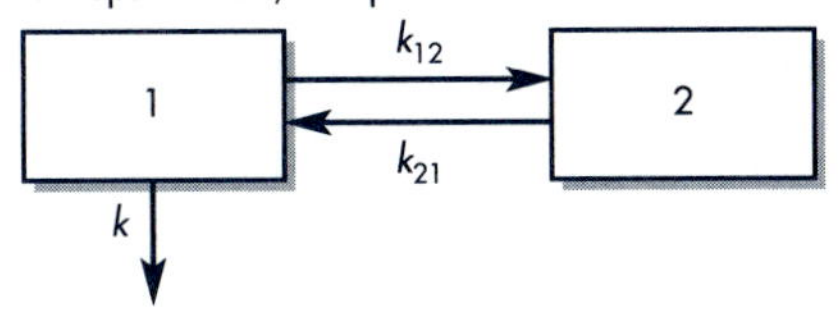

MODEL 4. Two-compartment open model with first-order absorption.

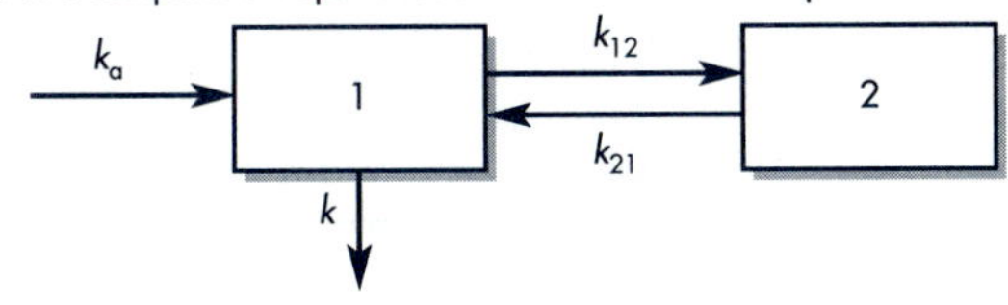

Figure 2-5. Various compartment models.

compartment. The drawing of models has three functions. The model (1) enables the pharmacokineticist to write differential equations to describe drug concentration changes in each compartment, (2) gives a visual representation of the rate processes, and (3) shows how many pharmacokinetic constants are necessary to describe the process adequately.

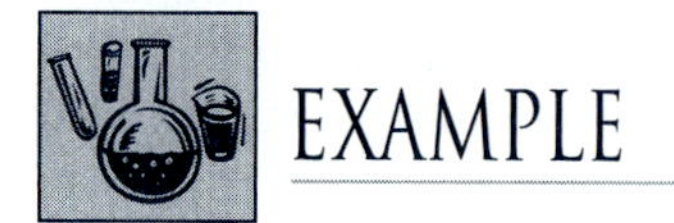

EXAMPLE

Two parameters are needed to describe model 1 (Fig. 2-5): the volume of the compartment and the elimination rate constant, k. In the case of model 4, the pharmacokinetic parameters consist of the volumes of compartments 1 and 2 and the rate constants—k_a, k, k_{12}, and k_{21}—for a total of six parameters.

In studying these models, it is important to know whether drug concentration data may be sampled directly from each compartment. For models 3 and 4 (Fig. 2-5), data concerning compartment 2 cannot be obtained easily because tissues are not easily sampled and may not contain homogeneous concentrations of drug. If the amount of drug absorbed and eliminated per unit time is obtained by sampling compartment 1, then the amount of drug contained in the tissue compartment 2 can be estimated mathematically. The appropriate mathematical equations for describing these models and evaluating the various pharmacokinetic parameters are given in the succeeding chapters.

Catenary Model

In pharmacokinetics, the mammillary model must be distinguished from another type of compartmental model called the *catenary* model. The catenary model consists of compartments joined to one another like the compartments of a train (Fig. 2-6). In contrast, the mammillary model consists of one or more compartments around a central compartment like satellites. Because the catenary model does not apply to the way most functional organs in the body are directly connected to the plasma, it is not used as often as the mammillary model.

Physiologic Pharmacokinetic Model (Flow Model)

Physiologic pharmacokinetic models, also known as blood flow or perfusion models, are pharmacokinetic models based on known anatomic and physiologic data. The models kinetically describe the data with the consideration that blood flow is

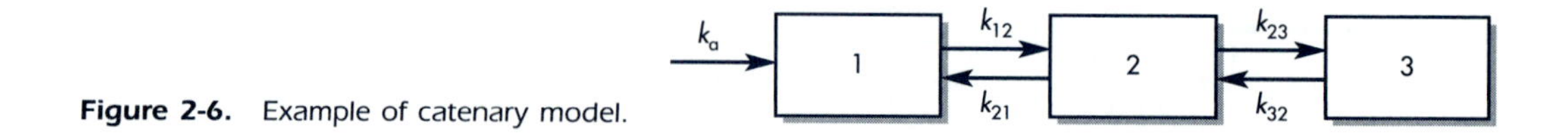

Figure 2-6. Example of catenary model.

responsible for distributing drug to various parts of the body. Uptake of drug into organs is determined by the binding of drug in these tissues. In contrast to an estimated tissue volume of distribution, the actual tissue volume is used. Because there are many tissue organs in the body, each tissue volume must be obtained and its drug concentration described. The model would potentially predict realistic tissue drug concentrations, which the two-compartment model fails to do. Unfortunately, much of the information required for adequately describing a physiologic pharmacokinetic model are experimentally difficult to obtain. In spite of this limitation, the physiologic pharmacokinetic model does provide a much better insight into how physiologic factors may change drug distribution from one animal species to another. Other major differences are described below.

First, no data fitting is required in the perfusion model. Drug concentrations in the various tissues are predicted by organ tissue size, blood flow, and experimentally determined drug tissue–blood ratios (ie, partition of drug between tissue and blood).

Second, blood flow, tissue size, and the drug tissue–blood ratios may vary due to certain pathophysiologic conditions. Thus, the effect of these variations on drug distribution must be taken into account in physiologic pharmacokinetic models.

Third, and most important of all, physiologically based pharmacokinetic models can be applied to several species, and, for some drugs, human data may be extrapolated. Extrapolation from animal data is not possible with the compartment models, because the volume of distribution in such models is a mathematical concept that does not relate simply to blood volume and blood flow. To date, numerous drugs (including digoxin, lidocaine, methotrexate, and thiopental) have been described with perfusion models. Tissue levels of some of these drugs cannot be predicted successfully with compartment models, although they generally describe blood levels well. An example of a perfusion model is shown in Figure 2-7.

The number of tissue compartments in a perfusion model varies with the drug. Typically, the tissues or organs that have no drug penetration are excluded from

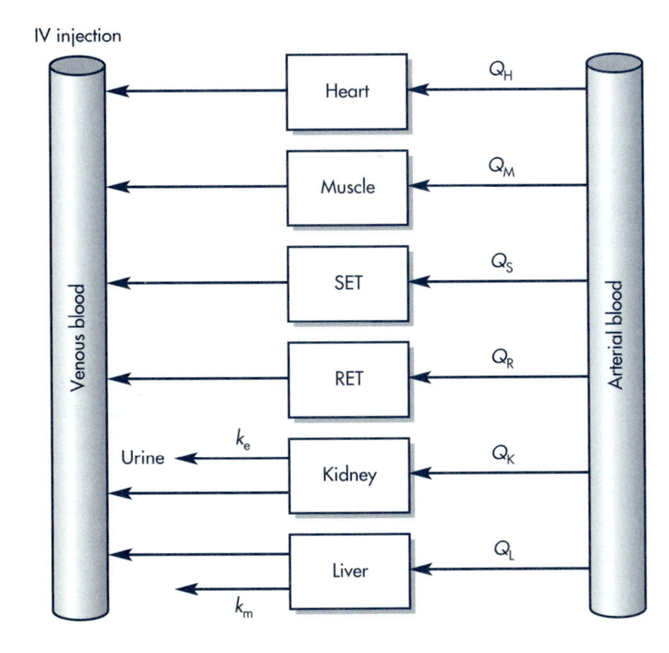

Figure 2-7. Pharmacokinetic model of drug perfusion. The *k*s represent kinetic constants: k_e is the first-order rate constant for urinary drug excretion and k_m is the rate constant for hepatic elimination. Each "box" represents a tissue compartment. Organs of major importance in drug absorption are considered separately, while other tissues are grouped as RET (rapidly equilibrating tissue) and SET (slowly equilibrating tissue). The size or mass of each tissue compartment is determined physiologically rather than by mathematical estimation. The concentration of drug in the tissue is determined by the ability of the tissue to accumulate drug as well as by the rate of blood perfusion to the tissue, represented by *Q*.

consideration. Thus, such organs as the brain, the bones, and other parts of the central nervous system are often excluded, as most drugs have little penetration into these organs. To describe each organ separately with a differential equation would make the model very complex and mathematically difficult. A simpler but equally good approach is to group all the tissues with similar blood perfusion properties into a single compartment. A perfusion model has been successfully used to describe the distribution of lidocaine in blood and various organs. In this case, organs such as lung, liver, brain, and muscle were individually described by differential equations, whereas other tissues were grouped as RET (rapidly equilibrating tissue) and SET (slowly equilibrating tissue), as shown in Figure 2-7. Figure 2-8 shows that the blood concentration of lidocaine declines biexponentially and was well predicted by the physiologic model based on blood flow. The tissue lidocaine level in the lung, muscle, and adipose and other organs is shown in Figure 2-9. The model shows that adipose tissue accumulates drugs slowly because of low blood supply. In contrast, vascular tissues, like the lung, equilibrate rapidly with the blood and start to decline as soon as drug level in the blood starts to fall. The physiologic pharmacokinetic model provides a realistic means of modeling tissue drug levels. Unfortunately, the simulated tissues levels in Figure 2-9 cannot be verified in humans because drug levels in tissues are not available. A criticism of physiologic pharmacokinetic models in general has been that there are fewer data points than parameters that one tries to fit. Consequently, the projected data are not well constrained.

The systems of different equations that describe drug distribution are usually solved by numerical integration. With the model as a base, the entire time course of drug levels in various tissue organs can be simulated.

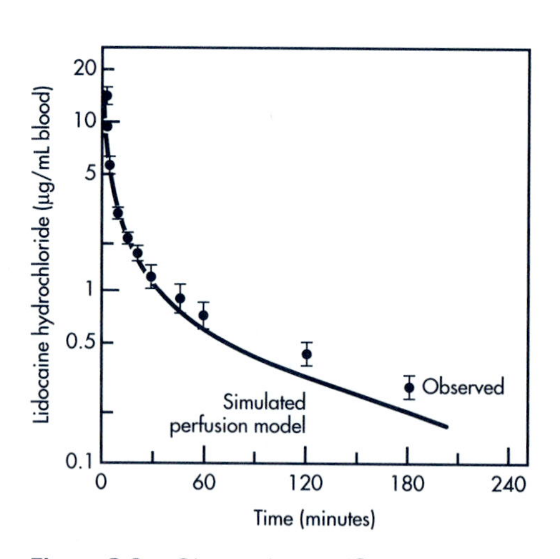

Figure 2-8. Observed mean (●) and simulated (—) arterial lidocaine blood concentrations in normal volunteers receiving 1 mg/kg per min constant infusion for 3 minutes.
(From Benowitz et al 1974, with permission; data from Tucker GT, Boas RA: *Anesthesiology* *34*:538, 1971.)

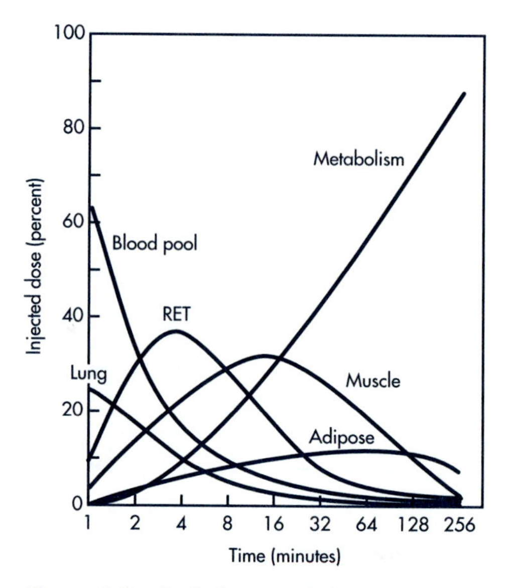

Figure 2-9. Perfusion model simulation of the distribution of lidocaine in various tissues and its elimination from humans following an intravenous infusion for 1 minute.
(From Benowitz et al 1974, with permission.)

The real significance of the physiologically based model is the potential application of this model in the prediction of human pharmacokinetics from animal data (Sawada et al, 1985). The mass of various body organs or tissues, extent of protein binding, drug metabolism capacity, and blood flow in humans and other species are often known or can be determined. Thus, physiologic and anatomic parameters can be used to predict the effects of drugs on humans from the effects on animals in cases where human experimentation is difficult or restricted.

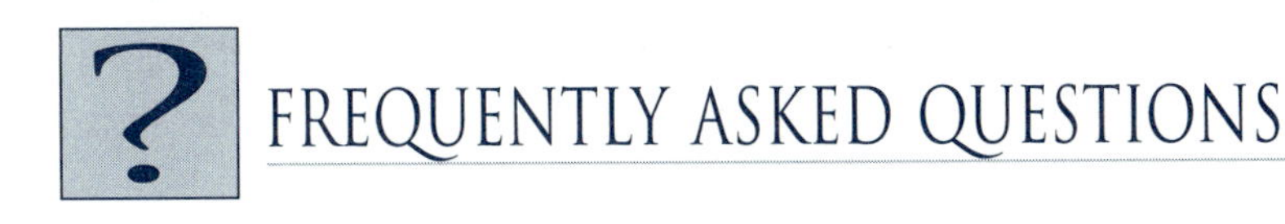

FREQUENTLY ASKED QUESTIONS

1. Why is plasma or serum drug concentration used to monitor drug concentration in the body rather than blood concentration?
2. What are reasons to use multicompartment model instead of physiologic model?
3. At what time should plasma drug concentration be taken in order to best predict drug response and side effect?

LEARNING QUESTIONS

1. What is the significance of the plasma level–time curve? How does the curve relate to the pharmacologic activity of a drug?
2. What is the purpose of pharmacokinetic models?
3. Draw a diagram describing a three-compartment model with first-order absorption and drug elimination from compartment 1.
4. The pharmacokinetic model presented in Figure 2-10 represents a drug that is eliminated by renal excretion, biliary excretion, and drug metabolism. The metabolite distribution is described by a one-compartment open model. The following questions pertain to Figure 2-10.
   a. How many parameters are needed to describe the model if the drug is injected intravenously (ie, the rate of drug absorption may be neglected)?
   b. Which compartment(s) can be sampled?
   c. What would be the overall elimination rate constant for elimination of drug from compartment 1?
   d. Write an expression describing the rate of change of drug concentration in compartment 1 (dC_1/dt).
5. Give two reasons for the measurement of the plasma drug concentration, C_p assuming (a) the C_p relates directly to the pharmacodynamic activity of the drug and (b) the C_p does *not* relate to the pharmacodynamic activity of the drug.

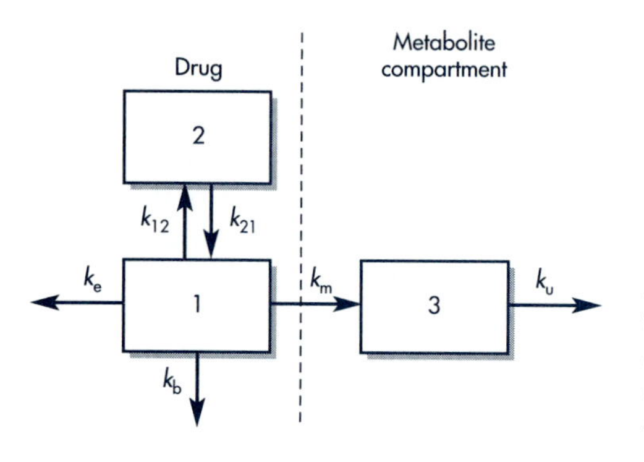

Figure 2-10. Pharmacokinetic model for a drug eliminated by renal and biliary excretion and drug metabolism. k_m = rate constant for metabolism of drug: k_u = rate constant for urinary excretion of metabolites; k_b = rate constant for biliary excretion of drug; and k_e = rate constant for urinary drug excretion.

6. Consider two biologic compartments separated by a biologic membrane. Drug A is found in compartment 1 and in compartment 2 in a concentration of c_1 and c_2, respectively.

a. What possible conditions or situations would result in concentration $c_1 > c_2$ at equilibrium?

b. How would you experimentally demonstrate these conditions given above?

c. Under what conditions would $c_1 = c_2$ at equilibrium?

d. The total amount of Drug A in each biologic compartment is A_1 and A_2, respectively. Describe a condition in which $A_1 > A_2$, but $c_1 = c_2$ at equilibrium.

Include in your discussion, how the physicochemical properties of Drug A or the biologic properties of each compartment might influence equilibrium conditions.

REFERENCES

Benowitz N, Forsyth R, Melmon K, Rowland M: Lidocaine disposition kinetics in monkey and man. *Clin Pharmacol Ther* **15:**87–98, 1974

Cone EJ, Darwin WD, Wang W-L: The occurrence of cocaine, heroin and metabolites in hair of drug abusers. *Forensic Sci Int* **63:**55–68, 1993

Leal M, Yacobi A, Batra VJ: Use of toxicokinetic principles in drug development: Bridging preclinical and clinical studies. In A Yacobi, JP Skelly, VP Shah, LZ Benet (eds), *Integration of Pharmacokinetics, Pharmacodynamics and Toxicokinetics in Rational Drug Development.* New York, Plenum Press, 1993, pp 55–67

Mallet A, Mentre F, Steimer JL, Lokiec F: Pharmacometrics: Nonparametric maximum likelihood estimation for population pharmacokinetics, with application to cyclosporine. *J Pharm Biopharm* **16:**311–327, 1988

Pippenger CE and Massoud N: Therapeutic drug monitoring. In Benet LZ et al (eds). *Pharmacokinetic Basis for Drug Treatment.* New York, Raven, 1984, chap 21

Rodman JH and Evans WE: Targeted systemic exposure for pediatric cancer therapy. In D'Argenio (ed), *Advanced Methods of Pharmacokinetic and Pharmacodynamic Systems Analysis.* New York, Plenum Press, 1991, pp 177–183

Sawada Y, Hanano M, Sugiyama Y, Iga T: Prediction of the disposition of nine weakly acidic and six weekly basic drugs in humans from pharmacokinetic parameters in rats. *J Pharmacokinet Biopharm* **13:**477–492, 1985

Shafer SL: Targeting the effect site with a computer controlled infusion pump. In D'Argenio (ed), *Advanced Methods of Pharmacokinetic and Pharmacodynamic Systems Analysis.* New York, Plenum Press, 1991, pp 185–195

Sheiner LB and Beal SL: Bayesian individualization of pharmacokinetics. Simple implementation and comparison with nonBayesian methods. *J Pharm Sci* **71:**1344–1348, 1982

Sheiner LB and Ludden TM: Population pharmacokinetics/dynamics. *Annu Rev Pharmacol Toxicol* **32:**185–201, 1992

BIBLIOGRAPHY

Benet LZ: General treatment of linear mammillary models with elimination from any compartment as used in pharmacokinetics. *J Pharm Sci* **61:**536–541, 1972

Bischoff K and Brown R: Drug distribution in mammals. *Chem Eng Med* **62:**33–45, 1966

Bischoff K, Dedrick R, Zaharko D, Longstreth T: Methotrexate pharmacokinetics. *J Pharm Sci* **60:**1128–1133, 1971

Chiou W: Quantitation of hepatic and pulmonary first-pass effect and its implications in pharmacokinetic study, I: Pharmacokinetics of chloroform in man. *J Pharm Biopharm* **3:**193–201, 1975

Colburn WA: Controversy III: To model or not to model. *J Clin Pharmacol* **28:**879–888, 1988

Cowles A, Borgstedt H, Gilles A: Tissue weights and rates of blood flow in man for the prediction of anesthetic uptake and distribution. *Anesthesiology* **35:**523–526, 1971

Dedrick R, Forrester D, Cannon T, et al: Pharmacokinetics of 1-B-D-arabinofurinosulcytosine (ARA-C) deamination in several species. *Biochem Pharmacol* **22:**2405–2417, 1972

Gerlowski LE and Jain RK: Physiologically based pharmacokinetic modeling: Principles and applications. *J Pharm Sci* **72:**1103–1127, 1983

Gibaldi M: *Biopharmaceutics and Clinical Pharmacokinetics,* 3rd ed. Philadelphia, Lea & Febiger, 1984

Gibaldi M: Estimation of the pharmacokinetic parameters of the two-compartment open model from post-infusion plasma concentration data. *J Pharm Sci* **58:**1133–1135, 1969

Himmelstein KJ and Lutz RJ: A review of the applications of physiologically based pharmacokinetic modeling. *J Pharm Biopharm* **7:**127–145, 1979

Lutz R, Dedrick R, Straw J, et al: The kinetics of methotrexate distribution in spontaneous canine lymphosarcoma. *J Pharm Biopharm* **3:**77–97, 1975

Lutz R and Dedrick RL: Physiologic pharmacokinetics: Relevance to human risk assessment. In Li AP (ed), *Toxicity Testing: New Applications and Applications in Human Risk Assessment.* New York, Raven, 1985, pp 129–149

Metzler CM: Estimation of pharmacokinetic parameters: Statistical considerations. *Pharmacol Ther* **13:**543–556, 1981

Montandon B, Roberts R, Fischer L: Computer simulation of sulfobromophthalein kinetics in the rat using flow-limited models with extrapolation to man. *J Pharm Biopharm* **3:**277–290, 1975

Rescigno A and Beck JS: The use and abuse of models. *J Pharm Biopharm* **15:**327–344, 1987

Ritschel WA and Banerjee PS: Physiologic pharmacokinetic models: Applications, limitations and outlook. *Meth Exp Clin Pharmacol* **8:**603–614, 1986

Rowland M, Thomson P, Guichard A, Melmon K: Disposition kinetics of lidocaine in normal subjects. *Ann NY Acad Sci* **179:**383–398, 1971

Rowland M and Tozer T: *Clinical Pharmacokinetics—Concepts and Applications,* 3rd ed. Philadelphia, Lea & Febiger, 1995

Segre G: Pharmacokinetics: Compartmental representation. *Pharm Ther* **17:**111–127, 1982

Tozer TN: Pharmacokinetic principles relevant to bioavailability studies. In Blanchard J, Sawchuk RJ, Brodie BB (eds), *Principles and Perspectives in Drug Bioavailability.* New York, S Karger, 1979, pp 120–155.

Wagner JG: Do you need a pharmacokinetic model, and, if so, which one? *J Pharm Biopharm* **3:**457–478, 1975

Welling P and Tse F: *Pharmacokinetics.* New York, Marcel Dekker, 1993.

Winters ME: *Basic Clinical Pharmacokinetics,* 3rd ed. Vancouver, WA, Applied Therapeutics Inc, 1994

3

ONE-COMPARTMENT OPEN MODEL

INTRAVENOUS ROUTE OF ADMINISTRATION OF DRUG

When a drug is given in the form of a rapid intravenous injection (IV bolus), the entire dose of drug enters the blood stream immediately, and the drug absorption process is considered to be instantaneous. In most cases, the drug distributes via the circulatory system to all the tissues in the body. Some uptake of drugs by various tissue organs will occur depending on the lipophilicity of the drug and its binding affinity for the tissue mass. Most drugs are eliminated from the body either through the kidney and/or metabolized in the liver. Due to rapid drug equilibration between the blood and tissue, drug elimination, in some sense, occurs as if the dose is all dissolved in a tank of uniform fluid from which the drug is eliminated. The one-compartment open model offers the simplest way to describe the process of drug distribution and elimination in the body. The volume in which the drug is assumed to be uniformly distributed is termed the *apparent volume of distribution*. The apparent volume of distribution is determined from the preinjected amount of the dose and the plasma drug concentration resulting immediately after the dose is injected.

The apparent volume of distribution is a parameter of the one-compartment model because the volume of distribution governs the plasma concentration of the drug after a given dose. A second parameter is the elimination constant k which governs the rate that the drug concentration declines over time. The one-compartment model that describes the distribution and elimination after a bolus dose is given in Figure 3-1.

The one-compartment open model does not predict actual drug levels in the tissues, but does imply that changes in the plasma levels of a drug will result in proportional changes in tissue drug levels since their kinetic profile is consistent with inclusion within the vascular compartment. The drug in the body (D_B) cannot be measured directly; however, accessible body fluids (such as blood) can be sampled to determine drug concentrations. The term, *apparent volume of distribution*, V_D, is the apparent volume in the body in which the drug is dissolved.

Figure 3-1. Pharmacokinetic model for a drug administered by rapid intravenous injection. D_B = drug in body; V_D = apparent volume of distribution; k = elimination rate constant.

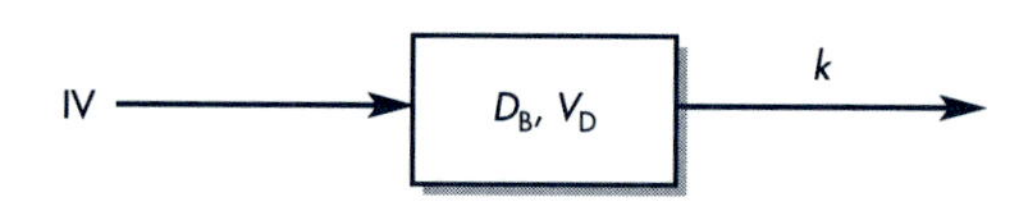

ELIMINATION RATE CONSTANT

The rate of elimination for most drugs is a first-order process. The elimination rate constant, k, is a first-order elimination rate constant with units of time^{-1} (eg, hr^{-1}). Generally, the parent or active drug is measured in the vascular compartment. Total removal or elimination of the parent drug from this compartment is effected by metabolism (biotransformation) and excretion. The elimination rate constant represents the sum of each of these processes:

$$k = k_m + k_e \tag{3.1}$$

where k_m = first-order rate process of metabolism and k_e = first-order rate process of excretion. There may be several routes of elimination of drug by metabolism or excretion. In such a case each of these processes has its own first-order rate constant.

A rate expression for Figure 3-1 is

$$\frac{dD_B}{dt} = -kD_B \tag{3.2}$$

This expression shows that the rate of elimination of drug in the body is a first-order process, depending on the elimination rate constant, k, and the amount of drug in the body, D_B, remaining. Integration of Equation 3.2 gives the following expression:

$$\log D_B = \frac{-kt}{2.3} + \log D_B^0 \tag{3.3}$$

where D_B = drug in body at time t and D_B^0 = drug in body at $t = 0$. When log D_B is plotted against t for this equation, a straight line is obtained (Fig. 3-2). In prac-

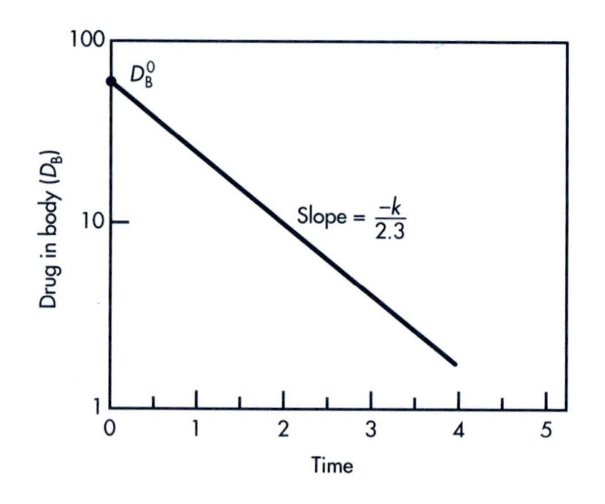

Figure 3-2. Semilog graph of the rate of drug elimination in a one-compartment model.

tice, instead of transforming values of D_B to their corresponding logarithms, each value of D_B is placed at logarithmic intervals on semilog paper.

Equation 3.3 can also be expressed as

$$D_B = D_B^0 e^{-kt} \tag{3.4}$$

APPARENT VOLUME OF DISTRIBUTION

The volume of distribution represents a volume that must be considered in estimating the amount of drug in the body from the concentration of drug found in the sampling compartment. The volume of distribution is also the apparent volume (V_D) in which the drug is dissolved (Eq. 3.5). Because the value of the volume of distribution does not have a true physiologic meaning in terms of an anatomic space, the term *apparent volume of distribution* is used.

In general, drug equilibrates rapidly in the body. However, each individual tissue in the body may contain a different concentration of drug due to differences in drug affinity for that tissue. The amount of drug in the body is not determined directly. Instead, a blood sample is removed at periodic intervals and analyzed for its concentration of drug. The V_D relates the concentration of drug in plasma (C_p) and the amount of drug in the body (D_B), as in the following equation:

$$D_B = V_D C_p \tag{3.5}$$

By substituting Equation 3.5 into Equation 3.3, a similar expression based on drug concentration in plasma is obtained for the first-order decline of drug plasma levels.

$$\log C_p = \frac{-kt}{2.3} + \log C_p^0 \tag{3.6}$$

where C_p = concentration of drug in plasma at time t and C_p^0 = concentration of drug in plasma at $t = 0$. Equation 3.6 can also be expressed as

$$C_p = C_p^0 e^{-kt} \tag{3.7}$$

The relationship between apparent volume, drug concentration, and total amount of drug may be better understood by the following example.

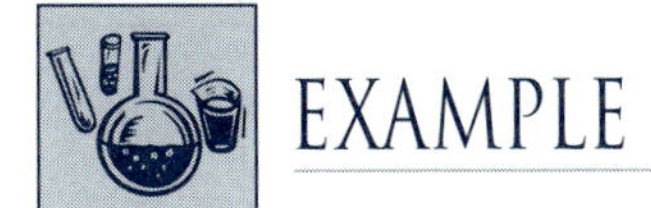

EXAMPLE

Exactly 1 g of a drug is dissolved in an unknown volume of water. Upon assay, the concentration of this solution is 1 mg/mL. What is the original volume of this solution?

The original volume of the solution may be obtained by the following proportion and remembering that 1 g = 1000 mg.

$$\frac{1000 \text{ mg}}{x \text{ mL}} = \frac{1 \text{ mg}}{\text{mL}} \qquad x = 1000 \text{ mL}$$

Therefore, the original volume was 1000 mL or 1 L.

If, in the above example, the volume of the solution is known to be 1 L, and the concentration of the solution is 1 mg/mL, then to calculate the total amount of drug present,

$$\frac{x \text{ mg}}{1000 \text{ mL}} = \frac{1 \text{ mg}}{\text{mL}} \qquad x = 1000 \text{ mg}$$

Therefore, the total amount of drug in the solution is 1000 mg, or 1 g.

From the preceding example, if the volume of solution in which the drug is dissolved and the drug concentration of the solution are known, then the total amount of drug present in the solution may be calculated. This relationship between drug concentration, volume in which the drug is dissolved, and total amount of drug present is given in the following equation.

$$D = VC \tag{3.8}$$

where D = total drug, V = total volume, and C = drug concentration. From Equation 3.8, which is similar to Equation 3.5, if any two parameters are known, then the third term may be calculated.

The body may be considered as a constant-volume system. Therefore, the apparent volume of distribution for any given drug is generally a constant. If both the concentration of drug in the plasma and the apparent volume of distribution for the drug are known, then the total amount of drug in the body (at the time in which the plasma sample was obtained) may be calculated from Equation 3.5.

Calculation of Volume of Distribution

In a one-compartment model (IV administration), the V_D is calculated with the following equation:

$$V_D = \frac{\text{dose}}{C_p^0} = \frac{D_B^0}{C_p^0} \tag{3.9}$$

with a rapid IV injection, the dose is identical to D_B^0. The term C_p^0 is the initial plasma concentration of drug at $t = 0$; its value can be obtained by extrapolation of the regression line to the y axis (Fig. 3-3).

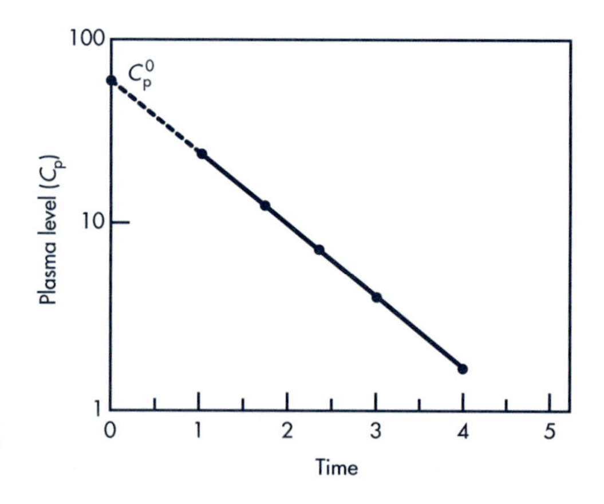

Figure 3-3. Semilog graph giving the value of C_p^0 by extrapolation.

When determined by extrapolation, C_p^0 represents the instantaneous drug concentration (concentration of drug at $t = 0$) after the drug has time for equilibration in the body. The dose of drug given by IV bolus (rapid IV injection) represents the amount of drug in the body, D_B^0, at $t = 0$. Because both D_B^0 and C_p^0 are known at $t = 0$, then the apparent volume of distribution, V_D, may be calculated from Equation 3.9.

The apparent V_D may also be calculated from knowledge of the dose, elimination rate constant, and AUC from $t = 0$ to $t = \infty$.

From Equation 3.2 (repeated here), the rate of drug elimination is

$$\frac{dD_B}{dt} = -kD_B$$

By substitution of Equation 3.5, $D_B = V_D C_p$, into Equation 3.2, the following expression is obtained:

$$\frac{dD_B}{dt} = -kV_D C_p \tag{3.10}$$

Rearrangement of Equation 3.10 gives

$$dD_B = -kV_D C_p \, dt \tag{3.11}$$

As both k and V_D are constants, Equation 3.10 may be integrated as follows:

$$\int_0^\infty dD_B = -kV_D \int_0^\infty C_p \, dt \tag{3.12}$$

Equation 3.12 shows that a small change in time (dt) results in a small change in the amount of drug in the body, D_B.

The integral $\int_0^\infty C_p \, dt$ represents the AUC_0^∞, which is the summation of the area under the curve from $t = 0$ to $t = \infty$. The AUC_0^∞ is usually estimated by the trapezoidal rule (Chapter 1). After integration, Equation 3.12 above becomes

$$D_o = kV_D \, [AUC]_0^\infty$$

which upon rearrangement yields the following equation:

$$V_D = \frac{D_0}{k[AUC]_0^\infty} \tag{3.13}$$

The calculation of the apparent V_D by means of Equation 3.13 is a *model-independent method* since no pharmacokinetic model is considered and the AUC is determined directly by the trapezoidal rule.

Significance of the Apparent Volume of Distribution

The apparent volume of distribution is not a true physiologic volume. Most drugs have an apparent volume of distribution smaller than, or equal to, the body mass. For some drugs, the volume of distribution may be several times the body mass. Equation 3.9 shows that the apparent V_D is dependent on C_p^0. For a given dose, a very small C_p^0 may occur in the body due to concentration of the drug in peripheral tissues and organs. For this dose, the small C_p^0 will result in a large V_D.

Drugs with a large apparent V_D are more concentrated in extravascular tissues and less concentrated intravascularly. If a drug is highly bound to plasma proteins or remains in the vascular region, then C_p^0 will be higher, resulting in a smaller apparent V_D. Consequently, binding of a drug to peripheral tissues or to plasma proteins will significantly affect V_D.

The apparent V_D is a volume term that can be expressed as a simple volume or in terms of percent of body weight. In expressing the apparent V_D in terms of percent body weight, a 1 L volume is assumed to be equal to the weight of 1 kg. For example, if the V_D is 3500 mL for a subject weighing 70 kg, the V_D expressed as percent of body weight would be

$$\frac{3.5 \text{ kg}}{70 \text{ kg}} \times 100 = 5\% \text{ of body weight}$$

If V_D is a very large number—ie, >100% of body weight—then it may be assumed that the drug is concentrated in certain tissue compartments. Thus, the apparent V_D is a useful parameter in considering the relative amounts of drug in the vascular and in the extravascular tissues.

Pharmacologists often attempt to conceptualize the apparent V_D as a true physiologic or anatomic fluid compartment. By expressing the V_D in terms of percent of body weight, values for the V_D may be found which appear to correspond to true anatomic volumes (Table 3.1). However, it may be only fortuitous that the value for the apparent V_D of a drug has the same value as a real anatomic volume. If a drug is to be considered to be distributed in a true physiologic volume, then an investigation is needed to test this hypothesis.

Given the apparent V_D for a particular drug, the total amount of drug in the body at any time after administration of the drug may be determined by the measurement of the drug concentration in the plasma (Eq. 3.5). Because the magnitude of the apparent V_D is a useful indicator for the amount of drug outside the sampling compartment (usually the blood), the larger the apparent V_D, the greater the amount of drug in the extravascular tissues.

For each drug, the apparent V_D is a constant. In certain pathologic cases, the apparent V_D for the drug may be altered if the distribution of the drug is changed. For example, in edematous conditions, the total body water and total extracellular water increase; this is reflected in a larger apparent V_D value for a drug that is highly water soluble. Similarly, changes in total body weight and lean body mass (which normally occur with age) may also affect the apparent V_D.

CLEARANCE

Clearance is a measure of drug elimination from the body without identifying the mechanism or process. Clearance is also discussed in subsequent chapters. Clearance (*drug clearance, systemic clearance, total body clearance, Cl_T*) considers the

TABLE 3.1 Fluid in the Body

WATER COMPARTMENT	PERCENT OF BODY WEIGHT	PERCENT OF TOTAL BODY WATER
Plasma	4.5	7.5
Total extracellular water	27.0	45.0
Total intracellular water	33.0	55.0
Total body water	60.0	100.0

entire body as a drug-eliminating system from which many elimination processes may occur.

Drug Clearance in the One-Compartment Model

The body is considered as a system of organs perfused by plasma and body fluids. Drug elimination from the body is an ongoing process due to both metabolism (biotransformation) and drug excretion through the kidney and other routes. The mechanisms of drug elimination are complex, but collectively drug elimination from the body may be quantitated using the concept of drug clearance. Drug clearance refers to the *volume of plasma fluid* that is cleared of drug per unit time. Clearance may also be considered as the fraction of drug removed per unit time. The rate of drug elimination may be expressed in several ways, each of which essentially describe the same process, but with different levels of insight and application in pharmacokinetics.

Drug Elimination Expressed as Amount Per Time Unit

The expression of drug elimination from the body in terms of mass per unit time (eg, mg/min, or mg/hr) is simple, absolute, and unambiguous. For a zero-order elimination process, expressing the rate of drug elimination as mass per unit time is convenient because the rate is constant (Fig. 3-4A). In contrast, the rate of drug elimination for a first-order elimination process is not constant and changes with respect to the drug concentration in the body. For a first-order elimination, drug clearance expressed as volume per unit time (eg, liters/hr or mL/min) is convenient because it is a constant.

Drug Elimination Expressed as Volume Per Time Unit

The concept of expressing a rate in terms of volume per unit time is common in pharmacy. For example, a patient may be dosed at the rate of 2 teaspoonsful (10 mL) of a liquid medicine (10 mg/mL) daily, or alternatively, a dose (weight) of 100 mg of the same drug daily.

Clearance is a concept that expresses "the rate of drug removal" in terms of volume of drug solution removed per unit time (at whatever drug concentration in the body prevailing at that time) (Fig. 3-4B). In contrast to a solution in a bottle, the drug concentration in the body will gradually decline such that the mass of

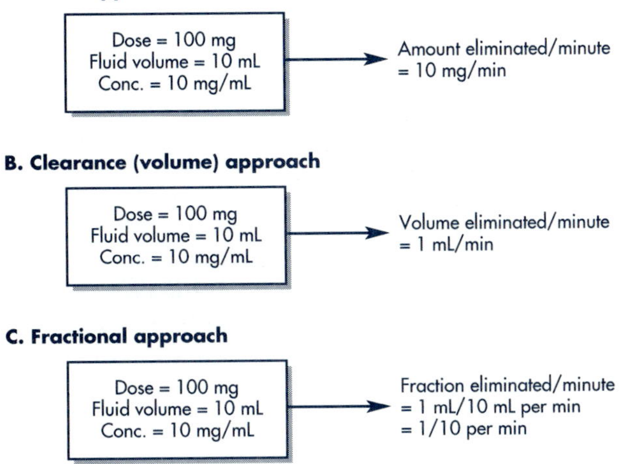

Figure 3-4. Diagram illustrating three different ways of describing drug elimination after a dose of 100 mg injected IV into a volume of 10 mL (a mouse, for example).

drug removed over time is not constant. The plasma volume in the healthy state is relatively constant because water lost through the kidney is rapidly replaced with fluid absorbed from the gastrointestinal tract.

Since a constant volume of plasma (about 120 mL per minute in humans) is filtered through the glomeruli of the kidneys, the rate of drug removal is dependent on the plasma drug concentration at all times. This observation leads to a simple basic rule (first-order process) governing drug elimination. For many drugs, the rate of drug elimination is dependent on the plasma drug concentration, multiplied by a constant factor k ($dC/dt = k\ C$). When the plasma drug concentration is high, the rate of drug removal is high and vice versa.

Clearance (volume of fluid removed of drug) for a first-order process is constant regardless of the drug concentration because clearance is expressed in volume per unit time rather than drug amount per unit time. Mathematically, the rate of drug elimination is similar to Equation 3.10.

$$\frac{dD_B}{dt} = -k\ C_p V_D \qquad \textbf{(3.2a)}$$

Dividing the expression on both sides by C_p yields Equation 3.14

$$\frac{dD_B/dt}{C_p} = \frac{-k\ C_p V_D}{C_p} \qquad \textbf{(3.14)}$$

$$\frac{dD_B/dt}{C_p} = -kV_D = Cl \qquad \textbf{(3.15)}$$

where dD_B/dt is the rate of drug elimination from the body (mg/hr), C_p is the plasma drug concentration (mg/L), k is a first-order rate constant (hr^{-1} or 1/hr) and V_D is the apparent volume of distribution (L). Cl is clearance and has the units L/hr in this example. In the example in Fig. 3-4B, Cl is in mL/min.

Clearance, Cl, is expressed as volume/time. Equation 3.15 shows that clearance is a constant because V_D and k are both constants. D_B is the amount of drug in the body, and dD_B/dt is the rate of change (of amount) of drug in the body with respect to time. The negative sign refers to the drug exiting from the body.

Drug Elimination Expressed as Fraction Eliminated Per Time Unit

Consider a compartment volume, containing V_D liters. If Cl is expressed in liters per minute (L/min), then the fraction of drug cleared per minute in the body is equal to Cl/V_D.

Expressing drug elimination as the fraction of total drug eliminated is applicable regardless or whether one is dealing with an amount or a volume (Fig. 3-4C). This approach is most flexible and convenient because of its dimensionless nature. Thus, it is valid to express drug elimination as a fraction (eg, 1/10 of the amount of drug in the body is eliminated or 1/10 of the drug volume is eliminated). Pharmacokineticists have incorporated this concept into the first-order equation (ie, k) that describes drug elimination from the one-compartment model. Indeed, the universal nature of many processes forms the basis of the first-order equation of drug elimination (eg, a fraction of the total drug molecules in the body will perfuse the glomeruli, a fraction of the filtered drug molecules will be reabsorbed at the renal tubules, and a fraction of the filtered drug molecules will be excreted from the body giving an overall first-order drug elimination rate constant, k). The rate of drug elimination is the product of k and the drug concentration (Equation

3.2a). The first-order equation of drug elimination can be also based on probability and a consideration of the statistical moment theory (Chapter 20).

Clearance and Volume of Distribution Ratio, Cl/V_D

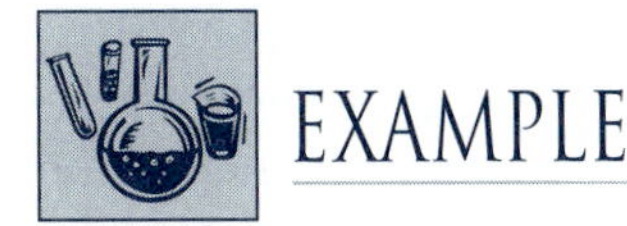

EXAMPLE

Consider that 100 mg of drug is dissolved in 10 mL of fluid and 10 mg of drug is removed in the first minute. The drug elimination process could be described as:

a. Number of mg of drug eliminated per minute (mg/min)

b. Number of mL of fluid cleared of drug per minute

c. Fraction of drug eliminated per minute.

The relationship of the three drug elimination processes is illustrated in Figure 3-4A–C. Note that in Figure 3-4C, the fraction Cl/V_D is dependent on both the volume of distribution and the rate of drug clearance from the body. This clearance concept forms the basis of classical pharmacokinetics and is later extended to flow models in pharmacologic modeling. If the drug concentration is C_p, the rate of drug elimination (in terms of rate of change in concentration, dC_p/dt) is:

$$-(Cl/V_D) \times C_p = \text{Rate of drug elimination} \tag{3.16}$$

For a first-order process,

$$-k\,C_p = \text{Rate of drug elimination} \tag{3.17}$$

Equating the two expressions yields:

$$k\,C_p = Cl/V_D \times C_p \tag{3.18}$$

$$k = Cl/V_D \tag{3.19}$$

Thus, a first-order rate constant is the fractional constant Cl/V_D. Some pharmacokineticists regard drug clearance and the volume of distribution as *independent* parameters that are necessary to describe the time course of drug elimination. Equation 3.19 is a rearrangement of Equation 3.15 given earlier.

One-Compartment Model Equation in Terms of *Cl* and V_D

This equation may be rewritten in terms of clearance and volume of distribution by substituting k with Cl/V. The clearance concept may also be applied a biologic system in physiologic modeling without the need of a theoretical compartment.

$$C_p = C_p^{0\,-kt} \tag{3.20}$$

$$C_p = D_0/V_D e^{-(Cl/V_D)t} \tag{3.21}$$

Equation 3.21 is applied directly in clinical pharmacy to determine clearance and volume of distribution in patients. When only one sample is available, ie, C_p is known at one sample time point, t after a given dose, the equation cannot be unambiguously determined because two unknown parameters must be solved, ie, Cl and V_D. In practice, the mean value for Cl and V_D of a drug are obtained from the population values in the literature. The values of Cl and V_D for the patient are adjusted using a computer program. Ultimately, a new pair of Cl and V_D values that better fit the observed plasma drug concentration is found. The process is repeated through iterations until the "best" parameters are obtained. Since many mathematical techniques (algorithms) are available for iteration, different results may be obtained using different iterative programs. An objective test to determine the accuracy of the estimated clearance and V_D values is to monitor how accurately those parameters will predict the plasma level of the drug after a new dose is given to the patient. In subsequent chapters, mean predictive error will be discussed and calculated in order to determine the performance of various drug monitoring methods in practice.

The ratio of Cl/V_D may be calculated regardless of compartment model type using minimal plasma samples. Clinical pharmacists have applied many variations of this approach to therapeutic drug monitoring and drug dosage adjustments in patients.

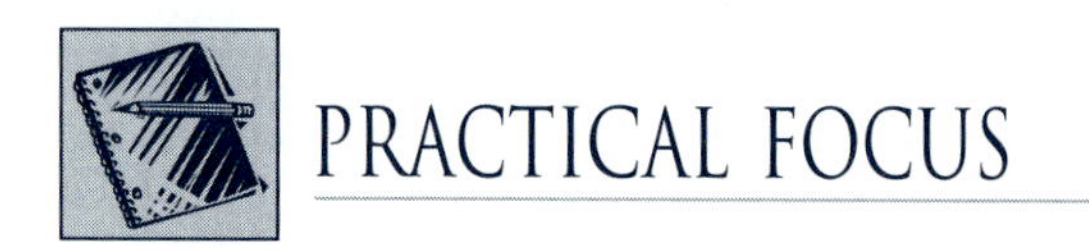

PRACTICAL FOCUS

The most accurate kinetic method to determine the volume of distribution and the distribution kinetic of a drug in a patient is to give the drug by a single IV bolus dose. An IV bolus dose avoids many variables such as delay, irregular and/or incomplete absorption compared to other routes of administration.

The IV single dose Equation 3.22 may be modified to calculate the elimination constant or half-life of a drug in a patient when two plasma samples and their time of collection are known:

$$\ln C_p = \ln C_p^0 - k\,t \tag{3.22}$$

If the first plasma sample is taken at t_1, instead of at zero and corresponds to plasma drug concentration, then C_2 is the concentration at time t_2 and t is set to $(t_2 - t_1)$.

$$C_2 = C_1 e^{-k(t_2 - t_1)} \tag{3.23}$$

$$\ln C_2 = \ln C_1 - k\,(t_2 - t_1)$$

Rearranging:

$$\ln C_2 = \ln C_1 - k\,(t_2 - t_1)$$

$$k = \frac{\ln C_1 - \ln C_2}{(t_2 - t_1)} \tag{3.24}$$

$$t_{1/2} = \frac{0.693\,(t_2 - t_1)}{\ln C_1 - \ln C_2} \tag{3.25}$$

t_1 = time of first sample collection
C_1 = plasma drug concentration at t_1
t_2 = time of second sample collection
C_2 = plasma drug concentration at t_2

In a clinical practice, several drug doses may have been given to the patient and the prior dosing times may not be accurately known. If the pharmacist judges that the drug in the body is in a declining phase (ie, absorption is completed), this equation may be used to determine the half-life of the drug in the patient by taking two plasma samples far apart and recording the times of sampling.

Clearance from Drug-Eliminating Tissues

Clearance may be applied to any organ that is involved in drug elimination from the body. As long as first-order elimination processes are involved, clearance represents the sum of the clearances for each drug-eliminating organ as shown in Equation 3.26:

$$Cl_T = Cl_R + Cl_{NR} \quad \textbf{(3.26)}$$

Where Cl_R is renal clearance or drug clearance through the kidney, Cl_{NR} is nonrenal clearance through other organs. Generally, clearance is considered as the sum of renal and nonrenal drug clearance, Cl_{NR}. Cl_{NR} is assumed to be primarily due to hepatic clearance (Cl_H) in the absence of other significant drug clearances, such as elimination through the lung or the bile, as shown in Equation 3.27.

$$Cl_T = Cl_R + Cl_H \quad \textbf{(3.27)}$$

Drug clearance considers that the drug in the body is uniformly dissolved in a volume of fluid (apparent volume of distribution, V_D) from which drug concentrations can be measured easily. Typically, plasma fluid concentration is measured and drug clearance is then calculated as the fixed volume of plasma fluid (containing the drug) cleared of drug per unit of time. The units for clearance are volume/time (eg, mL/min, L/hr).

Alternatively, Cl_T may be defined as the rate of drug elimination divided by the plasma drug concentration. Thus, clearance is expressed in terms of the volume of plasma containing drug that is eliminated per unit time. This clearance definition is equivalent to the previous definition and provides a practical way to calculate clearance based on plasma drug concentration data.

$$Cl_T = \frac{\text{Elimination rate}}{\text{Plasma concentration } (C_p)} \quad \textbf{(3.28)}$$

$$Cl_T = \frac{(dD_E/dt)}{C_p} = (\mu\text{g/min})/(\mu\text{g/mL}) = \text{mL/min} \quad \textbf{(3.29)}$$

where D_E is the amount of drug eliminated and dD_E/dt is the rate of drug elimination.

Rearrangement of Equation 3.29 gives Equation 3.30

$$\text{Drug elimination rate} = dD_E/dt = C_p\,Cl_T \quad \textbf{(3.30)}$$

Cl_T is a constant for a specific drug and represents the slope of the line obtained by plotting dD_E/dt versus C_p as shown in Equation 3.30.

For drugs that follow first-order elimination, the rate of drug elimination is dependent upon the amount of drug remaining in the body.

$$dD_E/dt = kD_B = kC_pV_D \quad \textbf{(3.31)}$$

Substituting the elimination rate in Equation 3.30 for kC_pV_D in Equation 3.31 and solving for Cl_T gives Equation 3.32.

$$Cl_T = kC_pV_D/Cp = kV_D \tag{3.32}$$

Equation 3.32 shows that clearance, Cl_T is the product of V_D and k, both of which are constant. This Equation 3.32 is similar to Equation 3.19 shown earlier. As the plasma drug concentration decreases during elimination, the rate of drug elimination, dD_E/dt, will decrease accordingly, but clearance will remain constant. Clearance will be constant as long as the rate of drug elimination is a first-order process.

For some drugs, the elimination rate process is more complex and a *noncompartment method* may be used to calculate certain pharmacokinetic parameters such as clearance.

Clearance can be determined directly from the plasma drug concentration versus time curve by

$$Cl_T = D_0/[\text{AUC}]_0^\infty \tag{3.33}$$

where D_0 is the dose and $[\text{AUC}]_0^\infty = \int_0^\infty C_p\, dt$.

Because $[\text{AUC}]_0^\infty$ is calculated from the plasma drug concentration versus time curve from 0 to infinity (∞) using the trapezoidal rule, no compartmental model is assumed. However, to extrapolate the data to infinity to obtain the residual $[\text{AUC}]_1^\infty$ or (C_{p_t}/k), first-order elimination is usually assumed. In this case, if the drug follows the kinetics of a one-compartment model, the Cl_T is numerically similar to the product of V_D and k obtained by fitting the data to a one-compartment model.

CALCULATION OF *k* FROM URINARY EXCRETION DATA

The elimination rate constant k may be calculated from urinary excretion data. In this calculation the excretion rate of the drug is assumed to be first order. The term k_e is the renal excretion rate constant, and D_u is the amount of drug excreted in the urine.

$$\frac{dD_u}{dt} = k_eD_B \tag{3.34}$$

From Equation 3.4, D_B can be substituted for $D_B^0e^{-kt}$:

$$\frac{dD_u}{dt} = k_eD_B^0e^{-kt} \tag{3.35}$$

Taking the natural logarithm of both sides and then transforming to common logarithms, the following expression is obtained:

$$\log\frac{dD_u}{dt} = \frac{-kt}{2.3} + \log k_eD_B^0 \tag{3.36}$$

A straight line is obtained from this equation by plotting semilog paper dD_u/dt against time (Figs. 3-5, 3-6). The slope of this curve is equal to $-k/2.3$ and the y intercept is equal to $k_eD_B^0$. For rapid intravenous administration, D_B^0 is equal to the dose D_0. Therefore, if D_B^0 is known, the renal excretion rate constant (k_e) can be

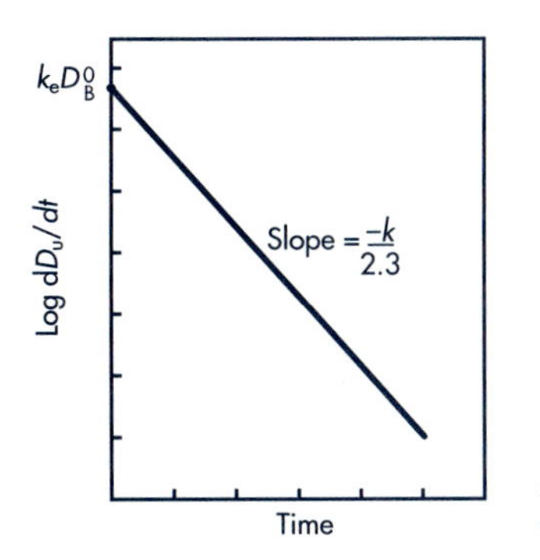

Figure 3-5. Graph of Equation 3.36: log rate of drug excretion vs t on regular paper.

obtained. Because both k_e and k can be determined by this method, the nonrenal rate constant (k_{nr}) for any route of elimination other than renal excretion can be found as follows:

$$k - k_e = k_{nr} \tag{3.37}$$

However, since elimination of a drug is usually effected by renal excretion and metabolism (biotransformation) of the drug,

$$k_{nr} \approx k_m \tag{3.38}$$

Substitution of k_m for k_{nr} in Equation 3.37 gives Equation 3.1. As the major routes of elimination for most drugs are renal excretion and metabolism (biotransformation), then k_{nr} is approximately equal to k_m.

The drug urinary excretion rate (dD_u/dt) cannot be determined experimentally for any given instant. Therefore, the average rate of urinary drug excretion, D_u/t is plotted against the average time, t^* for the collection of the urine sample. In practice, urine is collected over a specified time interval, and the urine specimen is analyzed for drug. An average urinary excretion rate is then calculated for that collection period. The average value of dD_u/dt is plotted on a semilogarithmic scale against the time which corresponds to the midpoint (average time) of the collection period.

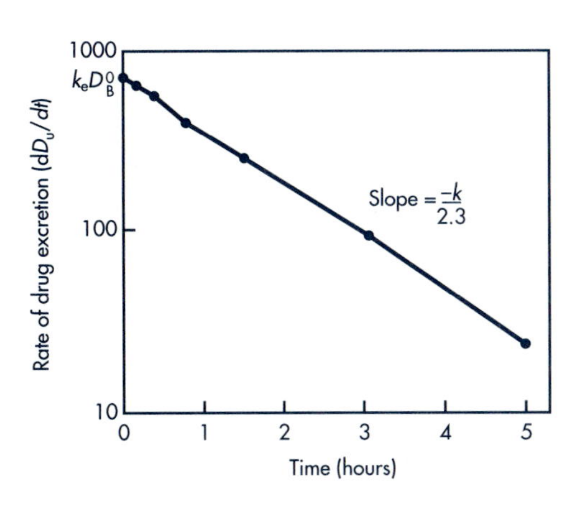

Figure 3-6. Semilog graph of rate of drug excretion versus time according to Equation 3.36 on semilog paper (Intercept = $k_eD_B^0$).

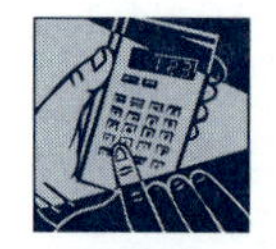

PRACTICE PROBLEM

A single IV dose of an antibiotic was given to a 50-kg woman at a dose level of 20 mg/kg. Urine and blood samples were removed periodically and assayed for parent drug. The following data were obtained:

Time (hr)	C_p (μg/mL)	D_u (mg)
0.25	4.2	160
0.50	3.5	140
1.0	2.5	200
2.0	1.25	250
4.0	0.31	188
6.0	0.08	46

Solution

Set up the following table:

Time (hr)	D_u (mg)	D_u/t	mg/hr	t^* (hr)
0.25	160	160/0.25	640	0.125
0.50	140	140/0.25	560	0.375
1.0	200	200/0.5	400	0.750
2.0	250	250/1	250	1.50
4.0	188	188/2	94	3.0
6.0	46	46/2	23	5.0

t^* = midpoint of collection period; t = time interval for collection of urine sample.

Construct a graph on a semilogarithmic scale of D_u/t versus t^*. The slope of this line should equal $-k/2.3$. The elimination $t_{1/2}$ is easier to determine directly from the curve and then calculate k from

$$k = \frac{0.693}{t_{1/2}}$$

In this problem, the $t_{1/2} = 1.0$ hr and $k = 0.693$ hr^{-1}. A similar graph of the C_p values versus t should yield a curve with a slope having the same value as that derived from the previous curve. Note that the slope of the log excretion rate constant is a function of elimination rate constant k and not of the urinary excretion rate constant k_e (Fig. 3-6).

An alternative method for the calculation of the elimination rate constant k from urinary excretion data is the *sigma-minus* method, or the *amount of drug remaining to be excreted* method. The *sigma-minus* method, is sometimes preferred over the previous method because fluctuations in the rate of elimination are minimized.

The amount of unchanged drug in the urine can be expressed as a function of time through the following equation:

$$D_u = \frac{k_e D_0}{k}(1 - e^{-kt}) \tag{3.39}$$

where D_u is the cumulative amount of unchanged drug excreted in the urine.

The amount of unchanged drug that is ultimately excreted in the urine, D_u^∞, can be determined by making time t equal to infinity. Thus, the term e^{-kt} becomes negligible and the following expression is obtained:

$$D_u^\infty = \frac{k_e D_0}{k} \quad \textbf{(3.40)}$$

Substitution of D_u^∞ for $k_e D_0/k$ in Equation 3.39 and rearrangement yields

$$D_u^\infty - D_u = D_u^\infty e^{-kt} \quad \textbf{(3.41)}$$

Equation 3.41 can be written in logarithmic form to obtain a linear equation:

$$\log(D_u^\infty - D_u) = \frac{-kt}{2.3} + \log D_u^\infty \quad \textbf{(3.42)}$$

Equation 3.42 describes the relationship for the amount of drug remaining to be excreted $(D_u^\infty - D_u)$ versus time.

A linear curve is obtained by graphing the logarithm scale of the amount of unchanged drug yet to be eliminated $\log(D_u^\infty - D_u)$ versus time. The slope of this curve is $-k/2.3$ and the y intercept is D_u^∞ on semilog paper (Fig. 3-7).

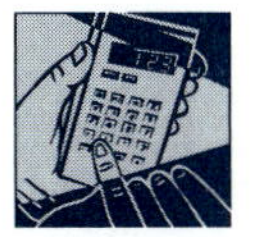

PRACTICE PROBLEM

Using the data in the preceding problem, determine the elimination constant.

Solution

Construct the following table:

Time (hr)	D_u (mg)	Cumulative D_u	$D_u^\infty - D_u$
0.25	160	160	824
0.50	140	300	684
1.0	200	500	484
2.0	250	750	234
4.0	188	938	46
6.0	46	984	0

Plot $\log(D_u^\infty - D_u)$ versus time. Use a semilogarithmic scale for $(D_u^\infty - D)$. Evaluate k and $t_{1/2}$ from the slope.

Comparison of the *Rate* and the *Sigma-Minus* Methods

The rate method does not require knowledge of D_u^∞, and the loss of one urine specimen does not invalidate the entire urinary drug excretion study. The sigma-minus method requires an accurate determination of D_u^∞ which requires the collection of urine until urinary drug excretion is complete. A small error in the assessment of D_u^∞ introduces an error in terms of curvature of the plot since each point is based

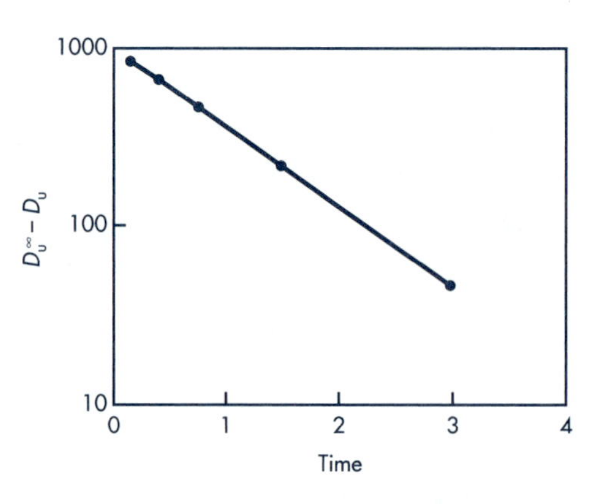

Figure 3-7. Sigma-minus method, or the amount of drug remaining to be excreted method, for the calculation of the elimination rate constant according to Equation 3.42.

on $\log(D_u^\infty - D_u)$ versus time. Fluctuations in the rate of drug elimination and experimental errors including incomplete bladder emptying for a collection period cause appreciable departure from linearity using the rate method, whereas the accuracy of the sigma-minus method is less affected. The rate method is applicable to zero-order drug elimination process, while the sigma-minus method is not. Lastly, the renal drug excretion rate constant may be obtained from the rate method but not from the sigma-minus method.

CLINICAL APPLICATION

The sigma-minus method and the excretion rate method was applied to the urinary drug excretion in subjects following the smoking of a single marijuana cigarette (Huestis et al, 1996). The urinary excretion curves of 11-nor-carboxy 9-tetrahydrocannabinol (THCCOOH), a metabolite of marijuana, in one subject from 24 to 144 hours after smoking one marijuana cigarette are shown in Figures 3-8 and 3-9. A total of 199.7 μg of THCCOOH was excreted in the urine over 7 days, which represents 0.54% of the total 9-tetrahydrocannabinol available in the cigarette. Using either urinary drug excretion method, the elimination half-life was determined to be about 30 hours. However, the urinary drug excretion rate method data were more scattered (variable) and the correlation coefficient r was equal to 0.744 (Fig. 3-9) compared to the correlation coefficient r of 0.992 using the sigma-minus method (Fig. 3-8).

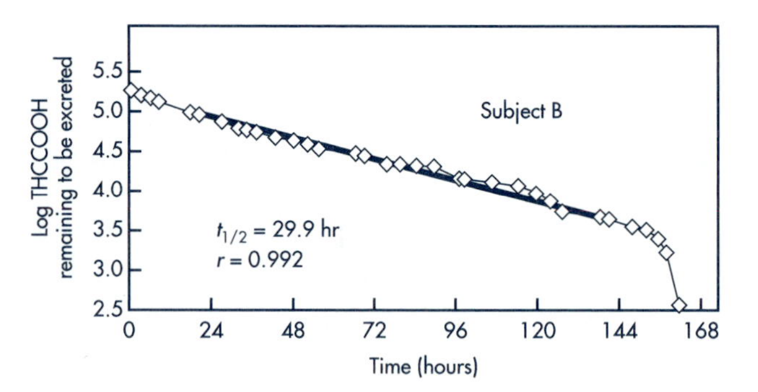

Figure 3-8. Amount remaining to be excreted method. The half-life of THCCOOH was calculated to be 29.9 hr from the slope of this curve; the correlation coefficient r was equal to 0.992. (Adapted from Huestis et al., 1996, with permission.)

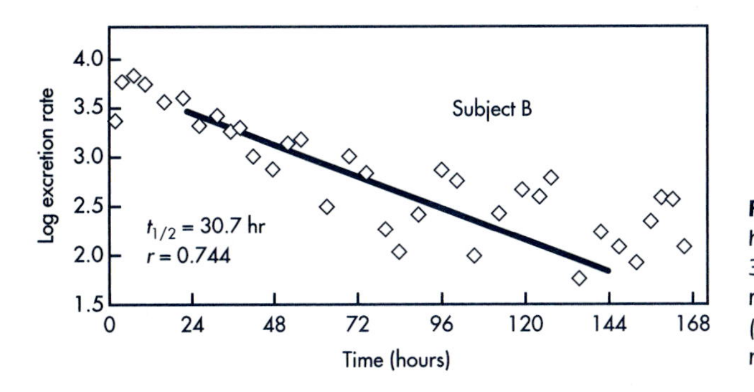

Figure 3-9. Excretion rate method. The half-life of THCCOOH was calculated to be 30.7 hr from the slope of this curve; the correlation coefficient r was equal to 0.744. (Adapted from Huestis et al., 1996, with permission.)

Problems in Obtaining Valid Urinary Excretion Data

Certain factors can make it difficult to obtain valid urinary excretion data. Some of these factors are as follows:

1. A significant fraction of the unchanged drug must be excreted in the urine.
2. The assay technique must be specific for the unchanged drug and must not have interference due to drug metabolites that have similar chemical structures.
3. Frequent sampling is necessary for a good curve description.
4. Urine samples should be collected periodically until almost all of the drug is excreted. A graph of the cumulative drug excreted versus time will yield a curve that approaches an asymptote at "infinite" time (Fig. 3-10). In practice, approximately seven elimination half-lives are needed for 99% of the drug to be eliminated.
5. Variations in urinary pH and volume may cause significant variation in urinary excretion rates.
6. Subjects should be carefully instructed as to the necessity of giving a complete urine specimen (ie, completely emptying the bladder).

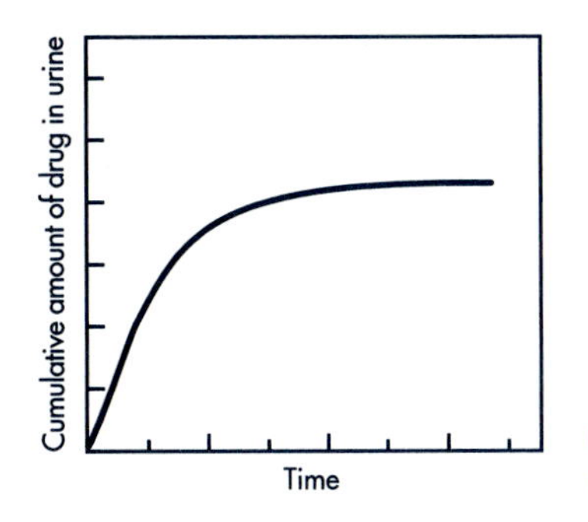

Figure 3-10. Graph showing the cumulative urinary excretion of drug as a function of time.

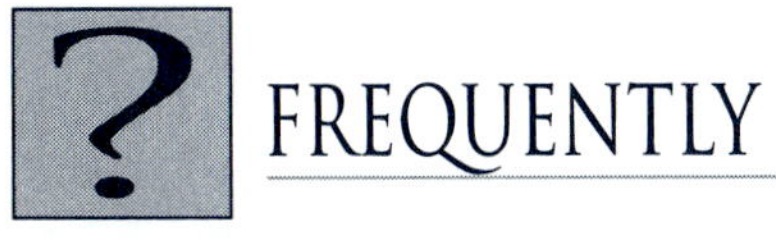

FREQUENTLY ASKED QUESTIONS

1. What is the difference between a rate and rate constant?
2. Why does k always have 1/time (eg, hr^{-1}) unit regardless of what the concentration unit is plotted?

3. If a drug is distributed in the one-compartment model, does it mean that there is no drug in the tissue?
4. How is clearance related to the volume of distribution and k?
5. If we use a physiologic model, are we dealing with actual volumes of blood and tissues? Why do we still use volumes of distribution that often are greater than the real physical volume?

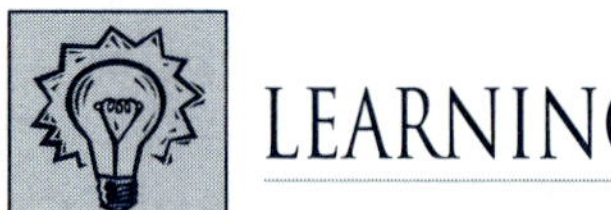

LEARNING QUESTIONS

1. A 70-kg volunteer is given an intravenous dose of an antibiotic, and serum drug concentrations were determined at 2 hours and 5 hours after administration. The drug concentrations were 1.2 and 0.3 μmg/mL, respectively. What is the biologic half-life for this drug, assuming first-order elimination kinetics?
2. A 50-kg woman was given a single IV dose of an antibacterial drug at a dose level of 6 mg/kg. Blood samples were taken at various time intervals. The concentration of the drug (C_p) was determined in the plasma fraction of each blood sample and the following data were obtained:

t (hr)	C_p (μg/mL)
0.25	8.21
0.50	7.87
1.0	7.23
3.0	5.15
6.0	3.09
12.0	1.11
18.0	0.40

   a. What are the values for V_D, k, and $t_{1/2}$ for this drug?
   b. This antibacterial agent is not effective at a plasma concentration of less than 2 μmg/mL. What is the duration of activity for this drug?
   c. How long would it take for 99.9% of this drug to be eliminated?
   d. If the dose of the antibiotic were doubled exactly, what would be the increase in duration of activity?
3. A new drug was given in a single intravenous dose of 200 mg to an 80-kg adult male patient. After 6 hours, the plasma drug concentration of drug was 1.5 mg/100 mL of plasma. Assuming that the apparent V_D is 10% of body weight, compute the total amount of drug in the body fluids after 6 hours. What is the half-life of this drug?
4. A new antibiotic drug was given in a single intravenous bolus of 4 mg/kg to 5 healthy male adults ranging in age from 23 to 38 years (average weight 75 kg). The pharmacokinetics of the plasma drug concentration–time curve for this drug fits a one-compartment model. The equation of the curve that best fits the data is

$$C_p = 78e^{-0.46t}$$

Determine the following (assume units of micrograms per milliliter for C_p and hours for t):

a. What is the $t_{1/2}$?

b. What is the V_D?

c. What is the plasma level of the drug after 4 hours?

d. How much drug is left in the body after 4 hours?

e. Predict what body water compartment this drug might occupy and explain why you made this prediction.

f. Assuming the drug is no longer effective when levels decline to less than 2 μmg/mL, when would you administer the next dose?

5. Define the term *apparent volume of distribution*. What criteria are necessary for the measurement of the apparent volume of distribution to be useful in pharmacokinetic calculations?

6. A drug has an elimination $t_{1/2}$ of 6 hours and follows first-order kinetics. If a single 200-mg dose is given to an adult male patient (68 kg) by IV bolus injection, what percent of the dose is lost in 24 hours?

7. A rather intoxicated young man (75 kg, age 21) was admitted to a rehabilitation center. His blood alcohol content was found to be 210 mg%. Assuming the average elimination rate of alcohol is 10 mL ethanol per hour, how long would it take for his blood alcohol concentration to decline to less than the legal blood alcohol concentration of 100 mg%? (*Hint:* Alcohol is eliminated by *zero*-order kinetics.) The specific gravity of alcohol is 0.8. The apparent volume of distribution for alcohol is 60% of body weight.

8. A single intravenous bolus injection containing 500 mg of cefamandole nafate (Mandol, Lilly) is given to an adult female patient (63 years, 55 kg) for a septicemic infection. The apparent volume of distribution is 0.1 L/kg and the elimination half-life is 0.75 hours. Assuming the drug is eliminated by first-order kinetics and may be described by a one-compartment model, calculate the following:

a. The C_p^0.

b. The amount of drug in the body at 4 hours after the dose is given.

c. The time for the drug to decline to 0.5 μg/mL, the minimum inhibitory concentration for streptococci.

9. If the amount of drug in the body declines from 100% of the dose (IV bolus injection) to 25% of the dose in 8 hours, what is the elimination half-life for this drug? (Assume first-order kinetics.)

10. A drug has an elimination half-life of 8 hours and follows first-order elimination kinetics. If a single 600-mg dose is given to an adult female patient (62 kg) by rapid IV injection, what *percent* of the dose is eliminated (lost) in 24 hours assuming the apparent V_D is 400 mL/kg? What is the expected plasma drug concentration (C_p) at 24 hours postdose?

11. For drugs that follow the kinetics of a one-compartment open model, must the tissues and plasma have the same drug concentration? Why?

12. An adult male patient (age 35 years, weight 72 kg) with a urinary tract infection was given a single intravenous bolus of an antibiotic (dose = 300 mg). The patient was instructed to empty his bladder prior to being medicated. After dose administration, the patient saved his urine specimens for drug analysis. The urine specimens were analyzed for both drug content and sterility (lack of bacteriuria). The drug assays gave the following results:

t (hr)	Amount of Drug in Urine (mg)
0	0
4	100
8	26

a. Assuming first-order elimination, calculate the elimination half-life for the antibiotic in this patient.

b. What are the practical problems in obtaining valid urinary drug excretion data for the determination of the drug elimination half-life?

REFERENCE

Huestis MA, Mitchell J, Cone EJ: Prolonged urinary excretion of marijuana metabolite (Abstract). Committee on Problems of Drug Dependence, San Juan, Puerto Rico, June 25, 1996.

BIBLIOGRAPHY

Gibaldi M, Nagashima R, Levy G: Relationship between drug concentration in plasma or serum and amount of drug in the body. *J Pharm Sci* **58:**193–197, 1969

Riegelman S, Loo JCK, Rowland M: Shortcomings in pharmacokinetic analysis by conceiving the body to exhibit properties of a single compartment. *J Pharm Sci* **57:**117–123, 1968

Riegelman S, Loo J, Rowland M: Concepts of volume of distribution and possible errors in evaluation of this parameter. *Science* **57:**128–133, 1968

Wagner JG, Northam JI: Estimation of volume of distribution and half-life of a compound after rapid intravenous injection. *J Pharm Sci* **58:**529–531, 1975

4

MULTICOMPARTMENT MODELS

Pharmacokinetic models may be used to represent drug distribution and elimination in the body. Ideally, a model should mimic closely the physiologic processes in the body. In practice, models seldom consider all the rate processes ongoing in the body and are, therefore, simplified mathematical expressions. The inability to measure all the rate processes in the body, including the lack of access to biological samples from the interior of the body, limit the sophistication of a model. Compartmental models are classical pharmacokinetic models that simulate the kinetic processes of drug absorption, distribution, and elimination with little physiologic detail. In contrast, the more sophisticated, physiologic model is discussed in Chapter 20. In compartmental models, drug tissue concentration is assumed to be uniform within a given hypothetical compartment. Hence, all muscle mass and connective tissues may be *lumped* into one hypothetical tissue compartment which equilibrates with drug from the central (or plasma) compartment. Since no data is collected on the tissue mass, the theoretical tissue concentration is unconstrained and cannot be used to forecast actual tissue drug levels. However, tissue drug uptake and tissue drug binding from the plasma fluid is kinetically simulated by considering the presence of a tissue compartment. Indeed, most drugs given by IV bolus dose decline rapidly soon after injection, and then decline moderately as some of the drug initially distributes into the tissue and back into the plasma.

Multicompartment models were developed to explain the observation that, after a rapid IV injection, the plasma level–time curve does not decline linearly as a single, first-order rate process. In a multicompartment model, the drug distributes at various rates into different tissue groups. Those tissues which have the highest blood flow may equilibrate with the plasma compartments. These highly perfused tissues and blood make up the central compartment. While this initial drug distribution is taking place, the drug is delivered concurrently to one or more peripheral compartments composed of groups of tissues with lower, but similar, blood flow and affinity for the drug. These distribution rate differences account for the appearance of a nonlinear log plasma drug concentration versus time curve. After drug equilibration within these peripheral tissues, the plasma level–time curve reflects first-order elimination of the drug from the body.

A drug will concentrate in a tissue in accordance with the affinity of the drug for that particular tissue. For example, lipid-soluble drugs tend to accumulate in fat tissues. Drugs that bind plasma proteins may be more concentrated in the plasma, because protein-bound drugs do not diffuse into the tissues. Drugs may also bind with tissue proteins and other macromolecules, such as DNA and melanin. Since sampling tissue is invasive and may not represent the entire organ, the tissue drug concentrations are usually projected from multicompartment models. Occasionally, tissue samples may be collected after a drug overdose episode. For example, the two-compartment model was used to describe the distribution of colchicine, but its toxic tissue levels after fatal overdoses was only recently described (Rochdi et al, 1992). The drug isotretinoin was found to have a long half-life because of substantial distribution into lipid tissues.

Kinetic analysis of a multicompartment model assumes that all transfer rate processes for the passage of drug into or out of individual compartments are first-order processes. On the basis of this assumption, the plasma level–time curve for a drug that follows a multicompartment model is best described by the summation of a series of exponential terms, each corresponding to first-order rate processes associated with a given compartment.

Because of these distribution factors, drugs will generally concentrate unevenly in the tissues, and different groups of tissues will accumulate the drug at different rates. A summary of the approximate blood flow to major human tissues is presented in Table 4.1. Many different tissues and rate processes are involved in the distribution of any drug. However, limited physiologic significance has been assigned to a few groups of tissues (Table 4.2)

The nonlinear profile of plasma drug concentration versus time is the result of many factors interacting together, including the permeability of the drug, the capacity of the tissues to accumulate drug, and the effect of disease factors on blood flow. Impaired cardiac function may produce a change in the drug distributive phase, whereas impairment of the kidney or the liver may prolong the elimination half-life as shown by a reduction in the slope of the terminal elimination phase of the curve. Frequently, multiple factors can complicate the distribution profile in such a way that the profile can only be described clearly with the assistance of a simulation model.

TABLE 4.1 Blood Flow to Human Tissues

TISSUE	PERCENT BODY WEIGHT	PERCENT CARDIAC OUTPUT	BLOOD FLOW (ml/100 g tissue per min)
Adrenals	0.02	1	550
Kidneys	0.4	24	450
Thyroid	0.04	2	400
Liver			
Hepatic	2.0	5	20
Portal		20	75
Portal-drained viscera	2.0	20	75
Heart (basal)	0.4	4	70
Brain	2.0	15	55
Skin	7.0	5	5
Muscle (basal)	40.0	15	3
Connective tissue	7.0	1	1
Fat	15.0	2	1

Adapted with permission from Butler (1972).

TABLE 4.2 General Grouping of Tissues According to Blood Supply[a]

BLOOD SUPPLY	TISSUE GROUP	PERCENT BODY WEIGHT
Highly perfused	Heart, brain, hepatic-portal system, kidney and endocrine glands	9
	Skin and muscle	50
	Adipose (fat) tissue and marrow	19
Slowly perfused	Bone, ligaments, tendons, cartilage, teeth and hair	22

[a]Tissue uptake will also depend on such factors as fat solubility, degree of ionization, partitioning, and protein binding of the drug.

Adapted from Eger (1993).

TWO-COMPARTMENT OPEN MODEL

Many drugs given in a single intravenous bolus dose demonstrate a plasma level–time curve that does not decline as a single exponential (first-order) process. The plasma level–time curve for a drug that follows a two-compartment model (Fig. 4-1) shows that the plasma drug concentration declines biexponentially as the sum of two first-order processes—distribution and elimination. A drug that follows the pharmacokinetics of a two-compartment model does not rapidly equilibrate throughout the body as is assumed for a one-compartment model. In this model, the drug distributes into two compartments, the central compartment and the tissue, or peripheral compartment. The *central compartment* represents the blood, extracellular fluid, and highly perfused tissues. The drug distributes rapidly and uniformly in the central compartment. A second compartment, known as the *tissue* or *peripheral compartment*, contains tissues in which the drug equilibrates more slowly. Drug transfer between the two compartments is assumed to take place by first-order processes.

There are several possible two-compartment models (Fig. 4-2). Model A is most often used and describes the plasma level–time curve observed in Figure 4-1. By convention, compartment 1 is the central compartment and compartment 2 is the tissue compartment. The rate constants k_{12} and k_{21} represent the first-order rate *transfer constants* for the movement of drug from compartment 1 to compartment 2 (k_{12}) and from compartment 2 to compartment 1 (k_{21}). The transfer constants

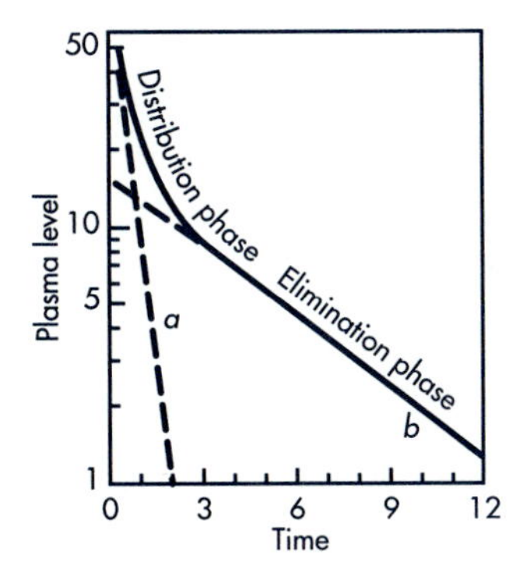

Figure 4-1. Plasma level–time curve for the two-compartment open model (single IV dose) described in Figure 4–2 (model A).

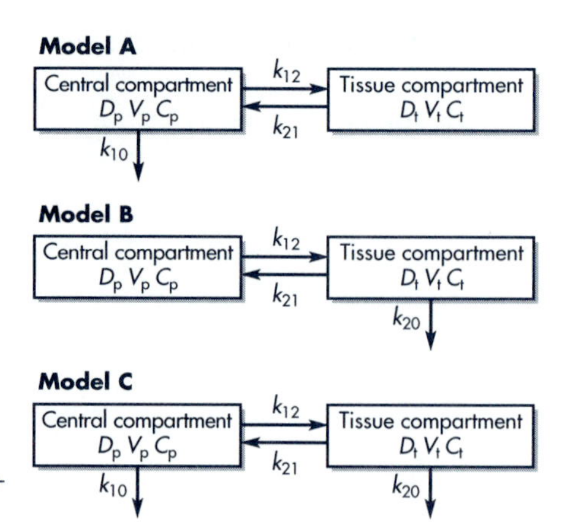

Figure 4-2. Two-compartment open models, intravenous injection.

are sometimes termed *microconstants*, and their values cannot be estimated directly. Most two-compartment models assume that elimination occurs from the central compartment model, as shown in Figure 4-2 (model A) unless other information about the drug is known. Drug elimination is presumed to occur from the central compartment, because the major sites of drug elimination (renal excretion and hepatic drug metabolism) occur in organs, such as the kidney and liver, which are highly perfused with blood.

The plasma level–time curve for a drug that follows a two-compartment model may be divided into two parts, a distribution (α) phase and an (β) elimination phase. After an intravenous bolus injection, drug rapidly equilibrates in the central compartment. The *distribution phase* of the curve represents the rapid decline of drug from the central compartment into the tissue compartment (Fig. 4-1, line *a*). Although some drug is eliminated during the distribution phase, there is a net transfer of drug from the central compartment to the tissue compartment. The fraction of drug in the tissue compartment during the distribution phase increases up to a maximum, at which time the fraction of drug in the tissue compartment is in equilibrium with the fraction of drug in the central compartment (Fig. 4-3). The maximum tissue drug concentration may be greater or less than the plasma drug concentration. After equilibration, the drug concentrations in both the central and tissue compartments decline more slowly as a first-order process during the elimination phase (Fig. 4-1, line *b*).

The two-compartment model assumes that, at $t = 0$, no drug is in the tissue compartment. After an intravenous dose, the drug is rapidly transferred into the tissue

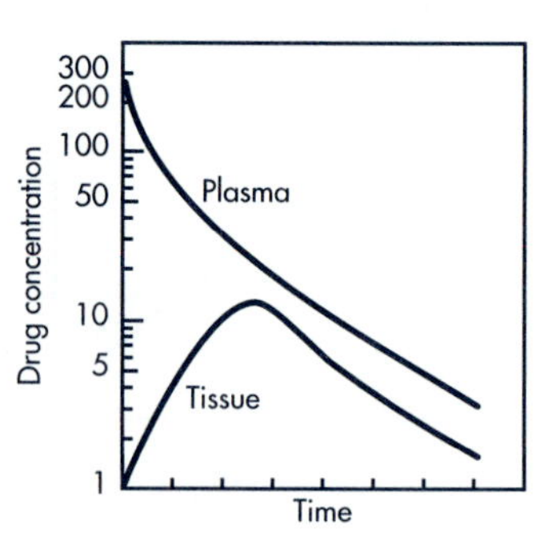

Figure 4-3. Relationship between tissue and plasma drug concentrations for a two-compartment open model. The maximum tissue drug concentration may be greater or less than the plasma drug concentration.

compartment while the blood level of drug declines rapidly due both to elimination of the drug and to transfer of the drug out of the central compartment into various tissues. A typical tissue drug level curve after a single intravenous dose is shown in Figure 4-3. The tissue drug level will eventually peak and then start to decline as the concentration gradient between the two compartments narrows.

The drug level in the theoretical tissue compartment can be calculated once the parameters for the model are determined. However, the drug concentration in the tissue compartment represents the average drug concentration in a group of tissues rather than any real anatomic tissue drug concentration. Real tissue drug concentration can sometimes be calculated by the addition of compartments to the model until a compartment that mimics the experimental tissue concentrations is found.

Tissue drug concentrations are theoretical only. Drug concentrations may vary among different tissues and possibly within an individual tissue. These varying tissue drug concentrations are due to differences in the partitioning of drug into the tissues, as discussed in Chapter 11. In terms of the pharmacokinetic model, the differences in tissue drug concentration is reflected in the k_{12}/k_{21} ratio. Thus, tissue drug concentration may be higher or lower than the plasma drug concentrations. Moreover, the elimination of drug from the tissue compartment may not be the same as the elimination from the central compartment. For example, if $k_{12}\cdot C_p$ is greater than $k_{21}\cdot C_t$ (rate in > rate out), then the tissue drug concentrations will increase and plasma drug concentrations will decrease.

In spite of the hypothetical nature of the tissue compartment, the theoretical tissue level is still valuable information for clinicians. The theoretical tissue concentration, together with the blood concentration, gives an accurate method of calculating the total amount of drug remaining in the body at any time (see digoxin example in Table 4.5). This information would not be available without pharmacokinetic models.

In practice, a blood sample is removed periodically from the central compartment and the plasma is analyzed for the presence of drug. The drug plasma level–time curve represents a phase of initial rapid equilibration with the central compartment (the distribution phase) followed by an elimination phase after the tissue compartment has also been equilibrated with drug. The distribution phase may take minutes or hours and may be missed entirely if the blood is sampled too late or at wide intervals after drug administration.

In the model depicted above, k_{12} and k_{21} are first-order rate constants that govern the rate of drug change in and out of the tissues:

$$\frac{dC_t}{dt} = k_{12}C_p - k_{21}C_t \tag{4.1}$$

The relationship between the amount of drug in each compartment and the concentration of drug in that compartment is shown by Equations 4.2 and 4.3:

$$C_p = \frac{D_p}{V_p} \tag{4.2}$$

$$C_t = \frac{D_t}{V_t} \tag{4.3}$$

where D_p = amount of drug in the central compartment, D_t = amount of drug in the tissue compartment, V_p = volume of drug in the central compartment, and V_t = volume of drug in the tissue compartment.

$$\frac{dC_p}{dt} = k_{21}\frac{D_t}{V_t} - k_{12}\frac{D_p}{V_p} - k\frac{D_p}{V_p} \tag{4.4}$$

$$\frac{dC_t}{dt} = k_{12}\frac{D_p}{V_p} - k_{21}\frac{D_t}{V_t} \tag{4.5}$$

Solving Equations 4.4 and 4.5 will give Equations 4.6 and 4.7, which describe the change in drug concentration in the blood and in the tissue with respect to time:

$$C_p = \frac{D_p^0}{V_p}\left[\frac{k_{21} - a}{b - a}e^{-at} + \frac{k_{21} - b}{a - b}e^{-bt}\right] \tag{4.6}$$

$$C_t = \frac{D_p^0}{V_t}\left[\frac{k_{12}}{b - a}e^{-at} + \frac{k_{12}}{a - b}e^{-bt}\right] \tag{4.7}$$

$$D_p = D_p^0\left[\frac{k_{21} - a}{b - a}e^{-at} + \frac{k_{21} - b}{a - b}e^{-bt}\right] \tag{4.8}$$

$$D_t = D_p^0\left[\frac{k_{12}}{b - a}e^{-at} + \frac{k_{12}}{a - b}e^{-bt}\right] \tag{4.9}$$

where D_p^0 = dose given intravenously, t = time after administration of dose, and a and b are constants that depend solely on k_{12}, k_{21}, and k. The amount of drug remaining in the plasma and tissue compartment at any time may be described realistically by Equations 4.8 and 4.9.

The rate constants for the transfer of drug between compartments are referred to as *microconstants* or *transfer constants*, and relate the amount of drug being transferred per unit time from one compartment to the other. The values for these microconstants cannot be determined by direct measurement but can be estimated by graphical method.

$$a + b = k_{12} + k_{21} + k \tag{4.10}$$

$$ab = k_{21}k \tag{4.11}$$

The constants a and b are hybrid first-order rate constants for the distribution phase and elimination phase, respectively. The mathematical relationship of a and b to the rate constants are given by Equations 4.10 and 4.11, which are derived after integration of Equations 4.4 and 4.5. Equation 4.6 can be transformed into the following expression:

$$C_p = Ae^{-at} + Be^{-bt} \tag{4.12}$$

The constants a and b are rate constants for the distribution phase and elimination phase, respectively. The constants A and B are intercepts on the y axis for each exponential segment of the curve in Equation 4.12. These values may be obtained graphically by the method of residuals or by computer. Intercepts A and B are actually hybrid constants, as shown in Equations 4.13 and 4.14.

$$A = \frac{D_0(a - k_{21})}{V_p(a - b)} \tag{4.13}$$

$$B = \frac{D_0(k_{21} - b)}{V_p(a - b)} \tag{4.14}$$

Method of Residuals

The method of residuals (also known as *feathering* or *peeling*) is a useful procedure for fitting a curve to the experimental data of a drug, which demonstrates the necessity of a multicompartment model. For example, 100 mg of a drug was administered by rapid IV injection to a 70-kg, healthy adult male. Blood samples were taken periodically after the administration of drug, and the plasma fraction of each sample was assayed for drug. The following data were obtained:

Time (hr)	Plasma Concentration (μg/mL)
0.25	43
0.5	32
1.0	20
1.5	14
2.0	11
4.0	6.5
8.0	2.8
12.0	1.2
16.0	0.52

When these data are plotted on semilogarithmic graph paper, a curved line is observed (Fig. 4-4). The curved-line relationship between the logarithm of the plasma concentration and time indicates that the drug is distributed in more than one compartment. From these data a biexponential equation, Equation 4.12, may be derived, either by computer or by the method of residuals.

As shown in the biexponential curve in Figure 4-4, the initial distribution rate is more rapid than the elimination rate. The rapid distribution phase is confirmed with the constant a being larger than the rate constant b. Therefore, at some later time the term Ae^{-at} will approach zero while Be^{-bt} will still have a value. At this later time Equation 4.12 will reduce to

$$C_p = Be^{-bt} \tag{4.15}$$

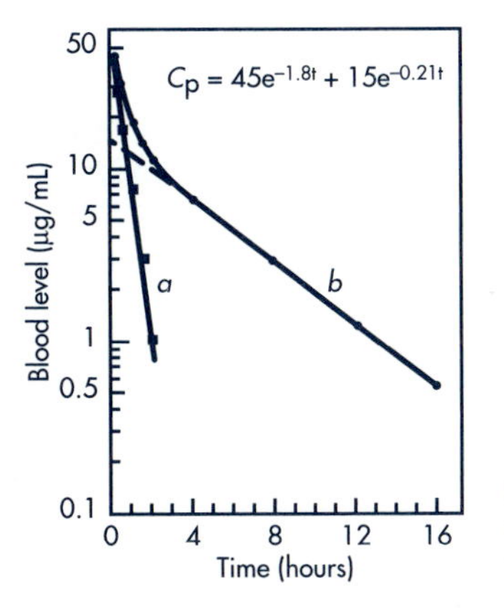

Figure 4-4. Plasma level–time curve for a two-compartment open model. The rate constants and intercepts were calculated by the method of residuals.

which, in common logarithms, is

$$\log C_p = \frac{-bt}{2.3} + \log B \qquad (4.16)$$

From Equation 4.16, the rate constant can be obtained from the slope $(-b/2.3)$ of a straight line representing the terminal exponential phase (Fig. 4-4). The $t_{1/2}$ for the elimination phase (beta half-life) can be derived from the following relationship:

$$t_{1/2_b} = \frac{0.693}{b} \qquad (4.17)$$

In the sample case considered here, b was found to be 0.21 hr^{-1}. From this information the regression line for the terminal exponential or b phase is extrapolated to the y axis; the y intercept is equal to B, or 15 μg/mL. Values from the extrapolated line are then subtracted from the original experimental data points (Table 4.3) and a straight line is obtained. This line represents the rapidly distributed a phase (Fig. 4-4).

The new line obtained by graphing the logarithm of the residual plasma concentration $(C_p - C'_p)$ against time represents the a phase. The value for a is 1.8 hr^{-1} and the y intercept is 45 μg/mL. The elimination $t_{1/2_b}$ is computed from b by use of Equation 4.17 and has the value of 3.3 hr.

A number of pharmacokinetic parameters may be derived by proper substitution of rate constants a and b and y intercepts A and B into the following equations:

$$k = \frac{ab(A + B)}{Ab + Ba} \qquad (4.18)$$

$$k_{12} = \frac{AB(b - a)^2}{(A + B)(Ab + Ba)} \qquad (4.19)$$

$$k_{21} = \frac{Ab + Ba}{A + B} \qquad (4.20)$$

Simulation of Plasma and Tissue Level of a Two-Compartment Model Drug—Digoxin in a Normal Patient and in a Renal Failure Patient

Once the pharmacokinetic parameters are determined for an individual, the amount of drug remaining in the plasma and tissue compartment may be calcu-

TABLE 4.3 Application of the Method of Residuals

TIME (hr)	C_p OBSERVED PLASMA LEVEL	C'_p EXTRAPOLATED PLASMA CONCENTRATION	$C_p - C'_p$ RESIDUAL PLASMA CONCENTRATION
0.25	43.0	14.5	28.5
0.5	32.0	13.5	18.5
1.0	20.0	12.3	7.7
1.5	14.0	11.0	3.0
2.0	11.0	10.0	1.0
4.0	6.5		
8.0	2.8		
12.0	1.2		
16.0	0.52		

TABLE 4.4 Two-Compartment Model Pharmacokinetic Parameters of Digoxin

PARAMETER	UNIT	NORMAL	RENAL IMPAIRED
k_{12}	hr^{-1}	1.02	0.45
k_{21}	hr^{-1}	0.15	0.11
k	hr^{-1}	0.18	0.04
V_p	L/kg	0.78	0.73
D	mcg/kg	3.6	3.6
a	1/hr	1.331	0.593
b	1/hr	0.019	0.007

lated using Equations 4.8 and 4.9. The pharmacokinetic data of digoxin was calculated in a normal and in a renal-impaired, 70-kg subject using the parameters in Table 4.4 as reported in the literature. The amount of digoxin remaining in the plasma and tissue compartment were tabulated in Table 4.5 and plotted in Figure 4-5. It can be seen that digoxin stored in the plasma declines rapidly during the initial distributive phase while drug amount in the tissue compartment take 3–4 hours ($5\ t_{1/2} = 5 \times 35$ minutes) to accumulate. It is interesting that clinicians have recommended that digoxin plasma samples be taken at least several hours after IV bolus dosing ($3–4^{+}$ hr, Winters, 1994, and 4–8 hr Schumacher, 1995) since the equilibrated level is more representative of myocardium digoxin level. In the simulation below, the amount of the drug in the plasma compartment at any time divided by V_p (54.6L for the normal subject) would yield the plasma digoxin level.

TABLE 4.5 Amount of Digoxin in Plasma and Tissue Compartment After an IV Dose of 0.252 mg in a Normal and Renal Failure Patient Weighing 70 kg[a]

	DIGOXIN AMOUNT			
	NORMAL RENAL FUNCTION		RENAL FAILURE (RF)	
Time (hr)	D_p (mcg)	D_t (mcg)	D_p (mcg)	D_t (mcg)
0.00	252.00	0.00	252.00	0.00
0.10	223.68	24.04	240.01	11.01
0.60	126.94	105.54	189.63	57.12
1.00	84.62	140.46	158.78	85.22
2.00	40.06	174.93	107.12	131.72
3.00	27.95	181.45	78.44	156.83
4.00	24.43	180.62	62.45	170.12
5.00	23.17	177.91	53.48	176.88
6.00	22.53	174.74	48.39	180.04
7.00	22.05	171.50	45.45	181.21
8.00	21.62	168.28	43.69	181.29
9.00	21.21	165.12	42.59	180.77
10.00	20.81	162.01	41.85	179.92
11.00	20.42	158.96	41.32	178.89
12.00	20.03	155.97	40.89	177.77
13.00	19.65	153.04	40.53	176.60
16.00	18.57	144.56	39.62	173.00
24.00	15.95	124.17	37.44	163.59

[a] D_p, drug in plasma compartment; D_t, drug in tissue compartment

Source: Data generated from parameters published by Harron (1989).

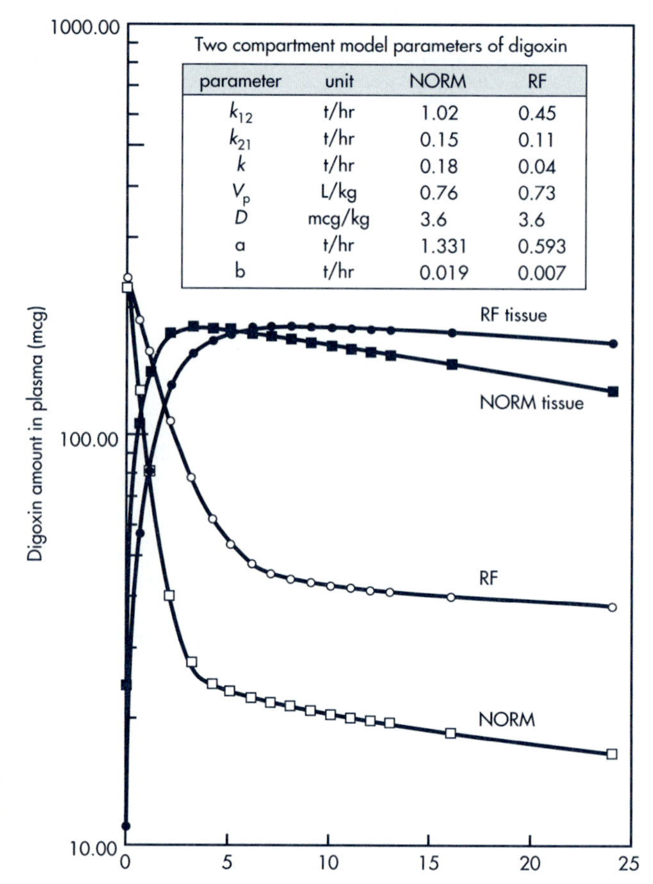

parameter	unit	NORM	RF
k_{12}	t/hr	1.02	0.45
k_{21}	t/hr	0.15	0.11
k	t/hr	0.18	0.04
V_p	L/kg	0.76	0.73
D	mcg/kg	3.6	3.6
a	t/hr	1.331	0.593
b	t/hr	0.019	0.007

Figure 4-5. Amount of digoxin (simulated) in plasma and tissue compartment after an IV dose to a normal and renal-failure (RF) patient.

At 4 hr after IV dose of 0.25 mg, $C_p = D_p/V_p = 24.43$ mcg/54.6 L = 0.45 ng/mL, corresponding to 3×0.45 ng/mL = 1.35 ng/mL if a full loading dose of 0.75 mg is given in a single dose. Although, the initial plasma drug levels were much higher than after equilibration, the digoxin plasma concentrations are generally regarded as not toxic since drug distribution is occurring rapidly. The tissue drug levels were not calculated. The tissue drug concentration represents the hypothetical tissue pool, which may not represent actual drug concentrations in the myocardium. In contrast, the amount of drug remaining in the tissue pool is real, since the amount of drug is calculated using mass balance. The rate of drug into the tissue in mcg/hr at any time is $k_{12}D_p$, while the rate of drug leaving the tissue is $k_{21}D_t$ in the same units. Both of these rates may be calculated from Table 4.5 using k_{12} and k_{21} from Table 4.4. Although some clinicians assume that tissue and plasma concentrations are equal when fully equilibrated, kinetic models only predict that the rate of drug transfer into and out of the compartments are equal at steady-state. In reality, tissue and plasma drug ratios are determined by the partition coefficient (a drug-specific physical ratio that measures the lipid/water affinity of a drug) and the extent of protein binding of the drug. Figure 4-5 shows that the time for the RF (renal failure or renal impaired) patient to reach stable tissue drug levels is longer than the time for the normal subject to reach steady-state due to changes in the elimination and transfer rate constants. As expected, a significantly higher amount of digoxin remains in both the plasma and tissue compartment in the renally impaired subject compared to the normal subject.

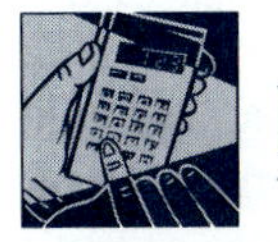

PRACTICE PROBLEM

From Figure 4-5 or Table 4.4, How many hours does it take for steady state to be reached in the normal and renal impaired patient?

Solution

At steady state, the rate of drug entering the tissue compartment is equal to the rate leaving (ie, at the peak of the tissue curve where the slope = 0 or not changing). This occurs at about 3 to 4 hours for the normal patient and 7 to 8 hours for the renal impaired patient. This may be verified by examining at what time $D_p k_{12} = D_t k_{21}$ using the data from Tables 4.4 and 4.5. Before steady state is reached, there is a net flux of drug into the tissue, ie, $D_p k_{12} > D_t k_{21}$ and beyond this point, there is a net flux of drug out the tissue compartment, ie, $D_t k_2 > D_p k_{12}$.

Apparent Volumes of Distribution

As discussed in Chapter 3, the apparent V_D is a useful parameter that relates plasma concentration to the amount of drug in the body. For drugs with large extravascular distribution, the apparent volume of distribution is generally large. Conversely, for polar drugs with low lipid solubility, the apparent V_D is generally small. Drugs with high peripheral tissue binding also contribute to a large apparent V_D. In multiple compartment kinetics, such as the two-compartment model, several volumes of distribution can be calculated. Volumes of distribution generally reflect the extent of drug distribution in the body on a relative basis, and the calculations depend on the availability of data. In general, it is important to refer to the same volume parameter when comparing kinetic changes in disease states. Unfortunately, values of apparent volumes of distribution of drugs from tables in the clinical literature are often listed without specifying the underlying kinetic processes, model parameter or method of calculation.

Volume of the Central Compartment

The volume of the central compartment is useful for determining the drug concentration directly after an IV injection into the body. In clinical pharmacy, this volume is also referred to as V_i or the initial volume of distribution as the drug distributes within the plasma and other accessible body fluids. This volume is generally smaller than the terminal volume of distribution after drug distribution to tissue is completed. The volume of the central compartment is generally greater than 3 liters, which is the volume of the plasma fluid for an average adult. For many polar drugs, an initial volume of 7 to 10 liters may be interpreted as rapid drug distribution within the plasma and some extracellular fluids. For example, the V_p of the moxalactam ranges from 0.14 to 0.15 L/kg, corresponding to about 9.8 L to 10.5 L for a typical 70-kg patient (Table 4.6). In contrast, V_p of hydromorphone is about 24 liters, possibly because of its rapid exit from the plasma into tissues even during the initial phase.

As in the case of the one-compartment model, V_p may be determined from the dose and the instantaneous plasma–drug concentration C_p^0. V_p is also useful in the determination of drug clearance if k is known, as in Chapter 3.

In the two-compartment model, V_p may also be considered as a mass balance factor as governed by the mass balance between dose and concentration, ie, drug concentration multiplied by the volume of the fluid must equal to the dose at time zero. At time zero, no drug is eliminated, $D_0 = V_p\ C_p$. The basic model assumption is: *plasma–drug concentration is representative of drug concentration within the distribution fluid.* If this statement is true, then the volume of distribution would be 3 liters; if not, it would indicate that distribution of drug also occur outside the vascular pool.

$$V_p = \frac{D_0}{C_p^0} \qquad \textbf{(4.21)}$$

At zero time ($t = 0$), all of the drug in the body is in the central compartment. C_p^0 can be shown to be equal to $A + B$ by the following equations.

$$C_p = Ae^{-at} + Be^{-bt} \qquad \textbf{(4.22)}$$

At $t = 0$, $e^0 = 1$. Therefore,

$$C_p^0 = A + B \qquad \textbf{(4.23)}$$

V_p is determined from Equation 4.24 by measuring A and B after feathering the curve, as discussed previously:

$$V_p = \frac{D_0}{A + B} \qquad \textbf{(4.24)}$$

Alternatively, the volume of the central compartment may be calculated from the $[AUC]_0^\infty$ in a manner similar to the calculation for the apparent V_D in the one-compartment model. For a one-compartment model

$$[AUC]_0^\infty = \frac{D_0}{kV_D} \qquad \textbf{(4.25)}$$

TABLE 4.6 Pharmacokinetic Parameters (mean ± SD) of Moxalactam in 3 Groups of Patients

GROUP	*A* mcg/mL	*B* mcg/mL	*a* hr^{-1}	*b* hr^{-1}	*k* hr^{-1}
1	138.9 ± 114.9	157.8 ± 87.1	6.8 ± 4.5	0.20 ± 0.12	0.38 ± 0.26
2	115.4 ± 65.9	115.0 ± 40.8	5.3 ± 3.5	0.27 ± 0.08	0.50 ± 0.17
3	102.9 ± 39.4	89.0 ± 36.7	5.6 ± 3.8	0.37 ± 0.09	0.71 ± 0.16

GROUP	*Cl* mL/min	V_P L/Kg	V_t L/Kg	$(V_D)_{ss}$ L/Kg	$(V_D)_\beta$ L/Kg
1	40.5 ± 14.5	0.12 ± 0.05	0.08 ± 0.04	0.20 ± 0.09	0.21 ± 0.09
2	73.7 ± 13.1	0.14 ± 0.06	0.09 ± 0.04	0.23 ± 0.10	0.24 ± 0.12
3	125.9 ± 28.0	0.15 ± 0.05	0.10 ± 0.05	0.25 ± 0.08	0.29 ± 0.09

In contrast, $[\mathrm{AUC}]_0^\infty$ for the two-compartment model is

$$[\mathrm{AUC}]_0^\infty = \frac{D_0}{kV_\mathrm{p}} \tag{4.26}$$

Rearrangement of this equation yields:

$$V_\mathrm{p} = \frac{D_0}{k[\mathrm{AUC}]_0^\infty} \tag{4.27}$$

Apparent Volume of Distribution at Steady State

At steady-state conditions, the rate of drug entry into the tissue compartment from the central compartment is equal to the rate of drug exit from the tissue compartment into the central compartment. These rates of drug transfer are described by the following expressions:

$$D_\mathrm{t}k_{21} = D_\mathrm{p}k_{12} \tag{4.28}$$

$$D_\mathrm{t} = \frac{k_{12}D_\mathrm{p}}{k_{21}} \tag{4.29}$$

Because the amount of drug in the central compartment D_p is equal to $V_\mathrm{p}C_\mathrm{p}$, by substitution in the above equation,

$$D_\mathrm{t} = \frac{k_{12}C_\mathrm{p}V_\mathrm{p}}{k_{21}} \tag{4.30}$$

The total amount of drug in the body at steady state is equal to the sum of the amount of drug in the tissue compartment, D_t, and the amount of drug in the central compartment, D_p. Therefore, the apparent volume of drug at steady state $(V_\mathrm{D})_\mathrm{ss}$ may be calculated by dividing the total amount of drug in the body by the concentration of drug in the central compartment at steady state:

$$(V_\mathrm{D})_\mathrm{ss} = \frac{D_\mathrm{p} + D_\mathrm{t}}{C_\mathrm{p}} \tag{4.31}$$

By substitution of Equation 4.30 into Equation 4.31, and by expressing D_p as $V_\mathrm{p}C_\mathrm{p}$, a more useful equation for the calculation of $(V_\mathrm{D})_\mathrm{ss}$ is obtained:

$$(V_\mathrm{D})_\mathrm{ss} = \frac{C_\mathrm{p}V_\mathrm{p} + k_{12}V_\mathrm{p}C_\mathrm{p}/k_{21}}{C_\mathrm{p}} \tag{4.32}$$

which reduces to

$$(V_\mathrm{D})_\mathrm{ss} = V_\mathrm{p} + \frac{k_{12}}{k_{21}}V_\mathrm{p} \tag{4.33}$$

In practice, Equation 4.33 is used to calculate $(V_\mathrm{D})_\mathrm{ss}$. The $(V_\mathrm{D})_\mathrm{ss}$ is a function of the transfer constants, k_{12} and k_{21}, which represent the rate constants of drug going into and out of the tissue compartment, respectively. The magnitude of $(V_\mathrm{D})_\mathrm{ss}$ is dependent on the hemodynamic factors responsible for drug distribution and on the physical properties of the drug, properties which, in turn, determine the relative amount of intra- and extravascular drug remaining in the body.

Extrapolated Volume of Distribution

The extrapolated volume of distribution $(V_D)_{exp}$ is calculated by the following equation:

$$(V_D)_{exp} = \frac{D_0}{B} \qquad \textbf{(4.34)}$$

where B is the y intercept obtained by extrapolation of the b phase of the plasma level curve to the y axis (Fig. 4-4). Because the y intercept is a hybrid constant, as shown by Equation 4.14, $(V_D)_{exp}$ may also be calculated by the following expression:

$$(V_D)_{exp} = V_p \frac{a - b}{k_{21} - b} \qquad \textbf{(4.35)}$$

This equation shows that a change in the distribution of a drug, which is observed by a change in the value for V_p, will be reflected in a change in $(V_D)_{exp}$.

Volume of Distribution by Area

The volume of distribution by area $(V_D)_{area}$, also known as $(V_D)_\beta$ is obtained through calculations similar to those used to find V_p, except that the rate constant b is used instead of the overall elimination rate constant k. $(V_D)_\beta$ is often calculated from total body clearance divided by b, unlike the steady state volume of distribution, $(V_D)_{ss}$, $(V_D)_\beta$ is influenced by drug elimination in the beta "b" phase. Reduced drug clearance from the body may increase AUC, such that $(V_D)_\beta$ is either reduced or unchanged depending on the value of b as shown in Equation 4.36.

$$(V_D)_\beta = (V_D)_{area} = \frac{D_0}{b[\text{AUC}]_0^\infty} \qquad \textbf{(4.36)}$$

Generally, reduced drug clearance is accompanied by a decrease in the constant, b (ie, an increase in the b elimination half-life). For example, in patients with renal dysfunction, the elimination half-life of the antibiotic, amoxacillin is longer because renal clearance is reduced.

Because total body clearance is equal to $D_0/[\text{AUC}]_0^\infty$, $(V_D)_\beta$ may be expressed in terms of clearance and the rate constant b:

$$(V_D)_\beta = \frac{\text{clearance}}{b} \qquad \textbf{(4.37)}$$

By substitution of kV_p for clearance in Equation 4.37, one obtains:

$$(V_D)_\beta = \frac{kV_p}{b} \qquad \textbf{(4.38)}$$

Theoretically, the value for b may remain unchanged in patients showing various degrees of moderate renal impairment. In this case, a reduction in $(V_D)_\beta$ may account for all the decrease in Cl while b is unchanged in Equation 4.37. Within the body, a redistribution of drug between the plasma and the tissue would mask the expected decline in b. The following example in two patients shows that the b elimination rate constant remains the same, while the distributional rate constants are changed. Interestingly, V_p is unchanged, while $(V_D)_\beta$ would be greatly changed in the simulated example. An example of a drug showing constant b slope while the renal function as measured by Cl_{cr} decreases from 107 to 56, 34, and 6 mL/min have been observed with the aminoglycoside drug, gentamicin in various patients after IV bolus dose (Schentag et al, 1977). Gentamicin follows polyexponential decline with a significant distributive phase. The following simulation problem may help to clarify the situation by changing k and clearance while keeping b constant.

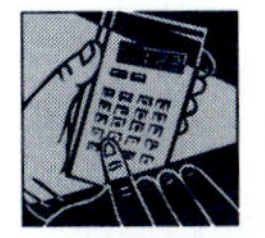

PRACTICE PROBLEM

Simulated plasma drug concentration after an IV bolus dose (100 mg) of an antibiotic in two patients—Patient 1 with a normal k, and Patient 2 with a reduced k is shown in Figure 4-6.

The data in the two patients were simulated with parameters using the two-compartment model equation. The parameters used are as follows:

Normal subject, $k = 0.3\ \text{hr}^{-1}$, $V\text{p} = 10$ L, $Cl = 3$ L/hr

$k_{12} = 5\ \text{hr}^{-1}$, $k_{21} = 0.2\ \text{hr}^{-1}$

Subject with moderate renal impairment, $k = 0.1\ \text{hr}^{-1}$, $V\text{p} = 10$ L, $Cl = 1$ L/hr.

$k_{12} = 2\ \text{hr}^{-1}$, $k_{21} = 0.25\ \text{hr}^{-1}$

Learning Questions

1. Is a reduction in drug clearance generally accompanied by increase in plasma drug concentration, regardless of which compartment model the drug follows?
2. Is a reduction in drug clearance generally accompanied by an increase in the b elimination half-life of a drug? (Find $(V_D)_\beta$ using Eq. 4.37, then b using Eq. 4.38)
3. Many antibiotics follow multiexponential plasma drug concentration profiles showing drug distribution into tissue compartments. In clinical pharmacokinetics, the terminal half-life was often determined with limited early data. Which patient has a greater terminal half-life based on the simulated data?

Solution

1. A reduction in drug clearance results in less drug being removed from the body per unit time. Drug clearance is model independent. Therefore, the plasma drug concentration should be higher in subjects with decreased drug clearance compared to subjects with normal drug clearance regardless of which compartment model is used (see Fig. 4-6).

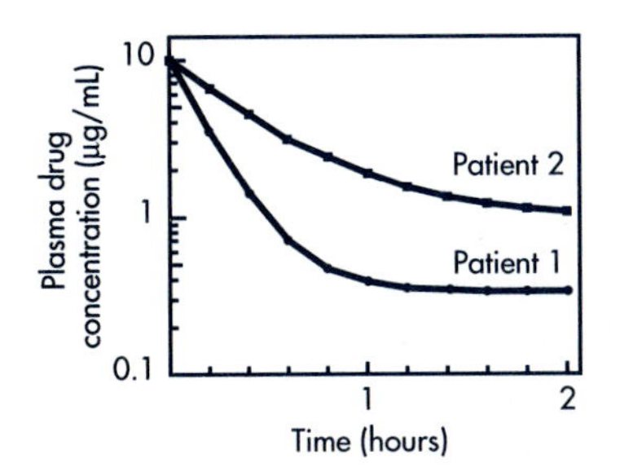

Figure 4-6. Simulation of plasma drug concentration after an IV bolus dose (100 mg) of an antibiotic in two patients—one with a normal k (Patient 1) and the other, reduced k (Patient 2).

2. Clearance in the two-compartment model is affected by the elimination rate constant, b, and the volume of distribution in the b phase which reflects the data. A decrease in the $(V_D)_\beta$ with b unchanged is possible, although this is not the common case. When this happens, the terminal data (see Fig. 4-6) concludes that the beta elimination half-life of patients 1 and 2 are the same due to a similar b. Actually, the real elimination half-life of the drug derived from k is a much better parameter since k reflects the changes in renal function, but not b which remains unchanged since it is masked by the changes in $(V_D)_\beta$.
3. Both patients have the same b value ($b = 0.011\ \text{hr}^{-1}$); the terminal slopes are identical. Ignoring early points by only taking terminal data would lead to an erroneous conclusion that the renal elimination process is unchanged, while the volume of distribution of the renally impaired patient is smaller. In this case, the renally impaired patient has a clearance of 1 L/hr compared with 3 L/hr for the normal subject, and yet the terminal slopes are the same. The rapid distribution of drug into the tissue in the normal subject causes a longer and steeper distribution phase. Later, redistribution of drug out of tissues masks the effect of rapid drug elimination through the kidney. In the renally impaired patient, distribution to tissue is reduced; as a result, little drug is redistributed out from the tissue in the b phase. Hence, it appears that the beta phases are identical in the two patients.

Significance of the Volumes of Distribution

From Equations 4.37 and 4.38 we can observe that $(V_D)_\beta$ is affected by changes in the overall elimination rate (ie, change in k) and by change in total body clearance of the drug. After the drug is distributed, the total amount of drug in the body during the elimination of b phase is calculated by using $(V_D)_\beta$.

In contrast, $(V_D)_{ss}$ is not affected by changes in drug elimination. $(V_D)_{ss}$ reflects the true distributional volume occupied by the plasma and the tissue pool when steady state is reached. Although this volume is not useful in calculating the amount of drug in the body during presteady state, $(V_D)_{ss}$ multiplied by the steady state plasma drug concentration, C_{ss} yields the amount of drug in the body. This volume is often used to determine the loading drug dose necessary to upload the body to a desired plasma drug concentration. As shown by Equation 4.33, $(V_D)_{ss}$ is several times greater than V_p, which represents the volume of the plasma compartment. V_p is sometimes called the initial volume of distribution and is useful in the calculation of drug clearance. The magnitude of the various apparent volumes of distribution have the following relationship to each other:

$$(V_D)_{exp} > (V_D)_\beta > V_p$$

$(V_D)_{ss}$ is much larger than V_p; it approximates $(V_D)_\beta$, but differs somewhat in value depending on the transfer constants. In a study involving a cardiotonic drug given intravenously to a group of normal and congestive heart failure (CHF) patients, the average AUC for CHF was 40% higher than in the normal subjects. The b elimination constant was 40% less in CHF patients, whereas the average $(V_D)_\beta$ remained essentially the same. In spite of the edematous conditions of these patients, the volume of distribution apparently remained constant. No change was found in the V_p or $(V_D)_\beta$. In this case, the volume of distribution was estimated by using Equation

4.33. In this study, a 40% increase in AUC in the CHF subjects was offset by a 40% smaller b elimination constant estimated by using computer methods. Because the dose was the same, the $(V_D)_\beta$ would not change unless the increase in AUC is not accompanied by a change in b elimination constant.

From Equation 4.37, the clearance of the drug in CHF patients was reduced by 40% and accompanied by a corresponding decrease in the b elimination constant, possibly due to a reduction in renal blood flow as a result of reduced cardiac output in CHF patients. In physiologic pharmacokinetics, clearance (Cl) and volume of distribution (V_D) are assumed to be independent parameters that explain the impact of disease factors on drug disposition. Thus, an increase in AUC of a cardiotonic, in CHF patient was assumed to be due to a reduction in drug clearance, since the volume of distribution is unchanged. The elimination half-life was reduced due to reduction in drug clearance. In reality, pharmacokinetic changes in a complex system is dependent on many factors that interact within the system. Clearance is affected by drug uptake, metabolism, binding, and more; all of these factors can also influence the drug distribution volume. Many parameters are assumed to be constant and independent for simplification of the model. Blood flow is an independent parameter that will affect both clearance and distribution. However, blood flow is, in turn, affected and regulated by many physiologic compensatory factors.

For drugs that follow two-compartment model kinetics, changes in disease states may not result in different pharmacokinetic parameters. Conversely, changes in pharmacokinetic parameters should not be attributed to physiologic changes without careful consideration of method of curve fitting and intersubject differences. Equation 4.38 shows that, unlike a simple one-compartment open model, $(V_D)_\beta$ may be estimated from k, b, and V_p. Errors in fitting are easily carried over to the other parameter estimates even if the calculations are performed by computer. The terms k_{12} and k_{21} often fluctuate due to minor fitting and experimental difference and may affect calculation of other parameters.

Drug in the Tissue Compartment

The apparent volume of the tissue compartment (V_t) is a conceptual volume only and does not represent true anatomic volumes. The V_t may be calculated from knowledge of the transfer rate constants and V_p.

$$V_t = \frac{V_p k_{12}}{k_{21}} \quad \textbf{(4.39)}$$

The calculation of the amount of drug in the tissue compartment does not entail the use of V_t. Calculation of the amount of drug in the tissue compartment provides an estimate for drug accumulation in the tissues of the body. This information is vital in estimating chronic toxicity and relating the duration of pharmacologic activity to dose. Tissue compartment drug concentration is an average estimate of the tissue pool and does not mean that all tissues have this concentration. The drug concentration in a tissue biopsy will provide an estimate for drug in that tissue sample. Due to differences in blood flow and drug partitioning into the tissue, and heterogenicity, even a biopsy from the same tissue may have different drug concentrations. Together with V_p and C_p, which calculate the amount of drug in the plasma, the compartment model provides mass balance information. Moreover, the pharmacodynamic activity may correlate better with the tissue drug concentration–time curve. To calculate the amount of drug in the tissue compartment D_t, the following expression is used:

$$D_t = \frac{k_{12} D_p^0}{a - b} (e^{-bt} - e^{-at}) \quad \textbf{(4.40)}$$

PRACTICE FOCUS

The therapeutic plasma concentration of digoxin is between 1 to 2 ng/mL; because digoxin has a long elimination half-life, digoxin takes a long time to reach a stable constant (steady state) level in the body. A loading dose is usually given with the initiation of digoxin therapy. Consider the implications of the loading dose of 1 mg suggested for a 70-kg subject. The clinical source cited an apparent volume of distribution of 7.3 L/kg for digoxin in determining the loading dose of digoxin. Use the pharmacokinetic parameters for digoxin in Table 4.4.

Solution:

The loading dose was calculated by considering the body as a one-compartment during steady state, at which time, the drug well penetrates the tissue compartment. The volume of distribution $(V_D)_\beta$ of digoxin is much larger than V_p, or the volume of the plasma compartment.

Using Equation (4.38),

$$(V_D)_\beta = \frac{kV_p}{b}$$

$$= 0.78 \text{ L/kg} \times 0.18/0.019 = 7.39 \text{ L/kg}$$

$$D_L = 7390 \text{ mL/kg} \times 70 \text{ kg} \times 1.5 \text{ ng/mL} = 775.95 \text{ mcg}$$

The loading dose is generally divided into 2 to 3 doses or administered 50% for the first dose and the remaining drug is given in 2 divided doses 6 to 8 hours apart to minimize potential side effects from overdigitization. If the entire loading dose were administered intravenously, the plasma level would be about 4 to 5 ng/mL after one hour, while the level would drop to about 1.5 ng/mL at about 4 hours. The exact level after a given IV dose may be calculated using Equation 4.6 at any time desired. The pharmacokinetic parameters for digoxin are available in Table 4.4.

Drug Clearance

The definition of clearance of a drug that follows a two-compartment model is similar to that of the one-compartment model. Clearance is the volume of plasma that is cleared of drug per unit time. Clearance may be calculated without consideration of the compartment model. Thus, clearance may be viewed as a physiologic concept for drug removal even though the development of clearance is rooted in classical pharmacokinetics.

Clearance is often calculated by a noncompartmental approach, as in Equation 4.41, in which the bolus IV dose is divided by the area under the plasma time concentration curve from zero to infinity, $[AUC]_0^\infty$. In evaluating the $[AUC]_0^\infty$, early time points must be collected frequently to observe the rapid decline in drug concentrations (distribution phase) for drugs with multicompartment pharmacokinetics. In the calculation of clearance using the noncompartmental approach, underestimating the area can inflate the calculated value of clearance.

$$Cl = \frac{D_0}{[\mathrm{AUC}]_0^\infty} \quad \textbf{(4.41)}$$

Equation 4.41 may be rearranged to Equation 4.36 to show that Cl in the two-compartment model is the product of $(V_D)_\beta$ and b. If both parameters are known, then calculation of clearance is simple and more accurate than using the trapezoidal rule to obtain area. Clearance calculations that use the two-compartment model are viewed as model dependent because more assumptions are required, and such calculations cannot be regarded as noncompartmental. However, the assumptions provide additional information and, in some sense, specifically describe the drug concentration versus time profile as biphasic. Clearance is a term that is useful in calculating average drug concentrations. With many drugs, a biphasic profile suggests a rapid tissue distribution phase followed by a slower elimination phase. Multicompartment pharmacokinetics is an important consideration in understanding drug permeation and toxicity. For example, the plasma time profile of aminoglycosides, such as gentamicin, are more useful in explaining toxicity than average plasma or drug concentration taken at peak or trough time.

$$Cl = (V_D)_\beta \mathrm{b} \quad \textbf{(4.42)}$$

Elimination Rate Constant

In the two-compartment model (IV administration), the elimination rate constant, k, represents the elimination of drug from the central compartment, whereas b represents drug elimination from the beta phase when distribution is mostly complete. Because of redistribution of drug out of the tissue compartment, the plasma–drug level in the b phase declines more slowly. Hence b is smaller than k; thus, k is a true elimination constant, whereas b is a hybrid elimination rate constant that is influenced by the rate of transfer of drug in and out of the tissue compartment. When it is impractical to determine k, b is calculated from the b slope. The $t_{1/2\beta}$ is often used to calculate the drug dose.

THREE-COMPARTMENT OPEN MODEL

The three-compartment model is an extension of the two-compartment model, with an additional deep tissue compartment. A drug that demonstrates the necessity of a three-compartment open model is distributed most rapidly to a highly perfused central compartment, less rapidly to the second or tissue compartment, and very slowly to the third or deep tissue compartment, containing such poorly perfused tissue as bone and fat. The deep tissue compartment may also represent tightly bound drug in the tissues. The three-compartment open model is shown in Figure 4-7.

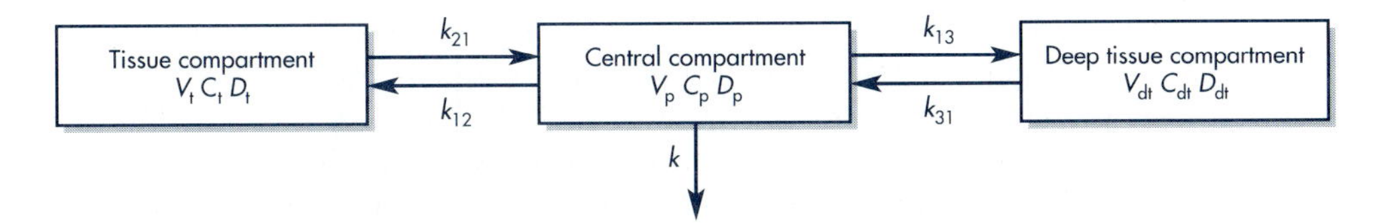

Figure 4-7. Three-compartment open model. This model, as with the previous two-compartment models, assumes that all drug elimination occurs via the central compartment.

A solution of the differential equation describing the rates of flow of drug into and out of the central compartment gives the following equation:

$$C_p = Ae^{-at} + Be^{-bt} + Ce^{-ct} \quad \textbf{(4.43)}$$

where A, B, and C are the y intercepts of extrapolated lines for the central, tissue, and deep tissue compartments, respectively, and a, b, and c are first-order rate constants for the central, tissue, and deep tissue compartments, respectively.

The parameters in Equation 4.45 may be solved graphically by the method of residuals (Fig. 4-8) or by computer. The calculations for the elimination rate constant k, volume of the central compartment, and area are shown in the following equations:

$$k = \frac{(A + B + C)\,abc}{Abc + Bac + Cab} \quad \textbf{(4.44)}$$

$$V_p = \frac{D_0}{A + B + C} \quad \textbf{(4.45)}$$

$$[\text{AUC}] = \frac{A}{a} + \frac{B}{b} + \frac{C}{c} \quad \textbf{(4.46)}$$

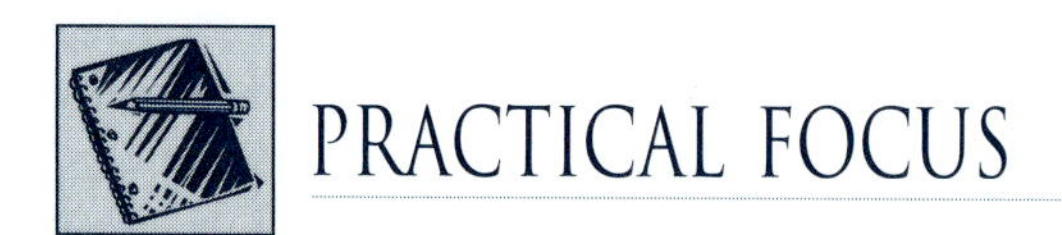

PRACTICAL FOCUS

Hydromorphone (Dilaudid)

Three independent studies on the pharmacokinetics of hydromorphone after a bolus intravenous injection reported that hydromorphone followed the pharma-

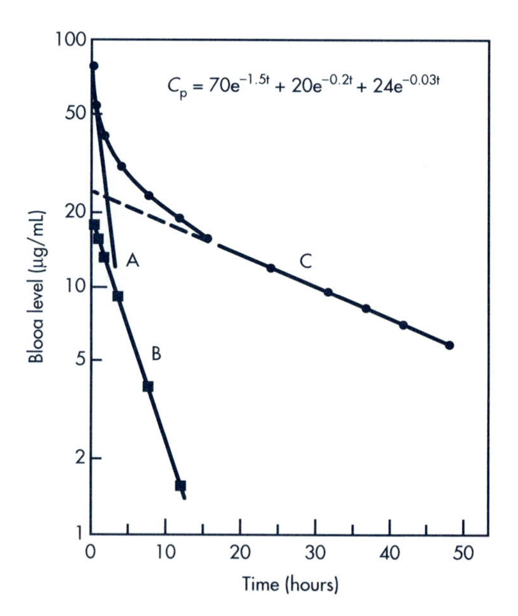

Figure 4-8. Plasma level-time curve for a three-compartment open model. The rate constants and intercepts were calculated by the method of residuals.

cokinetics of a one-compartment model (Vallner et al, 1981), a two-compartment model (Parab et al, 1988) or a three-compartment model (Hill et al, 1991), respectively. A comparison of these studies is listed in Table 4.7.

Comments

The adequacy of the pharmacokinetic model will depend upon the sampling intervals and the drug assay. The first two studies showed a similar elimination half-life. However, both Vallner et al (1981) and Parab et al (1988) did not observe a three-compartment pharmacokinetic model due to lack of appropriate description of the early distribution phases for hydromorphone. After an IV bolus injection, hydromorphone is very rapidly distributed into the tissues. Hill et al (1991) obtained a triexponential function by closely sampling early time periods after the dose. Average distribution half-lives were 1.27 min and 14.7 min, and the average terminal elimination was 184 min ($t_{1/2\beta}$). The average values for systemic clearance (Cl) was 1.66 L/min; the initial dilution volume was 24.4 L; and the steady-state volume of distribution, or $(V_D)_{ss}$ was 295 L. If distribution is rapid, the drug becomes distributed during absorption. Thus, hydromorphone pharmacokinetics follow a one-compartment model after a single oral dose.

Hydromorphone is administered to relieve acute pain in cancer or post-operative patients. Rapid pain relief is obtained by IV injection. Although the drug is effective orally, about 50% to 60% of the drug is cleared by the liver due to first-pass effects. The pharmacokinetics of hydromorphone after IV injection suggest a multicompartment model. The site of action is probably within the central nervous system, as part of the tissue compartment. The initial volume or initial dilution volume is V_p is the volume into which IV injections are injected and diluted. This volume is usually smaller than the $(V_D)_{ss}$, which is the steady-state volume of the drug in the body. Hydromorphone follows linear kinetics, ie, drug concentration is proportional to dose. Hydromorphone systemic clearance is much larger than the glomerular filtration rate GFR of 120 mL/min, hence the drug is probably me-

TABLE 4.7 Comparison of Hydromorphone Pharmacokinetics

STUDY	TIMING OF BLOOD SAMPLES	PHARMACOKINETIC PARAMETERS
6 Males, 25–29 yrs; mean weight, 76.8 kg Dose, 2 mg IV bolus Vallner, et al 1981	0, 15, 30, 45 min 1, 1.5, 2, 3, 4, 6, 8, 10, 12 hrs	One-Compartment Model Terminal $t_{1/2}$ = 2.64 (± 0.88) hr
8 Males, 20–30 yrs; weight, 50–86 kg Dose, 2 mg, IV bolus Parab, et al 1988	0, 3, 7, 15, 30, 45 min 1, 1.5, 2, 3, 4, 6, 8, 10, 12 hrs	Two-Compartment Model Terminal $t_{1/2}$ = 2.36 (± 0.58) hr
10 Males, 21–38 yrs; mean weight, 72.7 kg Dose, 10, 20, and 40 μg/kg, IV bolus Hill, et al 1991	1, 2, 3, 4, 5, 7, 10, 15, 20, 30, 45 min 1, 1.5, 2, 2.5, 3, 4, 5 hrs	Three-Compartment Model Terminal $t_{1/2}$ = 3.07 (± 0.25) hr

tabolized significantly by hepatic route. A clearance of 1.66 L/min is faster than the blood flow of 1.2 to 1.5 L/min to the liver. The drug must be rapidly extracted or, in addition, must have extrahepatic elimination. When the distribution phase is short, the distribution phase may be disregarded, provided that the targeted plasma concentration is sufficiently low and the terminal elimination phase is relatively long. If the drug has a sufficiently high target plasma drug concentration and the elimination half-life is short, the distributive phase must not be ignored. For example, lidocaine target effective concentration often lies close to the distributive phase, since its beta elimination half-life is very short; and ignoring the alpha phase will result in a large error in dosing projection.

DETERMINATION OF COMPARTMENT MODELS

Models based on compartmental analysis should always use the fewest number of compartments necessary to adequately describe the experimental data. Once an empirical equation is derived from the experimental observations, it becomes necessary to examine how well the theoretical values that are calculated from the derived equation fit the experimental data.

The observed number of compartments or exponential phases will depend upon (1) the route of drug administration, (2) the rate of drug absorption, (3) the total time for blood sampling, (4) the number of samples taken within the collection period, and (5) the assay sensitivity.

If drug distribution is rapid, then, after oral administration, the drug will become distributed during absorption, and the distribution phase will not be observed. For example, theophylline follows the kinetics of a one-compartment model after oral absorption, but, after intravenous bolus (given as aminophylline), theophylline follows the kinetics of a two-compartment model. Furthermore, if theophylline is given by a slow intravenous infusion rather than by intravenous bolus, the distribution phase will not be observed. Hydromorphone (Dilaudid), which follows a three-compartment model, also follows a one-compartment model after oral administration, since the first two distribution phases are rapid.

Depending upon the sampling intervals, a compartment may be missed because samples may be taken too late after administration of the dose to observe a possible distributive phase. For example, the data plotted in Figure 4-9 could easily be mistaken for those of a one-compartment model, because the distributive phase has been missed and extrapolation of the data to C_p^0 will give a lower value than was actually the case. Slower drug elimination compartments may also be missed if sampling is not performed at later sampling times when the dose or the assay for the drug cannot measure very low plasma drug concentrations.

The total time for collection of blood samples is usually estimated from the terminal elimination half-life of the drug. However, lower drug concentrations may not be measured if the sensitivity of the assay is not adequate. As the assay for the drug becomes more sensitive in its ability to measure lower drug concentrations, then another compartment with a smaller first-order rate constant may be observed.

In describing compartments, each new compartment requires an additional first-order plot. Compartment models having more than three compartments are rarely of pharmacologic significance. In certain cases, it is possible to "lump" a few com-

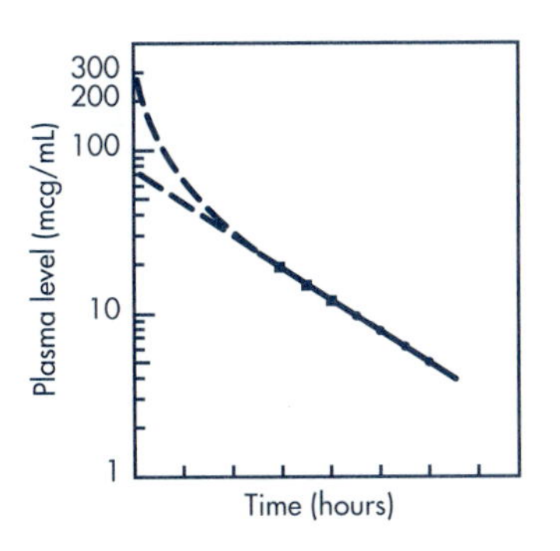

Figure 4-9. The samples from which data were obtained for this graph were taken too late to show the distributive phase; therefore, the value of C_p^0 obtained by extrapolation (straight broken line) is deceptively low.

partments together to get a smaller number of compartments, which, together, will describe the data adequately.

An adequate description of several tissue compartments can be difficult. When the addition of a compartment to the model seems necessary, it is important to realize that the drug may be retained or slowly concentrated in a deep tissue compartment.

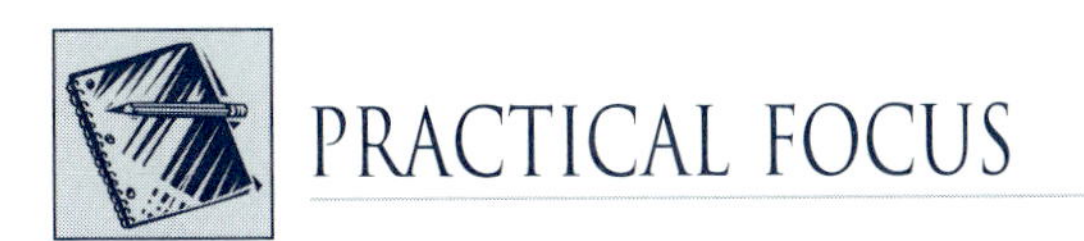

PRACTICAL FOCUS

Two-Compartment Model: Relation Between Distribution and Apparent (Beta) Half-Life

The distribution half-life of a drug is dependent upon the type of tissues the drug penetrates as well as by blood supply to those tissues. In addition, the capacity of the tissue to store drug is also a factor. Distribution half-life is generally short for many drugs because of the rapid blood supply and drug equilibration in the tissue compartment. However, there is some supporting evidence that a drug with a long elimination half-life is often associated with a longer distribution phase. It is conceivable that a tissue with little blood supply may not be equilibrated with significant drug to exert its impact and influence the overall plasma drug concentration profile in the presence of rapid elimination. In contrast, drugs such as digoxin have a long elimination half-life, and drug concentration declines slowly to allow more time for distribution to tissues. Human follicle stimulating hormone (hFSH) injected intravenously has a very long elimination half-life and its distribution half-life is also quite long. Drugs such as lidocaine, theophylline, and milrinone have short elimination half-lives and generally relatively short distributional half-lives.

In order to examine the effect of changing k (from 0.6 hr^{-1} to 0.2 hr^{-1}) on the distributional (alpha phase) and elimination (beta phase) half-lives of various drugs, four simulations based on a two-compartment model were generated (Table 4.8). The simulations show that a drug with a smaller k has a longer beta elimination half-life. Keeping all other parameters (k_{12}, k_{21}, V_p) constant, a smaller k will result in a smaller a, or a slower distributional phase. Examples of drugs with various distribution and elimination half-lives are shown in Table 4.8.

TABLE 4.8 Comparison of Beta Half-Life and Distributional Half-Life of Selected Drugs

DRUG	BETA HALF-LIFE	DISTRIBUTIONAL HALF-LIFE
Lidocaine	1.8 hr	8 min
Cocaine	1 hr	18 min
Theophylline	4.33	7.2 min
Ergometrine	2 hr	11 min
Hydromorphone	3 hr	14.7 min
Milrinone	3.6 hr	4.6 min
Procainamide	2.5–4.7 hr	6 min
Quinidine	6–8 hr	7 min
Lithium	21.39 hr	5 hr
Digoxin	1.6 day	35 min
Human FSH	1 day	60 min
IgG1 kappa MAB	9.6 day (monkey)	6.7 hr
Simulation 1	13.26 hr	36.24 min
Simulation 2	16.60 hr	43.38 min
Simulation 3	26.83 hr	53.70 min
Simulation 4	213.7 hr	1.12 hr

Simulation was performed using V_p of 10 L; dose = 100 mg; $k_{12} = 0.5\ hr^{-1}$; $k_{21} = 0.1\ hr^{-1}$; $k = 0.6$, 0.4, 0.2, and 0.02 hr for simulations 1–4, respectively (using Equations 4.10 and 4.11)

Source: from Manufacturer and Schumacher with permission (1995)

Clinical Example - Moxalactam, Effect of Changing Renal Function in Patients with Sepsis

The pharmacokinetics of moxalactam (see Table 4.6, p 78) was examined in 40 patients with abdominal sepsis (Swanson et al, 1983). The patients were grouped according to creatinine clearances into three groups:

Group 1—Average creatinine clearance = 35.5 mL/min/1.73 m^2
Group 2—Average creatinine clearance = 67.1 ± 6.7 mL/min/1.73 m^2
Group 3—Average creatinine clearance = 117.2 ± 29.9 mL/min/1.73 m^2

After intravenous bolus administration, the serum drug concentrations followed a biexponential decline (Fig. 4-10). The pharmacokinetics at steady state (2 g every 8 hr) was also examined in these patients. Mean steady-state serum concentrations ranged from 27.0 to 211.0 mcg/mL and correlated inversely with creatinine clearance ($r = 0.91$, $P < 0.0001$). The terminal half-life ranged from 1.27 to 8.27 hours and reflected the varying renal function of the patients. Moxalactam total body clearance (Cl) had excellent correlation with creatinine clearance ($r^2 = 0.92$). Cl determined by noncompartmental data analysis was in agreement with Cl determined by nonlinear least squares regression ($r = 0.99$, $P < 0.0001$). Moxalactam total body clearance was best predicted from creatinine clearance corrected for body surface area.

Questions (Refer to Table 4.6, p 78)

1. Calculate the beta half-life of moxalactam in the most renally impaired group.
2. What indicator is used to predict moxalactam clearance in the body?

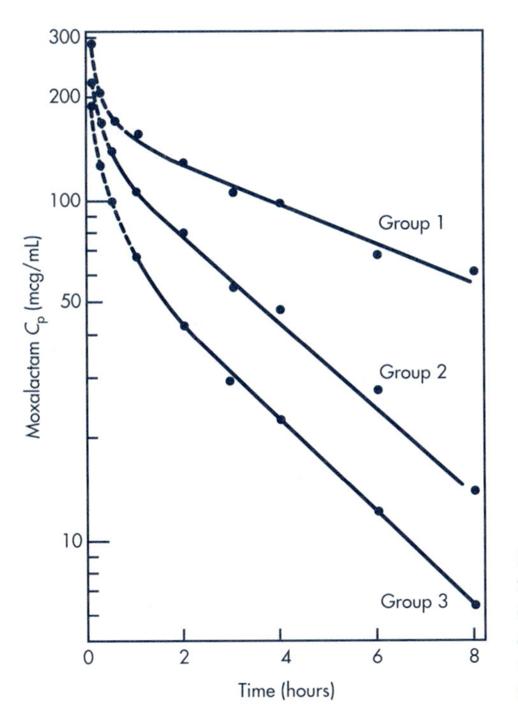

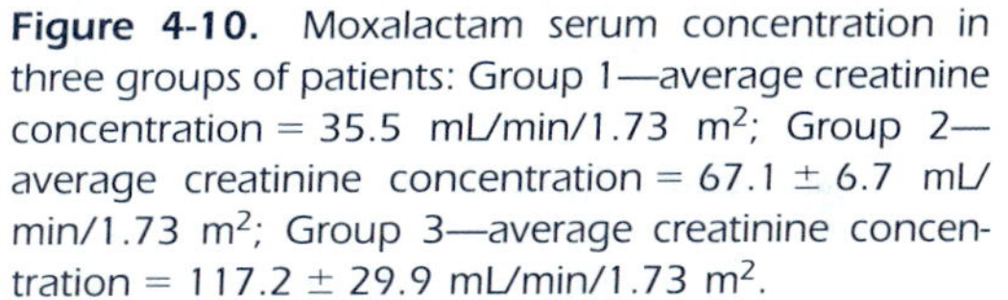
Figure 4-10. Moxalactam serum concentration in three groups of patients: Group 1—average creatinine concentration = 35.5 mL/min/1.73 m^2; Group 2—average creatinine concentration = 67.1 ± 6.7 mL/min/1.73 m^2; Group 3—average creatinine concentration = 117.2 ± 29.9 mL/min/1.73 m^2.

3. What is the beta volume of distribution of patients in group 3 with normal renal function?
4. What effect does variable renal clearance have on mean steady-state serum concentrations?
5. What is the initial volume (V_i) of moxalactam?

Solutions

1. Mean beta half life is 0.693/0.20 = 3.47 hours in the most renally impaired group.
2. Creatinine is mainly filtered through the kidney, and creatinine clearance is used as an indicator of renal glomerular filtration rate. Group 3 has normal renal function (average creatinine clearance = 117.2 mL/min/1.73 m^2).
3. Beta volume of distribution:
   Moxalactam clearance in group 3 subjects is 125.9 mL/min.

   From Equation 4.37, $(V_D)_\beta = \text{clearance}/b$

$$= \frac{125.9 \text{ mL/min} \times 60 \text{ min/hr}}{0.37 \text{ hr}^{-1}}$$

$$= 20416 \text{ mL or } (20.4 \text{ L})$$

4. Variable renal clearance may lead to erratic steady-state drug concentration.
5. The volume of the plasma compartment, V_p, is sometimes referred to as the initial volume. V_p ranges from 0.12 to 0.15 L/kg among the three groups and is considerably smaller than the steady state volume of distribution.

Clinical Example - Azithromycin Pharmacokinetics

Following oral administration, azithromycin is rapidly absorbed and widely distributed throughout the body. Azithromycin is rapidly distributed into tissues with high drug concentrations within cells, resulting in significantly higher azithromycin tissue concentrations than in plasma. The high values for apparent steady-state volume of distribution and plasma clearance (630 mL/min) suggests that the prolonged half-life is due to extensive uptake and subsequent release of drug from tissues.

Plasma concentrations of azithromycin decline in a polyphasic pattern resulting in an average terminal half-life of 68 hours. With this regimen, C_{min} and C_{max} remained essentially unchanged from day 2 through day 5 of therapy. However, without a loading dose, azithromycin C_{min} levels required 5 to 7 days to reach steady state.

The pharmacokinetic parameters of azithromycin in healthy elderly male subjects (65 to 85 years) were similar to those in young adults. Although higher peak drug concentrations (increased by 30% to 50%) were observed in elderly women, no significant accumulation occurred.

Questions

1. Do you agree with the following statements for *a* that is described by a two-compartment pharmacokinetic model? At steady state, the drug is well equilibrated between the plasma and the tissue compartment, $C_p = C_t$, and the rates of drug diffusion into and from the plasma compartment are equal. The steady-state volume of distribution is much larger than the initial volume, V_i, or the original plasma volume, V_p, of the central compartment. The loading dose is often calculated using the $(V_D)_{ss}$ instead of V_p.
2. Azithromycin may be described by a plasma and a tissue compartment model. "Rapid distribution of azithromycin into cells causes higher concentration in the tissues than in the plasma. . . ." Does this statement conflict with the steady-state concept?
3. Why is loading dose used?
4. What is V_i? How is this volume related to V_p?
5. What population factors could affect the concentration of azithromycin?

Solutions

1. For a drug that follows a multiple compartment model, the rates of drug diffusion into the tissues from the plasma and from the tissues into the plasma are equal at steady state. However, the tissue drug concentration is generally not equal to the plasma drug concentration.
2. When plasma drug concentration data is used alone to describe the disposition of the drug, no information on tissue drug concentration is known, and no model will predict actual tissue drug concentrations. To account for the mass balance (drug mass = volume × body drug concentration) of drug present in the body (tissue and plasma pool) at any time after dosing, the body drug concentration is assumed to be the plasma drug concentration. In reality, azithromycin tissue concentration is much higher. Therefore, the calcu-

lated volume of the tissue compartment is much bigger (31.1 L/kg) than its actual volume.

The product of the steady-state apparent $(V_D)_{ss}$ and the steady-state plasma drug concentration estimates the amount of drug present in the body. The amount of drug present in the body may be important information for toxicity considerations, but may be used as a therapeutic end point. In most cases, the therapeutic drug at the site of action accounts for only a small fraction of total drug in the tissue compartment. The pharmacodynamic profile may be described as a separate compartment (see effect compartment in Chapter 19). Based on pharmacokinetic and biopharmaceutic studies, the factors that account for high tissue concentrations include diffusion constant, lipid solubility, and tissue binding to cell components. A ratio measuring the relative drug concentration in tissue and plasma is the partition coefficient, which is helpful in predicting the distribution of a drug into tissues. Ultimately, studies of tissue drug distribution using radiolabeled drug are much more useful.

3. When drugs are given in a multiple dose regimen, a loading dose may be given to achieve steady-state drug concentrations more rapidly (see Chapter 15).
4. The volume of the plasma compartment, V_p, is sometimes referred to as the initial volume. V_p is smaller than the steady-state volume of distribution (see moxalactam discussion, above).
5. Age and gender may affect C_{max} level of the drug.

Clinical Example - Etoposide

Etoposide is a drug used for the treatment of lung cancer. Understanding the distribution of etoposide in normal and metastatic tissues is important to avoid drug toxicity. Etoposide follows a two-compartment model. The $(V_D)_\beta$ is 0.28 L/kg, and beta elimination half-life is 12.9 hr. Total body clearance is 0.25 mL/min/kg.

Questions

1. What is the $(V_D)_\beta$ in a 70-kg subject?
2. How is the $(V_D)_\beta$ different than the volume of the plasma fluid, V_p?
3. Why is the $(V_D)_\beta$ useful if it does not represent a real tissue volume?
4. How is $(V_D)_\beta$ calculated from plasma time concentration profile data for etoposide? Is $(V_D)_\beta$ related to total body clearance?

Solutions

1. $(V_D)_\beta$ of etoposide in a 70-kg subject = 0.28 L/kg × 70 kg = 19.6 L.
2. The plasma fluid volume is about 3 L in a 70-kg subject and is much smaller than $(V_D)_\beta$. The apparent volume of distribution, $(V_D)_\beta$, is also considerably larger than the volume of the plasma compartment (also referred to as the initial volume by some clinicians), which includes some extracellular fluid. $(V_D)_\beta$ is numerically closer to the steady-state volume of distribution and has

been listed as the apparent volume of distribution in some clinical literature.

3. Etoposide is a drug that follows a two-compartment model with a beta elimination phase. Within the first few minutes after an intravenous bolus dose, most of the drug is distributed in the plasma fluid. Subsequently, the drug will diffuse into tissues and drug uptake may occur. Eventually, plasma drug levels will decline due to elimination, and some redistribution as etoposide in tissue diffuses back into the plasma fluid. The volume of distribution at steady state, $(V_D)_{ss}$, is the "hypothetical space" in which the drug is assumed to be distributed. The product of the plasma drug concentration with $(V_D)_{ss}$ will give the total amount of drug in the body at that time period.

$$C_{pss} \times (V_D)_{ss} = \text{amount of drug in the body at steady state}$$

The real tissue drug level will differ from the plasma drug concentration depending on the partitioning of drug in tissues and plasma. $(V_D)_\beta$ is a volume of distribution often calculated because it is easier to calculate than $(V_D)_{ss}$. This volume of distribution, $(V_D)_\beta$, allows the area under the curve to be calculated, an area which has been related to toxicities associated with many cancer chemotherapy agents.

The two-compartment model allows continuous monitoring of the amount of the drug present in and out of the vascular system, including the amount of drug eliminated. This information is important in pharmacotherapy.

4. $(V_D)_\beta$ may be determined from the total drug clearance and beta:

$$\text{Clearance} = b \times (V_D)_\beta$$

$(V_D)_\beta$ is also calculated from Equation 4.36:

where

$$(V_D)_\beta = \frac{\text{Dose}}{b\,[\text{AUC}]_0^\infty}$$

This method for $(V_D)_\beta$ determination is popular because $[\text{AUC}]_0^\infty$ is easily calculated using the trapezoidal rule. Many values for apparent volumes of distribution reported in the clinical literature are obtained using the area equation. Some early pharmacokinetic literature only includes the steady-state volume of distribution, which approximates the $(V_D)_\beta$ but is substantially smaller in many cases. In general, both volume terms reflect extravascular drug distribution. $(V_D)_\beta$ appears to be much more affected by the dynamics of drug disposition in the beta phase, whereas $(V_D)_{ss}$ reflects more accurately the inherent distribution of the drug. In clinical practice, many potent drugs are not injected by bolus dose. Instead, these drugs are infused over a short interval, making it difficult to obtain accurate information on the distributive phase. As a result, many drugs following the two-compartment model are approximated using a single compartment. It should be cautioned that there are substantial deviations in some cases. When in doubt, the full equation with all parameters should be applied for comparison. A small bolus (test) dose may be injected to obtain the necessary data if a therapeutic dose injected rapidly causes side effects or discomfort to the subject. In the case of etoposide, the steady-state volume of distribution is listed as 7 to 17 L/m^2 by the manufacturer as compared with 19.6 L for the 70-kg subject under discussion and as determined above.

FREQUENTLY ASKED QUESTIONS

1. My preceptors and I both agree that the "hypothetical" or "mathematical" compartment models are just about useless in helping me with dosing in the clinical setting. Does "hypothetical" mean "not real"?
2. What is the apparent volume of distribution, and why are there so many different volumes of distribution?
3. If physiologic models are better than the compartment model, why not just use physiologic models?
4. Can I just learn clearance and forget about the other pharmacokinetic parameters, because clearance is the term most often used in clinical pharmacy?
5. What is the error if I assume a one-compartment model instead of the two-compartment or multicompartment model?
6. What kind of improvement in terms of patient care or drug therapy was made using the compartment model?

LEARNING QUESTIONS

1. A drug was administered by rapid IV injection into an 70-kg adult male. Blood samples were withdrawn over a 7-hour period and assayed for intact drug. The results are tabulated below. Using the method of residuals, calculate the values for intercepts A and B and slopes a, b, k, k_{12}, and k_{21}.

Time (hr)	C_p (μg/mL)	Time (hr)	C_p (μg/mL)
0.00	70.0	2.5	14.3
0.25	53.8	3.0	12.6
0.50	43.3	4.0	10.5
0.75	35.0	5.0	9.0
1.00	29.1	6.0	8.0
1.50	21.2	7.0	7.0
2.00	17.0		

2. A 70-kg male subject was given 150 mg of a drug by IV injection. Blood samples were removed and assayed for intact drug. Calculate the slopes and inter-

cepts of the three phases of the plasma level versus time plot from the results tabulated below. Give the equation for the curve.

Time (hr)	C_p (μg/mL)	Time (hr)	C_p (μg/mL)
0.17	36.2	3.0	13.9
0.33	34.0	4.0	12.0
0.50	27.0	6.0	8.7
0.67	23.0	7.0	7.7
1.0	20.8	18.0	3.2
1.5	17.8	23.0	2.4
2.0	16.5		

3. Mitenko and Ogilvie (1973) demonstrated that theophylline followed a two-compartment pharmacokinetic model in human subjects. After administering a single intravenous dose (5.6 mg/kg) in nine normal volunteers, these investigators demonstrated that the equation best describing theophylline kinetics in humans was as follows:

$$C_p = 12e^{-5.8t} + 18e^{-0.16t}$$

What is the plasma level of the drug 3 hours after the IV dose?

4. A drug has a distribution that can be described by a two-compartment open model. If the drug is given by IV bolus, then what is the cause of the initial or rapid decline in blood levels (a phase)? What is the cause of the slower decline in blood levels (b phase)?

5. What does it mean when a drug demonstrates a plasma level–time curve that indicates a three-compartment open model? Can this curve be described by a two-compartment model?

6. A drug that follows a multicompartment pharmacokinetic model is given to a patient by rapid intravenous injection. Would the drug concentration in each tissue be the same after the drug equilibrates with the plasma and all the tissues in the body? Explain.

7. Park and associates (1983) studied the pharmacokinetics of amrinone after a single IV bolus injection (75 mg) in 14 healthy adult male volunteers. The pharmacokinetics of this drug followed a two-compartment open model and fit the following equation:

$$C_p = Ae^{-at} + Be^{-bt}$$

where

$$A = 4.62 \pm 12.0\ \mu\text{g/mL}$$
$$B = 0.64 \pm 0.17\ \mu\text{g/mL}$$
$$a = 8.94 \pm 13\ \text{hr}^{-1}$$
$$b = 0.19 \pm 0.06\ \text{hr}^{-1}$$

From these data calculate:

a. The volume of the central compartment.
b. The volume of the tissue compartment.
c. The transfer constants k_{12} and k_{21}.
d. The elimination rate constant from the central compartment.
e. The elimination half-life of amrinone after the drug has equilibrated with the tissue compartment.

8. A drug may be described by a three-compartment model involving a central compartment and two peripheral tissue compartments. If you *could* sample the tissue compartments (organs), in which organs would you expect to find a drug level corresponding to the two theoretical peripheral tissue compartments?

9. A drug was administered to a patient at 20 mg by IV bolus dose and the time/plasma drug concentration is listed below. Use a suitable compartment model to describe the data and list the fitted equation and parameters. What are the statistical criteria used to describe your fit?

Hour	mg/L
0.20	3.42
0.40	2.25
0.60	1.92
0.80	1.80
1.00	1.73
2.00	1.48
3.00	1.28
4.00	1.10
6.00	0.81
8.00	0.60
10.00	0.45
12.00	0.33
14.00	0.24
18.00	0.13
20.00	0.10

10. The toxicokinetics of colchicine in seven cases of acute human poisoning was studied by Rochdi et al (1992). In three further cases, postmortem tissue concentrations of colchicine were measured. Colchicine follows the two-compartment model with wide distribution in various tissues. Depending on the time of patient admission, two disposition processes were observed. The first, in three patients, admitted early, showed a biexponential plasma colchicine decrease, with distribution half-lives of 30, 45, and 90 min. The second, in four patients, admitted late, showed a monoexponential decrease. Plasma terminal half-lives ranged from 10.6 to 31.7 hr for both groups.

Postmortem tissue analysis of colchicine showed that colchicine accumulated at high concentrations in the bone marrow (more than 600 ng/g), testicle (400 ng/g), spleen (250 ng/g), kidney (200 ng/g), lung (200 ng/g), heart (95 ng/g), and brain (125 ng/g).

The pharmacokinetic parameters of colchicine are:

Fraction of unchanged colchicine in urine = 30%

Renal clearance = 13 L/hr

Total body clearance = 39 L/hr

Apparent volume of distribution = 21 L/kg

a. Why is colchicine described by a monoexponential profile in some subjects and a biexponential in others?

b. What is the range of distribution of half-life of colchicine in the subjects?

c. Which parameter is useful in estimating tissue drug level at any time?

d. Some clinical pharmacists assumed that, at steady state when equilibration is reached between the plasma and the tissue, the tissue drug concentration would be the same as the plasma. Do you agree?

e. Which tissues may be predicted by the tissue compartment?

REFERENCES

Butler TC: The distribution of drugs. In LaDu BN et al (eds), *Fundamentals of Drug Metabolism and Disposition*. Baltimore, Williams & Wilkins, 1972

Eger E: In EM Papper and JR Kitz (eds), *Uptake and Distribution of Anesthetic Agents*. New York, McGraw Hill Book Co., 1963, p. 76

Harron DWG: Digoxin pharmacokinetic modelling—10 years later. *Intern J Pharm* **53**:181–188, 1989

Hill HF, Coda BA, Tanaka A, Schaffer R: Multiple-dose evaluation of intravenous hydromorphone pharmacokinetics in normal human subjects. *Anesth Analg* **72**:330–336, 1991

Mitenko PA, Ogilvie RI: Pharmacokinetics of intravenous theophylline. *Clin Pharmacol Ther* **14**:509, 1973

Parab PV, Ritschel WA, Coyle DE, Gree RV, Denson DD: Pharmacokinetics of hydromorphone after intravenous, peroral and rectal administration to human subjects. *Biopharm Drug Dispos* **9**:187–199, 1988

Park GP, Kershner RP, Angellotti J, et al: Oral bioavailability and intravenous pharmacokinetics of amrinone in humans. *J Pharm Sci* **72**:817, 1983

Rochdi M, Sabouraud A, Baud FJ, Bismuth C, Scherrmann JM: Toxicokinetics of colchicine in humans: Analysis of tissue, plasma and urine data in ten cases. *Hum Exp Toxicol* **11**(6):510–516, 1992

Schentag JJ, Jusko WJ, Plaut ME, Cumbo TJ, Vance JW, and Abutyn E: Tissue persistence of gentamicin in man. *JAMA* **238**:327–329, 1977

Schumacher GE: *Therapeutic Drug Monitoring*. Norwalk, CT, Appleton & Lange, 1995

Swanson DJ, Reitberg DP, Smith IL, Wels PB, Schentag JJ: Steady-state moxalactam pharmacokinetics in patients: Noncompartmental versus two-compartmental analysis. *J Pharmacokinet-Biopharm* **11**(4):337–353, 1983

Vallner JJ, Stewart JT, Kotzan JA, Kirsten EB, Honiger IL: Pharmacokinetics and bioavailability of hydromorphone following intravenous and oral administration to human subjects. *J Clin Pharmacol* **21**:152–156, 1981

Winters ME: *Basic Clinical Pharmacokinetics*, 3rd ed. Vancouver, WA, Applied Therapeutics Inc, 1994, p. 23

BIBLIOGRAPHY

Dvorchick BH, Vessell ES: Significance of error associated with use of the one-compartment formula to calculate clearance of 38 drugs. *Clin Pharmacol Ther* **23**:617–623, 1978

Jusko WJ, Gibaldi M: Effects of change in elimination on various parameters of the two-compartment open model. *J Pharm Sci* **61**:1270–1273, 1972

Loughman PM, Sitar DS, Oglivie RI, Neims AH: The two-compartment open-system kinetic model: A review of its clinical implications and applications. *J Pediatr* **88**:869–873, 1976

Mayersohn M, Gibaldi M: Mathematical methods in pharmacokinetics, II: Solution of the two-compartment open model. *Am J Pharm Ed* **35**:19–28, 1971

Riegelman S, Loo JCK, Rowland M: Concept of a volume of distribution and possible errors in evaluation of this parameter. *J Pharm Sci* **57**:128–133, 1968

Riegelman S, Loo JCK, Rowland M: Shortcomings in pharmacokinetics analysis by conceiving the body to exhibit properties of a single compartment. *J Pharm Sci* **57**:117–123, 1968

5

PHYSIOLOGIC FACTORS RELATED TO DRUG ABSORPTION

The systemic absorption of a drug is dependent upon (1) the physicochemical properties of the drug, (2) the nature of the drug product, and (3) the anatomy and physiologic functions at the site of drug absorption. All of these considerations are important in the manufacture and biopharmaceutic evaluation of drug products (Chapter 6). This chapter will focus on the anatomic and physiologic considerations for the systemic absorption of a drug. A thorough understanding of the physiologic and pathologic factors affecting drug absorption is important in drug product selection and in the avoidance of potential drug–drug and drug–nutrient interactions.

NATURE OF THE CELL MEMBRANE

For systemic absorption, a drug must pass from the absorption site through or around one or more layers of cells to gain access into the general circulation. The permeability of a drug at the absorption site into the systemic circulation is intimately related to the molecular structure of the drug and to the physical and biochemical properties of the cell membranes. For absorption into the cell, a drug must traverse the cell membrane.

Transcellular absorption is the process of a drug movement across a cell. Some polar molecules may not be able to traverse the cell membrane, but instead, go through gaps or "*tight junctions*" between cells, a process known as *paracellular drug absorption*. Figure 5-1 shows the difference of the two processes. Some drugs are probably absorbed by a mixed mechanism involving one or more processes.

Membranes are a major structure in cells, surrounding the entire cell (plasma membrane) and acting as a boundary between the cell and the interstitial fluid. In addition, membranes enclose most of the cell organelles (eg, the mitochondrion membrane). Functionally, membranes act as a selective barrier to the passage of molecules. Cell membranes are semipermeable membranes. Water, some selected small molecules, and lipid-soluble molecules pass through such membranes,

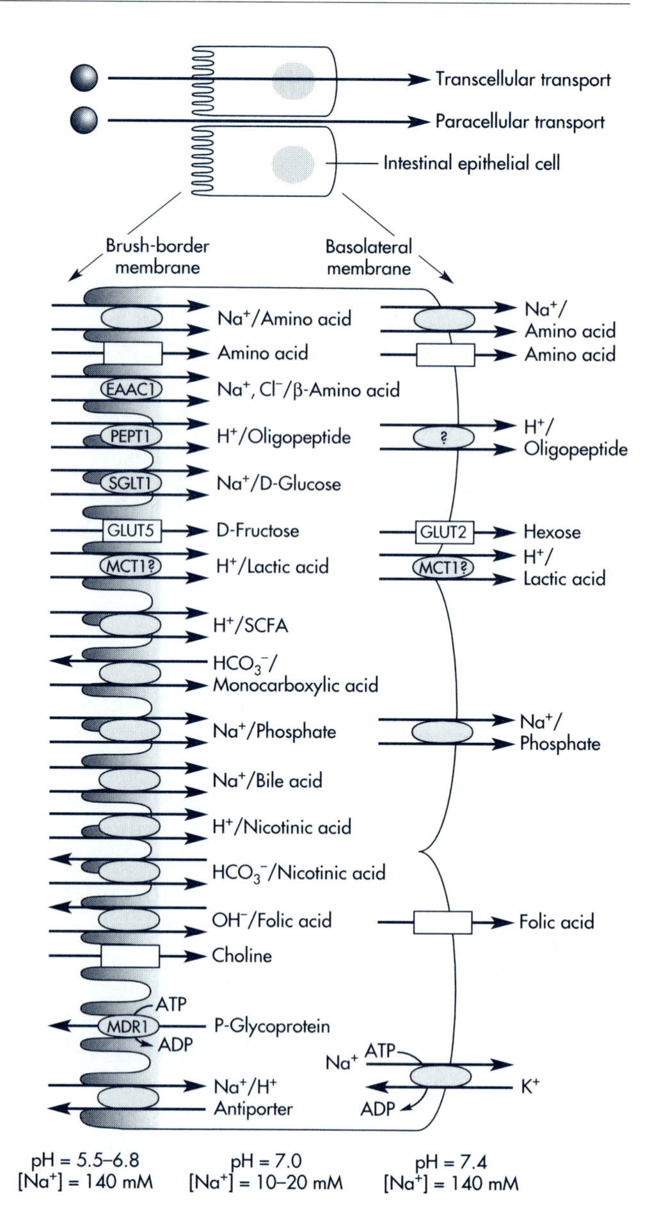

Figure 5-1. Summary of intestinal epithelial transporters. Transporters shown by square and oval shapes demonstrate active and facilitated transporters, respectively. Name of cloned transporters are shown with square or oval shapes. In the case of active transporter, arrows in the same direction represent symport of substance and the driving force. Arrows going in the reverse direction mean the antiport.
(From Tsuyi and Tamai, 1996, with permission.)

whereas highly charged molecules and large molecules, such as proteins and protein-bound drugs, do not.

The transmembrane movement of drugs is influenced by the composition and structure of the cell membranes. Cell membranes are generally thin, approximately 70 to 100Å in thickness. Cell membranes are primarily composed of phospholipids with interdispersed carbohydrates and integral protein groups in the form of a bilayer. There are several theories as to the structure of the cell membrane. The *lipid bilayer* or *unit membrane* theory, originally proposed by Davson and Danielli (1952), considers the cell membrane to be composed of two layers of phospholipid between two surface layers of proteins, with the hydrophilic "head" groups of the phospholipids facing the protein layers and the hydrophobic "tail" groups of the phospholipids aligned in the interior. The lipid bilayer theory explains the observation that lipid-soluble drugs tend to penetrate cell membranes more easily than polar molecules. However, the bilayer cell membrane structure does not account for the diffusion of water, small-molecular-weight molecules such as urea, and certain charged ions.

The *fluid mosaic model*, proposed by Singer and Nicolson (1972), explains the transcellular diffusion of polar molecules. According to this model, the cell membrane consists of globular proteins embedded in a dynamic fluid, lipid bilayer matrix (Fig. 5-2). These proteins provide a pathway for the selective transfer of certain polar molecules and charged ions through the lipid barrier. As shown in Figure 5-2, transmembrane proteins are interdispersed throughout the membrane. Two types of pores of about 10 nm and 50 to 70 nm were inferred to be present in membranes based on capillary membrane transport studies (Pratt and Taylor, 1990). These small pores provide a channel through which water, ions, and dissolved solutes such as urea may move across the membrane.

PASSAGE OF DRUGS ACROSS CELL MEMBRANES

Passive Diffusion

Passive diffusion is the process by which molecules spontaneously diffuse from a region of higher concentration to a region of lower concentration. This process is

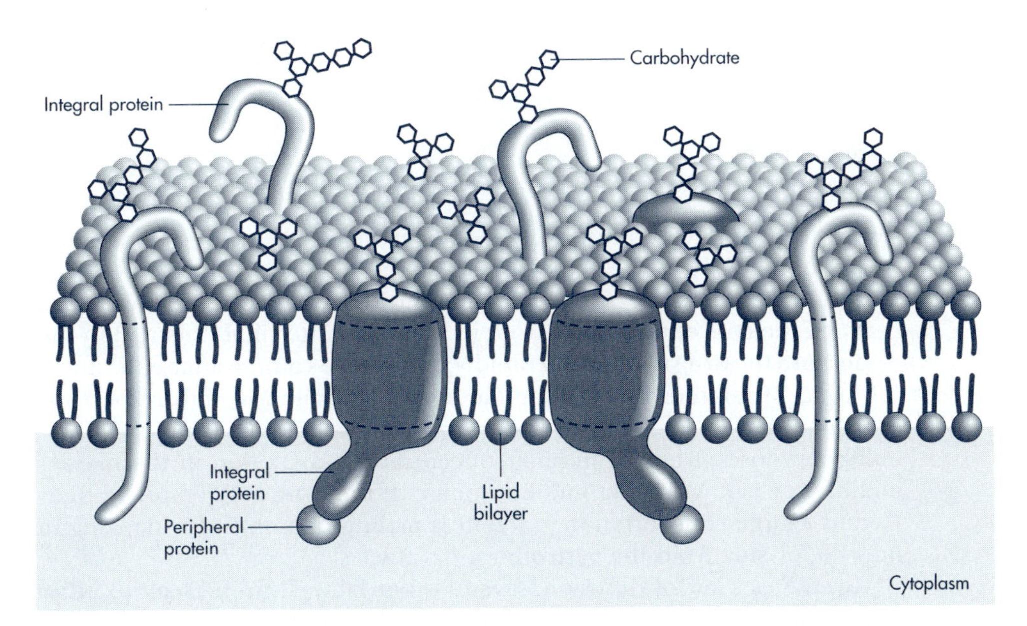

Figure 5-2. Model of the plasma membrane includes proteins and carbohydrates as well as lipids. Integral proteins are embedded in the lipid bilayer; peripheral proteins are merely associated with the membrane surface. The carbohydrate consists of monosaccharides, or simple sugars, strung together in chains that are attached to proteins (forming glycoproteins) or to lipids (forming glycolipids). The asymmetry of the membrane is manifested in several ways. Carbohydrates are always on the exterior surface and peripheral proteins are almost always on the cytoplasmic, or inner, surface. The two lipid monolayers include different proportions of the various kinds of lipid molecule. Most important, each species of integral protein has a definite orientation, which is the same for every molecule of that species.
(From Lodish and Rothman, 1979, with permission.)

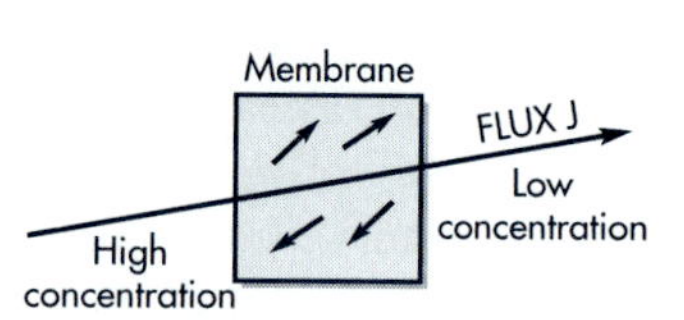

Figure 5-3. Passive diffusion of molecules. Molecules in solution diffuse randomly in all directions. As molecules diffuse from left to right and vice versa (small arrows), a net diffusion from the high-concentration side to the low-concentration side results. This results in a net flux (J) to the right side. Flux is measured in mass per unit area (eg, mg/cm^2).

passive because no external energy is expended. In Figure 5-3, drug molecules move forward and back across a membrane. If the two sides have the same drug concentration, forward-moving drug molecules will be balanced by molecules moving back, resulting in no net transfer of drug. When one side is higher in drug concentration, at any given time, the number of forward-moving drug molecules will be higher than the number of backward-moving molecules; the net result would be a transfer of molecules to the alternate side, as indicated in the figure by the big arrow. The rate of transfer is called *flux*, and is represented by a vector to show its direction in space. The tendency of molecules to move in all directions is natural because molecules possess kinetic energy and constantly collide with one another in space. Only left and right molecule movements are shown in Figure 5-3, because movement of molecules in other directions would not result in concentration changes because of the limitation of the container wall.

Passive diffusion is the major absorption process for most drugs. The driving force for passive diffusion is due to higher drug concentrations on the mucosal side over the blood. According to *Fick's law of diffusion*, drug molecules diffuse from a region of high drug concentration to a region of low drug concentration.

$$\frac{dQ}{dt} = \frac{DAK}{h}(C_{GI} - C_p) \tag{5.1}$$

where dQ/dt = rate of diffusion; D = diffusion coefficient; K = lipid water partition coefficient of drug in the biologic membrane that controls drug permeation; A = surface area of membrane; h = membrane thickness; and $C_{GI} - C_p$ = difference between the concentrations of drug in the gastrointestinal tract and in the plasma.

Because the drug distributed rapidly into a large volume after entering the blood, the concentration of drug in the blood will be quite low with respect to the concentration at the site of drug absorption. For example, a drug is usually given in milligram doses, whereas plasma concentrations are often in the microgram per milliliter or nanogram per milliliter range. If the drug is given orally, then $C_{GI} >> C_p$ and a large concentration gradient is maintained, thus driving drug molecules into the plasma from the gastrointestinal tract.

Given Fick's law of diffusion, several other factors can be seen to influence the rate of passive diffusion of drugs. For example, the degree of lipid solubility of the drug will influence the rate of drug absorption. The partition coefficient, K, represents the lipid–water partitioning of a drug across the hypothetical membrane in the mucosa. Drugs that are more lipid soluble will have a larger value for K. The surface area of the membrane also influences the rate of absorption. Drugs may be absorbed from most areas of the gastrointestinal tract. However, the duodenal area of the small intestine shows the most rapid drug absorption due to such anatomic features as villi and microvilli, which provide a large surface area. These villi are less abundant in other areas of the gastrointestinal tract.

The thickness of the hypothetical model membrane, h, is a constant for any particular absorption site. Drugs usually diffuse very rapidly through capillary cell membranes in the vascular compartments, in contrast to diffusion through cell membranes of capillaries in the brain. In the brain, the capillaries are densely lined with glial cells, so that a drug diffuses slowly into the brain as if a thick lipid membrane existed. The term *blood–brain barrier* is used to describe the poor diffusion of water-soluble molecules across capillary cell membranes into the brain. However, in certain disease states these cell membranes may be disrupted or become more permeable to drug diffusion.

The diffusion coefficient, D, is a constant for each drug and is defined as the amount of a drug that diffuses across a membrane of a given unit area per unit time when the concentration gradient is unity. The dimensions of D are area per unit time—for example, cm^2/sec.

Because D, A, K, and h are constants under usual conditions for absorption, a combined constant P or permeability coefficient may be defined.

$$P = \frac{DAK}{h} \tag{5.2}$$

Furthermore, in Equation 5.1 the drug concentration in the plasma, C_p, is extremely small compared to the drug concentration in the gastrointestinal tract, C_{GI}. If C_p is negligible and P is substituted into Equation 5.1, the following relationship for Fick's law is obtained:

$$\frac{dQ}{dt} = P(C_{GI}) \tag{5.3}$$

Equation 5.3 is an expression for a first-order process. In practice, the extravascular absorption of most drugs tends to be a first-order absorption process. Moreover, due to the large concentration gradient between C_{GI} and C_p, the rate of drug absorption is usually more rapid than the rate of drug elimination.

Many drugs have both lipophilic and hydrophilic chemical substituents. Those drugs that are more lipid soluble tend to traverse cell membranes more easily than less lipid-soluble or more water-soluble molecules. For drugs that act as weak electrolytes, such as weak acids and bases, the extent of ionization influences the rate of drug transport. The ionized species of the drug contains a charge and is more water soluble than the nonionized species of the drug, which is more lipid soluble. The extent of ionization of a weak electrolyte will depend on both the pK_a of the drug and the pH of the medium in which the drug is dissolved. *Henderson and Hasselbalch* used the following expressions pertaining to weak acids and weak bases to describe the relationship between pK_a and pH.

For weak acids,

$$\text{Ratio} = \frac{(\text{salt})}{(\text{acid})} = \frac{(A^-)}{(HA)} = 10^{(\text{pH} - \text{pKa})} \tag{5.4}$$

For weak bases,

$$\text{Ratio} = \frac{(\text{base})}{(\text{salt})} = \frac{(RNH_2)}{(RNH_3^+)} = 10^{(\text{pH} - \text{p}Ka)} \tag{5.5}$$

With Equations 5.4 and 5.5, the proportion of free acid or free base existing as the nonionized species may be determined at any given pH, assuming the pK_a for the drug is known. For example, at a plasma pH of 7.4, salicylic acid (pK_a 3.0) would exist mostly in its ionized or water-soluble form, as shown below:

$$\text{Ratio} = \frac{(\text{salt})}{(\text{acid})} = 10^{(7.4\,-\,3.0)}$$

$$\log \frac{(\text{salt})}{(\text{acid})} = 7.4 - 3.0 = 4.4$$

$$\frac{(\text{Salt})}{(\text{Acid})} = 2.51 \times 10^{4}$$

The total drug concentrations on either side of a membrane should be the same at equilibrium, assuming Fick's law of diffusion is the only distribution factor involved. For diffusible drugs, such as nonelectrolyte drugs or drugs that do not ionize, the drug concentrations on either side of the membrane are the same at equilibrium. However, for electrolyte drugs or drugs that ionize, the total drug concentrations on both sides of the membrane are not equal at equilibrium if the pH of the medium differs on respective sides of the membrane. For example, consider the concentration of salicylic acid (pK_a 3.0) in the stomach (pH 1.2) as opposed to its concentration in the plasma (pH 7.4) (Fig. 5-4).

According to the Henderson–Hasselbalch equation (Eq. 5.4) for weak acids, at pH 7.4 and at pH 1.2, salicylic acid would exist in the ratios that follow.

In the plasma, at pH 7.4:

$$\text{Ratio} = \frac{(\text{R COO}^-)}{(\text{R COOH})} = 2.51 \times 10^{4}$$

In gastric juice, at pH 1.2:

$$\text{Ratio} = \frac{(\text{R COO}^-)}{(\text{R COOH})} = 10^{(1.2\,-\,3.0)} = 1.58 \times 10^{-2}$$

The total drug concentration on either side of the membrane is determined as shown in Table 5.1. Thus, the pH affects distribution of salicylic acid (R COOH) and its salt (R COO^-) across cell membranes. It is assumed that the acid, R COOH, is freely permeable and the salt, R COO^-, is not permeable across the cell membrane. In this example the total concentration of salicylic acid at equilibrium is approximately 25,000 times greater in the plasma than in the stomach (Table 5.1). These calculations can also be applied to weak bases, using Equation 5.5.

According to the *pH–partition hypotheses*, if the pH on one side of a cell membrane differs from the pH on the other side of the membrane, then (1) the drug (weak acid or base) will ionize to different degrees on respective sides of the membrane; (2) the total drug concentrations (ionized plus nonionized drug) on either side of the membrane will be unequal; and (3) the compartment in which the drug is more highly ionized will contain the greater total drug concentration. For these

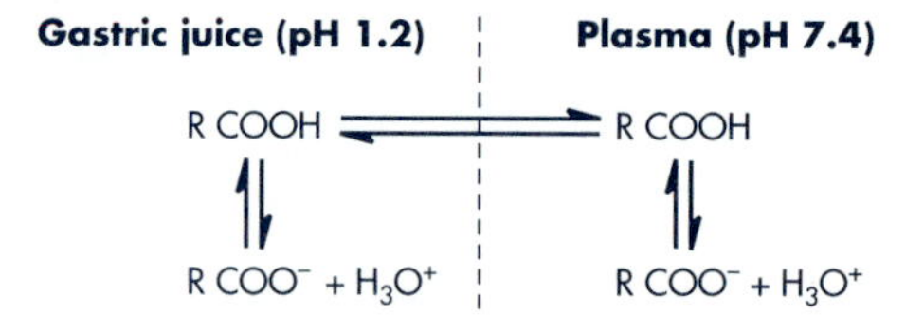

Figure 5-4. Model for the distribution of an orally administered weak electrolyte drug such as salicylic acid.

TABLE 5.1 Relative Concentrations of Salicylic Acid as Affected by pH

DRUG	GASTRIC JUICE (PH 1.2)	PLASMA (PH 7.4)
R COOH	1.0000	1
R COO^-	0.0158	25100
Total drug concentration	1.0158	25101

reasons, a weak acid (such as salicylic acid) would be rapidly absorbed from the stomach (pH 1.2), whereas a weak base (such as quinidine) would be poorly absorbed from the stomach.

Another factor that can influence drug concentrations on either side of a membrane is a particular *affinity* of the drug for a tissue component, which would prevent the drug from freely moving back across the cell membrane. For example, a drug may bind to plasma or tissue proteins. This drug–protein binding has been described for dicumarol, certain sulfonamides, and other drugs. Moreover, a drug such as chlordane, a lipid-soluble insecticide, might dissolve in the adipose (fat) tissue. In addition, a drug such as tetracycline might form a complex with calcium in the bones and teeth. Finally, a drug may concentrate in a tissue due to a specific uptake or active transport process. Such processes have been demonstrated for iodide in thyroid tissue, potassium in the intracellular water, and certain catecholamines in adrenergic storage sites.

Carrier-Mediated Transport

Theoretically, a lipophilic drug may pass through the cell or go around it. If the drug has a low molecular weight and is lipophilic, the lipid cell membrane is not a barrier to drug diffusion and absorption. In the intestine, molecules smaller than 500 MW may be absorbed by paracellular drug absorption. Numerous specialized carrier-mediated transport systems are present in the body, especially in the intestine for the absorption of ions and nutrients required by the body.

Active Transport

Active transport is a carrier-mediated transmembrane process that plays an important role in the gastrointestinal absorption and in renal and biliary secretion of many drugs and metabolites. A few lipid-insoluble drugs that resemble natural physiologic metabolites (such as 5-fluorouracil) are absorbed from the gastrointestinal tract by this process. Active transport is characterized by the transport of drug against a concentration gradient—that is, from regions of low drug concentrations to regions of high concentrations. Therefore, this is an energy-consuming system. In addition, active transport is a specialized process requiring a carrier that binds the drug to form a carrier–drug complex that shuttles the drug across the membrane and then dissociates the drug on the other side of the membrane (Fig. 5-5).

The carrier molecule may be highly selective for the drug molecule. If the drug structurally resembles a natural substrate that is actively transported, then it is likely to be actively transported by the same carrier mechanism. Therefore, drugs of similar structure may compete for sites of adsorption on the carrier. Furthermore, because only a fixed number of carrier is available, all the binding sites on the carrier may become saturated if the drug concentration gets very high. A comparison between the rate of drug absorption and the concentration of drug at the absorption

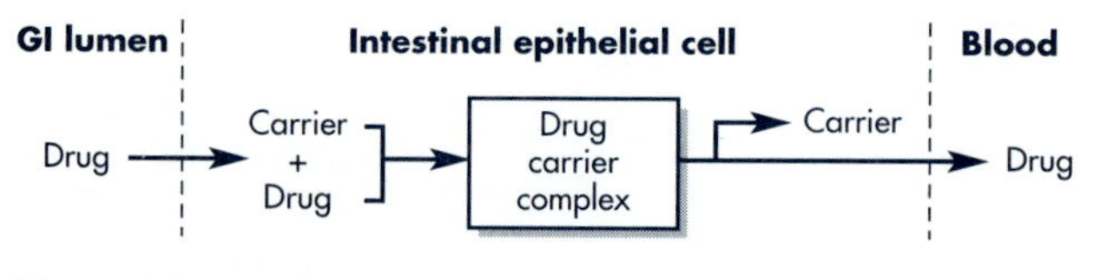

Figure 5-5. Hypothetical carrier-mediated transport process.

site is shown in Figure 5-6. Notice that for a drug absorbed by passive diffusion, the rate of absorption increases in a linear relationship to drug concentration. In contrast, when a drug is absorbed by a carrier-mediated process, the rate of drug absorption increases with drug concentration until the carrier molecules are completely saturated. At higher drug concentrations, the rate of drug absorption remains constant.

Facilitated Diffusion

Facilitated diffusion is also a carrier-mediated transport system, differing from active transport in that the drug moves along a concentration gradient (ie, moves from a region of high-drug concentration to a region of low-drug concentration). Therefore, this system does not require energy input. However, because this system is carrier mediated, it is saturable and structurally selective for the drug and shows competition kinetics for drugs of similar structure. In terms of drug absorption, facilitated diffusion seems to play a very minor role.

Carrier-Mediated Intestinal Transport

Various carrier mediated systems (*transporters*) are present at the intestinal brush border and basolateral membrane for the absorption of specific ions and nutrients essential for the body (Tsuji and Tamal, 1996). Many drugs are absorbed by these carriers because of the structural similarity to natural substrates (Table 5.2). A transmembrane protein, *P-glycoprotein* (P-gp) has been identified in the intestine. P-glycoprotein appears to reduce apparent intestinal epithelial cell permeability from lumen to blood for various lipophilic or cytotoxic drugs. Other transporters are present in the intestines (Tsuji and Tamal, 1996). For example, many oral cephalosporins are absorbed through the amino acid transporter. Cefazolin, a parenteral-only cephalosporin, is not available orally because it cannot be absorbed to a significant degree through this mechanism.

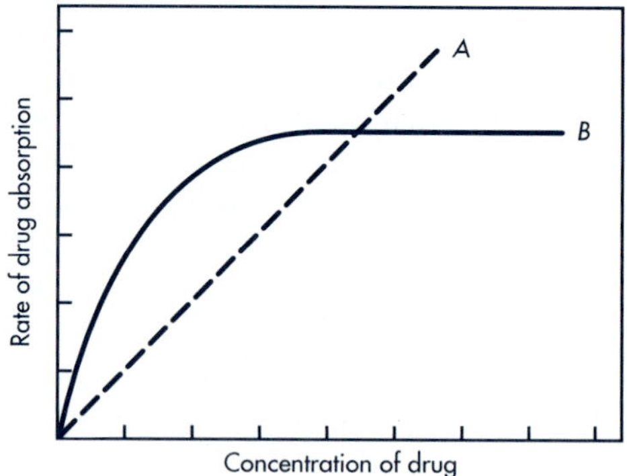

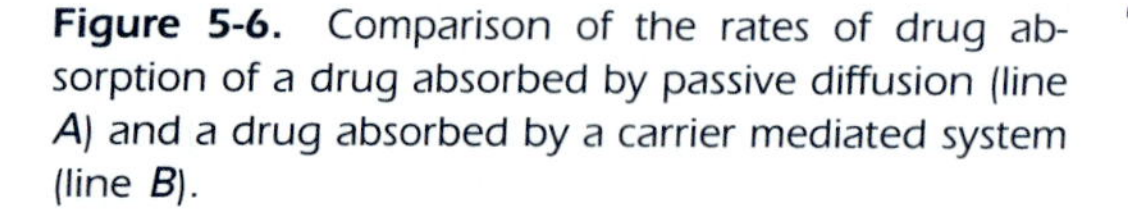
Figure 5-6. Comparison of the rates of drug absorption of a drug absorbed by passive diffusion (line *A*) and a drug absorbed by a carrier mediated system (line *B*).

TABLE 5.2 Intestine Transporters and Examples of Drugs Transported

TRANSPORTER	EXAMPLES	
Amino acid transporter	Gabapentin	D-cycloserine
	Methyldopa	Baclofen
	L-dopa	
Oligopeptide transporter	Cefadroxil	Cephradine
	Cefixime	Ceftibuten
	Cephalexin	Captopril
	Lisinopril	Thrombin inhibitor
Phosphate transporter	Fostomycin	Foscarnet
Bile acid transporter	S3744	
Glucose transporter	P-nitrophenyl-β-D-Glucopyranoside	
P-glycoprotein efflux	Etoposide	Vinblastine
	Cyclosporin A	
Monocarboxylic acid transporter	Salicylic acid	Benzoic acid
	Pravastatin	

Adapted from Tsuji and Tamai (1996).

Vesicular Transport

Vesicular transport is the process of engulfing particles or dissolved materials by the cell. *Pinocytosis* and *phagocytosis* are forms of vesicular transport that differ by the type of material ingested. Pinocytosis refers to the engulfment of small solutes or fluid, whereas phagocytosis refers to the engulfment of larger particles or macromolecules, generally by macrophages. *Endocytosis* and *exocytosis* are the processes of moving macromolecules into and out of a cell, respectively.

During pinocytosis or phagocytosis, the cell membrane invaginates to surround the material and then engulfs the material, incorporating it into the cell (Fig. 5-7).

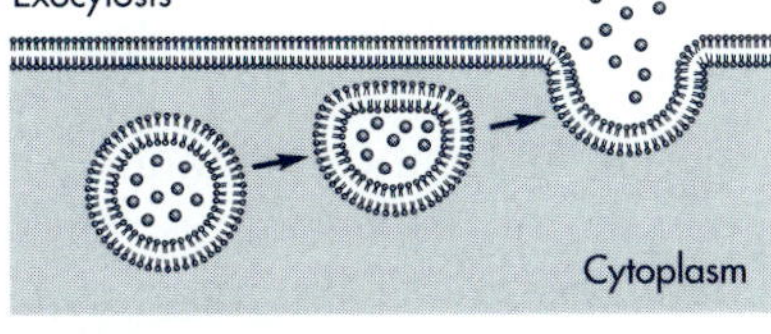

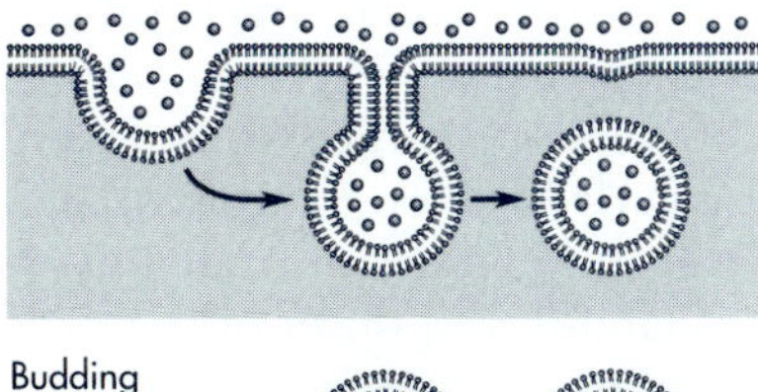

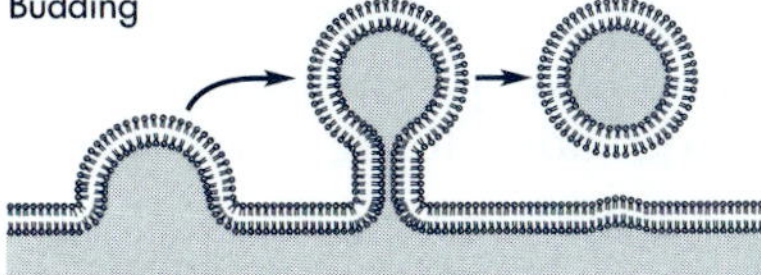

Figure 5-7. Diagram showing exocytosis and endocytosis. (From Alberts et al, 1988, with permission.)

Subsequently, the cell membrane containing the material forms a vesicle or vacuole within the cell. Vesicular transport is the proposed process for the absorption of orally administered Sabin polio vaccine and various large proteins.

An example of *exocytosis* is the transport of a protein such as insulin from insulin-producing cells of the pancreas into the extracellular space. The insulin molecules are first packaged into intracellular vesicles, which then fuse with the plasma membrane to release the insulin outside the cell.

Pore (Convective) Transport

Very small molecules (such as urea, water, and sugars) are able to rapidly cross cell membranes as if the membrane contained channels or pores. Although such pores have never been directly observed by microscopy, the model of drug permeation through aqueous pores is used to explain renal excretion of drugs and the uptake of drugs into the liver.

A certain type of protein called a transport protein may form an open channel across the lipid membrane of the cell (Fig. 5-1). Small molecules including drugs move through the channel by diffusion more rapidly than at other parts of the membrane.

Ion Pair Formation

Strong electrolyte drugs are highly ionized or charged molecules, such as quaternary nitrogen compounds with extreme pK_a values. Strong electrolyte drugs maintain their charge at all physiologic pH values and penetrate membranes poorly. When the ionized drug is linked up with an oppositely charged ion, an ion pair is formed in which the overall charge of the pair is neutral. This neutral drug complex diffuses more easily across the membrane. For example, the formation of ion pairs to facilitate drug absorption has been demonstrated for propranolol, a basic drug that forms an ion pair with oleic acid, and quinine, which forms ion pair with hexylsalicylate (Nienbert, 1989).

ROUTE OF DRUG ADMINISTRATION

Drugs may be given by parenteral, enteral, inhalation, transdermal (percutaneous), and intranasal routes for systemic absorption. Each route of drug administration has certain advantages and disadvantages. Some characteristics of the more common routes of drug administration are listed in Table 5.3. Many drugs are not administered orally because of instability in the gastrointestinal tract or the degradation by the digestive enzymes in the intestine. For example, erythropoietin and human growth hormone (somatrophin) are administered intramuscularly, and insulin is administered subcutaneously or intramuscularly because the potential of degradation of the drugs in the intestine. Drug absorption after subcutaneous injection is slower than intravenous injection. The availability and onset of the drug administered by parenteral routes may be affected by blood flow to the administration site and by disease factors. The bioavailability of these products is discussed in Chapter 10. Biotechnology products are often too labile to be administered orally.

TABLE 5.3 Common Routes of Drug Administration

ROUTE	BIOAVAILABILITY	ADVANTAGES	DISADVANTAGES
Parenteral Routes			
Intravenous bolus (IV)	Complete (100%) systemic drug absorption. Rate of bioavailability considered instantaneous.	Drug is given for immediate effect.	Increased chance for adverse reaction. Possible anaphylaxis.
Intravenous infusion (IV inf)	Complete (100%) systemic drug absorption. Rate of drug absorption controlled by infusion pump.	Plasma drug levels more precisely controlled. May inject large fluid volumes. May use drugs with poor lipid solubility and/or irritating drugs.	Requires skill in insertion of infusion set. Tissue damage at site of injection (infiltration, necrosis, or sterile abscess).
Intramuscular injection (IM)	Rapid from aqueous solution. Slow absorption from nonaqueous (oil) solutions.	Easier to inject than intravenous injection. Larger volumes may be used compared to subcutaneous solutions.	Irritating drugs may be very painful. Different rates of absorption depending upon muscle group injected and blood flow.
Subcutaneous injection (SC)	Prompt from aqueous solution. Slow absorption from repository formulations.	Generally, used for insulin injection.	Rate of drug absorption depends upon blood flow and injection volume.
Enteral Routes			
Buccal or sublingual (SL)	Rapid absorption from lipid-soluble drugs.	No "first-pass" effects.	Some drugs may be swallowed. Not for most drugs or drugs with high doses.
Oral (PO)	Absorption may vary. Generally, slower absorption rate compared to IV bolus or IM injection.	Safest and easiest route of drug administration. May use immediate-release and modified-release drug products.	Some drugs may have erratic absorption, be unstable in the gastointestinal tract, or be metabolized by liver prior to systemic absorption.
Rectal (PR)	Absorption may vary from suppository. More reliable absorption from enema (solution).	Useful when patient cannot swallow medication. Used for local and systemic effects.	Absorption may be erratic. Suppository may migrate to different position. Some patient discomfort.
Other Routes			
Transdermal	Slow absorption, rate may vary. Increased absorption with occlusive dressing.	Transdermal delivery system (patch) is easy to use. Used for lipid-soluble drugs with low dose and low MW.	Some irritation by patch or drug. Permeability of skin variable with condition, anatomic site, age, and gender. Type of cream or ointment base affects drug release and absorption.
Inhalation	Rapid absorption. Total dose absorbed is variable.	May be used for local or systemic effects.	Particle size of drug determines anatomic placement in respiratory tract. May stimulate cough reflex. Some drug may be swallowed.

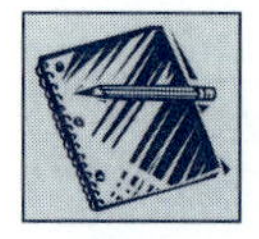

PRACTICAL FOCUS

The pharmacokinetics of erythropoietin (EPO) was investigated in uremic and healthy subjects (Jensen JD, 1994). After subcutaneous injection, the bioavailability was significantly lower in the patients (23.7 versus 38.5%; $P < 0.01$) than in the normal subjects, and the maximal s-EPO was lower (113 versus 153 U/L; $P < 0.05$) and delayed (15.4 versus 11.0 h; $P < 0.02$).

Subcutaneous administration offers an alternative route to oral administration for drugs with low bioavailability, for example, sumatriptine (Imitrex) has an oral bioavailability of about 14% due to extensive metabolism and low absorption. It is rapidly absorbed subcutaneously and gives prompt relief of migraine headache.

Oral Drug Absorption

Anatomic and Physiologic Considerations

The enteral system consists of the alimentary canal from the mouth to the anus (Fig. 5-8). The major physiologic processes that occur in the gastrointestinal (GI)

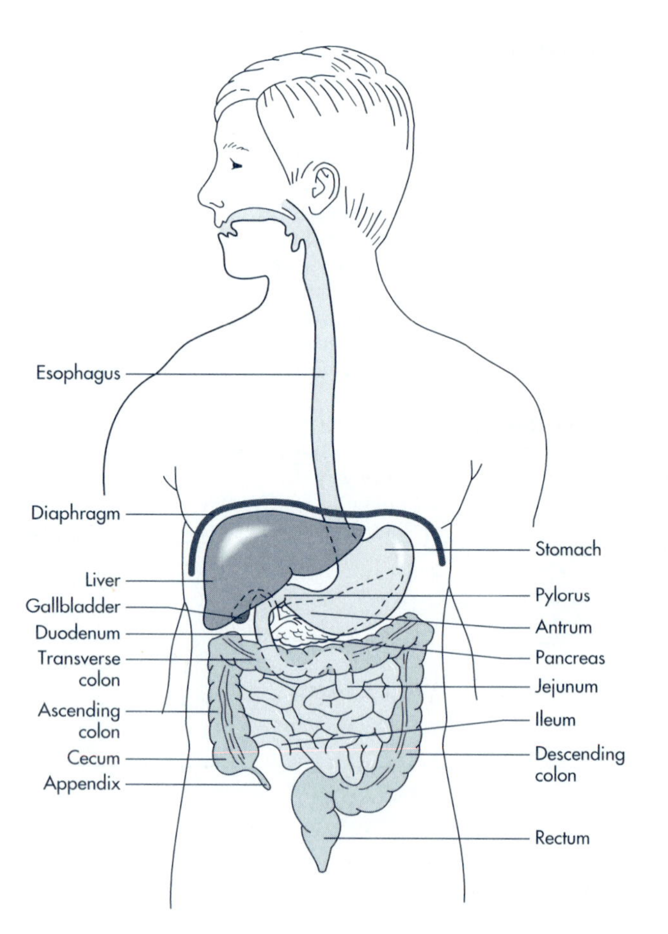

Figure 5-8. Gastrointestinal tract.

system are secretion, digestion, and absorption. *Secretion* includes the transport of fluid, electrolytes, peptides, and proteins into the lumen of the alimentary canal. Enzymes in saliva and pancreatic secretions are involved in the digestion of carbohydrates and proteins. Other secretions, such as mucus, protect the linings of the lumen of the GI tract. *Digestion* is the breakdown of food constituents into smaller structures in preparation for absorption. Food constituents are mostly absorbed in the proximal area (duodenum) of the small intestine. The process of *absorption* is the entry of constituents from the lumen of the gut into the body. Absorption may be considered as the net result of both lumen-to-blood and blood-to-lumen transport movements.

Drugs administered orally pass through various parts of the enteral canal, including the oral cavity, esophagus, and various parts of the gastrointestinal tract. Residues eventually exit the body through the anus. The total transit time, including gastric emptying, small intestinal transit, and colonic transit ranges from 0.4 to 5 days (Kirwan and Smith, 1974). The most important site for drug absorption is the small intestine. Small intestine transit time (SITT) ranges from 3 to 4 hours for most healthy subjects. If absorption is not completed by the time a drug leaves the small intestine, absorption may be erratic or incomplete. The small intestine is normally filled with digestive juices and liquids, keeping the lumen contents fluid. In contrast, the fluid in the colon is reabsorbed, and the lumenal content in the colon is either semisolid or solid, making further drug dissolution erratic and difficult. The lack of the solubilizing effect of the chyme and digestive fluid contributes to a less favorable environment for drug absorption.

The normal physiologic processes of the alimentary canal may be affected by diet, contents of the GI tract, hormones, the visceral nervous system, disease, and drugs. Thus, drugs given by the enteral route for systemic absorption may be affected by the anatomy, physiologic functions, and contents of the alimentary tract. Moreover, the physical, chemical, and pharmacologic properties of the drug itself will also affect its own absorption from the alimentary canal.

Oral Cavity. Saliva is the main secretion of the oral cavity, and has a pH of about 7. Saliva contains ptyalin (salivary amylase), which digests starches. Mucin, a glycoprotein that lubricates food, is also secreted and may interact with drugs. About 1500 mL of saliva is secreted per day.

Esophagus. The esophagus connects the pharynx and the cardiac orifice of the stomach. The pH of the fluids in the esophagus is between 5 and 6. The lower part of the esophagus ends with the esophageal sphincter, which prevents acid reflux from the stomach. Tablets or capsules may lodge in this area, causing local irritation. Very little drug dissolution occurs in the esophagus.

Stomach. The stomach is innervated by the vagus nerve. However, local nerve plexus, hormones, mechanoreceptors sensitive to the stretch of the GI wall, and chemoreceptors control the regulation of gastric secretions, including acid and stomach emptying. The fasting pH of the stomach is about 2 to 6. In the presence of food, the stomach pH is about 1.5 to 2, due to hydrochloric acid secreted by parietal cells. Stomach acid secretion is stimulated by gastrin and histamine. Gastrin is released from G cells, mainly in the antral mucosa and also in the duodenum. Gastrin release is regulated by stomach distension (swelling) and the presence of peptides and amino acids. A substance called intrinsic factor for vitamin B-12 absorption and various gastric enzymes, such as pepsin that initiate protein digestion, are secreted into the gastric lumen to initiate digestion.

Basic drugs are solubilized rapidly in the presence of stomach acid. Mixing is intense and pressurized in the antral part of the stomach, a process of breaking down large food particles described as *antral milling*. Food and liquid are emptied by opening the pyloric sphincter into the duodenum. Stomach emptying is influenced by the food content and osmolality. Fatty acids and mono- and diglycerides delay gastric emptying (Hunt and Knox, 1968). High-density foods generally are emptied from the stomach more slowly. The relation of gastric emptying time to drug absorption is discussed more fully in the next section.

Duodenum. A common duct from the pancreas and the gallbladder enters into the duodenum. The duodenal pH is about 6 to 6.5 due to the presence of bicarbonate that neutralizes the acidic chyme emptied from the stomach. The pH is optimum for enzymatic digestion of protein and peptide food. Pancreatic juice containing enzymes is secreted into the duodenum from the bile duct. Trypsin, chymotrypsin, and carboxypeptidase are involved in the hydrolysis of proteins into amino acids. Amylase is involved in the digestion of carbohydrates. Pancreatic lipase secretion hydrolyzes fats into fatty acid. The complex fluid medium in the duodenum helps to dissolve many drugs with limited aqueous solubility.

The duodenum is a site where many ester prodrugs are hydrolyzed during absorption. The presence of proteolytic enzymes also makes many protein drugs unstable in the duodenum, preventing adequate absorption.

Jejunum. The jejunum is the middle portion of the small intestine in between the duodenum and the ileum. Digestion of protein and carbohydrates continues after receiving pancreatic juice and bile in the duodenum. This portion of the small intestine generally has fewer contractions than the duodenum and is preferred for in vivo drug absorption studies.

Ileum. The ileum is the terminal part of the small intestine. This site has fewer contractions than the duodenum and may be blocked off by catheters with an inflatable balloon and perfused for drug absorption study. The pH is about 7, with the distal part as high as 8. Due to the presence of bicarbonate secretion, acid drugs will dissolve. Bile secretion helps to dissolve fats and hydrophobic drugs. The ileocecal valve separates the small intestine from the colon.

Colon. The colon lacks villi and has limited drug absorption also due to the more viscous and semisolid nature of the lumen contents. The colon is lined with mucin functioning as lubricant and protectant. The pH in this region is 5.5 to 7. A few drugs, such as theophylline and metoprolol, are absorbed in this region. Drugs that are absorbed well in this region are good candidates for an oral sustained-release dosage form. The colon contains both aerobic and anaerobic microorganisms that may metabolize some drugs. For example, L-dopa and lactulose are metabolized by enteric bacteria. Crohn's disease affects the colon and thickens the bowel wall. The microflora also become more anaerobic. Absorption of clindamycin and propranolol are increased, whereas other drugs have reduced absorption with this disease (Rubinstein et al, 1988).

Rectum. The rectum is about 15 cm long, ending at the anus. In the absence of fecal material, the rectum has a small amount of fluid (approximately 2 mL) with a pH about 7. The rectum is perfused by the superior, middle, and inferior hemorrhoidal veins. The inferior hemorrhoidal vein (closest to the anal sphincter) and the middle hemorrhoidal vein feed into the vena cava and back to the heart. The superior hemorrhoidal vein joins the mesenteric circulation, which feeds into the hepatic portal vein and then to the liver.

Drug absorption after rectal administration may be variable depending upon the placement of the suppository or drug solution within the rectum. A portion of the drug dose may be absorbed via the lower hemorrhoidal veins, from which the drug feeds directly into the systemic circulation; some drugs may be absorbed via the superior hemorrhoidal vein, which feeds into the mesenteric veins to the hepatic portal vein to the liver, and metabolized prior to systemic absorption.

Drug Absorption in the Gastrointestinal Tract

Drugs may be absorbed by passive diffusion from all parts of the alimentary canal including sublingual, buccal, GI, and rectal absorption. For most drugs, the optimum site for drug absorption after oral administration is the upper portion of the small intestine or duodenum region. The unique anatomy of the duodenum provides an immense surface area for the drug to passively diffuse (Fig. 5-9). The large

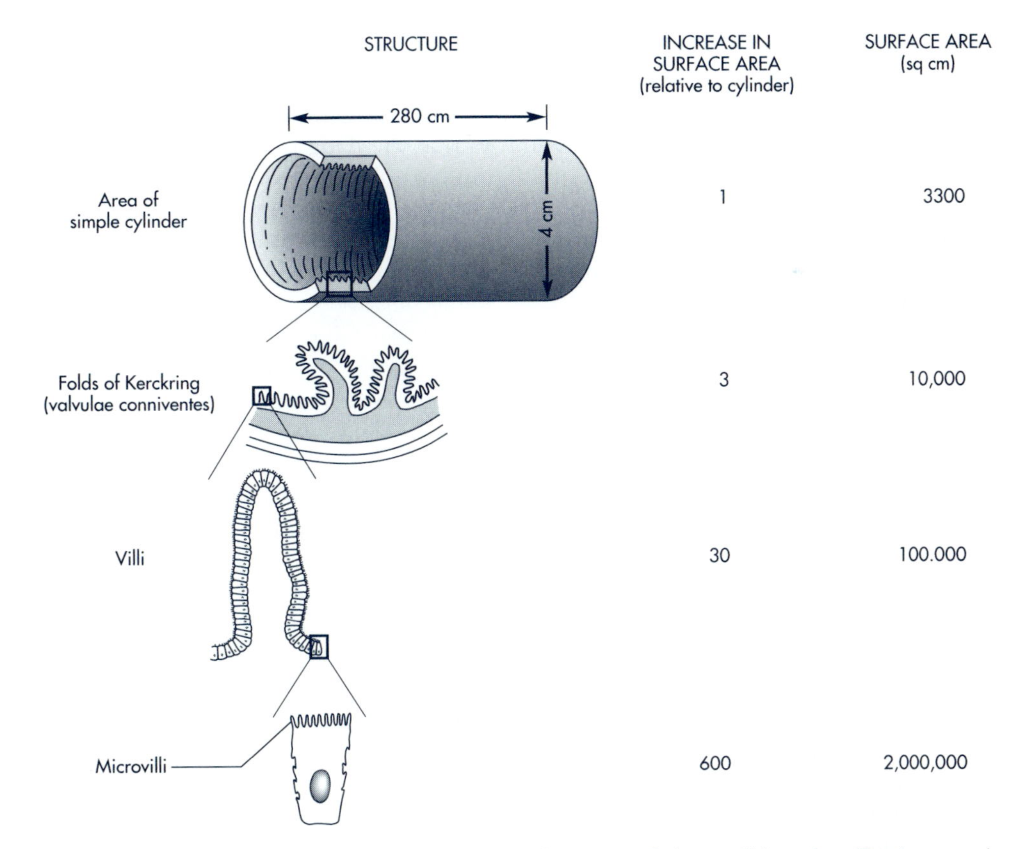

Figure 5-9. Three mechanisms for increasing surface area of the small intestine. The increase in surface area is due to folds of Kerkring, villi, and microvilli.
(From Wilson, 1962, with permission.)

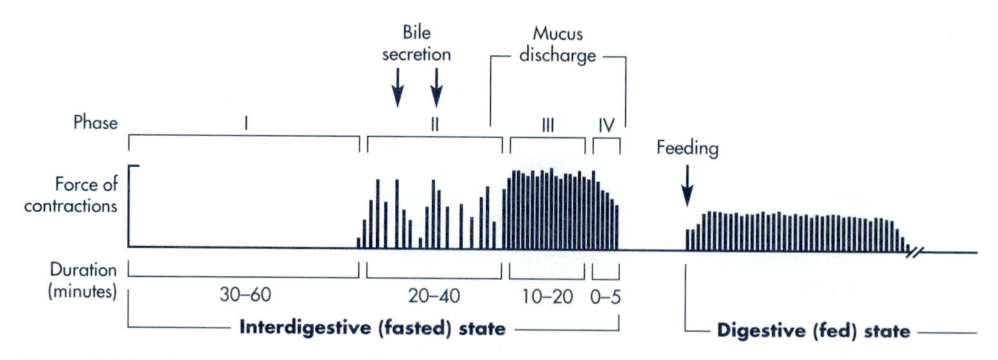

Figure 5-10. A pictorial representation of the typical motility patterns in the interdigestive (fasted) and digestive (fed) state.
(From Rubinstein et al, 1988, with permission.)

surface area of the duodenum is due to the presence of valvelike folds in the mucous membrane upon which are small projections known as *villi.* These villi contain even smaller projections known as *microvilli,* forming a brush border. In addition, the duodenal region is highly perfused with a network of capillaries, which helps to maintain a concentration gradient from the intestinal lumen and plasma circulation.

Gastrointestinal Motility

Once the drug is given orally, the exact location and/or environment of the drug product within the GI tract is difficult to discern. GI motility tends to move the drug through the alimentary canal so that the drug may not stay at the absorption site. For drugs given orally, an anatomic *absorption window* may exist within the GI tract in which the drug is efficiently absorbed. Drugs contained in a nonbiodegradable controlled-release dosage form must be completely released into this absorption window to be absorbed prior to the movement of the dosage form into the large bowel.

The transit time of the drug in the GI tract depends upon the pharmacologic properties of the drug, type of dosage form, and various physiologic factors. Physiologic movement of the drug within the GI tract depends upon whether the alimentary canal contains recently ingested food (*digestive* or *fed* state) or is in the *fasted* or *interdigestive* state (Fig. 5-10). During the fasted or interdigestive state, alternating cycles of activity known as the *migrating motor complex* (MMC) act as a propulsive movement that empties the upper GI tract to the cecum. Initially, the alimentary canal is quiescent. Then, irregular contractions followed by regular contractions with high amplitude (*housekeeper waves*) push any residual contents distally or farther down the alimentary canal. In the fed state, the migrating motor complex is replaced by irregular contractions, which have the effect of mixing intestinal contents and advancing the intestinal stream toward the colon in short segments (Table 5.4). The pylorus and ileocecal valves prevent regurgitation or movement of food from the distal to the proximal direction.

Gastric Emptying Time

Anatomically, the swallowed drug rapidly reaches the stomach. Eventually, the stomach empties its contents into the small intestine. Because the duodenum has the greatest capacity for the absorption of drugs from the GI tract, a delay in the *gas-*

TABLE 5.4 Characteristics of the Motility Patterns in the Fasted Dog

PHASE	DURATION	CHARACTERISTICS
Fasted State		
I	30–60 min	Quiescence.
II	20–40 min	▪ Irregular contractions. ▪ Medium amplitude but can be as high as phase III. ▪ Bile secretion begins. ▪ Onset of gastric discharge of administered fluid of small volume usually occurs before that of particle discharge. ▪ Onset of particle and mucus discharge may occur during the latter part of phase II.
III	5–15 min	▪ Regular contractions (4–5 contractions/min) with high amplitude. ▪ Mucus discharge continues. ▪ Particle discharge continues.
IV	0–5 min	▪ Irregular contractions. ▪ Medium descending amplitude. ▪ Sometimes absent.
Fed State		
One phase only	As long as food is present in the stomach	▪ Regular, frequent contractions. ▪ Amplitude is lower than phase III. ▪ 4–5 Contractions/min.

From Rubinstein et al (1988), with permission.

tric emptying time for the drug to reach the duodenum will slow the rate and possibly the extent of drug absorption, thereby prolonging the onset time for the drug. Some drugs, such as penicillin, are unstable in an acid and decompose if stomach emptying is delayed. Other drugs, such as aspirin, may irritate the gastric mucosa during prolonged contact.

A number of factors will affect gastric emptying time (Table 5.5). Some factors that tend to delay gastric emptying include consumption of meals high in fat, cold beverages, and anticholinergic drugs (Burks et al, 1985; Rubinstein et al, 1988). Liquids and small particles less than 1 mm are generally not retained in the stomach. These small particles are believed to be emptied due to a slightly higher basal pressure in the stomach over the duodenum. Different constituents of a meal will empty from the stomach at different rates. Feldman and associates (1984) observed that 10 ounces of liquid soft drink, scrambled egg (digestible solid), and a radiopaque (undigestible solid) were 50% emptied from the stomach in 30 minutes, 154 minutes, and 3 to 4 hours, respectively. Thus, liquids are generally emptied faster than digested solids from the stomach (Fig. 5-11). Large particles, including tablets and capsules, are delayed from emptying for 3 to 6 hours by the presence of food in the stomach. Indigestible solids empty very slowly, probably during the interdigestive phase, a phase in which food is not present and the stomach is less motile but periodically empties its content due to housekeeper wave contraction (Fig. 5-12).

Intestinal Motility

Normal peristaltic movements mix the contents of the duodenum, bringing the drug particles into intimate contact with the intestinal mucosal cells. The drug must have a sufficient time (*residence time*) at the absorption site for optimum absorption.

In the case of high motility in the intestinal tract, as in diarrhea, the drug has a very brief residence time and less opportunity for adequate absorption.

The average normal small intestine transit time (SITT) was about 7 hours in early studies using indirect methods based on the detection of hydrogen after an

TABLE 5.5 Factors Influencing Gastric Emptying

FACTOR	INFLUENCE ON GASTRIC EMPTYING
1. Volume	The larger the starting volume, the greater the initial rate of emptying; after this initial period, the larger the original volume, the slower the rate of emptying.
2. Type of meal	
Fatty acids	Reduction in rate of emptying is in direct proportion to their concentration and carbon chain length; little difference is detected from acetic to octanoic acids; major inhibitory influence is seen in chain lengths greater than 10 carbons (decanoic to stearic acids).
Triglycerides	Reduction in rate of emptying; unsaturated triglycerides are more effective than saturated ones; the most effective in reducing emptying rate were linseed and olive oils.
Carbohydrates	Reduction in rate emptying, primarily as a result of osmotic pressure; inhibition of emptying increases as concentration increases.
Amino acids	Reduction in rate of emptying to an extent directly dependent upon concentration, probably as a result of osmotic pressure.
3. Osmotic pressure	Reduction in rate of emptying to an extent dependent upon concentration for salts and nonelectrolytes; rate of emptying may increase at lower concentrations and then decrease at higher concentrations.
4. Physical state of gastric contents	Solutions or suspensions of small particles empty more rapidly than do chunks of material that must be reduced in size prior to emptying.
5. Chemicals	
Acids	Reduction in rate of emptying dependent upon concentration and molecular weight of the acid; lower molecular weight acids are more effective than those of higher molecular weight (in order of decreasing effectiveness: HCl, acetic, lactic, tartaric, citric acids).
Alkali ($NaHCO_3$)	Increased rate of emptying at low concentrations (1%), and decreased rate at higher concentrations (5%).
6. Drugs	
Anticholinergics	Reduction in rate of emptying.
Narcotic analgesics	Reduction in rate of emptying.
Metoclopramide	Increase in rate of emptying.
Ethanol	Reduction in rate of emptying.
7. Miscellaneous	
Body position	Rate of emptying is reduced in a patient lying on left side.
Viscosity	Rate of emptying is greater for less viscous solutions.
Emotional states	Aggressive or stressful emotional states increase stomach contractions and emptying rate; depression reduces stomach contraction and emptying.
Bile salts	Rate of emptying is reduced.
Disease states	Rate of emptying is reduced in some diabetics and in patients with local pyloric lesions (duodenal or pyloric ulcers; pyloric stenosis) and hypothyroidism; gastric emptying rate is increased in hyperthyroidism.
Exercise	Vigorous exercise reduces emptying rate.
Gastric surgery	Gastric emptying difficulties can be a serious problem after surgery.

From Mayersohn (1979), with permission.

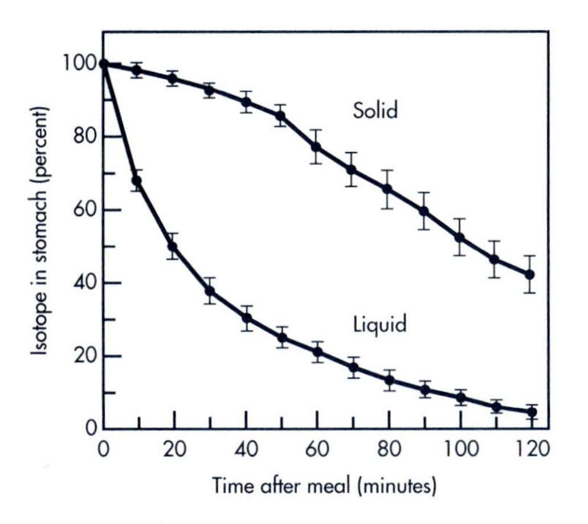

Figure 5-11. Gastric emptying of a group of normal subjects using the dual-isotope method. The mean and 1 SE of the fraction of isotope remaining in the stomach is depicted at various time intervals after ingestion of the meal. Note the exponential nature of liquid emptying and the linear process of solid emptying.
(From Minami and McCallum, 1984, with permission.)

oral dose of lactulose (fermentation of lactulose by colon bacteria yields hydrogen in the breath). Newer studies using gamma scintigraphy have shown SITT to be about 3 to 4 hours. Thus a drug may take about 4 to 8 hours to pass through the stomach and small intestine during the fasting state. During the fed state, SITT may take 8 to 12 hours. For modified-release or controlled-dosage forms, which slowly release the drug over an extended period of time, the dosage form must stay within a certain segment of the intestinal tract so that the drug contents are released and absorbed prior to loss of the dosage form in the feces. Intestinal transit is discussed further in the design of sustained-release products in Chapter 7.

Perfusion of the Gastrointestinal Tract

The blood flow to the GI tract is important in carrying the absorbed drug to the systemic circulation. A large network of capillaries and lymphatic vessels perfuse the duodenal region and peritoneum. The splanchnic circulation receives about 28% of the cardiac output and is increased after meals. Once the drug is absorbed from the small intestine, it enters via the mesenteric vessels to the hepatic–portal vein and the liver prior to reaching the systemic circulation. Any decrease in mesenteric blood flow, as in the case of congestive heart failure, will decrease the rate of drug removal from the intestinal tract, thereby reducing the rate of drug bioavailability (Benet et al, 1976).

The role of the lymphatic circulation in drug absorption is well established. Drugs are absorbed through the lacteal or lymphatic vessels under the microvilli. Absorption of drugs through the lymphatic system bypasses the first-pass effect due to liver metabolism, because drug absorption through the hepatic–portal vein is avoided. The lymphatics are important in the absorption of dietary lipids and may

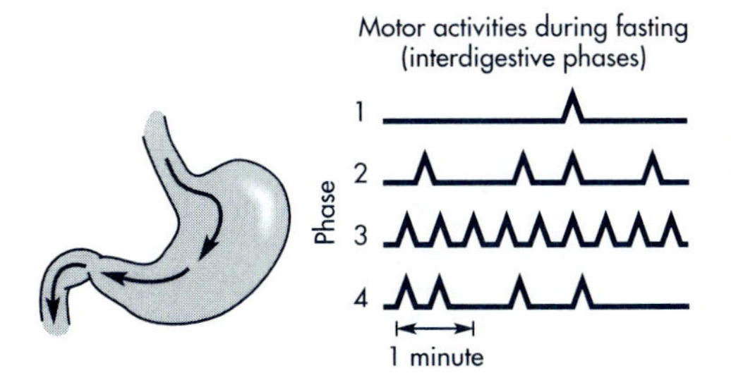

Figure 5-12. Motor activity responsible for gastric emptying of indigestible solids. Migrating myoelectric complex (MMC) usually initiated at proximal stomach or lower esophageal sphincter and contractions during phase 3 sweep indigestible solids through open pylorus.
(From Minami and McCallum, 1984, with permission.)

be partially responsible for the absorption for some lipophilic drugs. Many poorly water-soluble drugs are soluble in oil and lipids, which may dissolve in chylomicrons and be systemically absorbed via the lymphatic system. Bleomycin or aclarubicin were prepared in chylomicrons to improve oral absorption through the lymphatic system (Yoshikawa et al, 1983, 1989).

Effect of Food on Gastrointestinal Drug Absorption

The presence of food in the GI tract can affect the bioavailability of the drug. Digested foods contain amino acids, fatty acids, and many nutrients that may affect intestinal pH and solubility of drugs. The effects of food are not always predictable. The absorption of some antibiotics, such as penicillin and tetracycline, is decreased with food; whereas other drugs, such as griseofulvin, are better absorbed when given with food containing a high fat content (Fig. 5-13). The presence of food in the GI lumen stimulates the flow of bile. Bile contains bile acids, which are surfactants involved in the digestion and solubilization of fats, and also increases the solubility of fat-soluble drugs through micelle formation. For some basic drugs (eg, cinnarizine) with limited aqueous solubility, the presence of food in the stomach stimulates hydrochloric acid secretion, which lowers the pH, causing more rapid dissolution of the drug and better absorption. Absorption of this basic drug is reduced when gastric acid secretion is reduced (Ogata et al, 1986).

Generally, the bioavailability of drugs is better in patients in the fasted state and with a large volume of water (Fig. 5-14). However, drugs such as erythromycin, iron salts, aspirin, and nonsteroidal antiinflammatory agents (NSAID) are irritating to the GI mucosa and are given with food to reduce this irritation. For these drugs, the rate of absorption may be reduced in the presence of food, but the extent of absorption may be the same.

The dosage form of the drug may also be affected by the presence of food. Enteric-coated tablets may stay in the stomach for a longer period of time because food delays stomach emptying. Thus, the enteric-coated tablet does not reach the duodenum rapidly, delaying drug release and systemic drug absorption. In contrast, enteric-coated beads or microparticles disperse in the stomach, stomach emp-

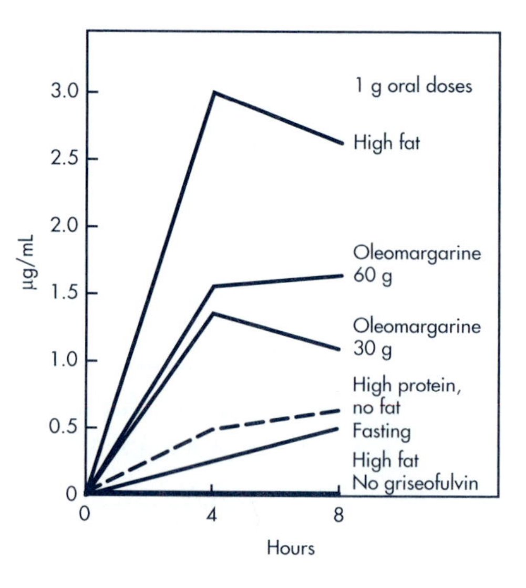

Figure 5-13. A comparison of the effects of different types of food intake on the serum griseofulvin levels following the 1.0-g oral dose.
(From Crounse, 1961, with permission.)

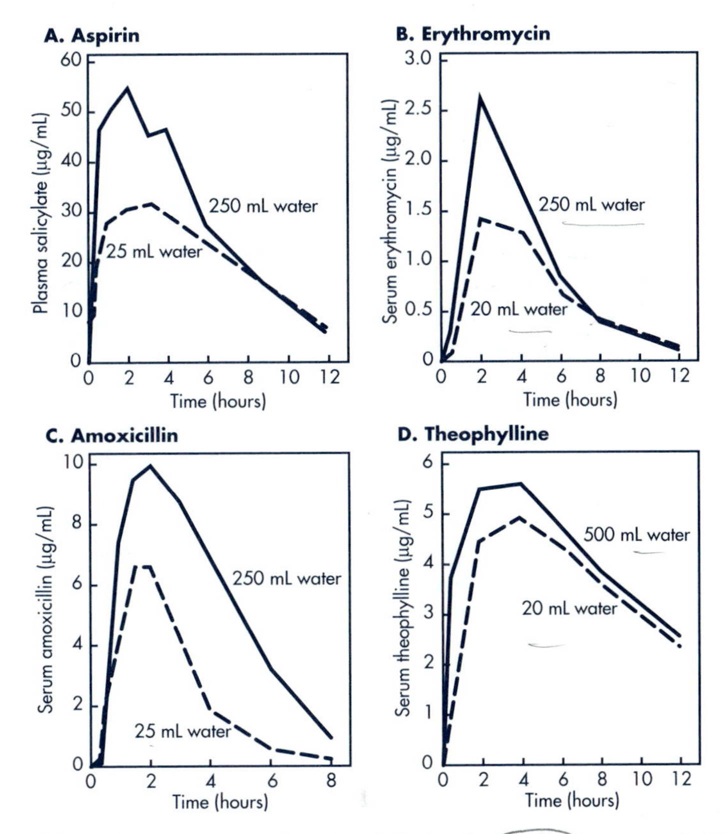

Figure 5-14. Mean plasma or serum drug levels in healthy, fasting human volunteers ($n = 6$ in each case) who received single oral doses of aspirin (650 mg) tablets, erythromycin stearate (500 mg) tablets, amoxicillin (500 mg) capsules, and theophylline (260 mg) tablets, together with large and small accompanying volumes of water.
(From Welling 1980, with permission.)

tying of the particles are less affected by food, and demonstrate more consistent drug absorption from the duodenum.

Food can also affect the integrity of the dosage form, causing an alteration in the release rate of the drug. For example, theophylline bioavailability from Theo-24 controlled-release tablets is much more rapid when given to a subject in the fed rather than fasted state (Fig. 5-15).

Double-Peak Phenomenon

Some drugs, such as ranitidine, cimetidine, and dipyridamole, after oral administration produce a blood concentration curve consisting of two peaks (Fig. 5-16). This double-peak phenomenon is generally observed after the administration of a single dose to fasted patients. The rationale for the double-peak phenomenon has been attributed to variability in stomach emptying, variable intestinal motility, presence of food, enterohepatic recycling, or failure of a tablet dosage form.

The double-peak phenomenon observed for cimetidine (Oberle and Amidon, 1987) may be due to variability in stomach emptying and intestinal flow rates during the entire absorption process after a single dose. For many drugs very little absorption occurs in the stomach. For a drug with high water solubility, dissolution

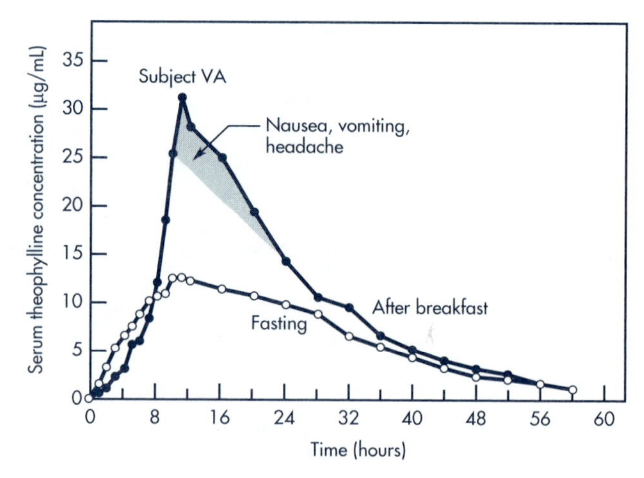

Figure 5-15. Theophylline serum concentrations in an individual subject after a single 1500 mg dose of Theo-24 taken during fasting and after breakfast. The shaded area indicates the period during which this patient experienced nausea, repeated vomiting, or severe throbbing headache. The pattern of drug release during the food regimen is consistent with "dose-dumping."
(From Hendeles et al 1985, with permission.)

of the drug occurs in the stomach, and partial emptying of the drug into the duodenum will result in the first absorption peak. A delay in stomach emptying results in a second absorption peak as the remainder of the dose is emptied into the duodenum.

In contrast, rantidine (Miller, 1984) produces a double peak after both oral or parenteral (IV bolus) administration. Ranitidine is apparently concentrated in the

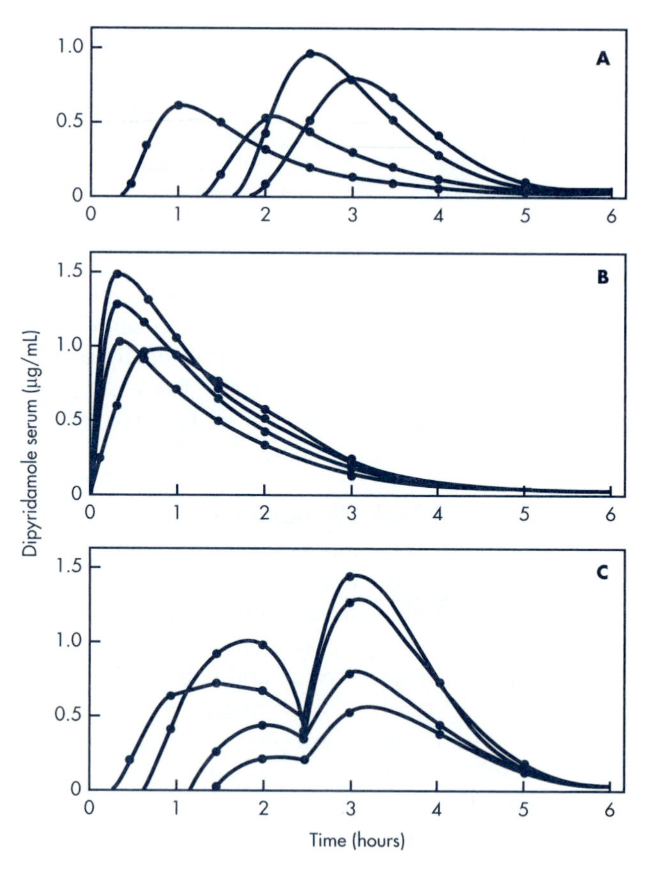

Figure 5-16. Serum concentrations of dipyridamole in 3 groups of 4 volunteers each. **A.** After taking 25 mg as tablet intact. **B.** As crushed tablet. **C.** As tablet intact 2 hours before lunch.
(From Mellinger and Bohorfoush 1966, with permission.)

bile within the gallbladder from the general circulation after IV administration. When stimulated by food, the gallbladder contracts and bile containing drug is released into the small intestine. The drug is then reabsorbed and recycled (enterohepatic recycling).

Tablet integrity may also be a factor in the production of double-peak phenomenon. Mellinger and Bohorfoush (1966) compared a whole tablet or a crushed tablet of dipyridamole in volunteers and showed that a tablet that does not disintegrate or incompletely disintegrates may have delayed gastric emptying, resulting in a second absorption peak.

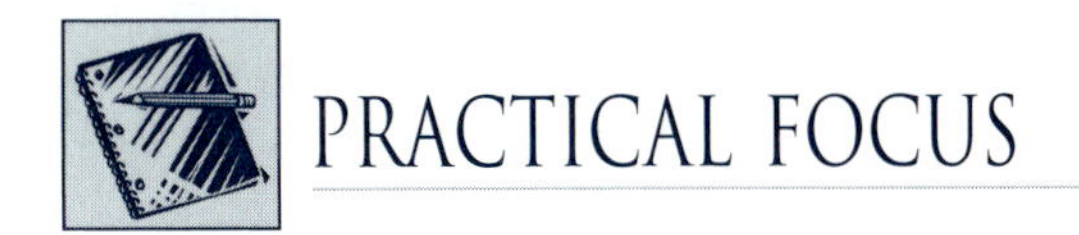

PRACTICAL FOCUS

Effect of Food on Drug Administration

Many antibiotics (Table 5.6), such as penicillin and tetracycline, have delayed or reduced absorption when taken orally with food. Pharmacists regularly advise patients to take a medication either 1 hour before or 2 hours after meals to avoid any delay in drug absorption. Since fatty foods may delay stomach emptying time

TABLE 5.6 Drugs With Absorption Reduced, Delayed, Increased, or Not Affected by the Presence of Food

REDUCED	DELAYED	INCREASED	NOT AFFECTED
Amoxicillin	Acetaminophen	Canrenone	Cephradine
Ampicillin	Amoxicillin	Dicoumarol	Chlorpropamide
Aspirin	Aspirin	Griseofulvin	Digoxin (elixir)
Demethylchlortetracycline	Cefaclor	Hydralazine	Glibenclamide
Ethanol	Cephalexin	Hydrochlorothiazide	Glipizide
Isoniazid	Cephradine	Metoprolol	Melperone
Levodopa	Digoxin (solid)	Oxazepam	Metronidazole
Furosemide	Nitrofurantoin	Phenytoin	Penicillin V (acid)
Methacycline	Potassium ion	Propoxyphene	Prednisone
Oxytetracycline	Sulfadiazine	Propranolol	Propylthiouracil
Penicillin G	Sulfadimethoxine	*Slightly Increased*	Theophylline
Penicillin V (K)	Sulfanilamide	Hetacillin	
Penicillin V (Ca)	Sulfisoxazole		
Pencillin V (acid)			
Phenacetin			
Phenethicillin			
Phenylmercaptomethyl-pencillin			
Pivampicillin			
Propantheline			
Rifampin			
Tetracycline			
Slightly Reduced			
Doxycycline			

From Welling (1980), with permission.

beyond 2 hours, patients who have just eaten a heavy, fatty meal should take these drugs 3 hours or more after the meal, whenever possible. The presence of food may delay stomach emptying of enteric-coated tablets or nondisintegrating dosage forms for several hours. Fine granules (smaller than 1 to 2 mm in size) and tablets that disintegrate are not significantly delayed from emptying from the stomach in the presence of food.

Fluid volume tends to distend the stomach and speed up stomach emptying; however, large volume of nutrients with high caloric content supersedes that faster rate and delays stomach emptying time. Reduction in drug absorption may be caused by several factors. For example, tetracyline hydrochloride absorption is well known to be reduced by milk and food that contains calcium due to chelation. However, significant reduction may simply be the result of reduced dissolution due to increased pH. Coadministration of sodium bicarbonate raises the stomach pH and reduces tetracycline dissolution and absorption. Calcium was absent in the well-controlled experiment reported by Barr and Garrettson (1971).

Food may enhance the absorption of a drug beyond 2 hours after meals. For example, the timing of a fatty meal on the absorption of cefpodoxime proxetil was studied in 20 healthy adults (Borin et al, 1995). The area under the plasma concentration–time curve and peak drug concentration were significantly higher after administration of cefpodoxime proxetil tablets with a meal and 2 hours after a meal relative to dosing under fasted conditions or 1 hour before a meal. The time to peak concentration was not affected by food, which suggests that food increased the extent but not the rate of drug absorption. These results indicate that absorption of cefpodoxime proxetil is enhanced with food or if the drug is taken closely after a heavy meal.

Ticlopidine (Ticlid) is an antiplatelet agent commonly used to prevent thromboembolic disorders. Ticlopidine has enhanced absorption after a meal. The absorption of ticlopidine was compared in subjects who received either an antacid or food or were in a control group (fasting). Subjects who received ticlopidine 30 minutes after a fatty meal had an average of 20% increase in concentration over fasting subjects, whereas antacid reduced ticlopidine concentration by approximately the same amount. There was a higher gastrointestinal complaint in the fasting group. Many other drugs have reduced gastrointestinal side effects when taken with food. The decreased gastrointestinal side effects may greatly improve tolerance and compliance in patients.

Medications that cause gastric irritation, such as aspirin and potassium chloride, may be taken with food. In the case of enteric-coated aspirin tablets, the presence of food may delay drug absorption for several hours due to slower stomach emptying time; taking a granular or pellet enteric-coated product will reduce the delay. The patient should be advised of possible delay in onset of action of the drug when taking a drug with food.

Erythromycin has been recommended to be taken on an empty stomach, although in practice some patients cannot tolerate the drug on an empty stomach and vomit the medication. The presence of food sometimes makes the patient less nauseous with some drugs. A therapeutic alternative may be necessary at times. Oral absorption of the macrolide antibiotic dirithromycin, unlike erythromycin, is not significantly affected by antacid or food, both of which seem to slightly increase absorption.

Some drugs are recommended to be taken with food for special therapeutic purposes. For example, the drug lovastatin (Mevacor) is recommended to be taken with food. Lovastatin inhibits (HMG-CoA reductase) cholesterol synthesis in the body and is taken long term to lower blood cholesterol.

Products that are used to curb stomach acid secretion are taken before meals in anticipation of acid secretion stimulated by food. Famotidine (Pepcid), and cimetidine (Tagamet) have been taken before meals to curb excessive acid production. Tagamet is recommended not to be taken with antacids since that may reduce its absorption. Iron supplements, and nonsteroidal antiinflammatory drugs (NSAIDS), such as ibuprofen, may be taken with food to decrease gastric irritation.

Timing of drug administration should not be based on absorption and onset information alone. Some drugs respond differently depending on the time of administration. Pravastatin is a drug for hypercholesterolemia recommended for twice a day (bid) or daily (qd) dosing. Interestingly, dosing once daily at bedtime is somewhat more effective than once in the morning. The observation is hypothesized to be related to peak cholesterol synthesis by the liver between midnight and 3 AM at night. With some anticancer drugs, time of administration may be critical, since responses have been shown to vary as related to the time of administration of the medication.

Most drugs should be taken with a full glass (approximately 8 fluid ounces) of water to ensure that drugs will wash down the esophagus. The solubility of many drugs is limited, and sufficient fluid is necessary for dissolution of the drug. Some patients may be on several drugs that are dosed frequently for months. These patients are often nauseous and are reluctant to take a lot of fluid. For example, HIV patients with active viral counts may be on an AZT or DDI combination with one or more of the protease inhibitors, Invirase (Hoffmann-La Roche), Crixivan (Merck), or Norvir (Abbott). These HIV treatments appear to be better than any previous treatment but depend on patient compliance in taking up to 12 to 15 pills daily for weeks. Any complications affecting drug absorption can influence the outcome of these therapies. With antibiotics, unabsorbed drug may influence the GI flora. Residual drug dose in the GI tract can potentially aggravate the incidence of diarrhea for drugs that cause GI disturbances.

Effect of Disease States on Drug Absorption

In theory, drug absorption may be affected by any disease that causes changes in (1) intestinal blood flow, (2) gastrointestinal motility, (3) changes in stomach emptying time, (4) gastric pH that affects drug solubility, (5) intestinal pH that affects the extent of ionization, (6) the permeability of the gut wall, (7) bile secretion, (8) digestive enzyme secretion, and (9) alteration of normal GI flora. Some factors may dominate, while other factors sometimes cancel the effect of each other. Pharmacokinetic studies comparing subjects with the disease to a control group is generally necessary to establish the effect of the disease on drug absorption.

Patients in an advanced stage of Parkinson's disease may have difficulty swallowing and greatly diminished gastrointestinal motility. A case was reported in which the patient could not be controlled with regular oral levodopa medication due to poor absorption. Infusion of oral levodopa solution using a *j*-tube gave adequate control of his symptoms. The patient was subsequently placed on this mode of therapy.

Patients on tricyclic antidepressants (imiprimine, amitriptyline, and nortriptyline) and antipsychotic drugs (phenothiazines) with anticholinergic side effects may have reduced gastrointestinal motility or even intestinal obstructions. Delay in drug absorption, especially with slow-release products have occurred.

Achlorhydric patients may not have adequate production of acids in the stomach; stomach HCl is essential for solubilizing insoluble free bases. Many weak base drugs that cannot form soluble salts will remain undissolved in the stomach when there is no hydrochloric acid present and are, therefore, unabsorbed. Salt forms of these drugs cannot be prepared since the free base readily precipitates out due to the weak basicity.

Crohn's Disease

Crohn's disease is an inflammatory disease of the distal small intestine and colon. The disease is accompanied by regions of thickening of the bowel wall, overgrowth of anaerobic bacteria, and sometimes obstruction and deterioration of the bowel occur. The effect on drug absorption is unpredictable, although impaired absorption may potentially occur because of reduced surface area and thicker gut wall for diffusion. In the case of propranolol administered orally, higher plasma propranolol concentration has been reported in patients with Crohn's disease. Alpha-1-acid glycoprotein level is increased in Crohn's disease patients. Higher alpha-1-acid glycoprotein may affect the protein binding and distribution of propranolol in the body and results in higher plasma concentration.

Celiac disease is an inflammatory disease affecting mostly the proximal small intestine. Celiac disease is caused by sensitization to gluten, a viscous protein found in cereals. Patients with celiac disease generally have an increased rate of stomach emptying and increased permeability of the small intestine. Cephalexin absorption appears to be increased in celiac disease although it is not possible to make general prediction in these patients. Other intestinal conditions that may potentially affect drug absorption include corrective surgery involving peptic ulcer, antrectomy with gastroduodenostomy, and selective vagotomy.

Drugs That Affect Absorption of Other Drugs

Propantheline bromide is an anticholinergic drug that may slow stomach emptying and motility of the small intestine. Anticholinergic drugs in general may reduce stomach acid secretion. Slower stomach emptying may cause delay in drug absorption. Tricyclic antidepressants and phenothiazines also have anticholinergic side effects that may cause slower peristalysis in the GI tract.

Metoclopramide is a drug that stimulates stomach contraction, relaxes the pyloric sphincter, and, in general, increases intestinal peristalsis which may reduce the effective time for the absorption of some drugs, and thereby reduce the peak drug concentration and the time for peak drug concentration. For example, digoxin absorption from a tablet is reduced due to metoclopramide but increased due to an anticholinergic drug, such as propantheline bromide. Allowing more time in the stomach for the tablet to dissolve generally helps with the dissolution and absorption of a poorly soluble drug but would not be helpful for a drug that is not soluble in stomach acid.

Cholestyramine is a nonabsorbable ion exchange resin for the treatment of hyperlipemia. Cholestyramine adsorbs warfarin, thyroxine, and loperamide similar to activated charcoal, thereby reducing absorption of these drugs.

Absorption of calcium in the duodenum is an active process facilitated by vitamin D, with calcium absorption as much as four times more than that in vitamin

D deficiency states. It is believed that a calcium-binding protein, which increases after vitamin D administration, binds calcium in the intestinal cell and transfers it out of the base of the cell to the blood circulation.

Nutrients That Interfere with Drug Absorption

Many nutrients substantially interfere with the absorption or metabolism of drugs in the body (Anderson, 1988; Kirk, 1995). Food intake has been reported to enhance the bioavailability of several common drugs such as propranolol, metoprolol, nitrofurantoin, and hydrochlorothiazide. In contrast, food reduces the absorption of many antibiotics such as ampicillin, tetracycline, and rifampicin. Oral drug-nutrient interactions are drug specific and can result in either an increased or decreased drug absorption. Some nutrients may reduce the gastrointestinal irritation of drugs during absorption. Knowing the nature of drug-nutrient interactions can help the clinician to avoid a high concentration of irritating medications. Diet can change the blood levels of some drugs without altering their absorption. For example, a high protein diet may cause reduced theophylline drug level due to increased liver metabolism of the drug rather than a change in the extent of absorption from the gastrointestinal tract.

Absorption of water-soluble vitamins, such as vitamin B-12 and folic acid, are aided by special absorption mechanisms. Vitamin B-12 absorption is facilitated by intrinsic factors in the stomach, where it forms a complex with the factor and is carried in the intestinal stream to the ileum, where it binds to a specific receptor. Vitamin B-12 then ultimately disassociates from the complex and is absorbed.

Grapefruit juice was found to increase the plasma level of many drugs (see Chapter 13) due to naringin that inhibits their metabolism. This is an important example showing that an increase in the blood level of a drug should not be automatically interpreted as an increase in absorption. Many substances reduce the decomposition/metabolism of drugs in the GI tract and, therefore, indirectly increase the amount absorbed.

? FREQUENTLY ASKED QUESTIONS

1. What is an "absorption window"?
2. Why are some drugs absorbed better with food and others retarded by food?
3. If a drug is administered orally as a solution, does it mean that all of the drug will be systemically absorbed?
4. What is the biggest biological factor that contributes to delay in drug absorption?

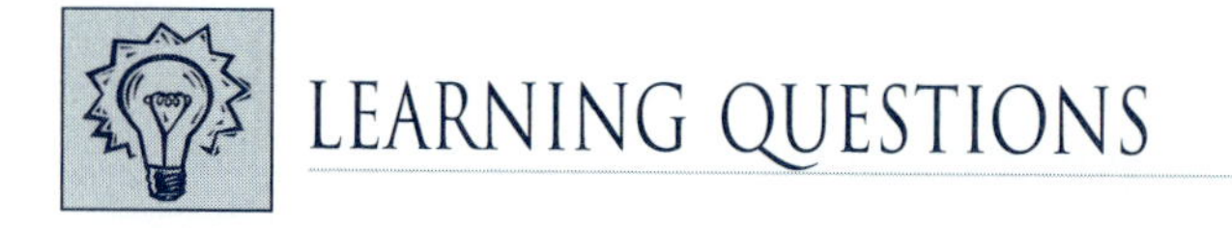

LEARNING QUESTIONS

1. A recent bioavailability study in adult human volunteers demonstrated that after the administration of a single enteric-coated aspirin granule product given with a meal, the plasma drug levels resembled the kinetics of a sustained-release drug product. In contrast, when the product was given to fasted subjects, the plasma drug levels resembled the kinetics of an immediate-release drug product. Give a plausible explanation for this observation.

2. The aqueous solubility of a weak base drug is poor. In an intubation (intestinal perfusion) study, the drug was not absorbed beyond the jejunum. Which of the following would be the correct strategy to improve drug absorption from the intestinal tract?

a. Give the drug as a suspension and recommend that the suspension be taken on an empty stomach.
b. Give the drug as a hydrochloride salt.
c. Give the drug with milk.
d. Give the drug as a suppository.

3. What is the primary reason that protein drugs like insulin are not given orally for systemic absorption?

4. Which of the following statements are true regarding an acidic drug with a pK_a of 4?

a. The drug is more soluble in the stomach when food is present.
b. The drug is more soluble in the duodenum than in the stomach.
c. The drug is more soluble when dissociated.

5. Which region of the gastrointestinal tract is most populated by bacteria? What types of drugs might affect the gastrointestinal flora?

6. Discuss methods by which the first-pass effect (presystemic absorption) may be circumvented.

7. Misoprostol (Cytotec, GD Searle) is a synthetic prostaglandin E_1 analog. According to the manufacturer, the following information was obtained when misoprostol was taken with an antacid or high-fat breakfast.

Condition	C_{max} (pg/mL)	$AUC_{0-4\,hr}$ (pg hr/mL)	t_{max} (min)
Fasting	811 ± 317[a]	417 ± 135	14 ± 8
With antacid	689 ± 315	349 ± 108[b]	20 ± 14
With high-fat breakfast	303 ± 176[b]	373 ± 111	64 ± 79[b]

[a] Results are expressed as the mean ± SD (standard deviation).
[b] Comparisons with fasting results statistically significant, $P < .05$.

What is the effect of *antacid* and *high-fat breakfast* on the bioavailability of misoprostol? Comment on how these factors affect the rate and extent of systemic drug absorption.

REFERENCES

Alberts B, Bray D, Lewis J, et al: *Molecular Biology of the Cell.* Garland, New York, Garland, 1988

Anderson KE: Influences of diet and nutrition on clinical pharmacokinetics. *Clin Pharm* **14:**325–346, 1988

Barr WH, Adir J, Garrettson L: Decrease in tetracycline absorption in man by sodium bicarbonate. *Clin Pharmacol Ther,* **12:**779–784, 1971

Benet LZ, Greither A, Meister W: Gastrointestinal absorption of drugs in patients with cardiac failure. In Benet LZ (ed), *The Effect of Disease States on Drug Pharmacokinetics.* Washington, DC, American Pharmaceutical Association, 1976, chap 3

Borin MT, Driver MR, Forbes KK: Effect of timing of food on absorption of cefpodoxime proxetil. *J Clin Pharmacol* May; **35**(5):505–509, 1995

Burks TF, Galligan JJ, Porreca F, Barber WD: Regulation of gastric emptying. *Fed Proc* **44:**2897–2901, 1985

Crounse RG: Human pharmacology of griseofulvin: The effect of fat intake on gastrointestinal absorption. *J Invest Derm* **37:**529–533, 1961

Davson H, Danielli JF: *The Permeability of Natural Membranes.* Cambridge, England, Cambridge University Press, 1952

Feldman M, Smith HJ, Simon TR: Gastric emptying of solid radiopaque markers: Studies in healthy and diabetic patients. *Gastroenterology* **87:**895–902, 1984

Hendeles L, Weinberger M, Milavetz G, et al: Food induced dumping from "once-a-day" theophylline product as cause of theophylline toxicity. *Chest* **87:**758–785, 1985

Hunt JN, Knox M: Regulation of gastric emptying. In Code CF (ed), *Handbook of Physiology. Section 6: Alimentary Canal.* American Physiological Society, Washington DC, 1968, pp 1917–1935

Jensen JD, Madsen JK, Jensen LW, Pedersen EB: Reduced production, absorption, and elimination of erythropoietin in uremia compared with healthy volunteers. *J Am Soc Nephrol* **5**(2):177–185, 1994

Kirk JK: Significant drug-nutrient interactions. *Am Fam Physician* **51**(5):1175–1182, 1185, 1995

Kirwan WO, Smith AN: Gastrointestinal transit estimated by an isotope capsule. *Scand J Gastroenterol* **9:**763–766, 1974

Lodish HF, Rothman JE: The assembly of cell membranes. *Sci Am* **240:**48–63, 1979

Mayersohn M: Physiological factors that modify systemic drug availability and pharmacologic response in clinical practice. In Blanchard J, Sawchuk RJ, Brodie BB (eds), *Principles and Perspectives in Drug Bioavailability.* Basel, Karger, 1979, chap 8

Mellinger TJ, Bohorfoush JG: Blood levels of dipyridamole (Persantin) in humans. *Arch Int Pharmacodynam Ther* **163:**465–480, 1966

Miller R: Pharmacokinetics and bioavailability of ranitidine in humans. *J Pharm Sci* **73:**1376–1379, 1984

Minami H, McCallum RW: The physiology and pathophysiology of gastric emptying in humans. *Gastroenterology* **86:**1592–1610, 1984

Nienbert R: Ion pair transport across membranes. *Phar Res* **6:**743–747, 1989

Oberle RL, Amidon GL: The influence of variable gastric emptying and intestinal transit rates on the plasma level curve of cimetidine: An explanation for the double-peak phenomenon, *J Pharmacokinet Biopharm* **15:**529–544, 1987

Ogata H, Aoyagi N, Kaniwa N, et al: Gastric acidity dependent bioavailability of cinnarizine from two commercial capsules in healthy volunteers. *Int J Pharm* **29:**113–120, 1986

Pratt P, Taylor P (eds): *Principles of Drug Action: The Basis of Pharmacology,* 3rd ed. New York, Churchill Livingstone, 1990, p 241

Rubinstein A, Li VHK, Robinson JR: Gastrointestinal–physiological variables affecting performance of oral sustained release dosage forms. In Yacobi A, Halperin-Walega E (eds), *Oral Sustained Release Formulations: Design and Evaluation.* New York, Pergamon, 1988, chap 6

Singer SJ, Nicolson GL: The fluid mosaic model of the structure of cell membranes. *Science* **175:**720–731, 1972

Tsuji A, Tamai I: Carrier-dedicated intestinal transport of drugs. *Pharm Res* **13**(7): 963–977, 1966

Welling PG: Drug bioavailability and its clinical significance. In Bridges KW, Chasseaud LF (eds): *Progress in Drug Metabolism,* vol 4. London, Wiley, 1980, chap 3

Wilson TH: *Intestinal Absorption.* Philadelphia, Saunders, 1962

Yoshikawa H, Muranishi S, Sugihira N, Seaki H: Mechanism of transfer of bleomycin into lymphatics by bifunctional delivery system via lumen of small intestine. *Chem Pharm Bull* **31:**1726–1732, 1983

Yoshikawa H, Nakao Y, Takada K, et al: Targeted and sustained delivery of aclarubicin to lymphatics by lactic acid oligomer microsphere in rat. *Chem Phar Bull* **37:**802–804, 1989

BIBLIOGRAPHY

Berge S, Bighley L, Monkhouse D: Pharmaceutical salts. *J Pharm Sci* **66:**1–19, 1977

Blanchard J: Gastrointestinal absorption, II. Formulation factors affecting bioavailability. *Am J Pharm* **150:**132–151, 1978

Davenport HW: *Physiology of the Digestive Tract,* 5th ed. Chicago, Year Book, 1982

Evans DF, Pye G, Bramley R, et al: Measurement of gastrointestinal pH profiles in normal ambulant human subjects. *Gut* **29:**1035–1041, 1988

Eye IS: A review of the physiology of the gastrointestinal tract in relation to radiation doses from radioactive materials. *Health Physics* **12:**131–161, 1966

Houston JB, Wood SG: Gastrointestinal absorption of drugs and other xenobiotics. In Bridges JW, Chasseaud LF (eds): *Progress in Drug Metabolism,* vol 4. London, Wiley, 1980, chap 2

Leesman GD, Sinko PJ, Amidon GL: Stimulation of oral drug absorption: Gastric emptying and gastrointestinal motility. In Welling PW, Tse FLS (eds), *Pharmacokinetics: Regulatory, Industry, Academic Perspectives.* New York, Marcel Dekker, 1988, chap 6

Mackowiak PA: The normal microbial flora. *N Engl J Med* **307:**83–93, 1982

Martonosi AN (ed): *Membranes and Transport,* vol 1. New York, Plenum, 1982

McElnay JC: Buccal absorption of drugs. In Swarbick J, Boylan JC (eds): *Encyclopedia of Pharmaceutical Technology,* vol 2. New York, Marcel Dekker, 1990, pp 189–211

Palin K: Lipids and oral drug delivery. *Pharma Int* November, 272–275, 1985

Palin K, Whalley D, Wilson C et al: Determination of gastric-emptying profiles in the rat: Influence of oil structure and volume. *Int J Pharm* **12:**315–322, 1982

Welling PG: Absorption of drugs. In Swarbrick J, Boylan JC (eds): *Encyclopedia of Pharmaceutical Technology,* vol 1. New York, Marcel Dekker, 1988, pp 1–32

Welling PG: Dosage route, bioavailability and clinical efficacy. In Welling PW, Tse FLS (eds), *Pharmacokinetics: Regulatory, Industry, Academic Perspectives.* New York, Marcel Dekker, 1988, chap 3

Welling PG: Interactions affecting drug absorption. *Clin Pharmacokinet* **9:**404–434, 1984

Wilson TH: *Intestinal Absorption.* Philadelphia, WB Saunders Co, 1962

6

BIOPHARMACEUTIC CONSIDERATIONS IN DRUG PRODUCT DESIGN

Drugs are not generally given as a pure chemical drug substance but formulated into a finished dosage form (drug product), such as a tablet, capsule, etc, before administering to a patient for therapy. A formulated drug product usually includes the active drug substance and selected ingredients (excipients) that make up the dosage form. Common pharmaceutical dosage forms include liquid, tablet, capsule, injection, suppository, transdermal systems, and topical products. Formulating a drug product requires a thorough understanding of the biopharmaceutic principles of drug delivery.

Biopharmaceutics is the study of the *in vitro* impact of the physicochemical properties of the drug and drug product on drug delivery to the body under normal or pathologic conditions. A primary concern in biopharmaceutics is the bioavailability of drugs. *Bioavailability* refers to the measurement of the rate and extent of active drug that reaches the systemic circulation. Because the systemic blood circulation delivers the therapeutically active drug to the tissues and to the site of action of the drug, changes in bioavailability affect changes in the pharmacodynamics and toxicity of the drug. The aim of biopharmaceutics is to adjust the delivery of drug from the drug product in such a manner as to provide optimal therapeutic activity and safety for the patient.

Biopharmaceutic studies allow for the rational design of drug products based on (1) the physical and chemical properties of the drug substance, (2) route of drug administration including the anatomic and physiologic nature of the application site (eg, oral, topical, injectable, implant, transdermal patch, etc), and (4) desired pharmacodynamic effect (eg, immediate or prolonged activity), (5) toxicologic properties of the drug, (6) safety of excipients, and (7) effect of excipients and dosage form on drug delivery. For example, some drugs are intended for topical or local therapeutic action at the site of administration. For these drugs, systemic absorption is undesirable. Drugs intended for local activity are designed to have a direct pharmacodynamic action without affecting other body organs. These drugs may be applied topically to the skin, nose, eye, mucous membranes, buccal cavity, throat, and rectum. A drug intended for local activity may be given intravaginally, into the urethral tract, intranasally, in the ear, on the eye, or orally. Examples of drugs used for local action include anti-infectives, antifungals, local anesthetics, antacids, astringents, vasoconstrictors, antihistamines, and corticosteroids. However, some systemic drug absorption may occur with drugs used for local activity.

Each route of drug application presents special biopharmaceutic considerations in drug product design. For example, the design of a vaginal tablet formulation for the treatment of a fungal infection must consider ingredients compatible with vaginal anatomy and physiology. An eye medication may require special biopharmaceutic considerations including appropriate pH, isotonicity, sterility, local irritation to the cornea, draining by tears, and concern for systemic drug absorption.

For a drug administered by extravascular route (eg, intramuscular injection), local irritation, drug dissolution, and drug absorption from the intramuscular site are some of the factors that must be considered. The systemic absorption of a drug from an extravascular site is influenced by the anatomic and physiologic properties of the site and the physicochemical properties of the drug and the drug product. If the drug is given by the intravascular route (eg, intravenous administration), systemic drug absorption is considered complete or 100% bioavailable because the drug is placed directly into the general circulation.

By carefully choosing the route of drug administration and properly designing the drug product, the bioavailability of the active drug can be varied from rapid and complete absorption to a slow, sustained rate of absorption or, even, virtually no absorption, depending on the therapeutic objective. Once the drug is systemically absorbed, normal physiologic processes for distribution and elimination occur, which usually are not influenced by the specific formulation of the drug. The rate of drug release from the product and the rate of drug absorption are important in determining the distribution, onset, intensity, and duration of the drug action.

Biopharmaceutic considerations often determine the ultimate *dose* and *dosage form* of a drug product. For example, the dosage for a drug intended for local activity, such as a topical dosage form, is often expressed in concentration or as percentage of the active drug in the formulation (eg, 0.5% hydrocortisone cream). The amount of drug applied is not specified because the concentration of the drug at the active site relates to the pharmacodynamic action. However, biopharmaceutic studies must be performed to ensure that the dosage form does not irritate, cause an allergic response, or allow systemic drug absorption. In contrast, the dosage of a drug intended for systemic absorption is given on the basis of mass, such as mg or g. In this case, dosage is based on the amount of drug that is absorbed systemically and dissolved in an apparent volume of distribution to produce a desired drug concentration at the target site. The dose may be based on the weight or surface area of the patient to account for the differences in the apparent volume of distribution. Thus, doses are expressed as mass per unit of body weight (mg/kg) or mass per unit of body surface area (mg/m^2).

RATE-LIMITING STEPS IN DRUG ABSORPTION

Systemic drug absorption from a drug product consists of a succession of rate processes (Fig. 6-1). For solid oral, immediate-release drug products (eg, tablet,

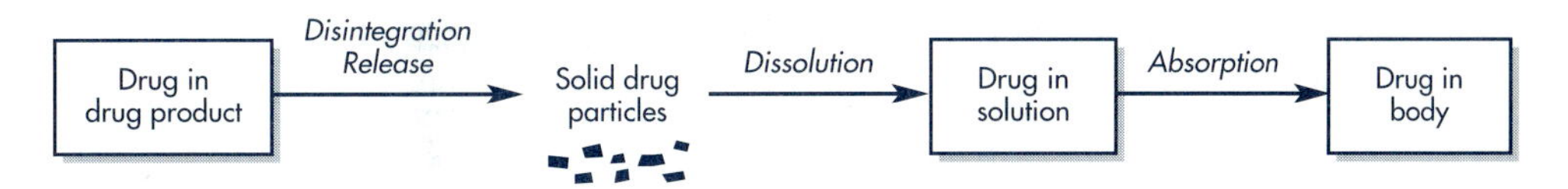

Figure 6-1. Rate processes of drug bioavailability.

capsule), the rate processes include (1) disintegration of the drug product and subsequent release of the drug; (2) dissolution of the drug in an aqueous environment; and (3) absorption across cell membranes into the systemic circulation. In the process of drug disintegration, dissolution, and absorption, the rate at which drug reaches the circulatory system is determined by the slowest step in the sequence.

The slowest step in a series of kinetic processes is called the *rate-limiting step*. Except for controlled release products, disintegration of a solid oral drug product is usually more rapid than drug dissolution and drug absorption. For drugs that have very poor aqueous solubility, the rate at which the drug dissolves (dissolution) is often the slowest step and, therefore, exerts a rate-limiting effect on drug bioavailability. In contrast, for a drug that has a high aqueous solubility, the dissolution rate is rapid, and the rate at which the drug crosses or permeates cell membranes is the slowest or rate-limiting step.

PHARMACEUTIC FACTORS AFFECTING DRUG BIOAVAILABILITY

Considerations in designing a drug product that will deliver the active drug with the desired bioavailability characteristics include (1) the type of drug product (eg, solution, suspension, suppository); (2) the nature of the excipients in the drug product; (3) the physicochemical properties of the drug molecule; and (4) the route of drug administration.

Disintegration

For immediate-release, solid oral dosage forms, the drug product must disintegrate into small particles and release the drug. For monitoring uniform tablet disintegration, the United States Pharmacopeia (USP) established an official disintegration test. Solid drug products exempted from disintegration tests include troches, tablets which are intended to be chewed, and drug products intended for sustained release or prolonged or repeat action. The process of disintegration does not imply complete dissolution of the tablet and/or the drug. Complete disintegration is defined by the USP (23rd edition) as "that state in which any residue of the tablet, except fragments of insoluble coating, remaining on the screen of the test apparatus in the soft mass have no palpably firm core." The official apparatus for the disintegration test and procedure is described in the USP. Separate specifications are given for uncoated tablets, plain coated tablets, enteric tablets, buccal tablets, and sublingual tablets.

Although disintegration tests allow for precise measurement of the formation of fragments, granules, or aggregates from solid dosage forms, no information is obtained from these tests on the rate of dissolution of the active drug. However, the disintegration test serves as a component in the overall quality control of tablet manufacture.

Dissolution

Dissolution is the process by which a chemical or drug becomes dissolved in a solvent. In biologic systems, drug dissolution in an aqueous medium is an important prior condition of systemic absorption. The rate at which drugs with poor aqueous solubility dissolve from an intact or disintegrated solid dosage form in the gastrointestinal tract often controls the rate of systemic absorption of the drug. Thus, dissolution tests are discriminating of formulation factors that may affect drug bioavailability.

Noyes and Whitney (1897) and other investigators studied the rate of dissolution of solid drugs. According to their observations, the steps in dissolution include the process of drug dissolution at the surface of the solid particle, thus forming a saturated solution around the particle. The dissolved drug in the saturated solution known as the *stagnant layer* diffuses to the bulk of the solvent from regions of high drug concentration to regions of low drug concentration (Fig. 6-2).

The overall rate of drug dissolution may be described by the *Noyes–Whitney equation* (Eq. 6.1).

$$\frac{dC}{dt} = \frac{DA}{h}(C_S - C) \tag{6.1}$$

where dC/dt = rate of drug dissolution at time t, D = diffusion rate constant, A = surface area of the particle, C_S = concentration of drug (equal to solubility of drug) in the stagnant layer, C = concentration of drug in the bulk solvent, and h = thickness of the stagnant layer.

The rate of dissolution, $\frac{dC}{dt}$ is the rate of drug dissolved per time expressed as concentration change in the dissolution fluid.

The Noyes–Whitney equation shows that dissolution in a flask may be influenced by the physicochemical characteristics of the drug, the formulation, and the solvent. Drug in the body, particularly in the gastrointestinal tract, is considered to be dissolving in an aqueous environment, permeation of drug across the gut wall (a model lipid membrane) is affected by the ability of the drug to diffuse (D) and to partition between the lipid membrane. A favorable partition coefficient ($K_{oil/water}$) will facilitate drug absorption.

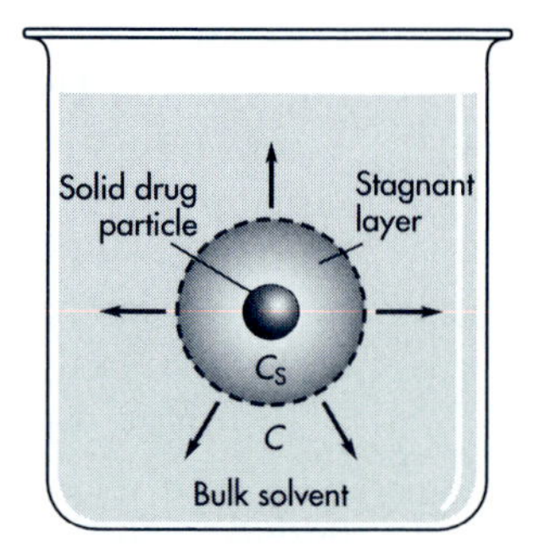

Figure 6-2. Dissolution of a solid drug particle in a solvent. (C_S = concentration of drug in the stagnant layer, C = concentration of drug in the bulk solvent.)

In addition to these factors, the temperature of the medium and the agitation rate also affect the rate of drug dissolution. *In vivo,* the temperature is maintained at a constant 37°C, and the agitation (primarily peristaltic movements in the gastrointestinal tract) is reasonably constant. In contrast, *in vitro* studies of dissolution kinetics require maintenance of constant temperature and agitation. Temperature is generally kept at 37°C, and the agitation or stirring rate is held to a specified rpm (revolutions per minute). An increase in temperature will increase the kinetic energy of the molecules and increase the diffusion constant, D. An increase in agitation of the solvent medium will reduce the thickness, h, of the stagnant layer, allowing for more rapid drug dissolution.

Factors that affect drug dissolution of a solid oral dosage form include (1) the physical and chemical nature of the active drug substance, (2) the nature of the ingredients, and (3) the method of manufacture.

PHYSICOCHEMICAL NATURE OF THE DRUG

The physical and chemical properties of the solid drug particles not only affect dissolution kinetics but are important considerations in designing the dosage form (Table 6.1). For example, intravenous solutions are difficult to prepare with drugs that have poor aqueous solubility. Drugs that are physically or chemically unstable may require special excipient, coating, or manufacturing process to protect the drug from degradation. The potent pharmacodynamic activity of drugs, such as estrogens and other hormones, penicillin antibiotics, cancer chemotherapeutic agents, and others, may cause adverse reactions to personnel who are exposed to these drugs during manufacture and also presents a problem.

Solubility, pH, and Drug Absorption

The *solubility–pH profile* is a plot of the solubility of the drug at various physiologic pH values. For designing oral dosage forms, the formulator must consider that the

TABLE 6.1 Physicochemical Properties for Consideration in Drug Product Design

pK_a and pH Profile	Necessary for optimum stability and solubility of the final product.
Particle Size	May affect the solubility of the drug and therefore the dissolution rate of the product.
Polymorphism	The ability of a drug to exist in various crystal forms may change the solubility of the drug. Also, the stability of each form is important, because polymorphs may convert from one form to another.
Hygroscopicity	Moisture absorption may affect the physical structure as well as stability of the product.
Partition Coefficient	May give some indication of the relative affinity of the drug for oil and water. A drug that has high affinity for oil may have poor release and dissolution from the foundation.
Excipient Interaction	The compatibility of the excipients with the drug and sometimes trace elements in excipients may affect the stability of the product. It is important to have specifications of all raw materials.
pH Stability Profile	The stability of solutions is often affected by the pH of the vehicle; furthermore, because the pH in the stomach and gut is different, knowledge of the stability profile would help to avoid or prevent degradation of the product during storage or after administration.

natural pH environment of the gastrointestinal tract varies from acidic in the stomach to slightly alkaline in the small intestine. A basic drug is more soluble in an acidic medium forming a soluble salt. Conversely, an acid drug is more soluble in the intestine, forming a soluble salt at the more alkaline pH. The solubility–pH profile gives a rough estimation of the completeness of dissolution for a dose of a drug in the stomach or in the small intestine. Solubility may be improved with the addition of an acidic or basic excipient. Solubilization of aspirin, for example, may be increased by the addition of an alkaline buffer. In the formulation of controlled-release drugs, buffering agents may be added to slow or modify the release rate of a fast-dissolving drug. To be effective, however, the controlled-release drug product must be a nondisintegrating dosage form. The buffering agent is released slowly rather than rapidly so that the drug does not dissolve immediately in the surrounding gastrointestinal fluid.

Stability, pH, and Drug Absorption

The *pH–stability profile* is a plot of the reaction rate constant for drug degradation versus pH. If drug decomposition occurs by acid or base catalysis, some prediction for degradation of the drug in the gastrointestinal tract may be made. For example, erythromycin has a pH-dependent stability profile. In acidic medium, as in the stomach, erythromycin decomposition occurs rapidly, whereas, in neutral or alkaline pH, the drug is relatively stable. Consequently, erythromycin tablets are enteric coated to protect against acid degradation in the stomach. This information also led subsequently to the preparation of a less water soluble erythromycin salt that is more stable in the stomach. The dissolution rate of erythromycin powder varied from 100% dissolved in 1 hour to less than 40% dissolved in 1 hour. The slow-dissolving raw drug material (active pharmaceutical ingredient) also resulted in slow-dissolving drug products. Therefore, the dissolution of powdered raw drug material is a very useful *in vitro* method for the prediction of a bioavailability problem of the erythromycin product in the body.

Particle Size and Drug Absorption

The effective surface area of the drug is increased enormously by a reduction in the particle size. Because dissolution is thought to take place at the surface of the solute (drug), the greater the surface area, the more rapid the rate of drug dissolution. The geometric shape of the particle also affects the surface area, and, during dissolution, the surface is constantly changing. In dissolution calculations, the solute particle is usually assumed to have retained its geometric shape.

Particle size and particle size distribution studies are important for drugs that have low water solubility. Many hydrophobic drugs are very active intravenously but are not very effective when given orally due to poor absorption. Griseofulvin, nitrofurantoin, and many steroids are drugs with low aqueous solubility; reduction of the particle size decreased by milling to a micronized form has improved the oral absorption of these drugs. Smaller particle size results in an increase in the total surface area of the particles, enhances water penetration into the particles, and increases the dissolution rates. With poorly soluble drugs, a disintegrant may be added to the formulation to ensure rapid disintegration of the tablet and release of the particles. The addition of surface-active agents may increase wetting as well as solubility of these drugs.

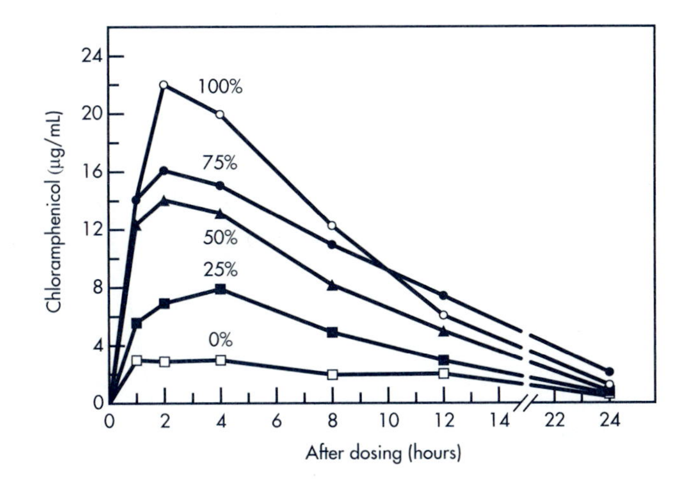

Figure 6-3. Comparison of mean blood serum levels obtained with chloramphenicol palmitate suspensions containing varying ratios of α and β polymorphs, following single oral dose equivalent to 1.5 g chloramphenicol. Percentage polymorph β in the suspension.
(From Aguiar et al, 1967, with permission.)

Polymorphic Crystals, Solvates, and Drug Absorption

Polymorphism refers to the arrangement of a drug in various crystal forms or polymorphs. Polymorphs have the same chemical structure but different physical properties, such as solubility, density, hardness, and compression characteristics. Some polymorphic crystals have much lower aqueous solubility than the amorphous forms, causing a product to be incompletely absorbed. Chloramphenicol, for example, has several crystal forms, and when given orally as a suspension, the drug concentration in the body was found to be dependent on the percent of β-polymorph in the suspension. The β-form is more soluble and better absorbed (Fig. 6-3). In general, the crystal form has the lowest free energy is the most stable polymorph. A drug that exists as an amorphous form (noncrystalline form) generally dissolves more rapidly than the same drug in a more structurally rigid crystalline form. Some polymorphs are metastable and may convert to a more stable form over time. A change in crystal form may cause problems in manufacturing the product. For example, a change in the crystal structure of the drug may cause cracking in a tablet or even prevent a granulation to be compressed into a tablet. Reformulation of a product may be necessary if a new crystal form of a drug is used. Some drugs interact with solvent during preparation to form a crystal called *solvate*. Water may form a special crystal with drugs called *hydrates*; for example, erythromycin hydrates have quite different solubility compared to the anhydrous form of the drug (Fig. 6-4). Ampicillin trihydrate, on the other hand, was reported to be less absorbed than the anhydrous form of ampicillin due to faster dissolution of the latter.

FORMULATION FACTORS AFFECTING DRUG DISSOLUTION

Excipients are added to a formulation to provide certain functional properties to the drug and dosage form. Some of these functional properties of the excipients are used

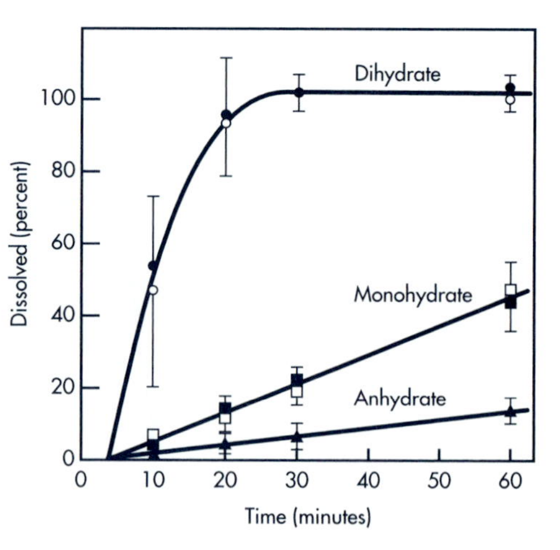

Figure 6-4. Dissolution behavior of erythromycin dihydrate, monohydrate, and anhydrate in phosphate buffer (pH 7.5) at 37°C.
(From Allen et al, 1978, with permission.)

to improve the compressibility of the active drug, stabilize the drug from degradation, decrease gastric irritation, control the rate of drug absorption from the absorption site, increase drug bioavailability, etc. Some of the excipients used in the manufacture of solid and liquid drug products are listed in Tables 6.2 and 6.3.

Excipients in the drug product may also affect dissolution kinetics of the drug either by altering the medium in which the drug is dissolving or by reacting with the drug itself. Some of the more common manufacturing problems that affect dissolution are listed on Table 6.2. Other excipients include suspending agents that increase the viscosity of the drug vehicle and thereby diminish the rate of drug dissolution from suspensions. Tablet lubricants, such as magnesium stearate, may repel water and reduce dissolution when used in large quantities. Coatings, particularly shellac upon aging can decrease the dissolution rate. However, surfactants may affect drug dissolution in an unpredictable fashion. Low concentrations of surfactants decrease the surface tension and increase the rate of drug dissolution, whereas higher surfactants concentrations tend to form micelles with the drug and thus decrease the dissolution rate. Large drug particles have a smaller surface area and dissolve more slowly than smaller particles. High compression of tablets without

TABLE 6.2 Common Excipients Used in Solid Drug Products

EXCIPIENT	PROPERTY IN DOSAGE FORM
Lactose	Diluent
Dibasic calcium phosphate	Diluent
Starch	Disintegrant, diluent
Microcrystalline cellulose	Disintegrant, diluent
Magnesium stearate	Lubricant
Stearic acid	Lubricant
Hydrogenated vegetable oil	Lubricant
Talc	Lubricant
Sucrose (solution)	Granulating agent
Polyvinyl pyrrolidone (solution)	Granulating agent
Hydroxypropylmethylcellulose	Tablet-coating agent
Titinium dioxide	Combined with dye as colored coating
Methylcellulose	Coating or granulating agent
Cellulose acetate phthalate	Enteric coating agent

TABLE 6.3 Common Excipients Used in Oral Liquid Drug Products

EXCIPIENT	PROPERTY IN DOSAGE FORM
Sodium carboxymethylcellulose	Suspending agent
Tragacanth	Suspending agent
Sodium alginate	Suspending agent
Xanthan gum	Thixotropic suspending agent
Veegum	Thixotropic suspending agent
Sorbitol	Sweetener
Alcohol	Solubilizing agent, preservative
Propylene glycol	Solubilizing agent
Methyl, propylparaben	Preservative
Sucrose	Sweetener
Polysorbates	Surfactant
Sesame oil	For emulsion vehicle
Corn oil	For emulsion vehicle

sufficient disintegrant may cause poor disintegration of a compressed tablet. Some excipients, such as sodium bicarbonate, may change the pH of the medium surrounding the active drug substance. Aspirin, a weak acid when formulated with sodium bicarbonate will form a water-soluble salt in an alkaline medium in which the drug rapidly dissolves. The term for this process is *dissolution in a reactive medium*. The solid drug dissolves rapidly in the reactive solvent surrounding the solid particle. However, as the dissolved drug molecules diffuse outward into the bulk solvent, the drug may precipitate out of solution with a very fine particle size. These small particles have enormous collective surface area, dispersing and redissolving readily for more rapid absorption upon contact with the mucosal surface.

Excipients in a formulation may interact directly with the drug to form a water-soluble or water-insoluble complex. For example, if tetracycline is formulated with calcium carbonate, an insoluble complex of calcium tetracycline is formed that has a slow rate of dissolution and poor absorption.

Excipients may be added intentionally to the formulation to enhance the rate and extent of drug absorption or to delay or slow the rate of drug absorption (Table 6.4). For example, excipients that increase the aqueous solubility of the drug generally increase the rate of dissolution and drug absorption. Excipients may increase the retention time of the drug in the gastrointestinal tract and therefore increase

TABLE 6.4 Effect of Excipients on the Pharmacokinetic Parameters of Oral Drug Products[a]

EXCIPIENTS	EXAMPLE	K_A	T_{MAX}	AUC
Disintegrants	Avicel, Explotab	↑	↓	↑/—
Lubricants	Talc, hydrogenated vegetable oil	↓	↑	↓/—
Coating agent	Hydroxypropylmethyl cellulose	—	—	—
Enteric coat	Cellulose acetate phthalate	↓	↑	↓/—
Sustained-release agents	Methylcellulose, ethylcellulose	↓	↑	↓/—
Sustained-release agents (waxy agents)	Castorwax, Carbowax	↓	↑	↓/—
Sustained-release agents (gum/viscous)	Veegum, Keltrol	↓	↑	↓/—

[a] This may be concentration and drug dependent. ↑ = Increase, ↓ = decrease, — = no effect, k_a = absorption rate constant, t_{max} = time for peak drug concentration in plasma, AUC = area under the plasma drug concentration time curve.

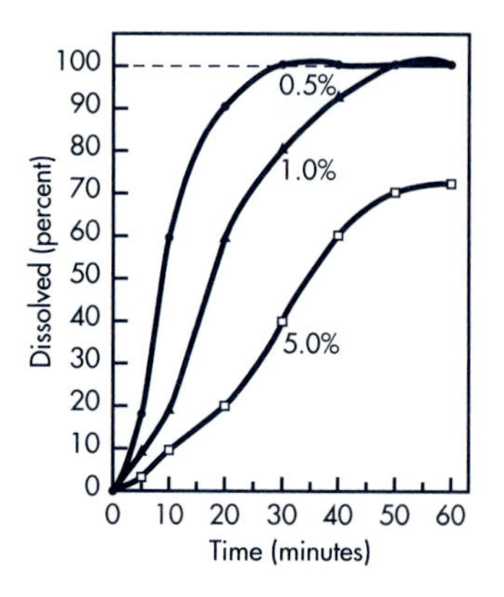

Figure 6-5. Effect of lubricant on drug dissolution. Percentage of magnesium stearate in formulation.

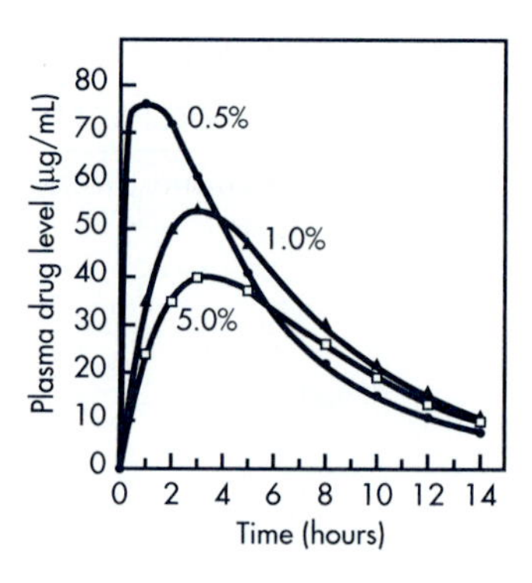

Figure 6-6. Effect of lubricant on drug absorption. Percentage of magnesium stearate in formulation. Incomplete drug absorption occurs for formulation with 5% magnesium stearate.

the total amount of drug absorbed. Excipients may act as carriers to increase drug diffusion across the intestinal wall. In contrast, many excipients may retard drug dissolution and thus reduce drug absorption. Common excipients found in oral drug products are listed in Table 6.2 and Table 6.3. Formulations contain various components (excipients) that are pharmacodynamically inert but that functionally enhance the drug and the dosage form. For solid oral dosage forms such as compressed tablets, excipients may include: (1) diluent (eg, lactose); (2) disintegrant (eg, starch); (3) lubricant (eg, magnesium stearate); and (4) other components such as binding and stabilizing agents. When improperly used in the formulation, the rate and extent of drug absorption may be affected. For example, Figure 6-5 shows that an excessive quantity of magnesium stearate (a hydrophobic lubricant) in the formulation may retard drug dissolution and slow the rate of drug absorption. The total amount of drug absorbed may also be reduced (Fig. 6-6). To prevent this problem, the lubricant level should be decreased or a different lubricant selected. Sometimes, increasing the amount of disintegrant may overcome the retarding effect of lubricants on dissolution. However, with some poorly soluble drugs an increase in disintegrant level has little or no effect on drug dissolution because the fine drug particles are not wetted. The influence of some common ingredients on drug absorption parameters is summarized in Table 6.4. These are general trends for typical preparations.

IN VITRO DISSOLUTION TESTING

Dissolution tests *in vitro* measure the rate and extent of dissolution of the drug in an aqueous medium in the presence of one or more excipients contained in the drug products. A bioavailability problem may be uncovered by a suitable dissolution method. However, the dissolution testing condition reveals that the bioavailability problem differs with each drug formulation. A reasonable approach involves selecting a dissolution method in which the acceptable and unacceptable drug formulation is distinguished by having different dissolution rates. Different agitation rates, different mediums (including different pH), and different types of dissolu-

TABLE 6.5 Dissolution of Erythromycin Stearate Bulk Drug and Corresponding Tablets

	PERCENT DISSOLUTION AFTER 1.0 HR		
CURVE NO.	***BULK DRUG***	***500-MG TABLET***	***250-MG TABLET***
4	49	44	
6	72	70	
7	75	70	
—	78	—	80
8	82	75	
9	92	85	

From Philip and Daly (1983), with permission.

tion apparatus should be tried. Once differences in dissolution rates are found, the formulation of the drug product may be matched with the dissolution rates to get an empirically acceptable criteria for the product. The composition and supplies of the raw materials may then be examined to reveal the problem. In one example, Philip and Daly (1983) devised a method using pH 6.6 phosphate buffer as the dissolution medium instead of 0.1 N HCL to avoid instability of the drug. Using the testing temperature at 22°C and the USP paddle method at 50 rpm, the dissolution of the various erythromycin tablets varied with the source of the bulk drug (as shown in Table 6.5 and Figure 6-7). There are a number of factors that must be considered when performing a dissolution test.

The size and shape of the dissolution vessel may affect the rate and extent of dissolution. For example, the vessel may range in size from several milliliters to several liters. The shape may be round-bottomed or flat, so that the tablet might lie in a different position in different experiments. The usual volume of the medium is 500 to 1000 mL. Drugs that are not very water soluble may require use of a very-large-capacity vessel (up to 2000 mL) to observe significant dissolution. *Sink con-*

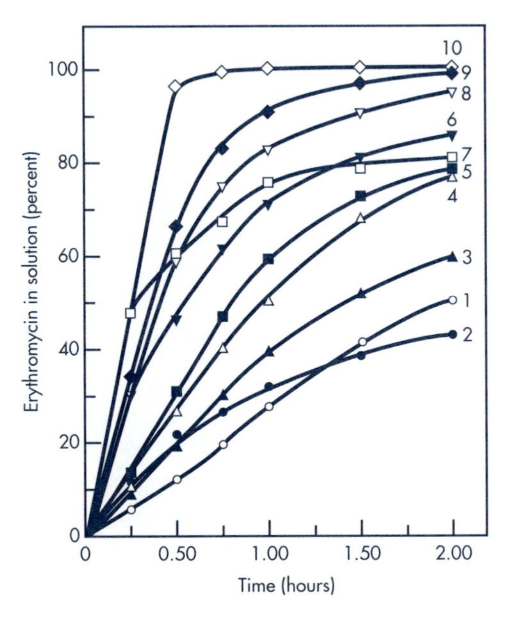

Figure 6-7. Dissolution profile of various lots of erythromycin stearate as a function of time (0.05 M pH 6.6 phosphate buffer).
(From Philip and Daly, 1983, with permission.)

ditions is a term referring an excess volume of medium that allows the solid drug to continuously dissolve. If the drug solution becomes saturated, no further net drug dissolution will take place. According to the USP (1995), "the quantity of medium used should be not less than 3 times that required to form a saturated solution of the drug substance."

The amount of agitation and the nature of the stirrer affect the dissolution rate. Stirring rates must be controlled, and specifications differ between drug products. Low stirring rates (50 to 100 rpm) are more discriminating of formulation factors affecting dissolution than higher stirring rates. The temperature of the dissolution medium must be controlled and variations in temperature must be avoided. Most dissolution tests are performed at 37°C.

The nature of the dissolution medium will also affect the dissolution test. The solubility of the drug must be considered as well as the amount of drug in the dosage form. The dissolution medium should not be saturated by the drug (ie, sink conditions are maintained). Usually, a volume of medium larger than the amount of solvent needed to completely dissolve the drug is used in such tests. Which medium is best is a matter of considerable controversy. The preferred dissolution medium in USP dissolution tests is deaerated water or if substantiated by the solubility characteristics of the drug or formulation, a buffered aqueous solution (typically pH 4 to 8) or dilute HCl may be used. The significance of deareation of the medium should be determined. Various investigators have used 0.1 N HCl, phosphate buffer, simulated gastric juice, water, and simulated intestinal juice, depending on the nature of the drug product and the location in the gastrointestinal tract where the drug is expected to dissolve.

The design of the dissolution apparatus, along with the factors described above, has a marked effect on the outcome of the dissolution test. No single apparatus and test can be used for all drug products. Each drug product must be tested individually with the dissolution test that best correlates to *in vivo* bioavailability.

Usually, the report on the dissolution test will state that a certain percentage of the labeled amount of drug product must dissolve within a specified period of time. In practice, the absolute amount of drug in the drug product may vary from tablet to tablet. Therefore, a number of tablets from each lot are usually tested to get a representative dissolution rate for the product.

COMPENDIAL METHODS OF DISSOLUTION

The USP-23 provides several official methods for carrying out dissolution tests of tablets, capsules and other special products such as transdermal preparations. Tablets are grouped into uncoated, plain-coated, and enteric-coated tablets. The selection of a particular method for a drug is usually specified in the monograph for a particular drug product. Buccal and sublingual tablets are tested applying the uncoated tablet procedure.

Rotating Basket Method (Apparatus 1)

The rotating basket method consists of a cylindrical basket held by a motor shaft. The basket holds the sample and rotates in a round flask containing the dissolution medium. The entire flask is immersed in a constant-temperature bath set at 37°C. The rotating speed and the position of the basket must meet specific requirements set forth in the current USP. The most common rotating speed for the basket method is 100 rpm. Dissolution calibration standards are available to make sure that these mechanical and operating requirements are met. Calibration tablets containing prednisone are made specially for dissolution tests requiring disintegrating tablets, whereas salicylic acid calibration tablets are used as a standard requiring nondisintegrating tablets. Apparatus 1 is generally preferred for capsules and for dosage forms that tend to float or disintegrate slowly.

Paddle Method (Apparatus 2)

The paddle method, or Apparatus 2, consists of a special, coated paddle that minimizes turbulence due to stirring (Fig. 6-8). The paddle is vertically attached to a variable-speed motor that rotates at a controlled speed. The tablet or capsule is placed into the round-bottom dissolution flask, which minimizes turbulence of the dissolution medium. The apparatus is housed in a constant-temperature water bath

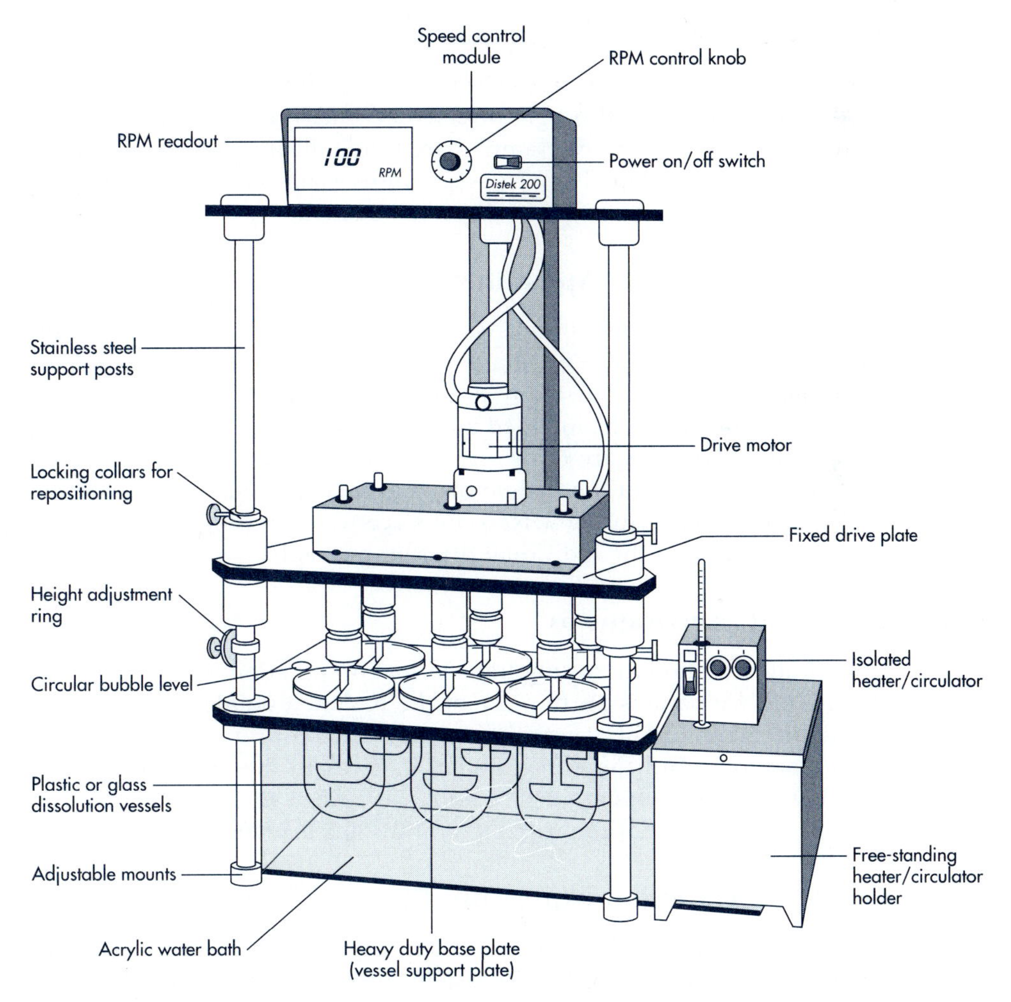

Figure 6-8. Typical set up for performing the USP dissolution test with the Distek 2000. The system is equipped with a height adjustment ring for easy adjustment of paddle height.
(Drawing courtesy of Distek Inc, Somerset, NJ.)

maintained at 37°C similar to that of the rotating-basket method. The position and alignment of the paddle are specified in the USP. The paddle method is very sensitive to tilting. Improper alignment may drastically affect the dissolution results with some drug products. The same set of dissolution calibration standards is used to check the equipment before tests are run. The most common operating speeds for Apparatus 2 are 50 rpm for solid oral dosage forms and 25 rpm for suspensions. Apparatus 2 is generally preferred for tablets. A *sinker* such as a few turns of platinum wire may be used to prevent a capsule from floating. The sinker should not alter the dissolution characteristics of the dosage form.

Reciprocating Cylinder Method (Apparatus 3)

This apparatus consists of a set of cylindrical, flat-bottomed glass vessels equipped with reciprocating cylinders for dissolution testing of extended release products, particularly the bead-type modified release dosage forms. Six units are tested and the dissolution media is maintained at 37°C.

Flow-Through Cell Method (Apparatus 4)

The apparatus consists of a reservoir for the dissolution medium and a pump forcing dissolution medium through the cell that holds the test sample. Flow rate ranges from 4 to 16 mL/minute. Six samples are tested during the dissolution testing and the medium is maintained at 37°C. Apparatus 4 may be used for modified release dosage forms that contain active ingredients having very limited solubility.

Paddle Over Disk Method (Apparatus 5)

The USP-23 lists a "paddle over disk" method for testing the release of drugs from transdermal products. The apparatus consists of a sample holder or disk assembly that holds the product. The entire preparation is placed in a dissolution flask filled with specified medium maintained at 32°C. The paddle is placed directly over the disk assembly. Samples are drawn midway between the surface of the dissolution medium and the top of the paddle blade at specified times. Similar to dissolution testing with capsules and tablets, 6 units are tested during each run. Acceptance criteria are stated in the individual drug monographs.

Cylinder Method (Apparatus 6)

The cylinder method for testing transdermal preparation is modified from the basket method (Apparatus 1). In place of the basket, a stainless steel cylinder is used to hold the sample. The sample is mounted onto cuprophan (an inert porous cellulosic material) and the entire system adheres to the cylinder. Testing is maintained at 32°C. Samples are drawn midway between the surface of the dissolution medium and the top of the rotating cylinder for analysis.

Reciprocating Disk Method (Apparatus 7)

With the reciprocating disk method for testing transdermal products, a motor drive assembly is used to reciprocate the system vertically, and the samples are placed on disk-shaped holders using cuprophan supports. The test is also carried out at 32°C and reciprocating frequency is about 30 cycles per minute. The acceptance criteria are listed in the individual drug monographs.

METHODS FOR TESTING ENTERIC-COATED PRODUCTS

For testing enteric-coated products, USP-23 lists two methods.

Method A

Dissolution is carried out in the apparatus specified in the drug monograph (usually Apparatus 2 or 1). The product is first tested with 0.1 N HCl for 2 hours and then changed to pH 6.8 by adding 0.2 M tribasic sodium phosphate, fine-tuning pH either with 2 N NaOH or HCl if necessary. The buffer stage generally runs for 45 minutes. The test objective involves making sure that no significant dissolution occurs in the acid phase (less than 10% for any sample unit), and specified percent of drug must be released in the buffer phase. Specifications are set in the individual drug monographs.

Method B

This method involves testing the product in 0.1 N HCl for 2 hours, and then draining the acid and replacing it with a pH 6.8 buffer medium formed by mixing 0.2 M tribasic sodium phosphate with 0.1 N HCl. The temperature of the replaced medium must be preequilibrated to 37°C. The acceptance criteria are similar to those for method A.

MEETING DISSOLUTION REQUIREMENTS

Dissolution test times and specifications are usually established on the basis of an evaluation of dissolution profile data. The dissolution test time points should be selected to characterize adequately the ascending and plateau phases of the dissolution curve.

The USP–NF sets dissolution requirements for many products (see Table 6.6). The requirements apply to both the basket and the paddle methods. Amount of drug dissolved within a given time period (Q) is expressed as a percentage of label content. The Q is generally specified in the monograph for a drug product to pass the dissolution test. For each dissolution run, 6 tablets or capsules are tested, and the dissolution test continues until the criteria are met or the stages are exhausted.

For many products the passing of Q is set at 75% in 45 minutes. Some products are set at Q of 85% in 30 minutes, others at 75% in 60 minutes. For a new drug

TABLE 6.6 Dissolution Acceptance

STAGE	NUMBER TESTED	ACCEPTANCE CRITERIA
S_1	6	Each unit is not less than $Q + 5\%$
S_2	6	Average of 12 units ($S_1 + S_2$) is equal to or greater than Q, and no unit is less than $Q - 15\%$
S_3	12	Average of 24 units ($S_1 + S_2 + S_3$) is equal to or greater than Q, not more than 2 units are less than $Q - 15\%$, and no unit is less than $Q - 25\%$

Adapted with permission from the United States Pharmacopeia (1995).

product, setting the dissolution specification requires a thorough consideration of the physical and chemical properties of the drug. In addition to the consideration that the dissolution test must ensure consistent bioavailability of the product, the test must provide for variation in manufacturing and testing variables so that a product may not be improperly rejected.

UNOFFICIAL METHODS OF DISSOLUTION TESTING

Rotating Bottle Method

This method was suggested in NF-XIII and has become less popular. The rotating bottle method was used mainly for controlled-release beads. For this purpose the dissolution media may be easily changed, such as from artificial gastric juice to artificial intestinal juice. The equipment consists of a rotating rack that holds the sample drug products in bottles. The bottles are capped tightly and rotated in a 37°C temperature bath. At various times, the samples are removed from the bottle, decanted through a 40-mesh screen, and the residues are assayed. To the remaining drug residues within the bottles are added an equal volume of fresh medium and the dissolution test is continued. A dissolution test with pH 1.2 medium for 1 hour, pH 2.5 medium for the next 1 hour, followed by pH 4.5 medium for 1.5 hours, pH 7.0 medium for 1.5 hours, and pH 7.5 medium for 2 hours was recommended to simulate condition of the gastrointestinal tract. The main disadvantage is that this procedure is manual and tedious. Moreover, it is not known if the rotating bottle procedure results in a better *in vitro–in vivo* correlation for drugs.

Flow-Through Dissolution Method

There are many variations of this method. Essentially, the sample is held in a fixed position while the dissolution medium is pumped through the sample holder dissolving the drug. Laminar flow of the medium is achieved by using a pulseless pump. Peristaltic or centrifugal pumps are not recommended. The flow rate is usually maintained between 10 and 100 mL/minute. The dissolution medium may be fresh or recirculated. In the case of fresh medium, the dissolution rate at any moment may be obtained, whereas in the official paddle or basket methods cumulative dissolution rates are monitored. A major advantage of the flow-through method is the easy maintenance of a sink condition for dissolution. A large volume of dissolution medium may also be used, and the mode of operation is easily adapted to automated equipment.

Intrinsic Dissolution Method

Most methods for dissolution deal with a finished drug product. Sometimes a new drug or substance may be tested for dissolution without the effect of excipients or the fabrication effect of processing. The dissolution of a drug powder by maintaining a constant surface area is called *intrinsic dissolution*. Intrinsic dissolution is usually expressed as mg/cm^2 min. In one method, the basket method is adapted to test dissolution of powder by placing the powder in a disk attached with a clipper to the bottom of the basket.

Peristalsis Method

This method attempts to simulate the hydrodynamic conditions of the gastrointestinal tract in an *in vitro* dissolution device. The apparatus consists of a rigid plastic cylindrical tubing fitted with a septum and rubber stoppers at both ends. The dissolution chamber consists of a space between the septum and the lower stopper. The apparatus is placed in a beaker containing the dissolution medium. The dissolution medium is pumped with peristaltic action through the dosage form.

PROBLEMS OF VARIABLE CONTROL IN DISSOLUTION TESTING

There are a number of equipment and operating variables associated with dissolution testing. Depending on the particular dosage form involved, the variables may or may not exert a pronounced effect on the rate of dissolution of the drug or drug product. Variations of 25% or more may occur with the same type of equipment and procedure. The centering and alignment of the paddle is critical in the paddle method. Turbulence can create increased agitation, resulting in a higher dissolution rate. Wobbling and tilting due to worn equipment should be avoided. The basket method is less sensitive to the tilting effect. However, the basket method is more sensitive to clogging due to gummy materials. Pieces of small particles can also clog up the basket screen and create a local nonsink condition for dissolution. Furthermore, dissolved gas in the medium may form air bubbles on the surface of the dosage form unit and can affect dissolution in both the basket and paddle methods.

The interpretation of dissolution data is probably the most difficult job for the pharmacist. In the absence of *in vivo* data, it is generally impossible to make valid conclusions about bioavailability from the dissolution data alone. The use of various testing methods makes it even more difficult to interpret dissolution results because there is no simple correlation among dissolution results obtained with various methods. For many drug products, the dissolution rates are higher with the paddle method. Dissolution results at 50 rpm with the paddle method may be equivalent to the dissolution at 100 rpm with the basket method. In a study of sustained theophylline tablets compressed at various degrees of hardness, Cameron et al (1983) found that, at 50 rpm, dissolution with the paddle method was faster than that of the basket method for tablets of 4.0 kg hardness. However, with tablets of 6.8 kg hardness, similar dissolution profiles were obtained at 125 rpm for the basket and paddle methods over a period of 6 hours. With both methods, increased dissolution rates were observed as the rates were increased. Apparently, the composition of the formulation as well as the process variables in manufacturing may be both important. No simple correlation can be made for dissolution results obtained with different methods.

In a comparison of the paddle and basket methods in evaluating sustained-release pseudoephedrine–guaifenesin preparation, Masih and coworkers (1983) found that the paddle method was more discriminating in demonstrating dissolution differences among drug products. At 100 rpm, the basket method failed to pick up formulation differences detected by the paddle method.

In the absence of *in vivo* data, the selection of the dissolution method is based on the type of drug product to be tested. For example, a low-density preparation may be poorly wetted in the basket method. A gummy preparation may clog up the basket screen; therefore the paddle method is preferred. A floating dosage form (eg, suppository) may be placed in a stainless steel coil so that the dosage form remains at the bottom of the dissolution flask. For many drugs, a satisfactory dissolution test may be obtained with more than one method by optimizing the testing conditions.

IN VITRO–IN VIVO CORRELATION OF DISSOLUTION

In vitro drug dissolution studies are most useful for monitoring drug product stability and manufacturing process control. Thus, dissolution testing is of immense value as a tool for quality control. Dissolution tests are discriminating of formulation factors that may affect bioavailability of the drug. In some cases, dissolution tests for immediate-release solid oral drug products are very discriminating and a clinically acceptable product might perform poorly in the dissolution test. When a proper dissolution method is chosen, the rate of dissolution of the product may be correlated to the rate of absorption of the drug into the body. Well defined *in vitro–in vivo* correlations have been reported for modified release drug products (Chapter 7) but have been more difficult to predict for immediate release preparations.

This dissolution test then becomes a part of the standard quality control procedure for the drug product. For example, USP-23 has separate and distinct dissolution test requirements for the two different phenytoin sodium capsules. Regarding the extended phenytoin sodium capsules, USP states that "not more than 35%, between 30% and 70% and not less than 85% of the labeled amount of $C_{15}H_{11}N_2NaO_2$ in the Extended Capsules dissolves in 30 minutes, 60 minutes, and 120 minutes, respectively, under the specified dissolution conditions." In contrast, about tolerances for the prompt phenytoin sodium capsules USP states that "not less than 85% of the labeled amount of $C_{15}H_{11}N_2NaO_2$ in the Prompt Capsules dissolves in 30 minutes." There are several ways of checking for *in vitro–in vivo* correlation. *In vitro–in vivo* correlation for modified release drug products is discussed in Chapter 7.

Biopharmaceutic Drug Classification System

A theoretical basis for correlating *in vitro* drug dissolution with *in vivo* bioavailability was developed by Amidon et al, 1995. This approach is based upon the aqueous solubility of the drug and the permeation of the drug through the gastrointestinal tract. This classification system was based on *Fick's First Law* applied to a membrane:

$$J_w = P_w C_w$$

where J_w is the drug flux (mass/area/time) through the intestinal wall at any position and time, P_w is the permeability of the membrane, and C_w is the drug concentration at the intestinal membrane surface.

This approach assumes that no other components in the formulation affect the membrane permeability and/or intestinal transport. Using this approach, Amidon et al (1995) studied the solubility and permeability characteristics of various representative drugs and obtained a biopharmaceutic drug classification (Table 6.7) for predicting the *in vitro* drug dissolution of immediate release solid oral drug products with *in vivo* absorption. As shown in Table 6.7, drugs that fall in class 1, *high solubility* and *high permeability* are drugs that are well absorbed after oral administration, whereas drugs that fall into class 4, *low solubility* and *low permeability* are drugs that present significant problems for complete oral absorption and an *in vitro–in vivo* correlation is not expected. Using this biopharmaceutics classification system, the FDA has developed a guidance "Dissolution Testing of Immediate Release Oral Dosage Forms" (August 1997). (FDA draft Guidances are available at *http://www.fda.gov/cder/index.html* on the Internet.) This draft guidance provides general recommendations for dissolution testing, approaches for setting dissolution specifications related to the biopharmaceutics characteristics of the drug substance, statistical methods for comparing dissolution profiles and a process to help determine when dissolution testing is sufficient to grant a waiver for an *in vivo* bioequivalence study.

Dissolution Rate Versus Absorption Rate

If dissolution of the drug is rate limiting, a faster dissolution rate may result in a faster rate of appearance of the drug in the plasma. It may be possible to establish a correlation between rate of dissolution and rate of absorption of the drug.

The absorption rate is usually more difficult to determine than peak-absorption time. Therefore, the absorption time may be used in correlating dissolution data to absorption data. In the analysis of *in vitro–in vivo* drug correlation, rapid drug absorption may be distinguished from the slower drug absorption by observation of the absorption time for the preparation. The absorption time refers to the time for a constant amount of drug to be absorbed. In one study involving three sustained-release aspirin products, the dissolution time for the preparations were linearly correlated to the absorption times for various amounts of aspirin absorbed (Fig. 6-9). The results from this study demonstrated that aspirin was rapidly absorbed and was very much dependent on the dissolution rate for absorption.

TABLE 6.7 Biopharmaceutic Drug Classification for Predicting the Correlation of *in Vitro* Drug Dissolution of Immediate Release Solid Oral Drug Products with *in Vivo* Bioavailability

CLASS	SOLUBILITY	PERMEABILITY	COMMENTS
1	High	High	*In vitro–in vivo* correlation expected if dissolution rate is slower than the gastric emptying rate
2	Low	High	*In vitro–in vivo* correlation expected if the *in vitro* dissolution rate is similar to the *in vivo* dissolution rate, unless dose is very high
3	High	Low	Drug absorption (permeability) is rate determining and an *in vitro–in vivo* correlation may not be demonstrated
4	Low	High	*In vitro–in vivo* correlation is not expected

Adapted from Amidon et al, 1995

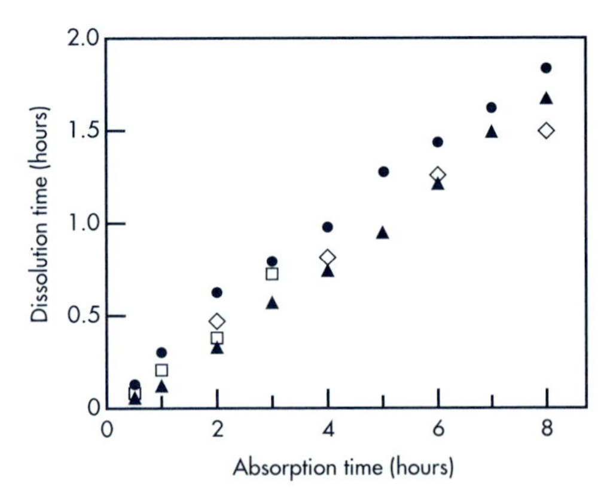

Figure 6-9. An example of correlation between time required for a given amount of drug to be absorbed and time required for the same amount of drug to be dissolved *in vitro* for three sustained-release aspirin products.
(From Wood, 1966, with permission.)

Percent of Drug Dissolved Versus Percent of Drug Absorbed

If a drug is absorbed completely after dissolution, a linear correlation may be obtained by comparing the percent of drug absorbed to the percent of drug dissolved. In choosing the dissolution method, one must consider the appropriate dissolution medium and use a slow dissolution stirring rate so that *in vivo* dissolution is approximated.

Aspirin is absorbed rapidly, and a slight change in formulation may be reflected in a change in the amount and rate of drug absorption during the period of observation (Figs. 6-9 and 6-10). If the drug is slow absorbing, which occurs when absorption is the rate-limiting step, a difference in dissolution rate of the product may not be observed. In this case, the drug would have been absorbed very slowly independent of the dissolution rate.

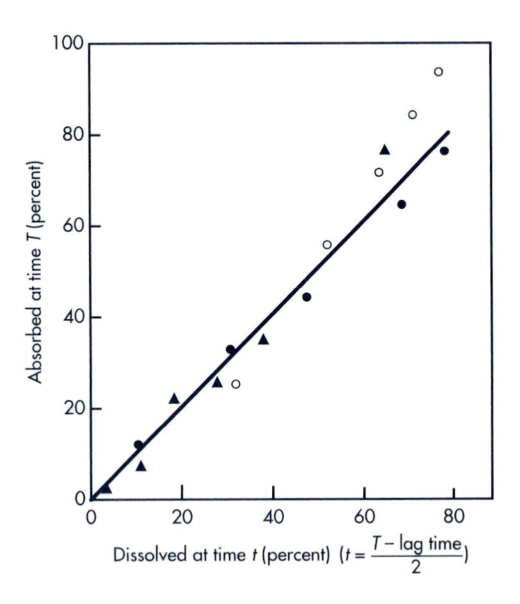

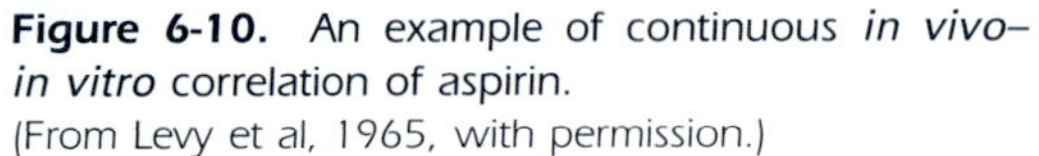

Figure 6-10. An example of continuous *in vivo–in vitro* correlation of aspirin.
(From Levy et al, 1965, with permission.)

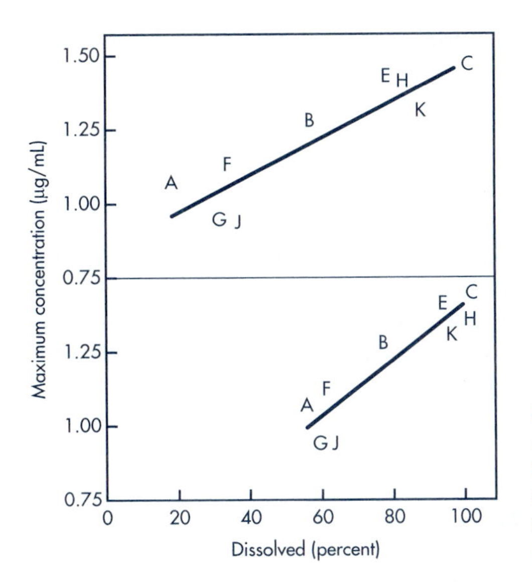

Figure 6-11. *In vitro–in vivo* correlation between C_{max} and percent drug dissolved. Top, 30 min (slope = 0.06, $r = 0.902$, $P < .001$). Bottom, 60 min (slope = 0.10, $r = 0.940$, $P < .001$). (Letters on graph indicate different products.)
(From Shah et al, 1983, with permission.)

Maximum Plasma Concentrations Versus Percent of Drug Dissolved *In Vitro*

When different drug formulations are tested for dissolution, a poorly formulated drug will not be completely dissolved and released, resulting in lower plasma drug concentrations. The percent of drug released at any time interval will be greater for the more available drug product. When such drug products are tested *in vivo*, the peak drug serum concentration will be higher for the drug product that shows the highest percent of drug dissolved. An example of *in vitro–in vivo* correlation for 100 mg phenytoin sodium capsules is shown in Figure 6-11. Several products were tested. A linear correlation was observed between the maximum drug concentration in the body and the percent of the drug dissolved *in vitro*.

The dissolution study on the phenytoin sodium products showed that the fastest dissolution rate was product *C*, for which about 100% of the labeled contents dissolved in the test (Fig. 6-12). Interestingly, these products also show the shortest time to reach peak concentration (t_{max}). The t_{max} is dependent on the absorption

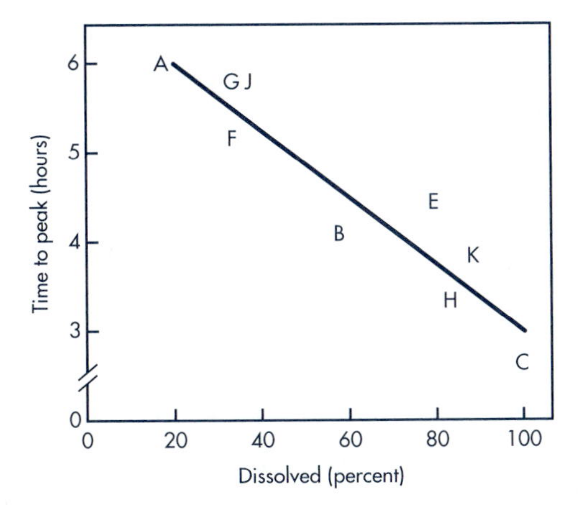

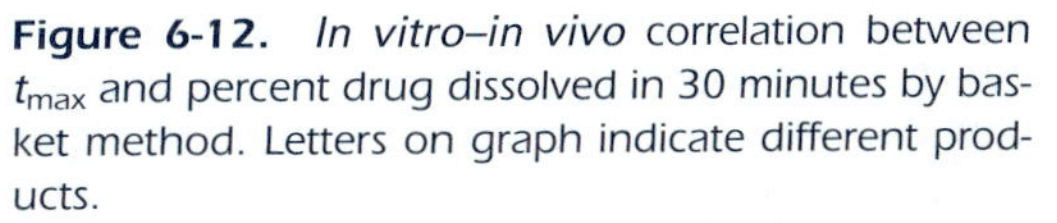

Figure 6-12. *In vitro–in vivo* correlation between t_{max} and percent drug dissolved in 30 minutes by basket method. Letters on graph indicate different products.
(From Shah et al, 1983, with permission.)

rate constant. In this case, the fastest absorption would also result in the shortest t_{max} (see Chapter 9).

Serum Drug Concentration Versus Percent of Drug Dissolved

In a study on aspirin absorption the serum concentration of aspirin was correlated to the percent of drug dissolved using an *in vitro* dissolution method. The dissolution medium was simulated gastric juice. Because aspirin is rapidly absorbed from the stomach, the dissolution of the drug is the rate-limiting step, and various formulations with different dissolution rates would cause differences in the serum concentration of aspirin by minutes (Fig. 6-13).

FAILURE OF CORRELATION OF *IN VITRO* DISSOLUTION TO *IN VIVO* ABSORPTION

Although there are many published examples of drugs with dissolution data that correlate well with drug absorption in the body, there are also many examples indicating poor correlation of dissolution to drug absorption. There are also instances where a drug has failed the dissolution test and yet is well absorbed. The problem of no correlation between bioavailability and dissolution may be due to the complexity of drug absorption and the weakness of the dissolution design. For example, a product that involves fatty components may be subjected to longer retention in the gastrointestinal tract. The effect of digestive enzymes may also play an important role in the dissolution of the drug *in vivo.* These factors may not be adequately simulated with a simple dissolution medium. An excellent example showing the importance of dissolution design is shown in Figure 6-14. Dissolution tests using four different dissolution media were performed for

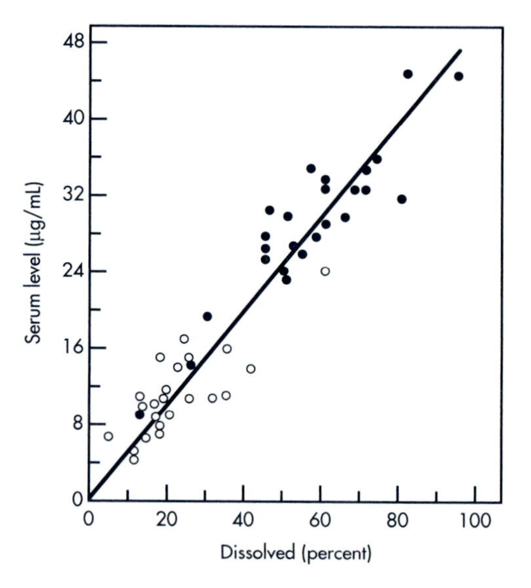

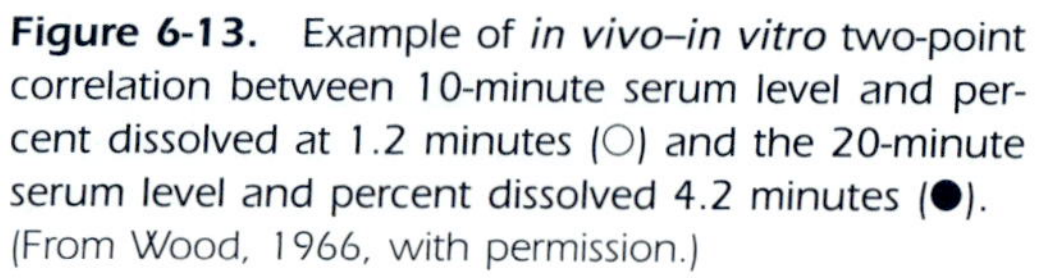
Figure 6-13. Example of *in vivo–in vitro* two-point correlation between 10-minute serum level and percent dissolved at 1.2 minutes (○) and the 20-minute serum level and percent dissolved 4.2 minutes (●). (From Wood, 1966, with permission.)

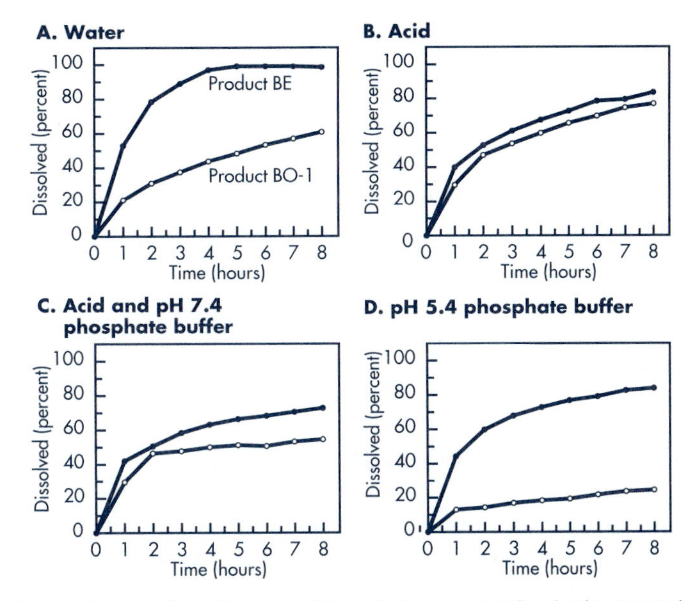

Figure 6-14. Dissolution profile of two quinidine gluconate sustained release products in different dissolution media. Each data point is the mean of 12 tablets. (● = product BE, ○ = product BO-1.) (From Prasad et al, 1983, with permission.)

two quinidine gluconate sustained-release tablets. Brand BE was known to be bioavailable, whereas product BO-1 was known to be incompletely absorbed. It is interesting to see that using acid media as well as acid followed by pH 7.4 buffer did not distinguish the two products well, whereas using water or pH 5.4 buffer as dissolution media clearly distinguishes the "good" product from the one that is not completely available. In this case, the use of an acid medium is consistent with the physiologic condition in the stomach, but this procedure would be misleading as a quality control tool. It is important that any new dissolution test be carefully researched before being adopted as a method for predicting drug absorption.

BIOPHARMACEUTIC CONSIDERATIONS

Some of the major biopharmaceutic considerations in the design of a drug product are given in Table 6.8. The prime considerations in the design of a drug product are safety and efficacy. The drug product must effectively deliver the active drug at an appropriate rate and amount to the target receptor site so that the intended therapeutic effect is achieved. The finished dosage form should not produce any additional side effects or discomfort due to the drug and/or excipients. Ideally, all excipients in the drug product should be inactive ingredients alone or in combination in the final dosage form.

The finished drug product is a compromise of various factors including therapeutic objectives, pharmacokinetics, physical and chemical properties, manufacturing, cost, and patient acceptance. Most importantly, the finished drug product should meet the therapeutic objective by delivering the drug with maximum bioavailability and minimum adverse effects.

TABLE 6.8 Biopharmaceutic Considerations in Drug Product Design

Pharmacodynamic Considerations	Patient Considerations
Therapeutic objective	Compliance and acceptability of drug product
Toxic effects	Cost
Adverse reactions	Manufacturing Considerations
Drug Considerations	Cost
Chemical and physical properties of drug	Availability of raw materials
Drug Product Considerations	Stability
Pharmacokinetics of drug	Quality control
Bioavailability of drug	
Route of drug administration	
Desired drug dosage form	
Desired dose of drug	

PHARMACODYNAMIC CONSIDERATIONS

Therapeutic considerations are concerned with the pharmacodynamic and pharmacologic properties of the drug, including the desired therapeutic response as well as the type and frequency of toxic and/or adverse reactions of the drug. The *therapeutic objective* will influence the type of drug product to be manufactured. A drug used to treat an acute illness should be formulated to release the drug rapidly, allowing for quick absorption and rapid onset. For example, nitroglycerin is formulated in a sublingual tablet for the treatment of angina pectoris. For prophylactic use in the treatment of certain chronic diseases such as asthma, an extended- or controlled-release dosage form is preferred. The extended-release dosage form releases the drug slowly, thereby controlling the rate of drug absorption and allowing for more constant plasma drug concentrations. In some cases, an immediate drug release component is included in the extended-release dosage form, to allow for both rapid onset followed by a slower sustained release of the drug. Controlled release and modified release dosage forms are discussed in Chapter 7.

DRUG CONSIDERATIONS

As discussed earlier, the *physicochemical properties* of the drug (Table 6.1) are major factors that are controlled or modified by the formulator. These physicochemical properties influence the type of dosage form and the process for the manufacture of the dosage form. Physical properties of the drug—such as dissolution, particle size, and crystalline form—are influenced by methods of processing and manufacturing. If the drug has low aqueous solubility and an intravenous injection is desired, then a soluble salt of the drug may be prepared. Chemical instability or chemical interactions with certain excipients will also affect the type of drug product and its method of fabrication. There are many creative approaches to improve the product. Only a few are discussed in this chapter.

DRUG PRODUCT CONSIDERATIONS

Pharmacokinetics of the Drug

Knowledge of the pharmacokinetic profile of the drug is important for the estimate of the appropriate amount (dose) of drug in the drug product and the release rate that will maintain a desired drug level in the body. The *therapeutic window* determines the desired or *target plasma drug concentration* that will be effective with minimal adverse effects. Drug concentrations higher than the therapeutic window (eg, minimum toxic concentration) may cause more intense pharmacodynamic and/or toxic response; drug concentrations below the therapeutic window (eg, minimum effective concentration) may be subtherapeutic. For drugs with a narrow therapeutic window, knowledge of the pharmacokinetic profile enhances drug therapy for many products through the development of an appropriate dosage regimen, including the *size of the dose* and the *dosing frequency*, that will achieve and maintain the target drug concentration.

Bioavailability of the Drug

The stability of the drug in the gastrointestinal tract, including the stomach and intestine, is another consideration. Some drugs, such as penicillin G, are unstable in the acid media of the stomach. The addition of buffering in the formulation or the use of an enteric coating on the dosage form protects the drug from degradation at a low pH. Some drugs have poor bioavailability because of first-pass effects (presystemic elimination). If oral drug bioavailability is poor due to metabolism by enzymes in the gastrointestinal tract or in the liver, then a higher dose may be needed, as in the case of propranolol or an alternative route of drug administration as in the case of insulin. Drugs which are only partially absorbed after oral administration usually leave residual drug in the gastrointestinal tract, which may cause local bowel irritation or alter the normal gastrointestinal flora. Unabsorbed drug always runs the risk of being completely absorbed under unusual situations (eg, change in diet or disease condition), leading to excessive drug bioavailability and toxicity. If the drug is not absorbed after the oral route or a higher dose causes toxicity, then the drug must be given by an alternate route of administration, and a different dosage form such as a parenteral drug product might be needed.

Dose Considerations

The size of the dose in the drug product is based on the inherent potency of the drug and its apparent volume of distribution which determines the target plasma drug concentration needed for the desired therapeutic effect. For some drugs, wide variation in the size of the dose is needed for different patients due to large intersubject differences in the pharmacokinetics and bioavailability of the drug. Therefore, the drug product must be available in several dose strengths to allow for individualized dosing. Some tablets are also scored for breaking to allow the administration of fractional doses.

The *size* and *shape* of the solid oral drug product are designed for easy swallowing. The total size of a drug product is determined by the dose of the drug and any additional excipients needed to manufacture the desired dosage form. For oral dosage forms, if the required dose is large (1 g or more), then the patient may have difficulty in swallowing the drug product. For example, many patients may find a capsule-shaped tablet (caplet) more easy to swallow than a large round tablet. Large or oddly shaped tablets, which may become lodged in the esophageal sphincter during swallowing, are generally not manufactured. Some esophageal injuries due to irritating drug lodged in the esophagus have been reported with potassium chloride tablets and other drugs. Older patients may have more difficulties in swallowing large tablets and capsules. Most of these swallowing difficulties may be overcome by taking the product with a large amount of fluid.

Dosing Frequency

The dosing frequency is related to the clearance of the drug and the target plasma drug concentration. If the pharmacokinetics show that the drug has a short duration of action due to a short elimination half-life or rapid clearance from the body, the drug must be given more frequently. To minimize fluctuating plasma drug concentrations and improve patient compliance, an extended release drug product may be preferred. An extended-release product contains two or more doses of the drug that are released over a prolonged period.

PATIENT CONSIDERATIONS

The drug product must be acceptable to the patient. Poor patient compliance may be the result of poor product attributes, such as difficulty in swallowing, disagreeable odor, bitter medicine taste, or two frequent and/or unusual dosage requirements. In recent years, creative packaging has allowed the patient to remove 1 tablet each day from a specially designed package so that the daily doses are not missed. This innovation improves compliance. Of course, pharmacodynamic factors, such as side effects of the drug or an allergic reaction, also influence patient compliance.

ROUTE OF DRUG ADMINISTRATION

The route of drug administration (Chapter 5) affects the bioavailability of the drug, thereby affecting the onset and duration of the pharmacologic effect. In the design of a drug dosage form, the pharmaceutical manufacturer must consider (1) the intended route of administration; (2) the size of the dose; (3) the anatomic and physiologic characteristics of the administration site, such as membrane permeability and blood flow; (4) the physicochemical properties of the site, such as pH, osmotic pressure, and presence of physiologic fluids; and (5) the interaction of the drug and dosage form at the administration site, including alteration of the administration site due to the drug and/or dosage form.

Although drug responses are quite similar with different routes of administration, there are examples where severe differences in response may occur. For example, with the drug isoproterenol, a difference in activity of a thousand-fold has been found, attributed to different routes of administration. Figure 6-15 shows the change in heart rate due to isoproterenol with different routes of administration. Studies have shown that isoproterenol is metabolized in the gut and during the passage through the liver. The rate and types of metabolite formed are found to be different depending on the routes of administration.

Oral Preparations

The major advantages of oral preparations are the convenience of administration, safety, and the elimination of discomforts involved with injections. The hazard of

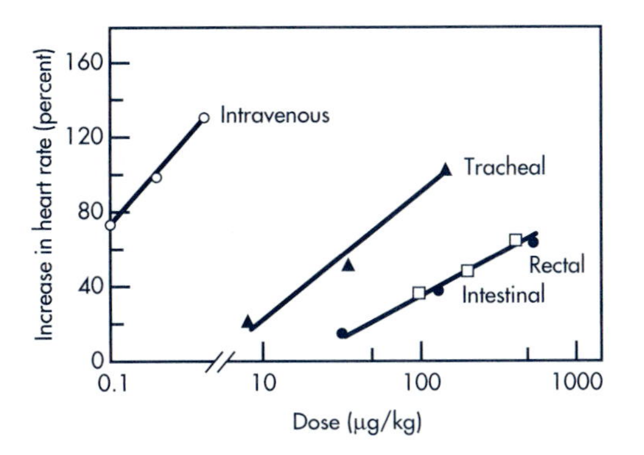

Figure 6-15. Dose response curve to isoproterenol by various routes in dogs.
(From Gillette and Mitchell, 1975, with permission.)

rapid intravenous administration causing toxic high concentration of drug in the blood is avoided. The main disadvantages of oral preparations are the potential problems of reduced and erratic bioavailability due to either incomplete absorption or drug interactions. Nausea or gastrointestinal discomfort may occur with some drugs that cause local irritation. Poor oral bioavailability or reduced absorption may be due to antacids or food interaction. Many drugs are adsorbed to antacids or food substances (see Chapter 5). These drugs would not diffuse effectively across the gastrointestinal tract to be absorbed. Drug molecules do not get absorbed easily when ionized. The ganglion-blocking drugs, hexamethonium, pentolinium, and bretylium, are ionized at intestinal pH. Therefore, they are not absorbed orally to be effective. Neomycin, gentamicin, and cefamandole are not well absorbed orally. In the case of neomycin, after oral administration the drug will concentration in the gastrointestinal tract to exert its local antibacterial effect.

Drugs with large molecular weights may not be well absorbed when given orally. There is some evidence that large drug molecules may be absorbed through the lymphatic system when formulated with a "carrier." The mechanism is not known. Some large molecules are absorbed when administered in solution with a surface-active agent. For example, the drug cyclosporin has been given orally with good absorption when formulated with a surfactant in oil. A possible role of the oil is to stimulate the flow of lymph as well as to delay the retention of the drug. Oily vehicles have been used to lengthen the gastrointestinal transit time of oral preparations.

Absorption of Lipid-Soluble Drugs

Most hydrophobic drugs are poorly soluble in water and generally are not well absorbed orally because of failure of the drug to dissolve in the fluids of the gastrointestinal (GI) tract. These lipophilic drugs are more soluble in lipids or oily vehicles. Lipid-soluble drugs given with fatty excipients mix with digested fatty acids, which are emulsified by bile in the small intestine. The emulsified drug is then absorbed through the GI mucosa or through the lymphatic system. A normal digestive function of the small intestine is the digestion and absorption of fats such as triglycerides. These fats are first hydrolyzed into monoglycerides and fatty acids by pancreatic lipase. The fatty acids then react with carrier lipoproteins to form *chylomicrons,* which are absorbed through the lymph. The chylomicrons eventually release the fatty acids and any lipophilic drugs are incorporated in the oil phase. Fat substances trigger receptors in the stomach to delay stomach emptying and reduce GI transit rates. Prolonged transit time would allow more contact time for increased drug absorption.

When griseofulvin or phenytoin was given orally in corn oil suspensions, an increase in drug absorption was demonstrated (Bates and Equeira, 1975). The increase in absorption was attributed to the formation of mixed micelles with bile secretions, which aid drug dissolution. In addition, stomach emptying may be delayed depending on the volume and nature of the oil. Long-chain fatty acids (above C-10) are more effective than short-chain acids in delaying stomach emptying. Unsaturated fatty acids are more effective than saturated straight-chain fatty acids; triglycerides are not as effective as fatty acids. Oleic acid, arachis oil, and myristic acid also delay stomach emptying. For example, the bioavailability of a water-insoluble antimalarial drug was increased in dogs when oleic acid was incorporated as part of a vehicle into a soft gelatin capsule (Stella et al, 1978).

Calcium carbonate, a source of calcium for the body, was only about 30% available in a solid dosage form, but was almost 60% bioavailable when dispersed in a special vehicle as a soft gelatin capsule (Fordtran et al, 1986). Bleomycin, an anticancer drug (MW 1500), is poorly absorbed orally and, therefore, was formulated for absorption through the lymphatic system. The lymphotropic carrier was dextran sulfate. Bleomycin was linked ionically to the carrier to form a complex. The carrier dextran (MW 500,000) was too large to be absorbed through the membrane and pass into the lymphatic vessels (Yoshikawa et al, 1989).

Gastrointestinal Side Effects

Many orally administered drugs are irritating to the stomach. These drugs may cause nausea or stomach pain when taken on an empty stomach. In some cases, food or antacids may be given together with the drug to reduce stomach irritation. Alternatively, the drug may be enteric-coated to reduce gastric irritation. A common drug that causes irritation is aspirin. Buffered aspirin tablets, enteric-coated tablets, and granules are available. However, enteric coating may sometimes delay or reduce the amount of drug absorbed. Furthermore, enteric coating may not abolish gastric irritation completely, because the drug may occasionally be regurgitated back to the stomach after the coating dissolves in the intestine. Enteric-coated tablets may be greatly affected by the presence of food in the stomach. The drug may not be released from the stomach for several hours when stomach emptying is delayed by food.

Buffering material or antacid ingredients have also been used with aspirin to reduce stomach irritation. When a large amount of antacid or buffering material is included in the formulation, dissolution of aspirin may occur quickly, leading to reduced irritation to the stomach. However, many buffered aspirin formulations do not contain sufficient buffering material to make a difference in dissolution in the stomach.

Certain drugs have been formulated into soft gelatin capsules to improve drug bioavailability and reduce gastrointestinal side effects. If the drug is formulated in the soft gelatin capsule as a solution, the drug may disperse and dissolve more rapidly, leaving less residual drug in the gut and causing less irritation. This approach may be useful for a drug that causes local irritation but would be ineffective if the drug is inherently ulcerogenic. Indomethacin, for example, may cause ulceration even when administered parenterally to animals.

There are many options available to the formulator to improve the tolerance of the drug and minimize gastric irritation. The nature of excipients and the physical state of the drugs are important and must be carefully assessed before a drug product is formulated. Some excipients may improve the solubility of the drug and facilitate absorption, whereas others may physically adsorb the drug to reduce irritation. Often, a great number of formulations must be tested before an acceptable one is chosen.

Buccal and Sublingual Tablets

A drug that diffuses and penetrates rapidly across mucosal membranes may be placed under the tongue and be rapidly absorbed. A tablet designed for release under the tongue is called a *sublingual tablet.* Nitroglycerin, isoproterenol, erythrityl tetranitrate and isosorbide dinitrate are common examples. Sublingual tablets usually dissolve rapidly.

A tablet designed for release and absorption of the drug in the buccal pouch is called a *buccal tablet.* The buccal (cheek) cavity refers to the space in between the mandibular arch and the oral mucosa, an area well supplied with blood vessels for efficient drug absorption. A buccal tablet may release drug rapidly or may be designed to release drug slowly for a prolonged effect. For example, Sorbitrate sublingual tablet, Sorbitrate chewable tablet, and Sorbitrate oral tablet (Zeneca) are three different dosage forms of isosorbide dinitrate for the relief and prevention of angina pectoris. The sublingual tablet is a lactose formulation that rapidly dissolves under the tongue and absorbed. The *chewable tablet* is chewed, and some drug is absorbed in the buccal cavity while the oral tablet is simply a conventional product for GI absorption. The chewable tablet contains flavor, confectioner's sugar, and mannitol, which are absent in both the oral and sublingual tablet. The sublingual tablet contains lactose and starch for rapid dissolution. The onset of sublingual nitroglycerin is rapid, much faster than when taken orally or absorbed through the skin. The duration of action, however, is shorter than with the other two routes. Drug absorbed through the buccal mucosa will not pass through the liver before general distribution. Consequently, for a drug with significant first-pass effect, buccal absorption may provide better bioavailability over oral administration. Some peptide drugs have been reported to be absorbed by buccal route, which provide a route of administration without the drug being destroyed by enzymes in the GI tract.

A newer approach to drug absorption from the oral cavity has been the development of a *translingual* nitroglycerin spray (Nitrolinqual). The spray, containing 0.4 mg per metered dose, is given by spraying 1 or 2 metered doses onto the oral mucosa at the onset of an acute angina attack.

Nasal Preparations

Nasal products provide a simple means of local and/or systemic drug delivery. The vehicle used for a nasal administration must be nonirritating and well tolerated. The most common drug products for local activity are the nasal vasoconstrictors phenylephrine and naphazoline. An example of a new nasal delivery for both local and systemic effect is ipratropium bromide, a drug used for rhinitis and the common cold. In patients with perennial rhinitis, about 10% of the drug was absorbed intranasally (Wood, 1995).

Nasacort AQ nasal spray (Rhone-Poulenc-Rorer) is triamcinolone acetonide delivered to the nasal area by spray. Each puff delivers about 50 mcg of the drug. It is useful for allergic rhinitis. The action is partially systemic and local. Another example is levocabastine, a histamine H_1-receptor antagonist developed as levocabastine nasal spray. Peak plasma concentrations (C_{max}) occur within 1 to 2 hours, with systemic availability ranging from 60% to 80% (Heykants, 1995). Benefits of levocabastine are predominantly mediated through local antihistaminic effects with some systemic contribution. Butorphanol tartrate nasal spray (Stadol NS) is an opioid analgesic available as a nasal spray for the treatment of pain as a preoperative or preanesthetic medication, as well as for pain relief during labor and migraine headache. The nasal route offers an alternative to injection. Some biological products such as peptides and proteins have been suggested for nasal delivery since they are not digested by enzymes as they were in the GI tract. The luteinizing hormone-releasing hormone agonist, buserelin, has been formulated with oleic acid for systemic nasal delivery in an experimental formulation. Therapeutic proteins, such as recombinant interferon-alpha/D, has also be been investigated for nasal delivery. Detectable levels of interferon-alpha β/D in the serum were achieved via nasal route and in the lung. Drug bioavailability was 6.8% from the lung in the rat, and 2.9% from the nasal cavity in the rabbit (Bayley et al, 1995). Other examples of nasal delivery drug products for systemic drug absorption are Nicotrol for the delivery of nicotine to aid smokers in quitting smoking and of Miacalcin for the delivery of calcitonin salmon, a parathyroid agent for the treatment of postmenopausal osteoporosis.

An *in vitro* human nasal model (De Fraissinettea et al, 1995) was developed as a tool to study the local tolerability of nasal powder forms using excised nasal mucosa in a diffusion chamber. The suitability of this model was tested using Sandostatin, an octapeptide analog of somatostatin. The drug is also used for ocular treatment of allergic rhinoconjunctivitis as eye drops; it was about 30 to 60% was available systemically by that route.

Colonic Drug Delivery

There has been considerable research in the delivery of drugs specifically to the colon after oral administration. Crohn's disease or chronic inflammatory colitis may be more effectively treated by direct drug delivery to the colon. One such drug, mesalamine ((5-aminosalicylic acid, Asacol) is available in a delayed-release tablet coated with an acrylic-based resin that delays the release of the drug until it reaches the distal ileum and beyond. Protein drugs are generally unstable in the acidic environment of the stomach and are also degraded by proteolytic enzymes present in the stomach and small intestine. Researchers are investigating the oral delivery of protein and peptide drugs by protecting them against enzymatic degradation for later release in the colon.

Over 500 different bacterial species inhabit the colon, although five frequent species dominate the microflora. Within the caecum and colon, anaerobic species dominate and bacterial counts of 10^{12}/mL has been reported. Drugs such as the β-blockers, oxprenolol and metoprolol, and isosorbide-5-mononitrate are well absorbed in the colon similar to absorption in the small intestine. Thus, these drugs are suitable candidates for colonic delivery. The nonsteroidal antiinflammatory drug, naproxen has been formed into a prodrug naproxen-detran that survives intestinal enzyme and intestinal absorption. The prodrug reaches the colon where it is enzymatically decomposed into naproxen and detran.

Rectal and Vaginal Drug Delivery

Products for rectal or vaginal drug delivery may be administered either in solid or liquid dosage forms. Rectal drug administration can be for either local or systemic drug delivery. Rectal drug delivery for systemic absorption is preferred to drugs that can not be tolerated orally (eg, when a drug causes nausea) or in situations where the drug cannot be given orally. A sustained-release preparation may be prepared for rectal administration. The rate of release of the drug from this preparation is dependent on the nature of the base composition and on the solubility of the drug involved. Rectal drug absorption may partially bypass the first-pass effects due to enzymes in the liver. The drug absorbed in the lower rectal region does not pass through the liver, whereas the drug absorbed in the upper rectal region passes through the hepatic portal vein. Release of drug from a suppository depends on the composition of the suppository base. A water-soluble base, such as PEG and glycerin, generally dissolve and release the drug; on the other hand, an oleaginous base with a low melting point may melt at body temperature and release the drug. Some suppositories contain an emulsifying agent that keeps the fatty oil emulsified and the drug dissolved in it.

Vaginal drug delivery is generally for local drug delivery, but some systemic drug absorption can occur. Progesterone vaginal suppositories have been evaluated for the treatment of premenstrual symptoms of anxiety and irritability. Antifungal agents are often formulated into suppositories for treating vaginal infections. Fluconazole, a triazole antifungal agent has been formulated to treat vulvovaginal candidiasis. The result of oral doses are compared with that of a clotrimazole vaginal suppository. Many vaginal preparations are used for the delivery of antifungal agents.

Parenteral Products

In general, intravenous (IV) bolus administration of a drug provides the most rapid onset of drug action. After IV bolus injection, the drug is distributed via the circulation to all parts of the body within a few minutes. After intramuscular (IM) injection, drug is absorbed from the injection site into the bloodstream (Figure 6-16). Plasma drug input after oral and IM administration involve an absorption phase in which the drug concentration rises slowly to a peak and then declines according to the elimination half-life of the drug. (Note that the systemic elimination of all products are essentially similar, only the rate and extent of absorption may be modified by formulation). The plasma drug level peaks instantaneously after an IV bolus injection so that a peak is usually not visible. After 3 hours, however, the plasma level of the drug after intravenous administration has declined to a lower level than that of the oral and intramuscular administration. In this example (Fig. 6-16), the areas under the plasma curves are all approximately equal, indicating that the oral and intramuscular preparations are both well formulated and are 100% available. Frequently, because of incomplete absorption or metabolism, oral preparations may have a lower area under the curve.

Drug absorption after an intramuscular injection may be faster or slower absorption than after oral drug administration. Intramuscular preparations are generally injected into a muscle mass such as in the buttocks (gluteus muscle) or in the deltoid muscle. Drug absorption occurs as the drug diffuses from the muscle into the surrounding tissue fluid and then into the blood. Different muscle tissues have different blood flow. For example, blood flow to the deltoid muscle is higher than blood flow to the gluteus muscle. Intramuscular injections may be formulated to have a faster or slower drug release by changing the vehicle of the injection

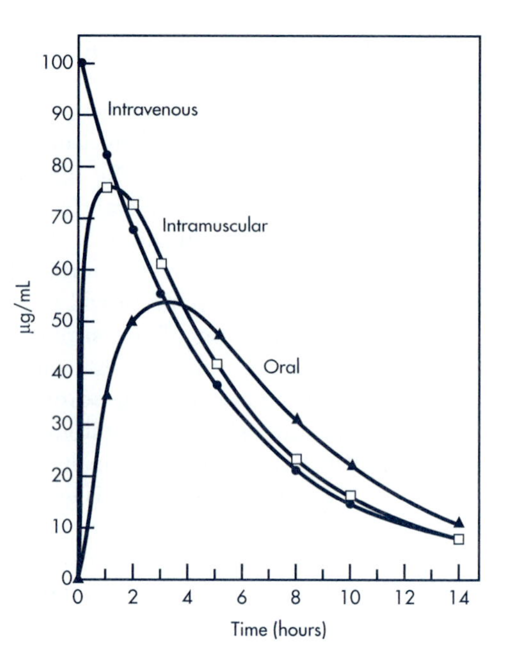

Figure 6-16. Plasma concentration of a drug after the same dose is administered by three different routes.

preparation. Aqueous solutions release drug more rapidly, and the drug more rapidly absorbed from the injection site, whereas a viscous, oily, or suspension vehicle may result in a slow drug release and consequently slow and sustained drug absorption. Viscous vehicles generally slow down drug diffusion and distribution. A drug in an oily vehicle must partition into an aqueous phase before systemic absorption. A drug that is very soluble in the oil and relatively insoluble in water may have a relatively long and sustained release from the absorption site because of slow partitioning.

CLINICAL EXAMPLE

Haloperidol (Haldol) is a butyrophenone antipsychotic agent with pharmacologic effects similar to the piperazine phenothiazines. Haloperidol is available for oral and IM administration. Two IM preparations of haloperidol are available, including haloperidol lactate in an aqueous vehicle and haloperidol deconate in a nonaqueous sesame oil vehicle. The following Table 6.9 shows the $T_{\max}$ and elimination half-life of haloperidol after the oral, IM, or IV administration.

Haloperidol lactate is in an aqueous solution and after intramuscular injection has a time for peak drug concentration of 20 minutes and an elimination half-life of 21 days. In contrast, haloperidol deconate, the deconate ester of the butyrophenone, is lipid soluble and is formulated in sesame oil. Due to the slow drug release from the oil after IM administration, the time for peak drug concentration is 4 to 11 days and the elimination half-life is about 3 weeks. Thus, the suggested dosage interval between intramuscular injections for haloperidol deconate is 4 weeks. Table 6.9 lists some of the pharmacokinetics of haloperidol after oral, IM and IV administration.

TABLE 6.9 Pharmacokinetic Parameters for Haloperidol After Oral and Parenteral Administration

ROUTE	PERCENT ABSORPTION	TIME FOR PEAK CONCENTRATION, t_{max}	ELIMINATION HALF-LIFE
Oral	60	3–5 hr	24 (12–38) hr
IM	75	0.33 hr	21 (13–36) hr
Deconate		6th day (4 to 11 days)	3 weeks
IV	100	immediate	14 (10–19) hr

Adapted from *Facts and Comparisons*, 1997

A major advantage of the intramuscular injection compared to intravenous bolus injection is the flexibility of formulation. A drug that is not water soluble cannot be easily administered by intravenous route. A nonaqueous injection for intravenous administration must be given very slowly to avoid any drug precipitation in the vein. Propylene glycol and PEG 400 in combination with other solvents have been used in intravenous preparations.

Parenteral dosage forms for intravenous administration containing suspensions, liposomes, or nanoparticles have been developed for the administration of antineoplastic drugs. In this case, the dosage form may alter the distribution of the drug, because small particles are engulfed by macrophages of the reticuloendothelial system resulting in drug concentration in the liver and spleen.

Inhalation Preparations

Drugs administered into the respiratory system, such as bronchodilators and corticosteroids, may be formulated as an aerosol or inhalation solution. An aerosol preparation with suitable propellant can administer drug rapidly into the bronchial region. The advantages of drugs given by inhalation include (1) rapid absorption and rapid onset of activity (eg, bronchodilators), (2) avoidance of first-pass effects or metabolism prior to systemic absorption (eg, isoproterenol, bitolterol), and (3) localize drug activity to the lung and minimize systemic toxicity (eg, dexamethasone).

The particle size of the suspension (or in the case of a solution, the size of the mist particles) is important in determining the extent of penetration into the bronchioles. For coarse particles, the inertia carries the drug for a short distance up the nasal cavity. Drugs with small particles move by sedimentation or brownian movements deeper into the bronchioles.

Many aerosol products are designed for drug therapy of chronic obstructive pulmonary disease (COPD), particularly asthma. For example, Intal (Rhone-Poulenc-Rorer) delivers sodium cromolyn to a patient through inhalation. The propellants for aerosols have been the chlorinated-fluorocarbons (CFCs, such as Freons—DuPont). Freons commonly used include dichlorodifluoromethane (Freon 12) and dichlortetrafluoroethane (Freon 114). However, these compounds deplete the ozone layer of the stratosphere and other propellants are now being investigated to replace CFCs. The new propellants include classes of hydrofluoroalkane (HFAs) which do not contain chlorines. HFA-227 and HFA-134a show promise as new propellents for medical inhalers since they are nonflammable, not chemically reactive,

TABLE 6.10 Examples of Aerosol Products

Alupent (metaproterenol sulfate)
Proventil (albuterol)
Alupent (metaproterenol)
Bronkosol (isoetharine)
Vaponefrin (racepinephrine)

and do not have ozone-depleting potential. Some examples of aerosol products are shown in Table 6.10.

Transdermal Preparations

Transdermal administration delivers a drug into the patient's systemic circulation through the skin for systemic activity. For example, scopolamine was delivered through the skin of the ear for motion sickness. Transdermal administration may release the drug over an extended period of several hours or days without the discomforts of gastrointestinal side effects or first-pass effects. For example, Estraderm delivers estradiol for estrogen replacement therapy in postmenopausal women and is applied twice a week. Many transdermal products deliver drug at a constant rate to the body similar to a zero-order infusion process. As a result, a stable, plateau level of the drug may be maintained. Many therapeutic categories of drugs are now available as transdermal products (Table 6.11).

Transdermal products vary in design. In general, the patch contains several parts: (1) a backing or support layer; (2) a drug layer (reservoir containing the dose); (3) a release-controlling layer (usually a semipermeable film), (4) a pressure sensitive adhesive (PSA); and (5) a protective strip, which must be removed prior to application. (See Fig. 7-13, Chapter 7.) The release controlling membrane could be a polymeric film such as ethylvinyl copolymer, which controls the release rate of the dose and its duration of action. The PSA layer is important for maintaining uninterrupted skin contact for drug diffusion through the skin. In some cases, the drug is directly blended into an adhesive, such as acrylate or silicone; performing the dual functions of release control and adhesion, this product is known as "drug in adhesive." In other products, the drug dose may be placed in a separate insoluble matrix layer which helps controlling the release rate. This is generally known as a "matrix patch," which gains a little more control of the release rate as com-

TABLE 6.11 Transdermal Products

DRUG	PRODUCT	DRUG CLASS
Estradiol	Vivelle	Estrogen
Fentanyl	Duragesic	Opiate agonist
Nicotine	Habitrol Tran	Smoking control
	Nicoderm	Smoking control
	Nicotrol	Smoking control
	Prostep patch	Smoking control
Naftifine HCl	Naftin	Antifungal
Nifedipine	Adalat	Calcium channel blocker
Nitroglycerin	Nitrodisc	Antiangina
	Nitro-Dur	Antiangina

pared with the simple "reservoir" type of patch. Multilayers of drugs may be involved in other transdermal products using the "laminate design." In many cases, drug permeation through the skin is the slowest step in the transdermal delivery of drug into the body. See Chapter 7 for modified-release patches.

Scale-Up and Post-Approval Changes (SUPAC)

Any changes in a drug product after it has been approved for marketing by the FDA is known as a *post-approval change.* A major concern by industry and FDA is that if a pharmaceutical manufacturer makes any change in the formulation; scales up the formulation to a larger batch size; changes the process, equipment, or manufacturing site; and whether these changes will affect the identity, strength, purity, quality, safety, and efficacy of the approved drug product. In addition any changes in the raw material (ie, active pharmaceutical ingredient), excipients or packaging (including container closure system) should also be shown not to affect the quality of the drug product.

FDA has been publishing draft guidances for the pharmaceutical industry that addresses the following issues:

- components and composition of the drug product
- manufacturing site change
- scale-up of drug product
- manufacturing equipment
- manufacturing process
- packaging
- active pharmaceutical ingredient

In these documents, FDA describes the (1) level of change, (2) recommended chemistry, manufacturing and controls tests for each level of change, (3) *in vitro* dissolution tests and/or bioequivalence tests for each level of change, and (4) documentation that should support the change. The level of change is classified as to the likelihood that a change in the drug product as listed above might affect the quality of the drug product. The level of changes as described by the FDA are listed in Table 6.12.

As noted in Table 6.12, a Level 1 change which could be a small change in the excipient amount (eg, starch, lactose) would be unlikely to alter the quality or performance of the drug product, whereas a Level 3 change which may be a qualitative or quantitative change in the excipients beyond an allowable range, particularly for drug products containing a narrow therapeutic drug, might require an *in vivo*

TABLE 6.12 FDA Definitions of Level of Changes That May Affect the Quality of an Approved Drug Product

CHANGE LEVEL	DEFINITION OF LEVEL
Level 1	Level 1 changes are those that are unlikely to have any detectable impact on the formulation quality and performance.
Level 2	Level 2 changes are those changes that could have a significant impact on formulation quality and performance.
Level 3	Level 3 changes are those changes that are likely to have a significant impact on formulation quality and performance.

bioequivalence study to demonstrate that drug quality and performance was not altered by the change.

FREQUENTLY ASKED QUESTIONS

1. What physical or chemical properties of a drug substance are important in designing a drug for **(a)** oral administration or **(b)** parenteral administration?
2. For a lipid soluble drug that has very poor aqueous solubility, what strategies could be used to make this drug more bioavailable after oral administration?
3. For a weak ester drug that is unstable in highly acid or alkaline solutions, what strategies could be used to make this drug more bioavailable after oral administration?
4. How do excipients in a drug product that are physically inert, chemically inert, and nontoxic change the bioavailability of the active drug substance?

LEARNING QUESTIONS

1. What are the two rate-limiting steps possible in the oral absorption of a solid drug product? Which one would apply to a soluble drug? Which one could be altered by the pharmacist? Give examples.
2. What is the physiologic transport mechanism for the absorption of most drugs from the gastrointestinal tract? What area of the gastrointestinal tract is most favorable for the absorption of drugs? Why?
3. Explain why the absorption rate of a soluble drug tends to be greater than the elimination rate of the drug.
4. What type of oral dosage form generally yields the greatest amount of systemically available drug in the least amount of time? (Assume that the drug can be prepared in any form.) Why?
5. What effect does the oral administration of an anticholinergic drug, such as atropine sulfate, have on the bioavailability of aspirin from an enteric-coated tablet? (Hint: Atropine sulfate decreases gastrointestinal absorption.)
6. Drug formulations of erythromycin, including its esters and salts, have significant differences in bioavailability. Erythromycin is unstable in an acidic medium. Suggest a method for preventing a potential bioavailability problem for this drug.

REFERENCES

Aguiar AJ, Krc J, Kinkel AW, Samyn JC: Effect of polymorphism on the absorption of chloramphenical from chloramphenical palmitate. *J Pharm Sci* **56:**847–853, 1967

Allen PV, Rahn PD, Sarapu AC, Vandewielen AJ: Physical characteristic of erythromycin anhydrate, and dihydrate crystalline solids. *J Pharm Sci* **67:**1087–1093, 1978

Amidon GL, Lennernas H, Shah VP, Crison JR: A theoretical basis for a biopharmaceutic drug classification: The correlation of *in vitro* drug product dissolution and *in vivo* bioavailability, *Pharm Res* **12:**413–420, 1995

Bates TR, Equeira JA: Bioavailability of micronized grieseofulvin from corn oil in water emulsion, aqueous suspension and commercial dosage form in humans. *J Pharm Sci* **64:**793–797, 1975

Bayley D, Temple C, Clay V, Steward A, Lowther N: The transmucosal absorption of recombinant human interferon-alpha B/D hybrid in the rat and rabbit. *J Pharm Pharmacol* **47**(9):721–724, 1995

Cameron CG, Cuff GW, McGinity J: Development and evaluation of controlled release theophylline tablet formulations containing acrylic resins: Comparison of dissolution test methodologies. American Pharmaceutical Association meeting, New Orleans, April 1983 (abstract)

De Fraissinette A, Kolopp M, Schiller I, Fricker G, Gammert C, Pospischil A, Vonderscher J, Richter F: *in vitro* tolerability of human nasal mucosa: Histopathological and scanning electron-microscopic evaluation of nasal forms containing Sandostatin. *Cell Biol Toxicol* **11**(5):295–301, 1995

Dressman JB, Amidon GL, Reppas C, Shah VP: Dissolution testing as a prognostic tool for oral drug absorption: Immediate release dosage forms, *Pharm Res* **15:**11–22, 1998

Fordtran J, Patrawala M, Chakrabarti S: Influence of vehicle composition on *in vivo* absorption of calcium from soft elastic gelatin capsule. *Pharm Res* **3**(suppl):645, 1986

Gillette JR, Mitchell JR: Routes of drug administration and response. In *Concepts in Biochemical Pharmacology.* Berlin, Springer-Verlag, 1975, chap 64

Heykants J, Van Peer A, Van de Velde V, Snoeck E, Meuldermans W, Woestenborghs R: The pharmacokinetic properties of topical levocabastine. A review. *Clin Pharmacokinet* **29**(4):221–230, 1995

Levy G, Leonards J, Procknal JA: Development of *in vitro* tests which correlate quantitatively with dissolution rate-limited drug absorption in man. *J Pharm Sci* **54:**1719, 1965

Masih SZ, Jacob KC, Majuh M, Fatmi A: Comparison of USP basket and paddle method for evaluation of sustained release formulation containing pseudoephedrine and guaifenesin. American Pharmaceutical Association (APhA) meeting, New Orleans, April 1983 (abstract)

Philip J, Daly RE: Test for selection of erythromycin stearate bulk drug for tablet preparation. *J Pharm Sci* **72:**979–980, 1983

Prasad V, Shah V, Knight P et al: Importance of media selection in establishment of *in vitro–in vivo* relationship for quinidine gluconate. *Int J Pharm* **13:**1–7, 1983

Shah VP, Prasad VK, Alston T, et al: Phenytoin I: *in vitro* correlation for 100 mg phenytoin sodium capsules. *J Pharm Sci* **72:**306–308, 1983

Stella V, Haslam J, Yata N, et al: Enhancement of bioavailability of a hydrophobic amine antimalarial by formulation with oleic acid in a soft gelatin capsule. *J Pharm Sci* **67:**1375–1377, 1978

The United States Pharmacopeial Convention: *The United States Pharmacopeia,* 23rd ed. Easton, PA, Mark, 1995

Wood CC, Fireman P, Grossman J, Wecker M, MacGregor T: Product characteristics and pharmacokinetics of intranasal ipratropium bromide. *J Allergy Clin Immunol* **95**(5 Pt 2):1111–1116, 1995

Wood JH: *in vitro* evaluation of physiological availability of compressed tablets. *Pharm Acta Helv* **42:**129, 1966

Yoshikawa H, Nakao Y, Takada K, et al: Targeted and sustained delivery of aclarubicin to lymphatics by lactic acid oligomer microsphere in rat. *Chem Pharm Bull* **37:**802–804, 1989

BIBLIOGRAPHY

Aguiar AJ: Physical properties and pharmaceutical manipulations influencing drug absorption. In Forth IW, Rummel W (eds), *Pharmacology of Intestinal Absorption: Gastrointestinal Absorption of Drugs.* New York, Pergamon, 1975, vol 1, Chap 6

Barr WH: The use of physical and animal models to assess bioavailability. *Pharmacology* **8:**88–101, 1972

Berge S, Bighley L, Monkhouse D: Pharmaceutical salts. *J Pharm Sci* **66:**1–19, 1977

Blanchard J: Gastrointestinal absorption, II. Formulation factors affecting bioavailability. *Am J Pharm* **150:**132–151, 1978

Blanchard J, Sawchuk RJ, Brodie BB: *Principles and Perspectives in Drug Bioavailability.* New York, Karger, 1979

Burks TF, Galligan JJ, Porreca F, Barber WD: Regulation of gastric emptying. *Fed Proc* **44:**2897–2901, 1985

Cabana BE, O'Neil R: FDA's report on drug dissolution. *Pharm Forum* **6:**71–75, 1980

Cadwalder DE: *Biopharmaceutics and Drug Interactions.* Nutley, NJ, Roche Laboratories, 1971

Christensen J: The physiology of gastrointestinal transit. *Med Clin North Am* **58:**1165–1180, 1974

Dakkuri A, Shah AC: Dissolution methodology: An overview. *Pharm Technol* **6:**28–32, 1982

Eye IS: A review of the physiology of the gastrointestinal tract in relation to radiation doses from radioactive materials. *Health Physics* **12:**131–161, 1966

Gilbaldi M: *Biopharmaceutics and Clinical Pharmacokinetics.* Philadelphia, Lea & Febiger, 1977

Hansen WA: *Handbook of Dissolution Testing.* Springfield, OR, Pharmaceutical Technology Publications, 1982

Hardwidge E, Sarapu A, Laughlin W: Comparison of operating characteristics of different dissolution test systems. *J Pharm Sci* **6:**1732–1735, 1978

Houston JB, Wood SG: Gastrointestinal absorption of drugs and other xenobiotics. In Bridges JW, Chasseaud LF (eds), *Progress in Drug Metabolism.* London, Wiley, 1980, vol 4, chap 2

Jollow DJ, Brodie BB: Mechanisms of drug absorption and drug solution. *Pharmacology* **8:**21–32, 1972

LaDu BN, Mandel HG, Way EL: *Fundamentals of Drug Metabolism and Drug Disposition.* Baltimore, Williams & Wilkins, 1971

Leesman GD, Sinko PJ, Amidon GL: Simulation of oral drug absorption: Gastric emptying and gastrointestinal motility. In Welling PW, Tse FLS (eds): *Pharmacokinetics: Regulatory, Industry, Academic Perspectives.* New York, Marcel Dekker, 1988, chap 6

Leeson LJ, Carstensen JT: Industrial pharmaceutical technology. In *Dissolution Technology.* Washington, DC, Academy of Pharmaceutical Sciences, 1974

Levine RR: Factors affecting gastrointestinal absorption of drugs. *Dig Dis* **15:**171–188, 1970

McElnay JC: Buccal absorption of drugs. In Swarbrick J, Boylan JC (eds), *Encyclopedia of Pharmaceutical Technology.* New York, Marcel Dekker, 1990, vol 2, pp 189–211

Mojaverian P, Vlasses PH, Kellner PE, Rocci ML Jr: Effects of gender, posture and age on gastric residence of an indigestible solid: Pharmaceutical considerations. *Pharm Res* **5:**639–644, 1988

Neinbert R: Ion pair transport across membranes. *Pharm Res* **6:**743–747, 1989

Niazi S: *Textbook of Biopharmaceutics and Clinical Pharmacokinetics.* New York, Appleton, 1979

Notari RE: *Biopharmaceutics and Pharmacokinetics: An Introduction.* New York, Marcel Dekker, 1975

Palin K: Lipids and oral drug delivery. *Pharm Int* November: 272–275, 1985

Palin K, Whalley D, Wilson C, et al: Determination of gastric-emptying profiles in the rat: Influence of oil structure and volume. *Int J Pharm* **12:**315–322, 1982

Parrott EL: *Pharmaceutical Technology.* Minneapolis, Burgess, 1970

Pernarowski M: Dissolution methodology. In Leeson L, Carstensen JT (eds), *Dissolution Technology.* Washington, DC, Academy of Pharmaceutical Sciences, 1975, p 58

Pharmacopeial Forum: FDA report on drug dissolution. *Pharm Forum* **6:**71–75, 1980

Prasad VK, Shah VP, Hunt J, et al: Evaluation of basket and paddle dissolution methods using different performance standards. *J Pharm Sci* **72:**42–44, 1983

Robinson JR: *Sustained and Controlled Release Drug Delivery Systems.* New York, Marcel Dekker, 1978

Robinson JR, Eriken SP: Theoretical formulation of sustained release dosage forms. *J Pharm Sci* **55:**1254, 1966

Rubinstein A, Li VHK, Robinson JR: Gastrointestinal–physiological variables affecting performance of oral sustained release dosage forms. In Yacobi A, Halperin-Walega E (eds), *Oral Sustained Release Formulations: Design and Evaluation.* New York, Pergamon, 1988, chap 6

Schwarz-Mann WH, Bonn R: Principles of transdermal nitroglycerin administration. *Eur Heart J* **10**(suppl A):26–29, 1989

Shaw JE, Chandrasekaran K: Controlled topical delivery of drugs for system in action. *Drug Metab Rev* **8:**223–233, 1978

Swarbrick J: *in vitro* models of drug dissolution. In Swarbrick J (ed), *Current Concepts in the Pharmaceutical Sciences: Biopharmaceutics.* Philadelphia, Lea & Febiger, 1970

Wagner JG: *Biopharmaceutics and Relevant Pharmacokinetics.* Hamilton, IL, Drug Intelligence Publications, 1971

Welling PG: Dosage route, bioavailability and clinical efficacy. In Welling PW, Tse FLS (eds): *Pharmacokinetics: Regulatory, Industry, Academic Perspectives.* New York, Marcel Dekker, 1988, chap 3

Wurster DE, Taylor PW: Dissolution rates. *J Pharm Sci* **54:**169–175, 1965

Yoshikawa H, Muranishi S, Sugihira N, Seaki H: Mechanism of transfer of bleomycin into lymphatics by bifunctional delivery system via lumen of small intestine. *Chem Pharm Bull* **31:**1726–1732, 1983

York P: Solid state properties of powders in the formulation and processing of solid dosage form. *Int J Pharm* **14:**1–28, 1983

Zaffaroni A: Therapeutic systems: The key to rational drug therapy. *Drug Metab Rev* **8:**191–222, 1978

7

MODIFIED-RELEASE DRUG PRODUCTS

MODIFIED-RELEASE DRUG PRODUCTS

Most conventional drug products, such as tablets and capsules, are formulated to release the active drug immediately after administration to obtain rapid and complete systemic drug absorption. In recent years, various modified drug products have been developed to release the active drug from the product at a controlled rate. The term *controlled-release drug product* was previously used to describe various types of oral extended-release-rate dosage forms, including sustained release, sustained action, prolonged action, long action, and retarded release. Many of these terms for controlled-release dosage forms were introduced by drug companies to reflect a special design for a controlled-release drug product or for use as a marketing term. Controlled-release drug products are designed for different routes of administration based on the physicochemical, pharmacologic, and pharmacokinetic properties of the drug and upon the properties of the materials used in the dosage form (Table 7.1). Several different terms are now defined to describe the available types of controlled-release drug products based on the drug release characteristics for the products.

The term *modified-release dosage form* is used to describe products that alter the timing and rate of release of the drug substance. A modified-release dosage form is defined "as one for which the drug-release characteristics of time course and/or location are chosen to accomplish therapeutic or convenience objectives not offered by conventional dosage forms such as solutions, ointments, or promptly dissolving dosage forms are presently recognized. (USP Subcommittee on Biopharmaceutics, 1985)." The USP/NF presently recognizes several types of modified-release dosage forms

1. *Extended-release dosage form.* A dosage form which allows at least a twofold reduction in dosage frequency as compared to that drug presented as an immediate-release (conventional) dosage form. Examples of extended-release dosage forms include controlled-release and sustained release drug products.
2. *Delayed-release dosage form.* A dosage form that releases a discrete portion or portions of drug at a time or at times other than promptly after administration, al-

TABLE 7.1 Modified-Release Dosage Forms

Oral Dosage Forms
Modified-release dosage forms
Extended release (eg, controlled release, sustained release, prolonged release)
Delayed release (eg, enteric coated)
Intramuscular Dosage Forms
Depot injections
Water-immiscible injections (eg, oil)
Subcutaneous Dosage Forms
Implants
Transdermal Delivery Systems
Patches, creams, etc
Targeted Delivery Systems

though one portion may be released promptly after administration. Enteric-coated dosage forms are the most common delayed-release products.

3. *Targeted-release dosage form.* A dosage form that releases drug at or near the intended physiologic site of action. Targeted-release dosage forms may have either immediate or extended-release characteristics.

Examples of Modified-Release Dosage Forms

An *enteric-coated* tablet is an example of a delayed-release type of modified-release dosage form designed to release drug in the small intestine. For example, aspirin irritates the gastric mucosal cells of the stomach. An enteric coating on the aspirin tablet prevents the tablet from dissolving and releasing its contents at the low pH in the stomach. The tablet will later dissolve and release the drug in the higher pH of the duodenum, where the drug is rapidly absorbed with less irritation to the mucosal cells. Mesalamine (5-aminosalicylic acid) tablets (Asacol, Proctor & Gamble) is a delayed-release tablet coated with an acrylic-based resin that delays the release of mesalamine until it reaches the terminal ileum and beyond. Mesalamine tablets could also be considered a *targeted-release* dosage form.

Other unofficial terms are used to describe drug products. *Repeat-action tablet* is

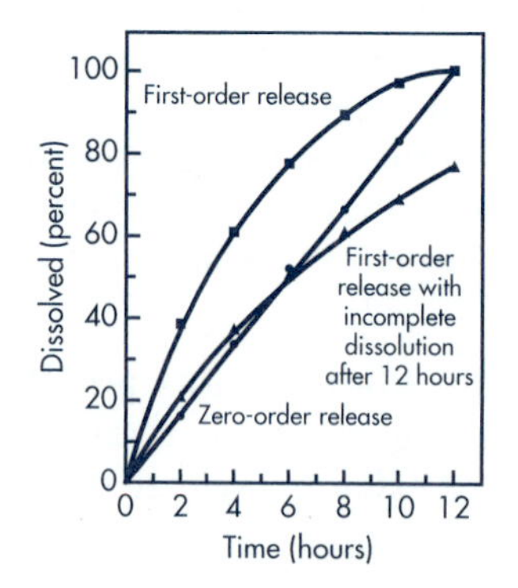

Figure 7-1. Drug dissolution rates of three different extended-release products *in vitro*.

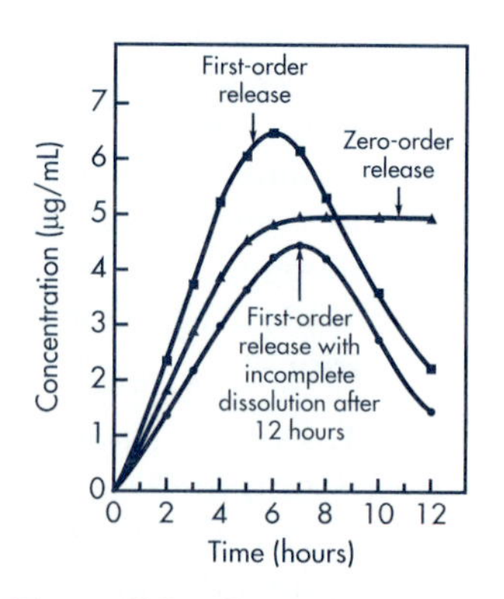

Figure 7-2. Simulated plasma–drug concentrations resulting from three different sustained-release products in Fig. 7-1.

a type of controlled-release drug product, which is designed to release one dose of drug initially and a second dose of drug at a later time. A *prolonged-action* drug product is designed to release the drug slowly and to provide a continuous supply of drug over an extended period. The prolonged-action drug product prevents very rapid absorption of the drug, which could result in extremely high peak plasma drug concentration. Most prolonged-release products extend the duration of action but do not release drug at a constant rate. A *sustained-release* drug product can be designed to deliver an initial therapeutic dose of the drug (loading dose) followed by a slower and constant release of drug. The rate of release of the maintenance dose is designed so that the amount of drug loss from the body by elimination is constantly replaced. With the sustained-release product, a constant plasma drug concentration is maintained with minimal fluctuations. Figure 7-1 shows the dissolution rate of three sustained-release products without loading dose. The plasma concentrations resulting from the sustained-release products are shown in Figure 7-2. A prolonged-action tablet is similar to the first-order release product except the peak is delayed differently. A prolonged-action tablet typically results in peak and trough drug level in the body. The product releases drug without matching the rate of drug elimination, resulting in uneven plasma drug levels in the body. Various other terms have been associated with extended-release drug products, including extended action, timed release, controlled release, drug delivery system, and programmed drug delivery.

The use of these various terms does not imply zero-order drug release. Many of these drug products release the drug at a first-order rate. Moreover, some drug products are formulated with materials that are more soluble at a specific pH, and the product may release the drug depending on the pH of the gastrointestinal tract. Ideally, the extended-release drug product should release the drug at a constant rate independent of both the pH and the ionic content within the entire segment of the gastrointestinal tract.

An extended-release dosage form with zero- or first-order drug absorption is compared to drug absorption from a conventional dosage form given in multiple doses in Figures 7-3 and 7-4, respectively. Drug absorption from conventional (immediate-release) dosage forms generally follow first-order drug absorption.

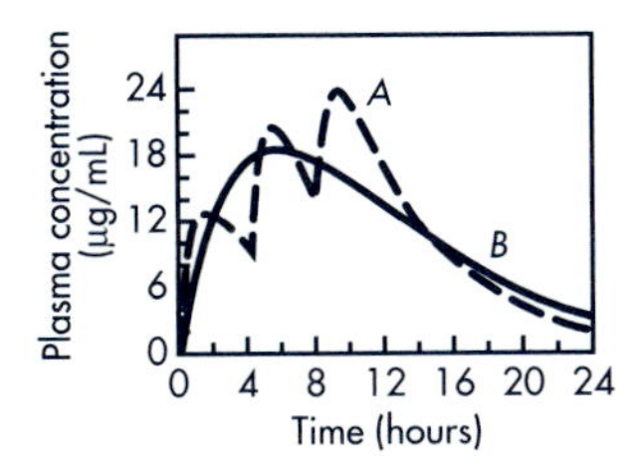

Figure 7-3. Plasma level of a drug from a conventional tablet containing 50 mg of drug given at 0 hr, 4 hr, and 8 hr (A) compared to a single 150-mg drug dose given in an extended-release dosage form (B). The drug absorption rate constant from each drug product is first order. The drug is 100% bioavailable and the elimination half-life is constant.

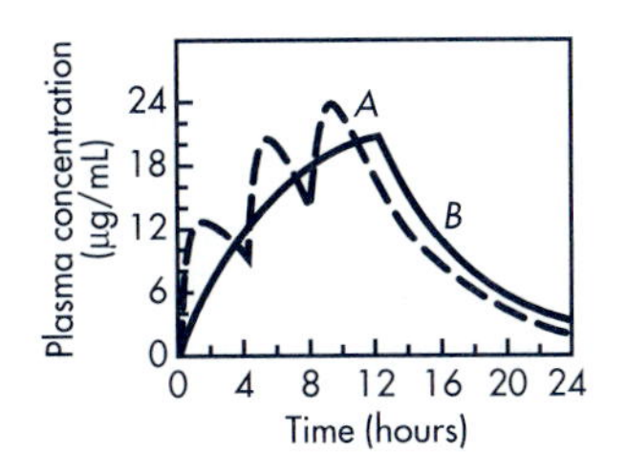

Figure 7-4. Bioavailability of a drug from an immediate-release tablet containing 50 mg of drug given at 0 hr, 4 hr, and 8 hr compared to a single 150-mg drug dose given in an extended-release dosage form. The drug absorption rate constant from the immediate-release drug product is first order, whereas the drug absorption rate constant from the extended-release drug product is zero order. The drug is 100% bioavailable and the elimination half-life is constant.

BIOPHARMACEUTIC FACTORS

The major objective of an extended-release drug product is to achieve a prolonged therapeutic effect while minimizing unwanted side effects due to fluctuating plasma drug levels. Ideally, the extended-release drug product should release the drug at a constant, or zero-order, rate. After release from the drug product, the drug is rapidly absorbed, and the drug absorption rate should follow zero-order kinetics similar to an intravenous drug infusion. In all cases, the drug product is designed so that the rate of systemic drug absorption is limited by the rate of drug release via the drug delivery system. Unfortunately, most extended-release drug products that release a drug by zero-order kinetics *in vitro* do not demonstrate zero-order drug absorption when given *in vivo*. The lack of zero-order drug absorption from these extended-release drug products after oral administration may be due to a number of unpredictable events happening in the gastrointestinal tract during absorption.

The Stomach

The stomach is a "mixing and secreting" organ where food is mixed with digestive juice and emptied periodically into the small intestine. However, the movement of food or drug product in the stomach and small intestine is very different depending on the physiologic state. In the presence of food, the stomach undergoes the digestive phase; in the absence of food, the stomach undergoes the interdigestive phase (Chapter 5). During the digestive phase, the food particles or solids larger than 2 mm are retained in the stomach, whereas smaller particles are emptied through the pyloric sphincter at a first-order rate depending on the content and size of the meals. During the interdigestive phase, the stomach rests for a period of up to 30 to 40 minutes, coordinated with an equal resting period in the small intestine. Peristaltic contractions then occur, which ends with strong "housekeeper contractions" that move everything in the stomach through to the small intestine. Similarly, large particles in the small intestine are moved along only in the housekeeper contraction period. A drug may remain for several hours in the stomach if administered during the digestive phase. Fatty material, nutrients, and osmolality may further extend the time the drug stays in the stomach. When the drug is administered during the interdigestive phase, the drug may be swept along rapidly into the small intestine. Dissolution of drugs in the stomach may also be affected by the presence or absence of food. When food is present, HCl is secreted and the pH is about 1 to 2. Although some food and nutrients can neutralize the acid and raise its pH. The fasting pH of the stomach is about 3 to 5. The release rates of some drugs are affected by food. For example, the extended-release drug product Theo-24 was shown to release drug at a higher rate in the presence of food. Whether this more rapid drug release rate is related to a change in pH or the stomach-emptying rate or a food–drug interaction is not known. A longer time of retention in the stomach may expose the drug to stronger agitation in the acid environment. The stomach has been described as having "jet mixing" action that sends mixture with up to 50 mm Hg pressure toward the pyloric sphincter, causing it to open and periodically release chyme to the small intestine.

The Small Intestine

The small intestine is about 10 to 14 feet in length. The first part is sterile, while the terminal part that connects the cecum contains some bacteria. The proximal part of the small intestine has a pH of about 6 due to neutralization of the acid by bicarbonates secreted by the duodenal mucosa and the pancreas. The small intestine provides an enormous surface area for drug absorption because of the presence of microvilli. The small intestine transit time of a solid preparation has been concluded to be about 3 hours or less in 95% of the population (Hofmann et al, 1983). Transit time for meals from mouth to cecum (beginning of large intestine) has been reviewed by the same authors. Various investigators have used the *lactulose hydrogen test*, which measures the appearance of hydrogen in a patient's breath (lactulose is metabolized by bacteria rapidly in the large intestine, yielding hydrogen that is normally absent in a person's breath), to estimate transit time. These results and gamma scintigraphy studies confirm a relatively short GI transit time from mouth to cecum of 4 to 6 hours. This interval was concluded to be too short for sustained-release preparations that last up to 12 hours, unless the drug is to be absorbed in the colon. The colon has little fluid and the abundance of bacteria may make drug absorption erratic and incomplete. The transit time for pellets has been studied in both disintegrating and nondisintegrating forms using both insoluble and soluble radiopaques. Most of the insoluble pellets were released from the capsule in 15 minutes. Scattering of pellets were seen in the stomach and along the entire length of the small intestine at 3 hours. At 12 hours most of the pellets were in the ascending colon, and at 24 hours the pellets were all in the descending colon ready to enter the rectum. With the disintegrating pellets, there was more scattering of the pellets along the GI tract. The pellets also varied widely in the rate of disintegration *in vivo* (Galeone et al, 1981).

The Large Intestine

The large intestine is about 4 to 5 feet long. This consists of the cecum and the ascending and descending colons eventually ending with the rectum. Little fluid is in the colon, and drug transit is slow. Not much is known about drug absorption in this area, although unabsorbed drug that reaches this region may be metabolized by bacteria. Incompletely absorbed antibiotics may affect the normal flora of the bacteria. The rectum has a pH of about 6.8 to 7.0 and contains more fluid. Drugs are absorbed rapidly when administered as rectal preparation. However, the transit rate is affected by the rate of defecation. Presumably, drugs formulated for 24 hours would remain in this region to be absorbed.

There are a number of sustained-release products formulated to take advantage of the physiologic conditions of the GI tract. Enteric-coated beads have been found to release drug over 8 hours when taken with food, due to the gradual emptying of the beads into the small intestine. Specially formulated "floating tablets" that remain in the top of the stomach have been used to extend the resident time of the product in the stomach. None of these methods, however, is consistent enough to perform reliably for potent medications. More experimental research is needed in this area.

DOSAGE FORM SELECTION

The selection of the drug and dosage is important in formulating a sustained-release product. In general, a drug with low solubility should not be formulated into a nondisintegrating tablet. The risk of incomplete dissolution is high. A drug with low solubility at neutral pH should be formulated so that most of the drug is released prior to reaching the colon. The lack of fluid in the colon may make complete dissolution difficult. Erosion tablets are more reliable because the entire tablet eventually dissolves. With most single-unit dosage forms, there is a risk of erratic performance due to variable stomach emptying and GI transit time. The selection of the pellet or bead dosage form may minimize the risk of erratic stomach emptying, because the pellets are usually scattered soon after ingestion. Disintegrating tablets have the same advantages because they are broken up soon after ingestion.

A drug highly soluble in the stomach but very insoluble at intestinal pH may be very difficult to formulate into a sustained-release product. Too much protection may result in low bioavailability, while too little protection may result in dose dumping in the stomach. A moderate extension of duration with enteric-coated beads may be possible. However, the risk of erratic performance is higher than that of the conventional dosage form. The osmotic type of controlled system may be more suitable for this type of drug.

DRUG RELEASE FROM MATRIX

A matrix is an inert solid vehicle in which a drug is uniformly suspended. A matrix may be formed simply by compressing or fusing the drug and the matrix material together. Generally, the drug is present in a smaller percent, so that the matrix gives extended protection against water and the drug diffuses out slowly over time. Most matrix materials are water insoluble, although some may swell slowly in water. Matrix type of drug release may be manufactured into a tablet or small beads depending on the formulation composition. Figure 7-5 shows three common approaches by which the matrix mechanisms are employed. In Figure 7-5A, the drug is coated with a soluble coating, so drug release solely relies on the regulation of the matrix material. If the matrix is porous, water penetration would be rapid and the drug would diffuse out rapidly. A less porous matrix may give a longer duration of release. Unfortunately, drug release from a simple matrix tablet is not zero order. The Higuchi equation below describes the release rate of a matrix tablet.

$$Q = DS(P/\lambda)[A - 0.5SP]^{1/2}\sqrt{t} \quad \textbf{(7.1)}$$

where Q = amount of drug release per cm^2 of surface at time t, S = solubility of drug in g/cm^3 in dissolution media, A = content of drug in insoluble matrix, P = porosity of matrix, D = diffusion coefficient of drug, and λ = tortuosity factor.

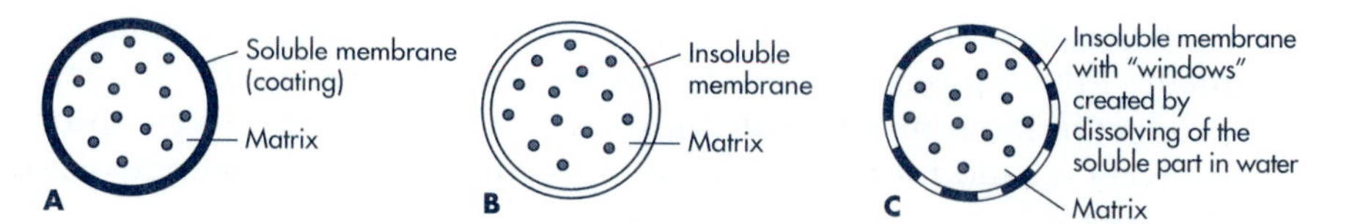

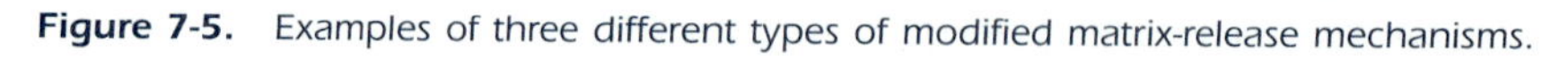
Figure 7-5. Examples of three different types of modified matrix-release mechanisms.

Figure 7-5B represents a matrix enclosed by an insoluble membrane, so that drug release rate is regulated by the permeability of the membrane as well as the matrix. Figure 7-5C represents a matrix tablet enclosed with a combined film. The film becomes porous after dissolution of the soluble part of the film. An example of this is the combined film formed by ethylcellulose and methylcellulose. Close to zero-order release has been obtained with this type of release mechanism.

ADVANTAGES AND DISADVANTAGES OF EXTENDED-RELEASE PRODUCTS

Extended-release drug products offer several important advantages over immediate-release dosage forms of the same drug. Extended release allows for sustained therapeutic blood levels of the drug; sustained blood levels provide for a prolonged and consistent clinical response in the patient. Moreover, if the drug input rate is constant, the blood levels should not fluctuate between a maximum and minimum, as in a multiple-dose regimen with an immediate-release drug product (Chapter 15). Highly fluctuating blood concentrations of drug may produce unwanted side effects in the patient if the drug level is too high, or may fail to exert the proper therapeutic effect if the drug level is too low. Another advantage of controlled release is patient convenience, which leads to better patient compliance. For example, if the patient only needs to take the medication once daily, he or she will not have to remember to take additional doses at specified times during the day. Furthermore, because the dosage interval is longer, the patient's sleep is not interrupted to take another drug dose; also, with the longer available dose, the patient awakes without having subtherapeutic drug levels. The patient may also derive an economic benefit in using a controlled-release drug product. A single dose of the controlled-release product may cost less than an equivalent drug dose given several times a day in rapid-release tablets. For patients under nursing care, the cost of nursing time required to administer medication is decreased if only one drug dosage is given to the patient each day.

For some drugs, such as chlorpheniramine, which have long elimination half-lives, the inherent duration of pharmacologic activity is long. Moreover, minimal fluctuations in blood concentrations of these drugs are observed after multiple doses are administered. Therefore, there is no rationale for controlled-release formulations of these drugs. However, such drug products are marketed with the justification that controlled-release products minimize toxicity, decrease adverse reactions, and provide patients with more convenience and, thus, better compliance.

There are also a number of disadvantages in using controlled-release medication. If the patient suffers from an adverse drug reaction or becomes accidentally intoxicated, the removal of drug from the system is more difficult with a controlled-release drug product. Orally administered controlled-release drug products may yield erratic or variable drug absorption due to various drug interactions with the contents of the GI tract and changes in GI motility. The formulation of controlled-release drug products may not be practical for drugs usually given in large doses (>500 mg) in conventional dosage forms. Because the controlled-release drug product may contain two or more times the dose given at more frequent intervals, the size of the controlled-release drug product would have to be quite large, too large for the patient to swallow easily.

The controlled-release dosage form contains the equivalent of two or more conventional drug doses given in a conventional dosage form. Therefore, the failure of the controlled-release dosage form may lead to dose dumping. *Dose dumping* can be defined either as the release of more than the usual fraction of drug or as the release of drug at a greater rate than the customary amount of drug per dosage interval, such that potentially adverse plasma levels may be reached (Dighe and Adams, 1988; Skelly and Barr, 1987). For delayed or enteric drug problems, two possible problems may occur if the enteric coating is poorly formulated. First, the enteric coating may become degraded in the stomach, allowing for early release of the drug, possibly causing irritation to the gastric mucosal lining. Second, the enteric coating may fail to dissolve at the proper site, and, therefore, the tablet may be lost prior to drug release, resulting in incomplete absorption.

KINETICS OF EXTENDED-RELEASE DOSAGE FORMS

The amount of drug required in a controlled-release dosage form to provide a sustained drug level in the body is determined by the pharmacokinetics of the drug, the desired therapeutic level of the drug, and the intended duration of action. In general, the total dose required (D_{tot}) is the sum of the *maintenance dose* (D_m) and the *initial dose* (D_I) immediately released to provide a therapeutic blood level.

$$D_{tot} = D_I + D_m \tag{7.2}$$

In practice, D_m (mg) is released over a period of time and is equal to the product of t_d (the duration of action per hr) and the zero-order rate k_r^0 (mg/hr). Therefore, Equation 7.2 can be expressed as

$$D_{tot} = D_I + k_r^0 t_d \tag{7.3}$$

Ideally, the maintenance dose (D_m) is released after D_I has produced a blood level equal to the therapeutic drug level (C_p). However, due to the limits of formulations, D_m actually starts to release at $t = 0$. Therefore, D_I may be reduced from the calculated amount to avoid "topping."

$$D_{tot} = D_I - k_r^0 t_p + k_r^0 t_d \tag{7.4}$$

Equation 7.4 describes the total dose of drug needed, with t_p representing the time needed to reach peak drug concentration after the initial dose.

For a drug that follows a one-compartment open model, the rate of elimination (R) needed to maintain the drug at a therapeutic level (C_p) is

$$R = kV_D C_p \tag{7.5}$$

where k_r^0 must be equal to R in order to provide a stable blood level of the drug. Equation 7.5 provides an estimation of the release rate (k_r^0) required in the formulation. Equation 7.5 may also be rewritten as

$$R = C_p Cl_T \tag{7.6}$$

where Cl_T is the clearance of the drug. In designing a controlled-release product, D_I would be the loading dose that would raise the drug concentration in the body to C_p, and the total dose needed to maintain therapeutic concentration in the body would simply be

$$D_{tot} = D_I + C_p Cl_T \cdot \tau \quad \textbf{(7.7)}$$

For many sustained-release drug products, there is no built-in loading dose (ie, $D_I = 0$). The dose needed to maintain a therapeutic concentration for τ hours would be

$$D_0 = C_p \tau Cl_T \quad \textbf{(7.8)}$$

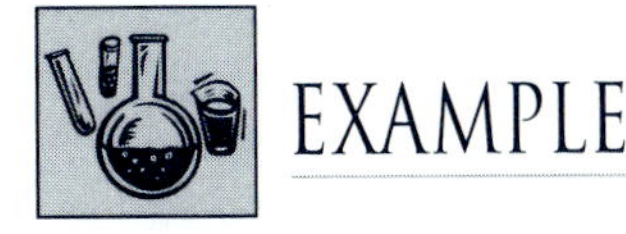

EXAMPLE

What dose is needed to maintain a therapeutic concentration of 10 μg/mL for 12 hours in a sustained-release product? 1. Assume $t_{1/2}$ of the drug is 3.46 hr and V_D is 10 L. 2. Assume $t_{1/2}$ of the drug is 1.73 hr and V_D is 5 L.

1.

$$k = 0.693/3.46 = 0.2/\text{hr}$$
$$Cl_T = kV_D = 0.2 \times 10 = 2\ \text{L/hr}$$

From Equation 7.8,

$$D_0 = (10\ \mu\text{g/mL})(1000\ \text{mL/L})(12\ \text{hr})(2\ \text{L/hr}) = 240{,}000\ \mu\text{g or } 240\ \text{mg}$$

2.

$$k = 0.693/1.73 = 0.4\ \text{hr}$$
$$Cl_T = 0.4 \times 5 = 2\ \text{L/hr}$$

From Equation 7.8,

$$D_0 = 10 \times 2 \times 1000 \times 12 = 240{,}000\ \mu\text{g or } 240\ \text{mg}$$

In this example, the amount of drug needed in a sustained-release product to maintain therapeutic drug concentration is dependent on both the V_D and the elimination half-life. In part 2 of the example, although the elimination half-life is shorter, the volume of distribution is also smaller. If the volume of distribution is constant, then the amount of drug needed to maintain C_p is simply dependent on the elimination half-life.

Table 7.2 shows the influence of $t_{1/2}$ on the amount of drug needed for an extended-release drug product. Table 7.2 was constructed by assuming that the drug has a desired serum concentration of 5 μg/mL and an apparent volume of distribution of 20,000 mL. The release rate R decreases as the elimination half-life increases. Because elimination is slower for a drug with a long half-life, the input rate should be slower. The total amount of drug needed in the extended-release drug product is dependent on both the release rate R and the desired duration of

TABLE 7.2 Release Rates for Extended-Release Drug Products as a Function of Elimination Half-Life[a]

			TOTAL (mg) TO ACHIEVE DURATION			
$t_{1/2}$ (hr)	k (hr^{-1})	R (mg/hr)	6 hr	8 hr	12 hr	24 hr
1	0.693	69.3	415.8	554.4	831.6	1663
2	0.347	34.7	208.2	277.6	416.4	832.8
4	0.173	17.3	103.8	138.4	207.6	415.2
6	0.116	11.6	69.6	92.8	139.2	278.4
8	0.0866	8.66	52.0	69.3	103.9	207.8
10	0.0693	6.93	41.6	55.4	83.2	166.3
12	0.0577	5.77	34.6	46.2	69.2	138.5

[a]Assume $C_{desired}$ is 5 μg/mL and the V_D is 20,000 mL; $R = kV_DC_p$; no immediate-release dose.

activity for the drug. For a drug with an elimination half-life of 4 hours and a release rate of 17.3 mg/hr, the extended-release product must contain 207.6 mg to provide a duration of activity of 12 hours. The bulk weight of the extended-release product will be greater than this amount due to the presence of excipients needed in the formulation. The values in Table 7.2 show that, in order to achieve a long duration of activity (≥12 hr) for a drug with a very short half-life (1 to 2 hr), the extended-release drug product becomes quite large and impractical for most patients to swallow.

PHARMACOKINETIC SIMULATION OF EXTENDED-RELEASE PRODUCTS

The plasma drug concentration profiles of many extended-release products fit an oral one-compartment model assuming first-order absorption and elimination. Compared to an immediate-release product, the extended-release product would typically show a smaller absorption rate constant due to the slower absorption of the extended-release product. The time for peak concentration (t_{max}) is usually longer (Fig. 7-6), and the peak drug concentration (C_{max}) is reduced. If the drug is properly formulated, the area under the plasma drug concentration curve should be the same. These parameters conveniently show how successfully the extended-release product performs *in vivo*. For example, a product with a t_{max} of 3 hours would not be very satisfactory if the product is intended to last 12 hours. Similarly, if the C_{max} is excessively high, it would be a sign of dose dumping due to inadequate formulation. The pharmacokinetic analysis of single- and multiple-dose plasma data has been used to evaluate many sustained-release products by regulatory agencies. The analysis is practical because many products can be fitted to this model even though the drug is not released in a first-order manner. The limitation of this type of analysis is that the absorption rate constant may not relate to the rate of drug dissolution *in vivo*. If the drug strictly follows zero-order release and absorption, the model may not fit the data. Various other models have been

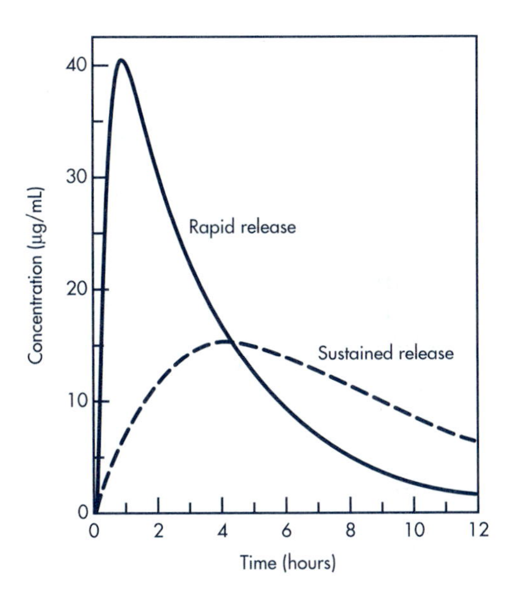

Figure 7-6. Plasma drug concentration of a sustained-release and a regular-release product. Note the difference of peak time and peak concentration of the two products.

used to simulate plasma drug levels of extended-release products (Welling, 1983). The plasma drug levels from a zero-order, extended-release drug product may be simulated with Equation 7.9 below. In the absence of a loading dose, the drug level in the body rises slowly to a plateau with minimum fluctuations (Fig. 7-7).

This simulation assumes that (1) rapid drug release occurs without delay, (2) perfect zero-order release and absorption of the drug takes place, and (3) the drug is given exactly every 12 hours. In practice, the above assumptions are not precise, and fluctuations in drug level do occur.

$$C_{\mathrm{p}} = \frac{D_{\mathrm{s}}}{V_{\mathrm{D}}k}(1 - e^{-kt}) \tag{7.9}$$

where D_s = maintenance dose or rate of drug release, mg/min; C_p = plasma drug concentration; k = overall elimination constant; and V_D = volume of distribution.

When a sustained-release drug product with a loading dose (rapid release) and

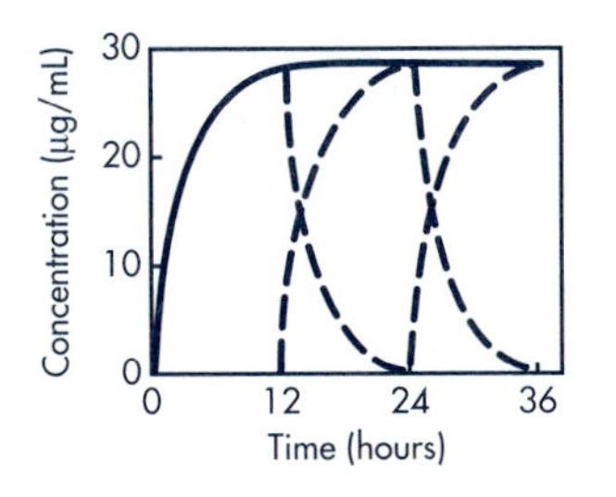

Figure 7-7. Simulated plasma drug level of a extended-release product administered every 12 hr. The plasma level shows a smooth rise to steady-state level with no fluctuations.

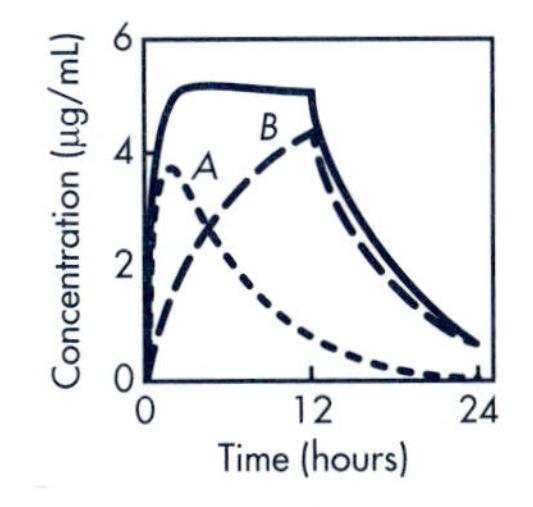

Figure 7-8. Simulated plasma drug level of a extended-release product with a fast-release component (A), and a maintenance component (B). The solid line represents total plasma drug level due to the two components.
(From Welling, 1983, with permission.)

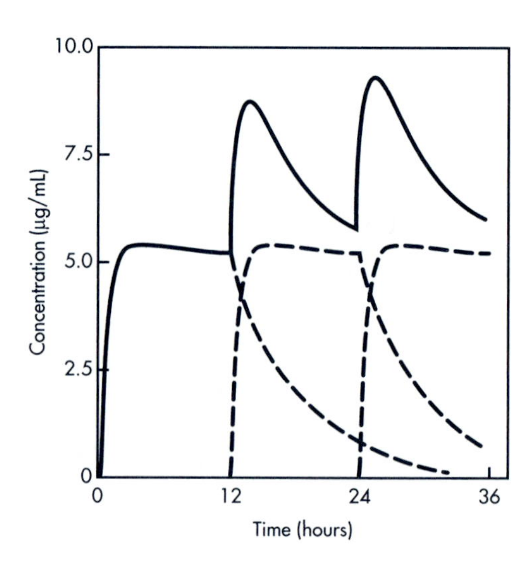

Figure 7-9. Simulated plasma level for a extended-release product given every 12 hr. The product has a built-in loading dose of 160 mg and a maintenance rate of 27.2 mg/hr. The plateau level was achieved rapidly after the first dose. Note the spiking peak following each dose due to the topping of the loading dose.
(From Welling, 1983, with permission.)

a zero-order maintenance dose is given, the resulting plasma drug concentrations are described by

$$C_{\mathrm{p}} = \frac{D_{\mathrm{i}} k_{\mathrm{a}}}{V_{\mathrm{D}}(k_{\mathrm{a}} - k)} (e^{-kt} - e^{-k_{\mathrm{a}}t}) + \frac{D_{\mathrm{s}}}{kV_{\mathrm{D}}} (1 - e^{-kt}) \tag{7.10}$$

where D_{i} = immediate-release (loading dose) dose and D_{s} = maintenance dose (zero-order). This expression is the sum of the oral absorption equation (first part) and the intravenous infusion equation (second part). An example of a zero-order release product with loading dose is shown in Figure 7-8. The contribution due to the loading and maintenance dose is shown by the dotted lines. The inclusion of a built-in loading dose in the extended-release product has only limited use.

With most extended-release products, the drug is administered for more than one dose, and there is no need for a built-in loading dose. Having a loading dose in the subsequent dosing would introduce more drug into the body than necessary due to the *"topping"* effect (Fig. 7-9). In situations where a loading dose is necessary, the rapid-release product is used to titrate a loading dose that would bring the plasma drug level to therapeutic level.

A pharmacokinetic model that assumes first-order absorption of the loading and maintenance dose has also been proposed. This model predicts spiking peaks due to loading dose when the drug is administered continuously (Fig. 7-9) in multiple doses.

TYPES OF EXTENDED-RELEASE PRODUCTS

Prior to the official adoption of the term, extended-release product, most products with controlled-release rates were described as controlled-release products. Table 7.3 shows some common extended-release product examples and the mechanisms for controlling drug release, and Table 7.4 lists the composition for some drugs.

Among the many types of commercial preparations available, none works by a single drug-release mechanism. Most extended-release products release drug by a combination of processes involving dissolution, permeation, and diffusion. The single most important factor is water permeation, without which none of the product release mechanisms would operate. Controlling the rate of water influx into the product generally dictates the rate at which the drug dissolves. Once the drug is dissolved, the rate of drug diffusion may be further controlled to a desirable rate.

Pellet-Type Sustained-Release Preparation

The pellet type of sustained-release preparation is often referred to as a *bead-type* preparation. In general, the beads are prepared by coating drug powder onto preformed cores called *nonpareil seeds*. The nonpareil seeds are made from slurry of starch, sucrose, and lactose. Preparation of the cores is tedious. The rough, core granules are rounded for hours on a coating pan and then classified according to size. The drug-coated beads generally provide a rapid-release carrier for the drug depending on the coating solution used. Commonly, sucrose solution provides a convenient way to coat the drug without impairing its rapid release. Once the drug beads are prepared, they may be further coated with a protective coating to allow a sustained or prolonged release of the drug.

The use of various amounts of coating solution can provide beads with various

TABLE 7.3 Examples of Oral Extended-Release Products

TYPE	TRADE NAME	RATIONALE
Erosion tablet	Constant-T	Theophylline
	Tenuate Dospan	Diethylpropion HCl dispersed in hydrophilic matrix
	Tedral SA	Combination product with a slow-erosion component (theophylline, ephedrine HCl) and an initial-release component theophylline, ephedrine HCl, phenobarbital)
Waxy matrix tablet	Kaon *Cl*	Slow release of potassium chloride to reduce GI irritation
Coated pellets in capsule	Ornade spansule	Combination phenylpropanolamine HCl and chlorpheniramine with initial- and extended-release component
Pellets in tablet	Theo-Dur	Theophylline
Leaching	Ferro-Gradumet (Abbott)	Ferrous sulfate in a porous plastic matrix that is excreted in the stool; slow release of iron decreases GI irritation
	Desoxyn gradumet tablet (Abbott)	Methamphetamine methylacrylate methylmethacrylate copolymer, povidone, magnesium stearate; the plastic matrix is porous
Coated ion exchange	Tussionex	Cation ion exchange resin complex of hydrocodone and phenyltoloxamine
Flotation–diffusion	Valrelease	Diazapam
Osmotic delivery	Acutrim	Phenylpropanolamine HCl (Oros delivery system)
	Procardia-XL	GITS–gastrointestinal therapeutic system with NaCl-driven (osmotic pressure) delivery system for nifedipine
Microencapsulation	Bayer timed-release	Aspirin
	Nitrospan	Microencapsulated nitroglycerin
	Micro-K Extencaps	Potassium chloride microencapsulated particles

TABLE 7.4 Composition and Examples of Some Modified-Release Products

K-Tab (Abbott)	750 mg or 10 meq of potassium chloride in a film-coated matrix tablet. The matrix may be excreted intact, but the active ingredient is released slowly without upsetting the GI tract. Inert ingredients: Cellulosic polymers, castor oil, colloidal silicon dioxide, polyvinyl acetate, paraffin. The product is listed as a waxy/polymer matrix tablet for release over 8–10 hr.
Toprol-XL tablets (Astra)	Contains metoprolol succinate for sustained release in pellets, providing stable beta-blockade over 24 hr with one daily dose. Exercise tachycardia was less pronounced compared to immediate-release preparation. Each pellet separately releases the intended amount of medication. Inert ingredients: Paraffin, PEG, povidone, acetyltributyl citrate, starch, silicon dioxide, and magnesium stearate.
Quinglute Dura tablet (Berlex)	Contains 320 mg quinidine gluconate in a prolonged-action matrix tablet lasting 8–12 hr and provides PVC protection. Inert ingredients: Starch, confection's sugar, and magnesium stearate.
Brontil Slow-Release capsules (Carnrick)	Phendimetrazine tartrate 105 mg sustained pellet in capsule.
Slow Fe tablet (Ciba)	Slow-release iron preparation (OTC medication) with 160 mg ferrous sulfate for iron deficiency. Inert ingredients: HPMC, PEG shellac, and cetostearyl alcohol.
Tegretol-XR tablets (Ciba Geneva)	Carbamazepine extended-release tablet. Inert ingredients: Zein, cetostearyl alcohol, PEG, starch, talc, gum tragacanth and mineral oil.
Sinemed CR tablet (Dupont pharma)	Contains a combination of carbidopa and levodopa for sustained release delivery. It is a special erosion polymeric tablet for Parkinson's disease treatment.
Pentasa capsule (Hoechst Marion/Roussel)	Contains mesalamine for ulcerative colitis in a sustained-release mesalamine coated with ethylcellulose. For local effect mostly, about 20% absorbed versus 80% otherwise.
Isoptin SR (Knoll)	Verapamil HCl sustained release tablet. Inert ingredients: PEG, starch, PVP, alginate, talc, HPMC, methylcellulose and microcrystalline cellulose.
Pancrease capsule (McNeil)	Enteric-coated microspheres of pancrelipase. Protects the amylase, lipase and protease from the action of acid in the stomach. Inert ingredients CAP, diethyl phthalate, sodium starch glycolate, starch, sugar, gelatin and talc.
Cotazym-S (Organon)	Enteric-coated microspheres of pancrelipase.
Eryc (erythromycin delayed-release capsule) (Warner-Chilcott)	Erythromycin enteric-coated tablet that protects the drug from instability and irritation.
Dilantin Kapseals (Parke-Davis)	Extended release phenytoin capsule which contains beads of sodium phenytoin, gelatin, sodium lauryl sulfate, glyceryl monooleate. PEG 200, silicon dioxide, and talc.
Micro-K Extencaps (Robbins)	Ethylcellulose forms semipermeable film surrounding granules by microencapsulation for release over 8–10 hr without local irritation. Inert ingredients: Gelatin, and sodium lauryl sulfate.
Quinidex Extentabs (Robbins)	300 mg dose, 100 mg release immediately in the stomach and is absorbed in the small intestine. The rest is absorbed later over 10–12 hr in a slow dissolving core as it moves down the GI tract. Inert ingredients: White wax, carnauba wax, acacia, acetylated monoglyceride, guar gum, edible ink, calcium sulfate, corn derivative, and shellac.

TABLE 7.4 Composition and Examples of Some Modified-Release Products (continued)

Compazine Spansule (SKB)	Initial dose of prochlorperazine release first, then release slowly over several hours. Inert Ingredients: Glycerylmonostearate, wax, gelatin, sodium lauryl sulfate.
Slo-bid Gyrocaps (Rhone-Poulenc Rorer)	A controlled release 12–24 hr theophylline product.
Theo-24 capsules (UCB Pharma)	A 24 hour sustained release theophylline product. Inert Ingredients: Ethylcellulose, edible ink, talc, starch, sucrose, gelatin, silicon dioxide, and dyes.
Sorbitrate SA (Zeneca)	The tablet contains isosorbide dinitrate 10 mg in the outer coat and 30 mg in the inner coat. Inert ingredients: Carbomer 934P, ethylcellulose, lactose magnesium stearate, and Yellow No. 10.

coating protection. A careful blending of beads may achieve any release profile desired. Alternatively, a blend of beads coated with materials of different solubility may also provide a means of controlling dissolution of the drug.

Some products take advantage of bead blending to provide two doses of drug in one formulation. For example, a blend of rapid-release beads with some pH-sensitive enteric-coated material may provide a second dose of drug release when the drug reaches the intestine.

The pellet dosage form can be prepared as a capsule or tablet. When pellets are prepared as tablets, the beads must be compressed lightly so that they do not break. Usually, a disintegrant is included in the tablet causing the beads to be released rapidly after administration. Formulation of a drug into pellet form may reduce gastric irritation, because the drug is released slowly over a period of time, therefore avoiding high drug concentration in the stomach. For example, theophylline has been formulated in a pellet-type controlled-release product (Gyrocap). Table 7.5 shows the frequency of adverse reactions after theophylline is administered as solution versus pellets.

If theophylline is administered as a solution, a high drug concentration may be reached in the body due to rapid drug absorption. Some side effects may be attributed to the high concentration of theophylline. Pellet dosage form allows drug to be absorbed gradually, therefore reducing the incidence of side effects by preventing high $C_{\max}$.

A second example involves the drug bitolterol mesylate (Tornalate). A study in dogs indicated that the incidence of tachycardia was reduced in a controlled-release bead preparation, whereas the bronchodilation effect was not reduced. Administering the drug as pellets apparently reduced excessively high drug concentration in the body and avoided stimulated increase in heart rate. Studies also reported reduced gastrointestinal side effects of the drug potassium chloride in pellet or microparticulate form. Potassium chloride is irritating to the GI tract. Formulation in pellet form reduces the chance of exposing high concentrations of potassium chloride to the mucosal cells in the GI tract.

Phenylpropanolamine HCl is used as a weight reducing drug (anorexiant) and is available in a sustained-release pellet capsule to curb appetite for 12 hours. Many long-acting cold products also employ the bead concept. A major advantage of the pellet dosage form is that the pellets are less affected by the effect of stomach emptying. Because numerous pellets are within a capsule, some pellets will gradually

TABLE 7.5 Incidence of Adverse Effects of Sustained-Release Theophylline Pellet Versus Theophylline Solution[a]

	VOLUNTEERS SHOWING SIDE EFFECTS	
SIDE EFFECTS	USING SOLUTION	USING SUSTAINED-RELEASE PELLETS
Nausea	10	0
Headache	4	0
Diarrhea	3	0
Gastritis	2	0
Vertigo	5	0
Nervousness	3	1

[a]After 5-day dosing at 600 mg theophylline/24 hr, adverse reaction points on fifth day: Solution, 135; pellets, 18. From Breimer 1980, with permission.

reach the small intestine each time the stomach empties, whereas a single enteric-coated tablet may be delayed in the stomach for a long time due to erratic stomach emptying. Stomach emptying is particularly important in the formulation of enteric-coated products. Enteric-coated tablets may be delayed for hours by the presence of food in the stomach, whereas enteric-coated pellets are relatively unaffected by the presence of food.

Prolonged-Action Tablet

A common way to prolong the action of a drug is to reduce the solubility of the drug, so that the drug dissolves slowly over a period of several hours. The solubility of a drug is dependent on the salt form used, and an examination of the solubility of the various salt forms of the drug should be the first step. In general, the base or acid form of the drug is usually much less soluble than the corresponding salt. For example, sodium phenobarbital is much more soluble than phenobarbital, the acid form of the drug. Diphenhydramine hydrochloride is more soluble than the base form, diphenhydramine.

In cases where it is inconvenient to prepare a less soluble form of the drug, the drug may be granulated with an excipient to slow dissolution of the drug. Often, fatty or waxy lipophilic materials are employed in formulations. Stearic acid, castor wax, high molecular weight polyethylene glycol (Carbowax), glyceryl monosterate, white wax, and spermaceti oil are useful ingredients in providing an oily barrier to slow water penetration and the dissolution of the tablet. Many of the lubricants used in tableting may also be used as lipophilic agents to slow dissolution. For example, magnesium stearate and hydrogenated vegetable oil (Sterotex) are actually used in high percentages to cause sustained drug release in a preparation. The major disadvantage of this type of preparation is the difficulty in maintaining a reproducible drug release from patient to patient, because oily materials may be subjected to digestion, temperature, and mechanical stress, which may affect the release rate of the drug.

Ion Exchange Preparation

Ion exchange preparations usually involve an insoluble resin capable of reacting with either an anionic or cationic drug. A cationic resin is negatively charged so that a positively charged cationic drug may react with the resin to form an insoluble nonabsorbable resin–drug complex. Upon exposure in the GI tract, cations in the gut, such as potassium and sodium, may displace the drug from the resin, releasing the drug, which is absorbed freely. The main disadvantage of ion exchange preparations is that the amount of cation–anion in the GI tract is not easily controllable and varies among individuals, making it difficult to be a consistent mechanism of drug release. A further disadvantage is that resins may provide a potential means of interaction with nutrients and other drugs.

Ion exchange may be used in a sustained-release liquid preparation. An added advantage is that the technique provides some protection for very bitter or irritating drugs. Recently, the ion exchange approach has been combined with a coating to obtain a more effective sustained-release product. For example, the drug dextromethorphan (Tussionex) has been formulated using the ion exchange principle to mask the bitter taste and to prolong the duration of action of the drug. In the past, amphetamine was formulated with ion exchange resins to provide prolonged release as an appetite suppressant in weight reduction.

A general mechanism for the formulation of *cationic* drugs is

$$\underset{\textit{Insoluble drug complex}}{H^+ + \text{resin–}SO_3^- \,\text{drug}^+} \rightleftarrows \underset{\textit{Soluble drug}}{\text{resin–}SO_3^-H^+ + \text{drug}^+}$$

For *anionic* drugs, the corresponding mechanism is

$$\underset{\textit{Insoluble drug complex}}{Cl^- + \text{resin–}N^+\,(CH_3)_3\,\text{drug}^-} \rightleftarrows \underset{\textit{Soluble drug}}{\text{resin–}N^+(CH_3)_3Cl^- + \text{drug}^-}$$

The insoluble drug complex containing the resin and drug dissociates in the GI tract in the presence of the appropriate counter ions. The released drug dissolves in the fluids of the GI tract and is rapidly absorbed.

Core Tablet

A core tablet is a tablet within a tablet. The core is usually for the slow drug-release component, and the outside shell contains a rapid-release dose of drug. Formulation of a core tablet requires two granulations. The core granulation is usually compressed lightly to form a loose core and then transferred to a second die cavity where a second granulation containing additional ingredients is compressed further to form the final tablet.

The core material may be surrounded by hydrophobic excipients so that the drug leaches out over a prolonged period of time. This type of preparation is sometimes called *slow erosion core* tablet, because the core generally contains either no disintegrant or insufficient disintegrant to fragment the tablet. The composition of the core may range from waxy to gummy or polymeric material. Numerous slow-erosion tablets have been patented and are commercially sold under various trade names.

The success of core tablets depends very much on the nature of the drug and the excipients used. As a general rule, this preparation is very much hardness dependent in its release rate. Critical control of hardness and processing variables are important in producing a tablet with a consistent release rate.

Core tablets are occasionally used to avoid incompatibility in preparations containing two physically incompatible ingredients. For example, buffered aspirin has been formulated into a core and shell to avoid a yellowing discoloration of the two ingredients upon aging.

Gum-Type Matrix Tablet

Some excipients have a remarkable ability to swell in the presence of water and form a gel-like consistency. When this happens, the gel provides a natural barrier to drug diffusion from the tablet. Because the gel-like material is quite viscous and may not disperse for hours, this provides a means for sustaining the drug for hours until all the drug has been completely dissolved and has diffused into the intestinal fluid. A common gelling material is gelatin. However, gelatin will dissolve rapidly after the gel is formed. Drug excipients such as methylcellulose, gum tragacanth, Veegum, and alginic acid will form a viscous mass and provide a useful matrix for controlling drug dissolution. Drug formulation with these excipients provides sustained drug release for hours. The drug diazepam, for example, has been formulated using methylcellulose to provide sustained release. In the case of sustained-release diazepam, claims were made that the hydrocolloid (gel) floated in the stomach to give sustained release. In other studies, material of various densities were emptied from the stomach without any difference as to whether the drug product was floating on top or sitting at the bottom of the stomach.

The most important consideration in this type of formulation appears to be the gelling strength of the gum material and the concentration of gummy material. Modification of the release rates of the product may further be achieved with various amounts of talc or other lipophilic lubricant.

Microencapsulation

Microencapsulation is a process of encapsulating microscopic drug particles with a special coating material, therefore making the drug particles more desirable in terms of physical and chemical characteristics. A common drug that has been encapsulated is aspirin. Aspirin has been microencapsulated with ethylcellulose, making the drug superior in its flow characteristics; when compressed into a tablet, the drug releases more gradually.

Many techniques are used in microencapsulating a drug. One process used in microencapsulating acetaminophen involves suspending the drug in an aqueous solution while stirring. The coating material, ethylcellulose, is dissolved in cyclohexane, and the two liquids are added together with stirring and heating. As the cyclohexane is evaporated by heat, the ethylcellulose coats the microparticles of the acetaminophen. The microencapsulated particles have a slower dissolution rate because the ethylcellulose is not water soluble and provides a barrier for diffusion of drug. The amount of coating material deposited on the acetaminophen will determine the rate of drug dissolution. The coating also serves as a means of reducing the bitter taste of the drug. In practice, microencapsulation is not consistent enough to produce a reproducible batch of product, and it may be necessary to blend the microencapsulated material in order to obtain a desired release rate.

Polymeric Matrix Tablet

The use of polymeric material in prolonging the release rate of drug has received increased attention. The most important characteristic of this type of preparation is that the prolonged release may last days and weeks rather than for a shorter duration (as with other techniques). The first example of an oral polymeric matrix tablet is Gradumet (Abbott Laboratories), which is marketed as an iron preparation. The plastic matrix provides a rigid geometric surface for drug diffusion so that a relatively constant rate of drug release is obtained. In the case of the iron preparation, the matrix reduces the exposure of the irritating drug to the GI mucosal tissues. The matrix is usually expelled unchanged in the feces after all the drug has been leached out.

The matrix tablets for oral use are generally quite safe. However, for certain patients with reduced GI motility caused by disease, the polymeric matrix tablet should be avoided, because accumulation or obstruction of the GI tract by the matrix tablet has been reported. As an oral sustained-release product, the matrix tablet has not been popular. In contrast, the use of the matrix tablet in implantation has been more popular.

The use of biodegradable polymeric material for controlled release has been the focus of intensive research. One such example is the use of polylactic acid copolymer, which degrades to natural lactic acid and eliminates the problem of retrieval after implantation.

The number of polymers available for drug formulations is increase and includes polyacrylate, methacrylate, polyester, ethylene–vinyl acetate copolymer (EVA), polyglycolide, polylactide, and silicone. Of these, the hydrophilic polymers, such as polylactic acid and polyglycolic acid, erode in water and release the drug gradually over time. A hydrophobic polymer such as EVA will release the drug over a longer duration time of weeks or months. The rate of release may be controlled by blending two polymers and increasing the proportion of the more hydrophilic polymer thus increasing the rate of drug release. The addition of a low-molecular-weight polylactide to a polylactide polymer formulation increased the release rate of the drug and enabled the preparation of a controlled-release system (Bodmeier et al, 1989). The type of plasticizer and the degree of cross-linking provide additional means for modifying the release rate of the drug. Many drugs are incorporated into the polymer as the polymer is chemically formed from its monomer. Light, heat, and other agents may affect the polymer chain length, degree of cross-linking, and other properties. This may provide a way to modify the release rate of the polymer matrices prepared. Drugs incorporated into polymers may have release rates that last over days, weeks, or even months. These vehicles have been often recommended for protein and peptide drug administration. For example, EVA is biocompatible and was shown to prolong insulin release in rats.

Hydrophobic polymers with water-labile linkages are prepared so that partial breakdown of the polymers allows for desired drug release without deforming the matrix during erosion. For oral drug delivery, the problem of incomplete drug release from the matrix is a major hurdle that must be overcome with polymeric matrix dosage form. Another problem is that the drug release rates may be affected by the amount of drug loaded. For implantation and other uses, the environment is more stable, so that a stable drug release from the polymer matrix may be attained for days or weeks.

Osmotic Controlled Release

The osmotic pump represents a newer concept in controlled-release preparations. Drug delivery is precisely controlled by the use of an osmotically controlled device that pumps a constant amount of water through the system, dissolving and releasing a constant amount of drug per unit time.

This device consists of an outside layer of semipermeable membrane filled with

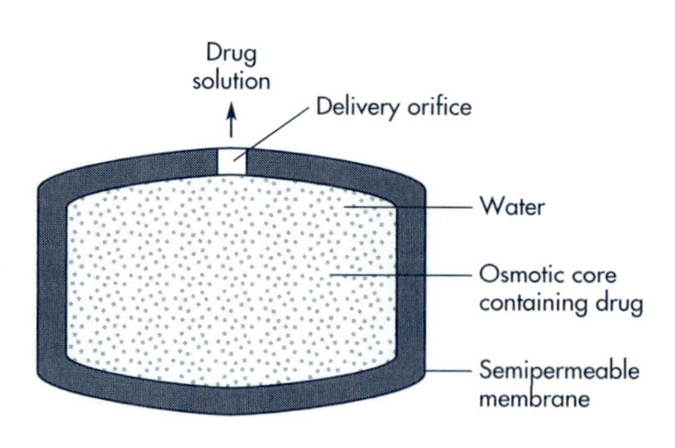

Figure 7-10. Cross-sectional diagram of simple osmotic delivery system (gastrointestinal therapeutic system).
(From Shaw and Chandrasekaran, 1978, with permission.)

a mixture of drug and osmotic agent (Fig. 7-10). When the device is placed in water, osmotic pressure generated by the osmotic agent within the core causes water to move into the device, which forces the dissolved drug to move out of the delivery orifice. The process continues until all the drug is released. The rate of drug delivery is relatively unaffected by the pH of the environment. The osmotic preparation available for implantation is known as the *osmotic minipump*. An improved "push and pull" osmotic system designed for oral use is the Gastrointestinal Therapeutic System (GITS) developed by Alza Corporation. The system consists of a semipermeable membrane and a two-layer core of osmotic ingredient and active drug respectively. As water enters the system, the osmotic pressure builds up from the inner layer pushing the drug out through a laser-drilled orifice in the drug layer. One example of GITS uses acetazolamide for the treatment of ocular hypertension in glaucoma. The drug was delivered from the system at zero-order rate for 12 hours at 15 mg/hr, as shown in Figure 7-11.

The frequency of side effects experienced by patients using GITS was considerably less than that of conventional tablet (Fig. 7-12). When the therapeutic system was compared to the regular 250-mg tablet given twice daily, ocular pressure was effectively controlled by the osmotic system. The blood level of acetazolanine using GITS, however, was considerably below that from the tablet. In fact, the therapeutic index of the drug was measurably increased by using the therapeutic system. The use of controlled-release drug products, which release drug consistently, may provide promise for administering many drugs that previously had frequent adverse side effects because of the drug's narrow therapeutic index. The osmotic drug delivery system has become a popular drug vehicle for many products that require extended period of drug delivery for 12 to 24 hours (Table 7.6).

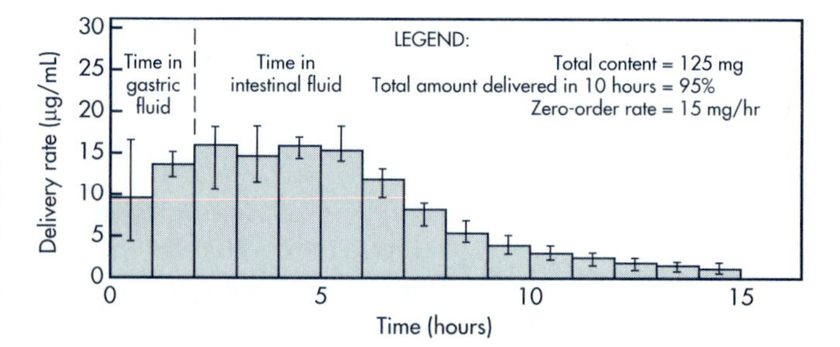

Figure 7-11. Pattern of delivery of acetazolamide from elementary osmotic pump therapeutic system delivering 70% of the total content (125 mg) at specified rate of 15 mg/hr in 6 hr and 80% in 8 hr.
(From Shaw and Chandrasekaran, 1978, with permission.)

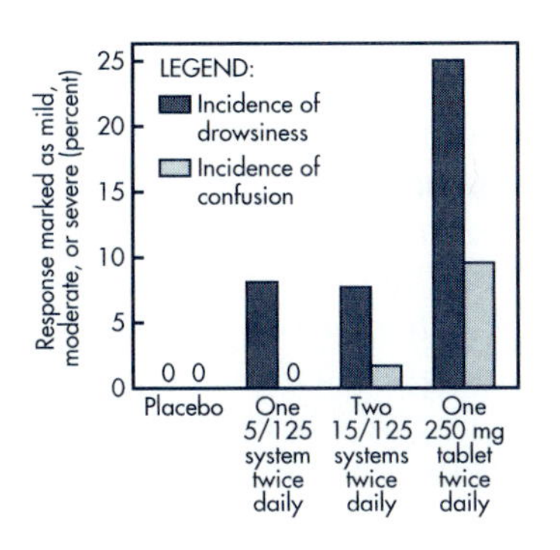

Figure 7-12. Incidence of drowsiness and confusion on acetazolamide given in three regimens. More frequent incidence of side effects were seen with the tablet over the osmotic system.
(From Shaw and Chandrasekaran, 1978, with permission.)

TABLE 7.6 OROS Osmotic Therapeutic Systems[a]

TRADE NAME	(MANUFACTURER)	GENERIC NAME	DESCRIPTION
Acutrim	(Ciba)	**(Phenylpropanolamine)**	Once-daily, over-the-counter appetite suppressant.
Covera-HS	(Searle)	**(Verapamil)**	Controlled-Onset Extended-Release (COER-24) system for hypertension and angina pectoris.
DynaCirc CR	(Sandoz Pharmaceuticals)	**(Isradipine)**	Treatment of hypertension.
Efidac 24	(Ciba Self-Medication)		Over-the-counter, 24-hour extended-release tablets providing relief of allergy and cold symptoms, Containing either chlorpheniramine maleate, pseudoephedrine hydrochloride or a combination of pseudoephedrine hydrochloride/brompheniramine maleate.
Glucotrol XL	(Pfizer)	**(Glipizide)**	Extended-release tablets indicated as an adjunct to diet for the control of hyperglycemia in patients with noninsulin dependent diabetes.
Minipress XL	(Pfizer)	**(Prazosin)**	Extended-release tablets for treatment of hypertension.
Procardia XL	(Pfizer)	**(Nifedipine)**	Extended-release tablets for the treatment of angina and hypertension.
Adalat CR	(Bayer AG)	**(Nifedipine)**	An Alza-based OROS system of nifedipine introduced internationally.
Volmax	(Glaxo-Wellcome)	**(Albuterol)**	An extended-release tablets for the relief of bronchospasm in patients with reversible obstructive airway disease.

[a]Alza's OROS Osmotic Therapeutic Systems use osmosis to deliver drug continuously at controlled rates for up to 24 hours.

Transdermal Drug Delivery Systems

A *transdermal drug delivery system* (or patch) is a drug-dose form intended for delivering a dose of medication across the skin for systemic drug absorption. The transdermal delivery system is popular with patients because it delivers the drug dose through the skin in a controlled rate over an extended period of time. Transdermal products allow a unique route of administration for drugs (Chapter 6, Table 6.11). More examples are listed in Tables 7.7 and 7.8. Transdermal products varies in the patch design, many units consist of drugs impregnated on a reservoir layer supported by a backing. Drug diffusion is controlled by a semipermeable membrane next to the reservoir layer. In general, the patch (Fig. 7-13) contains several parts: (1) a backing or support layer, (2) a drug layer (reservoir containing the dose), (3) a release-controlling layer (usually a semipermeable film), (4) a pressure sensitive adhesive (PSA), and (5) a protective strip, which must be removed prior to application. Nitroglycerin is commonly administered by transdermal delivery. Transdermal delivery systems of nitroglycerin may provide hours of protection against angina, whereas the duration of nitroglycerin given in a sublingual tablet may only last a few minutes. Several commercial transdermal preparations are available. These are Nitro-Disc (Searle), Transderm-Nitro (Novartis), and Nitro-Dur (Key Pharmaceuticals). These preparations are placed over the chest area and provide up to 12 hours of angina protection. In a study comparing these three dosage forms in patients, no substantial difference was observed among the three preparations. In all cases, the skin was found to be the rate-limiting step of nitroglycerin absorption. There were fewer variations among products than of the same product among different patients.

The skin is a natural barrier to prevent the influx of foreign chemicals (including water) into the body and the loss of water from the body (Guy, 1996). To be a suitable candidate for transdermal drug delivery, the drug must possess the right combination of physicochemical and pharmacodynamic properties. The drug must be highly potent so that only a small systemic drug dose is needed and the size of the patch (dose is also related to surface area) need not be exceptionally large, not greater than 50 cm^2 (Guy, 1996). Physicochemical properties of the drug include a small molecular weight (<500 Daltons) and highly lipid-soluble. The elimination half-life should not be too short to avoid having to apply the patch more frequently than once a day.

After the application of a transdermal patch, there is generally a lag time for the onset of the drug action, due to the drug's slow diffusion into the dermal lay-

TABLE 7.7 Examples of Transdermal Delivery Systems

TYPE	TRADE NAME	RATIONALE
Membrane-controlled system	Transderm-Nitro (Novartis)	Drug in reservoir, drug release through a rate-controlling polymeric membrane.
Adhesive diffusion-controlled system	Deponit system (PharmaSchwartz)	Drug dispersed in an adhesive polymer and in a reservoir.
Matrix dispersion system	Nitro-Dur (Key)	Drug dispersed into a rate-controlling hydrophilic or hydrophobic matrix molded into a transdermal system.
Microreservoir system	Nitro-Disc (Searle)	Combination reservoir and matrix-dispersion system.

TABLE 7.8 Transdermal Delivery Systems

TRADE NAME	(MANUFACTURER)	GENERIC NAME	DESCRIPTION
Catapres-TTS	(Boehringer Ingelheim)	**(Clonidine)**	Once weekly product for the treatment of hypertension.
Duragesic	(Janssen Pharmaceutical)	**(Fentanyl)**	Management of chronic pain in patients who require continuous opioid analgesia for pain that cannot be managed by lesser means.
Estraderm	(Ciba Geigy)	**(Estradiol)**	Twice weekly product for treating certain postmenopausal symptoms and preventing osteoporosis.
Nicoderm CQ	(Hoechst Marion)	**(Nicotine)**	An aid to smoking cessation for the relief of nicotine withdrawal symptoms.
Testoderm	(Alza)	**(Testosterone)**	Replacement therapy in males for conditions associated with a deficiency or absence of endogenous testosterone.
Transderm-Nitro	(Novartis)	**(Nitroglycerin)**	Once daily product for the prevention of angina pectoris due to coronary artery disease. It contains nitroglycerin in a proprietary, transdermal therapeutic system.
Transderm Scop		**(Scopolamine)**	Prevention of nausea and vomiting associated with motion sickness.

ers of the skin. When the patch is removed, diffusion of the drug from the dermal layer to the systemic circulation may continue for some time until the drug is depleted from the site of application. The solubility of drug in the skin rather than the concentration of drug in the patch layer is the most important factor controlling the rate of drug absorption through the skin. Humidity, temperature, and other factors have been shown to affect the rate of drug absorption through the skin. With most drugs, transdermal delivery provides a more stable blood level of the drug than oral application. However, with nitroglycerin, the sustained blood level of the drug provided by transdermal delivery is not desirable, due to induced tolerance to the drug not seen with sublingual tablets.

Transdermal Therapeutic Systems (TTS, Alza) consist of a thin, flexible composite of membranes, resembling a small adhesive bandage which is applied to the skin and delivers drug through intact skin into the bloodstream. Other examples of products delivered using this system are shown in Table 7.8. Transderm Nitro consists of several layers (1) an aluminized plastic backing that protects nitroglycerin from loss through vaporization, (2) a drug reservoir containing nitroglycerin adsorbed onto lactose, colloidal silicon dioxide, and silicone medical fluid, (3) a diffusion-controlling membrane consisting of ethylene-vinyl acetate copolymer, (4) a layer of silicone adhesive, and (5) a protective strip.

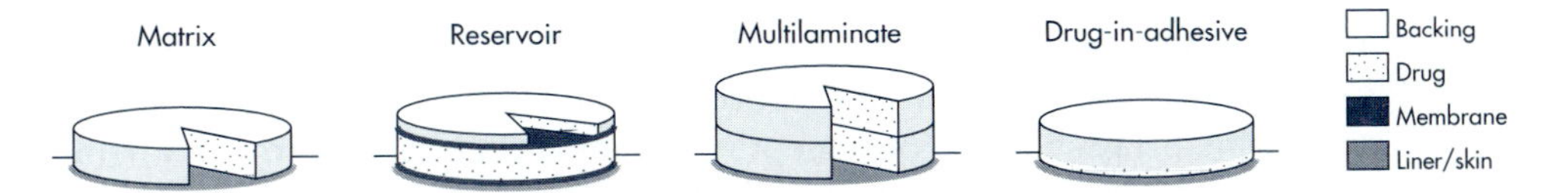

Figure 7-13. The four basic configurations for transdermal drug delivery systems.

Other transdermal delivery manufacturers have made transdermal systems in which the adhesive functions both as pressure sensitive adhesive and as a controlling matrix. Dermaflex (Elan) is a uniquely passive transdermal patch system which employs a hydrogel matrix into which the drug is incorporated. Dermaflex regulates both the availability and absorption of the drug in a manner which allows for controlled and efficient systemic delivery of many drugs.

An important limitation of transdermal preparation is quantitation of the dose. In general, drugs given at a dose of over 100 mg would require too large a patch to be used practically. However, new advances in pharmaceutic solvents may provide a mechanism for an increased amount of drug to be absorbed transdermally. Azone, a permeation enhancer, is a solvent that increases the absorption of many drugs through the skin. This solvent is relatively nontoxic.

For ionic drugs, absorption may be enhanced transdermally by *iontophoresis,* a method by which an electric field is maintained across the epidermal layer with special miniature electrodes. Some drugs, such as lidocaine, verapamil, insulin, and peptides, have been absorbed through the skin by iontophoresis. A process in which transdermal drug delivery is aided by high frequency sound is called *sonophoresis.* Sonophoresis has been used with hydrocortisone cream applied to the skin to enhance penetration for treating "tennis elbow" and other mildly inflamed muscular problems. Many such novel systems are being developed by drug delivery companies.

Panoderm XL patch technology (Elan) is a new system that delivers a drug through a concealed miniature probe which penetrates the stratum corneum. Panoderm XL is fully disposable and may be programmed to deliver drugs as a preset bolus, in continuous or pulsed regimen. The complexity of the device is hidden from the patient and is simple to use. Panoderm (Elan) is an electro-transdermal drug delivery system that overcomes the skin diffusion barriers through the use of low-level electric current to transport the drug through the skin. Several transdermal products, such as fentanyl, hydromorphone, calcitonin, and LHRH (luteinizing hormone–releasing hormone), are in clinical trial. More improvement in absorption enhancers and delivery systems will be available in the future for transdermal preparations.

Implants and Inserts

Polymeric drug implants can deliver and sustain drug levels in the body for an extended period of time. Both biodegradable and nonbiodegradable polymers can be impregnated with drugs in a controlled drug delivery system. For example, levonorgestrel implants (Norplant system, Wyeth-Ayerst) is a set of six flexible closed capsules made of silastic (dimethylsiloxane/methylvinylsiloxane copolymer), each containing 36 mg of the progestin, levonorgestrel. The capsules are sealed with silastic adhesive and sterilized. The Norplant system is available in an insertion kit to facilitate subdermal insertion of all six capsules in the mid-portion of the upper arm. The dose of levonorgestrel is about 85 μg/day, followed by a decline to about 50 μg/day by 9 months and to about 35 μg/day by 18 months, declining further to about 30 μg/day (Facts and Comparisons, 1997). The levonorgestrel implants are effective up to 5 years for contraception and then must be replaced. An intrauterine progesterone contraceptive system (Progestasert, Alza) is a T-shaped unit that contains a reservoir of 38 mg progesterone. Contraceptive effectiveness for

Progestasert is enhanced by continuous release of progesterone into the uterine cavity at an average rate of 65 μg/day for 1 year.

CONSIDERATIONS IN THE EVALUATION OF MODIFIED-RELEASE PRODUCTS

The two important requirements for preparing controlled-release products are: (1) demonstration of safety and efficacy and (2) demonstration of controlled drug release.

For many drugs, data are available demonstrating the safety and efficacy for those drugs given in a conventional dosage form. Bioavailability data demonstrating comparable blood level to an approved controlled-release product are acceptable. The bioavailability data requirements are specified in 21 CFR 320.25 (f). The important points are as follows.

1. The product should demonstrate sustained release, as claimed, without *dose dumping* (abrupt release of a large amount of the drug in an uncontrolled manner).
2. The drug should show steady-state levels comparable to those reached using a conventional dosage form given in multiple doses, and which was demonstrated to be effective.
3. The drug product should show consistent pharmacokinetic performance between individual dosage units.
4. The product should allow for the maximum amount of drug to be absorbed while maintaining minimum patient-to-patient variation.
5. The demonstration of steady-state drug levels after the recommended doses are given should be within the effective plasma drug levels for the drug.
6. An *in vitro* method and data that demonstrate the reproducible controlled-release nature of the product should be developed. The *in vitro* method usually consists of a suitable dissolution procedure that provides a meaningful *in vitro–in vivo* correlation.
7. *In vivo* pharmacokinetic data consist of single and multiple dosage comparing the controlled-release product to a reference standard (usually an approved non-sustained-release or a solution product).

The pharmacokinetic data usually consist of plasma drug data and/or urinary drug excreted. Pharmacokinetic analyses are performed to determine such parameters as $t_{1/2}$, V_D, t_{max}, AUC, and k.

Pharmacodynamic and Safety Considerations

Pharmacokinetic and safety issues must be considered in the development and evaluation of a modified-release dosage form. The most critical issue is to consider whether the modified-release dosage form truly offers an advantage over the same drug in an immediate-release (conventional) form. This advantage may be related to better efficacy, reduced toxicity, or better patient compliance. However, because the cost of manufacture of a modified-release dosage form is generally higher than the cost for a conventional dosage form, economy or cost savings for patients also may be an important consideration.

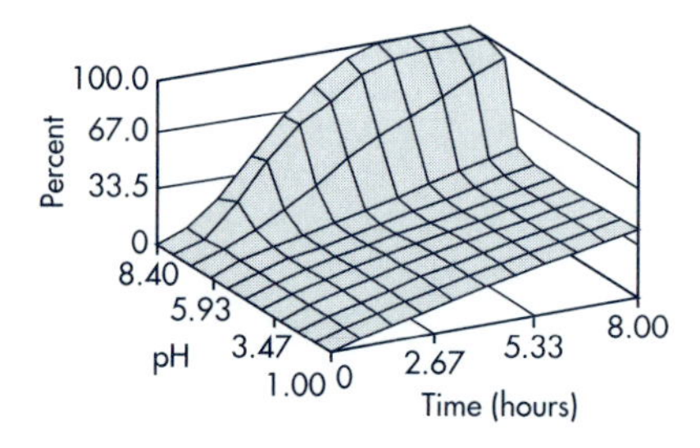

Figure 7-14. Topographical dissolution characterization of theophylline controlled release. Topographical dissolution characterization (as a function of time and pH) of Theo-24, a theophylline controlled-release preparation, which has been shown to have a greater rate and extent of bioavailability when dosed after a high-fat meal than when dosed under fasted conditions.
(From Skelly and Barr, 1987, with permission.)

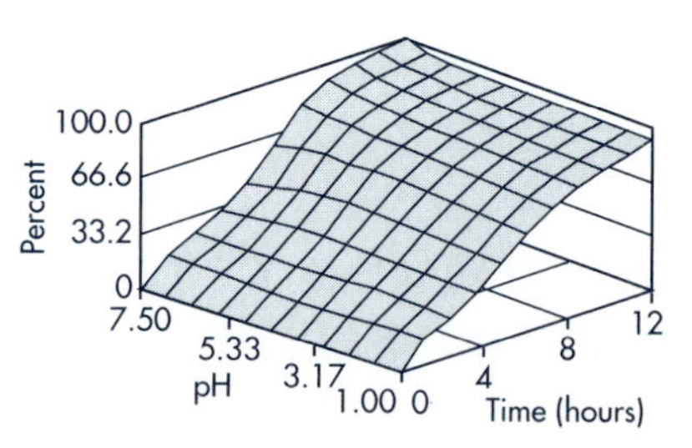

Figure 7-15. Topographical dissolution characterization of theophylline extended release. Topographical dissolution characterization (as a function of time and pH) of Theo-Dur, a theophylline controlled-release preparation, the bioavailability of which was essentially the same whether administered with food or under fasted conditions.
(From Skelly and Barr, 1987, with permission.)

Ideally, the extended-release dosage form should provide a more prolonged pharmacodynamic effect compared to the same drug given in the immediate release form. However, a controlled-release dosage form of a drug may have a different pharmacodynamic activity profile compared to the same drug given in an acute, intermittent, rapid-release dosage form. For example, transdermal patches of nitroglycerin, which produce prolonged delivery of the drug, may produce functional tolerance to the vasodilation activity that is not observed when nitroglycerin is given sublingually for acute angina attacks. Certain bactericidal antibiotics such as penicillin may be more effective when given in intermittent (pulsed) doses compared to continuous dosing. The continuous blood level of a hormone such as a corticosteroid might suppress adrenocorticotropic hormone (ACTH) release from the pituitary gland, resulting in atrophy of the adrenal gland. Furthermore, drugs that act indirectly or cause irreversible toxicity may be less efficacious when given in an extended-release rather than in conventional dosage form.

Because the modified-release dosage form may be in contact with the body for a prolonged period, the recurrence of sensitivity reactions or local tissue reactions due to the drug or constituents of the dosage form are possible. For oral modified-release dosage forms, prolonged residence time in the GI tract may lead to a variety of interactions with the contents of the GI tract, and the efficiency of absorption may be compromised as the drug moves distally from the duodenum to the large intestine. Moreover, dosage form failure due to dose dumping or failure due to the lack of drug release may have important clinical implications. Another unforeseen problem with modified-release dosage forms is an alteration in the metabolic fate of the drug, such as nonlinear biotransformation or site-specific disposition.

Design and selection of controlled-release products are often aided by dissolution tests carried out at different pH units for various time periods to simulate the condition of the GI tract. Topographical plots of the dissolution data may be used to graph the percent of drug dissolved versus two variables (time, pH) that may affect dissolution simultaneously. For example, Skelly and Barr (1987) have shown that controlled-release preparations of theophylline, such as Theo-24, have a more rapid dissolution rate at a higher pH of 8.4 (Fig. 7-14), whereas Theo-Dur is less affected by pH (Fig. 7-15). These dissolution tests *in vitro* may help to predict the *in vivo* bioavailability performance of the dosage form.

REGULATORY STUDIES FOR THE EVALUATION OF MODIFIED-RELEASE PRODUCTS

Dissolution Studies

Dissolution requirements for each of the three types of modified-release dosage form have also been defined by the USP. The clarification is useful for the submission of modified-release products for approval for marketing. Some of the key elements for the *in vitro* dissolution/drug release studies are listed in Table 7.9. Dissolution studies may be used together with bioavailability studies to predict *in vitro–in vivo* correlation of the drug release rate of the dosage forms.

In Vitro–In Vivo Correlations

A general discussion of correlating dissolution data to blood level data for immediate-release oral drug products was given in Chapter 6. Ideally, the *in vitro* drug release of the controlled-release product should relate to the bioavailability of the drug *in vivo,* so that changes in drug dissolution rates will be directly correlated to changes in drug bioavailability. Other methods of establishing *in vitro–in vivo* correlation were discussed by Skelly and coworkers (1990b) and in the USP Subcommittee on Biopharmaceutics (1988). The following is a brief summary of the various categories of dissolution showing different degrees of correlation to *in vivo* data.

Correlation Level A

Level A is the highest level of correlation, in which a 1:1 relationship between *in vitro* dissolution and *in vivo* bioavailability is demonstrated. Included in level A are extended-release dosage forms that demonstrate an *in vitro* drug release essentially independent of the dissolution medium. In this case, the *in vitro* dissolution curve is directly compared to the percentage of drug absorbed calculated from the plasma drug concentration–time curve using a pharmacokinetic model or a model-independent method.

Generally, the percentage of drug absorbed may be calculated by the Wagner–

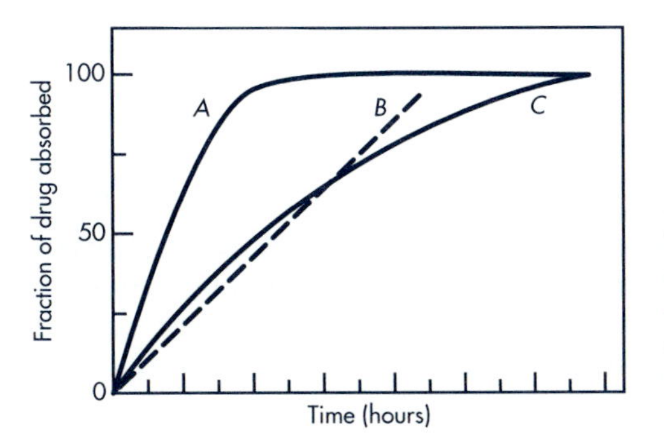

Figure 7-16. The fraction of drug absorbed using the Wagner–Nelson method may be used to distinguish between the first-order drug absorption rate of a conventional (immediate-release) dosage form (A) and an extended-release dosage form (C). Curve B represents an extended-release dosage form with zero-order absorption rate.

TABLE 7.9 Suggested Dissolution/Drug Release Studies for Modified-Release Dosage Forms

Dissolution Studies

1. Reproducibility of the method.
2. Proper choice of the media.
3. Maintenance of sink conditions.
4. Control of solution hydrodynamics.
5. Dissolution rate as a function of pH, ranging from pH 1 to pH 8 and including several intermediate values.
6. Selection of the most discriminating variables (media, pH, rotation speed, etc) as the basis for the dissolution test and specification.

Dissolution Procedures

1. Lack of dose dumping as indicated by a narrow limit on the 1-hour dissolution specification.
2. Controlled-release characteristics obtained by employing additional sampling windows over time. Narrow limits with an appropriate *Q* value system will control the degree of first-order release.
3. Complete drug release of the drug from the dosage form. A minimum of 75% to 80% of the drug should be released from the dosage form at the last sampling interval.
4. The pH dependence/independence of the dosage form as indicated by percent dissolution in water, appropriate buffer, simulated gastric juice, or simulated intestinal fluid.

Adapted from Skelly and Barr, 1987, with permission.

Nelson or Loo–Riegelman procedures or by direct mathematical deconvolution, a process of mathematical resolution of blood level into an input (absorption) and an output (disposition) component.

The main advantage of a level A correlation is that the quality control procedure of the *in vitro* dissolution test is predictive of the drug product performance *in vivo*.

Correlation Level B

Correlation level B is based on the principle of statistical moment analysis (see Chapter 20). The mean residence time of the drug in the body and mean dissolution time *in vitro* are determined and correlated. This level of correlation is less than a level A 1:1 correlation because the complete *in vivo* plasma drug concentration–time curve is not fully described by the mean residence time.

Correlation Level C

Correlation level C uses a single point in the dissolution curve to correlate to plasma drug concentration–time data. For example, a single dissolution time at $t_{50\%}$, $t_{90\%}$, and so forth, may be selected and correlated to pharmacokinetic parameters, such as AUC, t_{max}, or C_{max}. This is the weakest level of correlation because only partial relationship between absorption and dissolution is evident.

Pharmacokinetic Studies

Various types of pharmacokinetic studies may be required by the Food and Drug Administration (FDA) for marketing approval of the modified-release drug product, depending upon knowledge of the drug, its clinical pharmacokinetics, and its biopharmaceutics (Skelly et al, 1990a). Furthermore, the extended-release dosage form should be available in several dosage strengths to allow flexibility for the clinician to adjust the dose for the individual patient.

Both single- and multiple-dose steady-state crossover studies using the highest strength of the dosage form are required for a New Drug Application (NDA) and Abbreviated New Drug Application (ANDA). The reference dosage form may be a solution of the drug or the full NDA-approved conventional, immediate-release dosage form given in an equal daily dose as the extended-release dosage form. If the dosage strengths differ from each other only in the amount of the drug excipient blend, *but the concentration of the drug excipient blend is the same in each dosage form,* then the FDA may approve the NDA or ANDA on the basis of the single- and multiple-dose studies of the highest dosage strength, whereas the other lower-strength dosage forms may be approved on the basis of comparative *in vitro* dissolution studies.

At a workshop on controlled- and modified-release dosage forms (Skelly et al, 1990b) described several types of pharmacokinetic studies.

CASE ONE

The first case involves the controlled-release oral dosage form of a modified immediate-release drug for which extensive pharmacodynamic pharmacokinetic data exist. Both single- and multiple-dose steady-state crossover studies are required. In the case of the single-dose study, a well-controlled pharmacokinetic study must also be performed to define the effects of a concurrent high-fat meal on the extended-release dosage form. This food study, comparing fasting versus fed subjects, is to determine (1) whether there is any need for labeling specifications of special conditions for administration of the dosage form with respect to meals, and (2) whether the absorption pattern of the extended-release dosage compares to that for the immediate-release (conventional) form of the same drug.

CASE TWO

The second case concerns nonoral extended-release dosage forms. Pharmacokinetic studies for the evaluation of extended-release dosage forms designed for an alternate route of administration would require studies similar to case 1, but would not need a food-effect study. However, when the route of administration is changed from the oral route, other factors may need consideration. An alternate route of administration may alter the biotransformation pattern of active or inactive metabolites. For example, isoproterenol given orally forms a sulfate conjugation due to metabolism within the cells of the small intestine, whereas after IV administration, isoproterenol forms a 3-*O*-methylated metabolite via catechol *O*-methyltransferase (COMT). Clinical efficacy may be altered by an alternate route of administration when a drug is switched from the oral to the parenteral or transdermal route. In this case, possible risk factors, such as irritation or sensitivity at the site of applications, must also be studied.

CASE THREE

In case 3, studies involve the generic-equivalent of an NDA-approved, extended-release product. The same bioequivalence studies are required to establish the equivalence of the formulation used in efficacy studies if the formula is different from the one intended for marketing and generic approval. The establishment of bioequivalence is based on both pharmacokinetic and statistical analyses, as discussed elsewhere.

▶ CASE FOUR

Finally, case 4 addresses an extended-release dosage form as an NDA. For an NDA, the studies required for new extended-release dosage forms are clinical studies and pharmacokinetic studies including dose linearity, bioavailability, food effects, fluctuation of the plasma drug concentrations, and characterizations of the plasma drug concentration versus time profile.

The FDA's Center for Drug Evaluation and Research (CDER) maintains a website (*http://www.fda.gov/cder*) that lists regulatory guidances to provide the public with the FDA's latest submission requirements for NDAs and ANDAs.

EVALUATION OF *IN VIVO* BIOAVAILABILITY DATA

A properly designed bioavailability study is performed *in vivo*. The data is then evaluated using both pharmacokinetic and statistical analysis methods. The evaluation may include a pharmacokinetic profile, steady-state plasma drug concentrations, rate of drug absorption, occupancy time, and statistical evaluation of the computed pharmacokinetic parameters.

Pharmacokinetic Profile

The plasma drug concentration versus time curve should adequately define the bioavailability of the drug from the dosage form. The bioavailability data should include a profile of the fraction of drug absorbed (Wagner–Nelson) and should rule out dose dumping or lack of a significant food effect. The bioavailability data should also demonstrate the controlled-release characteristics of the dosage form compared to the reference or immediate-release drug product.

Steady-State Plasma Drug Concentration

The fluctuation between the C_{max}^{∞} (peak) and C_{min}^{∞} (trough) concentrations should be calculated:

$$\text{Fluctuation} = \frac{C_{max}^{\infty} - C_{min}^{\infty}}{C_{av}^{\infty}} \quad (7.11)$$

where C_{av}^{∞} is equal to $[\text{AUC}]/\tau$.

An ideal extended-release dosage form should have minimum fluctuation between C_{max} and C_{min}. A true zero-order release will have no fluctuation. In practice, the fluctuation in plasma drug levels after the extended-release dosage form should be less than the fluctuation after the same drug given in an immediate-release dosage form.

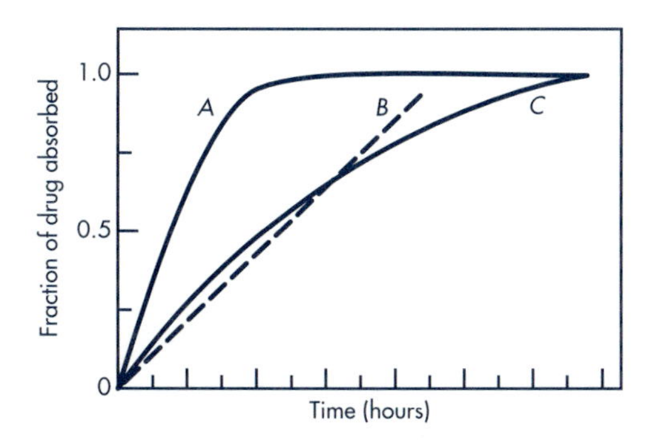

Figure 7-17. The fraction of drug absorbed using the Wagner–Nelson method may be used to distinguish among the first-order drug absorption rate of a conventional (immediate-release) dosage form (A) and a controlled-release dosage form (C). Curve B represents a controlled-release dosage form with zero-order absorption rate.

Rate of Drug Absorption

For the extended-release drug product to claim zero-order absorption, an appropriately calculated input function such as the Wagner–Nelson approach should substantiate this claim. The difference between first-order and zero-order absorption of a drug is shown in Figure 7-17. The rate of drug absorption from the conventional or immediate-release dosage form is generally first order, as shown by Fig. 7-17A, whereas drug absorption after an extended-release dosage form may be zero order (Fig. 7-17B), first order (Fig. 7-17C), or an indeterminate order. For many controlled-release dosage forms, the rate of drug absorption is first order, with an absorption rate constant k_a smaller than the elimination rate constant k. The pharmacokinetic model when $k_a < k$ is termed "*flip-flop pharmacokinetics*" and is discussed in Chapter 9.

Occupancy Time

For drugs for which the therapeutic window is known, the plasma drug concentrations should be maintained above the minimum effective drug concentration (MEC) and below the minimum toxic drug concentration (MTC). the time required for maintenance of the plasma drug levels within the therapeutic window is known as occupancy time (Fig. 7-18).

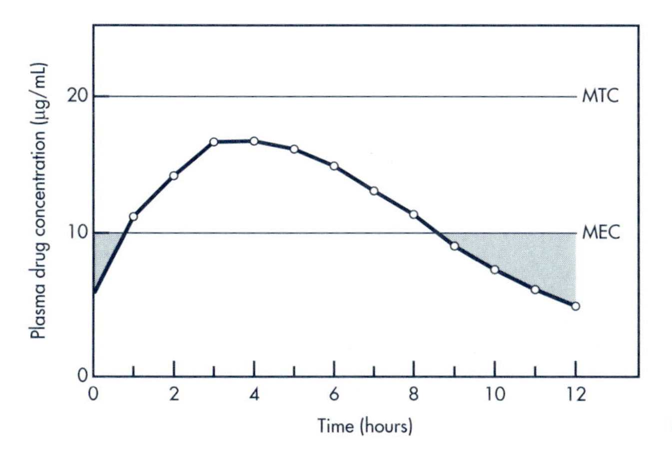

Figure 7-18. Occupancy time.

Bioequivalence Studies

Bioequivalence studies for controlled-release drug products are discussed in detail in Chapter 10. FDA presently requires three different bioavailability studies for an oral controlled-release drug product including (1) a fasting study, (2) a food intervention study, and (3) a multiple dose study.

Statistical Evaluation

Variables subjected to statistical analysis generally include plasma drug concentrations at each collection time, AUC (from zero to last sampling time), AUC (from zero to time infinity), $C_{\max}$, $t_{\max}$, and elimination half-life $t_{1/2}$. Statistical testing may include an analysis of variance (ANOVA), computation of 90% and 95% confidence intervals on the difference in formulation means, and the power of ANOVA to detect a 20% difference from the reference mean.

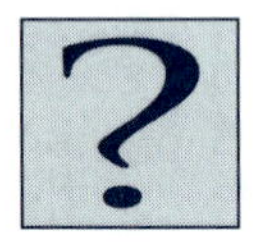

FREQUENTLY ASKED QUESTIONS

1. Are controlled-release drug products always more efficacious than immediate-release drug products containing the same drug?
2. What are the advantages and disadvantages of a zero-order rate for drug absorption?

LEARNING QUESTIONS

1. The design for most extended-release or sustained-release oral drug products allows for the slow release of the drug from the dosage form and subsequent slow absorption of the drug from the gastrointestinal tract.
   a. Why does the slow release of a drug from an extended-release drug product produce a longer-acting pharmacodynamic response compared to the same drug prepared in a conventional, oral, immediate-release drug product?
   b. Why do manufacturers of sustained-release drug products attempt to design this dosage form to have a zero-order rate of systemic drug absorption?
2. The dissolution profiles of three drug products are illustrated in Figure 7-19.
   a. Which of the drug products in Figure 7-19 release drug at a zero-order rate of about 8.3% every hour?
   b. Which of the drug products does not release drug at a zero-order rate?
   c. Which of the drug products has an almost zero-rate of drug release during certain hours of the dissolution process?

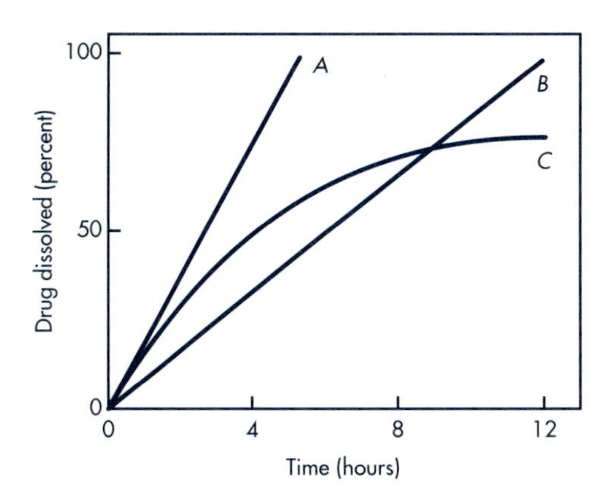

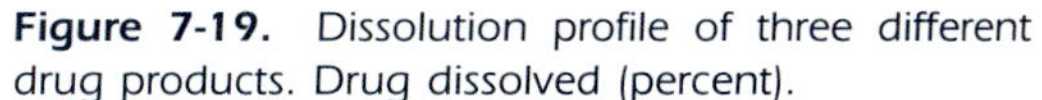
Figure 7-19. Dissolution profile of three different drug products. Drug dissolved (percent).

  d. Suggest a common cause of slowing drug dissolution rate of many rapid-release drug products toward the end of dissolution.
  e. Suggest a common cause of slowing drug dissolution of a sustained-release product toward the end of a dissolution test.

3. A drug is normally given at 10 mg four times a day. Suggest an approach for designing a 12-hour zero-order release product.
  a. Calculate the desired zero-order release rate.
  b. Calculate the concentration of the drug in an osmotic pump type of oral dosage form that delivers 0.5 mL/hr of fluid.

4. An industrial pharmacist would like to design a sustained-release drug product to be given every 12 hours. The active drug ingredient has an apparent volume of distribution of 10 L, an elimination half-life of 3.5 hours, and a desired therapeutic plasma drug concentration of 20 mg/mL. Calculate the zero-order release rate of the sustained-release drug product and the total amount of drug needed, assuming no loading dose is required.

REFERENCES

Arnon R: In Gregoriadis G, Senior J, Trouet A (eds), *Targeting of Drugs.* New York, Plenum, 1982, pp 31–54

Arnon R, Hurwitz E: In Goldberg EP (ed), *Targeted Drugs.* New York, Wiley, 1983, pp 23–55

Bodmeier R, Oh KH, Chen H: The effect of the addition of low molecular weight poly(DL-lactide) on drug release from biodegradable poly(DL-lactide) drug delivery systems. *Int J Pharm* **51:**1–8, 1989

Breimer DD, Dauhof M: *Towards Better Safety of Drugs and Pharmaceutical Products.* Amsterdam, Elsevier/North-Holland, 1980, pp 117–142

Chu BCF, Whiteley JM: High molecular weight derivatives of methotrexate as chemotherapeutic agents. *Mol Pharmacol* **13:**80, 1980

Dighe SV, Adams WP: Bioavailability and bioequivalence of oral controlled-release products: A regulatory perspective. In Welling PG, Tse FLS (eds), *Pharmacokinetics: Regulatory, Industrial, Academic Perspectives.* New York, Marcel Dekker, 1988

Fiume L, Busi C, Mattioli A: Targeting of antiviral drugs by coupling with protein carriers. *FEBS Lett* **153:**6, 1983

Fiume L, Busi C, Mattioli A, et al: In Gregoriadis G, Senior J, Trouet A (eds), *Targeting of Drugs.* New York, Plenum, 1982

Friend DR, Pangburn S: Site-specific drug delivery. *Medicinal Res Rev* **7:**53–106, 1987

Galeone M, Nizzola L, Cacioli D, Moise G: *In vivo* demonstration of delivery mechanisms from sustained-release pellets. *Curr Therapeut Res* **29:**217–234, 1981

Gros L, Ringsdorf H, Schupp H: *Angew Chem Int Ed Engl* **20:**312, 1981

Guy RH: Current status and future prospects of transdermal drug delivery. *Pharm Res* **13:**1765–1769, 1996

Hofmann FF, Pressman JH, Code CF, Witztum KF: Controlled entry of orally administered drugs: Physiological considerations. *Drug Dev Indust Pharm* **9:**1077, 1983

Joshi HN: Recent advances in drug delivery systems: Polymeric prodrugs. *Pharm Technol* **12:**118–125, 1988

Schechter B, Wilchek M, Arnon R: Increased therapeutic efficacy of *cis*-platinum complexes of poly L-glutamic acid against a murine carcinoma. *Int J Cancer* **39:**409–413, 1987

Shaw JE, Chandrasekaran SK: Controlled topical delivery systems for systemic action. *Drug Metab Rev* **8:**223–233, 1978

Skelly JP, Amidon GL, Barr WH, et al: *In vitro* and *in vivo* testing and correlation for oral controlled/modified-release dosage forms. *Pharm Res* **7:**975–982, 1990a

Skelly JP, Amidon GL, Barr WH, et al: Report of the workshop on *in vitro* and *in vivo* testing and correlation for oral controlled/modified-release dosage forms. *J Pharm Sci* **79:**849–854, 1990b

Skelly JP, Barr WH: Regulatory assessment. In Robinson JR, Lee VHL (eds), *Controlled Drug Delivery: Fundamentals and Applications,* 2nd ed. New York, Marcel Dekker, 1987

USP Subcommittee on Biopharmaceutics: In-vitro/in-vivo correlation for extended-release oral dosage forms. *Pharm Forum*: 4160–4161, 1988

Welling PG: Pharmacokinetic considerations of controlled release drug products. *Drug Dev Indust Pharm* **9:**1185–1225, 1983

BIBLIOGRAPHY

Akala EO, Collett JH: Influence of drug loading and gel structure on in-vitro release kinetics from photopolymerized gels. *Indust Pharm* **13:**1779–1798, 1987

Bayley H, Gasparro F, Edelson R: Photoactive drugs. *TIPS* **8:**138–144, 1987

Boxenbaum HG: Physiological and pharmacokinetic factors affecting performance of sustained release dosage forms. *Drug Dev Indust Pharm* **8:**1–25, 1982

Brodsky FM: Monoclonal antibodies as magic bullets. *Pharm Res* **5:**1–9, 1988

Bruck S (ed): *CRC Controlled Drug Delivery.* Boca Raton, CRC Press, 1983

Cabana BE: Bioavailability regulations and biopharmaceutic standard for controlled release drug delivery. *Proceedings of 1982 Research and Scientific Development Conference.* Washington, DC, The Proprietary Association, 1983, pp 56–69

Chien YW: Oral controlled drug administration. *Drug Dev Indust Pharm* **9:** 1983

Chien YW: *Novel Drug Delivery Systems.* New York, Marcel Dekker, 1982

Chien YW, Siddiqui O, Shi WM, et al: Direct current iontophoretic transdermal delivery of peptide and protein drugs. *J Pharm Sci* **78:**376–383, 1989

Heller J: Controlled drug release from monolithic bioerodible polymer devices. *Pharm Int* **7:**316–318, 1986

Hunter E, Fell JT, Sharma H: The gastric emptying of pellets contained in hard gelatin capsules. *Drug Dev Indust Pharm* **8:**151–157, 1982

Langer R: New methods of drug delivery. *Science* **249:**1527–1533, 1990

Levy G: Targeted drug delivery: Some pharmacokinetic considerations. *Pharm Res* **4:**3–4, 1987

Malinowski HJ: Biopharmaceutic aspects of the regulatory review of oral controlled release drug products. *Drug Dev Indust Pharm* **9:**1255–1279, 1983

Miyazaki S, Ishii K, Nadai T: Controlled release of prednisolone from ethylene-vinyl acetate copolymer matrix. *Chem Pharm Bull* **29:**2714–2717, 1981

Mueller-Lissner SA, Blum AL: The effect of specific gravity and eating on gastric emptying of slow-release capsules. *N Engl J Med* **304:**1365–1366, 1981

Okabe K, Yamoguchi H, Kawai Y: New ionotophoretic transdermal administration of the beta-blocker metoprolol. *J Control Release* **4:**79–85, 1987

Park H, Robinson JR: Mechanisms of mucoadhesion of poly(acrylic acid) hydrogels. *Pharm Res* **4:**457–464, 1987

Pozansky MJ, Juliano RL: Biological approaches to the controlled delivery of drugs: A critical review. *Pharmacol Rev* **36:**277–336, 1984

Robinson JR: Oral drug delivery systems. *Proceedings of 1982 Research and Scientific Development Conference.* Washington, DC, The Proprietary Association, 1983, pp 54–69

Robinson JR: *Sustained and Controlled Release Drug Delivery Systems.* New York, Marcel Dekker, 1978

Robinson JR, Eriksen SP: Theoretical formulation of sustained release dosage forms. *J Pharm Sci* **53:**1254–1263, 1966

Robinson JR, Lee VHL (eds): *Controlled Drug Delivery: Fundamentals and Applications,* 2nd ed. New York, Marcel Dekker, 1987

Rosement TJ, Mansdorf SZ: *Controlled Release Delivery Systems.* New York, Marcel Dekker, 1983

21 CFR 320.25 (B)

Urquhart J: *Controlled-Release Pharmaceuticals.* Washington, DC, American Pharmaceutical Association, 1981

8

TARGETED DRUG DELIVERY SYSTEMS AND BIOTECHNOLOGICAL PRODUCTS

TARGETED DRUG DELIVERY

Targeted drug delivery or *site-specific* drug delivery refers to drug carrier systems that place the drug at or near the receptor site. Most conventional dosage forms deliver drug into the body that eventually reaches the site of action by distribution and passive diffusion. Friend and Pangburn (1987) have classified site-specific drug delivery into three broad categories of drug targeting: (1) first-order targeting, which refers to drug delivery systems that deliver the drug to the capillary bed of the active site; (2) second-order targeting, which refers to the specific delivery of drug to a special cell type such as the tumor cells and not to the normal cells; and (3) third-order targeting, which refers to drug delivery specifically to the internal (intracellular) site of cells. An example of third-order drug targeting is the receptor-mediated entry of a drug complex into the cell by endocytosis followed by lysosomal release of the drug. Numerous techniques have been developed in the site-specific delivery areas. Ideally, site-specific carriers guide the drug to the intended target site (tissues or organ) in which the receptor is located without exposing the drug to other tissues, thereby avoiding adverse toxicity. Much of the research in targeted drug delivery has been in cancer chemotherapy.

Site-specific drug delivery has also been characterized as passive or active targeting (Takakura and Hashida, 1996). *Passive targeting* refers to the exploitation of the natural (passive) disposition profiles of a drug carrier which is passively determined by its physicochemical properties relative to the anatomic and physiologic characteristics of the body. *Active targeting* refers to the alterations of the natural disposition of a drug carrier, directing it to specific cells, tissues, or organs. One approach to active targeting is the use of ligands or monoclonal antibodies which can specifically target cells. Monoclonal antibodies are discussed more fully in this chapter. Active targeting employing receptor-mediated endocytosis is a saturable, nonlinear process dependent upon the drug–carrier concentration, whereas passive targeting is most often a linear process over a large range of doses.

General Considerations in Targeted Drug Delivery

Considerations in the development of the site-specific or targeted drug delivery systems include: (1) the anatomic and physiologic characteristics of the target site, including capillary permeability to macromolecules and cellular uptake of the drug (Molema et al, 1966); (2) the physicochemical characteristics of the therapeutically active drug; (3) the physical and chemical characteristics of the carrier; (4) the selectivity of the drug–carrier complex; (5) any impurities introduced during the conjugation reaction linking the drug and the carrier that may be immunogenic or toxic to the body and possible adverse immunologic reactions.

Target Site

The accessibility of the drug–carrier complex to the target site may present bioavailability and pharmacokinetic problems, which also include anatomic and/or physiologic considerations. For example, targeting a drug into a brain tumor requires a different route of drug administration (intrathecal injection) than targeting a drug into the liver or spleen. Moreover, the permeability of the tumor blood vessels to macromolecules or drug carrier complex may be a barrier preventing intracellular uptake of the these drugs (Molena et al, 1997).

Site-Specific Carrier

To target a drug or a drug–carrier complex to an active site, one must consider whether there is a unique property of the active site that makes the target site differ from other organs or tissue systems in the body. The next consideration is to take advantage of this unique difference so that the drug goes specifically to the site of action and not to other tissues in which adverse toxicity may occur. The application of macromolecules or a drug–carrier complex for site-specific drug delivery requires both the affinity of the drug–carrier complex for the targeted tissues as well as favorable pharmacokinetics for delivery of the drug–carrier complex to the organ, cells, and subcellular target site. An additional problem, particularly in the use of protein carriers, is the occurrence of adverse immunological reactions—an occurrence that is partially overcome by using less immunoreactive proteins (Takakura and Hashida, 1996).

Each of the carrier systems discussed in this chapter are approaches to the delivery of the active drug to the target site. The physicochemical properties of the carrier are chosen in order to favor uptake of the drug at the target site and diminish uptake of the drug in other tissues.

Drugs

Most of the drugs used for targeted drug delivery are highly reactive drugs with narrow therapeutic windows, and many of them are used in cancer chemotherapy. Many also have potent pharmacodynamic activities. These drugs may be derived from biologic sources, made by a semisynthetic process using a biologic source as a precursor, or produced by recombinant DNA techniques. The drugs may be large macromolecules, such as proteins, and are prone to instability and inactivation problems during processing, chemical manipulation, and storage.

Gene Therapy

Gene therapy is currently considered as a source of pharmaceutical products to produce the *in vivo* production of therapeutic proteins within somatic cells (Ledley, 1996). The therapeutic approach is the restoration of defective biologic function within cells. One example is the replacement of genetically defective gene functions in inherited disorders such as in cystic fibrosis. Three approaches (Ledley, 1996) to gene therapy have been considered. The first is a cell-based approach that involves the administration of genetically engineered cells to a patient. For example, the cells from the patient are removed; genes encoding a therapeutic product are introduced into these cells *ex vivo*, and then the cells are returned back into the patient. The second is a virus-based approach that involves the administration of genetically engineered or defective viruses to the patient. These viruses would carry therapeutic genes into the cells by the process of viral infection. The viruses themselves would not be capable of reproducing. One example that has been investigated is the use of retroviral vectors. These are RNA virions that have the ability to permanently insert their genes within the host cells. The third approach is a plasmid-based approach that involves the administration of purified DNA molecules or fragments of DNA into the cells of the patient.

Problems in gene therapy as a pharmaceutical product include the physical and chemical properties of DNA and RNA molecules including the size, shape, charge, surface characteristics, and chemical stability of these molecules. *In vivo*, problems may include bioavailability, distribution, and uptake of these macromolecules into cells. Furthermore, these molecules are rapidly degraded in the body (Ledley, 1996).

BIOTECHNOLOGY

Advances in biotechnology have resulted in the development of many naturally occurring biologically derived drugs for therapeutic use (Table 8.1). *Biotechnological products* broadly refers to biopharmaceutical drugs derived from discoveries and breakthrough in cell biology, genetics, and recombinant DNA chemistry. Some of these biologic drugs that are normally present in the body in small concentrations are now produced on a large scale by biotechnology and bioengineering. Treatments for many life-threatening diseases are now available with biotechnology products. Interferon Beta-1A (Bataseron—Berlex; Avonex—Biogen), for example, is produced by recombinant DNA techniques for the treatment of multiple sclerosis. Interferons are natural biochemical constituents consisting of proteins and glycoproteins produced by eukaryotic cells in response to viral infections and other biologic inducers. Other natural products such as cellular hormones known as *interleukins*, *lymphotoxins*, and tumor necrosis factor are under investigation to treat cancer and immune deficiency diseases. Epoetin (erythropoetin) alfa (Epogen—Amgen) is a glycoprotein that stimulates red blood cell production. New products aimed at preventing cell death/injury during a stroke include tirilazad (Freedox—Upjohn), a 21-aminosteroid antioxidant for treating strokes caused by blockages in blood vessels; selfotel (Ciba Pharmaceutical—Phase III), which blocks toxic brain

TABLE 8.1 Approved Recombinant and Other Biologic Products

DRUG	INDICATION	COMPANY (YEAR INTRODUCED)
Human insulin (Humulin)	Diabetes	Eli Lilly, Genentech (1982)
Somatrem for injection (Protropin)	hGH deficiency in children	Genentech (1985)
Interferon-α-2a (Roferon-A)	Hairy cell leukemia	Hoffmann-La Roche (1986)
Interferon-α-2b (Intron A)	Hairy cell leukemia	Schering-Plough; Biogen (1986)
Hepatitis B vaccine, MSD (Recombivax HB)	Hepatitis B prevention	Merck; Chiron (1986)
Muromonab-CD3 (Orthoclone OKT3)	Reversal of acute kidney transplant rejection	Ortho Biotech (1986)
Somatropin for injection (Humatrope)	hGH deficiency in children	Eli Lilly (1987)
Alteplase (Activase)	Acute myocardial infarction	Genetech (1987)
	Acute pulmonary embolism	(1990)
Interferon-α-2a (Roferon-A)	Aids-related Kaposi's sarcoma	Hoffmann-La Roche (1988)
Interferon-α-2b (Intron A)	Aids-related Kaposi's sarcoma	Schering-Plough, Biogen (1988)
	Genital warts	
	Hepatitis C	(1991)
Interferon-α-n3 (Alferon N injection)	Genital warts	Interferon Sciences (1989)
Hepatitis B vaccine (Engerix-B)	Hepatitis B prevention	Smith Kline Beecham; Biogen (1989)
Erythropoietin (Epogen)	Anemia associated with chronic renal failure	Amgen; Johnson & Johnson; Kirin (1989)
Erythropoietin (Procrit)	Anemia associated with AIDS/AZT	Amgen; Ortho Biotech (1990)
Erythropoietin (Procrit)	Anemia associated with chronic renal failure	Ortho Biotech (1990)
Erythropoietin (Procrit)	Chemotherapy-associated anemia in nonyloid malignancy patients	Amgen; Ortho Biotech (1993)
Erythropoietin (Procrit)	Anemia associated with cancer and chemotherapy	Ortho Biotech (1993)
PEG-adenosine	ADA-deficient SCID	Enzon; Eastman Kodak (1990)
Interferon-γ-1b (Actimmune)	Management of chronic granulomatous disease	Genentech (1990)
Alteplase (TPA) (Activase)	Acute pulmonary embolism	Genentech (1990)
CMV immune globulin (CytoGam)	CMV prevention in kidney transplant	Medimmune (1990)
Filgrastim; G-CSF (Neupogen)	Chemotherapy-induced neutropenia	Amgen (1991)
β-glucocerebrosidase (Ceredase)	Type I—Gaucher's disease	Genzyme (1991)
Glucocerebrosidase (Cerezyme)	Type I—Gaucher's disease	Genzyme (1994)

TABLE 8.1 Approved Recombinant and Other Biologic Products (continued)

DRUG	INDICATION	COMPANY (YEAR INTRODUCED)
Sargramostim (GM-CSF) (Prokine)	Autologous bone marrow transplantation	Hoechst-Roussel; Immunex (1991)
Sargramostim (GM-CSF) (Leukine)	Neutrophil recovery following bone marrow transplantation	Immunex; Hoechst-Roussel (1991)
Antihemophilic factor (Mononine)	Hemophilia B	Armour (1992)
Antihemophilic factor (Recombinate)	Hemophilia A	Genetics Institute; Baxter Healthcare (1992)
Aidesleukin (Interleukin-2) (Proleukin)	Renal cell carcinoma	Chiron (1992)
Indium-111 labeled antibody (OncoScint CR103)	Detection, staging, and follow-up of colon rectal cancer	Cytogen; Knoll (1992)
Indium-111 labeled antibody (OncoScint OV103)	Detection, staging, and follow-up of ovarian cancer	(1992)
Interferon-β (Betaseron)	Relapsing/remitting multiple sclerosis	Chiron; Berlex (1993)
DNase (Pulmozyme)	Cystic fibrosis	Genentech 1993
Factor VIII (Kogenate)	Hemophilia A	Genentech; Miles (1993)
Filgrastim (G-CSF) (Neupogen)	Bone marrow transplant	Amgen (1994)
PEG-L-asparaginase (Oncaspar)	Refractory childhood acute lymphoblastic leukemia	Enzon (1994)
Human growth hormone (Nutropin)	Short stature caused by human growth hormone deficiency	Genentech (1994)
Abciximab (ReoPro)	Antiplatelet prevention of blood clots	Centocor (1994)
Didanosine, ddl (Videx)	HIV/AIDS	Bristol-Myers Squibb (1991)
Zalcitabine, ddC (Hivid)	HIV/AIDS	Hoffmann La Roche (1992)
Lamivudine, 3 TC (Epivir)	HIV/AIDS	Glaxo Wellcome (11/1995)
Saquinavir (Invirase) Protease Inhibitor	HIV/AIDS	Hoffmann La Roche (12/1995)
Ritonavir (Norvir) Protease Inhibitor	HIV/AIDS	Abbott Laboratories (3/1996)
Indinovir (Crixivan) Protease Inhibitor	HIV/AIDS	Merck & Co, Inc. (3/1996)
Riluzole (Rilutek)	ALS (amyotrophic lateral sclerosis)	Rhône-Poulenc Rorer (12/1995)

Source: Yu and Fong, 1997, with permission

chemicals released after a stroke, and Cerestat (Cambridge NeuroScience—Phase II). Most biotechnological products must be specially delivered and be protected from enzymatic degradation. *Monoclonal antibodies (MAB)* can target and deliver toxins specifically to cancer cells and destroy them while sparing normal cells. Most of the preparations shown in Table 8.1 are delivered by intravenous, intramuscular, or subcutaneous injections. Additional biotechnology products include recombinant insulin and TPA (tissue plasmagen activator). Other products, such as human chorionic gonadotropin (hCG), recombinant erythropoietin (r-epo), atrial natriuretic factor (ANF), and adenosine deaminase (AD) are also delivered by parenteral injection.

Protein Drug Carriers

Research in immunology and cell biology have resulted in the commercialization of naturally produced active drug substances for therapy (Table 8.2). Until recently, many of these active drug substances were only produced *in vivo* in the body. Through genetic engineering these same substances have been produced *in vitro.* These substances hold great potential for more specific drug action with fewer side effects. However, several limitations must be overcome for the commercial production of these natural substances into drug dosage forms in order to provide reliable systemic bioavailability. Many naturally produced substances are complex molecules, such as large molecular weight proteins and peptides. In addition to the primary and secondary bonds that hold the amino acids together, tertiary and quaternary bonds are involved in keeping the protein chains together in preferred configurations. A change in quaternary structure, such as aggregation or deaggregation of the protein, may result in loss of activity. Therefore, extreme temperatures or oxidation can inactivate these drugs.

TABLE 8.2 Examples of Protein/Peptide Drugs

Interferon alpha-2a (Roferon-A)
Purified protein (MW about 19,000 d); prepared by recombinant DNA, stabilized with human serum albumin for hairless cell leukemia

Interferon alpha-2b (Intron-A)
For hairy cell leukemia treatment

Human growth hormone (Protropin)
For treatment of hormonal disorder

Human insulin (Humulin L)
Prepared by recombinant DNA technique using genetically altered *Escherichia coli*

Orthoclone OKT-3
Monoclonal antibody for kidney rejection

Vasopressin (Pitressin)
Synthetic vasopressin of the pituitary gland

Superoxide dismutase
Investigated for a variety of uses including infarction and shocks

Human epidermal growth factor
Investigated for treatment of skin disorders

Tissue plasmogen activator (TPA)
Potent blood clot dissolver produced by recombinant DNA technique

Erythropoietin
For the treatment of anemia associated with uremia

Common chemical inactivation reactions include deamidation of the amino acid chains, oxidation of chains with sulfhydryl groups, and cleavage by proteolytic enzymes that are present due to incomplete purification. Because of their complex structures, impurities are much harder to detect and quantify. Stability is a major consideration in formulating these drugs. Another problem with this carrier is the immunogenicity of many biologic proteins. Proteins may be recognized as foreign substances in the body and become actively phagocytized by the reticuloendothelial system (RES), resulting in the inability of these proteins to reach the intended target. Moreover, proteins have a high allergenic potential due to their antigenicity.

Monoclonal Antibodies

The formation of a monoclonal antibody (MAB) is one of the most powerful techniques for incorporating a drug into a *site-specific system*. Theoretically, an endless number of antibodies can be formed by inducing the body with suitable antigens. Nonprotein material or haptens may be conjugated to a protein to form an antigen. A large number of immunoassays for the specific analysis of low concentrations of drugs have been produced based on this immunologic principle. However, the techniques for the preparation of monoclonal antibodies are quite complicated.

Monoclonal antibodies are highly specific and recognize only one antigenic determinant or receptor site. This specific recognition provides an advantage over natural antibodies, which have both general (nonspecific) and specific binding affinities because natural antibodies are produced by clusters of cells. Antibodies are commonly isolated from the serum of an animal that has been stimulated for antibody production with periodic injections of an antigen. In monoclonal production, genetic engineering techniques are used to fuse a normal antibody-producing cell, such as a spleen cell, with a myeloma cell, allowing the hybrid cell to grow in a test tube. The nonfused cell will die, whereas the myeloma cell will be selectively destroyed with an antitumor drug such as aminopterin (Fig. 8-1). The resulting cell can then be cloned to produce many copies of itself for antibody production. Because all the cells originated from the same cell, the antibodies produced are specific. MABs are useful as drug delivery carriers and have therapeutic uses (Table 8.3).

Monoclonal antibody research holds great promise in the development of highly active drugs, such as cancer chemotherapeutic agents, that can be targeted to specific tissues while avoiding other tissues and reducing side effects. Properly applied, these techniques can improve the therapeutic index of many toxic drugs. However, MABs have not been the "magic bullet" many people had hoped for. One of the difficulties encountered is that the large molecule reduces the amount of active drug that can be easily dosed (ie, the ratio of drug to carrier). In contrast, conventional carriers that are not specific are often many orders of magnitude smaller in size, and a larger dose may be given more efficiently.

Some progress has been made. For example, a human IgM monoclonal antibody (HA-1A, Nebacumab) with specificity for the lipid A site of endotoxin was designed for septic shock treatment. The apparent volume of distribution at steady state (Romano-MJ, 1993) is small (0.11 ± 0.03 L/kg), possibly the result of specific targeting restricting random tissue distribution. The cytotoxic recombinant ricin A chain has been coupled to the monoclonal antibodies (Muraszko, 1993) specific for the human (454A12) transferrin receptors and evaluated in monkeys for targeted delivery and therapy in leptomeningeal carcinomatosis. The apparent vol-

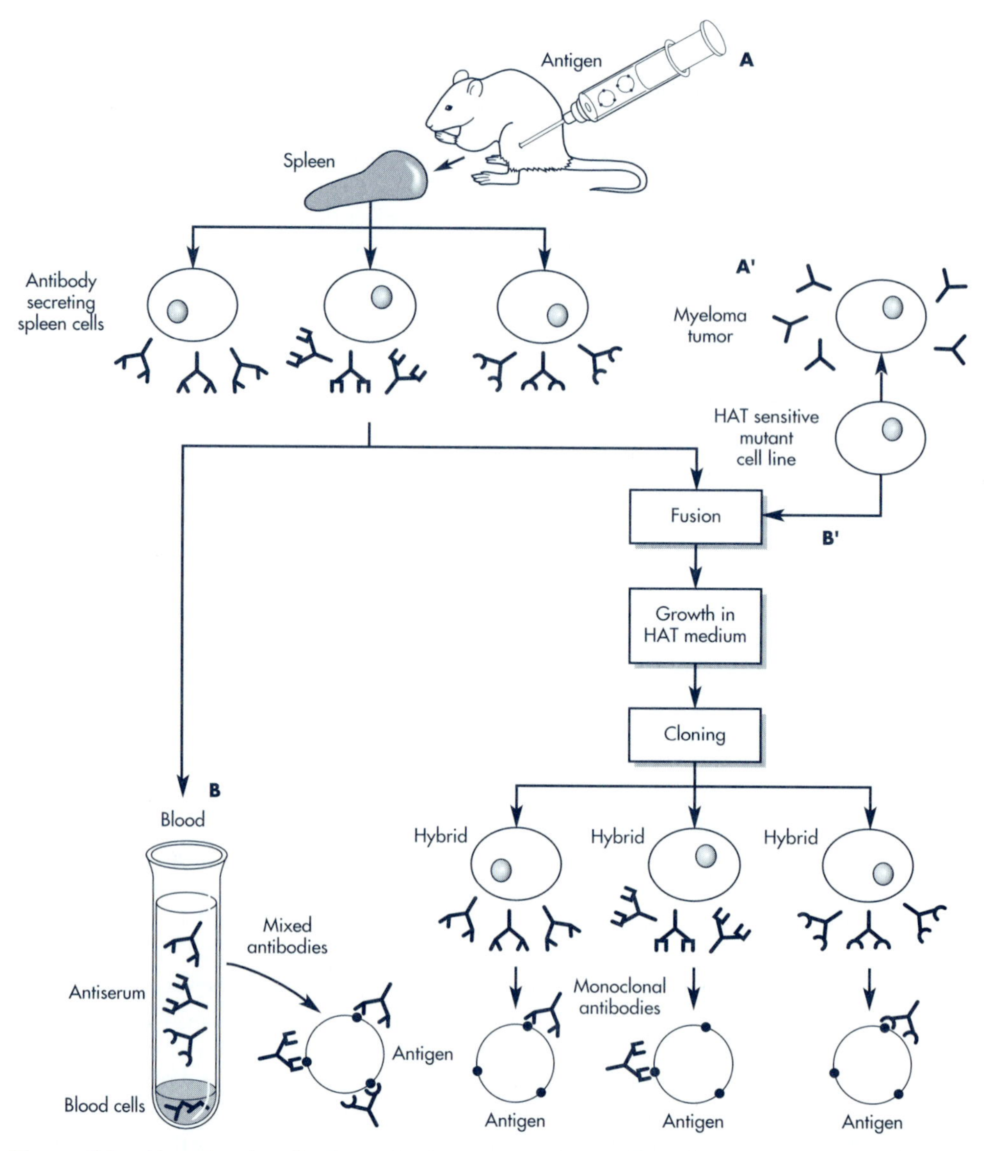

Figure 8-1. Monoclonal antibody production. **A.** A mouse is immunized with an antigen-bearing three antigenic determinants (distinct sites that can be recognized by an antibody). Antibodies to each determinant are produced in the spleen. One spleen cell produces a single type of antibody. A spleen cell has a finite lifetime and cannot be cultured indefinitely *in vitro*. **B.** In the mouse, the antibody-producing cells from the spleen secrete into the blood. The liquid portion of the blood (serum) therefore contains a mixture of antibodies reacting with all three sites on the antigen (antiserum). **A′.** A mutant cell derived from a mouse myeloma tumor of an antibody-producing cell that has stopped secreting antibody and is selected for sensitivity to the drug aminopterin (present in HAT medium). This mutant tumor cell can grow indefinitely *in vitro* but is killed by HAT medium. **B′.** The mutant myeloma cell is fused by chemical means with spleen cells from an immunized mouse. The resulting hybrid cells can grow indefinitely *in vitro* due to properties of the myeloma cell parent and can grow in HAT medium because of an enzyme provided by the spleen cell parent. The unfused myeloma cells die because of their sensitivity to HAT, and unfused spleen cells cannot grow indefinitely *in vitro*. The hybrid cells are cloned so that individual cultures are grown from a single hybrid cell. These individual cells produce a single type of antibody because they derive from a single spleen cell. The monoclonal antibody isolated from these cultures is specific for only one antigenic determinant on the original antigen. (From Milstein C. Sci Amer **243**(3):66–74, 1980 and Brodsky FM, Pharm Res **5**(1):1–9, 1988, with permission.)

TABLE 8.3 Applications of Monoclonal Antibodies

Cancer Treatment
MABS against leukemia and lymphomas have been used in treatment with variable results. Regression of tumor is produced in about 25%, although mostly transient.
Imaging Diagnosis
MABS may be used together with radioactive markers to locate and visualize the extent of the tumors.
Target-Specific Delivery
MABS may be conjugated to drugs to allow specific delivery to target sites. For example, urokinase was investigated for incorporation into an antifibrin MAB to dissolve fibrin clots. The carrier system would seek fibrin sites and activate the conversion of plasmogen to plasmin to cause fibrin to degrade.
Transplant Rejection Suppression
In kidney transplants, a MAB against CD3, a protein of cytotoxic T cells that causes rejection reaction, was found to be very useful in suppressing rejection and allowing the transplant to function. The drug was called OKT3. MAB uses were also reported for bone marrow transplants.

ume of distribution was 10.1 mL, or approximately three-fourths the total CSF volume of the monkey. The adverse side effects were moderate and reversible with time. There was evidence of minimal inflammation within the CSF, and there were no signs of systemic toxicity.

A common problem is the potential for immunogenic response elicited by the carrier or its derivative that may limit the drug for single use only. In addition, drug delivery is slow and variable in many cases. Cancer cells often have changed receptors, causing difficulties for such systems.

Still, the technology is only beginning to show its impact, and new research may overcome some of the current limitations in future. Several monoclonal antibodies with proven indications are listed in Table 8.1. ReoPro is a monoclonal antibody that targets the platelet specifically, with great promise for site-specific delivery of biological substances, particularly in cancer chemotherapy.

1. Zolimomab aritox (Orthozyme-CD5, Xoma/Ortho Biotech)

Zolimomab aritox is an immunoconjugate of monoclonal antiCD5 murine IgG and the ricin A-chain toxin. It is used in the treatment of steroid-resistant graft-versus-host disease after *allogeneic bone marrow transplants* for hematopoietic neoplasms, such as acute myelogenous leukemia.

2. Abciximab (c7E3 Fab)

Abciximab (c7E3 Fab) is a chimeric monoclonal antibody Fab fragment specific for platelet glycoprotein IIb-IIIa receptors. This drug was recently tested and found to be extremely effective in reducing fatalities (>50%) in subjects with unstable angina after angioplasty treatment.

3. Campath-1

Campath-1 are monoclonal antibodies which target human lymphocytes and monocytes. It is used for immunosuppression in organ transplants. Campath-1 have also been used to treat refractory autoimmune disorders, including rheumatoid arthritis and vasculitis experimentally.

4. Edobacomab

Edobacomab is an immune globulin directed against gram-negative bacterial endotoxins. For septic shock, single doses of 2 to 15 mg/kg intravenously every 24 hours have been used. The volume of distribution of Edobacomab ranges from 4 to 8 L and the elimination half-life is approximately 10 to 18 hours.

5. Muromonab-CD3

Muromonab-CD3 is an immunosuppressive agent with specific targeting. Muromonab-CD3 was demonstrated to be effective in reversing acute renal allograft rejection. The volume of distribution is approximately 6.5 L and the half-life is 18 hours.

6. Nebacumab

Nebacumab is an immune globulin directed against gram-negative bacterial endotoxins. The drug is being investigated for the treatment of gram-negative sepsis and septic shock. Its half-life is 15.9 hours and the volume of distribution is 48.5 mL/kg.

7. Satumomab

Satumomab pendetide is a monoclonal antibody conjugate produced from the murine monoclonal antibody B72.3. It is used as a diagnostic imaging agent in the staging of patients with known colorectal and ovarian carcinoma.

Antisense Drugs

Many diseases occur as a result of genetic defects or errors in the gene involved in producing essential enzymes or proteins in the body. Genetic information resides in chromosomes housing helical strands known as deoxyribonucleic acid (DNA) within the nucleus. The Human Genome Initiative was created several years ago to study all human genes. This national effort is now yielding information on many serious diseases involving congenital defects, cancer, AIDS, infection, and disorders involving the immune system. Strategies are now available to alter or block the transcriptional process in the DNA in order to moderate many disease processes. By altering the DNA sequence so that the complementary strand is transcribed instead of the normal "sense" gene, the DNA would not be able to make a copy of normal RNA which participates in protein synthesis. The aberrant copies of RNA may "pair up" (hybridize) with other RNAs that complement it and block protein synthesis. The process of targeting DNA or RNA using this technique is called *antisense* drug. Many oligonucleotides have been designed to target viral disease and cancer cells in the body. To further stabilize the drug, phosphodiesters are substituted with phosphothioates. Antisense drugs against HIV-1 as well as cytomegalovirus (CMV) infecting the eyes of AIDS victims are now in various phases of clinical trial.

When a gene's nucleotide base sequence that controls a specific body function is known, the antisense DNA strand can be synthesized. Such strands can then be introduced into cells where they attach themselves to the complementary sense DNA strands, thereby depressing transcription of these genes. This has been done successfully in cell culture, for the cancer-causing gene that produces human larynx squamous carcinoma.

If a duplicate copy of a gene is inserted into a chromosome in reverse orientation to the normal gene, the antisense DNA strand of this gene is transcribed. This yields an antisense messenger RNA strand that is complementary to the mRNA strand transcribed for the normal gene. The two RNAs, being complementary, bind to each other, thereby preventing the translation of the normal RNA strand which may control protein synthesis.

Albumin

A large protein (MW 69,000 d) distributed in the plasma and extracellular water, albumin has been experimentally conjugated with many drugs to improve site-specific drug delivery. Methotrexate, cytosine arabinoside, and 6-fluorodeoxyuridine have been conjugated respectively with albumin. Methotrexate albumin conjugates may increase the duration of drug action after conjugation (Chu and Whiteley, 1980). In general, the distribution of albumin is not site specific. Because albumin will concentrate in the liver, 5-fluorodeoxyuridine (Amanitin) albumin complex has been used to deliver drug to the Kupffer cells in the liver for treatment of ectromelia virus experimentally (Fiume et al, 1983).

Glycoproteins

Large molecules of protein and sacharrides, glycoproteins are not specific carriers but may be modified to have site-specific properties by the removal of the sugar group. For example, the removal of the sialo group resulted in the asialoglycoproteins that are recognized by various hepatocytes. Galactosyl-terminated fetuin (asialofetuin) has been investigated for potential use to deliver drug for hepatitis treatment (Fiume et al, 1982).

Lipoproteins

Lipoproteins are lipid protein complexes in the blood involved in the circulation and distribution of lipids in the body. The lipid components are polar phospholipids and cholesterol. Because of their various sizes, lipoproteins have been classified according to molecular weight based on centrifugation: (1) high-density lipoprotein (HDL, MW 300,000 to 600,000), (2) low-density lipoprotein (LDL, MW 2.3×10^6), and (3) very-low-density lipoprotein (VLDL, MW 10×10^6), and (4) chylomicrons (MW 10^9).

Low-density lipoproteins enter the cell by a receptor-mediated pathway through the process of *endocytosis*. Endocytosis is a potential means of transporting drugs into the cell in which the lipoprotein–drug complex is hydrolyzed by intracellular lysosomal enzymes, releasing the active drug.

More research is needed on the use of lipoproteins for drug targeting. For example, lipophilic drugs may be dissolved within the core of the lipoprotein. After oral administration, fatty substances incorporated into the chylomicron formed in the GI tract may be absorbed into the lymphatic system.

Dextrans and Polysaccharides

Dextrans are large polysaccharide molecules with good water solubility, stability, and low toxicity. Various molecular weight dextran fractions (MW 2000 to 1 million) are commercially available. Drugs with a free amino or hydroxyl group may be linked chemically to hydroxyl groups in dextrans by activation of the dextran with periodate, azide, or other agents. For example, daunomycin has been linked to dextran, resulting in improved drug activity in animal studies (Arnon, 1982; Arnon and Hurwitz, 1983). A targeted mitomycin C and a monoclonal antibody (A7) using dextran (MW 70,000) as the intermediate carrier resulted in a 10-fold increased activity against colon cancer cells due to improved target specificity. No *in vivo* test was performed (Joshi, 1988).

Deoxyribonucleic Acid

Deoxyribonucleic acid (DNA) has been used as a drug carrier involving anticancer drugs, such as daunorubicin and adriamycin. DNA drug conjugates gain entry into the cell through endocytosis. Different types of cells exhibit different endocytic activity, thereby allowing differential drug delivery. The reduced adverse effect of DNA daunorubicin conjugate was attributed to reduced myocardiac endocytosis and uptake of the drug compared to other cells. Reduced toxic effect allows a higher dose of daunorubicin to be administered compared to the free drug (Friend and Pangburn, 1987). Inside the cell, the DNA–drug complex in the presence of lysozyme, hydrolyzes the complex and releases the active drug. To improve efficacy, these drugs must be given locally or must be injected into the fluids flowing to the target. This method of drug administration may be required because DNA–drug complexes are actively taken up by the reticuloendothelial system.

Polymeric Drugs

Polymers have been used to prolong drug release in controlled-release dosage forms. The development of site-specific polymer or macromolecular carrier systems is a more recent extension of earlier research. The basic components of site-specific polymer carriers are (1) the polymeric backbone (Fig. 8-2), (2) a site-specific component (*homing device*) for recognizing the target, (3) the drug covalently attached to the polymer chain, and (4) functional chains to enhance the physical characteristics of the carrier system. Improved physical characteristics might include improved aqueous solubility. In the case of polymeric prodrugs, a *spacer* group may be present, bridging the drug and the carrier. The spacer chain may influence the rate at which the drug will hydrolyze from the prodrug system. At present, most site-specific polymeric drug carriers are limited to parenteral administration. Therefore, soluble polymers are advantageous.

Some commonly used polymers include poly(L-lysine), a homopolymer with repeating units of L-lysine; and polyglutamic acid (Fig. 8-3). For example, cisplatin was shown to have an improved therapeutic efficacy against murine carcinoma in mice when complexed to poly-L-glutamic acid (Schechter et al, 1987). Dextrans and poly-*N*-(2-hydroxypropyl) methacrylamide (HPMA) of about 25,000 d in molecular weight were also used as carrier (Joshi, 1988). The molecular weight of the polymer carrier is an important consideration in designing these dosage forms. Generally, large molecular weight polymers have longer residence time and diffuse more slowly. However, large polymers are also more prone to capture by the reticuloendothelial system. To gain specificity, a monoclonal antibody or a recognized sugar moiety may be incorporated into the system. The site-specific drugs discussed earlier are all candidates for inclusion. The site-recognition unit may also be a small cell-specific ligand.

For example, exposed galactose residues are recognized by hepatocytes; whereas with mannose or L-fructose in unreduced forms, exposed residues are recognized by surface receptors in macrophages. Insoluble polymers are used either as regu-

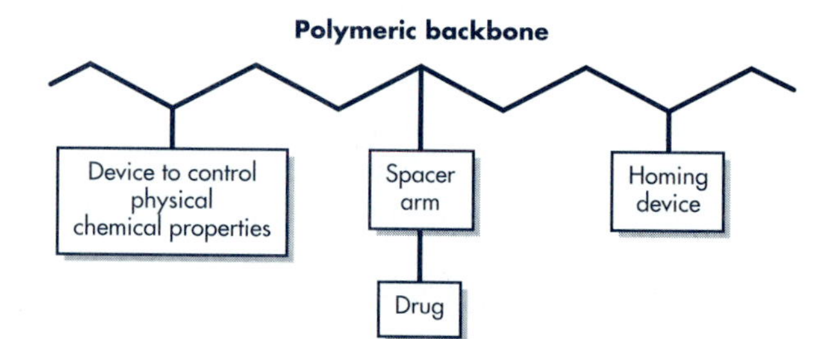

Figure 8-2. Site-specific polymeric carrier.

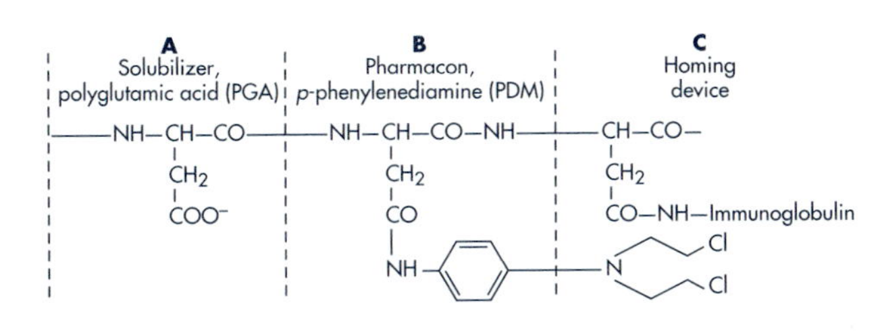

Figure 8-3. A = solubilizer, IG = immunoglobulin; polyglutamic acid [PGA]; B = Pharmacon, p-phenylenediamine [PDM]; C = homing device.
(Adapted from Gros et al, 1981.)

lar carriers or formulated into microparticles and nanoparticles. For example, 5-fluorouracil was formulated using polygluteraldehyde (PGL) into 450-nm nanospheres and administered to rats (Mukherji et al, 1987). Nanoparticles can be loaded with a high proportion of drug. The disadvantages of these systems are the high retention of the polymer complex in the reticuloendothelial system. Particles less than 0.5 μm (500 nm) move through the liver endothelial cells and deposit into the spleen and bone marrow. At 7 to 12 μm, particles are mechanically filtered by the lung. From 2 to 12 μm, particles are retained at the lung, spleen, or liver. At over 12 μm, particles will be lodged in the capillary bed at the site of the injection. Insoluble polymeric carriers are not easily disposed of by the body, unlike biodegradable polymer complexes. Administration of a large amount of insolute polymers may result in a disposal problem as most of the particles are engulfed by macrophages.

Liposomes

Bilayer microlipid vesicles with an aqueous interior surrounded by an exterior lipid bilayer, liposomes typically range from 0.5 to 100 μm. Formation of the liposome bilayer depends on the hydrophobic and hydrophilic orientation of the lipids (Fig. 8-4). Liposomes have different electrical surface charges dependent upon the type of material used. Common lipid materials are phosphatidyl choline and cholesterol. The phosphatidyl group is amphophilic with the choline being the polar group. This structure allows each molecule to attach to others through hydrophobic and hydrophilic interaction. Thermodynamically, liposomes are in equilibrium because of possible conversion to another form (lipid polymorphism). Thus, some seemingly stable liposome systems have leakage and generally do not have long shelf-lives. Some liposomes have reduced adverse effects and improved drug delivery when formulated with drugs. However, only a few liposomes are site specific.

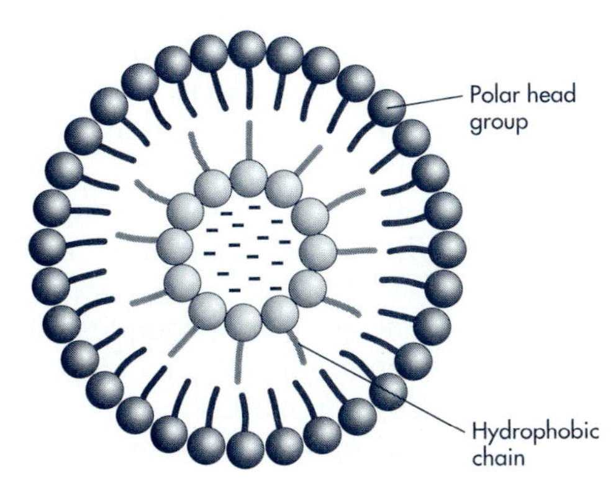

Figure 8-4. Diagrammatic representation of a liposome showing polar head group and hydrophobic chain.

Generally, site specificity is conferred by the type of lipid. Liposomes have been used successfully to reduce side effects of antitumor drugs and antibiotics. For example, doxorubicin liposomes have reduced cardiotoxicity and emetic side effects. Amphotericin B may have reduced nephrotoxicity side effects when formulated with liposomes. Liposome formulations have been prepared with gentamicin, cisplatin, and other drugs.

There are three general ways of preparing liposomes: (1) phase separation, (2) spray or shear method through orifice, and (3) coacervation. The choice of the method depends on the drug, the yield requirements, and the nature of the lipids. An innovative liposome-related product (Abelcet), amphotericin B, lipid complex with two phospholipids, L-α-dimyristoyl-phosphatidylcholine and L-α-dimyristoylphosphatidylglycerol, was developed by the Liposome Company. The lipid drug complex releases the drug at the site of infection and reduces renal toxicity of amphotericin B without altering its antifungal activity. Other liposomal products include TLC-C-53 (liposomal prostaglandin E1) for the treatment of acute respiratory distress syndrome (ARDS). TLC D-99, liposomal doxorubicin, is designed to target to tumor cells and spare healthy tissue, maintaining efficacy while reducing toxicity, particularly irreversible heart damage. TLC D-99 is on clinical trial against metastatic breast cancer (MBC). A more representative liposome product is AmBisome (NeXstar) which consists of very fine liposomes of amphotericin B. The product significantly reduces the side effects of amphotericin B.

Daunorubicin is an antineoplastic agent. Daunorubicin citrate liposomal (DaunoXome-NeXstar) is an aqueous solution of the citrate salt of daunorubicin encapsulated within lipid vesicles (liposomes) composed of a bilayer of distearoylphosphotidylcholine and cholesterol (2:1 molar ratio). The liposomal formulation attempts to maximize the selectivity of daunorubicin into solid brain tumors. Once in the tumor, daunorubicin is released and exerts its antineoplastic activity.

Formulation and Delivery of Protein Drugs

Conventional delivery of protein and peptide drugs is generally limited to injectables and implantable dosage forms. Insulin pumps for implantation have been developed for diabetes for precise control of sugar levels. Other conventional routes of protein drug administration include nasal, pulmonary, ocular, and rectal administration. Formulating protein drugs for systemic use by oral administration is extremely difficult due to instability and other delivery problems.

There are several requirements for effective oral drug delivery of protein and peptide drugs: (1) protection of the drug from degradation while in the harsh environment of the digestive tract, (2) consistent absorption of the drug in a manner that meets bioavailability requirements, (3) consistent release of the drug so that it enters the bloodstream in a reproducible manner, (4) nontoxicity, and (5) delivery of the drug through the GI tract and maintenance of its pharmacological effect similar to injecting.

Most approaches for oral formulation have not met all the requirements mentioned above. Some interesting protein delivery studies have been reported by researchers at Emisphere involving the Proteinoid Oral Drug Delivery System (PODDS). Researchers there have reported that protein drugs may be complexed with "prebiotic proteinoid" (apparently derived from prebiotic amino acid reaction mixtures) and may be absorbed when administered orally to animals. The protein drugs were not degraded during absorption. Studies have reported absorption in rats and in primates of various protein drugs including recombinant human growth hormone (rhGH), heparin, and interferon-a2b. In some cases, the drugs were encapsulated in derivatized amino acid microspheres and absorbed. Acylated amino acids were reported to be effective delivery agents for rhIFN, which appear to create a noncovalent complex between the delivery agent and the protein with physicochemical properties favorable for absorption from the gastrointestinal tract.

Oral Immunization

Antigens or fragmented antigenic protein may be delivered orally and stimulate gut-associated lymphoid tissue (GALT) in the gastrointestinal tract. This represents a promising approach for protecting many secretory surfaces against a variety of infectious pathogens. Immunization against salmonella and *E. coli* in chickens was investigated for agricultural purpose. Particulate antigen delivery systems, including several types of microspheres, have been shown to be effective at orally inducing various types of immune responses. Encapsulation of antigens with mucosal adjuvants can protect both the antigen and the adjuvant against gastric degradation and increase the likelihood that they will reach the site of absorption.

BIOEQUIVALENCE OF BIOTECHNOLOGY PRODUCTS

The dosage form or formulation of a drug product may change during the course of drug development. The initial drug formulation used in early clinical studies (eg, phase I/II) may not be the same formulation as the drug formulation used in later clinical trials (phase IV) or the marketed formulation. The demonstration of the bioequivalence of biotechnology products may be difficult (Mordenti et al, 1996). (See Chapter 10 for discussion on bioequivalence.) Some of the problems encountered include:

1. Subject selection—There may be a potential risk in exposing normal subjects to these potent biotechnologic drugs.
2. Endogenous concentration and drug analysis—Many of the biotechnologically derived drugs are normal endogenous compounds. The concentrations of the endogenous compounds in the body may vary substantially. The drug concentrations may be very low, and assay methods may lack the sensitivity and specificity to measure reliably. Thus, an adequate pharmacokinetic profile after administration of the biotechnology-derived drug product may be difficult to obtain.
3. Pharmacodynamic equivalence—Since drug concentrations for these products cannot be measured directly, a comparison of the pharmacodynamics of the drug products need to be employed. The pharmacodynamic measurement might be an *in vivo* response after drug administration or possibly the measurement of an *in vitro* response using tissue culture or biochemical endpoint.

The United States Food and Drug Administration (FDA) issued a guidance, *Concerning Demonstration of Comparability of Human Biological Products, Including Therapeutic Biotechnology-Derived Products* (April, 1996), recognizing that changes in the manufacturing process, equipment, or facilities could result in changes in the biologic product itself and sometimes require additional clinical studies to demonstrate the product's safety, identity, purity, and potency. The FDA advocates that for any manufacturing change, a *comparability* testing program including a combination of analytical testing, biologic assays (*in vitro* or *in vivo*), pharmacokinetic, pharmacodynamic, or toxicity assessment. Thus, for any manufacturing change, extensive chemical, physical, and bioactivity comparisons with side-by-side analyses of the "old" product and qualification lots of the "new" product are required.

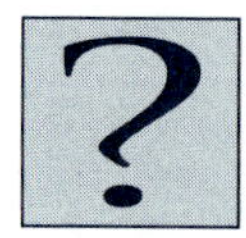

FREQUENTLY ASKED QUESTIONS

1. What is the most frequent route of administration of biologic compounds?
2. What is the effect of glycosylation on the activity of biologic compound? Give an example.
3. What are the major differences in drug distribution and elimination between conventional molecules and biotechnological compounds?
4. What is meant by targeted drug delivery? How does gene therapy differ from targeted drug delivery?
5. Why are macromolecular carrier systems used for targeted drug delivery?
6. What are monoclonal antibodies? What advantages do monoclonal antibodies have as carriers for site-specific drug delivery.

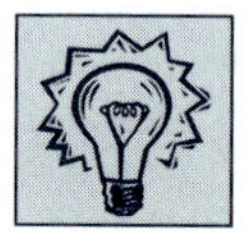

LEARNING QUESTIONS

1. Explain why most drugs produced by biotechnology cannot be given orally. What routes of drug administration would you recommend for these drugs? Why?
2. What is meant by site-specific drug delivery? Describe several approaches that have been used to target a drug to a specific organ.
3. Doxorubicin (Adriamycin) is available as a conventional solution and as a liposomal preparation. What effect would the liposomal preparation have on the distribution of doxorubicin compared to an injection of the conventional doxorubicin injection?

REFERENCES

Arnon R: In Gregoriadis G, Senior J, Trouet A (eds), *Targeting of Drugs*. New York, Plenum, 1982, pp 31–54

Arnon R, Hurwitz E: In Goldberg EP (ed), *Targeted Drugs*. New York, Wiley, 1983, pp 23–55

Bodmeier R, Oh KH, Chen H: The effect of the addition of low molecular weight poly(DL-lactide) on drug release from biodegradable poly(DL-lactide) drug delivery systems. *Int J Pharm* **51:**1–8, 1989

Breimer DD, Dauhof M: *Towards Better Safety of Drugs and Pharmaceutical Products.* Amsterdam, Elsevier/North-Holland, 1980, pp 117–142

Brester ME, Hora MS, Simpkins JW, Bodor N: Use of 2-hydroxypropyl-β-cyclodextrin as a solubilizing and stabilizing excipient for protein drugs. *Pharm Res* **8:**792–795, 1991

Chu BCF, Whiteley JM: High molecular weight derivatives of methotrexate as chemotherapeutic agents. *Mol Pharm* **13:**80, 1980

Dighe SV, Adams WP: Bioavailability and bioequivalence of oral controlled-release products: A regulatory perspective. In Welling PG, Tse FLS (eds), *Pharmacokinetics: Regulatory, Industrial, Academic Perspectives.* New York, Marcel Dekker, 1988

Eckhardt BM, Oeswein JQ, Bewley TA: Effect of freezing on aggregation of human growth hormone. *Pharm Res* **8:**1360–1364, 1991

Emisphere literature: Mucosal immunization with derivatized μ- and non-μ-amino acid delivery agents. Presented at the American Association of Pharmaceutical Scientists (AAPS) Annual Meeting, Seattle, WA, October, 1996

Emisphere literature: Oral delivery of interferon in rats and primates. Presented at the American Association of Pharmaceutical Scientists (AAPS) Annual Meeting, San Diego, CA, 1994. *Pharm Res* **11**(10):S-298, 1994

Fiume L, Busi C, Mattioli A: Targeting of antiviral drugs by coupling with protein carriers. *FEBS Lett* **153:**6, 1983

Fiume L, Busi C, Mattioli A, et al: In Gregoriadis G, Senior J, Trouet A (eds), *Targeting of Drugs.* New York, Plenum, 1982

Friend DR, Pangburn S: Site-specific drug delivery. *Med Res Rev* **7:**53–106, 1987

Galeone M, Nizzola L, Cacioli D, Moise G: *In vivo* demonstration of delivery mechanisms from sustained-release pellets. *Curr Ther Res* **29:**217–234, 1981

Gros L, Ringsdorf H, Schupp H: *Angew Chem Int Ed Engl* **20:**312, 1981

Jensen-JD; Jensen-LW; Madsen-JK; Poulsen-L: The metabolism of erythropoietin in liver cirrhosis patients compared with healthy volunteers. *Eur J Haematol* **54**(2):111–116, 1995

Joshi HN: Recent advances in drug delivery systems: Polymeric prodrugs. *Pharm Technol:* **12:**118–125, 1988

Le-Cotonnec JY, Porchet-HC et al: Comprehensive pharmacokinetics of urinary human follicle stimulating hormone in healthy female volunteers. *Pharm Res* **12**(6): 844–850, 1995

Ledley, FD: Pharmaceutical approaches to somatic cell therapy. *Pharm Res* **13:**1595–1614, 1996

Lee VH, Hashida M, Mizushima Y: *Trends and Future Perspectives in Peptide and Protein Drug Development.* Langhorne, PA, Harwood Academic, 1995

Molema G, de Leij LFMH, Meijer DKE: Tumor vascular endothelium: Barrier or target in tumor directed drug delivery and immunotherapy. *Pharm Res* **14:**2–10, 1997

Mordenti J, Cavagnaro JA, Green JD: Design of biological equivalence programs for therapeutic biotechnology products in clinical development: A perspective. *Pharm Res* **13:**1427–1437, 1996

Romano-MJ, Kearns-GL, Kaplan-SL, et al: Single-dose pharmacokinetics and safety of HA-1A, a human IgM anti-lipid-A monoclonal antibody, in pediatric patients with sepsis syndrome. *J Pediatr* **122**(6):974–984, 1993

Salmonson T, Danielson BG, Wikstrom B: The pharmacokinetics of recombinant erythropoietin after intravenous and subcutaneous administration to healthy subjects. *Br J Clin Pharm,* **29:**709, 1990

Sobel BE, et al: Coronary thrombolysis with facilitated absorption of intramuscular injected tissue-type plasminogen activator. *Proc Natl Acad Sci USA* **82:**4258, 1985

Takakura Y, Hashida M: Macromolecular carrier systems for targeted drug delivery: Pharmacokinetic considerations on biodistribution. *Pharm Res* **13:**820–831, 1996

Yu ABC, Fong GW: Biotechnologic products. In Shargel et al. (eds) *Comprehensive Pharmacy Review,* 3rd ed. Baltimore, Williams & Wilkins, 1997, chap 10

BIBLIOGRAPHY

Akala EO, Collett JH: Influence of drug loading and gel structure on in-vitro release kinetics from photopolymerized gels. *Indust Pharm* **13:**1779–1798, 1987

Bayley H, Gasparro F, Edelson R: Photoactive drugs. *TIPS* **8:**138–144, 1987

Body A, Aarons L: Pharmacokinetic and pharmacodynamic aspects of site specific drug delivery. *Adv Drug Deliv Rev* **3:**155–163, 1989

Borchardt RT, Repta AJ, Stella VJ (eds): *Directed Drug Delivery.* Clifton, NJ, Humana, 1985

Boxenbaum HG: Physiological and pharmacokinetic factors affecting performance of sustained release dosage forms. *Drug Dev Indust Pharm* **8:**1–25, 1982

Brodsky FM: Monoclonal antibodies as magic bullets. *Pharm Res* **5:**1–9, 1988

Bruck S (ed): *CRC Controlled Drug Delivery.* Boca Raton, CRC Press, 1983

Chien YW: *Novel Drug Delivery Systems.* New York, Marcel Dekker, 1982

Heller J: Controlled drug release from monolithic bioerodible polymer devices. *Pharm Int* **7:**316–318, 1986

Langer R: New methods of drug delivery. Science **249:**1527–1533, 1990

Levy G: Targeted drug delivery: Some pharmacokinetic considerations. *Pharm Res* **4:**3–4, 1987

Oeswein JA: Formulation considerations in polypeptide delivery. Presented at Biotech 87. Pinner, UK, Online Publications, 1987

Ostro MJ: *Liposome: From Biophysics to Therapeutics.* New York, Marcel Dekker, 1987

Park H, Robinson JR: Mechanisms of mucoadhesion of poly(acrylic acid) hydrogels. *Pharm Res* **4:**457–464, 1987

Pozansky MJ, Juliano RL: Biological approaches to the controlled delivery of drugs: A critical review. *Pharmacol Rev* **36:**277–336, 1984

Robinson JR: Oral drug delivery systems. In *Proceedings of 1982 Research and Scientific Development Conference.* Washington, DC, The Proprietary Association, 1983, pp 54–69

Rodwell JD (ed): *Antibody Mediated Delivery Systems,* New York, Marcel Dekker, 1988

Silverman HS, Becker LC, Siddoway LA, et al: Pharmacokinetics of human recombinant superoxide dismutase. *J Am Coll Cardiol* **11:**164A, 1988

Spenlehauer G, Vert M, Benoit JP, et al: Biodegradable cisplatin microspheres prepared by the solvent evaporation method: Morphology and release characteristics. *J Control Release* **7:**217–229, 1988

9

PHARMACOKINETICS OF ORAL ABSORPTION

PHARMACOKINETICS OF DRUG ABSORPTION

The systemic absorption of a drug from the gastrointestinal (GI) tract or any other extravascular site is dependent on the physicochemical properties of the drug, the dosage form used, and the anatomy and physiology of the absorption site. Such factors as surface area of the gut, stomach-emptying rate, GI mobility, and blood flow to the absorption site all affect the rate and the extent of drug absorption. In spite of these variations, the overall rate of drug absorption may be described mathematically as a first-order or zero-order input process. Most pharmacokinetic models assume first-order absorption unless an assumption of zero-order absorption improves the model significantly or has been verified experimentally.

The rate of change in the amount of drug in the body, dD_B/dt, is dependent on the rates of drug absorption and elimination (Fig. 9-1).

The rate of drug accumulation in the body at any time is equal to the rate of drug absorption less the rate of drug elimination.

$$\frac{dD_B}{dt} = \frac{dD_{GI}}{dt} - \frac{dD_e}{dt} \tag{9.1}$$

A plasma level–time curve showing drug adsorption and elimination rate processes is given in Figure 9-2. During the *absorption phase* of a plasma level–time curve (Fig. 9–2), the rate of drug absorption is greater than the rate of drug elimination.

$$\frac{dD_{GI}}{dt} > \frac{dD_e}{dt} \tag{9.2}$$

At the *time of peak drug concentration* in the plasma, which corresponds to the time of peak absorption in Figure 9-2, the rate of drug absorption just equals the rate of drug elimination, and there is no change in the amount of drug in the body.

$$\frac{dD_{GI}}{dt} = \frac{dD_e}{dt} \tag{9.3}$$

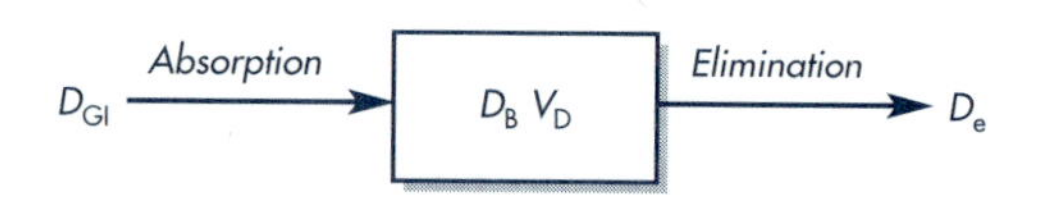

Figure 9-1. Model of drug absorption and elimination.

Immediately after the time of peak drug absorption, some drug may still be at the absorption site (ie, in the GI tract). However, the rate of drug elimination is, at this time, faster than the rate of absorption, as represented by the *postabsorption phase* in Figure 9-2.

$$\frac{dD_{GI}}{dt} < \frac{dD_e}{dt} \tag{9.4}$$

When the drug at the absorption site becomes depleted, the rate of drug absorption approaches zero, or $dD_{GI}/dt = 0$. The *elimination phase* of the curve then represents only the elimination of drug from the body, usually a first-order process. Therefore, during the elimination phase the rate of change in the amount of drug in the body is described as a first-order process.

$$\frac{dD_B}{dt} = -kD_B \tag{9.5}$$

where k is the first-order elimination rate constant.

ZERO-ORDER ABSORPTION MODEL

In this model, drug in the gastrointestinal tract, D_{GI}, is absorbed systemically at a constant rate, k_0. Drug is eliminated from the body by a first-order rate process with a first-order rate constant, k. This model is analogous to that of the administration of a drug by intravenous infusion (see Chapter 14). The pharmacokinetic model assuming zero-order absorption is described in Figure 9-3.

The rate of elimination at any time, by first-order process, is equal to D_Bk. The rate of input is simply k_0. Therefore, the net change per unit time in the body can be expressed as follows:

$$\frac{dD_B}{dt} = k_0 - kD_B \tag{9.6}$$

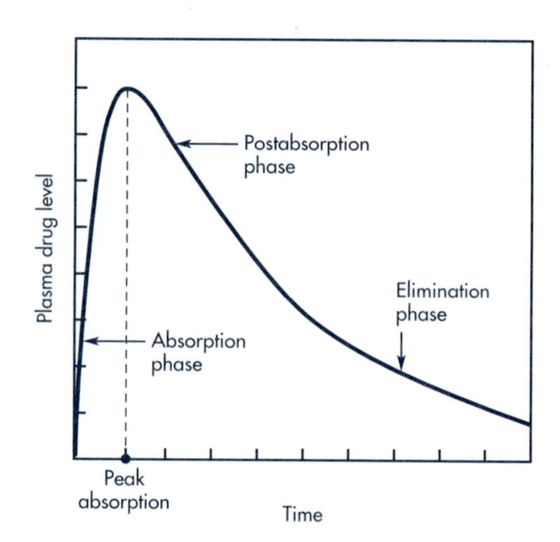

Figure 9-2. Plasma level–time curve for a drug given in a single oral dose. The drug absorption and elimination phases of the curve are shown.

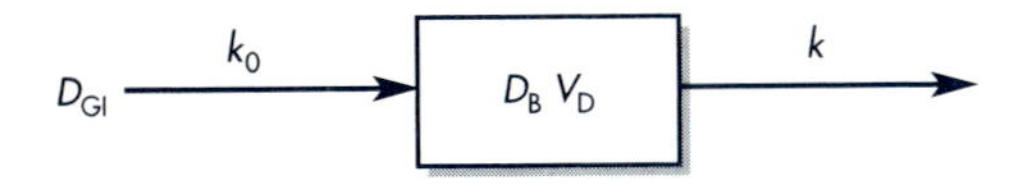

Figure 9-3. One-compartment pharmacokinetic model for zero-order drug absorption and first-order drug elimination.

Integration of this equation with substitution of $V_D C_p$ for D_B produces:

$$C_p = \frac{k_0}{V_D k}\,(1 - e^{-kt}) \tag{9.7}$$

The rate of drug absorption is constant and continues until the amount of drug in the gut, D_{GI}, is depleted. The time at which drug absorption is continuous is equal to D_{GI}/k_0. After this time, the drug is no longer available for absorption from the gut, and Equation 9.7 no longer holds. The drug concentration in the plasma will decline in accordance with a first-order elimination rate process.

FIRST-ORDER ABSORPTION MODEL

This model assumes a first-order input across the gut wall and first-order elimination from the body (Fig. 9-4). This model applies mostly to the oral absorption of drugs in solution or rapidly dissolving dosage (immediate release) forms such as tablets, capsules, and suppositories. In addition, drugs given by intramuscular aqueous injections may also be described using a first-order process.

After administration, the drug is absorbed from the absorption site by a first-order process. In the case of a drug given orally, the drug dissolves in the fluids of the GI tract and is absorbed into the body according to a first-order rate process. The rate of disappearance of drug from the gastrointestinal tract is described by the following:

$$\frac{dD_{GI}}{dt} = -k_a D_{GI} F \tag{9.8}$$

where k_a is the first-order absorption rate constant from the GI tract, F is the fraction absorbed, and D_{GI} is the amount of drug in solution in the GI tract at any time, t. Integration of the differential equation (9.8) gives

$$D_{GI} = D_0 e^{-k_a t} \tag{9.9}$$

where D_0 is the dose of the drug.

The rate of drug elimination is described by a first-order rate process for most drugs and is equal to $-kD_B$. The rate of drug change in the body, dD_B/dt, is therefore the rate of drug in, minus the rate of drug out—as given by the differential equation, Equation 9.10:

$$\frac{dD_B}{dt} = \text{Rate in} - \text{Rate out} \tag{9.10}$$

$$\frac{dD_B}{dt} = Fk_a D_{GI} - kD_B$$

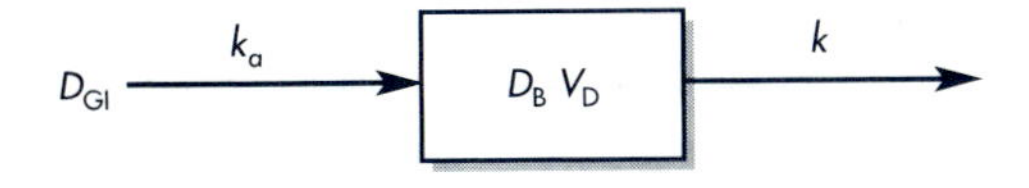

Figure 9-4. One-compartment pharmacokinetic model for first-order drug absorption and first-order elimination.

where F is the fraction of drug systemically absorbed. Since the drug in the gastrointestinal tract also follows a first-order decline process (ie, the drug is absorbed across the gastrointestinal wall), the amount of drug in the gastrointestinal tract is equal to $D_0e^{-k_a t}$.

$$\frac{dD_B}{dt} = Fk_aD_0{}^{-k_a t} - kD_B.$$

F may vary from 1 for a fully absorbed drug to zero for a drug completely unabsorbed. This equation can be integrated to give the general oral absorption equation for calculation of the drug concentration (C_p) in the plasma at any time t, as shown below.

$$C_p = \frac{Fk_aD_0}{V_D(k_a - k)}(e^{-kt} - e^{-k_a t}) \tag{9.11}$$

A typical plot of the concentration of drug in the body after a single oral dose is presented in Figure 9-5.

The maximum concentration is C_{max}, and the time needed to reach maximum concentration is t_{max}. The time needed to reach maximum concentration is independent of dose and is dependent on the rate constants for absorption (k_a) and elimination (k) (Equation 9.13a). At the maximum concentration, sometimes called peak concentration, the rate of drug absorbed is equal to the rate of drug eliminated. Therefore, the rate of concentration change is equal to zero. The rate of concentration change can be obtained by differentiating Equation 9.11, as follows:

$$\frac{dC_p}{dt} = \frac{k_aD_0F}{V_D(k_a - k)}(-ke^{-kt} + k_ae^{-k_a t}) = 0 \tag{9.12}$$

This can be simplified as follows:

$$-ke^{-kt} + k_ae^{-k_a t} = 0 \quad \text{or} \quad ke^{-kt} = k_ae^{-k_a t} \tag{9.13}$$

$$\ln k - kt = \ln k_a - k_at$$

$$t_{max} = \frac{\ln k_a - \ln k}{k_a - k} = \frac{\ln(k_a/k)}{k_a - k}$$

$$t_{max} = \frac{2.3 \log(k_a/k)}{k_a - k} \tag{9.13a}$$

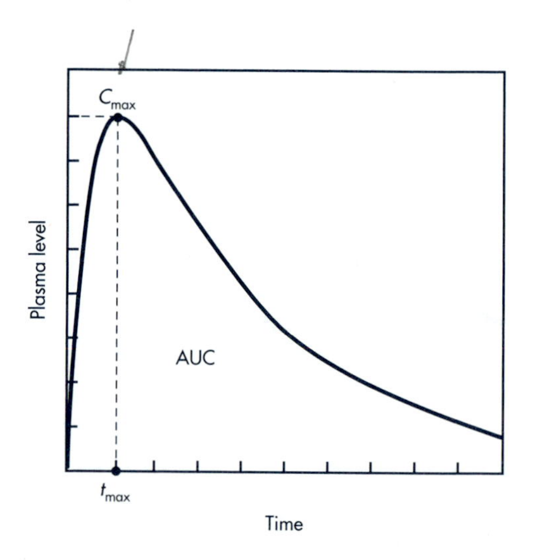

Figure 9-5. Typical plasma level–time curve for a drug given in a single oral dose.

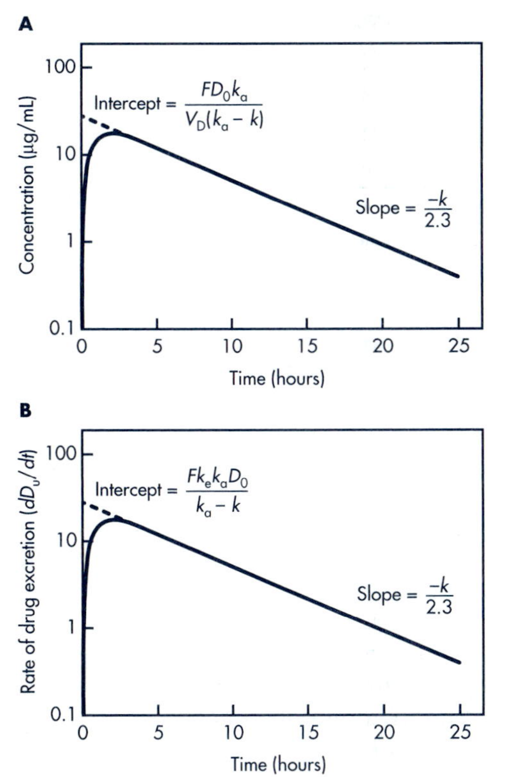

Figure 9-6. **A.** Plasma drug concentration versus time, single oral dose. **B.** Rate of urinary drug excretion versus time, single oral dose.

As shown in Equation 9.13a, the time for maximum drug concentration, t_{max}, is dependent only on the rate constants k_a and k. In order to calculate the peak plasma drug concentration, the value for t_{max} is determined via Equation 9.13a and then substituted into Equation 9.11, solving for C_{max}. Equation 9.11 shows that the C_{max} is directly proportional to the dose of drug given (D_0) and the fraction of drug absorbed (F). Calculation of t_{max} and C_{max} is usually necessary, since direct measurement of the maximum drug concentration may not be possible due to improper timing of the serum samples.

The first-order elimination rate constant may be determined from the elimination phase of the plasma level–time curve (Fig. 9-2). At the later time intervals, when drug absorption has been completed $e^{-k_a t} \approx 0$, and, Equation 9.11 reduces to the following expression:

$$C_p = \frac{Fk_aD_0}{V_D(k_a - k)} e^{-kt} \tag{9.14}$$

Taking the natural logarithm of this expression,

$$\ln C_p = \ln \frac{Fk_aD_0}{V_D(k_a - k)} - kt \tag{9.15}$$

Substitution of common logarithms gives

$$\log C_p = \log \frac{Fk_aD_0}{V_D(k_a - k)} - \frac{kt}{2.3} \tag{9.16}$$

With this equation, a graph constructed by plotting log C_p versus time will yield a straight line with a slope of $-k/2.3$ (Fig. 9-6A).

With a similar approach, *urinary drug excretion* data may also be used for calculation of the first-order elimination rate constant. The rate of drug excretion after a single oral dose of drug is given by

$$\frac{dD_u}{dt} = \frac{Fk_e k_a D_0}{k_a - k}(e^{-kt} - e^{-k_a t}) \tag{9.17}$$

where dD_u/dt = rate of urinary drug excretion, k_e = first-order renal excretion constant, and F = fraction of dose absorbed.

A graph constructed by plotting dD_u/dt versus time will yield a curve identical in appearance to the plasma level–time curve for the drug (Fig. 9-7B). After drug absorption is virtually complete, $-e^{k_a t}$ approaches zero, and Equation 9.17 reduces to the following expression:

$$\frac{dD_u}{dt} = \frac{k_e k_a F D_0}{k_a - k} e^{-kt} \tag{9.18}$$

Taking the natural logarithm of both sides of this expression and substituting in terms of common logarithms, Equation 9.18 becomes

$$\log \frac{dD_u}{dt} = \log \frac{k_e k_a F D_0}{k_a - k} - \frac{kt}{2.3} \tag{9.19}$$

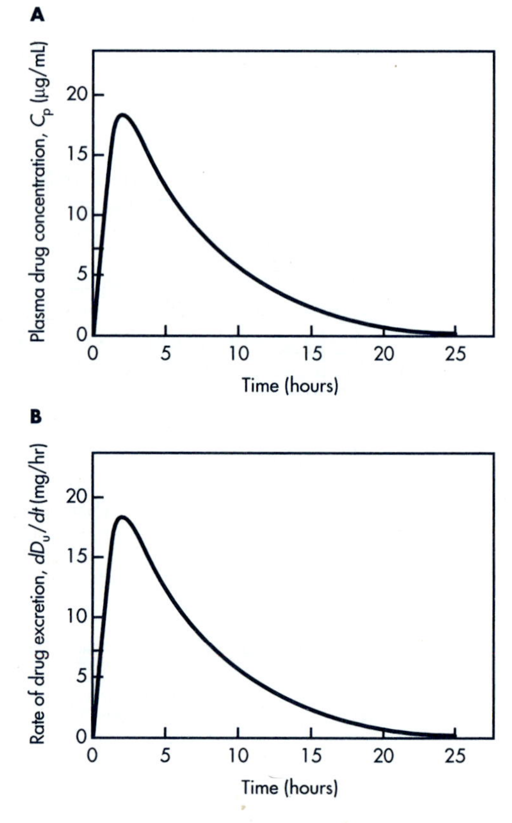

Figure 9-7. **A.** Plasma drug concentration versus time, single oral dose. **B.** Rate of urinary drug excretion versus time, single oral dose.

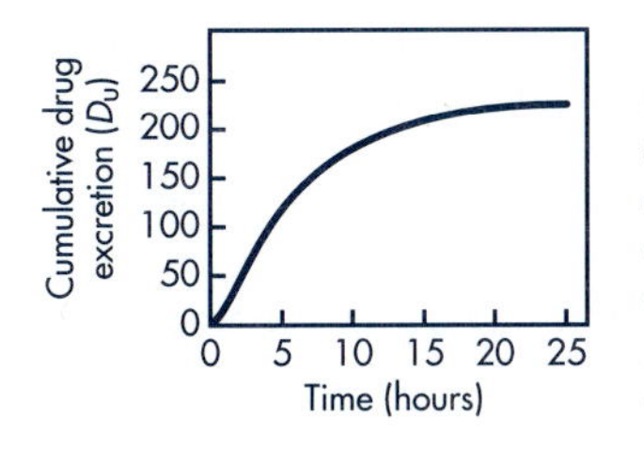

Figure 9-8. Cumulative urinary drug excretion versus time, single oral dose. Urine samples are collected at various time periods after the dose. The amount of drug excreted in each sample is added to the amount of drug recovered in the previous urine sample (cumulative addition). The total amount of drug recovered after all the drug is excreted is D_u^∞.

When log (dD_u/dt) is plotted against time, a graph of a straight line is obtained with a slope of $-k/2.3$ (Fig. 9-6B). Because the rate of urinary drug excretion, dD_u/dt, cannot be determined directly, an average rate of urinary drug excretion is obtained (see also Chapter 3), and this value is plotted against the midpoint of the collection period for each urine sample.

To obtain the *cumulative drug excretion* in the urine, Equation 9.17 must be integrated, as shown below.

$$D_u = \frac{Fk_e k_a D_0}{k_a - k}\left(\frac{e^{-k_a t}}{k_a} - \frac{e^{-kt}}{k}\right) + \frac{Fk_e D_0}{k} \qquad \textbf{(9.20)}$$

A plot of D_u versus time will give the urinary drug excretion curve described in Figure 9-8. When all of the drug has been excreted, at $t = \infty$, Equation 9.20 reduces to

$$D_u^\infty = \frac{Fk_e D_0}{k} \qquad \textbf{(9.21)}$$

where D_u^∞ is the maximum amount of active or parent drug excreted.

Determination of Absorption Rate Constants from Oral Absorption Data

Method of Residuals

Assuming $k_a \gg k$ in Equation 9.11, the value for the second exponential will become insignificantly small with time (ie, $e^{-k_a t} \approx 0$) and can therefore be omitted. When this is the case, drug absorption is virtually complete. Equation 9.11 then reduces to Equation 9.22.

$$C_p = \frac{Fk_a D_0}{V_D(k_a - k)} e^{-kt} \qquad \textbf{(9.22)}$$

From this, one may also obtain the intercept of the *y* axis (Fig. 9-9).

$$\frac{Fk_a D_0}{V_D(k_a - k)} = A$$

where A is a constant. Thus, Equation 9.22 becomes

$$C_p = Ae^{-kt} \qquad \textbf{(9.23)}$$

This equation, which represents first-order drug elimination, will yield a linear plot on semilog paper. The slope is equal to $-k/2.3$. The value for k_a can be obtained by using the method of *residuals* or a *feathering* technique, as described in Chapter 4. The value of k_a is obtained by the following procedure:

1. Plot the drug concentration versus time on semilog paper with the concentration values on the logarithmic axis (Fig. 9-9).
2. Obtain the slope of the terminal phase (line *BC*, Fig. 9-9) by extrapolation.
3. Take any points on the upper part of line *BC* (eg, x'_1, x'_2, x'_3, . . .) and drop vertically to obtain corresponding points on the curve (eg, x_1, x_2, x_3, . . .).
4. Read the values x_1 and x'_1, x_2 and x'_2, x_3 and x'_3, and so on. Plot the values of the differences at the corresponding time points Δ_1, Δ_2, Δ_3, ... A straight line will be obtained with a slope of $-k_a/2.3$ (Fig. 9-9).

When using the method of residuals, a minimum of three points should be used to define the straight line. Data points occurring shortly after t_{max} may not be accurate, because drug absorption is still continuing at that time. Because this portion of the curve represents the postabsorption phase, only data points from the elimination phase should be used to define the rate of drug absorption as a first-order process.

If drug absorption begins immediately after oral administration, the residual lines obtained by feathering the plasma level–time curve (as shown in Fig. 9-9) will intersect on the *y* axis at point *A*. The value of this *y* intercept, *A*, represents a hybrid constant composed of k_a, k, V_D, and FD_0. (See Equation 9.23.)

$$A = \frac{Fk_aD_0}{V_D(k_a - k)}$$

The value for *A*, as well as the values for *k* and k_a, may be substituted back into Equation 9.11 to obtain a general theoretical equation that will describe the plasma level–time curve.

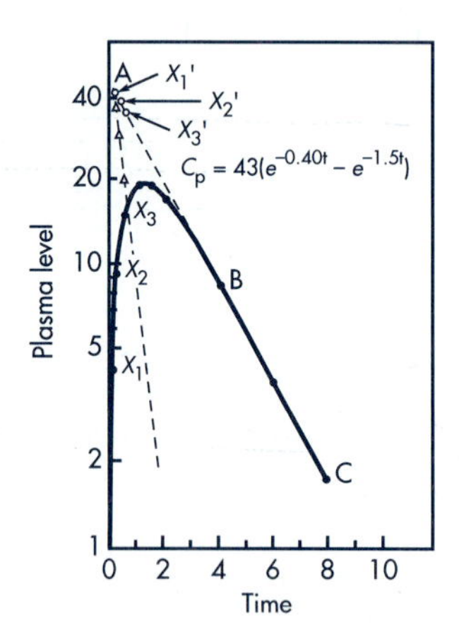

Figure 9-9. Plasma level–time curve for a drug demonstrating first-order absorption and elimination kinetics. The equation of the curve is obtained by the method of residuals.

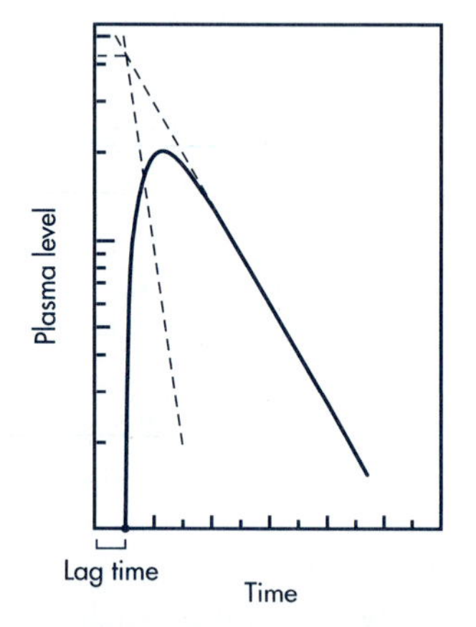

Figure 9-10. The lag time can be determined graphically if the two residual lines obtained by feathering the plasma level–time curve intersect at a point where $t > 0$.

Lag Time

In some individuals, absorption of drug after a single oral dose does not start immediately, due to such physiologic factors as stomach-emptying time and intestinal motility. The time delay prior to the commencement of first-order drug absorption is known as *lag time.*

The lag time for a drug may be observed if the two residual lines obtained by feathering the oral absorption plasma level—time curve intersect at a point after $t = 0$ on the x axis. The time at the point of intersection on the x axis is the lag time (Fig. 9-10).

The lag time, t_0, represents the beginning of drug absorption and should not be confused with the pharmacologic term, *onset time,* which represents latency, that is, the time required for the drug to reach minimum effective concentration.

Two equations can adequately describe the curve in Figure 9-10. In one, the lag time t_0 is subtracted from each time point, as shown in Equation 9.24.

$$C_p = \frac{Fk_aD_0}{V_D(k_a - k)}\left(e^{-k(t-t_0)} - e^{-k_a(t-t_0)}\right) \qquad \textbf{(9.24)}$$

where $Fk_aD_0/V_D\ (k_a - k)$ is the y value at the point of intersection of the residual lines in Figure 9-10.

The second expression that describes the curve in Figure 9-10 omits the lag time, as follows:

$$C_p = Be^{-kt} - Ae^{-k_at} \qquad \textbf{(9.25)}$$

where A and B represents the intercepts on the y axis after extrapolation of the residual lines for absorption and elimination, respectively.

Flip-flop of k_a *and* k

In using the method of residuals to obtain an estimate of k_a and k, the terminal phase of an oral absorption curve is usually represented by the elimination rate constant and the absorption rate constant is represented by the steeper slope (Fig. 9-11). In a few cases, the elimination rate constant k obtained from oral absorption data does not agree with that obtained after intravenous bolus injection. For example, the k obtained after an intravenous bolus injection of a bronchodilator was 1.72 hr^{-1}, whereas the k calculated after oral administration was 0.7 hr^{-1} (Fig. 9-11). When k_a was obtained by the method of residuals, the rather surprising result was that the k_a was 1.72 hr^{-1}.

Apparently, the k_a and k obtained by the method of residuals has been interchanged. This phenomenon is called *flip-flop* of the absorption and elimination rate constants. Flip-flop, or the reversal of the rate constants, may occur whenever k_a and k are estimated from oral drug absorption data. Use of computer methods does not ensure against flip-flop of the two constants estimated.

In order to unambiguously demonstrate that the steeper curve represents the elimination rate for a drug given extravascularly, the drug must be given by intravenous injection into the same patient. After intravenous injection, the decline in plasma drug levels over time represents the true elimination rate. The relationship between k_a and k on the shape of the plasma drug concentration–time curve for a constant dose of drug given orally is shown in Figure 9-11.

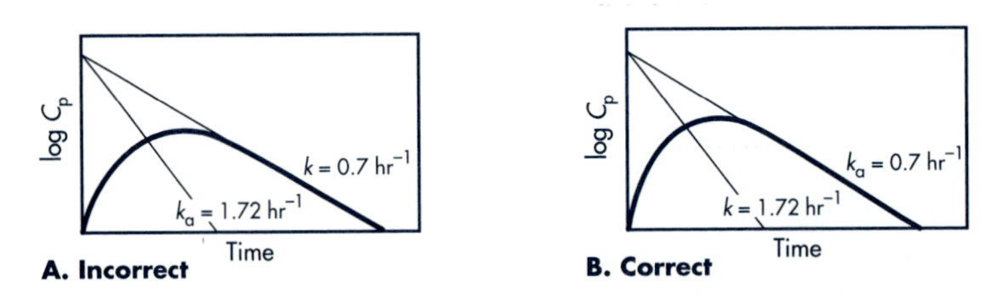

Figure 9-11. Flip-flop of k_a and k. Because $k > k_a$, the right-hand figure and slopes represent the correct values for k_a and k.

The only way to be certain of the estimates is to compare the k calculated after oral administration with the k from intravenous data.

Most of the drugs observed to have flip-flop characteristics are drugs with fast elimination (ie, $k > k_a$). Drug absorption of most drug solutions or fast dissolving products are essentially complete or at least half completed within an hour (ie, absorption half-life of 0.5 or 1 hr, corresponding to a k_a of 1.38 hr^{-1} or 0.69 hr^{-1}). Because most of the drugs used orally have longer elimination half-lives, the assumption that the smaller slope or smaller rate constant (ie, the terminal phase of the curve in Figure 9-11) should be used as the elimination constant is generally correct.

For drugs that have a large elimination rate constant ($k > 0.69$ hr^{-1}), the chance for flip-flop of k_a and k is much greater. The drug, isoproterenol, for example, has an oral elimination half-life of only a few minutes, and flip-flop of k_a and k has been noted (Portmann, 1970). Similarly, salicyluric acid was flip-flopped when oral data were plotted. The k for salicyluric acid was much larger than k_a (Levy et al, 1969). Many experimental drugs show flip-flop of k and k_a, whereas few of the marketed oral drugs do. The drugs with a large k are usually considered to be unsuitable for an oral drug product due to their large elimination rate constant, corresponding to a very short elimination half-life. An extended-release drug product may slow the absorption of a drug, such that the k_a is smaller than the k producing a flip-flop situation.

Determination of $\mathbf{k}_a$ by Plotting Percent of Drug Unabsorbed Versus Time (Wagner–Nelson Method)

After a single oral dose of a drug, the total should be completely accounted for in the amount present in the body, the amount present in the urine, and the amount present in the GI tract. Therefore, dose (D_0) is expressed as follows:

$$D_0 = D_{GI} + D_B + D_u \quad \textbf{(9.26)}$$

Let $Ab = D_B + D_u$ = amount of drug absorbed and Ab^∞ = amount of drug absorbed at $t = \infty$. At any time the fraction of drug absorbed would be Ab/Ab^∞, and the fraction of drug unabsorbed would be $1 - (Ab/Ab^\infty)$. The amount of drug excreted at any time t can be calculated as follows:

$$D_u = kV_D[AUC]_0^t \quad \textbf{(9.27)}$$

The amount of drug in the body (D_B), at any time, $= C_pV_D$. At any time t, the amount of drug absorbed (Ab) is as follows:

$$Ab = C_pV_D + kV_D[AUC]_0^t \quad \textbf{(9.28)}$$

At $t = \infty$, $C_p^{\infty} = 0$ (ie, plasma concentration is negligible), and the total amount of drug absorbed is

$$\mathrm{Ab}^{\infty} = 0 + kV_D[\mathrm{AUC}]_0^{\infty} \tag{9.29}$$

The fraction of drug absorbed at any time is

$$\frac{\mathrm{Ab}}{\mathrm{Ab}^{\infty}} = \frac{C_p V_D + kV_D[\mathrm{AUC}]_0^t}{kV_D[\mathrm{AUC}]_0^{\infty}} \tag{9.30}$$

$$\frac{\mathrm{Ab}}{\mathrm{Ab}^{\infty}} = \frac{C_p + k[\mathrm{AUC}]_0^t}{k[\mathrm{AUC}]_0^{\infty}} \tag{9.31}$$

The fraction unabsorbed at any time t is

$$1 - \frac{\mathrm{Ab}}{\mathrm{Ab}^{\infty}} = 1 - \frac{C_p + k[\mathrm{AUC}]_0^t}{k[\mathrm{AUC}]_0^{\infty}} \tag{9.32}$$

because the drug remaining in the GI tract at any time t is

$$D_{\mathrm{GI}} = D_0 e^{-k_a t} \tag{9.33}$$

Therefore, the fraction of drug remaining is

$$\frac{D_{\mathrm{GI}}}{D_0} = e^{-k_a t}, \qquad \log \frac{D_{\mathrm{GI}}}{D_0} = \frac{-k_a t}{2.3} \tag{9.34}$$

Because D_{GI}/D_0 is actually the fraction of drug unabsorbed—that is, $1 - (\mathrm{Ab}/\mathrm{Ab}^{\infty})$—a plot of $1 - (\mathrm{Ab}/\mathrm{Ab}^{\infty})$ versus time gives $-k_a/2.3$ as the slope (Fig. 9-12).

The following steps should be useful in determination of k_a:

1. Plot log concentration of drug versus time.
2. Find k from the terminal part of slope when the slope $= -k/2.3$.
3. Find $[\mathrm{AUC}]_0^t$ by plotting C_p versus t.
4. Find $k[\mathrm{AUC}]_0^t$ by multiplying each $[\mathrm{AUC}]_0^t$ by k.
5. Find $[\mathrm{AUC}]_0^{\infty}$ by adding up all the [AUC] pieces, from $t = 0$ to $t = \infty$.
6. Determine the $1 - (\mathrm{Ab}/\mathrm{Ab}^{\infty})$ value corresponding to each time point t by using Table 9.1.
7. Plot $1 - (\mathrm{Ab}/\mathrm{Ab}^{\infty})$ versus time on semilog paper, with $1 - (\mathrm{Ab}/\mathrm{Ab}^{\infty})$ on the logarithmic axis.

If the fraction of drug unabsorbed, $1 - \mathrm{Ab}/\mathrm{Ab}^{\infty}$, gives a linear regression line on a semilog graph, then the rate of drug absorption, dD_{GI}/dt, is a first-order process. Recall that $1 - \mathrm{Ab}/\mathrm{Ab}^{\infty}$ is equal to dD_{GI}/dt (Fig. 9-12).

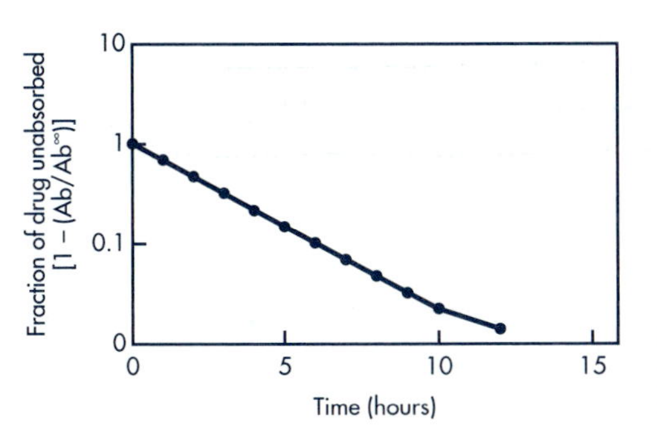

Figure 9-12. Semilog graph of data in Table 9.2, depicting the fraction of drug unabsorbed versus time using the Wagner–Nelson method.

As the drug approaches 100% absorption, C_p becomes very small and difficult to assay accurately. Consequently, the terminal part of the line described by $1 - Ab/Ab^{\infty}$ versus time tends to become scattered or nonlinear. This terminal part of the curve is excluded, and only the initial linear segment of the curve is used for the estimate of the slope.

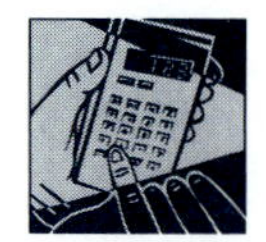

PRACTICE PROBLEM

Drug concentrations in the blood at various times are listed in Table 9.1. Assuming the drug follows a one-compartment model, find the k_a, and compare it with the k_a value obtained by the method of residuals.

Solution

The AUC is approximated by the *trapezoidal rule.* This method is fairly accurate when there are sufficient data points. The area between each time point is calculated as follows:

$$[\mathrm{AUC}]_{t_{n-1}}^{t_n} = \frac{C_{n-1} + C_n}{2}(t_n - t_{n-1}) \tag{9.35}$$

where C_n and C_{n-1} are concentrations. For example, at $n = 6$, the [AUC] is

$$\frac{6.28 + 6.11}{2}(6 - 5) = 6.20$$

To obtain $[\mathrm{AUC}]_0^{\infty}$, add all the area portions under the curve from zero to infinity. In this case, 48 hours is long enough to be considered as infinity, because the blood concentration at that point already has fallen to an insignificant drug concentration, 0.1 μg/mL. The rest of the needed information is given in Table 9.1. Notice that k is obtained from the plot of log C_p versus t; k was found to be 0.1 hr^{-1}. The plot of $1 - (Ab/Ab^{\infty})$ versus t on semilog paper is shown in Figure 9-12.

A more complete method of obtaining the $[\mathrm{AUC}]_0^{\infty}$ is to estimate the residual area from the last observed plasma concentration C_{pn} at t_n to time equal to infinity. This equation is

$$[\mathrm{AUC}]_t^{\infty} = \frac{C_{pn}}{k} \tag{9.36}$$

The total $[\mathrm{AUC}]_0^{\infty}$ is the sum of the areas obtained by the trapezoidal rule, $[\mathrm{AUC}]_0^t$, and the residual area $[\mathrm{AUC}]_t^{\infty}$, as described in the following expression:

$$[\mathrm{AUC}]_0^{\infty} = [\mathrm{AUC}]_0^t + [\mathrm{AUC}]_t^{\infty} \tag{9.37}$$

Estimation of k$_a$ *from Urinary Data*

The absorption rate constant may also be estimated from urinary excretion data, using a plot of percent of drug unabsorbed versus time. For a one-compartment model:

TABLE 9.1 Blood Concentrations and Associated Data for a Hypothetical Drug

TIME t_n (hr)	CONCENTRATION C_P (μg/mL)	$[AUC]_{tn-1}^{tn}$	$[AUC]_0^t$	$k[AUC]_0^t$	$C_P + k[AUC]_0^t$	$\frac{Ab}{Ab^\infty}$	$\left(1 - \frac{Ab}{Ab^\infty}\right)$
0	0.	0.	0.				
1	3.13	1.57	1.57	0.157	3.287	0.328	1.000
2	4.93	4.03	5.60	0.560	5.490	0.548	0.672
3	5.86	5.40	10.99	1.099	6.959	0.695	0.305
4	6.25	6.06	17.05	1.705	7.955	0.794	0.205
5	6.28	6.26	23.31	2.331	8.610	0.856	0.140
6	6.11	6.20	29.51	2.951	9.061	0.905	0.095
7	5.81	5.96	35.47	3.547	9.357	0.934	0.066
8	5.45	5.63	41.10	4.110	9.560	0.955	0.045
9	5.06	5.26	46.35	4.635	9.695	0.968	0.032
10	4.66	4.86	51.21	5.121			
12	3.90	8.56	59.77	5.977			
14	3.24	7.14	66.91	6.691			
16	2.67	5.92	72.83	7.283			
18	2.19	4.86	77.69	7.769			
24	1.20	10.17	87.85	8.785			
28	0.81	4.02	91.87	9.187			
32	0.54	2.70	94.57	9.457			
36	0.36	1.80	96.37	9.637			
48	0.10	2.76	99.13	9.913			

- Ab = total amount of drug absorbed—that is, the amount of drug in the body plus the amount of drug excreted.
- D_B = amount of drug in the body.
- D_u = amount of unchanged drug excreted in the urine.
- C_p = plasma drug concentration.
- C_B = body drug concentration.
- D_E = total amount of drug excreted (drug and metabolites).
- $Ab = D_B + D_E$ **(9.38)**

The differential of Equation 9.38 with respect to time gives

$$\frac{dAb}{dt} = \frac{dD_B}{dt} + \frac{dD_E}{dt} \tag{9.39}$$

Assuming first-order elimination kinetics with renal elimination constant, k_e,

$$\frac{dD_u}{dt} = k_e D_B = k_e V_D C_p \tag{9.40}$$

Assuming a one-compartment model,

$$V_D C_p = D_B$$

Substituting $V_D C_p$ into Equation 9.39,

$$\frac{dAb}{dt} = V_D \frac{dC_p}{dt} + \frac{dD_E}{dt} \tag{9.41}$$

And rearranging Equation 9.40,

$$C_p = \frac{1}{k_e V_D}\left(\frac{dD_u}{dt}\right) \quad \textbf{(9.42)}$$

$$\frac{dC_p}{dt} = \frac{d(dD_u/dt)}{dt\, k_e V_D} \quad \textbf{(9.43)}$$

Substituting for dC_p/dt into Equation 9.41 and kD_u/k_e for D_E,

$$\frac{dAb}{dt} = \frac{d(D_u/dt)}{k_e\, dt} + \frac{k}{k_e}\left(\frac{dD_u}{dt}\right) \quad \textbf{(9.44)}$$

When the above expression is integrated from zero to time t,

$$(\text{Ab})_t = \frac{1}{k_e}\left(\frac{dD_u}{dt}\right)_t + \frac{k}{k_e}(D_u)t \quad \textbf{(9.45)}$$

At $t = \infty$, all the drug that is ultimately absorbed is expressed as Ab^∞, and $dD_u/dt = 0$. The total amount of drug absorbed is as follows:

$$\text{Ab}^\infty = \frac{k}{k_e} D_u^\infty$$

where D_u^∞ is the total amount of unchanged drug excreted in the urine.

The fraction of drug absorbed at any time t is equal to the amount of drug absorbed at this time, $(\text{Ab})_t$, divided by the total amount of drug absorbed, Ab^∞.

$$\frac{(\text{Ab})_t}{\text{Ab}^\infty} = \frac{(dD_u/dt)_t + k(D_u)_t}{kD_u^\infty} \quad \textbf{(9.46)}$$

A plot of the fraction of drug unabsorbed $[1 - (\text{Ab}/\text{Ab}^\infty)]$ versus time gives $-k_a/2.3$ as the slope from which the absorption rate constant is obtained (Fig. 9-12).

When collecting urinary drug samples for the determination of pharmacokinetic parameters, one should obtain a valid urine collection as discussed in Chapter 3. If the drug is rapidly absorbed, it may be difficult to obtain multiple early urine samples to accurately describe the absorption phase. Moreover, drugs with very slow absorption will have low concentrations, which may present analytical problems.

Effect of k_a *and* k *on* C_{max}, t_{max}, *and AUC*

Changes in k_a and k may affect t_{max}, C_{max}, and AUC as shown in Table 9.2. If the values for k_a and k are reversed, then the same t_{max} is obtained, but the C_{max} and AUC are different. If the elimination rate constant is kept at 0.1 hr^{-1} and the k_a changes from 0.2 to 0.6 hr^{-1} (absorption rate increases), then the t_{max} becomes shorter (from 6.93 to 3.58 hr), the C_{max} increases (from 5.00 to 6.99 μg/mL), but the AUC remains constant (100 μg hr/mL). In contrast, when the absorption rate constant is kept at 0.3 hr^{-1} and k changes from 0.1 to 0.5 hr^{-1} (elimination rate increases), then the t_{max} decreases (from 5.49 to 2.55 hr), the C_{max} decreases (from 5.77 to 2.79 μg/mL), and the AUC decreases (from 100 to 20 μmg hr/mL). Graphical representations for the relationships of k_a and k on the time for peak absorption and the peak drug concentrations are shown in Figures 9-13 and 9-14.

TABLE 9.2 Effects of the Absorption Rate Constant and Elimination Rate[a]

ABSORPTION RATE CONSTANT k_a (hr^{-1})	ELIMINATION RATE CONSTANT k (hr^{-1})	t_{MAX} (hr)	C_{MAX} (μg/mL)	AUC (μg hr/mL)
0.1	0.2	6.93	2.50	50
0.2	0.1	6.93	5.00	100
0.3	0.1	5.49	5.77	100
0.4	0.1	4.62	6.29	100
0.5	0.1	4.02	6.69	100
0.6	0.1	3.58	6.99	100
0.3	0.1	5.49	5.77	100
0.3	0.2	4.05	4.44	50
0.3	0.3	3.33	3.68	33.3
0.3	0.4	2.88	3.16	25
0.3	0.5	2.55	2.79	20

[a] t_{max} = peak plasma concentration, C_{max} = peak drug concentration, AUC = area under the curve. Values are based on a single oral dose (100 mg) that is 100% bioavailable ($F = 1$) and has an apparent V_D of 10 L. The drug follows a one-compartment open model. t_{max} is calculated by Eq. 9.13 and C_{max} is calculated by Eq. 9.11. The AUC is calculated by the trapezoidal rule from 0 to 24 hours.

Determination of k_a from Two-Compartment Oral Absorption Data (Loo–Riegelman Method)

Plotting the percent of drug unabsorbed versus time to determine the k_a may be calculated for a drug exhibiting a two-compartment kinetic model. As in the method used previously to obtain an estimate of the k_a, no limitation is placed on the order of the absorption process. However, this method does require that the drug be given intravenously as well as orally to obtain all the necessary kinetic constants.

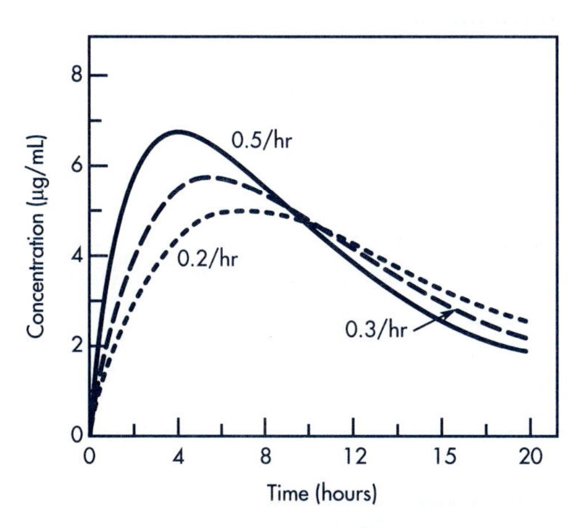

Figure 9-13. Effect of a change in the absorption rate constant, k_a, on the plasma drug concentration versus time curve. Dose of drug is 100 mg, V_D is 10 L, and k is 0.1 hr^{-1}.

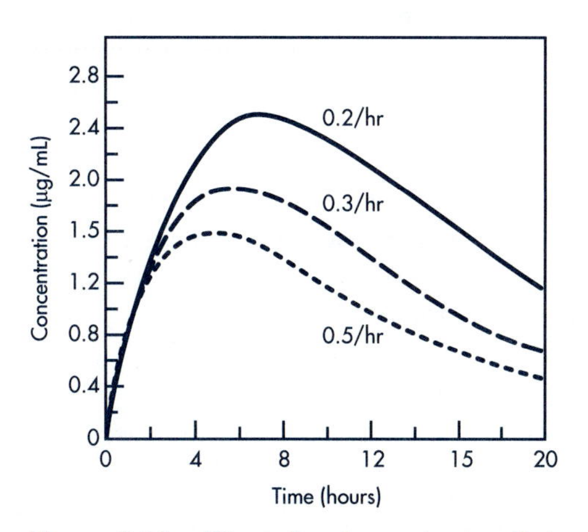

Figure 9-14. Effect of a change in the elimination rate constant, k, on the plasma drug concentration versus time curve. Dose of drug is 100 mg, V_D is 10 L, k_a is 0.1 hr^{-1}.

After oral administration of a dose of a drug that exhibits two-compartment model kinetics, the amount of drug absorbed is calculated as the sum of the amounts of drug in the central compartment (D_p) and in the tissue compartment (D_t) and the amount of drug eliminated by all routes (D_u) (Fig. 9-15).

$$\text{Ab} = D_p + D_t + D_u \tag{9.47}$$

Each of these terms may be expressed in terms of kinetics constants and plasma drug concentrations, as follows:

$$D_p = V_p C_p \tag{9.48}$$

$$D_t = V_t C_t \tag{9.49}$$

$$\frac{dD_u}{dt} = kV_p C_p \tag{9.50}$$

$$D_u = kV_p[\text{AUC}]_0^t$$

Substituting the above expression for D_p and D_u into Equation 9.46,

$$\text{Ab} = V_p C_p + D_t + kV_p[\text{AUC}]_0^t \tag{9.51}$$

By dividing this equation by V_p to express the equation on drug concentrations, we obtain

$$\frac{\text{Ab}}{V_p} = C_p + \frac{D_t}{V_p} + k[\text{AUC}]_0^t \tag{9.52}$$

At $t = \infty$ this equation becomes

$$\frac{\text{Ab}}{V_p} + k[\text{AUC}]_0^\infty \tag{9.53}$$

Equation 9.53 divided by Equation 9.54 gives the fraction of drug absorbed at any time.

$$\frac{\text{Ab}}{\text{Ab}^\infty} = \frac{C_p + \frac{D_t}{V_p} + k[\text{AUC}]_0^t}{k[\text{AUC}]_0^\infty} \tag{9.54}$$

A plot of the fraction of drug unabsorbed $[1 - (\text{Ab}/\text{Ab}^\infty)]$ versus time gives $-k_a/2.3$ as the slope from which the value for the absorption rate constant is obtained.

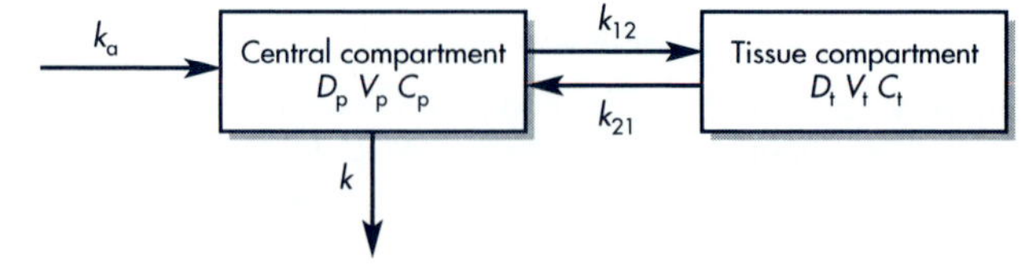

Figure 9-15. Two-compartment pharmacokinetic mode. Drug absorption and elimination occur from the central compartment.

C_p and $k[\mathrm{AUC}]_0^t$ are calculated from a plot of C_p versus time. Values for (D_t/V_p) can be approximated by the Loo–Riegelman method, as follows:

$$(C_t)_{tn} = \frac{k_{12}\Delta C_p \Delta t}{2} + \frac{k_{12}}{k_{21}}(C_p)_{t_{n-1}}(1 - e^{-k_{21}\Delta t}) + (C_t)_{t_{n-1}} e^{-k_{21}\Delta t} \tag{9.55}$$

where C_t is D_t/V_p, or apparent tissue concentration; t = time of sampling for sample n; t_{n-1} = time of sampling for the sampling point preceding sample n; and $(C_p)_{t_{n-1}}$ = concentration of drug at central compartment for sample $n-1$. Calculation of C_t values is shown in Table 9.3, using a typical set of oral absorption data. After calculation of C_t values, the percent of drug unabsorbed is calculated with Equation 9.54, as shown in Table 9.4. A plot of percent of drug unabsorbed versus time on a semilog graph gives a k_a of approximately 0.5 hr^{-1}.

For calculation of the k_a by this method, the drug must be given intravenously to allow evaluation of the distribution and elimination rate constants. For drugs that cannot be given by the IV route, the k_a cannot be calculated by the Loo–Riegelman method. For these drugs, given by the oral route only, the Wagner–Nelson method, which assumes a one-compartment model, may be used to provide an initial estimate of k_a. If the drug is given intravenously, there is no way of knowing whether there is any variation in the values for the elimination rate constant k and the distributive rate constants k_{12} and k_{21}. Such variations alter the rate constants. Therefore, a one-compartment model is frequently used to fit the plasma curves after an oral or intramuscular dose. The plasma level predicted from the k_a obtained by this method does deviate from the actual plasma level. However, in many instances, this deviation is not significant.

Cumulative Relative Fraction Absorbed

The fraction of drug absorbed at any time t (Eq. 9.31) may be summed or cumulated for each time period for which a plasma drug sample was obtained. From Equation 9.31 the term $\mathrm{Ab}/\mathrm{Ab}^\infty$ becomes the cumulative relative fraction absorbed (CRFA).

$$\mathrm{CRFA} = \frac{C_{p_t} + k[\mathrm{AUC}]_0^t}{k[\mathrm{AUC}]_0^\infty} \tag{9.56}$$

where C_{pt} is the plasma concentration at time t.

In the Wagner–Nelson equation, $\mathrm{Ab}/\mathrm{Ab}^\infty$ or CRFA will eventually equal unity, or 100%, even though the drug may not be 100% systemically bioavailable. The percent of drug absorbed is based on the total amount of drug absorbed (Ab^∞) rather than the dose D. Because the amount of the drug ultimately absorbed, Ab^∞, is equal to $k[\mathrm{AUC}]_0^\infty$, the numerator will always equal the denominator whether the drug is 10, 20, or 100% bioavailable. The percent of drug absorbed based on $\mathrm{Ab}/\mathrm{Ab}^\infty$ is therefore different from the real percent of drug absorbed unless $F = 1$. However, for the calculation of k_a, the method is acceptable.

To determine the real percent of drug absorbed, a modification of the Wagner–Nelson equation was suggested by Welling (1986). A reference drug product was administered and plasma drug concentrations were determined over time. CRFA was then estimated by dividing $\mathrm{Ab}/\mathrm{Ab}^\infty_{\mathrm{ref}}$ where Ab is the cumulative amount

TABLE 9.3 Calculation of C_t Values[a]

$(C_p)_{t_n}$	$(t)_{t_n}$	ΔC_p	Δt	$\frac{(k_{12}\Delta C_p \Delta t)}{2}$	$(C_p)_{t_{n-1}}$	$(k_{12}/k_{21}) \times (1 - e^{-k_{21}\Delta t})$	$(C_p)_{t_{n-1}} k_{12}/k_{21} \times (1 - e^{-k_{21}\Delta t})$	$(C_t)_{t_{n-1}} e^{-k_{21}\Delta t}$	$(C_t)t_n$
3.00	0.5	3.0	0.5	0.218	0	0.134	0.	0.	0.218
5.20	1.0	2.2	0.5	0.160	3.00	0.134	0.402	0.187	0.749
6.50	1.5	1.3	0.5	0.094	5.20	0.134	0.697	0.642	1.433
7.30	2.0	0.8	0.5	0.058	6.50	0.134	0.871	1.228	2.157
7.60	2.5	0.3	0.5	0.022	7.30	0.134	0.978	1.849	2.849
7.75	3.0	0.15	0.5	0.011	7.60	0.134	1.018	2.442	3.471
7.70	3.5	−0.05	0.5	−0.004	7.75	0.134	1.039	2.976	4.019
7.60	4.0	−0.10	0.5	−0.007	7.70	0.134	1.032	3.444	4.469
7.10	5.0	−0.50	1.0	−0.073	7.60	0.250	1.900	3.276	5.103
6.60	6.0	−0.50	1.0	−0.073	7.10	0.250	1.775	3.740	5.442
6.00	7.0	−0.60	1.0	−0.087	6.60	0.250	1.650	3.989	5.552
5.10	9.0	−0.90	2.0	−0.261	6.00	0.432	2.592	2.987	5.318
4.40	11.0	−0.70	2.0	−0.203	5.10	0.432	2.203	2.861	4.861
3.30	15.0	−1.10	4.0	−0.638	4.40	0.720	3.168	1.361	3.891

[a] Calculated with the following rate constants: $k_{12} = 0.29\ hr^{-1}$, $k_{21} = 0.31^{-1}$.

Adapted with permission from Loo and Riegelman (1968).

TABLE 9.4 Calculation of Percentage Unabsorbed[a]

TIME (hr)	$(C_P)_{t_n}$	$[AUC]_{t_{n-1}}^{t_n}$	$[AUC]_{t_0}^{t_n}$	$k[AUC]_{t_0}^{t_n}$	$(C_t)_{t_n}$	Ab/V_p	$\%Ab/V_p$	$100\%-Ab/V_p\%$
0.5	3.00	0.750	0.750	0.120	0.218	3.338	16.6	83.4
1.0	5.20	2.050	2.800	0.448	0.749	6.397	31.8	68.2
1.5	6.50	2.925	5.725	0.916	1.433	8.849	44.0	56.0
2.0	7.30	3.450	9.175	1.468	2.157	10.925	54.3	45.7
2.5	7.60	3.725	12.900	2.064	2.849	12.513	62.2	37.8
3.0	7.75	3.838	16.738	2.678	3.471	13.889	69.1	30.9
3.5	7.70	3.863	20.601	3.296	4.019	15.015	74.6	25.4
4.0	7.60	3.825	24.426	3.908	4.469	15.977	79.4	20.6
5.0	7.10	7.350	31.726	5.084	5.103	17.287	85.9	14.1
6.0	6.60	6.850	38.626	6.180	5.442	18.222	90.6	9.4
7.0	6.00	6.300	44.926	7.188	5.552	18.740	93.1	6.9
9.0	5.10	11.100	56.026	8.964	5.318	19.382	96.3	3.7
11.0	4.40	9.500	65.526	10.484	4.861	19.745	98.1	1.9
15.0	3.30	15.400	80.926	12.948	3.891	20.139	100.0	0

[a] $Ab/V_p = (C_p)t_n + k[AUC]_{t_0}^{t_n} + (C_t)_{t_n}$
$(C_t)_{t_n} = k_{12}\Delta C_p \Delta t/2 + k_{12}/k_{21}\ (C_p)_{t_{n-1}}(1 - e^{-k_{21}\Delta t} + (C_t)_{t_{n-1}}\ e^{-k_{21}\Delta t}$
$k = 0.16;\ k_{12} = 0.29;\ k_{21} = 0.31$

of drug absorbed from the drug product, and Ab_{ref}^{∞} is the cumulative final amount of drug absorbed from a reference dosage form. In this case, the denominator of Equation 9.56 is modified as follows:

$$\text{CRFA} = \frac{C_p + k[\text{AUC}]^{\infty}}{k_{ref}[\text{AUC}]_{ref}^{\infty}} \tag{9.57}$$

where k_{ref} and $[AUC]_{ref}^{\infty}$ are the elimination constant and the area under the curve determined from the reference product. The terms in the numerator of Equation 9.57 refer to the product, as in Equation 9.56.

Each fraction of drug absorbed is cumulated and plotted against the time interval in which the plasma drug sample was obtained (Fig. 9-16). An example of the relationship of CRFA versus time for the absorption of tolazamide from four different drug products is shown in Figure 9-17. The data for Figure 9-18 were obtained from

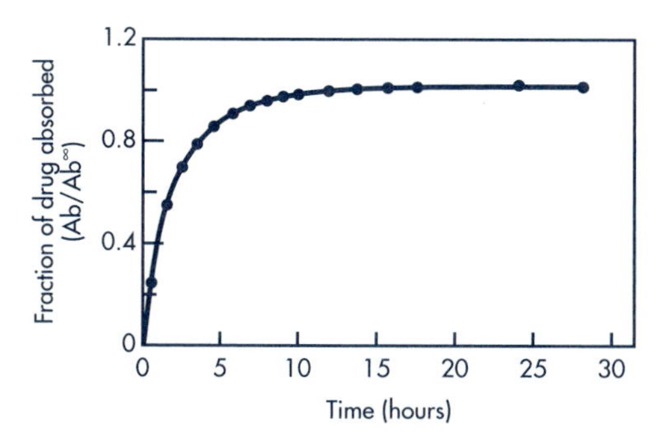

Figure 9-16. Fraction of drug absorbed. (Wagner–Nelson method).

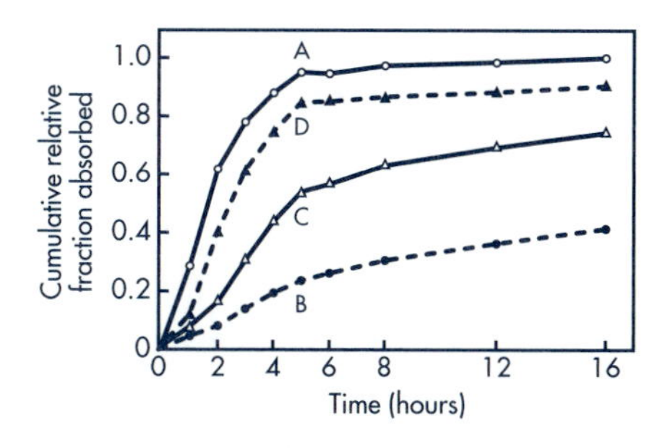

Figure 9-17. Mean cumulative relative fractions of tolazamide absorbed as a function of time.
(From Welling et al, 1982, with permission.)

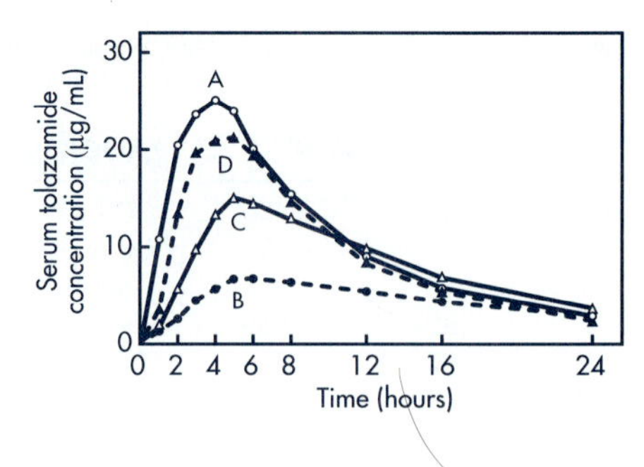

Figure 9-18. Mean serum tolazamide levels as a function of time.
(From Welling et al, 1982, with permission.)

the serum tolazamide levels versus time curves in Figure 9-17. The CRFA versus time graph provides a visual image of the relative rates of drug absorption from various drug products. If the CRFA versus time curve is a straight line, then the drug was absorbed from the drug product at an apparent zero-order absorption rate.

SIGNIFICANCE OF ABSORPTION RATE CONSTANTS

The overall rate of systemic drug absorption from an orally administered solid dosage form encompasses many individual rate processes, including dissolution of the drug, GI motility, blood flow, and transport of the drug across the capillary membranes and into the systemic circulation. The rate of drug absorption represents the net result of all these processes. The selection of a model with either first-order or zero-order absorption is generally empirical.

The actual drug absorption process may be zero-order, first-order, or a combination of rate processes that is not easily quantitated. For many immediate-release dosage forms, the absorption process is first order due to the physical nature of drug diffusion. For IV infusion and certain controlled-release drug products, the rate of drug absorption may be more appropriately described by a zero-order rate constant.

The calculation of k_a is useful in designing a multiple-dosage regimen. Knowledge of the k_a and k allows for the prediction of peak and trough plasma drug concentrations following multiple dosing. In bioequivalence studies, drug products are given in chemically equivalent (ie, pharmaceutical equivalents) doses, and the respective rates of systemic absorption may not differ markedly. Therefore, for these studies, t_{max}, or time of peak drug concentration, can be very useful in comparing the respective rates of absorption of a drug from chemically equivalent drug products.

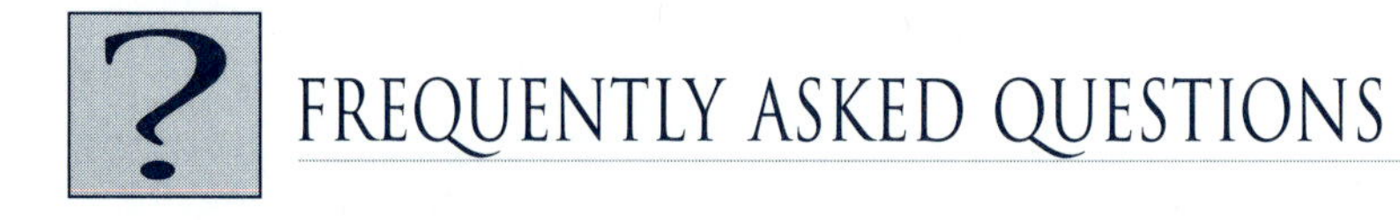

FREQUENTLY ASKED QUESTIONS

1. What is the absorption half-life of a drug and how is it determined?
2. When one simulates drug absorption with the oral one-compartment model, would a greater absorption rate constant result in a greater amount of drug absorbed?

3. How do you explain that k_a is often greater than k with most drugs?
4. Drug clearance is dependent on dose and area under the time–drug concentration curve. Would drug clearance be affected by the rate of absorption?
5. In switching a drug from IV to oral dosing, what is the most important consideration?

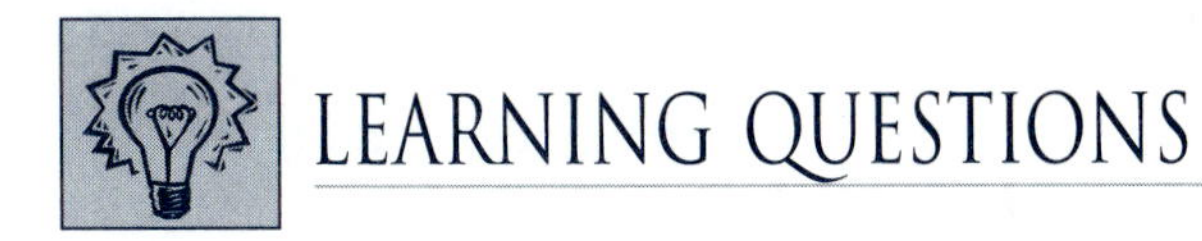

LEARNING QUESTIONS

1. Plasma samples from a patient were collected after an oral bolus dose of 10 mg of a new benzodiazepine solution as follows:

Time (hr)	**Concentration (ng/mL)**
0.25	2.85
0.50	5.43
0.75	7.75
1.00	9.84
2.00	16.20
4.00	22.15
6.00	23.01
10.00	19.09
14.00	13.90
20.00	7.97

   From the data above:
   a. Determine the elimination constant of the drug.
   b. Determine k_a by feathering.
   c. Determine the equation that describes the plasma drug concentration of the new benzodiazepine.
2. Assuming that the drug in Question 1 is 80% absorbed, find **(a)** the absorption constant, k_a; **(b)** the elimination half-life, $t_{1/2}$; **(c)** the t_{max}, or time of peak drug concentration; and **(d)** the volume of distribution of the patient.
3. Contrast the percent of drug-unabsorbed methods for the determination of rate constant for absorption, k_a, in terms of **(a)** pharmacokinetic model, **(b)** route of drug administration, and **(c)** possible sources of error.
4. What is the error inherent in the measurement of k_a for an orally administered drug that follows a two-compartment model when a one-compartment model is assumed in the calculation?
5. What are the main pharmacokinetic parameters that influence **(a)** time for peak drug concentration and **(b)** peak drug concentration?
6. Name a method of drug administration that will provide a zero-order input.
7. A single oral dose (100 mg) of an antibiotic was given to an adult male patient (43 years, 72 kg). From the literature, the pharmacokinetics of this drug fit a

one-compartment open model. The equation that best fits the pharmacokinetics of the drug is

$$C_p = 45(e^{-0.17t} - e^{-1.5t})$$

From the equation above, calculate **(a)** t_{max}, **(b)** C_{max}, and **(c)** $t_{1/2}$ for the drug in this patient. Assume C_p is in μg/mL and the first-order rate constants are in hours^{-1}.

8. Two drugs, *A* and *B*, have the following pharmacokinetic parameters after a single oral dose of 500 mg:

Drug	k_a (hr^{-1})	k (hr^{-1})	V_D (mL)
A	1.0	0.2	10,000
B	0.2	1.0	20,000

Both drugs follow a one-compartment pharmacokinetic model and are 100% bioavailable.

a. Calculate the t_{max} for each drug.
b. Calculate the C_{max} for each drug.

9. The bioavailability of phenylpropanolamine hydrochloride was studied in 24 adult male subjects. The following data represent the mean blood phenylpropanolamine hydrochloride concentrations (ng/mL) after the oral administration of a single 25-mg dose of phenylpropanolamine hydrochloride solution.

Time (hr)	Concentration (ng/mL)	Time (hr)	Concentration (ng/mL)
0	0	3	62.98
0.25	51.33	4	52.32
0.5	74.05	6	36.08
0.75	82.91	8	24.88
1.0	85.11	12	11.83
1.5	81.76	18	3.88
2	75.51	24	1.27

a. From the data, obtain the rate constant for absorption, k_a and the rate constant for elimination, k, by the method of residuals.
b. Is it reasonable to assume that $k_a > k$ for a drug in a solution? How would you determine unequivocally which rate constant represents the elimination constant k?
c. From the data, which method, Wagner–Nelson or Loo–Riegelman, would be more appropriate to determine the order of the rate constant for absorption?
d. From your values, calculate the theoretical t_{max}. How does your value relate to the observed t_{max} obtained from the subjects?
e. Would you consider the pharmacokinetics of phenylpropanolamine HCl to follow a one-compartment model? Why?

REFERENCES

Levy G, Amsel LP, Elliot HC: Kinetics of salicyluric acid elimination in man. *J Pharm Sci* **58:**827–829, 1969

Loo JCK, Riegelman S: New method for calculating the intrinsic absorption rate of drugs. *J Pharm Sci* **57:**918–928, 1968

Portmann G: Pharmacokinetics. In Swarbrick J (ed), *Current Concepts in the Pharmaceutical Sciences,* vol 1. Philadelphia, Lea & Febiger, 1970, Chap 1

Welling PG: *Pharmacokinetics: Processes and Mathematics.* ACS monograph 185. Washington, DC, American Chemical Society, 1986, pp 174–175

Welling PG, Patel RB, Patel UR, et al: Bioavailability of tolazamide from tablets: Comparison of in vitro and in vivo results. *J Pharm Sci* **71:**1259, 1982

Wagner JG: Use of computers in pharmacokinetics. *Clin Pharmacol Ther* **8:**201–218, 1967

BIBLIOGRAPHY

Boxenbaum HG, Kaplan SA: Potential source of error in absorption rate calculations. *J Pharmacokinet Biopharm* **3:**257–264, 1975

Boyes R, Adams H, Duce B: Oral absorption and disposition kinetics of lidocaine hydrochloride in dogs. *J Pharmacol Exp Ther* **174:**1–8, 1970

Dvorchik BH, Vesell ES: Significance of error associated with use of the one-compartment formula to calculate clearance of 38 drugs. *Clin Pharmacol Ther* **23:**617–623, 1978

Wagner JG, Nelson E: Kinetic analysis of blood levels and urinary excretion in the absorptive phase after single doses of drug. *J Pharm Sci* **53:**1392, 1964

Wagner JG, Nelson E: Percent absorbed time plots derived from blood level and/or urinary excretion data. *J Pharm Sci* **52:**610–611, 1963

10

BIOAVAILABILITY AND BIOEQUIVALENCE

Many drugs are marketed by more than one pharmaceutical manufacturer. The study of biopharmaceutics gives substantial evidence that the method of manufacture and the final formulation of the drug can markedly affect the bioavailability of the drug. Because of the plethora of drug products containing the same amount of active drug, physicians, pharmacists, and others who prescribe, dispense, or purchase drugs must select generic products that produce an equivalent therapeutic effect to the brand product. To facilitate such decisions, guidelines have been developed by the United States Food and Drug Administration (FDA). The guidelines are available on the Internet (http://www.fda.gov). Some of the guidelines also appear in the United States Pharmacopeia/National Formulary (USP-NF). These guidelines and methods for determining drug availability are discussed in this chapter.

DEFINITIONS

- *Bioavailability.* Indicates a measurement of the rate and extent (amount) of therapeutically active drug that reaches the systemic circulation and is available at the site of action.
- *Bioequivalence requirement.* A requirement imposed by the Food and Drug Administration (FDA) for *in vitro* and/or *in vivo* testing of specified drug products which must be satisfied as a condition for marketing.
- *Bioequivalent drug products.* Bioequivalent drug products are pharmaceutical equivalents that have similar bioavailability (ie, are not significantly different with respect to rate and extent of absorption) when given in the same molar dose and studied under similar experimental conditions. Some drugs may be considered bioequivalent that are equal in the extent of absorption but *not* in the rate of absorption; this is possible if the difference in the rate of absorption is considered clinically insignificant, is not essential for the attainment of effective body drug concentrations on chronic use, and is reflected in the proposed labeling. For example, aspirin and acetaminophen are well-absorbed drugs, and small differences in the rate of absorption are of very little clinical consequence. Bioequivalence

may sometimes be demonstrated using an *in vitro* bioequivalence standard, especially when such an *in vitro* test has been correlated with human in vivo bioavailability data. For some products, other *in vivo* tests may be appropriate, including comparative clinical trials or pharmacodynamic studies.

- *Brand name.* Trade name of the drug. This name is privately owned by the manufacturer or distributor and is used to distinguish the specific drug product from competitors' products (eg, Tylenol, McNeil Laboratories).
- *Chemical name.* Name used by the organic chemist to indicate the chemical structure of the drug (eg, N-acetyl-*p*-aminophenol).
- *Drug product.* The finished dosage form (eg, tablet, capsule or solution) that contains the active drug ingredient, generally, but not necessarily, in association with inactive ingredients.
- *Drug product selection.* The process of choosing or selecting the drug product in a specified dosage form.
- *Drug substance.* A drug substance is the active pharmaceutical ingredient (API) or component in the drug product that furnishes the pharmacodynamic activity.
- *Equivalence.* Relationship in terms of bioavailability, therapeutic response, or a set of established standards of one drug product to another.
- *Generic name.* The established, nonproprietary, or common name of the active drug in a drug product (eg, acetaminophen).
- *Generic substitution.* The process of dispensing a different brand or unbranded drug product in place of the prescribed drug product. The substituted drug product contains the same active ingredient or therapeutic moiety as the same salt or ester in the same dosage form but is made by a different manufacturer. For example, a prescription for Motrin brand of ibuprofen might be dispensed by the pharmacist as Advil brand of ibuprofen or as a nonbranded generic ibuprofen if generic substitution is permitted and desired by the physician.
- *Pharmaceutical alternatives.* Drug products that contain the same therapeutic moiety but as different salts, esters, or complexes. For example, tetracycline phosphate or tetracycline hydrochloride equivalent to 250 mg tetracycline base are considered pharmaceutical alternatives. Different dosage forms and strengths within a product line by a single manufacturer are pharmaceutical alternatives (eg, an extended-release dosage form and a standard immediate-release dosage form of the same active ingredient).
- *Pharmaceutical equivalents.* Drug products that contain the same active drug ingredient (same salt, ester, or chemical form) and are identical in strength or concentration, dosage form, and route of administration (eg, diazepam, 5 mg oral tablets). *Chemical equivalents* are pharmaceutical equivalents. Pharmaceutical equivalent drug products must meet the identical standards (strength, quality, purity, and identity), but may differ in such characteristics as color, flavor, shape, scoring configuration, packaging, excipients, preservatives, expiration time, and (within certain limits) labeling.
- *Pharmaceutical substitution.* The process of dispensing a pharmaceutical alternative for the prescribed drug product. For example, ampicillin suspension is dispensed in place of ampicillin capsules, or tetracycline hydrochloride is dispensed in place of tetracycline phosphate. Pharmaceutical substitution generally requires the physician's approval.
- *Therapeutic alternatives.* Drug products containing different active ingredients that are indicated for the same therapeutic or clinical objectives. Active ingredients in therapeutic alternatives are from the same pharmacologic class and are ex-

pected to have the same therapeutic effect when administered to patients for such condition of use. For example, ibuprofen is given instead of aspirin; cimetidine may be given instead of ranitidine.

- *Therapeutic equivalents.* Therapeutic equivalents are drug products that contain the same therapeutically active drug that should give the same therapeutic effect and have equal potential for adverse effects under conditions set forth in the labels of these drug products. Therapeutic drug products may differ in certain characteristics, such as color, scoring, flavor, configuration, packaging, preservatives, and expiration date. Therapeutic equivalent drug products must be (1) safe and effective, (2) pharmaceutical equivalents, (3) bioequivalent, (4) adequately labeled, and (5) manufactured in compliance with current good manufacturing practices.
- *Therapeutic substitution.* The process of dispensing a therapeutic alternative in place of the prescribed drug product. For example, amoxicillin is dispensed for ampicillin or acetaminophen is dispensed for aspirin.

PURPOSE OF BIOAVAILABILITY STUDIES

Bioavailability studies are performed for both approved active drug ingredients or therapeutic moieties not yet approved for marketing by the FDA. New formulations of active drug ingredients or therapeutic moieties must be approved prior to marketing by the FDA. In approving a drug product for marketing, the FDA must ensure that the drug product is safe and effective for its labeled indications for use. Moreover, the drug product must meet all applicable standards of identity, strength, quality, and purity. To ensure that these standards are met, the FDA requires bioavailability/pharmacokinetic studies and where necessary bioequivalence studies for all drug products.

For unmarketed drugs which do not have full new drug application (NDA) approval by the FDA, *in vitro* and/or *in vivo* bioequivalence studies must be performed on the drug formulation proposed for marketing as a generic drug product. Furthermore, the essential pharmacokinetics of the active drug ingredient or therapeutic moiety must be characterized. Essential pharmacokinetic parameters including the rate and extent of systemic absorption, elimination half-life, and rates of excretion and metabolism should be established after single- and multiple-dose administration. Data from these *in vivo* bioavailability studies are important to establish recommended dosage regimens and to support drug labeling.

In vivo bioavailability studies are performed also for new formulations of active drug ingredients or therapeutic moieties that have full NDA approval and are approved for marketing. The purpose of these studies is to determine the bioavailability and to characterize the pharmacokinetics of the new formulation, new dosage form, or new salt or ester relative to a reference formulation.

After the bioavailability and essential pharmacokinetic parameters of the active ingredient or therapeutic moiety are established, dosage regimens may be recommended in support of drug labeling.

In summary, clinical studies are useful in determining the safety and efficacy of the drug product. Bioavailability studies are used to define the effect of changes in the physicochemical properties of the drug substance and the effect of the drug product (dosage form) on the pharmacokinetics of the drug. Bioequivalence studies are used to compare the bioavailability of the same drug (same salt or ester) from various drug products. If the drug products are bioequivalent and therapeutically equivalent (as defined above), then the clinical efficacy and the safety profile of these drug products are assumed to be similar and may be substituted for each other.

RELATIVE AND ABSOLUTE AVAILABILITY

The area under the drug concentration–time curve (AUC) is used as a measure of the total amount of unaltered drug that reaches the systemic circulation. The AUC is dependent on the total quantity of available drug, FD_0, divided by the elimination rate constant, k, and the apparent volume of distribution, V_D. F is the fraction of the dose absorbed. After IV administration, F is equal to unity, because the entire dose is placed into the systemic circulation. Therefore, the drug is considered to be completely available after IV administration. After oral administration of the drug, F may vary from a value of 0 (no drug absorption) to 1 (complete drug absorption).

Relative Availability

Relative (apparent) availability is the availability of the drug from a drug product as compared to a recognized standard. The fraction of dose systemically available from an oral drug product is difficult to ascertain. The availability of drug in the formulation is compared to the availability of drug in a standard dosage formulation, usually a solution of the pure drug evaluated in a crossover study. The relative availability of two drug products given at the same dosage level and by the same route of administration can be obtained with the following equation:

$$\text{Relative availability} = \frac{[\text{AUC}]_A}{[\text{AUC}]_B} \tag{10.1}$$

where drug product B is the recognized reference standard. This fraction may be multiplied by 100 to give *percent* relative availability.

When different doses are administered, a correction for the size of the dose is made, as in the following equation:

$$\text{Relative availability} = \frac{[\text{AUC}]_A/\text{dose } A}{[\text{AUC}]_B/\text{dose } B}$$

Urinary drug excretion data may also be used to measure relative availability, as long as the total amount of intact drug excreted in the urine is collected. The percent relative availability using urinary excretion data can be determined as follows:

$$\text{Percent relative availability} = \frac{[D_u]_A^\infty}{[D_u]_B^\infty} \times 100 \tag{10.2}$$

where $[D_u]^\infty$ is the total amount of drug excreted in the urine.

Absolute Availability

The absolute availability of drug is the systemic availability of a drug after extravascular administration (eg, oral, rectal, transdermal, subcutaneous). The absolute availability of a drug is generally measured by comparing the respective AUCs after extravascular and IV administration. This measurement may be performed as long as V_D and k are independent of the route of administration. Absolute availability after oral drug administration using plasma data can be determined as follows:

$$\text{Absolute availability} = \frac{[\text{AUC}]_{\text{PO}}/\text{dose}_{\text{PO}}}{[\text{AUC}]_{\text{IV}}/\text{dose}_{\text{IV}}} = \frac{F}{z} \tag{10.3}$$

Absolute availability using urinary drug excretion data can be determined by the following:

$$\text{Absolute availability} = \frac{[D_u]_{\text{PO}}^{\infty}/\text{dose}_{\text{PO}}}{[D_u]_{\text{IV}}^{\infty}/\text{dose}_{\text{IV}}} \tag{10.4}$$

The absolute bioavailability is also equal to F, the fraction of the dose that is bioavailable. Absolute availability is sometimes expressed as a percent, ie, $F = 1$, or 100%. For drugs given intravascularly, such as by IV bolus injection, $F = 1$, because all the drug is completely absolved. For all extravascular routes of administration, $F \leq 1$. F is usually determined by Equations 10.3 or 10.4.

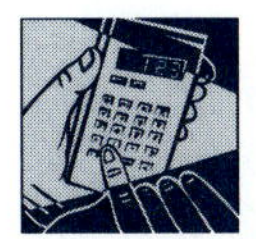

PRACTICE PROBLEM

The bioavailability of a new investigational drug was studied in 12 volunteers. Each volunteer received either a single oral tablet containing 200 mg of the drug, 5 mL of a pure aqueous solution containing 200 mg of the drug, or a single IV bolus injection containing 50 mg of the drug. Plasma samples were obtained periodically up to 48 hr after the dose and assayed for drug concentration. The average AUC values (0 to 48 hr) are given in the table below. From these data, calculate (1) the relative bioavailability of the drug from the tablet compared to the oral solution and (2) the absolute bioavailability of the drug from the tablet.

Drug Product	Dose (mg)	AUC(μg hr/mL)	Standard Deviation
Oral tablet	200	89.5	19.7
Oral solution	200	86.1	18.1
IV bolus injection	50	37.8	5.7

Solution

The relative bioavailability of the drug from the tablet is estimated using Equation 10.1. No adjustment for dose is necessary.

$$\text{Relative bioavailability} = \frac{89.5}{86.1} = 1.04$$

The relative bioavailability of the drug from the tablet is 1.04, or 104%, compared to the solution. In this study, the difference in drug bioavailability between tablet and solution was not statistically significant.

The absolute drug bioavailability from the tablet is calculated using Equation 10.3 and adjusting for the dose.

$$F = \text{absolute bioavailability} = \frac{89.5/200}{37.8/50} = 0.59$$

Because F, the fraction of dose absorbed from the tablet, was less than 1, the drug was not completely absorbed systemically either due to poor absorption or metabolism by first-pass effect. The relative bioavailability of the drug from the tablet was approximately 100% when compared to the oral solution. Results from bioequivalence studies may show that the relative bioavailability of the test oral product to be greater than, equal to, or less than 100% compared to the reference oral drug product. However, the results from these bioequivalence studies should not be misinterpreted to imply that the absolute bioavailability of the drug from the oral drug products is also 100% unless the oral formulation was compared to an intravenous injection of the drug.

METHODS FOR ASSESSING BIOAVAILABILITY

Direct and indirect methods may be used to assess drug bioavailability. The design of the bioavailability study depends on the objectives of the study, the ability to analyze the drug (and metabolites) in biological fluids, the pharmacodynamics of the drug substance, the route of drug administration and the nature of the drug product. Pharmacokinetic and/or pharmacodynamic parameters as well as clinical observations and in vitro studies may be used to determine drug bioavailability from a drug product (Table 10.1).

Plasma Drug Concentration

Measurement of drug concentrations in blood, plasma, or serum after drug administration is the most direct and objective data to determine systemic drug bioavailability. By appropriate blood sampling, an accurate description of the

TABLE 10.1 Methods for Assessing Bioavailability and Bioequivalence

Plasma Drug Concentration
The time for peak plasma (blood) concentration (t_{max})
The peak plasma drug concentration (C_{max})
The area under the plasma drug concentration versus time curve (AUC)
Urinary Drug Excretion
The cumulative amount of drug excreted in the urine (D_u)
The rate of drug excretion in the urine (dD_u/dt)
The time for maximum urinary excretion (t)
Acute Pharmacodynamic Effect
Maximum pharmacodynamic effect (E_{MAX})
Time for maximum pharmacodynamic effect
Area under the pharmacodynamic effect versus time curve
Onset time for pharmacodynamic effect
Clinical Observations
Well-controlled clinical trials
***In Vitro* Studies**
Drug dissolution

plasma drug concentration versus time profile of the therapeutically active drug substance(s) can be obtained using a validated drug assay (see Appendix).

t_{max}

The time of peak plasma concentration, t_{max}, corresponds to the time required to reach maximum drug concentration after drug administration. At t_{max}, peak drug absorption occurs and the rate of drug absorption exactly equals the rate of drug elimination (Fig. 10-5). Drug absorption still continues after t_{max} is reached, but at a slower rate. When comparing drug products, t_{max} can be used as an approximate indication of drug absorption rate. The value for t_{max} will become smaller (indicating less time required to reach peak plasma concentration) as the absorption rate for the drug becomes more rapid. Units for t_{max} are units of time (eg, hours, minutes).

C_{max}

The peak plasma drug concentration, C_{max}, represents the maximum plasma drug concentration obtained after oral administration of drug (Fig. 10-5). For many drugs, a relationship is found between the pharmacodynamic drug effect and the plasma drug concentration. C_{max} provides indications that the drug is sufficiently systemically absorbed to provide a therapeutic response. In addition, C_{max} provides warning of possibly toxic levels of drug. The units of C_{max} are concentration units (eg, μg/mL, ng/mL).

AUC

The area under the plasma level–time curve, AUC, is a measurement of the extent of drug bioavailability. The AUC reflects the total amount of active drug that reaches the systemic circulation. The AUC is the area under the drug plasma level–time curve from $t = 0$ to $t = \infty$, and is equal to the amount of unchanged drug reaching the general circulation divided by the clearance.

$$[\mathrm{AUC}]_0^\infty = \int_0^\infty C_p\,dt \tag{10.5}$$

$$[\mathrm{AUC}]_0^\infty = \frac{FD_0}{\text{clearance}} = \frac{FD_0}{kV_D} \tag{10.6}$$

where F = fraction of dose absorbed; D_0 = dose; k = elimination rate constant; and V_D = volume of distribution. The AUC is independent of the route of administration and processes of drug elimination as long as the elimination processes do not change. The AUC can be determined by a numerical integration procedure, such as the trapezoidal rule method. The units for AUC are concentration time (eg, μg hr/mL).

For many drugs, the AUC is directly proportional to dose. For example, if a single dose of a drug is increased from 250 to 1000 mg, the AUC will also show a fourfold increase (Figs. 10-1 and 10-2).

In some cases, the AUC is not directly proportional to the administered dose for all dosage levels. For example, as the dosage of drug is increased, one of the pathways for drug elimination may become saturated (Fig. 10-3). Drug elimination includes the processes of metabolism and excretion. Drug metabolism is an en-

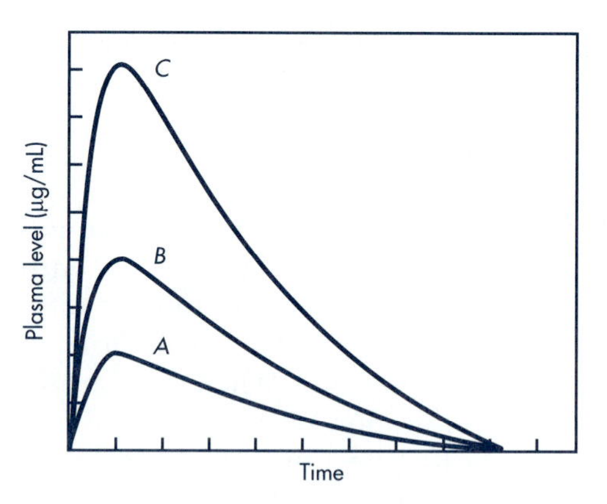

Figure 10-1. Plasma level–time curve following administration of single doses of **(A)** 250 mg, **(B)** 500 mg, and **(C)** 1000 mg of drug.

zyme-dependent process. For drugs such as salicylate and phenytoin, continued increase of the dose causes saturation of one of the enzyme pathways for drug metabolism and consequent prolongation of the elimination half-life. The AUC thus increases disproportionally to the increase in dose, because a smaller amount of drug is being eliminated (ie, more drug is retained). When the AUC is not directly proportional to the dose, bioavailability of the drug is difficult to evaluate because drug kinetics may be dose dependent.

Urinary Drug Excretion Data

Urinary drug excretion data is an indirect method for estimating bioavailability. The drug must be excreted in significant quantities as unchanged drug in the urine, timely urine samples must be collected and the total amount of urinary drug excretion must be obtained (see Chapter 3).

D_u^∞

The cumulative amount of drug excreted in the urine, D_u^∞ is directly related to the total amount of drug absorbed. Experimentally, urine samples are collected periodically after administration of the drug product. Each urine specimen is analyzed for free drug with a specific assay. A graph is constructed relating the cumulative drug excreted to the collection time interval (Figure 10-4B).

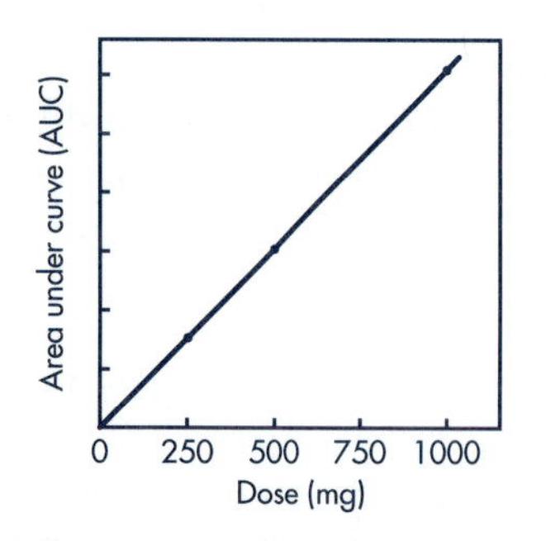

Figure 10-2. Linear relationship between AUC and dose (data from Fig. 10-1).

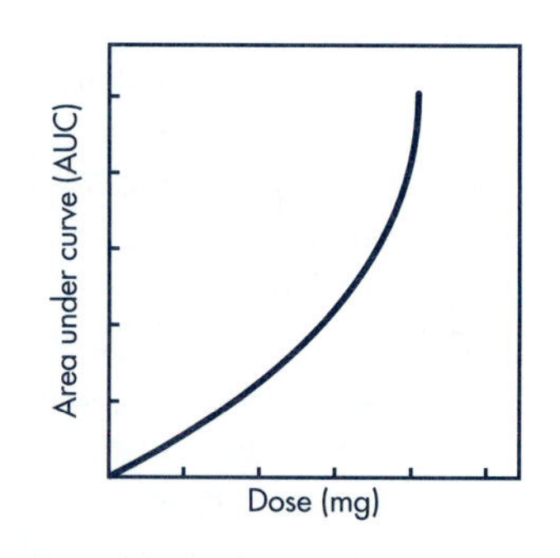

Figure 10-3. Relationship between AUC and dose when metabolism is saturable.

The relationship between the cumulative amount of drug excreted in the urine and the plasma level–time curve is shown in Figure 10-4. When the drug is almost completely eliminated (point *C*), the plasma concentration approaches zero and the maximum amount of drug excreted in the urine, D_u^∞, is obtained.

dD_u/dt

Because most drugs are eliminated by a first-order rate process, the rate of drug excretion is dependent on the first-order elimination rate constant k and the concentration of drug in the plasma C_p. In Figure 10-4, the maximum rate of drug excretion would be at point *B*, whereas the minimum rate of drug excretion would be at points *A* and *C*. Thus, a graph comparing the rate of drug excretion with respect to time should be similar in shape as the plasma level–time curve for that drug (Fig. 10-5).

t^∞

The total time for the drug to be excreted is t^∞. In Figures 10-4 and 10-5, the slope of the curve segment *A–B* is related to the rate of drug absorption, whereas point *C* is related to the total time required after drug administration for the drug to be absorbed and completely excreted ($t = \infty$). The t^∞ is a useful parameter in bio-equivalence studies that compare several drug products, as will be described later in this chapter.

Acute Pharmacodynamic Effect

In some cases, the quantitative measurement of a drug is not available, or it lacks sufficient accuracy and/or reproducibility. An acute pharmacodynamic effect—such as an effect on pupil diameter, heart rate, or blood pressure—can be used as an index of drug bioavailability. In this case, an acute pharmacodynamic effect–time curve is constructed. Measurements of the pharmacodynamic effect should be made with sufficient frequency to permit a reasonable estimate of the total area under

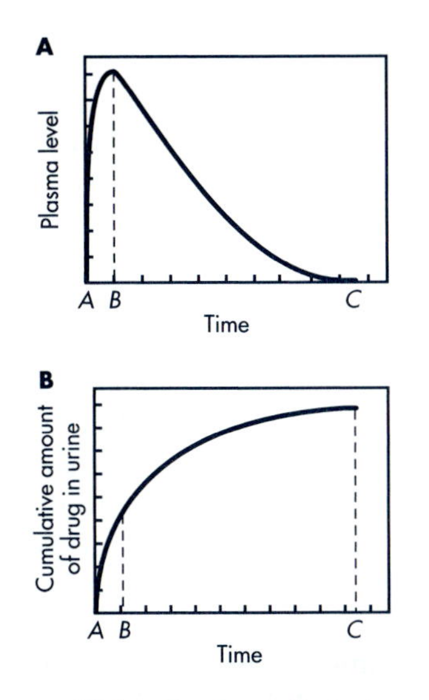

Figure 10-4. Corresponding plots relating the plasma level–time curve and the cumulative urinary drug excretion.

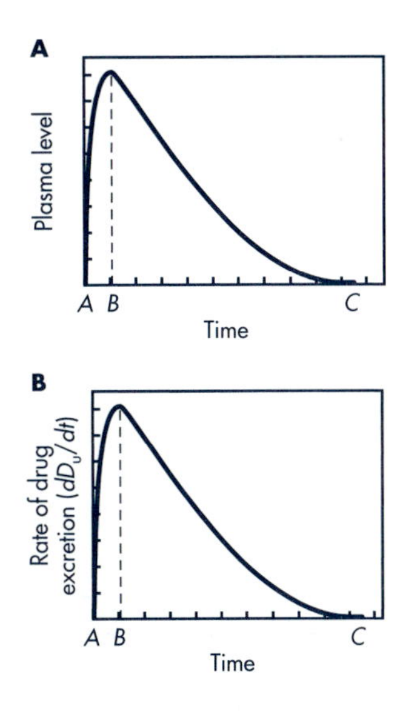

Figure 10-5. Corresponding plots relating the plasma level–time curve and the rate of urinary drug excretion.

the curve for a time period at least three times the half-life of the drug (Gardner, 1977).

The use of an acute pharmacodynamic effect to determine bioavailability generally requires demonstration of a dose-related response. Bioavailability is determined by characterization of the dose–response curve. Pharmacodynamic parameters that are obtained include the total area under the acute pharmacodynamic effect–time curve, peak pharmacodynamic effect, and time for peak pharmacodynamic effect. Onset time and duration of the pharmacokinetic effect may also be included in the analysis of the data.

Clinical Observations

Well-controlled clinical trials in humans that establish the safety and effectiveness of the drug product. The clinical trials approach is the least accurate, least sensitive and least reproducible of the general approaches for determining in vivo bioavailability. The FDA only considers this approach when analytical methods are not available to permit use of one of the approaches described above. An example of this approach is for the determination of the bioequivalence of two topical antifungal products by different manufacturers containing the same active antifungal agent (eg, ketoconazole)

In Vitro Studies

Drug dissolution studies may under certain conditions give an indication of drug bioavailability. Ideally, the *in vitro* drug dissolution rate should correlate with *in vivo* drug bioavailability. Dissolution studies are often performed on several test formulations of the same drug. The test formulation that demonstrates the most rapid rate of drug dissolution *in vitro* will generally have the most rapid rate of drug bioavailability *in vivo.*

BIOEQUIVALENCE STUDIES

For many years, medical practitioners have observed either lack of response (therapeutic failure), good therapeutic response, or toxicity in patients receiving similar drug products.

Differences in the predicted clinical response may be due to differences in both the pharmacokinetic and/or pharmacodynamic behavior of the drug among individuals. Bioequivalent drug products that have the same systemic drug bioavailability will have the same predictable drug response. However, variable clinical responses among individuals that are unrelated to bioavailability may be due to differences in the pharmacodynamics of the drug. Differences in pharmacodynamics, ie, the relationship between the drug and the receptor site, may be due to differences in receptor sensitivity to the drug. Various factors affecting pharmacodynamic drug behavior may include age, drug tolerance, drug interactions, and unknown pathophysiologic factors.

The bioavailability of a drug may be reproducible among fasted individuals in controlled studies who take the drug on an empty stomach. When the drug is used on a daily basis, however, the nature of an individual's diet may affect the plasma drug level due to variable absorption in the presence of food or even a change in the metabolic clearance of the drug. Feldman and associates (1982) reported that patients on a high-carbohydrate diet have a much longer elimination half-life of theophylline, due to the reduced metabolic clearance of the drug ($t_{1/2}$, 18.1 hr), compared to patients on normal diets ($t_{1/2}$, 6.76 hr). Previous studies demonstrated that the theophylline drug product was completely bioavailable. The higher plasma drug concentration resulting from a carbohydrate diet may subject the patient to a higher risk of drug intoxication with theophylline. The effect of food on the availability of theophylline has been reported by the FDA concerning the risk of higher theophylline plasma concentrations from a 24-hour sustained release drug product taken with food. Although most bioavailability drug studies use fasted volunteers, the diet of patients actually using the drug product may increase or decrease the bioavailability of the drug (Hendles et al, 1984).

Bases for Determining Bioequivalence

Bioequivalence is established if the *in vivo* bioavailability of a test drug product (usually the generic product) does not differ significantly (ie, statistically insignificant) in the product's rate and extent of drug absorption, as determined by comparison of measured parameters (eg, concentration of the active drug ingredient in the blood, urinary excretion rates, or pharmacodynamic effects), from that of the reference material (usually the brand name product). In addition, statistical techniques used should be of sufficient sensitivity to detect differences in the rate and extent of absorption that are not attributable to subject variability.

A drug product that differs from the reference material in its rate of absorption, but not in its extent of absorption, may be considered bioavailable if the difference in the rate of absorption is intentional and appropriately reflected in the labeling and/or the rate of absorption is not detrimental to the safety and effectiveness of the drug product.

Criteria for Establishing a Bioequivalence Requirement

Bioequivalence requirements may be imposed by the FDA on the basis of the following:

1. Evidence from well-controlled clinical trials or controlled observations in patients that various drug products do not give comparable therapeutic effects.
2. Evidence from well-controlled bioequivalence studies that such products are not bioequivalent drug products.
3. Evidence that the drug products exhibit a narrow therapeutic ratio and minimum effective concentrations in the blood and that safe and effective use of the drug products requires careful dosage titration and patient monitoring.
4. Competent medical determination that a lack of bioequivalence would have a serious adverse effect on the treatment or prevention of a serious disease or condition.
5. Physicochemical evidence of the following:
   - **a.** The active drug ingredient has a low solubility in water (eg, less than 5 mg/mL).
   - **b.** The dissolution rate of one or more such products is slow (eg, less than 50% in 30 min when tested with a general method specified by the FDA).
   - **c.** The particle size and/or surface area of the active drug ingredient is critical in determining its bioavailability.
   - **d.** Certain structural forms of the active drug ingredient (eg, polymorphic forms, conforms, solvates, complexes, and crystal modifications) dissolve poorly, thus affecting absorption.

e. Such drug products have a high ratio of excipients to active ingredients (eg, greater than 5 to 1).
f. Specific inactive ingredients (eg, hydrophilic or hydrophobic excipients and lubricants) either may be required for absorption of the active drug ingredient or of therapeutic moiety or may interfere with such absorption.

6. Pharmacokinetic evidence of the following:
   a. The active drug ingredient, therapeutic moiety, or its precursor is absorbed in large part in a particular segment of the GI tract or is absorbed from a localized site.
   b. The degree of absorption of the active drug ingredient, therapeutic moiety, or its precursor is poor (eg, less than 50%, ordinarily in comparison to an intravenous dose) even when it is administered in pure form (eg, in solution).
   c. There is rapid metabolism of the therapeutic moiety in the intestinal wall or liver during the absorption process (first-order metabolism), so that the rate of absorption is unusually important in the therapeutic effect and/or toxicity of the drug product.
   d. The therapeutic moiety is rapidly metabolized or excreted so that rapid dissolution and absorption are required for effectiveness.
   e. The active drug ingredient or therapeutic moiety is unstable in specific portions of the GI tract and requires special coatings or formulations (eg, buffers, enteric coatings, and film coatings) to ensure adequate absorption.
   f. The drug product is subject to dose-dependent kinetics in or near the therapeutic range, and the rate and extent of absorption are important to bioequivalence.

Criteria for Waiver of Evidence of *In Vivo* Bioavailability

For certain drug products, the *in vivo* bioavailability of the drug product may be self-evident or unimportant to the achievement of the product's intended purposes. The FDA will waive the requirement for submission of *in vivo* evidence demonstrating the bioavailability of the drug product if the product meets one of the following criteria:

1. The drug product (a) is a solution intended solely for intravenous administration and (b) contains an active drug ingredient or therapeutic moiety combined with the same solvent and in the same concentration as in an intravenous solution that is the subject of an approved, full, new drug application.
2. The drug product is a topically applied preparation (eg, a cream, ointment, or gel intended for local therapeutic effect). The FDA has released guidances for the performance of bioequivalence studies on topical corticosteroids and antifungal agents. The FDA is also considering performing dermatopharmacokinetic (DPK) studies on other topical drug products. In addition, *in vitro* drug release and diffusion studies may be required.
3. The drug product is in an oral dosage form that is not intended to be absorbed (eg, an antacid or a radiopaque medium). Specific *in vitro* bioequivalence studies may be required by the FDA. For example, the bioequivalence of cholestyramine resin is demonstrated *in vitro* by the binding of bile acids to the resin.

   The FDA has issued a guidance for establishing the bioequivalence of albuterol metered-dose inhalers using a pharmacodynamic effect study.

4. The drug product meets both of the following conditions:
   a. It is administered by inhalation as a gas or vapor (eg, as a medicinal or as an inhalation anesthetic).
   b. It contains an active drug ingredient or therapeutic moiety in the same dosage form as a drug product that is the subject of an approved, full, new drug application.
5. The drug product meets all of the following conditions:
   a. It is an oral solution, elixir, syrup, tincture, or similar other solubilized form.
   b. It contains an active drug ingredient or therapeutic moiety in the same concentration as a drug product that is the subject of an approved, full, new drug application.
   c. It contains no inactive ingredient that is known to significantly affect absorption of the active drug ingredient or therapeutic moiety.

DESIGN AND EVALUATION OF BIOEQUIVALENCE STUDIES

In the past, generic drug products that were pharmaceutical equivalents did not always give identical therapeutic effects *in vivo* in patients. Thus, bioequivalence studies are performed to compare the bioavailability of the generic drug product to the brand name product. Once bioequivalence is established, then it is likely that both the generic and brand name dosage forms will produce the same therapeutic effect. The FDA publishes guidances (*http://www.fda.gov/cder/guidance*) for bioequivalence studies. These guidances should be consulted for specific drugs. Sponsors may also request a meeting with the FDA to review the study design.

Design

The design and evaluation of well-controlled bioequivalence studies require the cooperative input from pharmacokineticists, statisticians, clinicians, bioanalytical chemists, and others. The basic design for a bioequivalence study is determined by (1) the scientific questions to be answered, (2) the nature of the reference material and the dosage form to be tested, (3) the availability of analytical methods, and (4) benefit-risk considerations with regard to testing in humans. For some generic drugs, the FDA offers general guidelines for conducting these studies. For example, *"Statistical Procedures for Bioequivalence Studies Using a Standard Two-Treatment Crossover Design"* is available from the FDA; the publication addresses three specific aspects, including (1) logarithmic transformation of pharmacokinetic data, (2) sequence effect, and (3) outlier consideration. However, even with the availability of such guidelines, the principal investigator should prepare a detailed protocol for the study. Some of the elements of a protocol for an *in vivo* bioavailability study are listed in Table 10.2. Bioavailability studies for controlled-release dosage forms are discussed in Chapter 7.

For bioequivalence studies, both the test and reference drug formulations contain the pharmaceutical equivalent drug in the same dose strength, in similar dosage forms (eg, immediate release or controlled release), and both are given by the same route of administration. Both a single dose and/or a multiple dose (steady-state) study may be required. Prior to initiation of the study, the *Institutional Review Board* (IRB) of the clinical facility in which the study is to be performed must ap-

TABLE 10.2 Elements of a Bioavailability Study Protocol

I. Title
  A. Principle investigator (study director)
  B. Project/protocol number and date
II. Study objective
III. Study design
  A. Design
  B. Drug products
    1. Test product(s)
    2. Reference product
  C. Dosage regimen
  D. Sample collection schedule
  E. Housing/confinement
  F. Fasting/meals schedule
  G. Analytical methods
IV. Study population
  A. Subjects
  B. Subject selection
    1. Medical history
    2. Physical examination
    3. Laboratory tests
  C. Inclusion/exclusion criteria
    1. Inclusion criteria
    2. Exclusion criteria
  D. Restrictions/prohibitions
V. Clinical procedures
  A. Dosage and drug administration
  B. Biological sampling schedule and handling procedures
  C. Activity of subjects
VI. Ethical considerations
  A. Basic principles
  B. Institutional review board
  C. Informed consent
  D. Indications for subject withdrawal
  E. Adverse reactions and emergency procedures
VII. Facilities
VIII. Data analysis
  A. Analytical validation procedure
  B. Statistical treatment of data
IX. Drug accountability
X. Appendix

prove the study. The IRB is composed of both professional and lay persons with diverse backgrounds who have clinical experience and expertise as well as sensitivity to ethical issues and community attitudes. The IRB is responsible for safeguarding the rights and welfare of human subjects.

The basic guiding principle in performing studies is that *no unnecessary human research be done.* Generally, the study is performed in normal, healthy male volunteers who have given informed consent to be in the study. The number of subjects in the study will depend upon the expected intersubject variability. Patient selection will be made according to certain established criteria for inclusion into, or exclusion from, the study. For example, the study might exclude any volunteers who are smokers, have known allergies to the drug, are overweight, or have taken any medication within a specified period (often 1 week) prior to the study. The subjects are generally fasted 10 to 12 hours (overnight) prior to drug administration and may continue to fast for a 2- to 4-hour period after dosing.

Reference Standard

In considering a bioequivalence study, one formulation of the drug is chosen as a reference standard against which all other formulations of the drug are compared. The reference material should be administered by the same route as the comparison formulations unless an alternative route or additional route is needed to answer specific pharmokinetic questions. For example, if an active drug is poorly bioavailable after oral administration, the drug may be compared to an oral solution or an intravenous injection. The reference standard is generally a formulation currently marketed with a fully approved NDA for which there are valid scientific safety and efficacy data. The reference formulation is usually the innovator's or original manufacturer's brand name product

Before beginning an *in vivo* bioequivalence study, the total content of the active drug substance in the test product (generally the generic product) must be within 5% of the reference product. Moreover, *in vitro* comparative dissolution or drug release studies under various specified conditions are usually performed for both test and reference products.

Study Designs

For many drug products, the FDA, Division of Bioequivalence, Office of Generic Drugs provides a guidance for the performance of in vitro dissolution and in vivo bioequivalence studies. Similar guidelines appear in the USP/NF. Currently, three different studies may be required for solid oral dosage forms, including (1) a fasting study, (2) a food intervention study and/or (3) a multiple dose (steady-state) study. Three other study designs have been proposed by FDA. For example, FDA published two draft guidelines in October and December of 1997 to consider the performance of individual bioequivalence using a replicate design and a two-way crossover food intervention study. Proper study design and statistical evolution are important considerations for the determination of bioequivalence. The designs listed above are summarized here.

Fasting Study

Bioequivalence studies are usually evaluated by a single dose, two-period, two treatment, two sequence, open label, randomized *crossover design* comparing equal doses of the test and reference products in fasted, adult, healthy subjects. This study is required for all immediate-release and modified-release oral dosage forms. Both male and female subjects may be used in the study. Blood sampling is performed just prior (zero time) to the dose and at appropriate intervals after the dose to obtain an adequate description of the plasma drug concentration versus time profile. The subjects should be in the fasting state (overnight fast) prior to drug administration and should continue to fast for up to 4-hour period after dosing. No other medication is normally given to the subject for at least one week prior to the study.

Food Intervention Study

This study is a single dose, randomized, three-treatment, three period, six sequence, crossover, limited food effects study comparing equal doses of the test product given under fasting conditions with those of the test and reference products given immediately after a standard, high fat content breakfast. This study is required for all modified-release dosage forms and may be required for immediate-release dosage forms if the bioavailability of the active drug ingredient is known to be affected by food (eg, ibuprofen, naproxen).

Multiple Dose (Steady-State) Study

A multiple dose, steady-state, randomized, two-treatment, two-way, crossover study comparing equal doses of the test and reference products in adult, healthy subjects is required for oral extended-release (controlled-release) drug products in addition to a single dose fasting study and a food intervention study. Three consecutive trough concentrations (C_{min}) on three consecutive days should be determined to ascertain that the subjects are at steady state. The last morning dose is given to the subject after an overnight fast with continual fasting for at least 2 hours following dose administration. Blood sampling is performed similarly to the single dose study.

Crossover Designs

Subjects who meet the inclusion and exclusion study criteria and have given informed consent are selected at random. A complete crossover design is usually employed, in which each subject receives the test drug product and the reference product. Examples of *Latin square* crossover designs for a bioequivalence study in

TABLE 10.3 Latin Square Crossover Design for a Bioequivalence Study of 3 Drug Products in 6 Human Volunteers

	DRUG PRODUCT		
SUBJECT	**STUDY PERIOD 1**	**STUDY PERIOD 2**	**STUDY PERIOD 3**
1	A	B	C
2	B	C	A
3	C	A	B
4	A	C	B
5	C	B	A
6	B	A	C

human volunteers, comparing three different drug formulations (*A, B, C*) or four different drug formulations (*A, B, C, D*), are described in Tables 10.3 and 10.4. The Latin square design plans the clinical trial so that each subject receives each drug product only once, with adequate time between medications for the elimination of the drug from the body. In this design, each subject is his own control, and subject-to-subject variation is reduced. Moreover, variation due to sequence, period, and treatment (formulation) are reduced, so that all patients do not receive the same drug product on the same day and in the same order. Possible carry-over effects from any particular drug product are minimized by changing the sequence or order in which the drug products are given to the subject. Thus, drug product *B* may be followed by drug product *A, D,* or *C* (Table 10.4). After each subject receives a drug product, blood samples are collected at appropriate time intervals so that a valid blood drug level–time curve is obtained. The time intervals should be spaced so that the peak blood concentration, the total area under the curve, and the absorption and elimination phases of the curve may be well described. In some cases, the measurement of drug in urine samples may be necessary.

TABLE 10.4 Latin Square Crossover Design for a Bioequivalency Study of 4 Drug Products in 16 Human Volunteers

	DRUG PRODUCT			
SUBJECT	**STUDY PERIOD 1**	**STUDY PERIOD 2**	**STUDY PERIOD 3**	**STUDY PERIOD 4**
1	A	B	C	D
2	B	C	D	A
3	C	D	A	B
4	D	A	B	C
5	A	B	D	C
6	B	D	C	A
7	D	C	A	B
8	C	A	B	D
9	A	C	B	D
10	C	B	D	A
11	B	D	A	C
12	D	A	C	B
13	A	C	D	B
14	C	D	B	A
15	D	B	A	C
16	B	A	C	D

Period refers to the time period in which a study is performed. A two-period study, sometimes referred to as a *two-legged* study, means that the study is performed on two different days (time periods) separated by a washout period during which most of the drug has been eliminated from the body—generally about 10 elimination half-lives. A *sequence* refers to the number of different orders in the treatment groups in a study. For example, a two-sequence, two-period study would be designed as follows:

	Period 1	**Period 2**
Sequence 1	T	R
Sequence 2	R	T

R = reference; T = treatment.

Table 10.4 shows a design for three different drug treatments groups given in a three-period study with six different sequences. The order in which the drug treatments are given should not stay the same in order to prevent any bias in the data due to a residual effect from the previous treatment.

EVALUATION OF THE DATA

Analytical Method

The analytical method for measurement of the drug must be validated for accuracy, precision, sensitivity, and specificity. The use of more than one analytical method during a bioequivalence study may not be valid, because different methods may yield different values. Data should be presented in both tabulated and graphical form for evaluation. The plasma drug concentration versus time curve for each drug product and each subject should be available.

Pharmacokinetic Evaluation of the Data

For single dose studies, including a fasting study or a food intervention study, the pharmacokinetic analyses include calculation for each subject of the area-under-the-curve to the last quantifiable concentration (AUC_{0-t}) and to infinity ($AUC_{0-\infty}$), T_{max} and C_{max}. Additionally, the elimination rate constant, k, the elimination half-life, $t_{1/2}$, and other parameters may be estimated. For multiple dose studies, pharmacokinetic analysis includes calculation for each subject of the steady-state area-under-the-curve, (AUC_{0-t}), T_{max}, C_{min}, C_{max}, and the percent fluctuation [$100 \times (C_{max} - C_{min})/C_{min}$]. Proper statistical evaluation should be performed on the estimated pharmacokinetic parameters.

Statistical Evaluation of the Data

To prove bioequivalence, there must be no statistical difference between the bioavailability of the test product and the reference product. Several statistical approaches are used to compare the bioavailability of drug from the test dosage form to the bioavailability of the drug from the reference dosage form. Many statistical approaches (parametric tests) assume that the data are distributed according to a normal distribution or "bell-shaped curve" (see Appendix A). The distribution of many biological parameters such as C_{max}, AUC have a longer right tail than would be observed in a normal distribution (Midha et al, 1993). Moreover, the true distribution of these biological parameters may be difficult to ascertain due to the small number of subjects used in a bioequivalence study. The distribution of data that has been transformed to log values resembles more closely a normal distribution compared to the distribution of non-log-transformed data. Therefore, log transformation of the bioavailability data (eg, C_{max}, AUC) is performed prior to statistical data evaluation for bioequivalence determination.

Analysis of Variance (ANOVA)

An *analysis of variance* (ANOVA) is a statistical procedure (Appendix A) used to test the data for difference within and between treatment and control groups. A bioequivalent product should produce no significant difference in all pharmacokinetic parameters tested. The parameters tested usually include AUC_{0-24}, $AUC_{0-\infty}$, t_{max}, and C_{max} obtained for each treatment or dosage form. Other metrics of bioavailability have also been used to compare the bioequivalence of two or more formulations. The ANOVA may evaluate variability in subjects, treatment groups, study period, formulation, and other variables depending on the study design. If the variability in the data is large, the difference in means for each pharmacokinetic parameter, such as AUC, may be masked, and the investigator might erroneously conclude that the two drug products are bioequivalent.

A statistical difference between the pharmacokinetic parameters obtained from two or more drug products is considered statistically significant if there is a probability of less than 1 in 20 times or .05 probability ($P \leq 0.05$) that these results would have happened on the basis of chance alone. The term *probability*, or *P*, is used to indicate the level of statistical significance. If $P > 0.05$, the differences between the two drug products are not considered statistically significant.

To reduce the possibility of failing to detect small differences between the test products, a *power test* is performed to calculate the probability that the conclusion of the ANOVA is valid. The power of the test will depend on the sample size, variability of the data, and desired level of significance. Usually the power is set at 0.80 with an $\alpha =$ 0.2 and a level of significance of 0.05. The higher the power, the more sensitive the test and the greater the probability that the conclusion of the ANOVA is valid.

Two One-Sided Tests Procedure

This procedure is also referred to as the *confidence interval* approach (Schuirmann, 1987). This statistical method is used to demonstrate if the bioavailability of the drug from the test formulation is too low or high in comparison to the reference drug product. The objective of the two one-sided tests statistical approach is to determine if there are large differences (ie, greater than 20%) between the mean parameters.

The 90% confidence limits are estimated for the sample means. The interval estimate is based on a Student's *t*-distribution of the data. In this test, presently required by the FDA, a 90% confidence interval about the ratio of means of the two drug products must be within ± 20% for measurement of the rate and extent of drug bioavailability. For most drugs, up to a 20% difference in AUC or C_{max} between two formulations would have no clinical significance. The lower 90% confidence interval for the ratio of means cannot be less than 0.80, and the upper 90% confidence interval for the ratio of the means cannot be greater than 1.20. When log-transformed data is used, the 90% confidence interval is set at 80 to 125%, since the log of 0.8 (except for sign) is 1.25 or 125%. These confidence limits have also been termed the *bioequivalence interval* (Midha et al, 1993). The 90% confidence interval is a function of sample size and study variability, including inter- and intrasubject variability.

For a single-dose, fasting study, an analysis of variance (ANOVA) is usually performed on the log-transformed AUC and C_{max}. There should be no statistical dif-

TABLE 10.5 Bioavailability Comparison of a Generic (Test) and Brand (Reference) Drug Product[a]

PARAMETER	TEST	REFERENCE	RATIO (%)T/R	90% CONFIDENCE LIMITS	ANOVA T vs R	POWER T vs R
AUC_{0-t} (μg hr/mL)	1466	1494	98.1	93.0–102.5	$P < 0.78$	>99.9%
$AUC_{0-\infty}$ (μg hr/mL)	1592	1606	99.1	94.5–104.1	$P < 0.76$	>99.7%
C_{max} (μg/mL)	11.6	12.5	92.8	88.5–98.6	$P < 0.65$	>87.9%
t_{max} (hr)	1.87	2.1	89.1			

[a] The results were obtained from a two-way crossover, single-dose, fasting study in 24 healthy adult volunteers. Mean values are reported. No statistical differences were observed between AUC and C_{max} values for the test and reference products.

ferences between the mean AUC and C_{max} parameters for the test (generic) and reference drug products. In addition, the 90% confidence intervals about the ratio of the means for AUC and C_{max} values of the test drug product should not be less than 0.80 (80%) nor greater than 1.25 (125%) of the reference product based on log-transformed data.

BIOEQUIVALENCE EXAMPLE

A simulated example of the results for a single dose, fasting study is shown in Table 10.5. As shown by the ANOVA, no statistical differences for the pharmacokinetic parameters AUC_{0-t} $AUC_{0-\infty}$, and C_{max} were observed between the test product compared to the brand product. The 90% confidence limits for the mean pharmacokinetic parameters of the test product were within the 0.80 to 1.25 (80–125%) of the reference product means based on log transformation of the data. The power test for the AUC measures were above 99%, showing good precision of the data. The power test for the C_{max} values was 87.9%, showing that this parameter was more variable.

For a single dose, three-way crossover food/fasting study, the mean values for the AUC and C_{max} for the test product when administered with food should be within 20% from the respective mean values of the reference product when given with food. No ANOVA is required by FDA.

For multiple dose studies, an ANOVA should be performed on the log transformed AUC and C_{max}. The AUC and C_{max} parameters for the test (generic) product should be within 80 to 125% of the reference product using the 90% confidence interval.

Table 10.6 shows the results for a hypothetical bioavailability study in which three different tablet formulations were compared to a solution of the drug given in the same dose. As shown in the table, the bioavailability from all three tablet formulations was greater than 80% of the solution. According to the ANOVA, the mean AUC values were not statistically different from each other or different from the solution. However, the 90% confidence interval for the AUC showed that for tablet A, the bioavailability was less than 80% (ie, 74%) compared to the solution at the low-range estimate.

For illustrative purposes, consider a drug that has been prepared at the same dosage level in three formulations, formulations *A*, *B*, and *C*. These formulations

TABLE 10.6 Summary of the Results of a Bioavailability Study[a]

DOSAGE FORM	C_{MAX} (μg/mL)	T_{MAX} (hr)	AUC_{0-24} (μg hr/mL)	F[b]	90% CONFIDENCE INTERVAL FOR AUC
Solution	16.1 ± 2.5	1.5 ± 0.85	1835 ± 235		
Tablet A	10.5 ± 3.2[c]	2.5 ± 1.0[c]	1523 ± 381	81	74–90%
Tablet B	13.7 ± 4.1	2.1 ± 0.98	1707 ± 317	93	88–98%
Tablet C	14.8 ± 3.6	1.8 ± 0.95	1762 ± 295	96	91–103%

[a] The bioavailability of a drug from 4 different formulations was studied in 24 healthy adult male subjects using a four-way Latin square crossover design. The results represent the mean ± standard deviation.
[b] Oral bioavailability relative to the solution.
[c] $P \leq .05$.

are given to a group of volunteers using a three-way, randomized crossover design. In this experimental design, all subjects receive each formulation once. From each subject, plasma drug level and urinary drug excretion data are obtained. With this data we can observe the relationship between plasma and urinary excretion parameters and drug bioavailability (Fig. 10-6). The rate of drug absorption from formulation *A* is more rapid than that from formulation *B*, because the t_{max} for formulation *A* is shorter. Because the AUC for formulation *A* is identical to the AUC for formulation *B*, the extent of bioavailability from both of these formulations is the same. Note, however, the C_{max} of *A* is higher than *B* because the rate of drug absorption is more rapid.

The C_{max} is generally higher when the extent of drug bioavailability is greater. The rate of drug absorption from formulation *C* is the same as that from formulation *A*, but the extent of drug available is less. The C_{max} for formulation *C* is less than for formulation *A*. The decrease in C_{max} for formulation *C* is proportional to the decrease in AUC in comparison to the drug plasma level data from formulation *A*. The corresponding urinary excretion data confirm these observations.

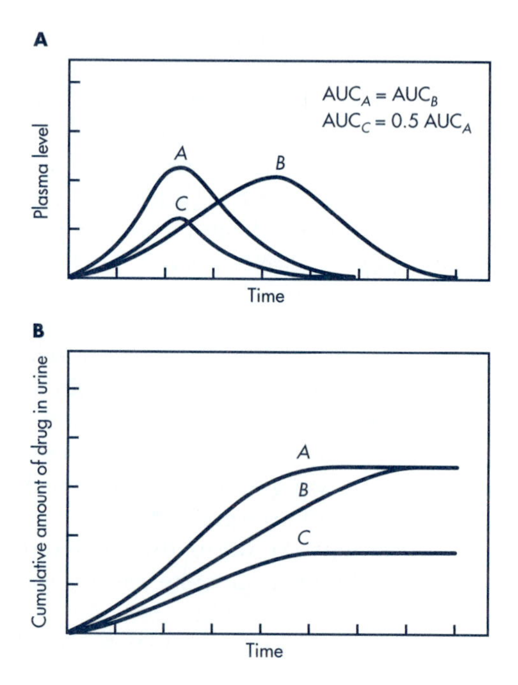

Figure 10-6. Corresponding plots relating plasma concentration and urinary excretion data.

TABLE 10.7 Relationship of Plasma Level and Urinary Excretion Parameters to Drug Bioavailability

EXTENT OF DRUG BIOAVAILABILITY DECREASES		RATE OF DRUG BIOAVAILABILITY DECREASES	
PARAMETER	**CHANGE**	**PARAMETER**	**CHANGE**
Plasma Data			
t_{max}	Same	t_{max}	Increase
C_{max}	Decrease	C_{max}	Decrease
AUC	Decrease	AUC	Same
Urine Data			
t^{∞}	Same	t^{∞}	Increase
$[dD_u/dt]_{max}$*	Decrease	$[dD_u/dt]_{max}$*	Decrease
D_u^{∞}	Decrease	D_u^{∞}	Same

*Maximum rate of urinary drug excretion.

These relationships are summarized in Table 10.7. The table illustrates how bioavailability parameters for plasma and urine change when the extent and rate of bioavailability is changed, respectively.

Study Submission

An outline for the submission of a completed bioavailability study for submission to the FDA is shown in Table 10.8. Before the study is performed, the investigator should be sure that the study has been properly designed, the objectives are clearly defined, and the method of analysis has been validated (ie, shown to measure precisely and accurately the plasma drug concentration). Moreover, the protocol for the study may be submitted to the FDA for discussion and approval prior to initiation of the investigation. After the study has been performed, the results are statistically and pharmacokinetically analyzed. These results, along with case reports and various data supporting the validity of the analytical method, are included in the submission. The Biopharmaceutics Branch of the FDA, after receiving the completed study, will review the study in detail according to the outline presented in Table 10.9. If necessary, an FDA investigator may inspect both the clinical and analytical facilities used for the study and audit the raw data used in support of the bioavailability study. The FDA then makes a decision to approve the bioavailability of the drug product.

Dissolution Testing in Lieu of Bioavailability Studies

Ideally, if there is a strong correlation between dissolution of the drug and the bioavailability of the drug, then the comparative dissolution tests comparing the test product to the reference product should be sufficient to demonstrate bioequivalence. For most drug products, especially the immediate-release tablets and capsules, no strong correlation exists, and the FDA requires an *in vivo* bioequivalence study. For oral solid dosage forms, an *in vivo* bioequivalence study may be required to support at least one dose strength of the product. Usually, an *in vivo* bioequivalence study is required for the highest dose strength. If the lower dose strength test product is proportionally similar in active and inactive ingredients, then only a comparison *in vitro* dissolution between the test and brand name formulations may be used. For example, if the drug product is available in 50 mg, 75

TABLE 10.8 Proposed Format and Contents of an In Vivo Bioequivalence Study Submission and Accompanying *In Vitro* Data

Title Page

- Study title
- Name of sponsor
- Name and address of clinical laboratory
- Name of principal investigator(s)
- Name of clinical investigator
- Name of analytical laboratory
- Dates of clinical study (start, completion)
- Signature of principal investigator (and date)
- Signature of clinical investigator (and date)

Table of Contents

I. Study Resume
- Product information
- Summary of bioequivalence study
- Summary of bioequivalence data
  - Plasma
  - Urinary excretion
- Figure of mean plasma concentration–time profile
- Figure of mean cumulative urinary excretion
- Figure of mean urinary excretion rates

II. Protocol and Approvals
- Protocol
- Letter of acceptance of protocol from FDA
- Informed consent form
- Letter of approval of Institutional Review Board
- List of members of Institutional Review Board

III. Clinical Study
- Summary of the study
- Details of the study
- Demographic characteristics of the subjects
- Subject assignment in the study
- Mean physical characteristics of subjects arranged by sequence
- Details of clinical activity
- Deviations from protocol
- Vital signs of subjects
- Adverse reactions report

IV. Assay Methodology and Validation
- Assay method description
- Validation procedure
- Summary of validation
- Data on linearity of standard samples
- Data on interday precision and accuracy
- Data on intraday precision and accuracy
- Figure for standard curve(s) for low/high ranges
- Chromatograms of standard and quality control samples
- Sample calculation

V. Pharmacokinetic Parameters and Tests
- Definition and calculations
- Statistical tests
- Drug levels at each sampling time and pharmacokinetic parameters
- Figure of mean plasma concentration–time profile
- Figures of individual subject plasma concentration—time profiles
- Figure of mean cumulative urinary excretion
- Figures of individual subject cumulative urinary excretion
- Figure of mean urinary excretion rates
- Figures of individual subject urinary excretion rates
- Tables of individual subject data arranged by drug, drug/period, drug/sequence

VI. Statistical Analyses
- Statistical considerations
- Summary of statistical significance
- Summary of statistical parameters
- Analysis of variance, least squares estimates and least squares means

VII. Appendices
- Randomization schedule
- Sample identification codes
- Analytical raw data
- Chromatograms of at least 20% of subjects
- Medical record and clinical reports
- Clinical facilities description
- Analytical facilities description
- *Curricula vitae* of the investigators

VIII. *In Vitro* Testing
- Dissolution testing
- Dissolution assay methodology
- Content uniformity testing
- Potency determination

IX. Batch Size and Formulation
- Batch record
- Quantitative formulation

From Dighe and Adams, 1991, with permission.

mg, and 100 mg dose strengths, an *in vivo* study is performed on the 100 mg dose strength, and comparative dissolution studies are performed on the 50 mg and 75 mg dose strengths. If these drug products have no known bioavailability problems, are well absorbed systemically, are well correlated with *in vitro* dissolution, and have a large margin of safety, then arguments for not performing an *in vivo* bioavailability study may be valid. Methods for correlation of *in vitro* dissolution of the drug with *in vivo* drug bioavailability are discussed in Chapters 6 and 7.

TABLE 10.9 General Elements of a Biopharmaceutics Review

Introduction	Determination of detectable differences
Study design	Determination of power to detect a 20% difference at alpha = .05
Study objective(s)	Comments
Assay description and validation	Deficiencies
Assay for individual samples checked	Recommendation
Summary and analysis of data	

From Purich (1980), with permission.

Clinical Significance of Bioequivalence Studies

Bioequivalence of different formulations of the same drug substance involves equivalence with respect to rate and extent of systemic drug absorption. Clinical interpretation is important in evaluating the results of a bioequivalence study. A small difference between drug products, even if statistically significant, may produce very little difference in therapeutic response. Generally, two formulations whose rate and extent of absorption differ by 20% or less are considered bioequivalent. The *Report by the Bioequivalence Task Force, 1988* considered that differences of less than 20% in AUC and C_{max} between drug products are "unlikely to be clinically significant in patients." The task force further states that "clinical studies of effectiveness have difficulty detecting differences in dose of even 50–100%." Therefore, normal variation is observed in medical practice and plasma drug levels may vary among individuals greater than 20%.

According to Westlake (1972), a small, statistically significant difference in drug bioavailability from two or more dosage forms may be detected if the study is well controlled and the number of subjects is sufficiently large. When the therapeutic objectives of the drug are considered, an equivalent clinical response should be obtained from the comparison dosage forms if the plasma drug concentrations remain above the minimum effective concentration (MEC) for an appropriate interval and do not reach the minimum toxic concentration (MTC). Therefore, the investigator must consider whether any statistical difference in bioavailability would alter clinical efficiency.

Special populations, such as the elderly or patients on drug therapy, are generally not used for bioequivalence studies. Normal healthy volunteers are preferred for bioequivalence studies, because these subjects are less at risk and may more easily endure the discomforts of the study, such as blood sampling. Furthermore, the objective of these studies is to evaluate the bioavailability of the drug from the dosage form, and use of healthy subjects should minimize both inter- and intrasubject variability. It is theoretically possible that the excipients in one of the dosage forms tested may pose a problem in the patient who uses the generic dosage form.

For the manufacture of a dosage form, specifications are set to provide uniformity of dosage forms. With proper specifications, quality control procedures should minimize product-to-product variability by different manufacturers and lot-to-lot variability with a single manufacturer.

Special Concerns in Bioavailability and Bioequivalence Studies

The general bioequivalence study designs and evaluation, such as the comparison of AUC, C_{max}, and t_{max}, may be used for systemically absorbed drugs and conventional oral dosage forms. However, for certain drugs and dosage forms, systemic bioavailability and bioequivalence are difficult to ascertain (Table 10.10).

TABLE 10.10 Problems in Bioavailability and Bioequivalence

Drugs with high intrasubject variability	Inhalation
Long elimination half-life drugs	Ophthalmic
Biotransformation of drugs	Intranasal
Stereoselective drug metabolism	Bioavailable drugs that should not produce peak drug levels
Drugs with active metabolites	Hormone replacement therapy
Drugs with polymorphic metabolism	Potassium supplements
Nonbioavailable drugs (drugs intended for local effect)	Biotechnology-derived drugs
Antacids	Erythropoietin interferon
Local anesthetics	Protease inhibitors
Antiinfectives	Complex drug substances
Antiinflammatory steroids	Conjugated estrogens
Dosage forms for nonoral administration	
Transdermal	

Drugs and drug products (eg, cyclosporine, chlorpromazine, verapamil, isosorbide dinitrate, sulindac) are considered to be highly variable if the intrasubject variability in bioavailability parameters is greater than 30% by analysis of variance coefficient of variation (Shah et al, 1996). The number of subjects required to demonstrate bioequivalence for these drug products may be excessive, requiring more than 48 subjects to meet the current FDA bioequivalence criteria. The intrasubject variability may be due to the drug itself or to the drug formulation or to both. The FDA has held public forums to determine whether the current bioequivalence guidelines need to be changed for these highly variable drugs (Shah et al, 1996).

For drugs with very long elimination half-lives or a complex elimination phase, a complete plasma drug concentration versus time curve (ie, three elimination half-lives or an AUC representing >90% of the total AUC) may be difficult to obtain for a bioequivalence study using a crossover design. For these drugs, a truncated (shortened) plasma drug concentration versus time curve (AUC_{0-t}) may be more practical. The use of a truncated AUC allows for the measurement of peak absorption and would decrease the time and cost for performing the bioequivalence study.

Many drugs are stereoisomers, and each isomer may give a different pharmacodynamic response and may have a different rate of biotransformation. The bioavailability of the individual isomers may be difficult to measure due to problems in analysis. Some drugs have active metabolites, which should be quantitated as well as the parent drug. Drugs such as thioridazine and selegilene have two active metabolites. The question for such drugs is whether bioequivalence should be proven by matching the bioavailability of both metabolites and the parent drug. Assuming both biotransformation pathways follow first-order-reaction kinetics, then the metabolites should be in constant ratio to the parent drug. In contrast, some drugs, such as procainamide, have an active metabolite, N-acetylprocainamide. The acetylation of procainamide demonstrates genetic polymorphism with two groups of subjects consisting of either rapid acetylators or slow acetylators. To decrease intersubject variability, a bioequivalence study may be performed only on one phenotype, such as the rapid acetylators.

Some drugs (eg, benzocaine, hydrocortisone, antiinfectives, antacids) are intended for local effect; formulated as topical ointments, oral suspensions, or rectal suppositories. These drugs should not have significant systemic bioavailability from the site of administration. The bioequivalence determination for drugs that are not absorbed systemically from the site of application can be difficult to assess. For these nonsystemic absorbable drugs, a *"surrogate"* marker is needed for bio-

TABLE 10.11 Possible Surrogate Markers for Bioequivalence Studies

DRUG PRODUCT	DRUG	POSSIBLE SURROGATE MARKER FOR BIOEQUIVALENCE
Metered dose inhaler	Albuterol	Forced expiratory volume (FEV_1)
Topical steroid	Hydrocortisone	Skin blanching
Anion exchange resin	Cholestyramine	Binding to bile acids
Antacids	Magnesium and aluminum hydroxide gel	Neutralization of acid
Topical antifungal	Ketoconazole	Drug uptake into stratum corneum

equivalence determination (Table 10.11). For example, the acid neutralizing capacity of an oral antacid and the binding of bile acids to cholestyramine resin have been used as surrogate markers in lieu of *in vivo* bioequivalence studies.

Various drug-delivery systems and newer dosage forms are designed to deliver the drug by a nonoral route, which may produce only partial systemic bioavailability. For the treatment of asthma, inhalation of the drug (eg, albuterol, beclomethasone dipropionate) has been used to maximize drug in the respiratory passages and to decrease systemic side effects. Drugs such as nitroglycerin given transdermally may differ in release rates, in the amount of drug in the transdermal delivery system, and in the surface area of the skin to which the transdermal delivery system is applied. Thus, the determination of bioequivalence among different manufactures of transdermal delivery systems for the same active drug is difficult. *Dermatokinetics* are pharmacokinetic studies that investigate drug uptake into skin layers after topical drug administration. The drug is applied topically, the skin is peeled at various time periods after the dose, using transparent tape, and the drug concentrations are measured in the skin.

Drugs such as hormonal replacement (estrogen, levothyroxine) or potassium supplements are given orally and may not produce the usual bioavailability parameters of AUC, C_{max}, and t_{max}. For these drugs, more indirect methods must be used to ascertain bioequivalence. For example, urinary potassium excretion parameters are more appropriate for the measurement of bioavailability of potassium supplements. However, for certain hormonal replacement drugs (eg, levothyroxine), the steady-state hormone concentration in hypothyroid individuals, the thyroidal stimulating hormone level, and pharmacodynamic endpoints may be more appropriate to measure.

GENERIC SUBSTITUTION

To contain drug costs, most states have adopted generic substitution laws to allow the pharmacist to dispense a generic drug product for a brand name drug product that has been prescribed. Some states have adopted a *positive formulary*, which lists therapeutically equivalent or interchangeable drug products that the pharmacist may dispense. Other states use a *negative formulary*, which lists drug products that are not therapeutically equivalent, and/or the interchange of which is prohibited. If the drug is not in the negative formulary, the unlisted generic drug products are assumed to be therapeutically equivalent and may be interchanged.

Due to public demand, the FDA Center for Drug Evaluation and Research publishes annually a listing of approved drug products, *Approved Drug Products with*

TABLE 10.12 Therapeutic Equivalence Evaluation Codes

A Codes

Drug products considered to be therapeutically equivalent to other pharmaceutically equivalent products.

AA	Products in conventional dosage forms not presenting bioequivalence problems.
AB	Products meeting bioequivalence requirements.
AN	Solutions and powders for aerosolization.
AO	Injectable oil solutions.
AP	Injectable aqueous solutions.
AT	Topical products.

B Codes

Drug products that the FDA does not consider to be therapeutically equivalent to other pharmaceutically equivalent products.

BC	Extended-release tablets, extended-release capsules, and extended-release injectables.
BD	Active ingredients and dosage forms with documented bioequivalence problems.
BE	Delayed-release oral dosage forms.
BN	Products in aerosol–nebulizer drug delivery systems.
BP	Active ingredients and dosage forms with potential bioequivalence problems.
BR	Suppositories or enemas for systemic use.
BS	Products having drug standard deficiencies.
BT	Topical products with bioequivalence issues.
BX	Insufficient data.

Adapted from USP DI, vol 3, Approved Drug Products and Legal Requirements, 1998.

Therapeutic Equivalence Evaluations (commonly known as the "Orange Book"). This monograph is also reproduced in the *United States Drug Information* publication (USP DI, vol 3), entitled *Approved Drug Products and Legal Requirements.* The Orange Book is available on the Internet at http://www.fda.gov/cder/drug.htm.

The Orange Book contains therapeutic equivalence evaluations for approved drug products made by various manufacturers. These marketed drug products are evaluated according to specific criteria. The evaluation codes used for these drugs are listed in Table 10.12. The drug products are divided into two major categories: "A" codes apply to drug products considered to be therapeutically equivalent to other pharmaceutically equivalent products, and "B" codes apply to drug products that the FDA does not at this time consider to be therapeutically equivalent to other pharmaceutically equivalent products. A list of therapeutic-equivalence-related terms and their definitions is also given in the monograph. According to the FDA, evaluations do not mandate that drugs be purchased, prescribed, or dispensed, but provide public information and advice. The FDA evaluation of the drug products should be used as a guide only, with the practitioner exercising professional care and judgment.

FREQUENTLY ASKED QUESTIONS

1. Why are preclinical animal toxicology studies and clinical efficacy drug studies in human subjects not required by FDA to approve a generic drug product as a therapeutic equivalent to the brand name drug product?

2. What does sequence, washout period, and period mean in a crossover bioavailability study?
3. Why does FDA require a food intervention (food effect) study for some generic drug products prior to approval? For which drug products are food effect studies required?
4. What type of bioequivalence studies are required for drugs that are not systemically absorbed or for those drugs in which the C_{max} and AUC cannot be measured in the plasma?
5. How does inter- and intrasubject variability affect the statistical demonstration of bioequivalence for a drug product?
6. Can chemically equivalent drug products that are *not* bioequivalent (ie, *bioinequivalent*) to each other have similar clinical efficacy?

LEARNING QUESTIONS

1. An antibiotic was formulated into two different oral dosage forms, *A* and *B*. Biopharmaceutic studies revealed different antibiotic blood level curves for each drug product (Fig. 10-7). Each drug product was given in the same dose as the others. Explain how the various possible formulation factors could have caused the differences in blood levels. *Give examples* where possible. How would the corresponding urinary drug excretion curves relate to the plasma level–time curves?
2. Assume that you have just made a new formulation of acetaminophen. Design a protocol to compare your drug product against the acetaminophen drug products on the market. What criteria would you use for proof of bioequivalence for your new formulation? How would you determine if the acetaminophen was completely (100%) systemically absorbed?
3. The data in Table 10.13 represent the average findings in antibiotic plasma samples taken from 10 humans (average weight 70 kg), tabulated in a four-way crossover design.

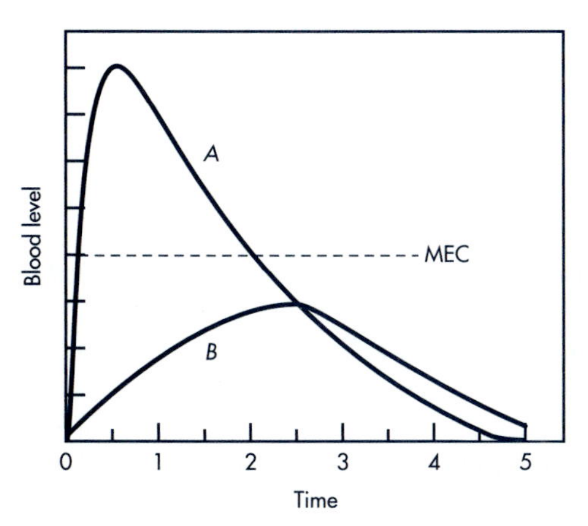

Figure 10-7. Blood level curves for two different oral dosage forms of a hypothetical antibiotic.

TABLE 10.13 Comparison of Plasma Concentrations of Antibiotic, as Related to Dosage Form and Time

TIME AFTER DOSE (hr)	PLASMA CONCENTRATION (μg/mL)			
	IV SOLUTION (2 mg/kg)	ORAL SOLUTION (10 mg/kg)	ORAL TABLET (10 mg/kg)	ORAL CAPSULE (10 mg/kg)
0.5	5.94	23.4	13.2	18.7
1.0	5.30	26.6	18.0	21.3
1.5	4.72	25.2	19.0	20.1
2.0	4.21	22.8	18.3	18.2
3.0	3.34	18.2	15.4	14.6
4.0	2.66	14.5	12.5	11.6
6.0	1.68	9.14	7.92	7.31
8.0	1.06	5.77	5.00	4.61
10.0	0.67	3.64	3.16	2.91
12.0	0.42	2.30	1.99	1.83
AUC $\left(\frac{\mu g}{mL} \times hr\right)$	29.0	145.0	116.0	116.0

a. Which of the four drug products in Table 10.13 would be preferred as a reference standard for the determination of relative bioavailability? Why?
b. From which oral drug product is the drug absorbed more rapidly?
c. What is the absolute bioavailability of the drug from the oral solution?
d. What is the relative bioavailability of the drug from the oral tablet compared to the reference standard?
e. From the data in Table 10.13 determine:
(1) Apparent V_D
(2) Elimination $t_{1/2}$
(3) First-order elimination rate constant k
(4) Total body clearance
f. From the data above, graph the cumulative urinary excretion curves that would correspond to the plasma concentration time curves.

4. Aphrodisia is a new drug manufactured by the Venus Drug Company. When tested in humans, the pharmacokinetics of the drug assumes a one-compartment open model with first-order absorption and first-order elimination:

$$D_{GI} \xrightarrow{k_a} D_B V_D \xrightarrow{k}$$

The drug was given in a single oral dose of 250 mg to a group of college students 21 to 29 years of age. Mean body weight was 60 kg. Samples of blood were obtained at various time intervals after the administration of the drug, and the plasma fractions were analyzed for active drug. The data is summarized in Table 10.14.

a. The minimum effective concentration of Aphrodisia in plasma is 2.3 μg/mL. What is the *onset* time of this drug?
b. The minimum effective concentration of Aphrodisia in plasma is 2.3 μg/mL. What is the *duration* of activity of this drug?
c. What is the elimination half-life of Aphrodisia in college students?
d. What is the time for peak drug concentration (t_{max}) of Aphrodisia?
e. What is the peak drug concentration (C_{max})?
f. Assuming that the drug is 100% systemically available (ie, fraction of drug absorbed equals unity), what is the AUC for Aphrodisia?

TABLE 10.14 Data Summary of Active Drug Concentration in Plasma Fractions

TIME (hr)	C_P (μg/mL)	TIME (hr)	C_P (μg/mL)
0	0	12	3.02
1	1.88	18	1.86
2	3.05	24	1.12
3	3.74	36	0.40
5	4.21	48	0.14
7	4.08	60	0.05
9	3.70	72	0.02

5. You wish to do a bioequivalence study on three different formulations of the same active drug. Lay out a Latin square design for the proper sequencing of these drug products in 6 normal healthy volunteers. What is the main reason for using a crossover design in a bioequivalence study? What is meant by a "random" population?

6. Four different drug products containing the same antibiotic were given to 12 volunteer adult males (age 19 to 28 years, average weight 73 kg) in a four-way crossover design. The volunteers were fasted 12 hours prior to taking the drug product. Urine samples were collected up to 72 hours after the administration of the drug to obtain the maximum urinary drug excretion, D_u^∞. The data are presented in Table 10.15.

a. What is the *absolute* bioavailability of the drug from the *tablet*?

b. What is the *relative* bioavailability of the capsule compared to the oral solution?

7. According to the prescribing information for cimetidine (Tagamet, SKF Lab Co), following IV or IM administration, 75% of the drug is recovered from the urine after 24 hours as the parent compound. Following a single oral dose, 48% of the drug is recovered from the urine after 24 hours as the parent compound. From this information, determine what fraction of the drug is absorbed systemically from the oral dose after 24 hours.

8. Define the term "*bioequivalence requirement.*" Why does the FDA require a bioequivalence requirement for the manufacture of a generic drug product?

9. Why can we use the time for peak drug concentration (t_{max}) in a bioequivalence study for an estimate of the *rate* of drug absorption rather than calculating the k_a?

10. Ten male volunteers (18 to 26 years of age) weighing an average of 73 kg were given either 4 tablets each containing 250 mg of drug (drug product *A*) or 1

TABLE 10.15 Urinary Drug Excretion Data Summary

DRUG PRODUCT	DOSE (mg/Kg)	CUMULATIVE URINARY DRUG EXCRETION (D_U^∞), 0–72 hr (mg)
IV solution	0.2	20
Oral solution	4	380
Oral tablet	4	340
Oral capsule	4	360

TABLE 10.16 Blood Level Data Summary for Two Drug Products

		DRUG PRODUCT		
KINETIC VARIABLE	UNIT	A 4 × 250 MG TABLET	B 1000 MG TABLET	STATISTIC
Time for peak drug concentration (range)	hr	1.3 (0.7–1.5)	1.8 (1.5–2.2)	$P < 0.05$
Peak concentration (range)	μg/mL	53 (46–58)	47 (42–51)	$P < 0.05$
AUC (range)	μg hr/mL	118 (98–125)	103 (90–120)	NS
$t_{1/2}$	hr	3.2 (2.5–3.8)	3.8 (2.9–4.3)	NS

tablet containing 1000 mg of drug (drug product *B*). Blood levels of the drug were obtained and the data are summarized in Table 10.16.

a. State a possible reason for the difference in the time for peak drug concentration ($t_{\max,A}$) after drug product *A* compared to the $t_{\max,B}$ after drug product *B*. (Assume that all the tablets were made from the same formulation—that is, the drug is in the same particle size, same salt form, same excipients, and same ratio of excipients to active drug.)

b. Draw a graph relating the cumulative amount of drug excreted in urine of patients given drug product *A* compared to the cumulative drug excreted in urine after drug product *B*. *Label axes!*

c. In a second study using the same 10 male volunteers, a 125-mg dose of the drug was given by intravenous bolus and the AUC was computed as 20 μg hr/mL. Calculate the fraction of drug systemically absorbed from drug product *B* (1 × 1000 mg) tablet using the data in Table 10.13.

11. After performing a bioequivalence test comparing a generic drug product to a brand name drug product, it was observed that the generic drug product had a greater bioavailability than the brand name drug product.

a. Would you approve marketing the generic drug product, claiming it was superior than the brand name drug product?

b. Would you expect *identical* pharmacodynamic responses to *both* drug products?

c. What therapeutic problem might arise in using the generic drug product that might not occur when using the brand name drug product?

12. The following study is from Welling and associates (1982):

Tolazamide Formulations. Four tolazamide tablet formulations were selected for this study. The tablet formulations were labeled *A*, *B*, *C*, and *D*. Disintegration and dissolution tests were performed by standard USP-23 procedures.

Subjects. Twenty healthy adult male volunteers between the ages of 18 and 38 (mean, 26 years) and weighing between 61.4 and 95.5 kg (mean, 74.5 kg) were selected for the study. The subjects were randomly assigned to 4 groups of 5 each. The four treatments were administered according to 4 × 4 Latin square design. Each treatment was separated by 1-week intervals. All subjects fasted overnight prior to receiving the tolazamide tablet the following morning. The tablet was given with 180 mL of water. Food intake was allowed at 5 hours post dose. Blood samples (10 mL) were taken just prior to the dose and periodically

TABLE 10.17 Disintegration Times and Dissolution Rates of Tolazamide Tablets[a]

TABLET	MEAN DISINTEGRATION TIME[b] MIN (RANGE)	PERCENT DISSOLVED IN 30 MIN[c] (RANGE)
A	3.8 (3.0–4.0)	103.9 (100.5–106.3)
B	2.2 (1.8–2.5)	10.9 (9.3–13.5)
C	2.3 (2.0–2.5)	31.6 (26.4–37.2)
D	26.5 (22.5–30.5)	29.7 (20.8–38.4)

[a] $N = 6$.
[b] By the method of USP-23.
[c] Dissolution rates in pH 7.6 buffer.

From Welling et al, 1982, with permission.

after dosing. The serum fraction was separated from the blood and analyzed for tolazamide by high-pressure liquid chromatography.

Data Analysis. Serum data were analyzed by a digital computer program using a regression analysis and by the percent of drug unabsorbed by the method of Wagner and Nelson. AUC was determined by the trapezoidal rule and an analysis of variance was determined by Tukey's method.

a. Why was a *Latin square crossover design* used in this study?
b. Why were the subjects *fasted* prior to taking the tolazamide tablets?
c. Why did the authors use the Wagner–Nelson method rather than the Loo-Riegelman method for measuring the amount of drug absorbed?
d. From the data in Table 10.17 *only*, from which tablet formulation would you expect the greatest bioavailability? *Why?*
e. From the data in Table 10.14, did the disintegration times correlate with the dissolution times? *Why?*
f. Do the data in Table 10.17 appear to correlate with the data in Table 10.18? *Why?*
g. Draw the expected cumulative urinary excretion versus time curve for formulations *A* and *B*. *Label axes* and identify each curve.
h. Assuming formulation *A* is the *reference* formulation, what is the *relative* bioavailability of formulation *D*?
i. Using the data in Table 10.18 for formulation *A*, calculate the elimination half-life ($t_{1/2}$) for tolazamide.

13. If *in vitro* drug dissolution and/or release studies for an oral solid dosage form (eg, tablet) does not correlate with the bioavailability of the drug *in vivo*, why should the pharmaceutical manufacturer continue to perform *in vitro* release studies for each production batch of the solid dosage form?

14. Is it possible for two pharmaceutically equivalent solid dosage forms containing different inactive ingredients (ie, excipients) to demonstrate bioequivalence *in vivo* even though these drug products demonstrate differences in drug dissolution tests *in vitro*?

15. For bioequivalence studies, t_{max}, C_{max}, and AUC, along with an appropriate statistical analysis are the parameters generally used to demonstrate the bioequivalence of two similar drug products containing the same active drug.

a. Why are the parameters, t_{max}, C_{max}, and AUC acceptable for proving that two drug products are bioequivalent?

TABLE 10.18 Mean Tolazamide Concentrations[a] in Serum

	TIME (hr)	TREATMENT, μg/mL				
		A	B	C	D	STATISTIC[b]
	0	10.8 ± 7.4	1.3 ± 1.4	1.8 ± 1.9	3.5 ± 2.6	$A\overline{DCB}$
	1	20.5 ± 7.3	2.8 ± 2.8	5.4 ± 4.8	13.5 ± 6.6	$AD\overline{CB}$
	3	23.9 ± 5.3	4.4 ± 4.3	9.8 ± 5.6	20.0 ± 6.4	$\overline{AD}CB$
	4	25.4 ± 5.2	5.7 ± 4.1	13.6 ± 5.3	22.0 ± 5.4	$\overline{AD}CB$
	5	24.1 ± 6.3	6.6 ± 4.0	15.1 ± 4.7	22.6 ± 5.0	$\overline{AD}CB$
	6	19.9 ± 5.9	6.8 ± 3.4	14.3 ± 3.9	19.7 ± 4.7	$\overline{AD}CB$
	8	15.2 ± 5.5	6.6 ± 3.2	12.8 ± 4.1	14.6 ± 4.2	$\overline{ADC}B$
	12	8.8 ± 4.8	5.5 ± 3.2	9.1 ± 4.0	8.5 ± 4.1	$\overline{CAD}B$
	16	5.6 ± 3.8	4.6 ± 3.3	6.4 ± 3.9	5.4 ± 3.1	$C\overline{ADB}$
	24	2.7 ± 2.4	3.1 ± 2.6	3.1 ± 3.3	2.4 ± 1.8	$\overline{CBAD}$
C_{max}[c], μg/mL		27.8 ± 5.3	7.7 ± 4.1	16.4 ± 4.4	24.0 ± 4.5	$\overline{AD}CB$
t_{max}[d], hr		3.3 ± 0.9	7.0 ± 2.2	5.4 ± 2.0	4.0 ± 0.9	$BC\overline{DA}$
AUC_{0-24}[e], μg hr/mL		260 ± 81	112 ± 63	193 ± 70	231 ± 67	$\overline{AD}CB$

[a] Concentrations ± 1 SD, $n = 20$.
[b] For explanation see text.
[c] Maximum concentration of tolazamide in serum.
[d] Time of maximum concentration.
[e] Area under the 0–24-hr serum tolazamide concentration curve calculated by trapezoidal rule.

From Welling et al (1982), with permission.

b. Are pharmacokinetic models needed in the evaluation of bioequivalence?
c. Is it necessary to use a pharmacokinetic model to completely describe the plasma drug concentration versus time curve for the determination of t_{max}, C_{max}, and AUC?
d. Why are log-transformed data used for the statistical evaluation of bioequivalence?
e. What is an *add-on study*?

REFERENCES

Approved Drug Products and Legal Requirements, USP DI, 18th ed. Rockville, MD, The United States Pharmacopeial Convention, Inc, 1998, vol 3.

Code of Federal Regulation: *Bioavailability and Bioequivalence Requirements,* vol 21, part 320 (CFR320). Washington DC, US Government Printing Office, 1991

Dighe SV, Adams WP: Bioequivalence: A United States regulatory perspective. In Welling PG, Tse FLS, Dighe SV (eds), *Pharmaceutical Bioequivalence.* New York, Marcel Dekker, 1991, chap 12

Feldman CH, Hutchinson VE, Sher TH, et al: Interaction between nutrition and theophylline metabolism in children. *Ther Drug Monit* **4:**69–76, 1982

Gardner S: Bioequivalence requirements and in vivo bioavailability procedures. *Fed Reg* **42:**1651, 1977

Hendles L, Iafrate RP, Weinberger M: A clinical and pharmacokinetic basis for the selection and use of slow release theophylline products. *Clin Pharmacokinet* **9:**95–135, 1984

Midha KA, Ormsby ED, Hubbard JW, McKay G, Hawes EM, Gavalas, McGilvery IJ: Logarithmic transformation in bioequivalence: Application with two formulations of perphenazine. *J Pharm Sci* **82:**138–144, 1993.

Mordenti J, Cavagnaro JA, Green JD: Design of biological equivalence programs for therapeutic biotechnology products in clinical development: A perspective. *Pharm Res* **13:**1427–37, 1996.

Purich E: Bioavailability/bioequivalence regulations: An FDA perspective. In Albert KS (ed), *Drug Absorption and Disposition, Statistical Considerations.* Washington, DC, American Pharmaceutical Association, 1980

Report by the Bioequivalence Task Force 1988 on Recommendations from the Bioequivalence Hearings Conducted by the Food and Drug Administration, Sept 29–Oct 1, 1986. Rockville, MD, FDA, 1988

Schuirmann DJ: A comparison of the two one-sided tests procedure and the power approach for assessing the equivalence of average bioavailability. *J Pharmacokinet Biopharm* **15:**657–680, 1987

Shah P, Yacobi A, Barr WH, Benet LZ, Breimer D, et al: Evaluation of orally administered highly variable drugs and drug formulations. *Pharm Res* **13:**1590–1595, 1996

Welling PG, Patel RB, Patel UR, et al: Bioavailability of tolazamide from tablets: Comparison of in vitro and in vivo results. *J Pharm Sci* **71:**1259–1263, 1982

Westlake WJ: Use of confidence intervals in analysis of comparative bioavailability trials. *J Pharm Sci* **61:**1340–1341, 1972

BIBLIOGRAPHY

Abdou HM: *Dissolution, Bioavailability and Bioequivalence.* Easton, PA, Mack, 1989

Bennett RW, Popovitch NG: Statistical inferences as applied to bioavailability data: A guide for the practicing pharmacist. *Am J Hosp Pharm* **34:**712–723, 1977

Chodes DJ, DiSanto AR: *Basics of Bioavailability.* Kalamazoo, MI, Upjohn, 1974

Dighe SV: Biopharmaceutics program. *Clin Res Pract Drug Res Aff* **1:**61–76, 1983

DiSanto AR, Desante KA: Bioavailability and pharmacokinetics of prednisone in humans. *J Pharm Sci* **64:**109–112, 1975

Hendeles L, Wienberger M, Bighley L: Absolute bioavailability of oral theophylline. *Am J Hosp Pharm* **34:**525–527, 1977

Kennedy D: Therapeutically equivalent drugs. *Fed Reg* **44:**2932–2952, 1979

Martin A, Dolusio JT (eds): *Industrial Bioavailability and Pharmacokinetics: Guidelines, Regulations and Controls.* Austin, TX, Austin Drug Dynamics Institute, University of Texas, 1977

Metzler CM: Bioavailability: A problem in equivalence. *Biometrics* **30:**309–317, 1974

Report of the Blue Ribbon Committee on Generic Medicines. *Generic Medicines: Restoring Public Confidence.* Rockville, MD, FDA, 1990

Schumacher GE: Interpretation of bioavailability data by practitioners. *J Clin Pharmacol* **16:**554–559, 1976

Schumacher GE: Use of bioavailability data by practitioners, I. Pitfalls in interpreting the data. *Am J Hosp Pharm* **32:**839–842, 1975

Wagner JG: An overview of the analysis and interpretation of bioavailability studies in man. *Pharmacology* **8:**102–117, 1972

Welling PG, Tse FLS, Dighe SV (eds): *Pharmaceutical Bioequivalence.* New York, Marcel Dekker, 1991

Westlake WJ: The design and analysis of comparative blood level trials. In Swarbrick J (ed), *Current Concepts in Pharmaceutical Sciences: Dosage Form Design and Bioavailability.* Philadelphia, Lea & Febiger, 1973, chap 5

Westlake WJ: Use of statistical methods in evaluation of in vivo performance of dosage forms. *J Pharm Sci* **62:**1579–1589, 1973

11

PHYSIOLOGIC DRUG DISTRIBUTION AND PROTEIN BINDING

PHYSIOLOGIC FACTORS

Once a drug is absorbed or injected into the bloodstream, the drug molecules are distributed throughout the body by systemic circulation. The drug molecules are carried by the blood to the target site (receptor) for drug action and to other (nonreceptor) tissues as well. Drug concentration in untargeted sites may cause side effects. Some drug molecules are distributed to eliminating organs, such as the liver and kidney; others are distributed to tissues, such as the brain, skin, and muscle. Some drugs will cross the placenta and may affect the developing fetus; other drugs will be secreted in milk in the mammillary glands. A substantial portion of the drug may be bound to proteins in the plasma and/or tissues. Lipophilic drugs will deposit in fat from which the drug may be slowly released.

The circulatory system consists of a series of blood vessels; these include the arteries, which carry blood to tissues, and veins, which return the blood back to the heart. An average subject (70 kg) has about 5 liters of blood, which is equivalent to 3 liters of plasma (Fig. 11-1). About 50% of the blood is in the large veins or venous sinuses. The volume of blood pumped by the heart per minute—the *cardiac output*—is the product of the stroke volume of the heart and the number of heartbeats per minute. An average cardiac output is 0.08 L/min × 69 beats/min, or about 5.5 L/min in subjects at rest. The cardiac output may be 5 to 6 times higher during exercise. Left ventricular contraction may produce a systolic blood pressure of 125 mm Hg, and moves blood at a linear speed of 300 mm/sec through the aorta. Mixing of a drug solution in the blood occurs rapidly at this flow rate. Drug molecules rapidly diffuse through a network of fine capillaries to the tissue spaces filled with *interstitial fluid* (Fig. 11-2). The interstitial fluid plus the plasma water is termed the *extracellular water* because they are outside the cells. Drug molecules may further diffuse from the interstitial fluid across the cell membrane into the cell cytoplasm.

Drug distribution is generally rapid, and most small drug molecules permeate capillary membranes easily. The passage of drug molecules across a cell membrane

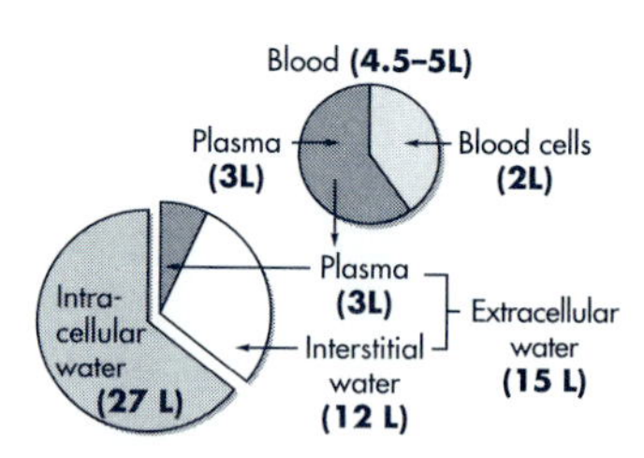

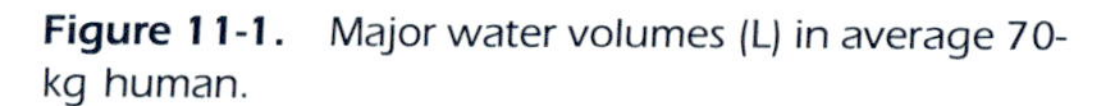

Figure 11-1. Major water volumes (L) in average 70-kg human.

depends upon the physicochemical nature of both the drug and the cell membrane. Cell membranes are composed of protein and a bilayer of phospholipid, which act as a lipid barrier to drug uptake. Thus, lipid-soluble drugs generally diffuse across cell membranes more easily than highly polar or water-soluble drugs. Small drug molecules generally diffuse more rapidly across cell membranes than large drug molecules. If the drug is bound to a plasma protein such as albumin, the drug–protein complex becomes too large for easy diffusion across the cell membrane. A comparison of diffusion rates for water-soluble molecules is illustrated in Table 11.1.

Diffusion and Hydrostatic Pressure

The processes by which drugs transverse capillary membranes include passive diffusion and hydrostatic pressure. Passive diffusion is the main process by which most drugs cross cell membranes. Passive diffusion (Chapter 5) is the process by which drug molecules move from an area of high concentration to an area of low concentration. Passive diffusion is described by *Fick's law of Diffusion:*

$$\text{Rate of drug diffusion} = \frac{dQ}{dt} = \frac{-DKA}{h}(C_p - C_t) \qquad \textbf{(11.1)}$$

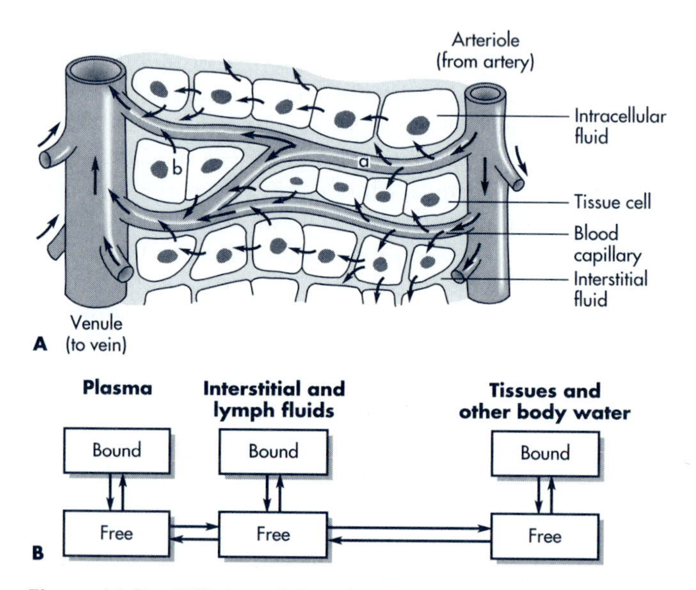

Figure 11-2. Diffusion of drug from capillaries to interstitial spaces.

TABLE 11.1 Permeability of Molecules of Various Sizes to Capillaries

	MOLECULAR WEIGHT	RADIUS OF EQUIVALENT SPHERE (A)	DIFFUSION COEFFICIENT	
			IN WATER $(cm^2/sec) \times 10^5$	ACROSS CAPILLARY $(cm^2/sec \times 100\ g)$
Water	18		3.20	3.7
Urea	60	1.6	1.95	1.83
Glucose	180	3.6	0.91	0.64
Sucrose	342	4.4	0.74	0.35
Raffinose	594	5.6	0.56	0.24
Inulin	5,500	15.2	0.21	0.036
Myoglobin	17,000	19	0.15	0.005
Hemoglobin	68,000	31	0.094	0.001
Serum albumin	69,000		0.085	<0.001

From Goldstein et al (1974).

where $C_p - C_t$ is the difference in drug concentration in the plasma (C_p) and tissue (C_t), respectively; A is the surface area of the membrane; h is the thickness of the membrane; K is the lipid-water partition coefficient; and D is the diffusion constant. The negative sign denotes net transfer of drug from inside the capillary lumen into the tissue and extracellular spaces. Diffusion is spontaneous and temperature dependent. Diffusion is distinguished from blood-flow-initiated mixing, which involves hydrostatic pressure.

Hydrostatic pressure represents a pressure gradient between the arterial end of the capillaries entering the tissue and the venous capillaries leaving the tissue. Hydrostatic pressure is responsible for penetration of water-soluble drugs into spaces between endothelial cells and possibly into lymph. In the kidneys, high arterial pressure creates a filtration pressure that allows small drug molecules to be filtered in the glomerulus of the renal nephron.

Flow-induced drug distribution is rapid and efficient, but requires pressure. As blood pressure gradually decreases when arteries branch into the small arterioles, the speed of flow slows and diffusion into the interstitial space becomes diffusion or concentration driven and facilitated by the large surface area of the capillary network. The average pressure of the blood capillary is higher (+18 mm Hg) than the mean tissue pressure (−6 mm Hg), resulting in a net total pressure of 24 mm Hg higher in the capillary over the tissue. This pressure difference is offset by an average osmotic pressure in the blood of 24 mm Hg, pulling the plasma fluid back into the capillary. Thus, on average, the pressures in the tissue and most parts of the capillary are equal, with no net flow of water. At the arterial end, as the blood newly enters the capillary (Fig. 11-2 A), however, the pressure of the capillary blood is slightly higher (about 8 mm Hg) than that of the tissue causing fluid to leave the capillary and enter the tissues. This pressure is called *hydrostatic* or *filtration pressure.* This filtered fluid (filtrate) is later returned to the venous capillary (Fig. 11-2 B) due to a lower venous pressure of about the same magnitude. The lower pressure of the venous blood compared with the tissue fluid is termed *absorptive pressure.* A small amount of fluid returns to the circulation through the lymphatic system. Because the process of drug transfer from the capillary into the tissue fluid is mainly diffusional, the membrane thickness, diffusion coefficient of the drug, and concentration gradient across the capillary membrane are important factors in determining the rate of drug diffusion. Kinetically, if a drug diffuses rapidly across the membrane in such a way that blood flow is the rate limiting step in the distribution of drug, then the process is *perfusion* or *flow-limited.* In contrast, if drug distribution is limited by the slow diffusion of drug across the membrane in the tissue, then the process is termed *diffusion* or *permeability limited.* A person with congestive heart failure has decreased cardiac output resulting in impaired blood flow that may reduce the volume of distribution through reduced filtration pressure and blood flow. Drugs that are permeability limited may have an increased distribution in disease conditions that cause inflammation and increased capillary membrane permeability. The delicate osmotic pressure balance may be altered due to albumin and/or blood loss or due to changes in electrolyte levels in renal and hepatic disease, resulting in net flow of plasma water into the interstitial space (edema). This change in fluid distribution may partially explain the increased extravascular drug distribution during some diseased states.

Distribution Half-Life, Blood Flow and Drug Uptake by Organs

After the drug molecules enter the bloodstream, drug distribution to various body organs is governed by the rate of blood flow (perfusion) to each organ and the ability of the drug to diffuse across the membrane into the tissue of that organ. Tissues that have good permeability to drug are generally called *perfusion limited* because flow determines the rate by which the drug reaches the tissue; in contrast, a second type of drug distribution is characterized by poor permeation and slow diffusion of drug into the tissue regardless of the rate of blood flow to the organ (Fig. 11-3).

For perfusion limited drugs, drug distribution will be rapid in tissues or organs that receive a high blood flow; whereas, drug distribution will be slower in tissues that are poorly perfused (low blood flow). Table 11.2 lists the blood flow and tissue mass for many tissues in the human body. In addition to blood flow, tissue size and tissue storage are also important in determining the time it takes the drug to become fully distributed. *Drug affinity* for a tissue or organ refers to the partitioning and accumulation of the drug in the tissue. The time for drug distribution is generally measured by the *distribution half-life* or the time for 50% distribution. The factors that determine the distribution constant of a drug into an organ are related to the blood flow to the organ, the volume of

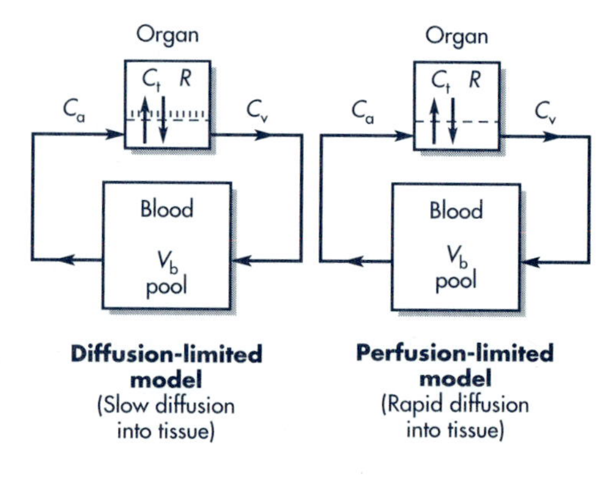

Figure 11-3. Drug distribution to body organs by blood flow (perfusion). **Right.** Tissue with rapid permeability; **Left.** Tissue with slow permeability.

TABLE 11.2 Blood Flow to Human Tissues

TISSUE	PERCENT BODY WEIGHT	PERCENT CARDIAC OUTPUT	BLOOD FLOW (mL/100 g TISSUE/min)
Adrenals	0.02	1	550
Kidneys	0.4	24	450
Thyroid	0.04	2	400
Liver			
Hepatic	2.0	5	20
Portal		20	75
Portal-drained viscera	2.0	20	75
Heart (basal)	0.4	4	70
Brain	2.0	15	55
Skin	7.0	5	5
Muscle (basal)	40.0	15	3
Connective tissue	7.0	1	1
Fat	15.0	2	1

Adapted with permission from Butler (1972).

the organ and the partitioning of the drug into the organ tissue as shown in Equation 11.2.

$$k_d = \frac{Q}{VR} \tag{11.2}$$

where, k_d = first order distribution constant, Q = blood flow to the organ, V = volume of the organ, R = ratio of drug concentration in the organ tissue to drug concentration in the blood (venous).

The distribution half-life of the drug to the tissue, $t_{d1/2}$ may easily be determined from the distribution constant. The distribution half-life of the drug, $t_{d1/2} = 0.693/k_d$.

The ratio, R, must be determined experimentally from tissue samples. With many drugs, however, only animal tissue data are available. Pharmacokineticists have estimated the ratio R based on knowledge of the partition coefficient of the drug. The *partition coefficient* is a physical property that measures the ratio of the solubility of the drug in the oil phase and in aqueous phase. The *partition coefficient* ($P_{o/w}$) is defined as a ratio of the drug concentration in the oil phase (usually represented by octanol) divided by the drug concentration in the aqueous phase measured at equilibrium under specified temperature *in vitro* in an oil/water two-layer system (Fig. 11-4). The *partition coefficient* is one of the most important factors that determine the tissue distribution of a drug.

If each tissue has the same ability to store the drug, then the distribution half-life is governed by the blood flow, Q, and volume (size), V, of the organ. A large blood flow, Q, to the organ decreases the distribution time; whereas, a large organ size or volume, V, increases the distribution time because a longer time is needed to fill a large organ volume with drug. Figure 11-5 illustrates the distribution time (for 0, 50, 90 and 95% distribution) for the adrenal gland, kidney, muscle (basal), skin, and fat tissue in an average human subject (IBW = 70 kg). In this illustration, the blood drug concentration be equally maintained at 100 mcg/mL, and the drug is assumed to have equal distribution between all the tissues and blood, ie, when fully equilibrated, the partition or drug concentration ratio (R) between the tissue

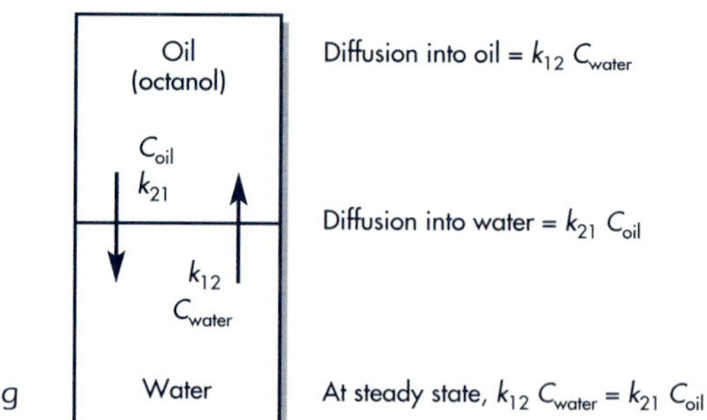

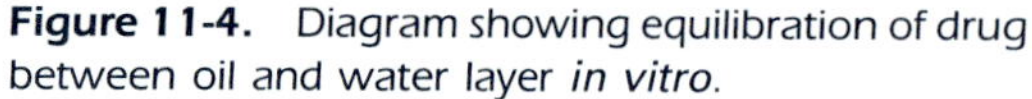

Figure 11-4. Diagram showing equilibration of drug between oil and water layer *in vitro*.

and the plasma will equal 1. Vascular tissues such as the kidneys and adrenal glands achieve 95% distribution in less than 2 minutes. In contrast, drug distribution time in fat tissues takes 4 hours, while less vascular tissues, such as the skin and muscles, take between 2 and 4 hours (Fig. 11-5). When drug partition of the tissues is the same, the distribution time is dependent only on the tissue volume and its blood flow.

Figure 11-6 illustrates the distribution of a drug to three different tissues when the partition of the drug for each tissue varies. For example, the adrenal glands has 5 times the concentration over the plasma ($R = 5$), while drug partition for the kidney, ($R = 3$), and that of the basal muscle ($R = 1$). In this illustration, the adrenal gland and kidney now take 5 and 3 times as long to be equilibrated with drug. Thus, it can be seen that even for vascular tissues, high drug partition can take much more time for the tissue to become fully equilibrated. Some tissues have great ability to store and accumulate drug, as is shown by the large R values. For example, the antiandrogen drug, flutamide, and its active metabolite are highly concentrated in the prostate. The prostate drug concentration is 20 times that of the plasma drug concentration; thus, the antiandrogen effect of the drug is not

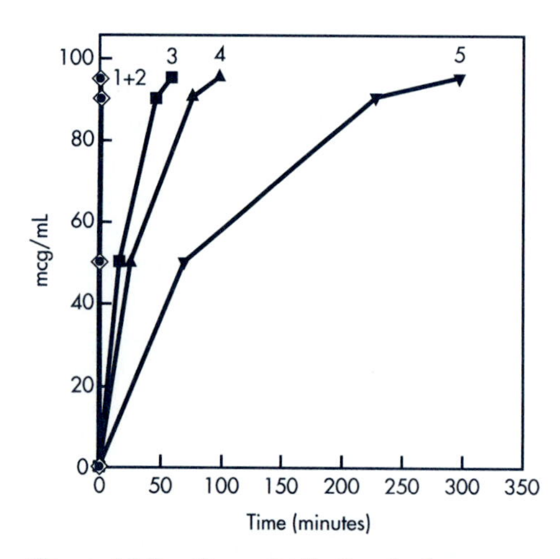

Figure 11-5. Drug distribution in five groups of tissues at various rate of equilibration. (1 = adrenal, 2 = kidney, 3 = skin, 4 = muscle (basal), 5 = fat.)

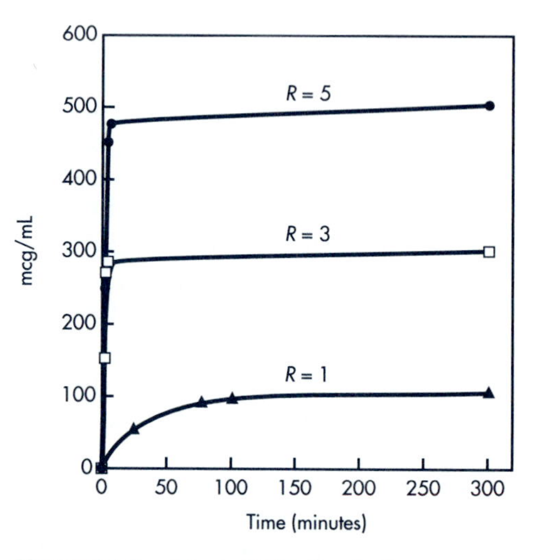

Figure 11-6. Drug distribution in three groups of tissues with various ability to store drug (R). (**Top** = Adrenal; **Middle** = Kidney; **Bottom** = Muscle)

fully achieved until distribution to this receptor site is complete. Digoxin is highly bound to myocardial membranes. Digoxin has a high tissue/plasma concentration ratio ($R = 60$ to 130) in the myocardium. This high R ratio for digoxin leads to a long distributional phase (see Chapter 4) despite abundant blood flow to the heart. It is important to note that if a tissue has a long distribution half-life, a long time is needed for the drug to leave the tissue when blood level decreases. Understanding drug distribution is important because the activities of many drugs are not well correlated with plasma drug level. Kinetically, both protein binding or favorable solubility in the tissue site will lead to a longer distribution time.

Chemical knowledge in molecular structure often helps to estimate the lipid solubility of a drug, and a drug with large oil/water partition coefficient tends to have high R values in vivo. A reduction in the partition coefficient of a drug often reduces the rate of drug uptake into the brain. This may decrease drug distribution to the central nervous system and decrease undesirable central nervous system side effects. Extensive tissue distribution is kinetically evidenced by an increase in the volume of distribution, while a secondary effect is a prolonged elimination half-life of the drug distributed over a larger volume (thus, more diluted) and, therefore, less efficiently removed by the kidney or the liver. For example, etretinate (a retinoate derivative) for acne treatment has an unusually long elimination half-life of about 100 days (Chien et al, 1992) due to its extensive distribution to body fats. Newly synthesized agents were designed to reduce lipophilicity and distribution. These new agents have less accumulation and less potential for teratogenicity.

Relationship Between Drug Distribution and Drug Elimination Half-Life

Drug elimination is mainly governed by renal and other metabolic processes in the body. However, extensive drug distribution has the effect of diluting the drug in a large volume, making it harder for the kidney to filter the drug by glomerular filtration. Thus, the $t_{1/2}$ of the drug is prolonged if clearance is constant and V_D is increased according to Equation 11.4. Cl is related to apparent volume of distribution, V_D and the elimination constant k as shown in Equation 11.3 (see also Chapter 3). For a first order process, Cl is the product of V_D and the elimination rate constant, k, according to Equation 11.3. The equation is derived for a drug given after a given dose is distributed in a single volume of body fluid without protein binding. The equation basically describes the empirical observation that a large clearance or large volume of distribution both lead to low plasma drug concentration after a given dose. Mechanistically, a low plasma drug concentration may be due to (1) extensive distribution into tissues due to favorable lipophilicity, (2) extensive distribution into tissues due to protein binding in peripheral tissues, (3) lack of drug plasma protein binding.

$$Cl = kV_D \quad \textbf{(11.3)}$$

$$t_{1/2} = 0.693\ V_D/Cl \quad \textbf{(11.4)}$$

Two drug examples are selected to further illustrate the relationship between elimination half-life, clearance and the volume of distribution. Although the kinetic relationship is straightforward, there is more than one way of explaining the observations.

Clinical Examples

Drug with a Large Volume of Distribution and a Long Elimination $t_{1/2}$

The macrolide antibiotic, dirithromycin (Lilly) is extensively distributed in the tissues resulting in a large steady-state volume of distribution of about 800 liters (range, 504 to 1041 L). The elimination $t_{1/2}$ in humans is about 44 hours (range, 16–65 hr). The drug has a relatively large total body clearance of 226 to 1040 mL/min (13.6–62.4 L/hr) and is given once daily. In this case, even clearance is big due to a large V_D. k is relatively small. Equation 11.4 shows that a small clearance generally leads to a longer $t_{1/2}$. In this case, Cl is large but the elimination half-life is longer because of the large V_D. Intuitively, the drug will take a long time to be removed when the drug is extensively distributed over a large volume, despite a relatively large clearance, $t_{1/2}$ accurately describes drug elimination alone.

Drug with a Small Volume of Distribution and a Long Elimination $t_{1/2}$

Tenoxicam is a nonsteroidal antiinflammatory drug (Nilsen, 1994) that is about 99% bound in human plasma protein. The drug has low lipophilicity, is highly ionized (approximately 99%), and is distributed in blood. Because tenoxicam is very polar, the drug penetrates cell membranes slowly. The synovial fluid peak drug level is only one-third that of the plasma drug concentration and occurs 20 hours (range, 10–34 hr) later than the peak plasma drug level. In addition, the drug is poorly distributed to body tissues and has an apparent volume of distribution, V_D, of 9.6 L (range, 7.5–11.5 L). Tenoxicam has a low total plasma clearance of 0.106 L/h (0.079–0.142 L/h) and an elimination half-life of 67 hours (range, 49–81 hr), undoubtedly related to the extensive drug binding to plasma proteins.

According to Equation 11.3, drug clearance from the body is small if V_D is small and k is not too large, this is consistent with a small Cl and a small V_D observed for tenoxicam. Equation 11.4, however, predicts that a small V_D would result in a small elimination $t_{1/2}$. In this case, the actual elimination half-life is long (67 hr) because the plasma tenoxicam clearance is so small that it dominates in Equation 11.4. The long elimination half-life of tenoxicam is better explained by restrictive drug clearance due to its binding to plasma protein, making it difficult for the drug to clear rapidly.

Clearance and Volume of Distribution

Cl and V_D are regarded as independent model variables by some physiologic pharmacokineticists based on Equation 11.4. Actually, Equation 11.3 and its Equivalent 11.4 are rooted in classical pharmacokinetics. Initially, it may be difficult to understand why a drug with a rapid clearance of 226 to 1040 mL/min, such as dirithromycin has a long half-life. In pharmacokinetics, the elimination constant, $k = 0.0156\ \text{hr}^{-1}$ implies that 1/64 of the drug is cleared per hour (a low efficiency elimination factor). From k, one can estimate that it takes 44 hours ($t_{1/2} = 44$ hr) to eliminate half the drug in the body regardless of V_D. While $t_{1/2}$ is dependent on clearance and V_D as shown by Equation 11.4, clearance is clearly affected by the volume of distribution and by many variables of the drug in the biological system also.

These examples show that partitioning of drugs into tissues, drug protein binding, and the extent of drug ionization are factors that influence drug distribution and elimination. The extent of drug binding to tissues and blood proteins is discussed later in this chapter. These factors are considered in the calculation of the apparent volume of distribution of the drug using the physiological model.

Drug Accumulation

The deposition or uptake of the drug into the tissue is generally controlled by the diffusional barrier of the capillary membrane and other cell membranes. For example, the brain is well perfused with blood, but many drugs with good aqueous solubility have high kidney, liver, and lung concentration and yet little or negligible brain drug concentration. The brain capillaries are surrounded by a layer of tightly joined glial cells that impede the diffusion of polar or highly ionized drugs. A diffusion-limited model may be necessary to describe the pharmacokinetics of these drugs that are not adequately described by perfusion models.

Tissues receiving high blood flow equilibrate quickly with the drug in the plasma. However, at steady state, the drug may or may not accumulate (concentrate) within the tissue. The accumulation of drug into tissues is dependent upon both the blood flow and the affinity of the drug for the tissue. Drug uptake into a tissue is generally reversible. The drug concentration in a tissue with low capacity equilibrates rapidly with the plasma drug concentration and then declines rapidly as the drug is eliminated from the body. Drugs with high tissue affinity tend to accumulate or concentrate in the tissue. Drugs with a high lipid/water partition coefficient are very fat soluble and tend to accumulate in lipid or adipose (fat) tissue. In this case, the lipid-soluble drug partitions from the aqueous environment of the plasma into the fat. This process is reversible, but the extraction of drug out of the tissue is so slow that the drug may remain for days or even longer in adipose tissues long after the drug is depleted from the blood. Because the adipose tissue is poorly perfused with blood, drug accumulation is slow. However, once the drug is concentrated in fat tissue, drug removal from fat may also be slow. For example, the chlorinated hydrocarbon DDT (dichlorodiphenyltrichloroethane) is highly lipid soluble and remains in fat tissue for years.

Drugs may accumulate in tissues by other processes. For example, drugs may accumulate by binding to proteins or other macromolecules in a tissue. Digoxin is highly bound to proteins in cardiac tissue leading in a large volume of distribution (440 L/70 kg) and long elimination $t_{1/2}$ (approximately 40 hr). Some drugs may complex with melanin in the skin and eye, as observed after long-term administration of high doses of phenothiazine to chronic schizophrenic patients. The antibiotic, tetracycline, forms an insoluble chelate with calcium. In growing teeth and bones, tetracycline will complex with the calcium and remain in these tissues. Some tissues have enzyme systems that actively transport natural biochemical substances into the tissues. For example, various adrenergic tissues have a specific uptake system for catecholamines, such as norepinephrine. Thus, amphetamine, which has a phenylethylamine structure similar to norepinephrine, is actively transported into adrenergic tissue. Other examples of drug accumulation are well documented. For some drugs, the actual mechanism for drug accumulation may not be clearly understood.

In a few cases, the drug is irreversibly bound into a particular tissue. *Irreversible binding* of drug may occur when the drug or a reactive intermediate metabolite becomes covalently bound to a macromolecule within the cell, such as to a tissue protein. Many purine and pyrimidine drugs used in cancer chemotherapy are incorporated into nucleic acids, causing destruction of the cell.

Drug Distribution and Pharmacodynamics

The onset of drug action depends upon the rate of the free (unbound) drug that reaches the receptor at a minimum effective concentration (MEC) to produce a pharmacodynamic response (see Chapter 2). The onset time is often dependent upon the rate of drug uptake and distribution to the receptor site. The intensity of a drug action depends upon the total drug concentration of the receptor site and the number of receptors occupied by drug. To achieve a pharmacodynamic response with the initial (priming) dose, the amount (mass) of drug when dissolved in the volume of distribution must give a drug concentration ≥ MEC at the receptor site. Subsequent drug doses maintain the pharmacodynamic effect by sustaining the drug concentration at the receptor site. Subsequent doses are given at a dose rate (eg, 250 mg every 6 hr) that replaces drug loss from the receptor site, usually by elimination. However, redistributional factors may also contribute to the loss of drug from the receptor site.

Drug protein binding in plasma and tissue are important considerations. Only free drug may diffuse from the capillaries into tissue sites, whereas protein bound drugs are generally too large to cross the biological membranes. For many drugs, the free drug concentration in the plasma is used as an indicator for pharmacodynamic activity if the target site is well equilibrated with blood. For example, the free concentration of serum propranolol (a beta blocker) is related to the decrease in exercise induced heart rate (Fig. 11-7). The free plasma drug concentration may be estimated by multiplying the unbound fraction (f_u) in the plasma with the total plasma drug concentration, C_p. The fraction of drug unbound will change in a patient in certain diseases, especially renal and hepatic disease. The total plasma drug concentration may not be a good indicator of overall drug activity because simultaneous drug binding to blood and tissue proteins ultimately determines the free drug concentration.

Effect of Changing Plasma Protein: An Example

The effect of increasing the plasma α_1-acid glycoprotein (AAG) level on drug penetration into tissues may be verified with cloned animals that have high blood AAG level. In an experiment investigating the activity of the tricyclic antidepressant drug, imipramine, equal drug doses were administered to both normal and transgenic rats. The transgenic rat has 8.6 times the normal serum protein level of α_1-acid glycoprotein (AAG). Since imipramine is highly bound to AAG, the steady-state imipramine serum level was greatly increased in the blood due to protein binding:

Imipramine serum level (transgenic rat)	859 ng/mL
Imipramine serum level (normal rat)	319.9 ng/mL
Imipramine brain level (transgenic rat)	3862.6 ng/mL
Imipramine brain level (normal rat)	7307.7 ng/mL

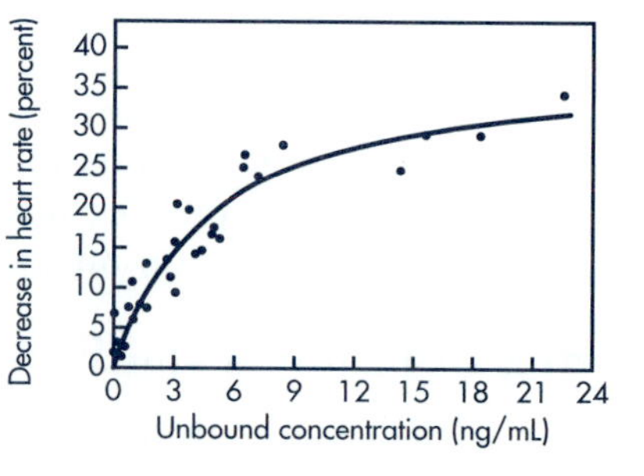

Figure 11-7. Relationship between unbound propranolol and decrease in heart rate.
From Holladay et al (1996).

However, the imipramine concentration was greatly reduced in the brain tissue because of higher binding to AAG in the serum, resulting in reduced drug penetration into the brain tissue. The antidepressant effect was observed to be lower in the transgenic rats due to lower brain imipramine level. This experiment illustrates that high drug protein binding in the serum can reduce drug penetration to tissue receptors for some drugs.

Clinically, the pharmacodynamic response is influenced by the distribution of the drug and the concentration of the unbound drug fraction. The drug dose and the dosage form must be chosen to provide sufficiently high unbound drug concentrations so that an adequate amount of drug reaches the site of drug action (receptor). Blood flow is an important consideration in determining how rapid and how much drug reaches the receptor site.

Under normal conditions, limited blood flow reaches the muscles. During exercise, the increase in blood flow may change the fraction of drug reaching the muscle tissues. Diabetic patients receiving intramuscular injection of insulin may experience the effects of changing onset of drug action during exercise. Normally, the blood reserve of the body stays mostly in the large veins and sinuses in the abdomen. During injury or when blood is lost, constriction of the large veins redirect more blood to needed areas and, therefore, affect drug distribution. Accumulation of carbon dioxide may lower the pH of certain tissues and may affect the level of drugs reaching those tissues. Drug distribution may be changed in many disease and physiologic states, making it difficult to predict the amount of drug that reaches the site of drug action (receptor).

Permeability of Cell and Capillary Membranes

Cell membranes vary in their permeability characteristics depending upon the tissue. For example, capillary membranes in the liver and kidneys are more permeable to transmembrane drug movement than capillaries in the brain. The sinusoidal capillaries of the liver are very permeable and allow the passage of large-molecular-weight molecules. In the brain and spinal cord, the capillary endothelial cells are surrounded by a layer of *glial cells*, which have tight intercellular junctions. This added layer of cells around the capillary membranes acts to effectively slow the rate of drug diffusion into the brain by acting as a thicker lipid barrier. This lipid barrier, which slows the diffusion and penetration of water-soluble and polar drugs into the brain and spinal cord, is called the *blood–brain barrier.*

Under certain pathophysiologic conditions, the permeability of the cell membrane may be altered. For example, burns will alter the permeability of skin and allow drugs and larger molecules to permeate inward or outward. In meningitis, which involves the inflammation of the membranes of the spinal cord or brain, drug uptake into the brain will be enhanced.

The diameters of the capillaries are very small and the capillary membranes are very thin. The high blood flow within a capillary allows for intimate contact of the drug molecules with the cell membrane, providing for rapid drug diffusion. For capillaries that perfuse the brain and spinal cord, the layer of glial cells functions to effectively increase the thickness term h in Equation 11.1, thereby slowing the diffusion and penetration of water-soluble and polar drugs into the brain and spinal cord.

Mass Balance of Drug and Apparent Volume Distribution

The apparent volume of distribution, V_D, is used to estimate the extent of drug distribution in the body. Although the apparent volume of distribution does not represent the physical size of the tissues, the V_D represents the result of dynamic drug distribution between the blood and the tissues. The V_D accounts for the mass balance of the drug in the body. To illustrate the use of V_D, consider an example of a drug dissolved in a simple solution. A volume term is needed to relate drug concentration in the system (or human body) to the amount of drug present in that system. The volume of the system may be estimated if the amount of drug added to the system and the drug concentration after equilibrium in the system are known.

$$\text{Volume (L)} = \frac{\text{amount (mg) of drug added to system}}{\text{drug concentration (mg/L) in system after equilibration}} \tag{11.5}$$

Equation 11.5 describes the relationship of concentration, volume, and mass, as shown in Equation 11.6.

$$\text{Concentration (mg/L)} \times \text{volume (L)} = \text{mass (mg)} \tag{11.6}$$

Considerations in the Calculation of Volume of Distribution: A Simulated Example

Assume that 3 beakers are each filled with 100 mL of water. Then, 100 mg of drug is added to each beaker (Fig. 11-8). Beaker 1 contains water only; beakers 2 and 3 each contain water and a small compartment filled with cultured cells. The cells in beaker 2 can bind the drug while the cells in beaker 3 can metabolize the drug. One hundred mg of drug is added to each beaker, and the concentration of drug in the water (fluid) compartment is sampled and assayed. After the amount of drug is added and the fluid concentration of drug in each beaker is at equilibration the volume of water may be computed. The objective of this exercise is to determine how to calculate the volume in each case and to compare the calculated volume to the real volume of water in the beaker. The three beakers represent the following, respectively:

Beaker 1. Drug distribution in a fluid (water) compartment only without drug binding and metabolism.

Beaker 2. Drug distribution in a fluid compartment containing cell clusters that reversibly bind drugs.

Beaker 3. Drug distribution in a fluid compartment containing cell clusters (similar to tissues *in vivo*) in which the drug may be metabolized and the metabolites bound to cells.

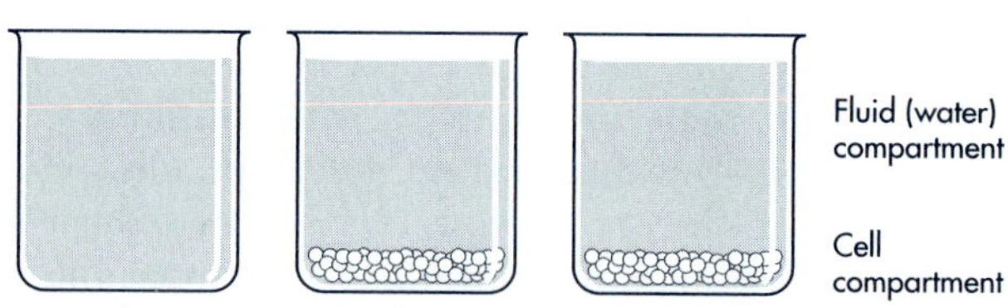

Figure 11-8. Experiment simulating drug distribution in the body. Three beakers each contain 100 mL of water (fluid compartment) and 100 mg of a water-soluble drug. Beakers 2 and 3 also contain 5 mL of cultured cell clusters.

CASE ONE

The volume of water in beaker 1 is calculated from the amount of drug added (100 mg) and the equilibrated drug concentration using Equation 11.5. After equilibration, the drug concentration was measured to be 1 mg/mL.

Volume = 100 mg/1 mg/mL = 100 mL

The calculated volume in beaker 1 confirms that the system is a simple, homogeneous system and, in this case, represents the "true" fluid volume of the beaker.

CASE TWO

Beaker 2 contains cell clusters stuck to the bottom of the beaker. Binding of drug to the proteins of the cells occurs on the surface and within the cytoplasmic interior. This case represents a heterogeneous system consisting of a well-stirred fluid compartment and a tissue (cell). To correctly determine the volume of this system, more information is needed than in Case 1:

1. The amount of drug dissolved in the fluid compartment must be determined. Because some of the drug will be bound within the cell compartment, the amount of drug in the fluid compartment will be less than the 100 mg placed in the beaker.
2. The amount of drug taken up by the cell cluster must be known to account for the entire amount of drug in the beaker. Therefore, both the cell and the fluid compartments must be sampled and assayed to determine the drug concentration in each compartment.
3. The volume of the cell cluster must be determined.

Assume that the above measurements were made and that the following information was obtained:

- Drug concentration in fluid compartment = 0.5 mg/mL.
- Drug concentration in cell cluster = 10 mg/mL.
- Volume of cell cluster = 5 mL.
- Amount of drug added = 100 mg.
- Amount of drug taken up by the cell = 10 mg/mL × 5 mL = 50 mg.
- Amount of drug dissolved in the fluid (water) compartment = 100 mg (total) − 50 mg (in cells) = 50 mg (in water).

Using the above information, the true volume of the fluid (water) compartment is calculated using Equation 11.5.

Volume of fluid compartment = 50 mg/0.5 mg/uL = 100 mL

The value of 100 mL agrees with the volume of fluid we put into the beaker. If the tissue cells were not accessible for sampling as in the case of in vivo drug administration, the volume of the fluid (water) compartment is calculated using Equation 11.5 assuming the system is homogenous:

Apparent volume = 100 mg/0.5 mg/mL = 200 mL

The value of 200 mL is a substantial overestimation of the true volume (100 mL) of the system. When a heterogeneous system is involved, the real or true volume of the system may not be accurately calculated by monitoring only one compartment. Therefore, an apparent volume of distribution is calculated and the infrastructure of the system is ignored. The term *apparent volume of distribution* refers to the lack of true volume characteristics. The apparent volume of distribution is used in pharmacokinetics because the tissue (cellular) compartments are not easily sampled and the true volume is not known. When the experiment in beaker 2 is performed with an equal volume of cultured cells that have different binding affinity for the drug, then the apparent volume of distribution is very much affected by the extent of cellular drug binding (Table 11.3).

As shown in Table 11.3, as the amount of drug in the cell compartment increases (column 3), the apparent V_D of the fluid compartment increases (column 6). Extensive cellular drug binding effectively pulls drug molecules out of the fluid compartment, decreases the drug concentration in the fluid compartment, and increases V_D. In biological systems, the quantity of cells, cell compartment volume, and extent of drug binding within the cells will affect V_D. A large cell volume and/or extensive drug binding in the cells reduces the drug concentration in the fluid compartment and increases the apparent volume of distribution.

In this example, the fluid compartment is comparable to the central compartment and the cell compartment is analogous to the peripheral or tissue compartment. If the drug is distributed widely into the tissues or concentrates unevenly into the tissues, the V_D for a drug may exceed the physical volume of the body (about 70 L of total volume or 42 L of body water for a 70-kg subject). Besides cellular protein binding, partitioning of drug into lipid cellular components may greatly inflate V_D. Many drugs have oil/water partition coefficients above 10,000. These lipophilic drugs are mostly concentrated in the lipid phase of adipose tissue, resulting in a very low drug-concentration in the extracellular water. Generally, drugs with very large V_D values will have very low drug concentrations in the plasma.

A large V_D is often interpreted as broad drug distribution for a drug, even though many other factors also lead to the calculation of a large apparent volume of distribution. A true V_D that exceeds the volume of the body is physically impossible. Only if the drug concentrations in both the tissue and plasma compartments are sampled and the volumes of each compartment are clearly defined, can a true physical volume be calculated.

▶ CASE THREE

The drug in the cell compartment in beaker 3 decreases due to undetected metabolism because the metabolite formed is bound to the peripheral cells. Thus, the apparent volume of distribution would also be greater than 100 mL. Any unknown source that decreases the drug concentration in the fluid compartment will in-

TABLE 11.3 Relationship of Volume of Distribution and Amount of Drug in Tissue (Cellular) Compartment[a]

TOTAL DRUG (mg)	VOLUME OF CELLS (mL)	DRUG IN CELLS (mg)	DRUG IN WATER (mg)	DRUG CONCENTRATION IN WATER (mg/mL)	V_D IN WATER (mL)
100	15	75	25	0.25	400
100	10	50	50	0.50	200
100	5	25	75	0.75	133
100	1	5	95	0.95	105

[a]For each condition, the true water (fluid) compartment is 100 mL. Apparent volume of distribution (V_D) is calculated according to Equation 11.5.

crease the V_D, resulting in an overestimated apparent volume of distribution. This is illustrated with the experiment in beaker 3. In beaker 3, the cell cluster metabolizes the drug and binds the metabolite to the cells. Therefore, the drug is effectively removed from the fluid concentration. The data for this experiment (note that metabolite is expressed as equivalent intact drug) are as follows:

- Total drug placed in beaker = 100 mg.
- Cell compartment:
  Drug concentration = 0.2 mg/mL.
  Metabolite-bound concentration = 9.71 mg/mL.
  Metabolite-free concentration = 0.29 mg/mL.
  Cell volume = 5 mL.
- Fluid (water) compartment:
  Drug concentration = 0.2 mg/mL.
  Metabolite concentration = 0.29 mg/mL.

To calculate the total amount of drug and metabolite in the cell compartment, Equation 11.5 is rearranged as shown:

Total drug and metabolite in cells = 5 mL × (0.2 + 9.71 + 0.29 mg/mL) = 51 mg

Therefore, the total drug in the fluid compartment is 100 − 51 mg = 49 mg. If only the intact drug is considered, V_D is calculated using Equation 11.5.

$$V_D = 100 \text{ mg}/0.2 \text{ mg/mL} = 500 \text{ mL}$$

Considering that only 100 mL of water was placed into beaker 3, the calculated apparent volume of distribution of 500 mL is an overestimate of the true fluid volume of the system.

The distribution of drug in a biological system is illustrated by Figure 11-9. Within the plasma pool, albumin is present at about 4.4 g/dL. Albumin concentration is lower in the extracellular fluid at about 60% of the plasma level. Only free drug diffuses between the plasma and tissue fluids. The tissue fluid, in turn, equilibrates with the intracellular water inside the tissue cells. The tissue drug concentration is influenced by the partition coefficient (lipid/water affinity) of the drug and tissue protein drug binding. Figure 11-10 lists the steady-state volume of distribution of 10 common drugs in ascending order. Drugs with lower distribution within the extracellular water are more extensively distributed inside the tissues. Most of these drugs follow multicompartment kinetics with various tissue distribution phases (Chapter 4). The physiologic volume of an ideal 70-kg subject are also plotted for comparison: (1) the plasma (3L), (2) the extracellular fluid (15 L), and (3) the

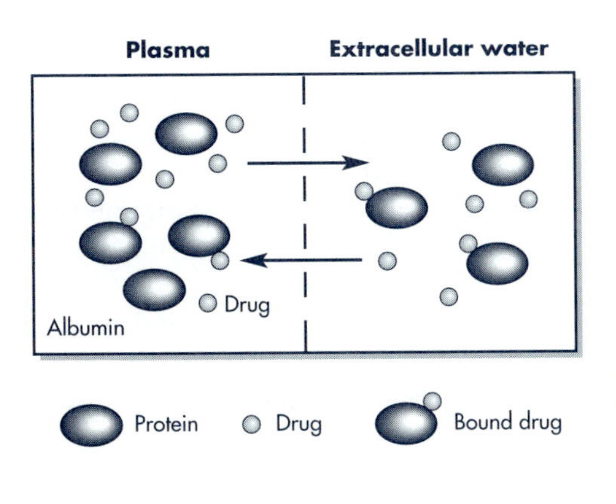

Figure 11-9. Diagram showing bound drugs will not diffuse across membrane but free drug will diffuse freely between the plasma and extracellular water.

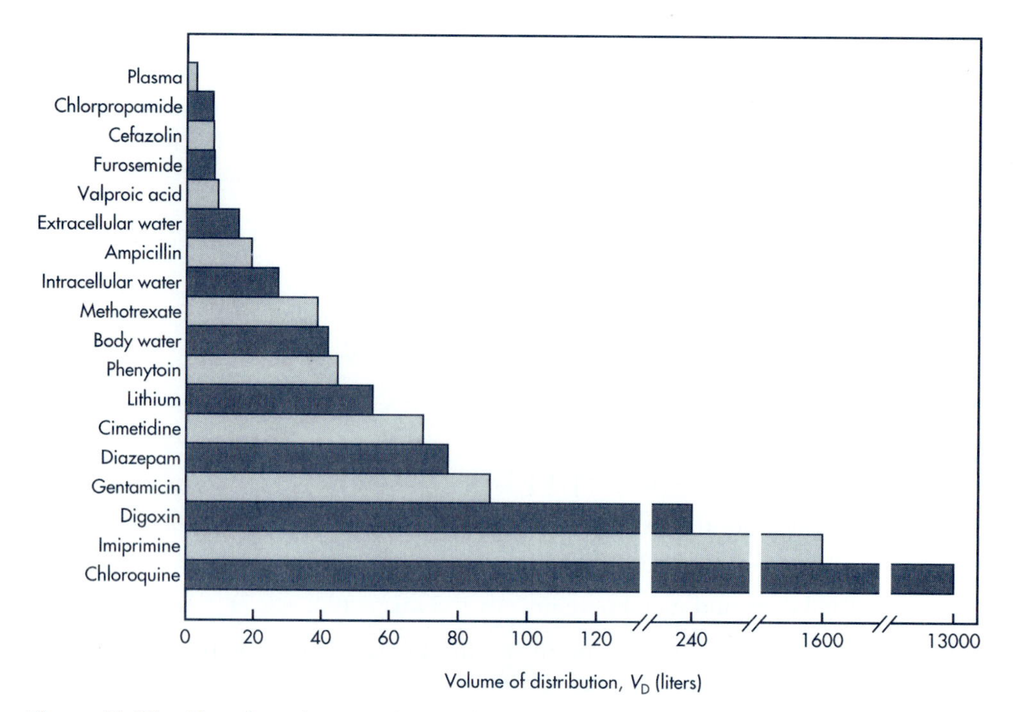

Figure 11-10. Lists of steady-state volumes of distribution of 10 common drugs in ascending order showing various factors affect V_D. Drugs with high V_D generally has high tissue affinity or low binding to serum albumin. Polar or hydrophilic drugs tend to have V_D similar to the volume of extracellular water.

intracellular fluid (27L). Drugs such as penicillin, cephalosporin, valproic acid, and furosemide are polar compounds that stay mostly within the plasma and extracellular fluids. Any unusual tissue drug level is most likely influenced by protein binding or the presence of a special carrier or efflux system. An excessively high volume of distribution (> than the body volume of 70 L) is mostly due to special tissue storage which removes drug from the plasma fluid. Digoxin, for example, is bound to myocardial membrane which has drug levels that are 60 and 130 times the serum drug level, in adults and children, respectively (Park et al, 1982). The high tissue binding is responsible for the large steady-state volume of distribution (Chapter 4). The greater drug affinity also results in longer distribution (alpha) half-life in spite of the heart's great vascular blood perfusion. Imipramine is a drug that is highly protein bound and concentrated in the plasma, yet its favorable tissue partition and binding accounts for a large volume of distribution. Several tricyclic antidepressants (TCA) also have large volumes of distribution due to tissue (CNS) penetration and binding.

The following conclusions can be drawn from the beaker exercise above:

1. Drug must be at equilibrium in the system before any drug concentration is measured. In nonequilibrium conditions, the sample removed from the system for drug assay does not represent all parts of the system.
2. Drug binding distorts the true physical volume of distribution when all components in the system are not properly sampled and assayed. Extravascular drug binding increases the apparent V_D.
3. Both intravascular and extravascular drug binding must be determined to calculate meaningful volumes of distribution.
4. The apparent V_D is essentially a measure of the relative extent of drug distri-

bution outside the plasma compartment. Greater tissue drug binding and drug accumulation increases V_D, whereas greater plasma protein drug binding decreases the V_D distribution.

5. Undetected cellular drug metabolism increases V_D.
6. An apparent V_D larger than the combined volume of plasma and body water is indicative of (4) and (5), or both, listed above.
7. Although the V_D is not a true physiologic volume, the V_D is useful to relate the plasma drug concentration to the amount of drug in the body (Eq. 11.5). This relationship of the product of the drug concentration and volume to equal the total mass of drug is important in pharmacokinetics.

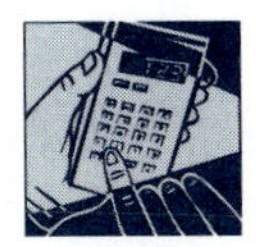

PRACTICE PROBLEM

Table 11.3 (p. 294) shows the amount of drug in the system calculated from V_D and the drug concentration in the fluid compartment. Calculate the amount of drug in the system using the true volume and the drug concentration in the fluid compartment.

Solution

In each case, the product of the drug concentration (column 5) times the apparent volume of distribution (column 6) yields 100 mg of drug, accurately accounting for the total amount of drug present in the system. For example, 0.25 mg/mL × 400 mL = 100 mg. Notice that the total amount of drug present cannot be determined using the true volume and the drug concentration (column 5).

The physiologic approach requires more information, including (1) cell drug concentration, (2) cell compartment volume, and (3) fluid compartment volume. Using the physiologic approach, the total amount of drug is equal to the amount of drug in the cell compartment and the amount of drug in the fluid compartment.

$$(15 \text{ mg/mL} \times 5 \text{ mL}) + (100 \text{ mL} \times 0.25 \text{ mg/mL}) = 100 \text{ mg}$$

The two approaches shown above each correctly account for the amount of drug present in the system. However, the second approach requires more information than is commonly available. The second approach does, however, make more physiologic sense. Most physiologic compartment spaces are not clearly defined for measuring drug concentrations.

Effect of Protein Binding on the Apparent Volume of Distribution

The extent of drug protein binding in the plasma or tissue will affect V_D. Drugs highly bound to plasma proteins will have a low fraction of free drug (f_u = unbound fraction) in the plasma water, harder to diffuse, and less extensively distributed to tissues (Fig. 11-9). Drugs with low plasma protein binding have greater f_u and thus generally easier diffusion and greater volume of distributions. Since the apparent volume of distribution is influenced by lipid solubility besides protein binding, there are some exceptions to the rule. However, when several drugs are selected from a single family with close physical and lipid partition characteristics, the apparent volume of distribution may be explained by the relative degree of drug binding to tissue and plasma proteins. The V_D of four cephalosporin antibiotics (Fig. 11-11) in man and rat (Sawada et al, 1984) demonstrated that the differences in volume of distribution of cefazolin, cefotetan, moxalactam, and cefoperazone are mostly due to differences in the degree of protein binding. For example, the fraction of unbound drug f_u in the plasma is the highest for cefoperazone in man and mouse, and the volume of distribution is also the highest among the four drugs in both man and mouse. Conversely, cefazolin has the lowest f_u in humans and is correlated with the lowest volume of distribution. Interestingly, the volume of distribution per kg in man (V_{man}) is generally higher than that in rat (V_{rat}) since the fraction of unbound drug is also greater, resulting in a greater volume of distribution. Differences in V_D and $t_{1/2}$ among various species may be due to differences in drug protein binding. An equation (see Eq. 11.13 on p. 300) relating quantitatively the effect of protein binding on apparent volume of distribution is derived in the next section.

Drugs such as furosemide, sulfisoxazole, tolbutamide, and warfarin are bound greater than 90% to plasma proteins and have a V_D value ranging from 7.7 to 11.2 L/70 kg body weight (see Appendix E). Basic drugs such as imipramine, nortriptyline, and propranolol are extensively bound to both tissue and plasma proteins and have very large V_D values. As discussed earlier, displacement of drugs from plasma proteins can affect the pharmacokinetics of a drug in several ways: (1) directly increase the free (unbound) drug concentration as a result of reduced binding in the blood; (2) increase the free drug concentration that reaches the receptor sites directly, causing a more intense pharmacodynamic (or toxic) response; (3) increase the free drug concentration causing a transient increase in V_D and decreasing partly some of the increase in free plasma drug concentration; (4) increase the free drug concentration resulting in more drug diffusion into tissues of eliminating organs, particularly the liver and kidney, resulting in a transient increase in drug elimination. The ultimate drug concentration reaching the target depends on one or more of these four factors dominating in the clinical situation. The effect of drug protein binding must be evaluated carefully before dosing changes are made.

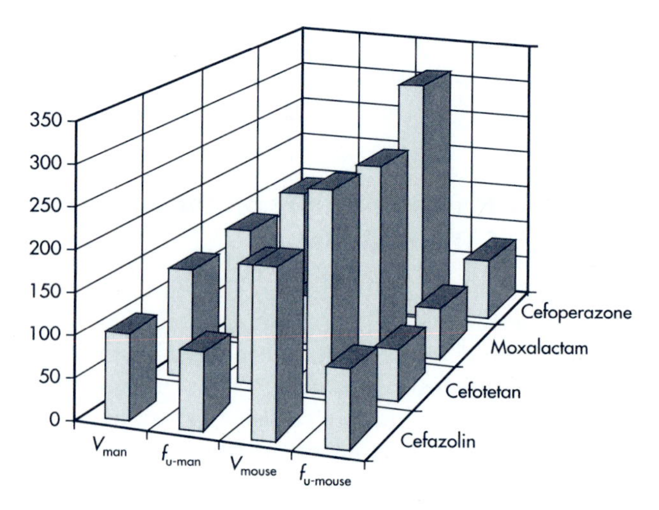

Figure 11-11. Plot of V_D of four cephalosporin antibiotics in man and rat showing the relationship between the fraction of unbound drug (f_u) and the volume of distribution. (Sawada et al, 1984)

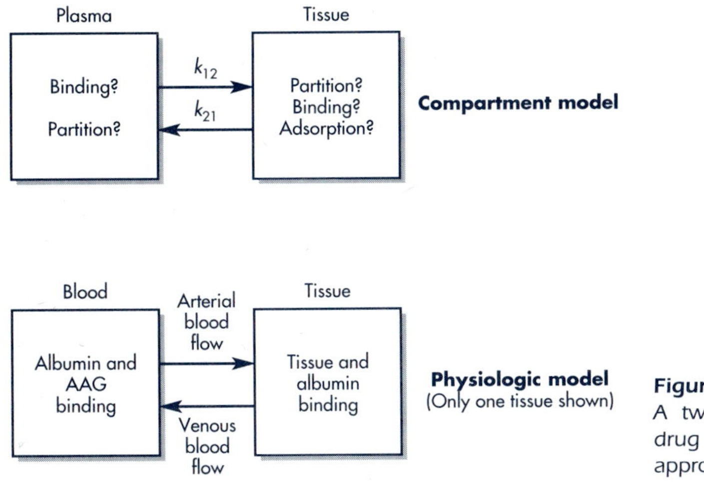

Figure 11-12. A diagram showing: **Top.** A two-compartment model approach to drug distribution. **Bottom.** A physiologic approach to drug distribution.

CALCULATION OF APPARENT VOLUME OF DISTRIBUTION

Steady-State Apparent Volume of Distribution

The apparent volume of distribution, V_{app}, relates the plasma drug concentration to the amount of drug present in the body. V_{app} is determined at steady state when the drug concentration in the tissue compartment is at equilibrium with the drug concentration in the plasma compartment (Fig. 11-12). The derivation is based on Equation 11.5, as shown below.

$$V_{app} = D_B / C_p \tag{11.7}$$

$$D_B = V_p C_p + V_t C_t \tag{11.8}$$

where D_B is the amount of drug in the body, V_p is the plasma compartment volume, V_t is the tissue compartment volume, C_p is the plasma drug concentration, and C_t is the tissue drug concentration.

Because drug may bind to both plasma and tissue proteins, the bound and unbound drug concentrations must be considered. At steady state, unbound drug in plasma and tissue are in equilibration.

$$C_u = C_{ut}$$

Alternatively,

$$C_p f_u = C_t f_{ut} \tag{11.9}$$

or

$$C_t = C_p f_u / f_{ut} \tag{11.10}$$

where $= f_u$ is the unbound (free) drug *fraction* in the plasma, $= f_{ut}$ is the unbound drug *fraction* in the tissue, C_u is the unbound drug *concentration* in the plasma, and C_{ut} is the unbound drug *concentration* in the tissues. Substituting Equation 11.10 into 11.8, will result in the following:

$$D_B = V_p C_p + V_t [C_p (f_u / f_{ut})] \tag{11.11}$$

Rearranging

$$D_B/C_p = V_p + V_t[f_u/f_{ut}] \qquad \textbf{(11.12)}$$

Because $D_B/C_p = V_{app}$ (Eq. 11.7), by substitution into Equation 11.12, V_{app} may be estimated by Equation 11.13:

$$V_{app} = V_p + V_t[f_u/f_{ut}] \qquad \textbf{(11.13)}$$

Equation 11.13 relates the amount of drug in the body to plasma volume, tissue volume, and fraction of free plasma and tissue drug in the body. Equation 11.13 may be expanded to include several tissue organs with V_{ti} each with unbound tissue fraction f_{uti}.

$$V_{app} = V_p + \sum V_{ti}[f_u/f_{uti}] \qquad \textbf{(11.14)}$$

where, V_{ti} = tissue volume of the ith organ and f_{uti} = unbound fraction of the ith organ.

The following are important considerations in the calculation of V_{app}:

1. The volume of distribution is a constant only when the drug concentrations are in equilibrium between the plasma and tissue.
2. Values of $= f_u$ and $= f_{ut}$ are concentration dependent and must be determined also at equilibrium conditions.
3. Equation 11.13 shows that V_{app} is an indirect measure of drug binding in the tissues rather than a measurement of a true anatomical volume.
4. When $= f_u$ and $= f_{ut}$ are both unity, Equation 11.13 is simplified to

$$D_B/C_p = V_p + V_t \qquad \textbf{(11.15)}$$

When no drug binding occurs in tissue and plasma, the volume of distribution will not exceed the real anatomical volume. Only at equilibrium, does the free drug concentration $C_p = C_t$. At other time points, C_p is not equal to C_t. The value of D_B cannot be calculated easily from V_{app} and C_p under nonequilibrium conditions.

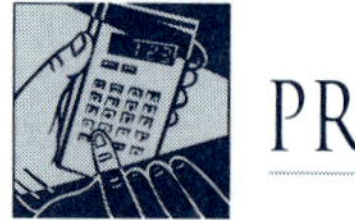

PRACTICE PROBLEM

Two drugs, *A* and *B*, have a V_{app} of 20 and 100 L, respectively. Both drugs have a V_p of 4 L and a V_t of 10 L, and they are 60% bound to plasma protein. What is the fraction of tissue binding of the two drugs? Assume that V_p is 4 L and V_t is 10 L.

Solution

Drug A

Applying Equation 11.13

$$V_{app} = V_p + V_t[f_u/f_{ut}]$$

Because drug A is 60% bound, then the drug is 40% free, or $f_u = 0.4$.

$$20 = 4 + 10(0.4/f_{ut})$$

$$f_{ut} = \frac{4}{16} = 0.25$$

The fraction of drug bound to tissues is $1 - 0.25 = 0.75$ or 75%.

Drug B

$$100 = 4 + 10(0.4/f_{ut})$$

$$f_{ut} = 0.042$$

The fraction of drug bound to tissues is $1 - 0.042 = 0.958 = 95.8\%$.

The percent drug free (unbound) for drug A is 25% and the percent free for drug B is 4.2% in plasma fluid. Drug B is more highly bound to tissue, which results in a larger apparent volume of distribution. This approach assumes a pooled tissue group because it is not possible to physically identify the tissue group to which the drug is bound.

Equation 11.13 may explain the wide variation in the apparent volumes of distribution for drugs observed in the literature (Table 11.4 to Table 11.6). Drugs in Table 11.4 have small apparent volumes of distribution due to plasma drug binding (less than 10 L when extrapolated to a 70-kg subject). Drugs in Table 11.5 show that in general, as the fraction of unbound drug, f_u, in the plasma increases, the apparent volume is increased. Reduced drug binding in the plasma results in an increased free drug concentration which diffuses into the extracellular water. Drugs showing exceptionally large volumes of distribution may have unusual tissue binding. Some drugs move into the interstitial fluid but are unable to diffuse across the cell membrane into the intracellular fluids, thereby reducing the volume of distribution.

Drugs in Table 11.6 apparently do not obey the general binding rule, because their volumes of distribution are not related to plasma drug binding. These drugs have very large volumes of distribution and may have undiscovered tissue binding or tissue metabolism. Based on their pharmacologic activities, presumably all of these drugs penetrate into the intracellular space.

Relationship of Plasma Drug–Protein Binding to Distribution and Elimination

The relationship of reversible drug–protein binding in the plasma and drug distribution and elimination is shown in Figure 11-13. A decrease in protein binding

TABLE 11.4 Relationship Between Affinity for Serum Albumin and the Volume of Distribution for Some Acidic Drugs

DRUG	PLASMA FRACTION BOUND (%)	AFFINITY CONSTANT (M^{-1})	V_D (L/kg)
Clofibric acid	97	300,000	0.09
Fluorophenindione	95	3,000,000	0.09
Phenylbutazone	99	230,000	0.09
Warfarin	97	230,000	0.13

From Houin (1985), with permission.

TABLE 11.5 Examples of Drugs Where Diffusion Is Limited by Binding to Protein

DRUG	PLASMA FRACTION UNBOUND (%)	V_D (L/kg)
Carbenoxolone	1	0.10
Ibuprofen	1	0.14
Phenylbutazone	1	0.10
Naproxen	2	0.09
Fusidic acid	3	0.15
Clofibrate	3	0.09
Warfarin	3	0.10
Bumetanide	4	0.18
Dicloxacillin	4	0.29
Furosemide	4	0.20
Tolbutamide	4	0.14
Nalidixic acid	5	0.35
Cloxacillin	5	0.34
Sulfaphenazole	5	0.29
Chlorpropramide	8	0.20
Oxacillin	8	0.44
Nafcillin	10	0.63

From Houin (1985), with permission.

that results in free drug concentration will allow more drug to cross cell membranes and distribute into all tissues. More drug will therefore be available to interact at a receptor site to produce a more intense pharmacologic effect. Furthermore, more drug will be available to those tissues involved in drug elimination, including the liver and kidney.

The elimination half-lives of some drugs like the cephalosporins, which are excreted mainly by renal excretion, are generally increased when the percent of drug bound to plasma increases (Table 11.7). Protein-bound drug acts as larger molecules that cannot easily diffuse through the capillary membranes in the glomeruli. Some cephalosporins are excreted by both renal and biliary secretion. The half-lives of drugs that are significantly excreted in the bile do not correlate well with the extent of plasma protein binding. For a drug metabolized mainly by the liver, binding to plasma proteins prevents the drug from entering the hepatocytes, resulting in reduced drug metabolism by the liver. In addition, molecularly bound drugs may not be available as a substrate for liver enzymes, thereby further reducing the rate of metabolism. In general, drugs that are highly bound to plasma protein have reduced overall drug clearance. When some drugs with different fractions

TABLE 11.6 Examples of Drugs for Which Tissue Distribution Is Apparently Independent of Plasma Protein Binding

DRUG	PLASMA FRACTION BOUND (%)	V_D (L/kg)
Desipramine	92	40
Imipramine	95	30
Nortriptyline	94	39
Vinblastine	70	35
Vincristine	70	11

From Houin (1985), with permission.

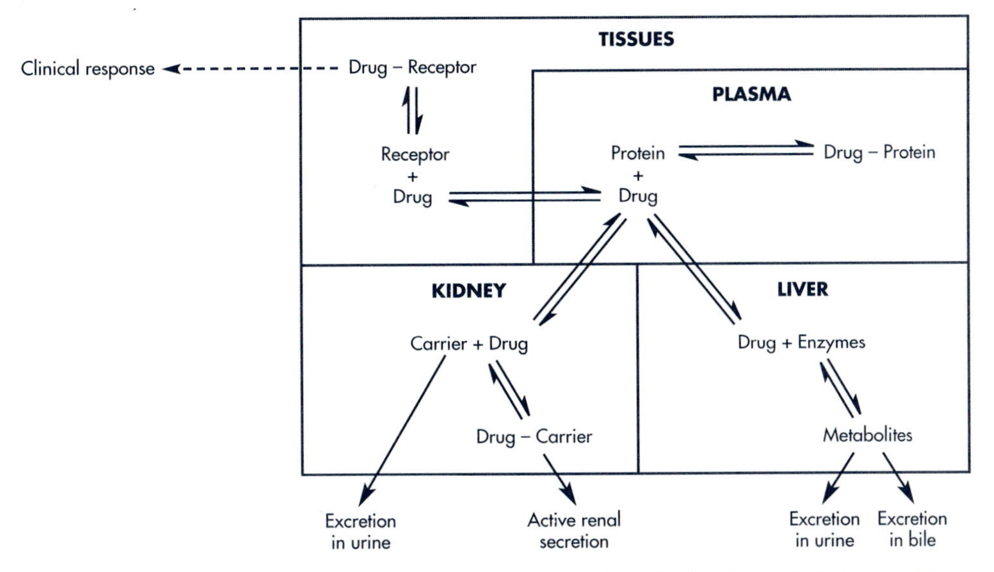

Figure 11-13. Effect of reversible drug–protein binding on drug distribution and elimination. Drugs may reversibly bind with proteins. Free (nonbound) drugs penetrate cell membranes distributing into various tissues including those tissues involved in drug elimination, such as kidney and liver. Active renal secretion, which is a carrier-mediated system, may have a greater affinity for free-drug molecules compared to the plasma protein. In this case, active renal drug excretion allows for rapid drug excretion despite drug protein binding. If a drug is displaced from the plasma proteins, more free drug is available for distribution into tissues and interaction with the receptors responsible for the pharmacologic response. Moreover, more free drug is available for drug elimination.

of plasma protein binding are examined, the expected reduction in clearance is sometimes absent or very minor because some drugs are nonrestrictively cleared (p. 386, Chapter 13).

PROTEIN BINDING OF DRUGS

Many drugs interact with plasma or tissue proteins or with other macromolecules, such as melanin and DNA, to form a drug–macromolecule complex. The forma-

TABLE 11.7 Influence of Protein Binding on the Pharmacokinetics of Primarily Glomerular Filtrated Cephalosporins

	PROTEIN BOUND (%)	$t_{1/2}$ (hr)	RENAL CLEARANCE (mL/min/1.73 m^2)
Ceftriaxone	96	8.0	10
Cefoperazone	90	1.8	19
Cefotetan	85	3.3	28
Ceforanide	81	3.0	44
Cefazolin	70	1.7	56
Moxalactam	52	2.3	64
Cefsulodin	26	1.5	90
Ceftazidime	22	1.9	85
Cephaloridine	21	1.5	125

From Houin (1985), with permission.

tion of a drug protein complex is often named *drug–protein binding.* Drug–protein binding may be a reversible or an irreversible process. *Irreversible drug–protein binding* is usually a result of chemical activation of the drug, which then attaches strongly to the protein or macromolecule by covalent chemical bonding. Irreversible drug binding accounts for certain types of drug toxicity that may occur over a long time period, as in the case of chemical carcinogenesis, or within a relatively short time period, as in the case of drugs that form reactive chemical intermediates. For example, the hepatotoxicity of high doses of acetaminophen is due to the formation of reactive metabolite intermediates which interact with liver proteins.

Most drugs bind or complex with proteins by a reversible process. *Reversible drug–protein binding* implies that the drug binds the protein with weaker chemical bonds, such as hydrogen bonds or van der Waals forces. The amino acids that compose the protein chain have hydroxyl, carboxyl, or other sites available for reversible drug interactions.

Drugs may bind to various macromolecular components in the blood including albumin, α_1-acid glycoprotein, lipoproteins, immunoglobulins (IgG), and erythrocytes (RBC). *Albumin* is a protein synthesized by the liver with a molecular weight of 65,000 to 69,000 d. Albumin is the major component of plasma proteins responsible for reversible drug binding (Table 11.8). In the body, albumin is distributed in the plasma and in the extracellular fluids of skin, muscle, and various other tissues. Interstitial fluid albumin concentration is about 60% of that in the plasma. The elimination half-life of albumin is 17 to 18 days. Normally, albumin concentration is maintained at a relatively constant level of 3.5% to 5.5% (weight per volume) or 4.5 mg/dL. Albumin is responsible for maintaining osmotic pressure of the blood and for the transport of endogenous and exogenous substances. As a transport protein for endogenous substances, albumin complexes with free fatty acids (FFA), bilirubin, various hormones (such as cortisone, aldosterone, and thyroxine), tryptophan, and other compounds. Many weak acidic (anionic) drugs bind to albumin by electrostatic and hydrophobic bonds. Weak acidic drugs such as salicylates, phenylbutazone, and penicillins are highly bound to albumin. However, the strength of the drug binding is different for each drug.

α_1-acid glycoprotein (orosomucoid) is a globulin with a molecular weight of about 44,000 d. The plasma concentration of α_1-acid glycoprotein is low (0.4 to 1%) and binds primarily basic (cationic) drugs such as propranolol, imipramine, and lidocaine. *Globulins* (α, β, γ globulins) may be responsible for the transport of certain endogenous substances such as corticosteroids. These globulins have a low capacity but high affinity for the binding of these endogenous substances.

TABLE 11.8 Major Proteins to Which Drugs Bind in Plasma

		NORMAL RANGE OF CONCENTRATIONS	
PROTEIN	**MOLECULAR WEIGHT (D)**	**(g/L)**	**(mol/L)**
Albumin	65,000	35–50	$5\text{–}7.5 \times 10^{-4}$
α_1-Acid glycoprotein	44,000	0.4–1.0	$0.9\text{–}2.2 \times 10^{-5}$
Lipoproteins	200,000–3,400,000	Variable	

From Tozer (1984), with permission.

TABLE 11.9 Methods for Studying Drug–Protein Binding

• Equilibrium dialysis	• Gel chromatography
• Dynamic dialysis	• Spectrophotometry
• Diafiltration	• Electrophoresis
• Ultrafiltration	• Optical rotatory dispersion and circulatory dichroism

Lipoproteins are macromolecular complexes of lipids and proteins and are classified according to their density and separation in the ultracentrifuge. The terms VLDL, LDL, and HDL are abbreviations for *very-low-density, low-density,* and *high-density lipoproteins,* respectively. Lipoproteins are responsible for the transport of plasma lipids and may be responsible for the binding of drugs if the albumin sites become saturated.

Erythrocytes, or red blood cells (RBCs), may bind both endogenous and exogenous compounds. RBCs consist of about 45% of the volume of the blood. Phenytoin, pentobarbital, and amobarbital are known to have RBC/plasma water ratio of 4 to 2, indicating preferential binding of drug to the erythrocytes over plasma water. Penetration into RBC is dependent on the free concentration of the drug. In the case of phenytoin, RBC drug level increases linearly with an increase in the plasma-free drug concentration (Borondy et al, 1973). Increased drug binding to plasma albumin reduced RBC drug concentration. With most drugs, however, binding of drug to RBC generally does not significantly affect the volume of distribution, because the drug is often bound to albumin in the plasma water. Even though the phenytoin has a great affinity for RBC, only about 25% of the blood drug concentration is present in the blood cells, and 75% is present in the plasma because the drug is also strongly bound to albumin. For drugs with strong erythrocyte binding, the hematocrit will influence the total amount of drug in the blood. For these drugs, the total whole blood drug concentration should be measured.

Reversible drug–protein binding is of major interest in pharmacokinetics. The protein-bound drug is a large complex that cannot easily cross cell membranes and therefore has a restricted distribution. Moreover, the protein-bound drug is usually pharmacologically inactive. In contrast, the free or unbound drug crosses cell membranes and is therapeutically active. Studies that critically evaluate drug–protein binding are usually performed in vitro using a purified protein such as albumin. Methods for studying protein binding, including equilibrium dialysis and ultrafiltration, make use of a semipermeable membrane that separates the protein and protein-bound drug from the free or unbound drug (Table 11.9). By these methods, the concentrations of bound drug, free drug, and total protein may be determined.

Each method for the investigation of drug–protein binding *in vitro* has advantages and disadvantages in terms of cost, ease of measurement, time, instrumentation, and other considerations. Various experimental factors for the measurement of protein binding are listed in Table 11.10. Drug–protein binding kinetics yield valuable information concerning proper therapeutic use of the drug and predictions of possible drug interactions.

Drug–protein binding is influenced by a number of important factors, including the following:

1. The drug
   Physicochemical properties of the drug.
   Total concentration of the drug in the body.

TABLE 11.10 Considerations in the Study of Drug–Protein Binding

- Equilibrium between bound and free drug must be maintained.
- The method must be valid over a wide range of drug and protein concentrations.
- Extraneous drug binding or drug adsorption onto the apparatus walls, membranes, or other components must be avoided or considered in the method.
- Denaturation of the protein or contamination of the protein must be prevented.
- The method must consider pH and ionic concentrations of the media and Donnan effects due to the protein.
- The method should be capable of detecting both reversible and irreversible drug binding, including fast- and slow-phase associations and dissociations of drug and protein.
- The method should not introduce interfering substances, such as organic solvents.
- The results of the *in vitro* method should allow extrapolation to the *in vivo* situation.

Adapted with permission from Bridges and Wilson (1976).

2. The protein
   Quantity of protein available for drug–protein binding.
   Quality or physicochemical nature of the protein synthesized.
3. The affinity between drug and protein
   Includes the magnitude of the association constant.
4. Drug interactions
   Competition for the drug by other substances at a protein-binding site.
   Alteration of the protein by a substance that modifies the affinity of the drug for the protein; for example, aspirin acetylates lysine residues of albumin.
5. The pathophysiologic condition of the patient
   For example, drug–protein binding may be reduced in uremic patients and in patients with hepatic disease.

Plasma drug concentrations are generally reported as the total drug concentration in the plasma, including both protein-bound drug and unbound (free) drug concentrations. Most literature values for the therapeutic effective drug concentrations refer to the total plasma or serum drug concentration. For therapeutic drug monitoring, the total plasma drug concentrations are generally used in the development of the appropriate drug dosage regimen for the patient. In the past, measurement of free drug concentration was not routinely performed in the laboratory. More recently, free drug concentrations may be measured quickly using ultrafiltration. Because of the high plasma protein binding of phenytoin and the narrow therapeutic index of the drug, more hospital laboratories are measuring both free and total phenytoin plasma levels.

KINETICS OF PROTEIN BINDING

The kinetics of reversible drug–protein binding for a protein with one simple binding site can be described by the *law of mass action*, as follows:

$$\text{Protein} + \text{drug} \rightleftarrows \text{drug–protein–complex}$$

or

$$(\text{P}) + (\text{D}) \rightleftarrows (\text{PD}) \quad \textbf{(11.16)}$$

From Equation 11.16 and the law of mass action, an association constant, K_a, can be expressed as the ratio of the molar concentration of the products and the molar concentration of the reactants. This equation assumes only one-binding site per protein molecule.

$$K_a = \frac{(PD)}{(P)(D)} \tag{11.17}$$

The extent of the drug–protein complex formed is dependent on the association binding constant K_a. The magnitude of K_a yields information on the degree of drug protein binding. Drugs strongly bound to protein have a very large K_a and exist mostly as the drug–protein complex. With such drugs, a large dose may be needed to obtain a reasonable therapeutic concentration of free drug.

Most kinetic studies *in vitro* use purified albumin as a standard protein source, because this protein is responsible for the major portion of plasma drug–protein binding. Experimentally, both the free drug (D) and the protein-bound drug (PD), as well as the total protein concentration $(P) + (PD)$, may be determined. To study the binding behavior of drugs, a determinable ratio r is defined, as follows:

$$r = \frac{\text{moles of drug bound}}{\text{total moles of protein}}$$

Because moles of drug bound is (PD) and the total moles of protein is $(P) + (PD)$, this equation becomes:

$$r = \frac{(PD)}{(PD) + (P)} \tag{11.18}$$

According to Equation 11.17, $(PD) = K_a(P)(D)$; by substitution into Equation 11.18, the following expression is obtained:

$$r = \frac{K_a(P)(D)}{K_a(P)(D) + (P)}$$

$$r = \frac{K_a(D)}{1 + K_a(D)}$$

This equation describes the simplest situation, in which 1 mole of drug binds to 1 mole of protein in a 1:1 complex. This case assumes only one independent binding site for each molecule of drug. If there are n identical independent binding sites per protein molecule, then the following is used:

$$r = \frac{nK_a(D)}{1 + K_a(D)} \tag{11.20}$$

Protein molecules are quite large compared to drug molecules and may contain more than one type of binding site for the drug. If there is more than one type of binding site and the drug binds independently on each binding site with its own association constant, then Equation 11.20 expands to the following:

$$r = \frac{n_1K_1(D)}{1 + K_1(D)} + \frac{n_2K_2(D)}{1 + K_2(D)} + \cdots \tag{11.21}$$

where the numerical subscripts represent different types of binding sites, the *K*s represent the binding constants, and the *n*s represent the number of binding sites per molecule of albumin.

These equations assume that each drug molecule binds to the protein at an independent binding site, and the affinity of a drug for one binding site does not influence binding to other sites. In reality, drug–protein binding sometimes exhibits a phenomenon of *cooperativity*. For these drugs, the binding of the first drug molecule at one site on the protein molecule influences the successive binding of other drug molecules. The binding of oxygen to hemoglobin is an example of drug cooperativity.

In terms of K_d, which is $1/K_a$, the Equation 11.20 reduces to:

$$r = \frac{n(D)}{K_d + (D)} \tag{11.22}$$

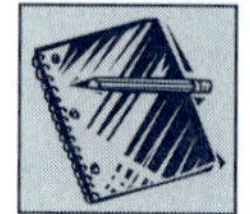

PRACTICAL FOCUS

1. How is r related to the fraction of drug bound (f_u), a term that is often of clinical interest?

Solution

r is the *ratio of number of moles of drug bound/number of moles of albumin.* r determines the extent to which the binding sites in albumin (or another protein) are occupied by the drug and the saturation drug concentration. f_u is based on the total concentration of drug and is used to determine the free drug concentration from total plasma level. The value of f_u is often assumed to be fixed. However, f_u may change, especially with drugs that have therapeutic levels close to the *Kd.* (See examples on diazoxide.)

2. At maximum binding, the number of binding sites is n (see Eq 11.22). The drug disopyramide has a $K_d = 1 \times 10^{-6}$ M/L. How close to saturation is the drug when the free drug concentration is 1×10^{-6} M/L?

Solution

Substitution for $D = 1 \times 10^{-6}$ M/L and $K_d = 1 \times 10^{-6}$ M/L in Equation 11.22 gives:

$$r = \frac{n}{2}$$

When $n = 1$ and the unbound (free) drug concentration equals to K_d, the protein binding of the drug is half saturated. Interestingly, when (D) is much greater than K_d, K_d is negligible in Equation 11.22, and $r = n$, (ie, r is independent of concentration or fully saturated).

When $K_d > (D)$, (D) is negligible in the denominator of Equation 11.22, and r is dependent on n/K_d (D), or nK_a (D). In this case, the dissociation constant, K_d is greater than the drug concentration, (D), the number of sites bound is directly proportionally to the number of binding sites, the association binding constant (also called affinity constant), and the free drug concentration. This relationship also explains why a drug with a higher K_a may not necessarily have a higher percent of drug bound since the number of binding sites n may be different from one drug to another.

DETERMINATION OF BINDING CONSTANTS AND BINDING SITES BY GRAPHIC METHODS

In Vitro Methods (Known Protein Concentration)

A plot of the ratio r (moles of drug bound per mole of protein) versus free drug concentration (D) is shown in Figure 11-14. Equation 11.20 shows that as free drug concentration increases, the number of moles of drug bound per mole of protein becomes saturated and plateaus. Thus, drug protein binding resembles a Langmuir adsorption isotherm, which is also similar to adsorption of a drug to an adsorbent becoming saturated as the drug concentration increases. Due to nonlinearity in drug–protein binding, Equation 11.20 is rearranged for the estimation of n and K_a, using various graphical methods as discussed in the next section.

The values for the association constants and the number of binding sites are obtained by various graphic methods. The reciprocal of Equation 11.20 gives the following equation:

$$\frac{1}{r} = \frac{1 + K_a(D)}{nK_a(D)} \tag{11.23}$$

$$\frac{1}{r} = \frac{1}{nK_a(D)} + \frac{1}{n}$$

A graph of $1/r$ versus $1/(D)$ is called a *double reciprocal plot*. The y intercept is $1/n$ and the slope is $1/nK_a$. From this graph (Fig. 11-15), the number of binding sites may be determined from the y intercept, and the association constant may be determined from the slope, if the value for n is known.

If the graph of $1/r$ versus $1/(D)$ does not yield a straight line, then the drug–protein binding process is probably more complex. Equation 11.20 assumes one type

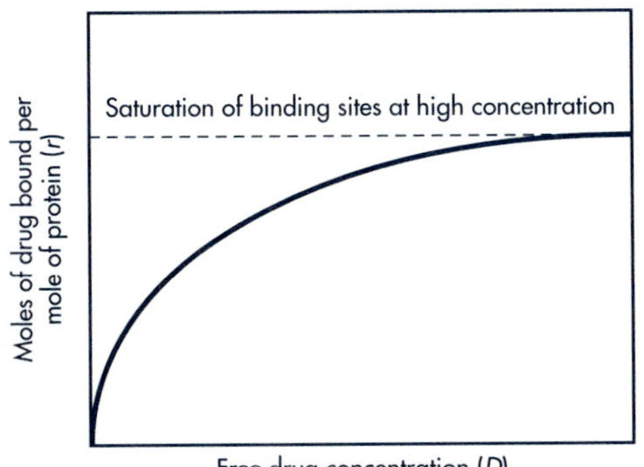

Figure 11-14. Graphical representation of Equation 11.15, showing saturation of protein at high drug concentrations.

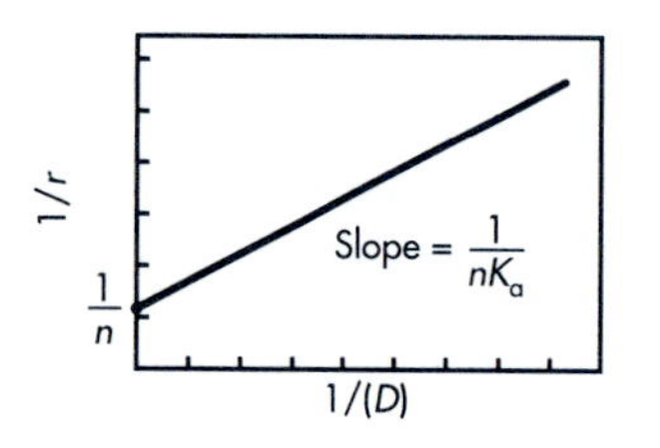

Figure 11-15. Hypothetical binding of drug to protein. The line was obtained with the double reciprocal equation.

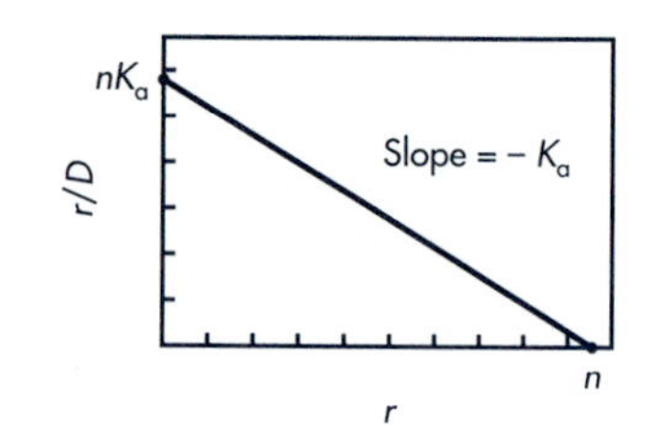

Figure 11-16. Hypothetical binding of drug to protein. The line was obtained with the Scatchard equation.

of binding site and no interaction among the binding sites. Frequently, Equation 11.23 is used to estimate the number of binding sites and binding constants, using computerized iteration methods.

Another graphic technique called the *Scatchard plot* is a rearrangement of Equation 11.20. The Scatchard plot spreads the data to give a better line for the estimation of the binding constants and binding sites. From Equation 11.20 we obtain:

$$r = \frac{nK_a(D)}{1 + K_a(D)} \tag{11.24}$$

$$r + rK_a(D) = nK_a(D)$$

$$r = nK_a(D) - rK_a(D)$$

$$\frac{r}{(D)} = nK_a - rK_a$$

A graph constructed by plotting $r/(D)$ versus r yields a straight line with the intercepts and slope shown in Figures 11-16 and 11-17.

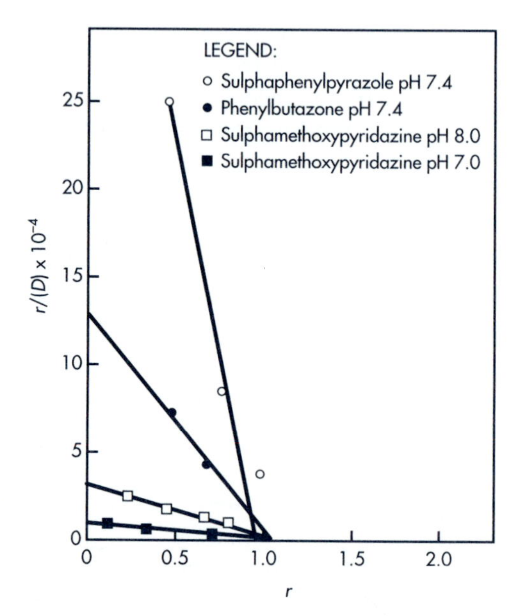

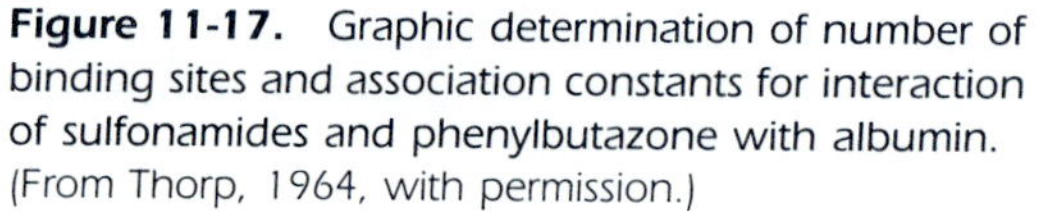
Figure 11-17. Graphic determination of number of binding sites and association constants for interaction of sulfonamides and phenylbutazone with albumin. (From Thorp, 1964, with permission.)

Some drug–protein binding data produce Scatchard graphs of curvilinear lines (Figs. 11-18 and 11-19). The curvilinear line represents the summation of two straight lines that collectively form the curve. The binding of salicylic acid to albumin is an example of this type of drug–protein binding in which there are at least two different, independent binding sites (n_1 and n_2), each with its own independent association constant (k_1 and k_2). Equation 11.21 best describes this type of drug–protein interaction.

In Vivo Methods (Unknown Protein Concentration)

Reciprocal and Scatchard plots cannot be used if the exact nature and amount of protein in the experimental system is unknown. The percent of drug bound is often used to describe the extent of drug–protein binding in the plasma. The fraction of drug bound, β, can be determined experimentally and is equal to the ratio of the concentration of bound drug, D_β, and the total drug concentration of, D_T, in the plasma, as follows:

$$\beta = \frac{D_\beta}{D_T} \tag{11.25}$$

The value of the association constant can be determined, even though the nature of the plasma proteins binding the drug is unknown, by rearranging Equation 11.25 into Equation 11.26:

$$r = \frac{D_\beta}{P_T} = \frac{nK_a(D)}{1 + K_a(D)} \tag{11.26}$$

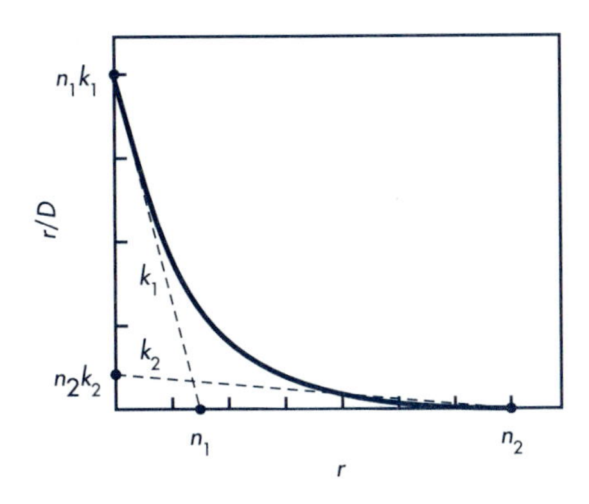

Figure 11-18. Hypothetical binding of drug to protein. The *k*s represent independent binding constants and the *n*s represent the number of binding sites per molecule of protein.

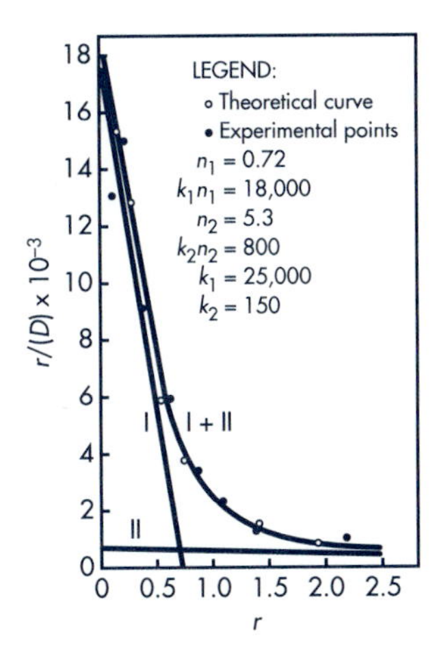

Figure 11-19. Binding curves for salicylic acid to crystalline bovine serum albumin. Curve I, plot for one class, $n_1 = 0.72$, $k_1 = 25{,}000$. Curve II, plot for second class, $n_2 = 5.3$, $k_2 = 150$. Curve I + II, plot for both binding sites, sum of the above.
(From Davison, 1971, with permission.)

where D_β is the bound drug concentration; D is the free drug concentration; and P_T is the total protein concentration. Rearrangement of this equation gives the following expression, which is analogous to the Scatchard equation:

$$\frac{D_\beta}{(D)} = nK_aP_T - K_aD_\beta \quad \textbf{(11.27)}$$

Concentrations of both free and bound drug may be found experimentally, and a graph obtained by plotting $D_\beta/(D)$ versus D_β will yield a straight line from which the slope is the association constant K_a. Equation 11.27 shows that the ratio of bound C_p to free C_p is influenced by the affinity constant, the protein concentration, P_T, which may change during disease states and with the drug concentration in the body.

The values for n and K_a give a general estimate of the affinity and binding capacity of the drug, as plasma contains a complex mixture of proteins. The drug–protein binding in plasma may be influenced by competing substances such as ions, free fatty acids, drug metabolites, and other drugs. Measurements of drug–protein binding should be obtained over a wide drug concentration range, because at low drug concentrations a high-affinity, low-capacity binding site might be missed or, at a higher drug concentration, saturation of the protein-binding sites might occur.

Relationship Between Protein Concentration and Drug Concentration in Drug–Protein Binding

The drug concentration, the protein concentration, and the association (affinity) constant, K_a influence the fraction of drug bound (Eq. 11.25). At a constant protein concentration (which is normally the case), the fraction of drug bound will decrease with an increase in drug concentration (Fig. 11-20).

With a constant concentration of protein, only a certain number of binding sites are available for a drug. At low drug concentrations, most of the drug may be bound to the protein, whereas, at high drug concentrations, the protein-binding sites may become saturated, with a consequent rapid increase in the free drug concentrations.

To demonstrate the relationship of the drug concentration, protein concentration, and K_a, the following expression can be derived from Equations 11.25 and 11.26.

$$\beta = \frac{1}{1 + \dfrac{(D)}{nP_T} + \dfrac{1}{nK_aP_T}} \quad \textbf{(11.28)}$$

From Equation 11.28, both the free drug concentration, (D), and the total protein concentration, P_T, will have important effects on the fraction of drug bound. Any factors that suddenly increase the fraction of free drug concentration in the plasma will cause a change in the pharmacokinetics of the drug.

Because protein binding is nonlinear in most cases, the percent of drug bound is dependent on the concentrations of both the drug and proteins in the plasma. In disease situations, the concentration of protein may vary, thus affecting the percent of drug bound. The effect of protein concentration is demonstrated in Figure 11-21. As the protein concentration increases, the percent of drug bound increases to a maximum. The shapes of the curves are determined by the association constant of the drug–protein complex and the drug concentration.

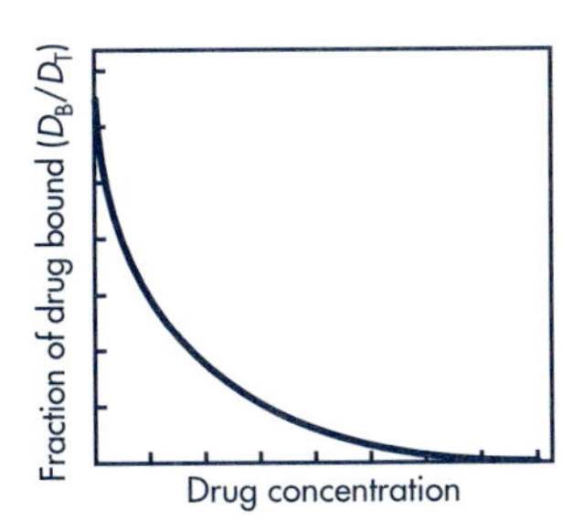

Figure 11-20. Fraction of drug bound versus drug concentration at constant protein concentration.

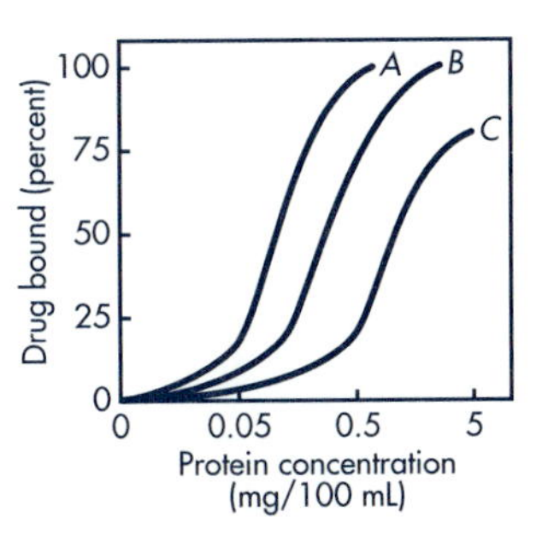

Figure 11-21. Effect of protein concentration on the percentage of drug bound. A, B, and C represent hypothetical drugs with respectively decreasing binding affinity.

CLINICAL SIGNIFICANCE OF DRUG–PROTEIN BINDING

Most drugs bind reversibly to plasma proteins to some extent. When the clinical significance of the fraction of drug bound is considered, it is important to know whether the study was performed using pharmacologic or therapeutic plasma drug concentrations. As mentioned previously, the fraction of drug bound can change with plasma drug concentration and dose of drug administered. In addition, the patient's plasma protein concentration should be considered. If a patient has a low plasma protein concentration, then, for any given dose of drug, the concentration of free (unbound) bioactive drug may be higher than anticipated. The plasma protein concentration is controlled by a number of variables, including (1) protein synthesis, (2) protein catabolism, (3) distribution of albumin between intravascular and extravascular space, and (4) excessive elimination of plasma protein, particularly albumin. A number of diseases, age, trauma, and related circumstances affect the plasma protein concentration (Tables 11.11 to 11.13).

For example, liver disease results in a decrease in plasma albumin concentration due to decreased protein synthesis. In nephrotic syndrome, an accumulation of waste metabolites, such as urea and uric acid, as well as an accumulation of drug metabolites, may alter protein binding of drugs. Severe burns may cause an increased distribution of albumin into the extracellular fluid, resulting in a smaller plasma albumin concentration. In certain genetic diseases, the *quality* of the protein that is in the plasma synthesized may be altered due to a change in the amino acid sequence. Both chronic liver disease and renal disease, such as uremia, may cause an alteration in the quality of plasma protein synthesized. An alteration in the protein quality may be demonstrated by an alteration in the association constant or affinity of the drug for the protein.

TABLE 11.11 Factors That Decrease Plasma Protein Concentration

MECHANISM	DISEASE STATE
Decreased protein synthesis	Liver disease
Increased protein catabolism	Trauma, surgery
Distribution of albumin into extravascular space	Burns
Excessive elimination of protein	Renal disease

TABLE 11.12 Physiologic and Pathologic Conditions Altering Protein Concentrations in Plasma[a]

	ALBUMIN	α_1-GLYCOPROTEIN	LIPOPROTEIN
Decreasing	Age (geriatric, neonate)	Fetal concentrations	Hyperthyroidism
	Bacterial pneumonia	Nephrotic syndrome	Injury
	Burns	Oral contraceptives	Liver disease?
	Cirrhosis of liver		Trauma
	Cystic fibrosis		
	GI disease		
	Histoplasmosis		
	Leprosy		
	Liver abscess		
	Malignant neoplasms		
	Malnutrition (severe)		
	Multiple myeloma		
	Nephrotic syndrome		
	Pancreatitis (acute)		
	Pregnancy		
	Renal failure		
	Surgery		
	Trauma		
Increasing	Benign tumor	Age (geriatric)	Diabetes
	Exercise	Celiac disease	Hypothyroidism
	Hypothyroidism	Crohn's disease	Liver disease?
	Neurological disease?	Injury	Nephrotic syndrome
	Neurosis	Myocardial infarction	
	Paranoia	Renal failure	
	Psychosis	Rheumatoid arthritis	
	Schizophrenia	Stress	
		Surgery	
		Trauma	

[a] In the conditions listed, the protein concentrations are altered, on average, by 30% or more, and in some cases by more than 100%.

From Tozer (1984), with permission.

When a highly protein-bound drug is displaced from binding by a second drug or agent, a sharp increase in the free drug concentration in the plasma may occur, leading to toxicity. For example, an increase in free warfarin level was responsible for an increase in bleeding when warfarin was coadministered with phenylbutazone, which competes for the same protein-binding site (O'Reilly, 1973; Udall, 1970).

Albumin has two known binding sites that share the binding of many drugs (MacKichan, 1992). Binding site I is shared by phenylbutazone, sulfonamides, phenytoin, and valproic acid. Binding site II is shared by the semisynthetic penicillins, probenecid, medium chain fatty acids, and the benzodiazepines. Some drugs bind to both sites. *Displacement* occurs when a second drug is taken that competes for the same binding site in the protein as the initial drug. Although it is generally assumed that binding sites are preformed, there is some evidence pointing to the *allosteric* nature of protein binding. This means that the binding of a drug modifies the conformation of protein in such a way that the drug binding influences the nature of binding of further molecules of the drug. The binding of oxygen to hemoglobin is a well studied biochemical example in which the initial binding of

TABLE 11.13 Protein Binding in Normal (Norm) Renal Function, End-Stage Renal Disease (ESRD), During Hemodialysis (HD), and in Nephrotic Syndrome (NS)

	NORM (% BOUND)	ESRD (% BOUND)	HD (% BOUND)	NS (% BOUND)
Azlocillin	28	25		
Bilirubin		Decreased		
Captopril	24	18		
Cefazolin	84	73	22	
Cefoxitin	73	20		
Chloramphenicol	53	45	30	
Chlorpromazine	98	98		
Clofibrate	96		89	
Clonidine	30	30		
Congo red		Decreased		
Dapsone		Normal		
Desipramine	80	Normal		
N-desmethyldiazepam	98	94		
Desmethylimipramine	89	88		
Diazepam	99	94		
Diazoxide (30 μg/mL)	92	86	83	
(300 μg/mL)	77	72		
Dicloxacillin	96	91		
Diflunisal	88	56		39
Digitoxin	97	96	90	96
Digoxin	25		22	
Doxycycline	88	71		
Erythromycin	75	77		
Etomidate	75	57		
Fluorescein	86	Decreased		
Furosemid	96	94		93
Indomethacin		Normal		
Maprotiline	90	Normal		
β-methyldigoxin	30		19	
Methyl orange		Decreased		
Methyl red		Decreased		
Morphine	35	31		
Nafcillin	88	81		
Naproxen	75	21		
Oxazepam	95	88		
Papaverine	97	94		
Penicillin G	72	36		
Pentobarbital	66	59		
Phenobarbital	55	Decreased		
Phenol red		Decreased		
Phenylbutazone	97	88		
Phenytoin	90	80	93	81
Pindolol	41	Normal		
Prazosin	95	92		
Prednisolone (50 mg)	74		65	64
(15 mg)	87	88		85
D-propoxyphene	76	80		
Propranolol	88	89	90	
Quinidine	88	86	88	
Salicylate	94	85		
Sulfadiazine		Decreased		
Sulfamethoxazole	74	50		
Sulfonamides		Decreased		

(*continued*)

TABLE 11.13 Protein Binding in Normal (Norm) Renal Function, End-Stage Renal Disease (ESRD), During Hemodialysis (HD), and in Nephrotic Syndrome (NS) *(Continued)*

	NORM (% BOUND)	ESRD (% BOUND)	HD (% BOUND)	NS (% BOUND)
Strophantin	1		2	
Theophylline	60	Decreased		
Thiopental	72	44		
Thyroxine		Decreased		
Triamterene	81	61		
Trimethoprim	70	68		70
Tryptophan	75	Decreased		
D-tubocurarine	44	41		
Valproic acid	85	Decreased		
Verapamil	90	Normal		
Warfarin	99	98		

From Keller et al (1984), with permission.

other oxygen to the iron in the heme portion influences the binding of other oxygen molecules.

A less understood aspect of protein binding is the effect of binding on the intensity and pharmacodynamics of the drug after intravenous administration. Rapid IV injection may increase the free drug concentration of some highly protein-bound drugs and therefore increase its intensity of action. Sellers and Koch-Weser (1973) reported a dramatic increase in hypotensive effect when diazoxide was injected rapidly IV in 10 seconds versus a slower injection of 100 seconds. Diazoxide was 9.1 and 20.6% free when the serum levels were 20 and 100 $\mu g/mL$, respectively. Figure 11-22 shows a transient high free diazoxide concentration, which resulted after a rapid IV injection causing maximum arterial dilation and hypotensive effect due to initial saturation of the protein-binding sites. In contrast, when dia-

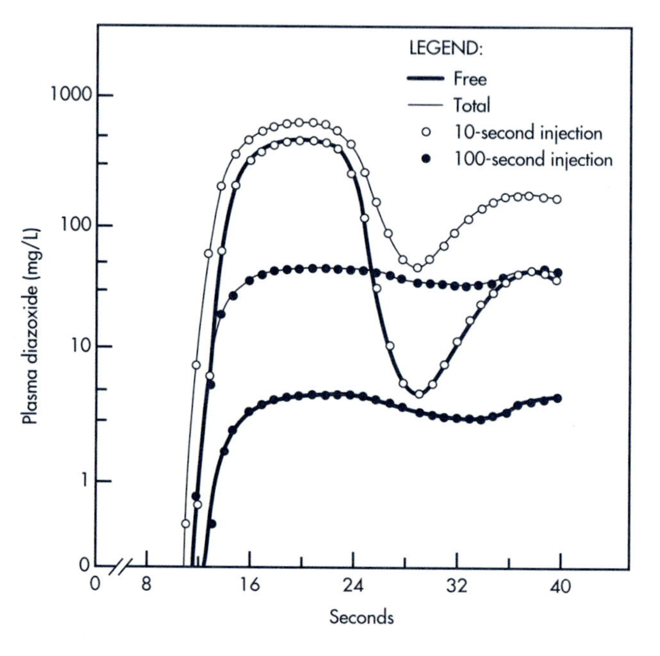

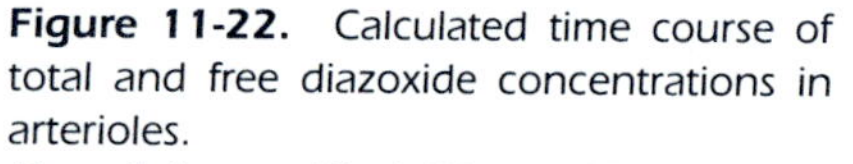

Figure 11-22. Calculated time course of total and free diazoxide concentrations in arterioles.
(From Sellers and Koch-Weser, 1973, with permission.)

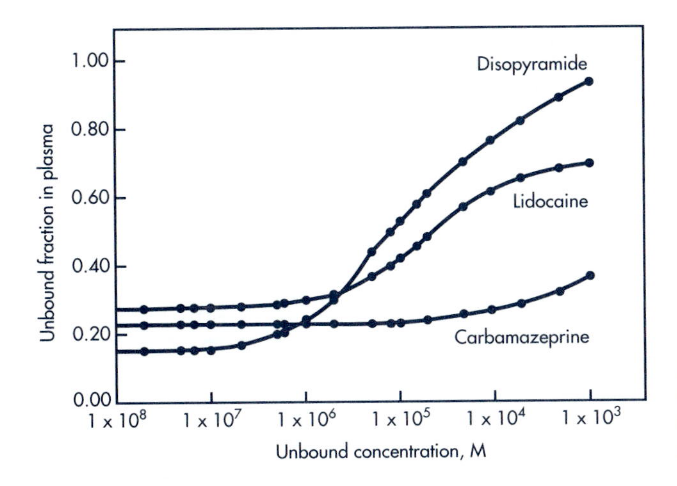

Figure 11-23. Simulation showing changes in fraction of free (unbound) drug over various molar drug concentrations for three drugs with protein binding.

zoxide was injected more slowly over 100 seconds, free diazoxide serum level was low, due to binding and drug distribution. The slower injection of diazoxide produced a smaller fall in blood pressure, even though the total drug dose injected was the same. Although most drugs have linear binding at therapeutic dose, in some patients, free drug concentration can increase rapidly with rising drug concentration as binding sites become saturated. An example is illustrated in Figure 11-23 for lidocaine (MacKichan, 1991).

The nature of drug–drug and drug–metabolite interactions is also important in drug–protein binding. In this case, one drug may displace a second bound drug from the protein, causing a sudden increase in pharmacologic response due to an increase in free drug concentration.

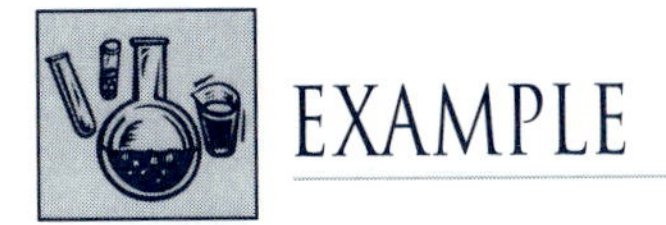

EXAMPLE

Compare the percent of change in free drug concentration when two drugs, *A* (95% bound) and *B* (50% bound), are displaced by 5% from their respective binding sites by the administration of another drug (Table 11.14). For a highly bound drug *A*, a displacement of 5% of free drug is actually a 100% increase in free drug level. For a weakly bound drug like drug *B*, a change of 5% in free concentration due to displacement would only cause a 10% increase in free drug level over the initially high (50%) free drug concentration. For a patient medicated with drug *B*, a 10% increase in free drug level would probably not affect the therapeutic outcome. However, a 100% increase in active drug, as occurs with drug *A*, may be toxic. Although this example is based on one drug displacing another drug, nutrients, physiologic products, and the waste products of metabolism may cause displacement from binding in a similar manner.

As illustrated by this example, displacement is most important with drugs that are more than 95% bound and have a narrow therapeutic index. Under normal circumstances, only a small proportion of the total drug is active. Consequently, a

TABLE 11.14 Comparison of Effects of 5% Displacement from Binding on Two Hypothetical Drugs

	BEFORE DISPLACEMENT	AFTER DISPLACEMENT	PERCENT INCREASE IN FREE DRUG
Drug *A*			
Percent drug bound	95	90	
Percent drug free	5	10	+100
Drug *B*			
Percent drug bound	50	45	
Percent drug free	50	55	+10

small displacement of bound drug causes a disproportionate increase in the free drug concentration, which may cause drug intoxication.

With drugs that are not as highly bound to plasma proteins, a small displacement from the protein causes a transient increase in the free drug concentration, which may cause a transient increase in pharmacologic activity. However, more free drug is available for both renal excretion and hepatic biotransformation, which may be demonstrated by a transient decreased elimination half-life. Drug displacement from protein by a second drug can occur by competition of the second drug for similar binding sites. Moreover, any alteration of the protein structure may also change the capacity of the protein to bind drugs. For example, aspirin acetylates the lysine residue of albumin, which changes the binding capacity of this protein for certain other antiinflammatory drugs, such as phenylbutazone.

The displacement of endogenous substances from plasma proteins by drugs is usually of little consequence. Some hormones, such as thyroid and cortisol, are normally bound to specific plasma proteins. A small displacement of these hormones rarely causes problems because physiologic feedback control mechanisms take over. However, in infants, the displacement of bilirubin by drugs can cause mental retardation and even death due to the difficulty of bilirubin elimination in newborns.

Finally, the bindings of drugs to proteins can affect the duration of action of the drug. A drug that is extensively but reversibly bound to protein may have a long duration of action due to a depot effect of the drug–protein complex.

The effect of serum protein binding on the renal clearance and elimination half-life on several tetracycline analogs is shown in Table 11.15. For example, doxycycline, which is 93% bound to serum proteins, has an elimination half-life of 15.1

TABLE 11.15 Comparison of Serum Protein Binding of Several Tetracycline Analogs with Their Half-Life in Serum Renal Clearance and Urinary Recovery After Intravenous Injection

TETRACYCLINE ANALOGS	SERUM BINDING (%)	HALF-LIFE (hr)	RENAL CLEARANCE (mL/min)	URINARY RECOVERY (%)
Oxytetracycline	35.4	9.2	98.6	70
Tetracycline	64.6	8.5	73.5	60
Demeclocycline	90.8	12.7	36.5	45
Doxycycline	93.0	15.1	16.0	45

From Kunin CM et al (1973), with permission.

hours, whereas oxytetracycline, which is 35.4% bound to serum proteins, has an elimination half-life of 9.2 hours.

In contrast, a drug that is both extensively bound and actively secreted, such as penicillin, has a short elimination half-life, because active secretion takes preference in removing or stripping the drug from the proteins as the blood flows through the kidney.

Elimination of Protein-Bound Drug: Restrictive Versus Nonrestrictive Elimination

When a drug is tightly bound to a protein, only the unbound drug is assumed to be metabolized; drugs belonging to this category are described as restrictively eliminated. On the other hand, some drugs may be eliminated even when they are protein bound; drugs in this category are described as nonrestrictively eliminated. In practice, the molecular effect of protein binding on elimination is not always predictable. Drugs with restrictive elimination are recognized by very small plasma clearances and extensive plasma protein binding. The hepatic extraction ratios (ER) for drugs that are restrictively eliminated are generally small due to strong protein binding. Their hepatic extraction ratios are generally smaller than their unbound fractions in plasma, (ie, ER $< f_u$). For example, phenylbutazone, the oxicams, including piroxicam, isoxicam, and tenoxicam all have hepatic extraction ratios smaller than their unbound fraction in plasma (Verbeeck and Wallace, 1994). The hepatic elimination for these drugs is, therefore, restrictive. A series of nonsteroid antiinflammatory drugs (NSAIDs) were reported by the same authors to be nonrestrictive with the following characteristics: (1) drug elimination is exclusively hepatic, (2) bioavailability of the drug from an oral dosage form is complete and (3) these drugs do not undergo extensive reversible biotransformation or enterohepatic circulation.

Propranolol is a drug that has low bioavailability with a hepatic extraction ratio (ER) of 0.7 to 0.9. Propranolol is 89% bound, ie, 11% free (or $f_u = 0.11$) so that the ER $> f_u$. Thus, propranolol is considered to be nonrestrictively eliminated. The bioavailability of propranolol is very low because of the large first-pass effect and its elimination half-life is relatively short. In contrast, diazepam is 98% bound ($f_u =$ 0.02). Diazepam has a small ER of 0.1 due to extensive drug protein binding. Therefore, diazepam is considered to be restrictively eliminated. Diazepam has a long elimination half-life of 37 hours (Appendix E).

Effect of Displacement

Plasma binding drug displacement will lead to an increased apparent volume of distribution and an increased half-life, but clearance will remain unaffected. If administered by multiple doses, the mean steady state concentration will remain unchanged; however, the mean steady-state free drug level will be increased due to displacement. The therapeutic effect will therefore increase.

$$Cl = \frac{0.693\ V_D}{t_{1/2}}$$

In patients with ascites, the increase in clearance with no increase in half-life was a reflection of the increase in volume of distribution in patients with ascites (Stoeckel et al, 1983).

Tissue Drug Binding and Binding to Other Macromolecules

Most studies on the kinetics of drug–protein binding consider binding to plasma proteins. However, certain drugs may also bind specific tissue proteins or other macromolecules, such as melanin or DNA. As discussed earlier in this chapter, a high degree of tissue binding results in lower plasma drug levels and a larger apparent volume of distribution.

Studies on the binding of drugs to intracellular components *in vivo* are more difficult to perform. However, recent studies have shown that drugs may also be displaced from tissue binding sites. For example, digoxin, a cardiac glycoside, binds strongly to the myocardial tissue of the heart. If patients who are on digoxin take quinidine, steady-state digoxin plasma levels increase, possibly due to displacement of the tissue-bound digoxin (Reifell et al, 1979).

? FREQUENTLY ASKED QUESTIONS

1. Do all drugs that bind proteins lead to clinically significant interactions?
2. What macromolecules participate in drug protein binding?
3. How does drug protein binding affect drug elimination?
4. How does a physical property, such as partition coefficient, affect drug distribution?
5. What are the factors to consider when adjusting the drug dose for a patient whose plasma protein concentration decreases to half that of normal?
6. How does one distinguish between the distribution phase and the elimination phase after an IV injection of a drug?
7. What are the causes of a long distribution half-life for a body organ if blood flow to the tissue is rapid?
8. How long does it take for a tissue organ to be fully equilibrated with the plasma? How long for a tissue organ to be half equilibrated?
9. When a body organ is equilibrated with drug from the plasma, the drug concentration in that organ should be the same as that of the plasma. True or false?
10. What is the parameter that tells when half of the protein binding sites are occupied?

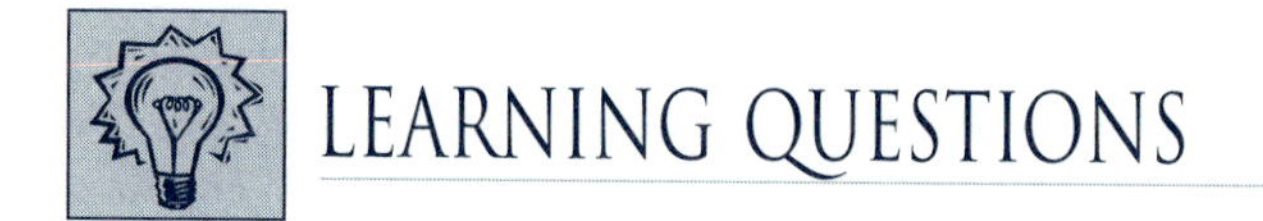

LEARNING QUESTIONS

1. Why is the zone of inhibition in an antibiotic disc assay larger for the same drug concentration (10 μg/mL) in water than in serum? See Figure 11-24.

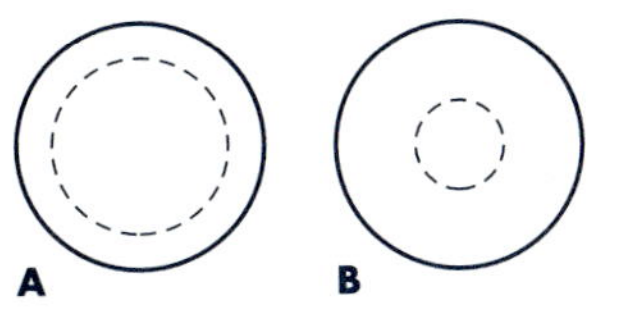

Figure 11-24. Antibiotic disc assay. **A.** Antibiotic in water (10 μg/mL). **B.** Antibiotic in serum (10 μg/mL).

2. Determine the number of binding sites (n) and the association constant (K_a) from the following data using the Scatchard equation.

r	$(D \times 10^{-4}\ M)$	$r/(D)$
0.40	0.33	
0.80	0.89	
1.20	2.00	
1.60	5.33	

Can n and K_a have fractional values? Why?

3. Discuss the clinical significance of drug protein binding on the following:
a. Drug elimination
b. Drug–drug interactions
c. *"Percent of drug-bound"* data
d. Liver disease
e. Kidney disease

4. Vallner (1977) reviewed the binding of drugs to albumin or plasma proteins. The following data were reported:

Drug	Percent Drug Bound
Tetracycline	53
Gentamycin	70
Phenytoin	93
Morphine	38

Which drug(s) listed above might be predicted to cause an adverse response due to the concurrent administration of a second drug such as sulfisoxazole (Gantrisin)? Why?

5. What are the main factors that determine the uptake and accumulation of a drug into tissues? Which tissues would have the most rapid drug uptake? Explain your answer.

6. As a result of edema, fluid may leave the capillary into the extracellular space. What effect does edema have on osmotic pressure in the blood and on drug diffusion into extracellular space?

7. Explain the effects of plasma drug–protein binding and tissue drug–protein binding on (a) the apparent volume of distribution and (b) drug elimination.

8. Naproxen (Naprosyn—Syntex) is a nonsteroidal anti-inflammatory drug (NSAID) which is highly bound to plasma proteins, >99%. Explain why the plasma concentration of *free* (unbound) naproxen *increases* in patients with chronic alcoholic liver disease and probably other forms of cirrhosis; whereas, the *total* plasma drug concentration *decreases.*

9. Most literature references give an average value for the percentage of drug bound to plasma proteins.
a. What factors influence the percentage of drug bound?

b. How does renal disease affect protein binding of drugs?

c. How does hepatic disease affect protein binding of drugs?

10. It is often assumed that linear binding occurs at therapeutic dose, what are the potential risks of this assumption?

11. When a drug is 99% bound, it means that there is a potential risk of saturation. True or false?

12. Adenosine is a drug used for termination of tachycardia. The $t_{1/2}$ after IV dose is only 20 to 30 seconds according to product information, suggest a reason for such a short half life based on your knowledge of drug distribution and elimination?

REFERENCES

Borondy P, Dill WA, Chang T, et al: Effect of protein binding on the distribution of 5, 5-diphenylhydantoin between plasma and red cells. *Ann NY Acad Sci* **226**:293, 1973

Bridges JW, Wilson AGE: Drug–serum protein interactions and their biological significance. In Bridges JW, Chasseaud LF (eds), *Progress in Drug Research,* vol 1. New York, Wiley, 1976

Butler TC: The distribution of drugs. In LaDu BN, Mandel HG, Way EL, (eds), *Fundamentals of Drug Metabolism and Disposition.* Baltimore, Williams & Wilkins, 1972

Davison C: Protein binding. In LaDu BN, Mandel HG, Way EL (eds), *Fundamentals of Drug Metabolism and Drug Disposition.* Baltimore, Williams & Wilkins, 1971

Gillette JR: Overview of drug-protein binding. *Ann N Y Acad Sci* **226**:6, 1973

Goldstein A, Aronow L, Kalman SM: *Principles of Drug Action. The Basis of Pharmacology,* 2nd ed. New York, Wiley, 1974, p 166

Holladay JW, Dewey MJ, Yoo SD: Steady state kinetics of imipramine in transgenic mice with elevated serum AAG levels. *Pharm Res* 1313, 1996

Houin G: Drug binding and apparent volume of distribution. In Tillement JP, Lindenlaub E (eds), *Protein Binding and Drug Transport.* Stuttgart, Schattauer, 1985

Keller F, Maiga M, Neumayer HH, et al: Pharmacokinetic effects of altered plasma protein binding of drugs in renal disease. *Eur J Drug Metab Pharmacokinet* **9**:275–282, 1984

Kunin CM, Craig WA, Kornguth M, Monson R: Influence of binding on the pharmacologic activity of antibiotics. *NY Acad Sci* **226**:214–224, 1973

Limbert M, Siebert G: Serum protein binding and pharmacokinetics of cephalosporins. In Tillement JP, Lindenlaub E (eds), *Protein Binding and Drug Transport.* Stuttgart, Schattauer, 1985

MacKichan JJ: Influence of protein binding. In Evans WE, Schentag JJ, Jusko WJ (eds), *Applied Pharmacokinetics—Principles of Drug Monitoring,* 3rd ed. Vancouver, WA, Applied Therapeutics, 1992, Chap 5

O'Reilly RA: The binding of sodium warfarin to plasma albumin and its displacement by phenylbutazone, *Ann NY Acad Sci* **226**:319–331, 1973

Park MK, Ludden T, Arom KV, et al: Myocardial vs serum concentration in infants and children. *J Dis Child* **136**:418–420, 1982

Reifell JA, Leahy EB, Drusin RE et al: A previously unrecognized drug interaction between quinidine and digoxin. *Clin Cardiol* **2**:40–42, 1979

Sellers EM, Koch-Weser J: Influence of intravenous injection rate on protein binding and vascular activity of diazoxide. *Ann NY Acad Sci* **226**:214–224, 1973

Thorp JM: The influence of plasma proteins on the action of drugs. In Binns TB (ed), *Absorption and Distribution of Drugs.* Baltimore, Williams & Wilkins, 1964

Tozer TN: Implications of altered plasma protein binding in disease states. In Benet LZ, Massoud N, Gambertoglio JG (eds), *Pharmacokinetic Basis for Drug Treatment.* New York, Raven Press, 1984

Udall JA: Drug interference with warfarin therapy. *Clin Med* **77**:20, 1970

Vallner JJ: Binding of drugs by albumin and plasma proteins. *J Pharm Sci* **66**:447–465, 1977

BIBLIOGRAPHY

Anton AH, Solomon HM (eds): Drug protein binding. *Ann NY Acad Sci* **226:**1–362, 1973

Barza M, Samuelson T, Weinstein L: Penetration of antibiotics into fibrin loci in vivo, II. Comparison of nine antibiotics: Effect of dose and degree of protein binding. *J Infect Dis* **129:**66, 1974

Bergen T: Pharmacokinetic properties of the cephalosporins *Drugs* **34**(suppl 2):89–104, 1987

Birke G, Liljedahl SO, Plantin LO, Wetterfors J: Albumin catabolism in burns and following surgical procedures. *Acta Chir Scand* **118:**353–366, 1959–1960

Chien DS, Sandri RB, Tang-Liu DS: Systemic pharmacokinetics of acitretin, etretinate, isotretinoin, and acetylenic retinoids in guinea pigs. *Drug Metab Dispos* **20**(2):211–217, 1992

Coffey CJ, Bullock FJ, Schoenemann PT: Numerical solution of nonlinear pharmacokinetic equations: Effect of plasma protein binding on drug distribution and elimination. *J Pharm Sci* **60:**1623, 1971

D'Arcy PF, McElnay JC: Drug interactions involving the displacement of drugs from plasma protein and tissue binding sites. *Pharm Ther* **17:**211–220, 1982

Gibaldi M, Levy G, McNamara PJ: Effect of plasma protein and tissue binding on the biologic half-life of drugs. *Clin Pharmacol Ther* **24:**1–4, 1978

Grainger-Rousseau TJ, McElnay JC, Collier PS: The influence of disease on plasma protein binding of drugs. *Int J Pharm* **54:**1–13, 1989

Greenblatt DJ, Sellers EM, Koch-Weser J: Importance of protein binding for the interpretation of serum or plasma drug concentration. *J Clin Pharmacol* **22:**259–263, 1982

Hildebrandt P, Birch K, Mehlsen J: The relationship between the subcutaneous blood flow and the absorption of Lente type insulin. *Acta Endocrinol* **112**(suppl):275, 1986

Jusko WJ: Pharmacokinetics in disease states changing protein binding. In Benet LZ (ed), *The Effects of Disease States on Drug Pharmacokinetics.* Washington, DC, American Pharmaceutical Association, 1976

Jusko WJ, Gretch M: Plasma and tissue protein binding of drugs in pharmacokinetics. *Drug Metab Rev* **5:**43–140, 1976

Koch-Wester J, Sellers EM: Binding of drugs to serum albumin. *N Engl J Med* **294:**311, 1976

Kremer JMH, Wilting J, Janssen LHM: Drug binding to alpha-1-acid glycoprotein in health and disease. *Pharmacol Rev* **40:**1–47, 1988

Kunin CM, Craig WA, Kornguth M, Monson R: Influence of binding on the pharmacologic activity of antibiotics. *Ann NY Acad Sci* **226:**214–224, 1973

Levy R, Shand D (eds): Clinical implications of drug–protein binding. Proceedings of a symposium sponsored by Syva Company. *Clin Pharmacokin* **9**(suppl 1), 1984

MacKichan JJ: Influences of protein binding and use of unbound (free) drug concentrations. In Evans, WE, Schentag JJ, Jusko WJ (eds) *Applied pharmacokinetics—Principles of Therapeutic Drug Monitoring,* 3rd ed. Vancouver, WA, Applied Therapeutics, 1992, chap 5

MacKichan JJ: Pharmacokinetic consequences of drug displacement from blood and tissue proteins. *Clin Pharmacokin* **9**(suppl 1):32–41, 1984

Meijer DKF, van der Sluijs P: Covalent and noncovalent protein binding of drugs: Implication for hepatic clearance, storage and cell-specific drug delivery. *Pharm Res* **6:**105–118, 1989

Meyer MC, Gutlman DE: The bindings of drugs by plasma proteins. *J Pharm Sci* **57:**895–918, 1968

Nilsen OG: Clinical pharmacokinetics of tenoxicam. *Clin Pharmacokinet* **26**(1):16–43, 1994

Oie S: Drug distribution and binding, *J Clin Pharmacol* **26:**583–586, 1986

Pardridge WM: Recent advances in blood—brain barrier transport. *Annu Rev Pharmacol Toxicol* **26:**25–39, 1988

Rothschild MA, Oratz M, Schreiber SS: Albumin metabolism. *Gastroenterology* **64:**324–331, 1973

Rowland M: Plasma protein binding and therapeutic monitoring. *Ther Drug Monitor* **2:**29–37, 1980

Rowland M, Tozer TN: *Clinical Pharmacokinetics.* New York, Marcel Dekker, 1985, chap 25

Sawada Y, Hanano M, Sugiyama Y, Iga T: Prediction of the disposition of β-lactam antibiotics in human from pharmacokinetic parameters in animals. *J Pharmacokinet Biopharm* **12:**241–261, 1984

Stoeckel K, Trueb V, Tuerk H: Minor changes in biological half-life of ceftriaxone in functionally anephric and liver diseased patients: Explanations and consequences. In Armengaud and Fernex (eds), *Long-Acting Cephalosporins: Ceftriaxone,* Part 28. Proceedings of the 13th International Congress of Chemotherapy, Vienna, 1983, pp 9–13, ss 4.2/1

Tillement JP, Houin G, Zini R, et al: The binding of drugs to blood plasma macromolecules: Recent advances and therapeutic significance. *Adv Drug Res* **13:**59–94, 1984

Tillement JP, Lhoste F, Guidicelli JF: Diseases and drug protein binding. *Clin Pharmacokinet* **3:**144–154, 1978

Tillement JP, Zini R, d'Athier P, Vassent G: Binding of certain acidic drugs to human albumin: Theoretical and practical estimation of fundamental parameters. *Eur J Clin Pharmacol* **7**:307–313, 1974

Upton RN: Regional pharmacokinetics, I. Physiological and physicochemical basis. *Biopharm Drug Dispos* **11**:647–662, 1990

Wandell M, Wilcox-Thole WL: Protein binding and free drug concentrations. In Mungall DR (ed), *Applied Clinical Pharmacokinetics.* New York, Raven, 1983, pp 17–48

Zini R, Riant P, Barre J, Tillement JP: Disease-induced variations in plasma protein levels. Implications for drug dosage regimens, (Parts 1 and 2). *Clin Pharmacokinet* **19**:147–159, 218–229, 1990

12

DRUG ELIMINATION AND CLEARANCE CONCEPTS

DRUG ELIMINATION

Drug elimination refers to the irreversible removal of drug from the body by all routes of elimination. Drug elimination may be divided into two major components: excretion and biotransformation.

Drug excretion is the removal of the intact drug. Nonvolatile drugs are excreted mainly by *renal excretion*, a process in which the drug passes through the kidney to the bladder and ultimately into the urine. Other pathways for drug excretion may include the excretion of drug into bile, sweat, saliva, milk (via lactation), or other body fluids. Volatile drugs, such as gaseous anesthetics or drugs with high volatility, are excreted via the lungs into expired air.

Biotransformation or *drug metabolism* is the process by which the drug is chemically converted in the body to a metabolite. Biotransformation is usually enzymatic, but some of the drug may be chemically changed by a nonenzymatic process, as in the case of ester hydrolysis. Enzymes involved in the biotransformation of drugs are mainly located in the liver (Chapter 13). However, other tissues such as kidney, lung, small intestine, and skin also contain biotransformation enzymes.

Drug elimination in the body involves many complex rate processes. In Chapter 3, all forms of elimination were modeled by a first-order elimination rate process. In this chapter, drug elimination is described in terms of clearance. The term *clearance* describes the process of drug elimination from the body or from a single organ without identifying the individual processes involved. Clearance may be defined as the volume of fluid cleared of drug from the body per unit of time. The units for clearance are mL/min or L/hr. The volume concept is simple and convenient, because all drugs are dissolved and distributed in the fluids of the body. The advantage of the clearance approach is that clearance applies to all elimination rate processes. For example, clearance considers that a certain portion or percent of the distribution volume is cleared of drug over a given time period. This basic concept (see Chapter 3 also) will be elaborated upon after a review of the anatomy and physiology of the kidney.

THE KIDNEY

The kidney is the main excretory organ for the removal of metabolic waste products and plays a major role in maintaining the normal fluid volume and composition in the body. To maintain salt and water balance, the kidney excretes excess electrolytes, water, and waste products while conserving solutes necessary for proper body function. In addition, the kidney has two endocrine functions: (1) the secretion of renin, which regulates blood pressure; and (2) secretion of erythropoietin, which stimulates red blood cell production.

Anatomic Considerations

The kidneys are located in the peritoneal cavity. A general view is shown in Figure 12-1 and a longitudinal view in Figure 12-2. The outer zone of the kidney is called the *cortex*, and the inner region is called the *medulla*. The *nephrons* are the basic functional units, collectively responsible for the removal of metabolic waste and the maintenance of water and electrolyte balance. There are 1 to 1.5 million nephrons in each kidney. The glomerulus of each nephron starts in the cortex. *Cortical nephrons* have short loops of Henle that remain exclusively in the cortex; *juxtamedullary nephrons* have long loops of Henle that extend into the medulla (Fig. 12-3). The longer loops of Henle allow for a greater ability of the nephron to reabsorb water, thereby producing a more concentrated urine.

Blood Supply

The kidneys represent about 0.5% of the total body weight and receive approximately 20 to 25% of the cardiac output. The kidney is supplied by blood via the renal artery, which subdivides into the interlobar arteries penetrating within the kidney and branching further into the afferent arterioles. Each afferent arteriole carries blood toward a single nephron into the glomerular portion of the nephron (Bowman's capsule). The filtration of blood occurs in the glomeruli in Bowman's capsule. From the capillaries (*glomerulus*) within Bowman's capsule, the blood flows out via the efferent arterioles and then into a second capillary network that sur-

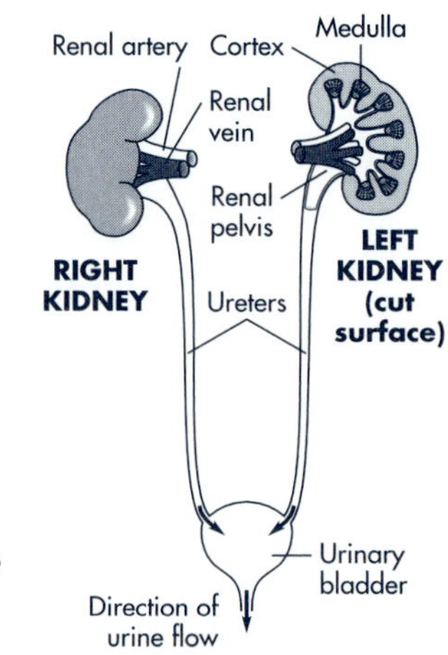

Figure 12-1. The general organizational plan of the urinary system.
(From Guyton (1991), with permission.)

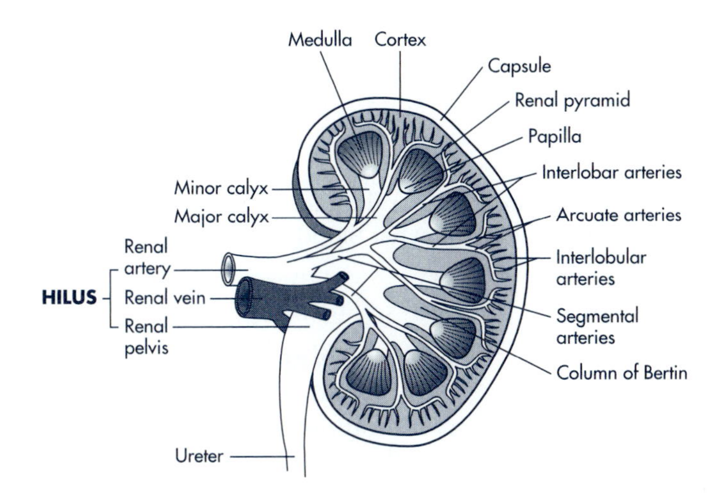

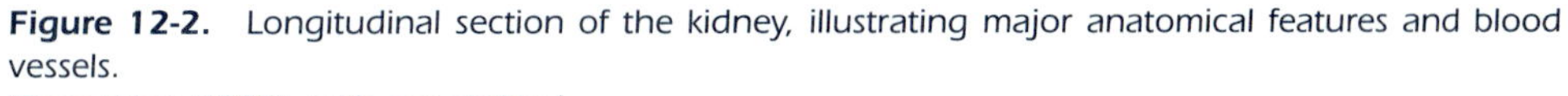

Figure 12-2. Longitudinal section of the kidney, illustrating major anatomical features and blood vessels.
(From West (1985), with permission.)

rounds the tubules (*peritubule capillaries* and *vasa recti*), including the loop of Henle, where some water is reabsorbed.

The *renal blood flow* (RBF) is the volume of blood flowing through the renal vasculature per unit time. Renal blood flow exceeds 1.2 L/min or 1700 L/day. *Renal plasma flow* (RPF) is the renal blood flow minus the volume of red blood

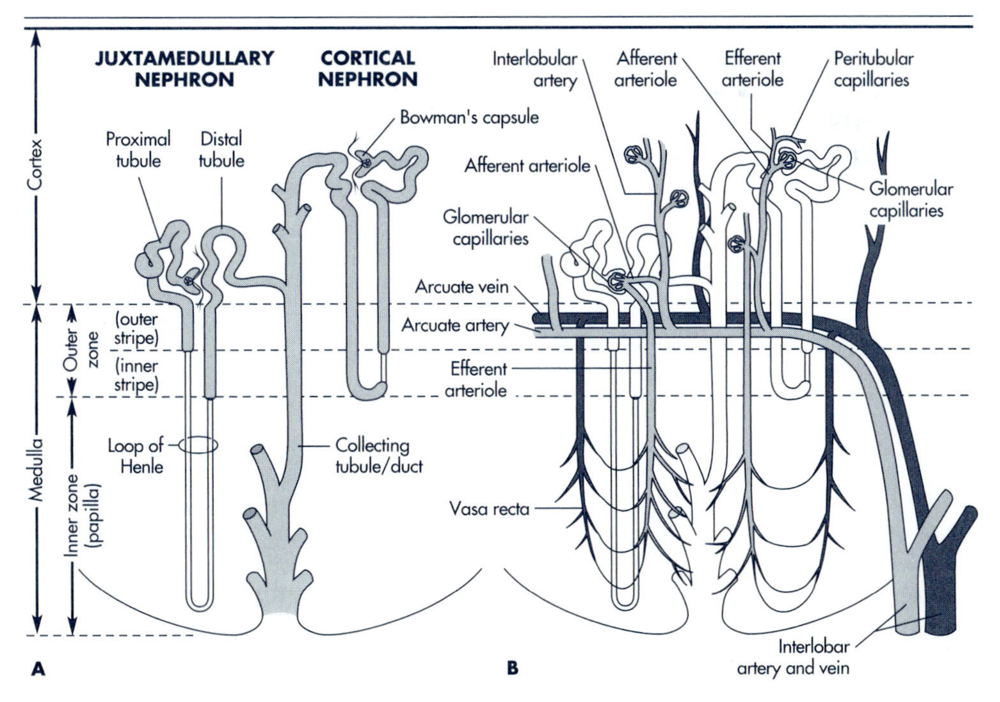

Figure 12-3. Cortical and juxtamedullary nephrons and their vasculature.
(From West (1985), with permission.)

cells present. Renal plasma flow is an important factor in the rate of drug filtration at the glomerulus.

$$RPF = RBF - (RBF \times \text{Hct}) \tag{12.1}$$

where Hct is the hematocrit.

Hct is the fraction of blood cells in the blood, about 45% of the total blood volume, or 0.45. The relationship of renal blood flow to renal plasma flow is given by a rearrangement of Equation 12.1.

$$RPF = RBF(1 - \text{Hct}) \tag{12.2}$$

Assuming a hematocrit of 0.45 and RBF of 1.2 L/min, using the above equation, RPF = 1.2 − (1.2 × 0.45) = 0.66 L/min or 660 mL/min, approximately 950 L/day. The glomerular filtration rate (GFR) is about 125 mL/min in an average adult, or about 20% of the RPF. The ratio of GFR/RPF is the *filtration fraction.*

Regulation of Renal Blood Flow

Blood flow to an organ is directly proportional to the arteriovenous pressure difference (perfusion pressure) across the vascular bed and indirectly proportional to the vascular resistance. The normal renal arterial pressure (Fig. 12-4) is approximately 100 mm Hg and falls to approximately 45 to 60 mm Hg in the glomerulus (glomerular capillary hydrostatic pressure). This pressure difference is probably due to the increasing vasculature resistance provided by the small diameters of the capillary network. Thus, the GFR is controlled by changes in the glomerular capillary hydrostatic pressure.

In the normal kidney, RBF and the GFR remain relatively constant even with large differences in mean systemic blood pressure (Fig. 12-5). The term *autoregulation* refers to the maintenance of a constant blood flow in the presence of large fluctuations in arterial blood pressure. Because autoregulation maintains a relatively constant blood flow, the filtration fraction (GFR/RPF) also remains fairly constant in this pressure range.

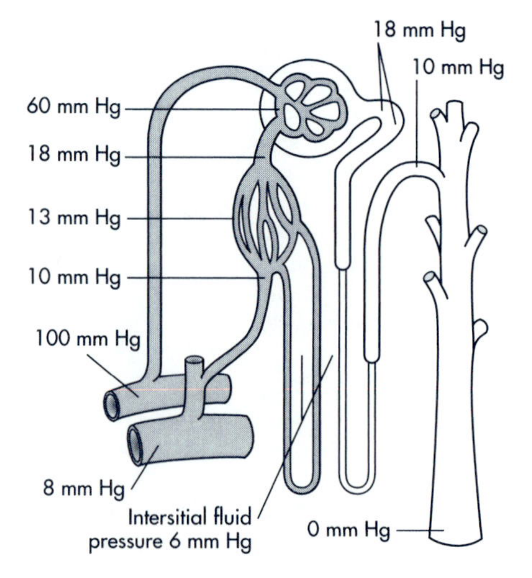

Figure 12-4. Approximate pressures at different points in the vessels and tubules of the functional nephron and in the interstitial fluid.
(From Guyton (1991), with permission.)

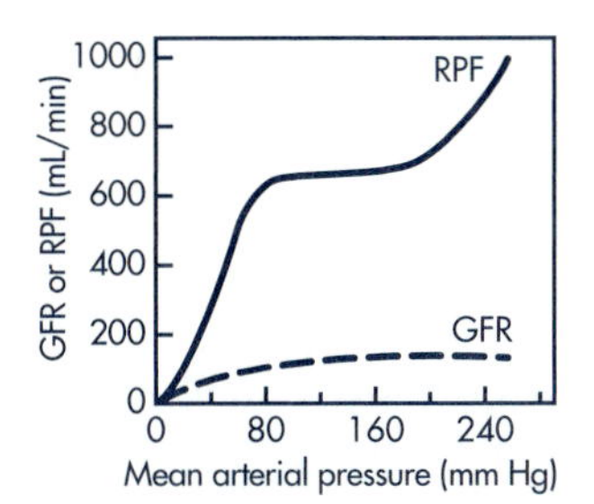

Figure 12-5. Schematic representation of the effect of mean arterial pressure on GFR and RPF, illustrating the phenomenon of autoregulation.
(From West (1985), with permission.)

Glomerular Filtration (GFR) and Urine Formation

A normal adult male subject has a GFR of approximately 125 mL/min. About 180 liters of fluid per day are filtered through the kidneys. In spite of this large filtration volume, the average urine volume is 1 to 1.5 L. Up to 99% of the fluid volume filtered at the glomerulus is reabsorbed. Besides fluid regulation, the kidney also regulates the retention or excretion of various solutes and electrolytes (Table 12.1). With the exception of proteins and protein-bound substances, most small molecules are filtered through the glomerulus from the plasma. The filtrate contains some ions, glucose, and essential nutrients as well as waste products, such as urea, phosphate, sulfate, and other substances. The essential nutrients and water are reabsorbed at various sites, including the proximal tubule, loops of Henle, and distal tubules. Both active reabsorption and secretion mechanisms are involved. The urine volume is reduced, and the urine generally contains a high concentration of metabolic wastes and eliminated drug products.

RENAL DRUG EXCRETION

Renal excretion is a major route of elimination for many drugs. Drugs that are nonvolatile, water soluble, have a low molecular weight, or are slowly biotransformed

TABLE 12.1 Quantitative Aspects of Urine Formation[a]

	PER 24 HOURS				
SUBSTANCE	**FILTERED**	**REABSORBED**	**SECRETED**	**EXCRETED**	**PERCENT REABSORBED**
Sodium ion (mEq)	26,000	25,850		150	99.4
Chloride ion (mEq)	18,000	17,850		150	99.2
Bicarbonate ion (mEq)	4,900	4,900		0	100
Urea (mM)	870	460[b]		410	53
Glucose (mM)	800	800		0	100
Water (mL)	180,000	179,000		1,000	99.4
Hydrogen ion			Variable	Variable[c]	
Potassium ion (mEq)	900	900[d]	100	100	100[d]

[a]Quantity of various plasma constituents filtered, reabsorbed, and excreted by a normal adult on an average diet.
[b]Urea diffuses into, as well as out of, some portions of the nephron.
[c]pH or urine is on the acid side (4.5 to 6.9) when all bicarbonate is reabsorbed.
[d]Potassium ion is almost completely reabsorbed before it reaches the distal nephron. The potassium ion in the voided urine is actively secreted into the urine in the distal tubule in exchange for sodium ion.

From Levine 1990, with permission.

by the liver will be eliminated by renal excretion. The processes by which a drug is excreted via the kidneys may include any combination of the following:

- Glomerular filtration
- Active tubular secretion
- Tubular reabsorption

Glomerular filtration is a unidirectional process that occurs for most small molecules (MW < 500), including undissociated (nonionized) and dissociated (ionized) drugs. Protein-bound drugs behave as large molecules and do not get filtered at the glomerulus. The major driving force for glomerular filtration is the hydrostatic pressure within the glomerular capillaries. The kidneys receive a large blood supply (approximately 25% of the cardiac output) via the renal artery with very little decrease in the hydrostatic pressure.

Glomerular filtration rate (GFR) is measured by using a drug that is eliminated by filtration only (ie, the drug is neither reabsorbed nor secreted). Examples of such drugs are inulin and creatinine. Therefore, the clearance of inulin will be equal to the GFR, which is equal to 125 to 130 mL/min. The value for the GFR correlates fairly well with body surface area. Glomerular filtration of drugs is directly related to the free or nonprotein-bound drug concentration in the plasma. As the free drug concentration in the plasma increases, the glomerular filtration for the drug will increase proportionately, thus increasing renal drug clearance for some drugs.

Active renal secretion is an active transport process. As such, active renal secretion is a carrier-mediated system that requires energy input, because the drug is transported against a concentration gradient. The carrier system is capacity limited and may be saturated. Drugs with similar structures may compete for the same carrier system. Two active renal secretion systems have been identified, systems for (1) weak acids and (2) weak bases. For example, probenecid will compete with penicillin for the same carrier system (*weak acids*). Active tubular secretion rate is dependent on renal plasma flow. Drugs commonly used to measure active tubular secretion include *p*-amino-hippuric acid (PAH) and iodopyracet (Diodrast). These substances are both filtered by the glomeruli and secreted by the tubular cells. Active secretion is extremely rapid for these drugs, and practically all the drug carried to the kidney is eliminated in a single pass. The clearance for these drugs therefore reflects the *effective renal plasma flow* (ERPF), which varies from 425 to 650 mL/min. For a drug that is excreted solely by glomerular filtration, the elimination half-life may change markedly in accordance with the binding affinity of the drug for plasma proteins. In contrast, protein binding has very little effect on the elimination half-life of a drug excreted mostly by active secretion. Because drug protein binding is reversible, the bound drug and free drug are excreted by active secretion during the first pass through the kidney. For example, some of the penicillins are extensively protein bound, but their elimination half-lives are short due to rapid elimination by active secretion.

Tubular reabsorption occurs after the drug is filtered through the glomerulus and can be active or passive. If a drug is completely reabsorbed (eg, glucose), then the value for the clearance of the drug is approximately zero. For drugs that are partially reabsorbed, clearance values will be less than the GFR of 125 to 130 mL/min.

The reabsorption of drugs that are acids or weak bases is influenced by the pH of the fluid in the renal tubule (ie, urine pH) and the pK_a of the drug. Both of these factors together determine the percentage of dissociated (ionized) and undissociated (nonionized) drug. Generally, the undissociated species is more lipid soluble (less water soluble) and has greater membrane permeability. The undissociated drug is easily reabsorbed from the renal tubule back into the body. This process of drug reabsorption can significantly reduce the amount of drug excreted, depending on the pH of the urinary fluid and the pK_a of the drug. The pK_a of the drug is a constant, but the normal urinary pH may vary from 4.5 to 8.0, depending on diet, pathophysiology, and drug intake. Vegetable diets or diets rich in carbohydrates will result in higher urinary pH, whereas diets rich in protein will result in lower urinary pH. Drugs such as ascorbic acid and antacids such as sodium carbonate may decrease (acidify) or increase (alkalinize) the urinary pH, respectively, when administered in large quantity. By far the most important changes in urinary pH are caused by fluids administered intravenously. Intravenous fluids, such as solutions of bicarbonate or ammonium chloride, are used in acid-base therapy. Excretion of these solutions may drastically change urinary pH and alter drug reabsorption and drug excretion.

The percentage of ionized weak acid drug corresponding to a given pH can be obtained from the *Henderson–Hesselbalch equation.*

$$pH = pK_a + \log \frac{[\text{ionized}]}{[\text{nonionized}]} \tag{12.3}$$

Rearrangement of this equation yields

$$\frac{[\text{ionized}]}{[\text{nonionized}]} = 10^{pH - pK_a} \tag{12.4}$$

$$\text{Fraction of drug ionized} = \frac{[\text{ionized}]}{[\text{ionized}] + [\text{nonionized}]} \tag{12.5}$$

$$= \frac{10^{pH - pK_a}[\text{nonionized}]}{[\text{nonionized}] + 10^{pH - pK_a}[\text{nonionized}]}$$

$$= \frac{10^{pH - pK_a}}{1 + 10^{pH - pK_a}}$$

The fraction or percent of weak acid drug ionized in any pH environment may be calculated with Equation 12.5. For acidic drugs with pK_a values of from 3 to 8, a change in urinary pH will affect the extent of dissociation (Table 12.2). The extent of dissociation is more greatly affected by changes in urinary pH with a pK_a of 5 than with a pK_a of 3. Weak acids with pK_a values of less than 2 are highly ionized at all urinary pH values and are only slightly affected by pH variations.

TABLE 12.2 Effect of Urinary pH and pK_a on the Ionization of Drugs

pH OF URINE	PERCENT OF DRUG IONIZED: $pK_a{}^{-3}$	PERCENT OF DRUG IONIZED: $pK_a{}^{-5}$
7.4	100	99.6
5	99	50.0
4	91	9.1
3	50	0.99

For a weak base drug, the Henderson–Hasselbalch equation is given as

$$\text{pH} = \text{pK}_a + \log \frac{[\text{nonionized}]}{[\text{ionized}]} \quad \textbf{(12.6)}$$

and

$$\text{Percent of drug ionized} = \frac{1 + 10^{\text{pH} - \text{pK}_a}}{10^{\text{pH} - \text{pK}_a}} \quad \textbf{(12.7)}$$

The greatest effect of urinary pH on reabsorption occurs with weak base drugs with pK_a values of 7.5 to 10.5.

From the Henderson–Hesselbalch relationship, a concentration ratio for the distribution of a weak acid or basic drug between urine and plasma may be derived. The urine–plasma (*U/P*) ratios for these drugs are as follows.

For weak acids

$$\frac{U}{P} = \frac{1 + 10^{\text{pH}_{\text{urine}} - \text{pK}_a}}{1 + 10^{\text{pH}_{\text{plasma}} - \text{pK}_a}} \quad \textbf{(12.8)}$$

For weak bases

$$\frac{U}{P} = \frac{1 + 10^{\text{pK}_a - \text{pH}_{\text{urine}}}}{1 + 10^{\text{pK}_a - \text{pH}_{\text{plasma}}}} \quad \textbf{(12.9)}$$

For example, amphetamine, a weak base, will be reabsorbed if the urine pH is made alkaline and more lipid-soluble nonionized species are formed. In contrast, acidification of the urine will cause the amphetamine to become more ionized (form a salt). The salt form is more water soluble and less likely to be reabsorbed and has a tendency to be excreted into the urine more quickly. In the case of weak acids (such as salicylic acid), acidification of the urine causes greater reabsorption of the drug and alkalinization of the urine causes more rapid excretion of the drug.

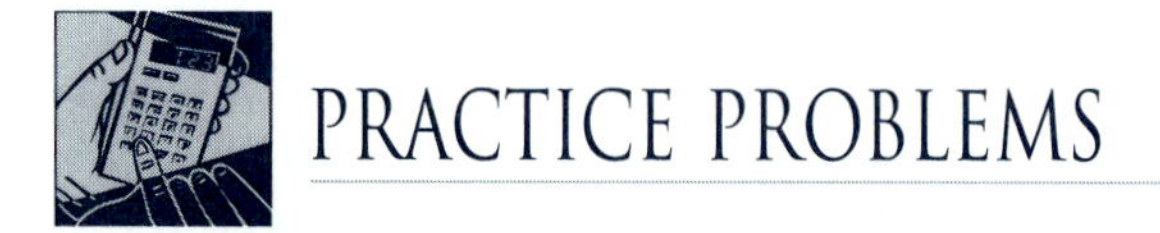

PRACTICE PROBLEMS

Let $\text{pK}_a = 5$ for an acidic drug. Compare the *U/P* at urinary pH (a) 3, (b) 5, and (c) 7.

Solution

a. At pH = 3:

$$\frac{U}{P} = \frac{1 + 10^{3-5}}{1 + 10^{7.4-5}} = \frac{1.01}{1 + 10^{2.4}}$$

$$= \frac{1.01}{252} = \frac{1}{252}$$

b. At pH = 5:

$$\frac{U}{P} = \frac{1 + 10^{5-5}}{1 + 10^{7.4-5}} = \frac{2}{1 + 10^{2.4}} = \frac{2}{252}$$

c. At pH = 7:

$$\frac{U}{P} = \frac{1 + 10^{7-5}}{1 + 10^{7.4-5}} = \frac{101}{1 + 10^{2.4}} = \frac{101}{252}$$

In addition to the pH of the urine, the rate of urine flow will influence the amount of filtered drug that is reabsorbed. The normal flow of urine is approximately 1 to 2 mL/min. Nonpolar and nonionized drugs, which are normally well reabsorbed in the renal tubules, are sensitive to changes in the rate of urine flow. Drugs that increase urine flow, such as ethanol, large fluid intake, and methylxanthines (such as caffeine or theophylline), will decrease the time for drug reabsorption and promote their excretion. Thus, forced diuresis through the use of diuretics may be a useful adjunct for removing excessive drug in an intoxicated patient by increasing renal drug excretion.

DRUG CLEARANCE

Drug clearance is a pharmacokinetic term for describing drug elimination from the body without identifying the mechanism of the process. Drug clearance (*body clearance, total body clearance,* or Cl_T) considers the entire body as a single drug-eliminating system from which many unidentified elimination processes may occur. Instead of describing drug elimination rate in terms of amount of drug removed per time unit, drug clearance is described in terms of volume of fluid clear of drug per time unit.

There are several definitions of clearance, which are similarly based on volume of drug removed per unit time. The simplest concept of clearance regards the body as a space that contains a definite volume of body fluid (apparent volume of distribution, V_D) in which the drug is dissolved. Drug clearance is defined as the fixed volume of fluid (containing the drug) cleared of drug per unit of time. The units for clearance are volume/time (eg, mL/min, L/hr). For example, if the Cl_T of penicillin is 15 mL/min in a patient and penicillin has a V_D of 12 L, then from the clearance definition, 15 mL of the 12 L would be cleared of drug per minute.

Alternatively, Cl_T may be defined as the rate of drug elimination divided by the plasma drug concentration. This definition expresses drug elimination in terms of the volume of plasma eliminated of drug per unit time. This definition is a practical way to calculate clearance based on plasma drug concentration data.

$$Cl_T = \frac{\text{Elimination rate}}{\text{Plasma concentration } (C_p)} \tag{12.10}$$

$$Cl_T = \frac{dD_E/dt}{C_p} = \frac{\mu g/\text{min}}{\mu g/\text{mL}} = \text{mL/min} \tag{12.11}$$

where D_E is the amount of drug eliminated and dD_E/dt is the rate of elimination.

Rearrangement of Equation 12.11 gives Equation 12.12.

$$\text{Elimination rate} = dD_E/dt = C_p\ Cl_T \tag{12.12}$$

The two definitions for clearance are similar because dividing the elimination rate by the C_p yields the volume of plasma cleared of drug per minute, as shown in Equation 12.10.

As discussed in previous chapters, a first-order elimination rate, dD_E/dt, is equal to kD_B or kC_pV_D. Based on Equation 12.10, substituting elimination rate of kC_pV_p

$$Cl_T = \frac{kC_pV_D}{C_p} = kV_D \tag{12.13}$$

Equation 12.13 shows that clearance is the product of V_D and k, both of which are constant. As the plasma drug concentration decreases during elimination, the rate of drug elimination, dD_E/dt, will decrease accordingly, but clearance will remain constant. Clearance will be constant as long as the rate of drug elimination is a first-order process.

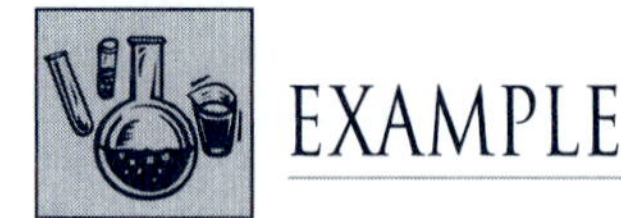

EXAMPLE

Penicillin has a Cl_T of 15 mL/min. Calculate the elimination rate for penicillin when the plasma drug concentration, C_p, is 2 μg/mL.

Solution

Elimination rate = $C_p \times Cl_T$ (from Eq. 12.12)

$$dD_E/dt = 2\ \mu\text{g/mL} \times 15\ \text{mL/min} = 30\ \mu\text{g/min}$$

Using the previous penicillin example, assume that the plasma penicillin concentration is 10 μg/mL. From Equation 12.11, the rate of drug elimination is

$$dD_E/dt = 10\ \mu\text{g/mL} \times 15\ \text{mL/min} = 150\ \mu\text{g/min}$$

Thus, 150 μg/min of penicillin is eliminated from the body when the plasma penicillin concentration is 10 μg/mL.

Clearance may be used to estimate the rate of drug elimination at any given concentration. Using the same example, if the elimination rate of penicillin was measured as 150 μg/min when the plasma penicillin concentration was at 10 μg/mL, then the clearance of penicillin is calculated from Equation 12.11.

$$Cl_{\text{penicillin}} = \frac{150\ \mu\text{g/min}}{10\ \mu\text{g/mL}} = 15\ \text{mL/min}$$

Just as the elimination rate constant (k) represents the sum total of all the rate constants for drug elimination, including excretion and biotransformation, Cl_T is the sum total of all the clearance processes in the body, including clearance through the kidney (renal clearance), lung, and liver (hepatic clearance).

Renal clearance = $k_e V_D$
Lung clearance = $k_l V_D$
Hepatic clearance = $k_m V_D$
Body clearance = $k_e V_D + k_l V_D + k_m V_D$

$$Cl_T = V_D (k_e + k_l + k_m) = V_D k \tag{12.14}$$

From Equation 12.14, Cl_T of a drug is the product of two constants, k and V_D, which reflect all the distribution and elimination processes of the drug in the body. The volume of distribution and elimination rate constant are affected by blood flow, which will be considered using a physiologic model.

Clearance values are often normalized on a per-kilogram body weight basis, such as mL/min per kg. This approach is similar to the method for expressing V_D, because both pharmacokinetic parameters vary with body weight. The clearance for an individual patient is estimated as the product of the clearance per kilogram multiplied by the body weight (kg) of the patient.

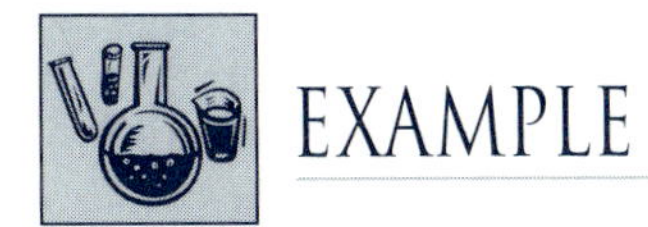

EXAMPLE

Determine the total body clearance for a drug in a 70-kg male patient. The drug follows the kinetics of a one-compartment model and has an elimination half-life of 3 hours with an apparent volume of distribution of 100 mL/kg.

Solution

First determine the elimination rate constant (k) and then substitute properly into Equation 12.13.

$$k = 0.693/t_{1/2} = 0.693/3 = 0.231 \text{ hr}^{-1}$$
$$Cl_T = 0.231 \text{ hr}^{-1} \times 100 \text{ mL/kg} = 23.1 \text{ mL/kg hr}$$

For a 70-kg patient:

$$Cl_T = 23.1 \text{ mL/kg hr} \times 70 \text{ kg} = 1617 \text{ mL/hr}$$

PHYSIOLOGIC APPROACH TO CLEARANCE

The calculation of clearance from k and V_D assumes (sometimes incorrectly) a defined model, whereas clearance estimated directly from the plasma drug concentration versus time curve does not assume any model. Although clearance may be regarded as the product of k and V_D, Equation 12.10 is far more general because the reaction order for the rate of drug elimination, dD_E/dt, is not specified, and the elimination rate may or may not follow first-order kinetics. Nevertheless, any elimination process other than first order would be complex, and it would be difficult to relate clearance to a compartment model.

Organ Drug Clearance

Clearance may be calculated for any organ involved in the irreversible removal of drug from the body. Many organs in the body have the capacity for drug elimination, including drug excretion and biotransformation. The kidneys and liver are the most common organs involved in excretion and metabolism, respectively.

Physiologic pharmacokinetic models are based on drug clearance through individual organs or tissue groups (Fig. 12-6).

For any organ, clearance may be defined as the fraction of blood volume containing drug that flows through the organ and is eliminated of drug per unit time. From this definition, clearance is the product of the blood flow (Q) to the organ, and the extraction ratio (ER). The ER is the fraction of drug extracted by the organ as drug passes through.

$$\text{Clearance} = Q\,(\text{ER}) \tag{12.15}$$

If the drug concentration in the blood (C_a) entering the organ is greater than the drug concentration of blood (C_v) leaving the organ, then some of the drug has been extracted by the organ (Fig. 12-6). The ER is $C_a - C_v$ divided by the entering drug concentration (C_a), as shown in Equation 12.16.

$$\text{ER} = (C_a - C_v)/C_a \tag{12.16}$$

ER is a ratio with no units. The value of ER may range from 0 (no drug removed by the organ) to 1 (100% of the drug is removed by the organ). An ER of 0.25 indicates that 25% of the incoming drug concentration is removed by the organ as the drug passes through.

Substituting for ER into Equation 12.14 yields

$$Cl = Q[(C_a - C_v)/C_a] \tag{12.17}$$

The physiologic approach to clearance shows that clearance depends upon the blood flow rate and the ability of the organ to eliminate drug, whereas the classical definitions of clearance is that a constant or static fraction of the volume in which the drug is contained is removed per unit time by the organ. However, clearance measurements using the physiologic approach require invasive techniques to obtain measurements of blood flow and extraction ratio. The physiologic approach has been used to describe hepatic clearance, which is discussed under hepatic elimination (Chap. 13). More classical definitions of clearance have been applied to renal clearance because direct measurements of plasma drug concentration and urinary drug excretion may be obtained.

RENAL CLEARANCE

Renal clearance, Cl_R, is defined as the volume of plasma that is cleared of drug per unit of time through the kidney. Similarly, renal clearance may be defined as a constant fraction of the V_D in which the drug is contained that is excreted by the kidney per unit of time. More simply, renal clearance is defined as

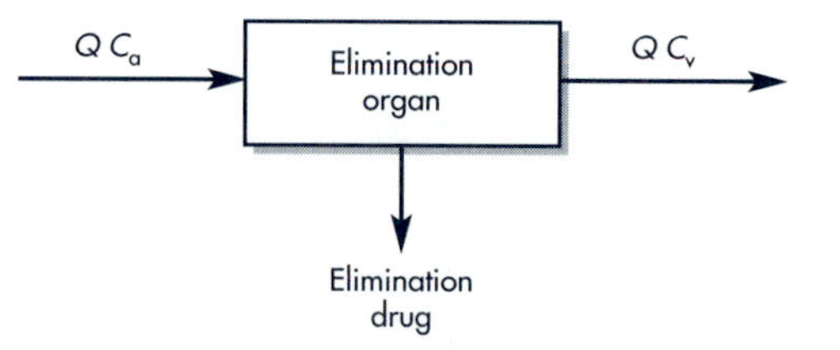

Figure 12-6. Drug clearance model. (Q = blood flow, C_a = incoming drug concentration [usually arterial drug concentration], C_v = outgoing drug concentration [venous drug concentration]).

the urinary drug excretion rate (dD_u/dt) divided by the plasma drug concentration C_p.

$$Cl_R = \frac{\text{Excretion rate}}{\text{Plasma concentration}} = \frac{dD_u/dt}{C_p} \tag{12.18}$$

An alternative approach to obtaining Equation 12.18 is to consider the mass balance of drug cleared by the kidney and ultimately excreted in the urine. For any drug cleared through the kidney, the rate of the drug passing through kidney (via filtration, reabsorption, and/or active secretion) must equal the rate of drug excreted in the urine.

Rate of drug passing through kidney = Rate of drug excreted

$$Cl_R \times C_p = Q_u \times C_u \tag{12.19}$$

$$\text{mL/min} \times \mu\text{g/mL} = \text{mL/min} \times \mu\text{g/mL}$$

where Cl_R is renal clearance, C_p is plasma drug concentration, Q_u is the rate of urine flow, and C_u is the urine drug concentration.

If the Cl_R of the drug is by glomerular filtration only, as in the case of inulin, then Cl_R = GFR. Otherwise, Cl_R represents all the processes by which the drug is cleared through the kidney, including any combination of filtration, reabsorption, and active secretion. Rearrangement of Equation 12.19 gives

$$Cl_R = \frac{Q_u C_u}{C_p} = \frac{\text{Excretion rate}}{C_p} \tag{12.20}$$

where Cl_R is renal clearance, C_p is plasma drug concentration, Q_u is the rate of urine flow (mL/min), and C_u is the urine drug concentration (μg/mL).

Because the excretion rate = $Q_u C_u = dD_u/dt$, Equation 12.20 is the equivalent of Equation 12.18.

Clearance Ratio

Renal clearance may be measured without regard to the physiologic mechanisms involved in this process. From a physiologic viewpoint, however, renal clearance may be considered as the ratio of the sum of the glomerular filtration and active secretion rates less the reabsorption rate divided by the plasma drug concentration:

$$Cl_R = \frac{\text{filtration rate} + \text{secretion rate} - \text{reabsorption rate}}{C_p} \tag{12.21}$$

The actual renal clearance of a drug is not generally obtained by direct measurement. The clearance value for the drug is compared to that of a standard reference, such as inulin, which is cleared completely through the kidney by glomerular filtration only; the clearance ratios show the mechanism of renal excretion of the drug (Table 12.3).

RENAL DRUG EXCRETION

Compartment Versus Physiologic Model

The process of renal drug excretion by the kidney is affected by the body physiology and involves many variables. A realistic method to quantify renal drug excre-

TABLE 12.3 Comparison of Clearance of a Sample Drug to Clearance of a Reference Drug, Inulin

CLEARANCE RATIO	PROBABLE MECHANISM OF RENAL EXCRETION
$\frac{Cl_{drug}}{Cl_{inulin}} < 1$	Drug is partially reabsorbed
$\frac{Cl_{drug}}{Cl_{inulin}} = 1$	Drug is filtered only
$\frac{Cl_{drug}}{Cl_{inulin}} > 1$	Drug is actively secreted

tion is to consider the kinetic nature of the elimination processes. For this consideration, some of the detailed steps in the elimination process may be omitted or simplified. For example, assume that the body fluid volume is the V_D and that the plasma drug concentration, C_p, is changing after an intravenous bolus injection. If glomerular filtration is the sole process for drug excretion and no drug is reabsorbed, then the amount of drug filtered at any time (t) would always be the $C_p \times$ GFR (Table 12.4).

Note that the quantity of drug excreted per minute is always the plasma concentration (C_p) multiplied by a constant (125 mL/min), which in this case is also the renal clearance for the drug. The glomerular filtration rate may be treated as a first-order process relating to C_p. The rate of drug excretion using a compartment approach and physiologic approach are compared in Equations 12.22 and 12.23.

$$dD_u/dt = k_R V_D C_p \quad \text{(compartment)} \tag{12.22}$$

$$dD_u/dt = Cl_R C_p \quad \text{(physiologic)} \tag{12.23}$$

Equating 12.22 with 12.23,

$$k_R V_D C_p = Cl_R C_p \tag{12.24}$$

$$k_R = Cl_R / V_D$$

Equation 12.24 shows that, in the absence of other processes of drug elimination, the excretion rate constant is a fractional constant reflecting the volume pumped out per unit time due to GFR relative to the volume of the body compartment (V_D). For a drug with a reabsorption fraction of fr, the drug excretion rate would be reduced, and Equation 12.23 is restated as Equation 12.25.

$$dD_u/dt = Cl_R\,(1 - fr)\,C_p \quad \text{(physiologic)} \tag{12.25}$$

Equating the right sides of Equations 12.25 and 12.22 indicates that the first-order rate constant (k_R) in the compartment model is equivalent to $Cl_R\,(1 - fr)/V_D$.

TABLE 12.4 Urinary Drug Excretion Rate[a]

TIME (min)	C_P (μg/mL)	EXCRETION RATE (μg/min) (Drug filtered by GFR per min)
0	$(C_p)_0$	$(C_p)_0 \times 125$
1	$(C_p)_1$	$(C_p)_1 \times 125$
2	$(C_p)_2$	$(C_p)_2 \times 125$
t	$(C_p)_t$	$(C_p)_t = 125$

[a]Assumes that the drug is excreted by filtration only and that the GFR is 125 mL/min.

Compartment model

Static volume and first-order elimination is assumed.
Plasma flow is not considered. $Cl_T = k\ V_D$.

Physiologic model

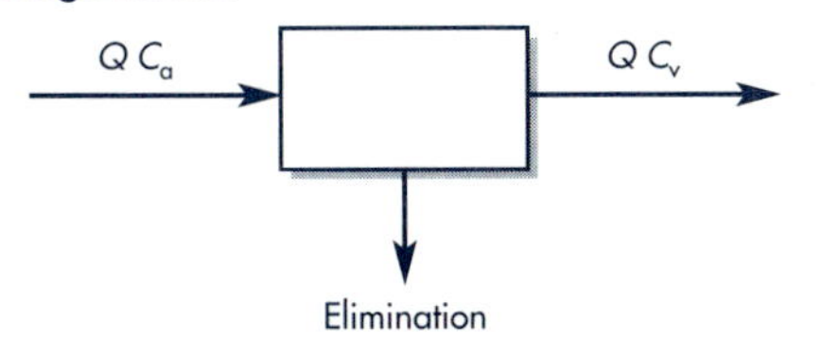

Clearance is the product of the plasma flow (Q) and the extraction ratio (ER).
Thus $Cl_T = Q$ ER

Model independent

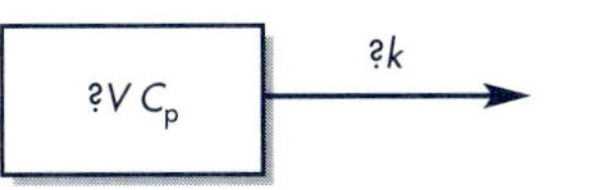

Volume and elimination rate constant not defined. $Cl_T = \text{Dose}/[\text{AUC}]_0^\infty$.

Figure 12-7. General approaches to clearance. Volume and elimination rate constant not defined.

In this case, the excretion rate constant is affected by the reabsorption fraction (*fr*) and the GFR. Because these two parameters generally remain constant, the general adoption of a first-order elimination process to describe renal drug excretion is a reasonable approach. The power of the kinetic approach is that, even when lacking any knowledge of GFR, active secretion, or the reabsorption process, modeling the data allows the process of drug elimination to be described quantitatively. If a change to a higher-order elimination rate process occurs, then an additional process besides GFR may be involved. The compartmental analysis aids the ultimate development of a model consistent with physiologic functions of the body.

In the one-compartment model, a drug is assumed to be uniformly and instantly equilibrated. However, the renal plasma drug concentration entering the kidney is always higher than the plasma drug concentration leaving the kidney. In spite of this inconsistency, the rate of drug elimination is properly adjusted in the estimation of the first-order elimination rate constant (k) given in Equation 12.23 if the overall plasma drug concentration profile is adequately described. If the pharmacokinetic parameters are properly calculated to fit the data, the parameters k and V_D reflect the underlying kinetic processes. Figure 12-7 summarizes the various approaches to estimating clearance.

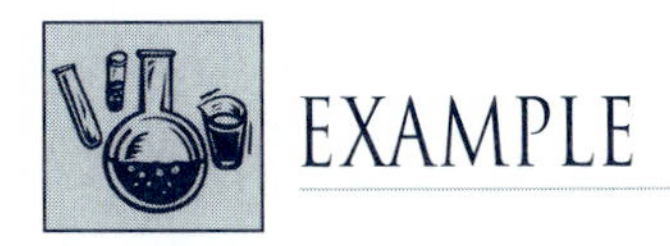

EXAMPLE

Two drugs, *A* and *B*, are entirely eliminated through the kidney by glomerular filtration (125 mL/min) with no reabsorption. Drug *A* has half the distribution volume of drug *B*, and the V_D of drug *B* is 20 Liters. What are the drug clearances for each drug based on the classical and physiologic approach?

Solution

Since glomerular filtration of the two drugs are the same, and both drugs are not eliminated by other means. Clearance for both drugs will depend on renal plasma flow and extraction by the kidney only.

Basing the clearance calculation on the physiologic definition and using Equation 12.17 results in the following:

$$Cl = Q\,(C_a - C_v)/C_a = 125 \text{ mL/min.}$$

Interestingly, known drug clearance tells little about the dosing differences of the two drugs, although it helps to identify the mechanism of drug elimination. In this example, both drugs have the same clearance.

Basing the calculation on the elimination concept, and applying Equation 12.14, *k* is easily determined, resulting in an obvious difference in $t_{1/2}$ between the two drugs—in spite of similar drug clearance.

$$k_{\text{Drug }A} = Cl/V_D = \frac{125 \text{ mL/min}}{10 \times 1000 \text{ mL}} = 0.0125 \text{ min}^{-1}$$

$$k_{\text{Drug }B} = Cl/V_D = \frac{125 \text{ mL/min}}{20 \times 1000 \text{ mL}} = 0.00625 \text{ min}^{-1}$$

Note *k* is dimensionless in the numerator, min^{-1}; *k* specifies the fraction of drug eliminated regardless of distributional differences of the drug.

In spite of identical drug clearances, *k* for drug *A* is twice that of drug *B*. Drug *A* has an elimination half-life of 80 minutes while that of drug *B* is 160 minutes, much longer due to a bigger volume of distribution.

DRUG CLEARANCE

Model-Independent Method

Clearance is commonly used to describe first-order drug elimination from compartment models in which the distribution volume and elimination rate constant are well defined. However, for some drugs, the elimination rate process is more complex and a noncompartment or model-independent method may be used.

Model-independent methods are noncompartment model approaches used to calculate certain pharmacokinetic parameters such as clearance and bioavailability (F). The major advantage of model-independent methods is that no assumption for a specific compartment model is required to analyze the data. The volume of distribution and the elimination rate constant need not be determined directly from the equation that best fits the plasma drug concentration versus time curve. In fact, for some drugs, these two parameters may not be constant during the course of drug distribution. Clearance can be determined directly from the plasma–time concentration curve by

$$Cl = \int_0^\infty \frac{D_0}{C(t)\,dt} \quad \textbf{(12.26)}$$

where D_0 is the dose and $C(t)$ is an unknown function that describes the declining plasma drug concentrations.

For example, in a one-compartment model, $C(t) = C_p = C_p^0 e^{-kt}$, from which clearance is most often calculated. In practice, $C(t)$ can be different mathematical functions that describe the individual pharmacokinetics of the drug. The more general equation uses area under the curve of the plasma drug concentration curve for the calculation of clearance.

$$Cl_T = \frac{D_0}{[AUC]_0^\infty} \quad \textbf{(12.27)}$$

where D_0 is the dose and $[AUC]_0^\infty = \int_0^\infty C_p \, dt$.

Because $[AUC]_0^\infty$ is calculated from the plasma drug concentration versus time curve from 0 to infinity using the trapezoidal rule, no compartmental model is assumed. However, to extrapolate the data to infinity to obtain the residual $[AUC]_t^\infty$ or (C_{p_t}/k), first-order elimination is usually assumed. This calculation of Cl_T is referred to as a noncompartment or model-independent method. In this case, if the drug follows the kinetics of a one-compartment model, the Cl_T is numerically similar to the product of V_D and k obtained by fitting the data to a one-compartment model.

DETERMINATION OF RENAL CLEARANCE

The clearance is given by the slope of the curve obtained by plotting the rate of drug excretion in urine (dD_u/dt) against C_p (Eq. 12.28). For a drug that is excreted rapidly, dD_u/dt is large, the slope is steeper, and clearance is greater (Fig. 12-8, line *A*). For a drug that is excreted slowly through the kidney, the slope is smaller (Fig. 12-8, line *B*).

From Equation 12.18

$$Cl_R = \frac{dD_u/dt}{C_p}$$

Multiplying both sides by C_p gives

$$Cl_R C_p = \frac{dD_u}{dt} \quad \textbf{(12.28)}$$

By rearranging Equation 12.28 and integrating, one obtains

$$\int_0^{Du} dD_u = Cl_R \int_0^t C_p \, dt \quad \textbf{(12.29)}$$

$$[D_u]_0^t = Cl_R [AUC]_0^t \quad \textbf{(12.30)}$$

A graph is then plotted of cumulative drug excreted in the urine versus the area under the concentration–time curve (Fig. 12-9). Clearance is obtained from the slope of the curve. The area under the curve can be estimated by the trapezoidal rule or by other measurement methods. The disadvantage of this method is that if a data point is missing, the cumulative amount of drug excreted in the urine is difficult to obtain. However, if the data are complete, then the determination of clearance is more accurate by this method.

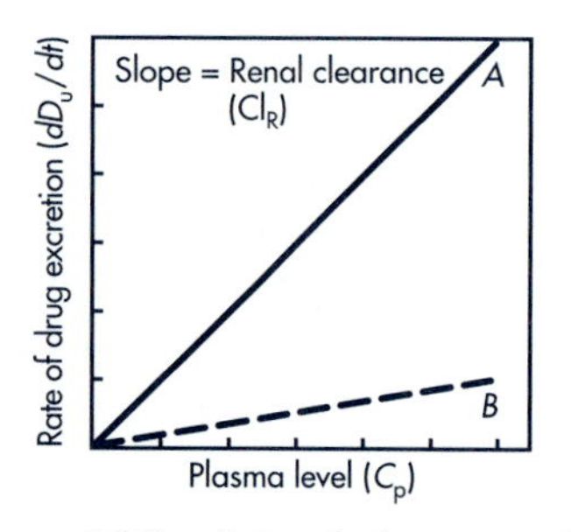

Figure 12-8. Rate of drug excretion versus concentration of drug in the plasma. Drug A has a higher clearance than drug B, as shown by the slopes of line A and line B.

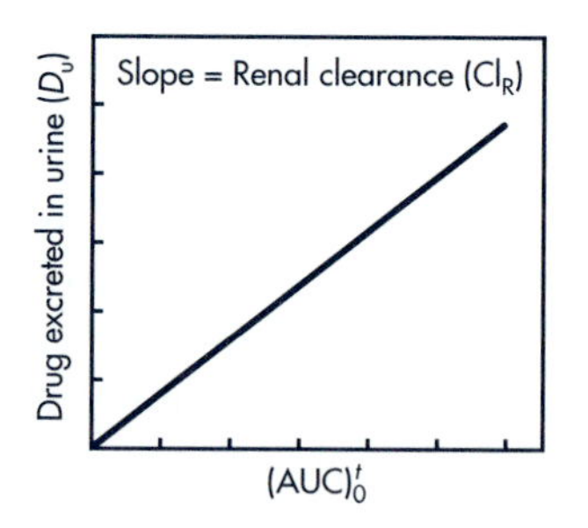

Figure 12-9. Cumulative drug excretion versus AUC. The slope is equal to Cl_R.

By plotting cumulative drug excreted in the urine from t_1 to t_2, $[D_u]_{t1}^{t2}$ versus $[\text{AUC}]_{t1}^{t2}$, one obtains an equation similar to that presented previously.

$$\int_{D_u^1}^{D_u^2} dD_u = Cl_R \int_{t1}^{t2} C_p \, dt \tag{12.31}$$

$$[D_u]_{t1}^{t2} = Cl_R[\text{AUC}]_{t1}^{t2} \tag{12.32}$$

The slope is equal to the clearance (Fig. 12-10).

Clearance rates may also be estimated by a single (nongraphical) calculation from knowledge of the $[\text{AUC}]_0^\infty$, the total amount of drug absorbed, FD_0, and the total amount of drug excreted in the urine, D_u^∞. For example, if a single IV bolus drug injection is given to a patient and the $[\text{AUC}]_0^\infty$ is obtained from the plasma drug level–time curve, then total body clearance is estimated by

$$Cl_T = \frac{D_0}{[\text{AUC}]_0^\infty} \tag{12.33}$$

If the total amount of drug excreted in the urine, D_u^∞, has been obtained, then renal clearance is calculated by

$$Cl_R = \frac{D_u^\infty}{[\text{AUC}]_0^\infty} \tag{12.34}$$

The calculations using Equations 12.33 and 12.34 allow for rapid and easily obtainable estimates of drug clearance. However, only a single dose estimate is ob-

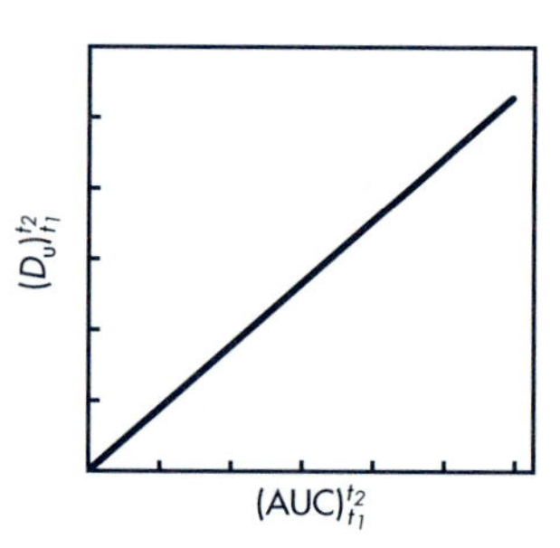

Figure 12-10. Drug excreted versus $(\text{AUC})_{t1}^{t2}$. The slope is equal to Cl_R.

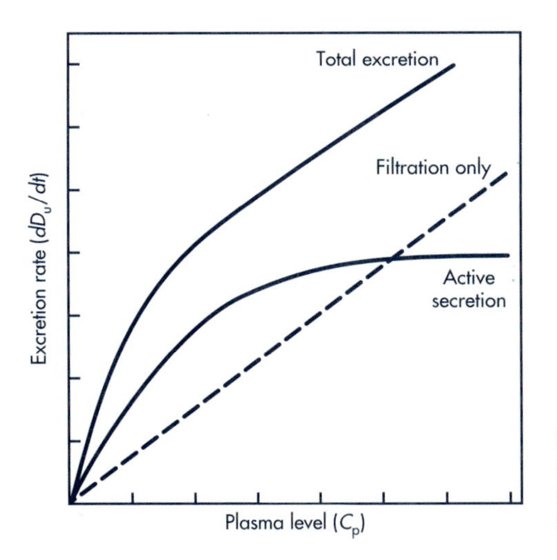

Figure 12-11. Excretion rate versus plasma level curves for a drug that demonstrates active tubular secretion and a drug that is secreted by glomerular filtration only.

tained; therefore, the calculations will not reflect nonlinear changes in the clearance rates, as indicated in Figure 12-11.

Clearance can also be calculated from fitted parameters. If the volume of distribution and elimination constants are known, body clearance (Cl_T), renal clearance (Cl_R), and hepatic clearance (Cl_h) can be calculated according to the following expressions.

$$Cl_T = kV_D \quad \textbf{(12.35)}$$

$$Cl_R = k_e V_D \quad \textbf{(12.36)}$$

$$Cl_h = k_m V_D \quad \textbf{(12.37)}$$

Total body clearance (Cl_T) is equal to the sum of renal clearance and hepatic clearance and is based on the concept that the entire body acts as a drug-eliminating system.

$$Cl_T = Cl_R + Cl_h \quad \textbf{(12.38)}$$

By substitution of Equations 12.35 and 12.36 into Equation 12.38,

$$kV_D = k_e V_D + k_m V_D \quad \textbf{(12.39)}$$

Dividing by V_D on both sides of Equation 12.39,

$$k = k_e + k_m \quad \textbf{(12.40)}$$

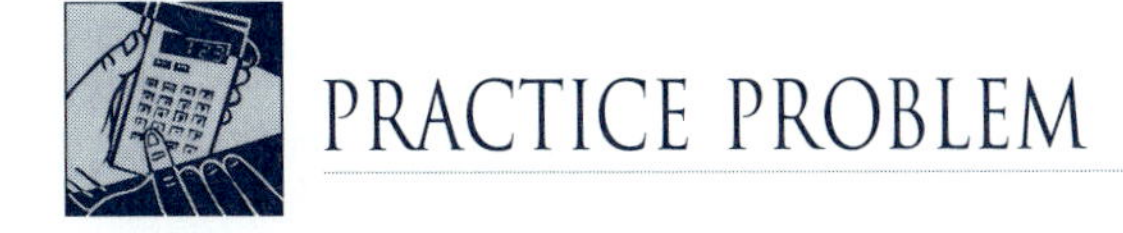

PRACTICE PROBLEM

Consider a drug that is eliminated by first-order renal excretion and hepatic metabolism. The drug follows a one-compartment model and is given in a single intravenous or oral dose (Fig. 12-12).

Working with the model presented in Figure 12-12, assume that a single dose (100 mg) of this drug is given orally. The drug is 90% systemically available. The total amount of unchanged drug recovered in the urine is 60 mg, and the total amount of metabolite recovered in the urine is 30 mg (expressed as mg equivalents to the parent drug). According to the literature, the elimination half-life for this drug is 3.3 hr and its apparent volume of distribution is 1000 mL. From the information given, find (a) the total body clearance, (b) the renal clearance, and (c) the nonrenal clearance of the drug.

Solution

a. Total body clearance:

$$Cl_T = kV_D$$

$$Cl_T = \frac{0.693}{3.3}(1000) = 210 \text{ mL/hr}$$

b. Renal clearance. First find k_e:

$$\frac{k_e}{k} = \frac{D_u^\infty}{FD_0} = \frac{D_u^\infty}{M_u^\infty + D_u^\infty} \tag{12.41}$$

$$k_e = \left(\frac{0.693}{3.3}\right)\left(\frac{60}{30 + 60}\right) = 0.14 \text{ hr}^{-1}$$

Then, from Equation 12.36,

$$Cl_R = k_e V_D$$
$$Cl_R = (0.14)\ (1000) = 140 \text{ mL/hr}$$

c. Nonrenal clearance:

$$Cl_h = Cl_T - Cl_R$$
$$Cl_h = 210 - 140 = 70 \text{ mL/hr}$$

Alternatively,

$$\begin{aligned} k_m &= k - k_e \\ &= 0.21 - 0.14 = 0.07 \text{ hr}^{-1} \\ &= k\left(\frac{M_u^\infty}{M_u^\infty + D_u^\infty}\right) \\ &= 0.21\left(\frac{30}{30 + 60}\right) = 0.07 \text{ hr}^{-1} \end{aligned}$$

Because (Eq. 12.37)

$$Cl_h = k_m V_D$$
$$Cl_h = (0.07)(1000) = 70 \text{ mL/hr}$$

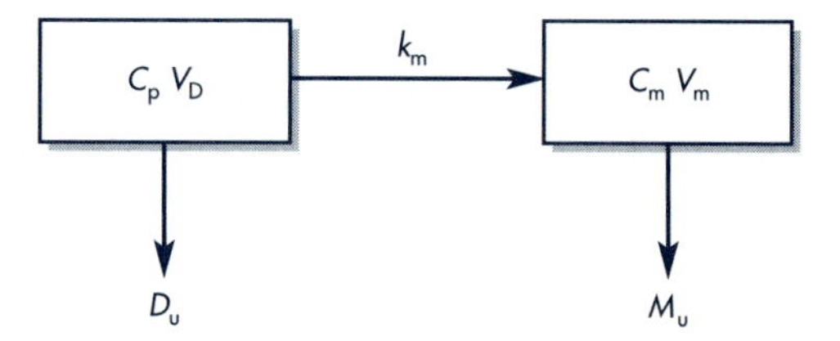

Figure 12-12. Model of a drug eliminated by first-order renal excretion and hepatic metabolism. (k_e = renal excretion rate constant of parent drug, k_m = metabolism rate constant [conversion of parent drug to metabolite], k_u = renal excretion rate constant of metabolite, D_u = amount of unchanged drug in urine, M_u = amount of metabolite in urine, C_m = plasma concentration of the metabolite, C_p = plasma concentration of the parent drug, V_D = apparent volume of distribution of parent drug, V_m = apparent volume of distribution of metabolite.)

Protein-Bound Drugs

Protein-bound drugs are not eliminated by glomerular filtration. Therefore, Equation 12.18 for the calculation of renal clearance must be modified, because only the free drug is excreted by a linear process. The bound drugs are usually excreted by active secretion, following capacity-limited kinetics. The determination of clearance that separates the two components would result in a hybrid clearance. There is no simple way to overcome this problem. Clearance values for the protein-bound drug are therefore calculated with the following equation.

$$Cl_R = \frac{\text{rate of unbound drug excretion}}{\text{concentration of unbound drug in the plasma}} \quad \textbf{(12.42)}$$

In practice, this equation is not easily applied because the rate of drug excretion is usually determined after collecting urine samples. The drug excreted in the urine is the sum of drug excreted by active tubular secretion and by passive glomerular filtration. However, it is not possible to distinguish the amount of bound drug actively secreted from the amount of drug excreted by glomerular filtration. Equation 12.42 can be used for drugs that are protein bound but not actively secreted. Nonlinear drug binding would make clearance less useful due to model complication.

Equation 12.42 is also used in the calculation of free drug concentration in the plasma, where α is the fraction of bound drug and $1 - \alpha$ is the fraction of free drug.

$$(1 - \alpha)\, C_{p,\text{total}} = C_{p,\text{free}} \quad \textbf{(12.43)}$$

For most drug studies, the total plasma drug concentration (free plus bound drug) is used in clearance calculations. If renal clearance is corrected for the fraction of drug bound to plasma proteins using Equation 12.43, then the renal clearance for the free drug concentration will have a higher value compared to the uncorrected renal clearance using the total plasma drug concentrations.

Plasma protein binding has very little effect on the renal clearance of actively secreted drugs such as penicillin. For these drugs the free drug fraction is filtered at the glomerular; whereas the protein-bound drug appears to be stripped from the binding sites and actively secreted into the renal tubules.

Body Clearance for Drugs That Follow the Two-Compartment Model

Clearance is a direct measure of elimination from the central compartment regardless of the number of compartments. The central compartment consists of the plasma and highly perfused tissues in which drug equilibrates rapidly. The tissues for drug elimination, namely kidney and liver, are considered integral parts of the central compartment.

The first-order elimination rate constant k is a useful measurement for drug elimination in a one-compartment model. In multicompartment models, several methods for the estimation of clearance are possible, as shown by Equations 12.44 and 12.45. The overall elimination rate constant k represents elimination from the central compartment, and total body clearance is the product of k times the volume of the central compartment, V_p. Alternatively, total body clearance may be estimated according to Equation 12.45 as the product by the elimination rate constant b times $V_{D\beta}$. This latter method gives the same value for clearance. Other methods for calculating total body clearance considers either instantaneous clearance or steady-state clearance depending on which volume of distribution is chosen. Generally, the various calculations of total body clearance for drugs characterized by multicompartment pharmacokinetics are useful for comparison purposes. For the two-compartment model drug, body clearance can be calculated with the following equation:

$$Cl_T = kV_p \tag{12.44}$$

or, alternatively,

$$Cl_T = bV_{D\beta} \tag{12.45}$$

To obtain renal clearance for drugs demonstrating two-compartment kinetics with metabolism and excretion, the following equation is used:

$$Cl_R = k_e V_p \tag{12.46}$$

Fraction of Drug Excreted

For many drugs the total amount of unchanged drug, D_u^∞, excreted in the urine may be obtained by direct assay. The ratio of D_u^∞, to the fraction of the dose absorbed, FD_0, is equal to the fraction of drug excreted unchanged in the urine and is also equal to k_e/k.

$$\text{Fraction of drug excreted unchanged in the urine} = fe = \frac{D_u^\infty}{FD_0} = \frac{k_e}{k} \tag{12.47}$$

Renal clearance may be determined from the fraction of unchanged drug excreted in the urine and the total body clearance.

$$Cl_R = \frac{D_u^\infty}{FD_0} Cl_T = f_e Cl_T \tag{12.48}$$

Equation 12.48 can also be expressed as

$$Cl_R = \frac{k_e}{k} Cl_T \tag{12.49}$$

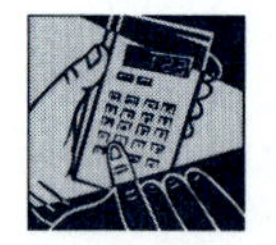

PRACTICE PROBLEM

An antibiotic is given by IV bolus injection at a dose of 500 mg. The apparent volume of distribution was 21 liters and the elimination half-life was 6 hours. Urine was collected for 48 hours, and 400 mg of unchanged drug was recovered. What is the fraction of the dose excreted unchanged in the urine? Calculate k, k_e, Cl_T, Cl_R, and Cl_h.

Solution

Since the elimination half-life, $t_{1/2}$, for this drug is 6 hours, a urine collection for 48 hours represents $8t_{1/2}$, which allows for greater than 99% of the drug to be eliminated from the body. The fraction of drug excreted unchanged in the urine, f_e, is obtained by using Equation 12.47 and recalling that $F = 1$ for drugs given by IV bolus injections.

$$f_e = \frac{400}{500} = 0.8$$

Therefore, 80% of the absorbed dose is excreted in the urine unchanged. Calculations for k, k_e, Cl_T, Cl_R, and Cl_h are given here.

$$k = \frac{0.693}{6} = 0.1155\ \text{hr}^{-1}$$

$$k_e = f_e k = (0.8)(0.1155) = 0.0924\ \text{hr}^{-1}$$

$$Cl_T = (0.1155)(21) = 2.43\ \text{L/hr}$$

$$Cl_R = f_e Cl_T = (0.8)(2.43) = 1.94\ \text{L/hr}$$

Alternatively,

$$Cl_R = k_e V_D = (0.0924)\ (21) = 1.94\ \text{L/hr}$$

$$Cl_h = Cl_T - Cl_R = 2.43 - 1.94 = 0.49\ \text{L/hr}$$

Total Body Clearance of Drugs After Intravenous Infusion

When drugs are administered by intravenous infusion (Chapter 14), the total body clearance is obtained with the following equation.

$$Cl_T = \frac{R}{C_{ss}} \quad \textbf{(12.50)}$$

where C_{ss} is the steady-state plasma drug concentration and R is the rate of infusion. Equation 12.50 is valid for drugs that follow either the one- or two-compartment open model (see Chapter 14).

Clearance for Drugs Involving Active Secretion

At low drug plasma concentrations, active secretion is not saturated, and the drug is excreted by filtration and active secretion. At high concentrations, the percentage of drug excreted by active secretion decreased due to saturation. Clearance decreases because excretion rate decreases (Fig. 12-11). Clearance decreases since the total excretion rate of the drug increases to the point where it is approximately equal to the filtration rate (Fig. 12-13).

RELATIONSHIP OF CLEARANCE ELIMINATION HALF-LIFE, AND VOLUME OF DISTRIBUTION

The half-life of a drug can be determined if the clearance and V_D are known. From Equation 12.35 we obtain

$$Cl_T = kV_D$$

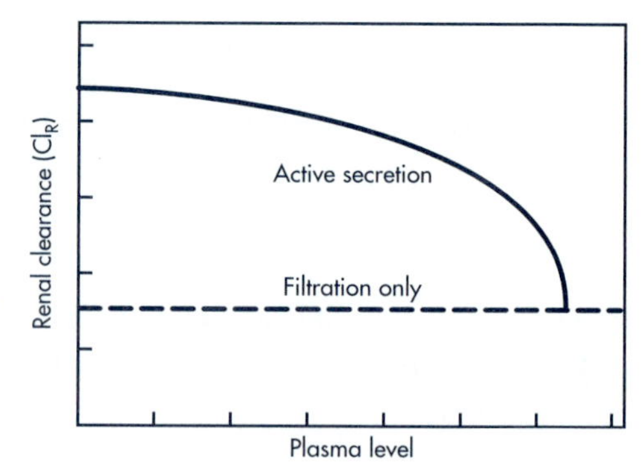

Figure 12-13. Graph representing the decline of renal clearance. As the drug plasma level increases to a concentration that saturates the active tubular secretion, glomerular filtration becomes the major component for renal clearance.

and

$$k = \frac{0.693}{t_{1/2}}$$

Therefore, by substitution,

$$Cl_T = \frac{0.693\, V_D}{t_{1/2}} \quad \textbf{(12.51)}$$

$$t_{1/2} = \frac{0.693\, V_D}{Cl_T}$$

From Equation 12.51, as Cl_T decreases, which might happen in the case of renal insufficiency, the $t_{1/2}$ for the drug increases. A good relationship of V_D, k, and $t_{1/2}$ is shown in Table 12.5.

Total body clearance, Cl_T, is a more useful index of measurement of drug removal compared to the elimination half-life, $t_{1/2}$. Total body clearance takes into account changes in both the apparent volume of distribution, V_D, and the $t_{1/2}$. In overt obesity or edematous conditions, the V_D may change without a marked change in the $t_{1/2}$. As will be shown in Chapters 14 and 15, the V_D is important in the calculation of the loading dose, whereas the Cl_T is important in the calculation of the maintenance dose.

TABLE 12.5 Relationships of Clearance, Rate Constant of Elimination, and Elimination Half-Life

	MEDIUM OF DISTRIBUTION		
CLEARANCE[a]	**PLASMA WATER (3000 mL)**	**EXTRACELLULAR FLUID (12,000 mL)**	**BODY WATER (41,000 mL)**
Partial reabsorption (eg, 30 mL/min)	1.00×10^{-2} (69 min)	2.50×10^{-3} (277 min)	7.32×10^{-4} (947 min)
Glomerular filtration (eg, 130 mL/min)	4.33×10^{-2} (16 min)	1.08×10^{-2} (64 min)	3.17×10^{-3} (219 min)
Tubular secretion (eg, 650 mL/min)	2.17×10^{-1} (3 min)	5.42×10^{-2} (13 min)	1.59×10^{-2} (44 min)

[a]Entries are values for k_e, the rate constant of elimination (in units of min^{-1}); parenthetic entries are corresponding values of the elimination half-life. The clearance given under "partial reabsorption" is arbitrary; any clearance between 0 (complete reabsorption) and 650 mL/min is possible.

From Goldstein et al (1974), with permission.

Total body clearance may be calculated by the ratio $FD_0/[\text{AUC}]_0^\infty$, which is considered a *model-independent method* and assumes no particular pharmacokinetic model for drug elimination.

$$Cl_T = \frac{FD_0}{[\text{AUC}]_0^\infty} \tag{12.52}$$

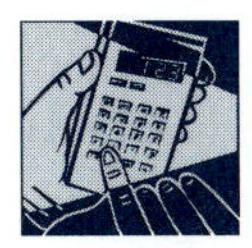

PRACTICE PROBLEMS

A new antibiotic is actively secreted by the kidney and V_D is 35 L in the normal adult. The clearance of this drug is 650 mL/min.

1. What is the usual $t_{1/2}$ for this drug?

$$t_{1/2} = \frac{0.693(35000 \text{ mL})}{650 \text{ mL/min}}$$

$$t_{1/2} = 37.3 \text{ min}$$

2. What would be the new $t_{1/2}$ for this drug in an adult with partial renal failure whose clearance of the antibiotic was only 75 mL/min?

Solution

$$t_{1/2} = \frac{0.693(35000 \text{ mL})}{75 \text{ mL/min}}$$

$$t_{1/2} = 323 \text{ min}$$

In patients with renal impairment the $t_{1/2}$ generally changes more drastically than the V_D. The clearance given under partial reabsorption in Table 12.5 is arbitrary; any clearance between 0 (complete reabsorption) and 650 mL/min is possible.

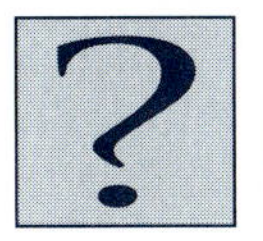

FREQUENTLY ASKED QUESTIONS

1. Is clearance a better parameter to describe drug elimination than half-life? Why is it necessary to use both parameters in the literature?

2. What is an independent parameter in a model? Is clearance an independent parameter of the physiologic model? How is clearance related to parameters in the compartment model?

3. What is the difference between drug clearance and creatinine clearance?

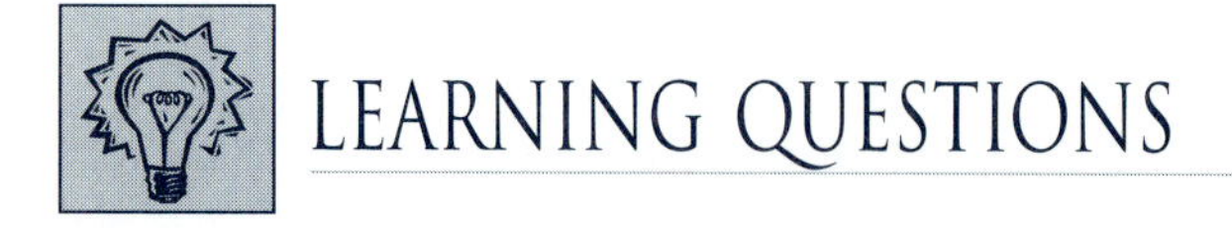

LEARNING QUESTIONS

1. Explain why plasma protein binding will prolong the renal clearance of a drug that is excreted only by glomerular filtration but does not affect the renal clearance of a drug excreted by both glomerular filtration *and* active tubular secretion.

2. Explain the effect of alkalization or acidification of the urine on the renal clearance of dextroamphetamine sulfate. Dextroamphetamine sulfate is a weak base with a pK_a of 9.4.

3. Theophylline is effective in the treatment of bronchitis at a blood level of 10 to 20 μg/mL. At therapeutic range, theophylline follows first-order kinetics. The average $t_{1/2}$ is 3.4 hours, and the range is 1.8 to 6.8 hours. The average volume of distribution is 30 liters.
   a. What are the average, upper, and lower clearance limits for theophylline?
   b. The renal clearance of theophylline is 0.36 L/hr. What are the k_m and k_e, assuming all nonrenal clearance (Cl_{NR}) is due to metabolism?

4. A single 250-mg oral dose of an antibiotic is given to a young man (age 32 years, creatinine clearance 122 mL/min, 78 kg). From the literature, the drug is known to have an apparent V_D equal to 21% of body weight and an elimination half-life of 2 hours. The dose is normally 90% bioavailable. Urinary excretion of the unchanged drug is equal to 70% of the absorbed dose.
   a. What is the total body clearance for this drug?
   b. What is the renal clearance for this drug?
   c. What is the probable mechanism for renal clearance of this drug?

5. A drug with an elimination half-life of 1 hour was given to a male patient (80 kg) by intravenous infusion at a rate of 300 mg/hr. At 7 hours after infusion, the plasma drug concentration was 11 μg/mL.
   a. What is the total body clearance for this drug?
   b. What is the apparent V_D for this drug?
   c. If the drug is not metabolized and is eliminated only by renal excretion, what is the renal clearance of this drug?
   d. What is the probable mechanism for renal clearance of this drug?

6. In order to rapidly estimate the renal clearance of a drug in a patient, a 2-hour postdose urine sample was collected and found to contain 200 mg of drug. A midpoint plasma sample was taken (1 hr postdose) and the drug concentration in plasma was found to be 2.5 mg%. Estimate the renal clearance for this drug in the patient.

7. According to the manufacturer, the antibiotic, cephradine (Velosef, Squibb), when given by IV infusion at rate of 5.3 mg/kg hr to 9 adult male volunteers (average weight, 71.7 kg), a steady-state serum concentration of 17 μg/mL was measured. Calculate the average total body clearance for this drug in adults.

8. Cephradine is completely excreted unchanged in the urine, and studies have shown that probenecid given concurrently causes elevation of the serum cephradine concentration. What is the probable mechanism for the interaction of probenecid with cephradine?

9. Why is clearance used as a measurement of drug elimination rather than the excretion rate of the drug?

10. What is the advantage of using total body clearance as a measurement of drug elimination compared to using the elimination half-life of the drug?

11. A patient was given 2500 mg of a drug by IV bolus dose, and periodic urinary data was collected. (1) Determine the renal clearance of the drug using urinary data. (2) Determine total body clearance using area method. (3) Is there any nonrenal clearance of the drug in this patient? What would be the nonrenal clearance if any? How would you determine clearance using a compartmental approach and compare that with the area method?

Time (hr)	Plasma Concentration (μg/mL)	Urinary Volume (mL)	Urinary Concentration (μg/mL)
0	250.00	100.00	0.00
1	198.63	125.00	2880.00
2	157.82	140.00	1901.20
3	125.39	100.00	2114.80
4	99.63	80.00	2100.35
5	79.16	250.00	534.01
6	62.89	170.00	623.96
7	49.97	160.00	526.74
8	39.70	90.00	744.03
9	31.55	400.00	133.01
10	25.06	240.00	176.13

REFERENCES

Goldstein A, Aronow L, Kalman SM: *Principles of Drug Action.* New York, Wiley, 1974

Guyton AC: *Textbook of Medical Physiology,* 8th ed. Philadelphia, Saunders, 1991

Levine RR: *Pharmacology: Drug Actions and Reactions,* 4th ed. Boston, Little, Brown, 1990

West JB (ed): *Best and Taylor's Physiological Basis of Medical Practice,* 11th ed. Baltimore, Williams & Wilkins, 1985, p 451

BIBLIOGRAPHY

Cafruny EJ: Renal tubular handling of drugs. *Am J Med* **62:**490–496, 1977

Hewitt WR, Hook JB: The renal excretion of drugs. In Bridges VW, Chasseaud LF (eds), *Progress in Drug Metabolism,* vol. 7. New York, Wiley, 1983, chap 1

Renkin EM, Robinson RR: Glomerular filtration. *N Engl J Med* **290:**785–792, 1974

Rowland M, Benet LZ, Graham GG: Clearance concepts in pharmacokinetics. *J Pharm Biopharm* **1:**123–136, 1973

Smith H: *The Kidney: Structure and Function in Health and Disease.* New York, Oxford, 1951

Thomson P, Melmon K, Richardson J, et al: Lidocaine pharmacokinetics in advanced heart failure, liver disease and renal failure in humans. *Ann Intern Med* **78:**499–508, 1973

Tucker GT: Measurement of the renal clearance of drugs. *Br J Clin Pharm* **12:**761–770, 1981

Weiner IM, Mudge GH: Renal tubular mechanisms for excretion and organic acids and bases. *Am J Med* **36:**743–762, 1964

Wilkinson GR: Clearance approaches in pharmacology. *Pharmacol Rev* **39:**1–47, 1987

13

HEPATIC ELIMINATION OF DRUGS

The elimination of most drugs from the body involves the processes of both metabolism (biotransformation) and excretion. The rate constant of elimination (k) is the sum of the first-order rate constant for metabolism (k_{m}) and the first-order rate constant for excretion (k_{e}).

$$k = k_{\mathrm{e}} + k_{\mathrm{m}} \tag{13.1}$$

Because a drug may be biotransformed to several metabolites (metabolite A, metabolite B, metabolite C, etc), the metabolism rate constant (k_{m}) is the sum of the rate constants for the formation of each metabolite.

$$k_{\mathrm{m}} = k_{\mathrm{m}A} + k_{\mathrm{m}B} + k_{\mathrm{m}C} + \cdots + k_{\mathrm{m}I} \tag{13.2}$$

The relationship in this equation assumes that the process of metabolism is first order and that the substrate (drug) concentration is very low. Drug concentrations at therapeutic plasma levels for most drugs are much lower than the Michaelis–Menten constant and do not saturate the enzymes involved in metabolism.

Because these rates of elimination are considered first-order processes, the percentage of total drug metabolized may be found by the following expression:

$$\%\ \text{drug metabolized} = \frac{k_m}{k} \times 100 \tag{13.3}$$

In practice, the excretion rate constant (k_{e}) is easily evaluated for drugs that are primarily renal excreted. *Nonrenal drug elimination* is usually assumed to be due for the most part to hepatic metabolism. The rate constant for metabolism (k_{m}) is difficult to measure directly and is usually found by the difference of k and k_{e}.

$$k_{\mathrm{m}} = k - k_{\mathrm{e}}$$

FRACTION OF DRUG EXCRETED UNCHANGED (f_e) AND FRACTION OF DRUG METABOLIZED ($1 - f_e$)

For most drugs, the fraction of dose eliminated unchanged (f_e) and the fraction eliminated as metabolites can be determined. For example, consider a drug that has two major metabolites and is also eliminated by renal excretion (Fig. 13-1). Assume that 100 μM of the drug was given to a patient and the drug was completely absorbed (bioavailability factor, $F = 1$). A complete (cumulative) urine collection was obtained, and the quantities in parentheses indicate the amounts of each metabolite and unchanged drug that were recovered. The overall elimination half-life ($t_{1/2}$) for this drug was 2.0 hrs ($k = 0.347\ \text{hr}^{-1}$).

To determine the renal excretion rate constant, the following relationship is used.

$$\frac{k_e}{k} = \frac{D_u^\infty}{\text{total dose absorbed}} = \frac{D_u^\infty}{FD_0} \tag{13.4}$$

where D_u^∞ is the total amount of unchanged drug recovered in the urine. In this example, k_e is found by proper substitution into Equation 13.4.

$$k_e = (0.347)\frac{70}{100} = 0.243\ \text{hr}^{-1}$$

To find the percent of drug eliminated by renal excretion, the following approach may be used:

$$\%\ \text{drug excretion} = \frac{k_e}{k} \times 100$$
$$= \frac{0.243}{0.347} \times 100 = 70\%$$

Alternatively, because 70 μM of unchanged drug was recovered from a total dose of 100 μM, the percent of drug excretion may be found by:

$$\%\ \text{drug excretion} = \frac{70}{100} \times 100 = 70\%$$

Therefore, the percent of drug metabolized is 100% minus 70%, or 30%.

For many drugs, approximate literature values are available for the fraction of drug (f_e) excreted unchanged in the urine. In this example, the value of k_e may

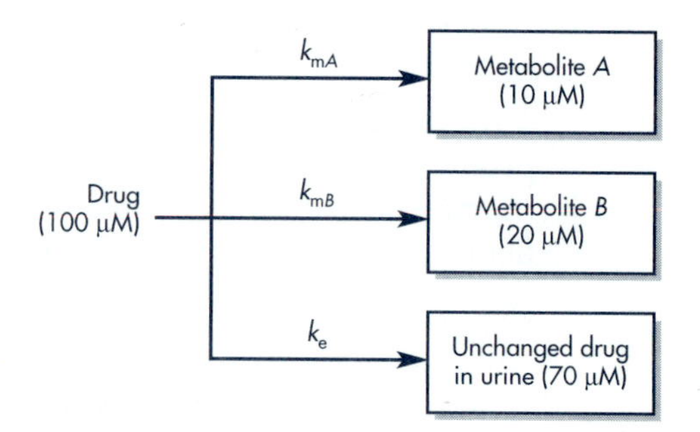

Figure 13-1. Model of a drug that has two major metabolites and is also eliminated by renal excretion.

be estimated from the literature values for the elimination half-life of the drug and $= f_e$, respectively. Assuming the elimination half-life of the drug is 2 hrs and f_e is 0.7, then k_e is estimated by Equation 13.5.

$$k_e = f_e k \tag{13.5}$$

Because $t_{1/2}$ is 2 hrs, k is $0.693/2$ hr $= 0.347$ hr^{-1}, and k_e is

$$k_e = (0.7)(0.347) = 0.243 \text{ hr}^{-1}$$

CLINICAL FOCUS

The percentages of drug excretion and metabolism are clinically useful information. If the renal excretion pathway becomes impaired as in the case of certain kidney disorders, then less drug will be excreted renally and hepatic metabolism may become the primary drug elimination route. The reverse is true if liver function declines. For example, if in the above situation renal excretion becomes totally impaired ($k_e \approx 0$), the elimination $t_{1/2}$ can be determined as follows.

$$k = k_m + k_e$$

but

$$k_e \approx 0$$

Therefore,

$$k \approx k_m \approx 0.104 \text{ hr}^{-1}$$

The new $t_{1/2}$ (after complete renal shutdown) is:

$$t_{1/2} = \frac{0.693}{0.104} = 6.7 \text{ hr}$$

In this example, renal impairment caused the drug elimination $t_{1/2}$ to be prolonged from 2 to 6.7 hours. Clinically, the dosage of this drug must be lowered to prevent the accumulation of toxic drug levels. Methods for adjusting the dose for renal impairment are discussed in Chapter 18.

PHARMACOKINETICS OF DRUGS AND METABOLITES

Enzyme Kinetics

The process of *biotransformation* or *metabolism* is the enzymatic conversion of a drug to a metabolite. In the body, the metabolic enzyme concentration is constant at a given site, and the drug (substrate) concentration may vary. When the drug concentration is low relative to the enzyme concentration, there are abundant enzymes to catalyze the reaction, and the rate of metabolism is a first-order process. *Saturation* of the enzyme occurs when the drug concentration is high, all the enzyme molecules become complexed with drug, and the reaction rate is at a maximum rate; the rate process then becomes a zero-order process (Fig. 13-2). The maximum reaction rate is known as the V_{max}, and the substrate or drug concen-

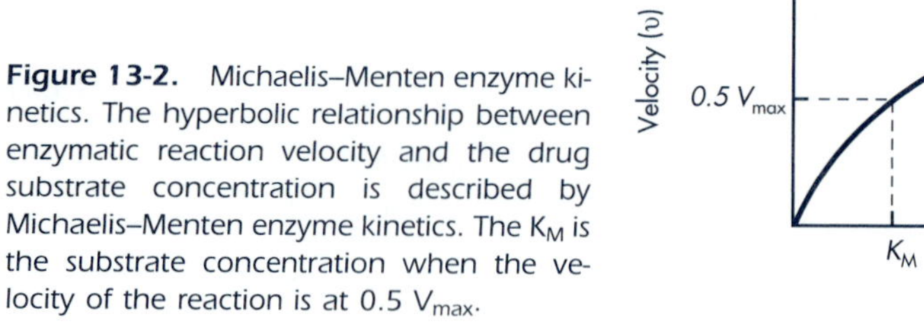
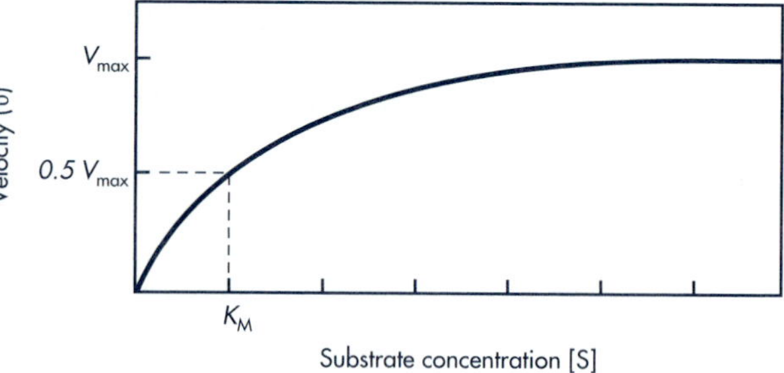

Figure 13-2. Michaelis–Menten enzyme kinetics. The hyperbolic relationship between enzymatic reaction velocity and the drug substrate concentration is described by Michaelis–Menten enzyme kinetics. The K_M is the substrate concentration when the velocity of the reaction is at $0.5\ V_{max}$.

tration at which the reaction occurs at half the maximum rate is known as K_M. These two parameters determine the profile of a simple enzyme reaction rate at various drug concentrations. The relationship of these parameters is described by the *Michaelis–Menten equation.*

Enzyme kinetics generally considers that one mole of drug interacts with one mole of enzyme to form an enzyme–drug (ie, enzyme–substrate) intermediate. The enzyme–drug intermediate further reacts to yield a reaction product or a drug metabolite (Fig. 13-3). The rate process for drug metabolism is described by the Michaelis–Menten equation, which assumes that the rate of an enzymatic reaction is dependent upon the concentrations of both the enzyme and the drug and that an energetically favored drug–enzyme intermediate is initially formed which is followed by the formation of the product and regeneration of the enzyme.

Each rate constant in Figure 13-3 is a first-order reaction rate constant. The following rates may be written.

Rate of intermediate (ED) formation $= k_1(E)(D)$

Rate of intermediate (ED) decomposition $= k_2(ED) + k_3(ED)$

$$d(ED)/dt = k_1(E)(D) - k_2(ED) - k_3(ED)$$

$$= k_1(E)(D) - (k_2 + k_3)(ED) \quad \textbf{(13.6)}$$

By mass balance, the total enzyme concentration (E_t) is the sum of the free enzyme concentration (E) and the enzyme–drug intermediate (ED).

$$(E_t) = (E) + (ED) \quad \textbf{(13.7)}$$

Rearranging,

$$(E) = (E_t) - (ED) \quad \textbf{(13.8)}$$

Substituting for (E) into Equation 13.6,

$$d(ED)/dt = k_1[(E_t) - (ED)(D)] - (k_2 + k_3)(ED) \quad \textbf{(13.9)}$$

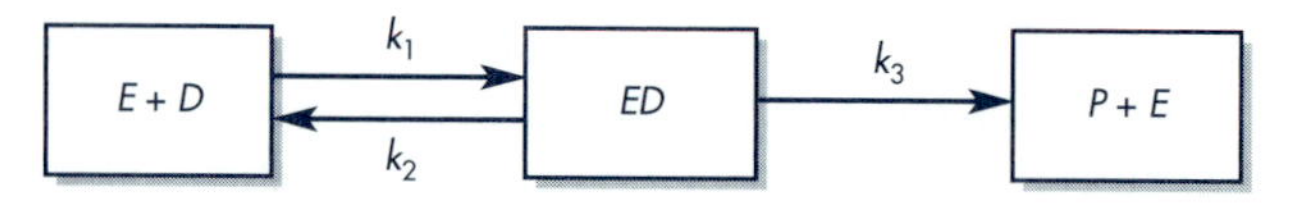

Figure 13-3. (D) = drug; (E) = enzyme; (ED) = drug–enzyme intermediate; (P) = metabolite or product; k_1, k_2, and k_3 = first-order rate constants. Parentheses denote concentration.

At steady state, the *ED* concentration is constant with respect to time, because the rate of formation of the drug–enzyme intermediate equals the rate of decomposition of the drug–enzyme intermediate. Thus, $d(ED)/dt = 0$, and

$$k_1(E_t)(D) = (ED)(k_1(D) + (k_2 + k_3)) \quad \textbf{(13.10)}$$

$$(E_t)(D) = (ED)(D + (k_2 + k_3)/k_1) \quad \textbf{(13.11)}$$

Let

$$K_M = (k_2 + k_3)/k_1 \quad \textbf{(13.12)}$$

$$(E_t)(D) = (ED)((D) + K_M) \quad \textbf{(13.13)}$$

Solve for (ED)

$$(ED) = (D)(E_t)/((D) + K_M) \quad \textbf{(13.14)}$$

Multiply by k_3 on both sides,

$$k_3(E_t)(D)/((D) + K_M) = k_3(ED) \quad \textbf{(13.15)}$$

When all the enzyme is saturated (ie, all the enzyme is in the form of the *ES* intermediate) due to a large drug concentration, the reaction is dependent upon the availability of free enzyme, and the reaction proceeds at the maximum velocity, V_{max}.

$$V_{max} = k_3 E_t \quad \textbf{(13.16)}$$

The velocity or rate (v) of the reaction is the rate for the formation of the product (metabolite), which is also the forward rate of decomposition of the *ES* intermediate (Fig. 13-3).

$$v = k_3(ED) \quad \textbf{(13.17)}$$

Therefore, the velocity of metabolism is given by the equation:

$$v = V_{max}(D)/((D) + K_M) \quad \textbf{(13.18)}$$

Equation 13.18 describes the rate of metabolite formation, or the Michaelis–Menten equation. The maximum velocity (V_{max}) corresponds to the rate when all of the available enzyme is in the form of the drug enzyme (ED) intermediate. At V_{max}, the drug (substrate) concentration is in excess, and the forward reaction, $k_3(ED)$, is dependent on the availability of more free enzyme molecules. The *Michaelis constant*, K_M, is defined as the substrate concentration when the velocity (v) of the reaction is equal to one-half maximal velocity, or 0.5 V_{max} (Fig. 13-2). The K_M is a useful parameter that reveals the concentration of the substrate at which the reaction occurs at half V_{max}. In general, for a drug with a large K_M, a greater concentration will be necessary before saturation is reached.

The Michaelis–Menten equation assumes that one drug molecule is catalyzed sequentially by one enzyme at a time. However, enzymes may catalyze more than one drug molecule at a time, which may be demonstrated *in vitro*. In the body, drug may be eliminated by enzymatic reactions (metabolism) to one or more metabolites and by the excretion of the unchanged drug via the kidney. In Chapter 16, the Michaelis–Menton equation is used for modeling drug conversion in the body.

The relationship of the rate of metabolism to the drug concentration is a nonlinear, hyperbolic curve (Fig. 13-3). To estimate the parameters V_{max} and K_M, the reciprocal of the Michaelis–Menten equation is used to obtain a linear relationship.

$$\frac{1}{v} = \frac{K_M}{V_{max}}\frac{1}{(D)} + \frac{1}{V_{max}} \tag{13.19}$$

Equation 13.19 is known as the *Lineweaver–Burk equation*, in which the K_M and V_{max} may be estimated from a plot of $1/v$ versus $1/(D)$ (Fig. 13-4). Although the Lineweaver–Burk equation is widely used, other rearrangements of the Michaelis–Menten equation have been used to obtain more accurate estimates of V_{max} and K_M. In Chapter 16, drug concentration (D) is replaced by C, which represents drug concentration in the body.

Kinetics of Enzyme Inhibition

Many compounds (eg, cimetidine) may inhibit the enzymes that metabolize other drugs in the body. An inhibitor may decrease the rate of drug metabolism by several different mechanisms. The inhibitor may combine with a cofactor such as $NADPH_2$ needed for enzyme activity, interact with the drug or substrate, or interact directly with the enzyme. Enzyme inhibition may be reversible or irreversible. The type of enzyme inhibition is usually classified by enzyme kinetic studies and observing changes in the K_M and V_{max} (Fig. 13-4).

In the case of *competitive enzyme inhibition*, the inhibitor and drug–substrate compete for the same active center on the enzyme. Both the drug and inhibitor may have similar chemical structures. An increase in the drug–substrate concentration may displace the inhibitor from the enzyme and partially or fully reverse the

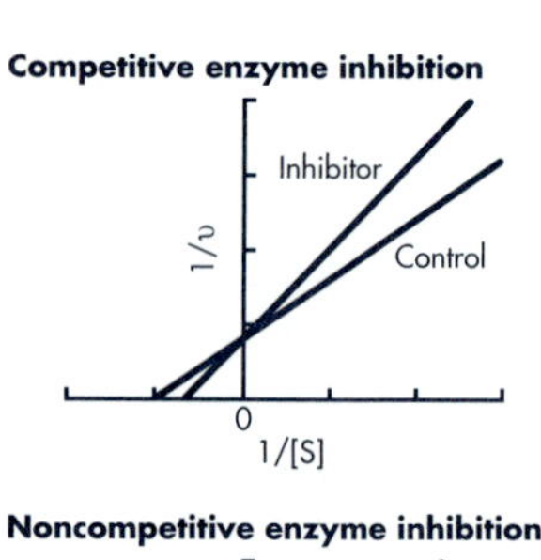

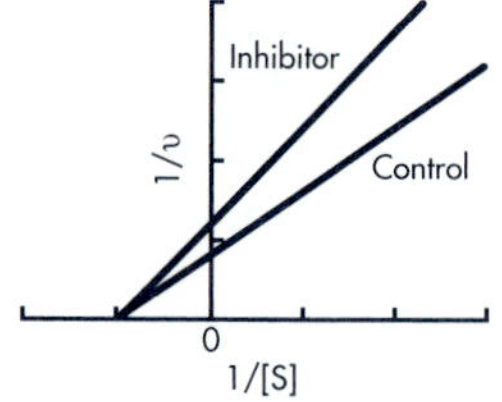

Uncompetitive enzyme inhibition

Inhibitor

Control

1/v

0

1/[S]

Figure 13-4. Lineweaver–Burk plots. The Lineweaver–Burk equation, which is the reciprocal of the Michaelis–Menten equation, is used to obtain estimates of V_{max} and K_M and to distinguish between various types of enzyme inhibition. $[S]$ is the substrate concentration equal to $[D]$ or drug concentration.

inhibition. Competitive enzyme inhibition is usually observed by a change in the K_M, but the V_{max} remains the same.

The equation of competitive inhibition is

$$v = \frac{V_{max}(D)}{(D) + K_M(1 + (I)/k_i)} \tag{13.20}$$

where (I) is the inhibitor concentration and k_i is the inhibition constant.

In *noncompetitive enzyme inhibition*, the inhibitor may inhibit the enzyme by combining at a site on the enzyme that is different from the active site (ie, an allosteric site). In this case, enzyme inhibition depends only upon the inhibitor concentration. In noncompetitive enzyme inhibition, K_M is not altered, but V_{max} is lower. Noncompetitive enzyme inhibition cannot be reversed by increasing the drug–substrate concentration.

For a noncompetitive reaction

$$v = \frac{V_{max}(D)/(1 + (I)/k_i)}{K_M + (D)} \tag{13.21}$$

Other types of enzyme inhibition, such as mixed enzyme inhibition and enzyme uncompetitive inhibition, have been described by observing changes in K_M and V_{max}.

Metabolite Pharmacokinetics for Drugs that Follow a One-Compartment Model

If a drug is given by intravenous bolus injection and the drug is metabolized by more than one parallel pathway (Fig. 13-5), the one-compartment model may be used to estimate simultaneously both metabolite formation and drug decline in the plasma. This method assumes that both metabolites and drug concentrations follow linear (first-order) pharmacokinetics at therapeutic concentrations. The elimination rate constant and the volume of distribution for each metabolite and the parent drug are obtained from curve fitting of the plasma drug concentration versus time and each metabolite concentration versus time curves. If the metabolites are available, each metabolite should be administered IV separately and the pharmacokinetic parameters verified independently.

The rate of elimination of the metabolite may be faster or slower than the rate of formation of the metabolite from the drug. Generally, metabolites, such as glucuronide, sulfate, or glycine conjugates that are more polar or more water soluble than the parent drug, will be eliminated more rapidly than the parent drug. Therefore, the rate of elimination of the metabolite is more rapid than the rate of formation of the metabolite. In contrast, if the drug is acetylated or metabolized to a less polar or less water-soluble metabolite, then the rate of elimination of the metabolite is slower than the rate of formation of the metabolite.

Compartment modeling of drug and metabolites is relatively simple and practical. The major shortcoming of compartment modeling is the lack of realistic physiologic information when compared to more sophisticated models that take into account spatial location of enzymes and flow dynamics. Deterministic compartment models are useful for predicting drug and metabolite plasma levels.

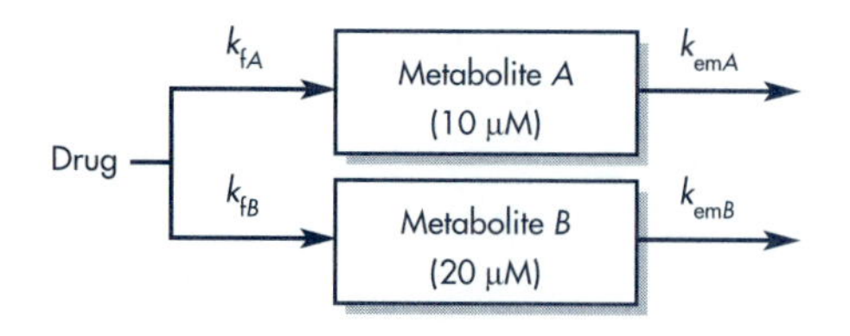

Figure 13-5. Parallel pathway for the metabolism of a drug to metabolite *A* and metabolite *B*. Each metabolite may be excreted and/or further metabolized.

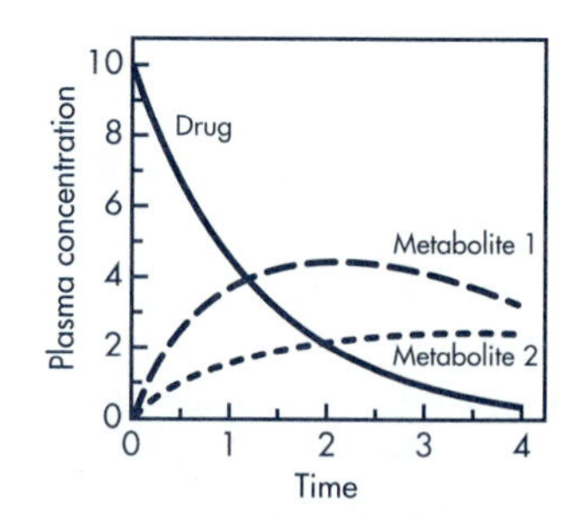

Figure 13-6. Simulation showing an IV bolus with formation of two metabolites.

For a drug given by IV bolus injection, the metabolite concentration may be predicted from the following equation.

$$C_m = \frac{k_f D_0}{V_m (k_f - k_{em})} (e^{-k_{em}t} - e^{-k_f t}) \tag{13.22}$$

where C_m is the metabolite concentration in plasma, k_{em} is the metabolite elimination rate constant, k_f is the metabolite formation rate constant, V_m is the metabolite volume of distribution, D_0 is the dose of drug, and V_D is the apparent volume of distribution of drug. All rate constants are first order.

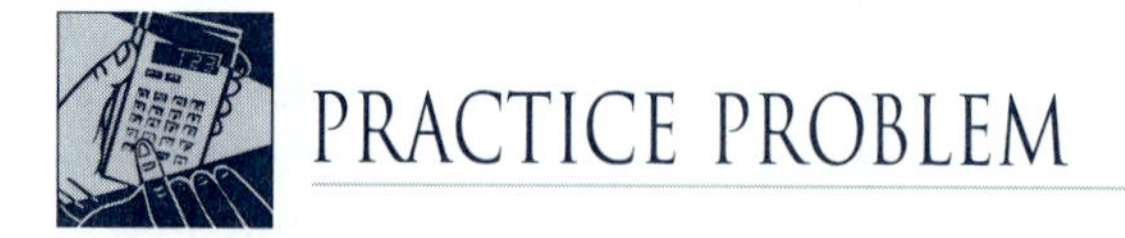

PRACTICE PROBLEM

A drug is eliminated primarily by biotransformation (metabolism) to a glucuronide conjugate and a sulfate conjugate. A single dose (100 mg) of the drug is given by IV bolus injection, and all elimination processes of the drug follow first-order kinetics. The V_D is 10 L and the elimination rate constant for the drug is 0.9 hr^{-1}. The rate constant (k_f) for the formation of the glucuronide conjugate is 0.6 hr^{-1}, and the rate constant for the formation of the sulfate conjugate is 0.2 hr^{-1}.

1. Predict the drug concentration 1 hour after the dose.
2. Predict the concentration of glucuronide and sulfate metabolites at 1 hour after the dose, if the V_m for both metabolites is the same as the parent drug and the k_{em} for both metabolites is 0.4 hr^{-1}. (Note: V_m and k_{em} for each metabolite are usually different and not the same as for the parent drug.) In this example, V_m and k_{em} are assumed to be the same, so that the concentration of the two metabolites may be compared by examining the formation constants.

Solution

The plasma drug concentration at 1 hour after the dose may be estimated using the following equation for a one-compartment model, IV bolus administration:

$$C_p = C_p^0 e^{-kt} = (D_0/V_D)(e^{-kt})$$
$$C_p = (100/10)(e^{-(0.9)(1)}) = 4.1 \text{ mg/L}$$

The plasma concentrations for the glucuronide and sulfate metabolites at 1 hour postdose are estimated after substitution into Equation 13.22.

Glucuronide:

$$C_m = \frac{(0.6)(100)}{10(0.6 - 0.4)}(e^{-(0.4)(1)} - e^{-(0.6)(1)})$$

$$C_m = 3.6 \text{ mg/L}$$

Sulfate:

$$C_m = \frac{(0.2)(100)}{10(0.2 - 0.4)}(e^{-(0.4)(1)} - e^{-(0.2)(1)})$$

$$C_m = 1.5 \text{ mg/L}$$

After an IV bolus dose of a drug, the equation describing metabolite concentration formation and elimination by first-order processes is kinetically analogous to drug absorption after oral administration (Chapter 9). Simulated plasma concentration–time curves were generated using Equation 13.22 for the glucuronide and sulfate metabolites, respectively (Fig. 13-6). The rate constant for the formation of the glucuronide is faster than the rate constant for the formation of the sulfate. Therefore, the time for peak plasma glucuronide concentrations is shorter compared to the time for peak plasma sulfate conjugate concentrations. Equation 13.22 cannot be used if drug metabolism is nonlinear due to enzyme saturation (ie, if metabolism follows Michaelis–Menten kinetics).

Metabolite Pharmacokinetics for Drugs that Follow a Two-Compartment Model

Cephalothin is an antibiotic drug that is metabolized rapidly by hydrolysis in both man and rabbit. The metabolite, desacetylcephalothin, has less antibiotic activity than the parent drug. In urine, 18 to 33% of the drug was recovered as desacetylcephalothin metabolite in man. The time course of both the drug and the metabolite may be predicted after a given dose from the distribution kinetics of both the drug and the metabolite. Cephalothin follows a two-compartment model after IV bolus injection in a rabbit, whereas the desacetylcephalothin metabolite follows a one-compartment model (Figure 13-7). After a single IV bolus dose of cephalothin (20 mg/kg) to a rabbit, cephalothin declines due to excretion and metabolism to desacetylcephalothin. The plasma levels of both cephalothin and desacetylcephalothin may be calculated using the equations based on a model with linear metabolism and excretion.

The equations for cephalothin plasma and tissue levels are the same as those derived in Chapter 4 for a simple two-compartment model, except that the elimination constant k for the drug now consist of $k_e + k_f$, representing excretion and formation constant for metabolite, respectively.

$$C_p = D_0\left[\frac{k_{21} - a}{V_p(b - a)}e^{-at} + \frac{k_{21} - b}{V_p(a - b)}e^{-bt}\right] \quad \textbf{(13.23)}$$

$$C_t = D_0\left[\frac{k_{12}}{V_t(b - a)}e^{-at} + \frac{k_{12}}{V_t(a - b)}e^{-bt}\right] \quad \textbf{(13.24)}$$

$$a + b = k + k_{12} + k_{21} \quad \textbf{(13.25)}$$

$$ab = k_{21}k \quad (13.26)$$
$$k = k_f + k_e \quad (13.27)$$

The equation for metabolite plasma concentration C_m is triexponential, with three preexponential coefficients (C_5, C_6, and C_7) calculated from the various kinetic constants, V_m, and dose of drug.

$$C_m = C_5 e^{-k_u t} + C_6 e^{-at} + C_7 e^{-bt} \quad (13.28)$$
$$C_5 = (k_f D_0 k_{21} - k_f D_0 k_u)/V_m(b - k_u)(a - k_u) \quad (13.29)$$
$$C_6 = (k_f D_0 k_{21} - k_f D_0 a)/V_m(b - a)(k_u - a) \quad (13.30)$$
$$C_7 = (k_f D_0 k_{21} - k_f D_0 b)/V_m(k_u - b)(a - b) \quad (13.31)$$

For example, after the IV administration of cephalothin to a rabbit, both metabolite and plasma cephalothin concentration may be fitted to Equations 13.23 and 13.28 simultaneously (Fig. 13-8), with the following parameters obtained using a regression computer program (all rate constants in min^{-1}).

$k_{12} = 0.052$ $\quad k_{21} = 0.009$ $\quad V_m = 285$ mL/kg
$k_u = 0.079$ $\quad k = 0.067$ $\quad D_0 = 20$ mg/kg
$k_f = 0.045$ $\quad V_p = 548$ mL/kg $\quad k_e = 0.022$

ANATOMY AND PHYSIOLOGY OF THE LIVER

The liver is the major organ responsible for drug metabolism. However, intestinal tissues, lung, kidney, and skin also contain appreciable amounts of biotransformation enzymes, as reflected by animal data (Table 13.1). The liver consists of a large right and left lobe that merges in the middle. The liver is perfused by blood from the hepatic artery; in addition, the large hepatic portal vein that collects blood from various segments of the GI tract also perfuses the liver (Fig. 13-9). The hepatic artery carries oxygen to the liver and accounts for about 25% of the blood supply. The hepatic portal vein carries nutrients and accounts for about 75% of liver blood flow. The terminal branches of the hepatic artery and portal vein fuse within the liver and mix with the sinusoids (Fig. 3-10). Blood leaves the liver via the hepatic vein, which empties into the vena cava (Fig. 13-9). The liver also secretes bile acids within the liver lobes that flow through a network of channels, eventually emptying into the common bile duct (Figs. 13-10 and 13-11). The common bile duct drains bile and biliary excretion products from both lobes into the gallbladder.

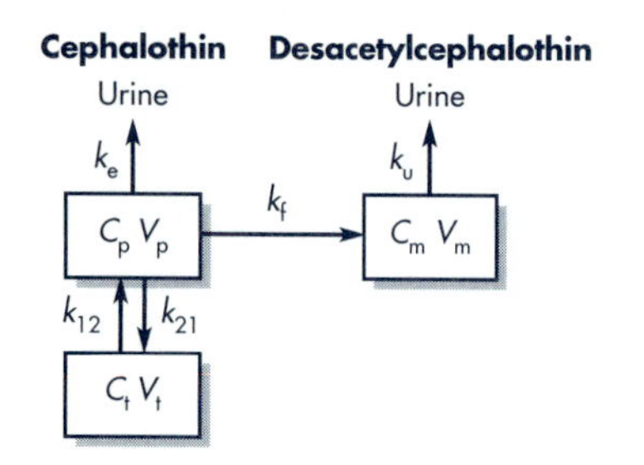

Figure 13-7. Pharmacokinetic model of cephalothin and desacetylcephalothin (metabolite) after an IV bolus dose.

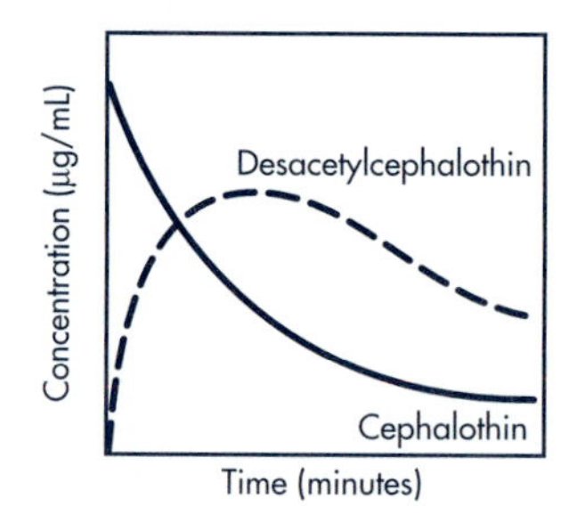

Figure 13-8. Formation of desacetylcephalothin from cephalothin in the rabbit after an IV bolus dose of cephalothin.

TABLE 13.1 Distribution of Cytochrome P-450 and Glutathione S-Transferase in the Rat

TISSUE	CYT P-450[a]	GSH TRANSFERASE[b]
Liver	0.73	599
Lung	0.046	61
Kidney	0.135	88
Small intestine	0.042	103
Colon	0.016	—[c]
Skin	0.12	—[c]
Adrenal gland	0.5	308

[a]Cytochrome P-450, nmole/mg microsome protein.
[b]Glutathione S-transferase, nmole conjugate formed/min/mg cytosolic protein.
[c]Values not available.

Adapted from Wolf (1984), with permission.

The liver is both a synthetic and excreting organ. The basic unit of liver is the liver lobule, which contains parenchymal cells, a network of interconnected lymph and blood vessels. Large vascular capillaries known as sinusoids form a large reservoir of blood, facilitating drug and nutrient removal prior to entering the general circulation. The sinusoids are lined with endothelial cells, or Kupffer cells. *Kupffer cells* are phagocytic tissue macrophages that are part of the reticuloendothelial system (RES). Kupffer cells engulf worn-out red blood cells and foreign material. Drug metabolism in the liver has been shown to be "flow and site dependent." Some enzymes are reached only when blood flow travels from a given direction. The quantity of enzyme involved in metabolizing drug is not uniform throughout the liver.

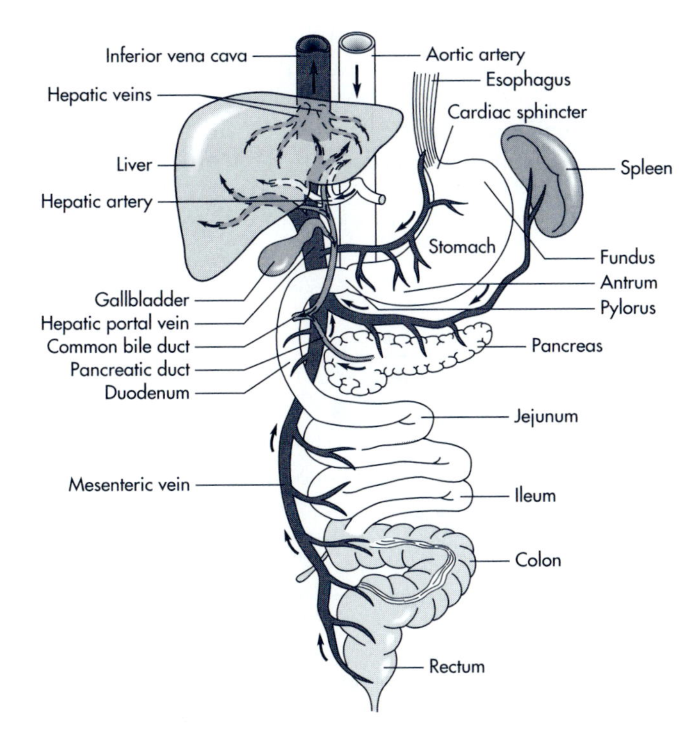

Figure 13-9. The large hepatic portal vein that collects blood from various segments of the GI tract also perfuses the liver.

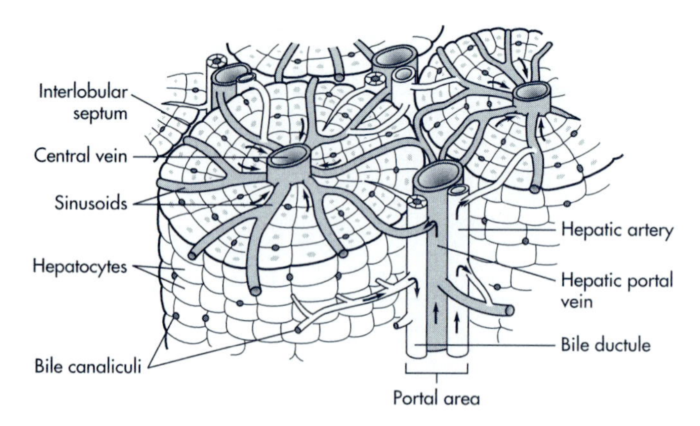

Figure 13-10. Intrahepatic distribution of the hepatic and portal veins.

Consequently, changes in blood flow can greatly affect the fraction of drug metabolized. Clinically, hepatic diseases, such as liver cirrhosis, can cause tissue fibrosis, necrosis, and hepatic shunt, resulting in changing blood flow and changing bioavailability of drugs. For this reason and, in part, because of genetic differences in enzyme levels among different subjects, the half-lives of drugs eliminated by drug metabolism are generally very variable. Realistically, a pharmacokinetic model simulating hepatic metabolism must involve several elements including the heterogenicity of the liver, the hydrodynamics of hepatic blood flow, the nonlinear kinetics of drug metabolism, and any unusual or pathological condition of the subject. Most models in practical use are simple or incomplete models because insufficient information is available on individual patient. For example, the average hepatic blood flow is cited as 1.3 L/min. Actually, hepatic arterial blood flow and hepatic venous (portal) blood enter the liver at different flow rates and their drug concentrations are different. It is possible that a toxic metabolite may be transiently higher in some liver tissues and not in others. The pharmacokinetic challenge is to build models that predict regional (organ) changes from easily accessible data, such as plasma drug concentration.

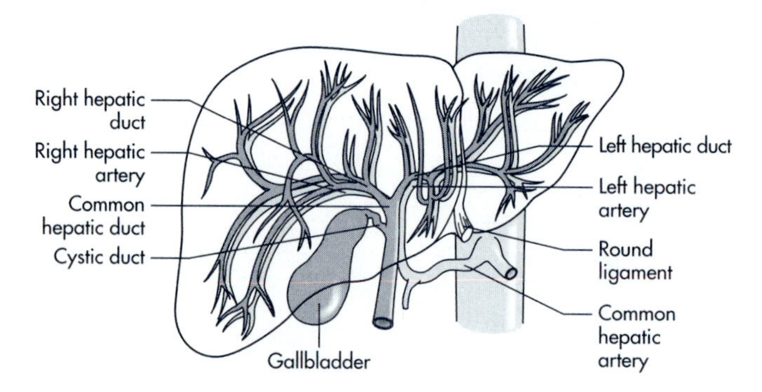

Figure 13-11. Intrahepatic distribution of the hepatic artery, portal vein, and biliary ducts. (From Lindner HH: *Clinical Anatomy*. Norwalk, CT, Appleton & Lange, 1989, with permission.)

HEPATIC ENZYMES INVOLVED IN THE BIOTRANSFORMATION OF DRUGS

Mixed-Function Oxidases

The liver is the major site of drug metabolism, and the type of metabolism is based on the reaction involved. Oxidation, reduction, hydrolysis, and conjugation are the most common reactions, as discussed under phase I and phase II reactions in the next two sections. The enzymes responsible for oxidation and reduction of drugs (*xenobiotics*) and certain natural metabolites, such as steroids, are monoxygenase enzymes known as the *mixed-function oxidases* (MFOs). The hepatic parenchymal cells contain the MFOs in association with the *endoplasmic reticulum*, a network of lipoprotein membranes within the cytoplasm and continuous with the cellular and nuclear membranes. If hepatic parenchymal cells are fragmented and differentially centrifuged in an ultracentrifuge, a microsomal fraction, or *microsome*, is obtained from the postmitochondrial supernatant. The microsomal fraction contains fragments of the endoplasmic reticulum.

The mixed-function oxidase enzymes are structural enzymes that constitute an electron transport system that requires reduced NADPH ($NADPH_2$), molecular oxygen, cytochrome P-450, NADPH-cytochrome P-450 reductase, and phospholipid. The phospholipid is involved in the binding of the drug molecule to the cytochrome P-450 and coupling the NADPH-cytochrome P-450 reductase to the cytochrome P-450. Cytochrome P-450 is a heme protein with iron protoporphyrin IX as the prosthetic group. Cytochrome P-450 is the terminal component of an electron transfer system in the endoplasmic reticulum and acts as both oxygen and substrate binding locus for drugs and endogenous substrates in conjunction with a flavoprotein reductase, NADPH-cytochrome P-450 reductase. Many lipid-soluble drugs bind to cytochrome P-450, resulting in oxidation (or reduction) of the drug. Cytochrome P-450 consists of closely related isoenzymes (isozymes) that differ somewhat in amino acid sequence and drug specificity. A general scheme for MFO drug oxidation is described in Figure 13-12.

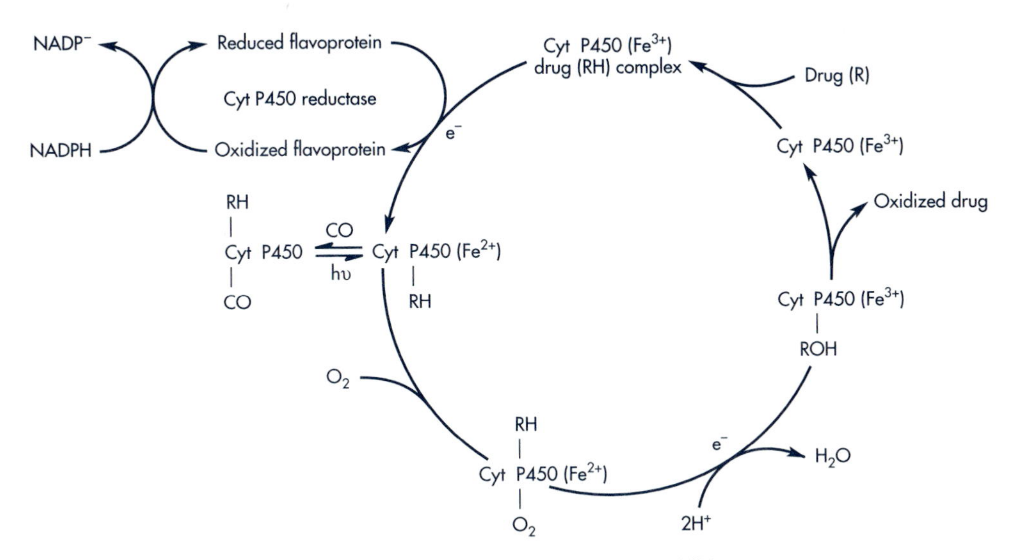

Figure 13-12. Electron flow pathway in the microsomal drug-oxidizing system. (From Alvares & Pratt, 1990, with permission.)

DRUG BIOTRANSFORMATION REACTIONS

The hepatic biotransformation enzymes play an important role for the inactivation and subsequent elimination of drugs not easily cleared through the kidney. For these drugs—such as theophylline, phenytoin, acetaminophen, and others—there is a direct relationship between the rate of drug metabolism (biotransformation) and the elimination half-life for the drug.

For most biotransformation reactions, the metabolite of the drug is more polar than the parent compound. The conversion of a drug to a more polar metabolite enables the drug to be eliminated more quickly than if the drug remained lipid soluble. A lipid-soluble drug crosses cell membranes and is easily reabsorbed by the renal tubular cells, exhibiting a consequent tendency to remain in the body. In contrast, the more polar metabolite does not cross cell membranes easily, is filtered through the glomerulus, is not readily reabsorbed, and is more rapidly excreted in the urine.

The biotransformation of drugs may be classified according to the pharmacologic activity of the metabolite or according to the biochemical mechanism for each biotransformation reaction. For most drugs, biotransformation results in the formation of a more polar metabolite that is pharmacologically inactive and is eliminated more rapidly than the parent drug (Table 13.2). For some drugs the metabolite may be pharmacologically active or produce toxic effects. *Prodrugs* are inactive and must be biotransformed in the body to metabolites that have pharmacologic activity. Initially, prodrugs were discovered by serendipity, as in the case of prontosil, which is reduced to the antibacterial agent sulfanilamide. More recently, prodrugs have been intentionally designed to improve drug stability, increase systemic drug absorption, or to prolong the duration of activity. For example, the antiparkinsonian agent, levodopa, crosses the blood–brain barrier and is then decarboxylated in the brain to L-dopamine, an active neurotransmitter. L-dopamine

TABLE 13.2 Biotransformation Reactions and Pharmacologic Activity of the Metabolite

REACTION		EXAMPLE
	Active Drug to Inactive Metabolite	
Amphetamine	Deamination →	Phenylacetone
Phenobarbital	Hydroxylation →	Hydroxyphenobarbital
	Active Drug to Active Metabolite	
Codeine	Demethylation →	Morphine
Procainamide	Acetylation →	N-acetylprocainamide
Phenylbutazone	Hydroxylation →	Oxyphenbutazone
	Inactive Drug to Active Metabolite	
Hetacillin	Hydrolysis →	Ampicillin
Sulfasalazine	Azoreduction →	Sulfapyridine + 5-aminosalicylic acid
	Active Drug to Reactive Intermediate	
Acetaminophen	Aromatic Hydroxylation →	Reactive metabolite (hepatic necrosis)
Benzo[a]pyrene	Aromatic Hydroxylation →	Reactive metabolite (carcinogenic)

TABLE 13.3 Some Common Drug Biotransformation Reactions

PHASE I REACTIONS	PHASE II REACTIONS
Oxidation	Glucuronide conjugation
Aromatic hydroxylation	Ether glucuronide
Side chain hydroxylation	Ester glucuronide
N-, O-, and S-dealkylation	Amide glucuronide
Deamination	
Sulfoxidation, N-oxidation	Peptide conjugation
N-hydroxylation	
Reduction	Glycine conjugation (hippurate)
Azoreduction	
Nitroreduction	Methylation
Alcohol dehydrogenase	*N*-methylation
Hydrolysis	*O*-methylation
Ester hydrolysis	
Amide hydrolysis	Acetylation
	Sulfate conjugation
	Mercapturic acid synthesis

does not easily penetrate the blood–brain barrier into the brain and therefore cannot be used as a therapeutic agent.

Pathways of drug biotransformation may be divided into two major groups of reactions, phase I and phase II reactions. *Phase I,* or asynthetic reactions, include oxidation, reduction, and hydrolysis. *Phase II,* or synthetic reactions, include conjugations. A partial list of these reactions is presented in Table 13.3. In addition, a number of drugs that resemble natural biochemical molecules are able to utilize the metabolic pathways for normal body compounds. For example, isoproterenol is methylated by catechol O-methyl transferase (COMT), and amphetamine is deaminated by monamine oxidase (MAO). Both COMT and MAO are enzymes involved in the metabolism of noradrenaline.

Phase I Reactions

Usually phase I biotransformation reactions occur first and introduce or expose a functional group on the drug molecules. For example, oxygen is introduced into the phenyl group on phenylbutazone by aromatic hydroxylation to form oxyphenbutazone, a more polar metabolite. Codeine is demethylated to form morphine. In addition, the hydrolysis of esters, such as aspirin or benzocaine, will yield more polar products, such as salicylic acid and *p*-aminobenzoic acid, respectively. For some compounds, such as acetaminophen, benzo[*a*]pyrene, and other drugs containing aromatic rings, reactive intermediates, such as epoxides, are formed during the hydroxylation reaction. These aromatic epoxides are highly reactive and will react with macromolecules, possibly causing liver necrosis (acetaminophen) or cancer (benzo[*a*]pyrene). The biotransformation of salicylic acid (Fig. 13-13) demonstrates the variety of possible metabolites that may be formed. It should be noted that salicylic acid is also conjugated directly (phase II reaction) without a preceding phase I reaction.

Conjugation (Phase II) Reactions

Once a polar constituent is revealed or placed into the molecule, then a phase II or conjugation reaction may occur. Common examples include the conjugation of

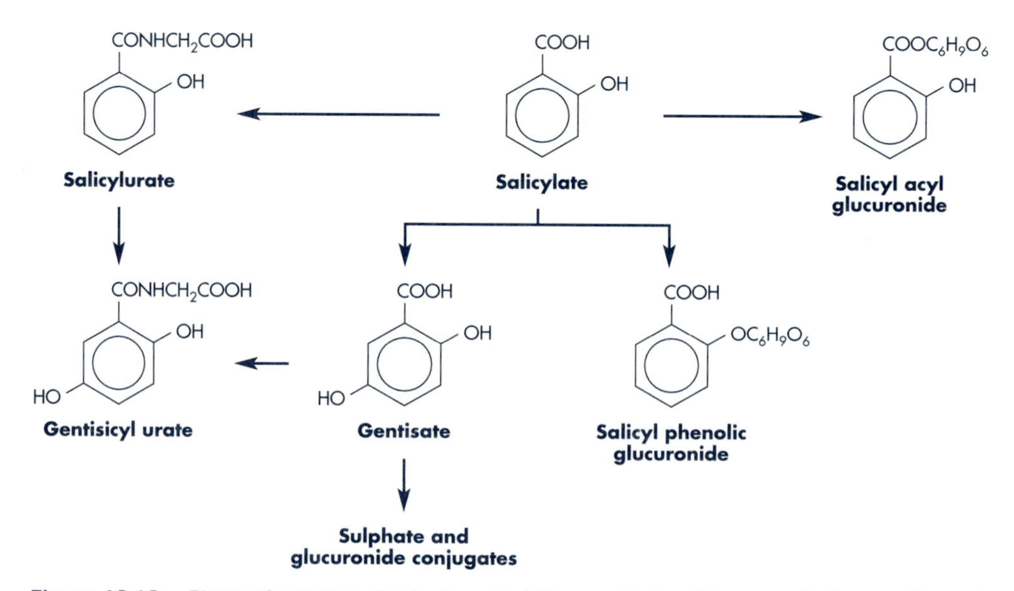

Figure 13-13. Biotransformation of salicylic acid. (GA = gentisate, GU = gentisicyl urate, SA = salicylate, SAG = salicyl acyl glucuronide, SPG = salicyl phenolic glucuronide, SU = salicylurate.) (From Hucker et al, 1980, with permission.)

salicyclic acid with glycine to form salicyluric acid or glucuronic acid to form salicylglucuronide (Fig. 13-13).

Conjugation reactions use conjugating reagents, which are derived from biochemical compounds involved in carbohydrate, fat, and protein metabolism. These reactions may include an active, high-energy form of the conjugating agent, such as uridine diphosphoglucuronic acid (UDPGA), acetyl CoA, 3′-phosphoadenosine-5′-phosphosulfate (PAPS), or *S*-adenosylmethionine (SAM), which in the presence of the appropriate transferase enzyme, combines with the drug to form the conjugate. Conversely, the drug may be activated to a high energy compound that then reacts with the conjugating agent in the presence of a transferase enzyme (Fig. 13-14). The major conjugation (phase II) reactions are listed in Tables 13.3 and 13.4. Some of the conjugation reactions may have limited capacity at high drug concentrations, leading to nonlinear drug metabolism. In most cases, enzyme activity follows first-order kinetics with low drug (substrate) concentrations. At high doses, the drug concentration may rise above the Michaelis–Menten rate constant (K_M), and the reaction rate approaches a zero-order rate (V_{max}). Glucuronidation reactions have a high capacity and may demonstrate nonlinear (saturation) kinetics at very high drug concentrations. In contrast, glycine, sulfate, and glutathione conjugations show lesser capacity and demonstrate nonlinear kinetics at therapeutic drug concentrations (Caldwell, 1980). The limited capacity of certain conjugation pathways may be due to several factors, including (1) limited amount of the conjugate transferase, (2) limited ability to synthesize the active nucleotide intermediate, or (3) limited amount of conjugating agent, such as glycine. In addition, the *N*-acetylated conjugation reaction shows genetic polymorphism in which, for certain drugs, the human population may be divided into fast and slow acetylators. Finally, some of these conjugation reactions may be diminished or defective in cases of inborn errors of metabolism.

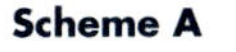

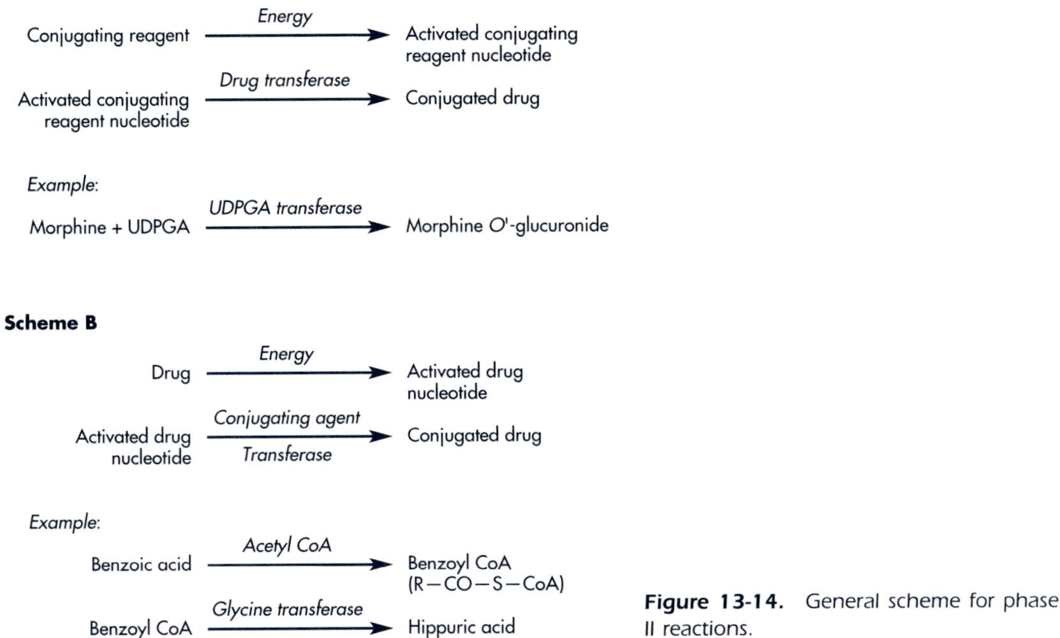

Figure 13-14. General scheme for phase II reactions.

Glucuronidation and sulfate conjugation are very common phase II reactions that result in water-soluble metabolites rapidly excreted in bile (for some high MW glucuronides) and/or urine. Acetylation and mercapturic acid synthesis are conjugation reactions often implicated in the toxicity of the drug; they will now be discussed more fully.

TABLE 13.4 Phase II Conjugation Reactions

CONJUGATION REACTION	CONJUGATING AGENT	HIGH ENERGY INTERMEDIATE	FUNCTIONAL GROUPS COMBINED WITH
Glucuronidation	Glucuronic acid	UDPGA[a]	—OH, —COOH, —NH_2, SH
Sulfation	Sulfate	PAPS[b]	—OH, —NH_2
Amino acid conjugation	Glycine[c]	Coenzyme A thioesters	—COOH
Acetylation	Acetyl CoA	Acetyl CoA	—OH, —NH_2
Methylation	CH_3 from S-adenosylmethionine	S-adenosylmethionine	—OH, —NH_2
Glutathione (mercapturine acid conjugation)	Glutathione	Arene oxides, epoxides	Aryl halides, epoxides, arene oxides

[a]UDPGA = uridine diphosphoglucuronic acid.
[b]PAPS = 3′-phosphoadenosine-5′-phosphosulfate.
[c]Glycine conjugates are also known as hippurates.

Acetylation

The acetylation reaction is an important conjugation reaction for several reasons. First, the acetylated product is usually less polar than the parent drug. The acetylation of such drugs as sulfanilamide, sulfadiazine, and sulfisoxazole produces metabolites that are less water soluble and that in sufficient concentration will precipitate in the kidney tubules, causing kidney damage and crystaluria. In addition, a less polar metabolite will be reabsorbed in the renal tubule and have a longer elimination half-life. For example, procainamide (elimination half-life of 3 to 4 hr) has an acetylated metabolite, *N*-acetylprocainamide, which is biologically active and has an elimination half-life of 6 to 7 hrs. Lastly, the *N*-acetyltransferase enzyme responsible for catalyzing the acetylation of isoniazid and other drugs demonstrates a genetic polymorphism. Two distinct subpopulations have been observed to inactivate isoniazid, including the "slow inactivators" and the "rapid inactivators" (Evans, 1968). Therefore, the former group may demonstrate an adverse effect of isoniazide, such as peripheral neuritis, due to the longer elimination half-life and accumulation of the drug.

Glutathione and Mercapturic Acid Conjugation

Glutathione (GSH) is a tripeptide of glutamyl-cysteine-glycine that is involved in many important biochemical reactions. GSH is the main intracellular molecule for protection of the cell against reactive electrophilic compounds. Through the nucleophilic sulfhydryl group of the cysteine residue, GSH reacts nonenzymatically and enzymatically via the enzyme glutathione *S*-transferase, with reactive electrophilic oxygen intermediates of certain drugs, particularly aromatic hydrocarbons formed during oxidative biotransformation. These reactive electrophilic intermediates may react with nucleophilic macromolecules, such as proteins in the cell, leading to cell injury and cellular necrosis. Thus, GSH is important in the detoxification of reactive oxygen intermediates into nonreactive metabolites. The resulting GSH conjugates are precursors for a group of drug conjugates known as mercapturic acid (*N*-acetylcysteine) derivatives. The formation of a mercapturic acid conjugate is shown in Figure 13-15.

The enzymatic formation of GSH conjugates is saturable. High doses of drugs such as acetaminophen (APAP) may form electrophilic intermediates and deplete GSH in the cell. The reactive intermediate covalently bonds to hepatic cellular macromolecules, resulting in cellular necrosis. The suggested antidote for intoxication (overdose) of acetaminophen is the administration of *N*-acetylcysteine (Mucomyst), a drug molecule that contains available sulfhydryl (R-SH) groups.

Metabolism of Enantiomers

Many drugs are given as mixtures of stereoisomers. Each isomeric form may have different pharmacologic actions and different side effects. For example, the natural thyroid hormone is L-thyroxine; whereas the synthetic D-enantiomer, D-thyroxine, lowers cholesterol but does not stimulate basal metabolic rate like the L-form. Since enzymes as well as drug receptors demonstrate stereoselectivity, isomers of drugs may show differences in biotransformation and in its pharmacokinetics (Tucker and Lennard, 1990). With improved techniques for isolating mixtures of enantiomers, many drugs are now available as pure enantiomers. The rate of drug metabolism and the extent of drug protein binding are often differ-

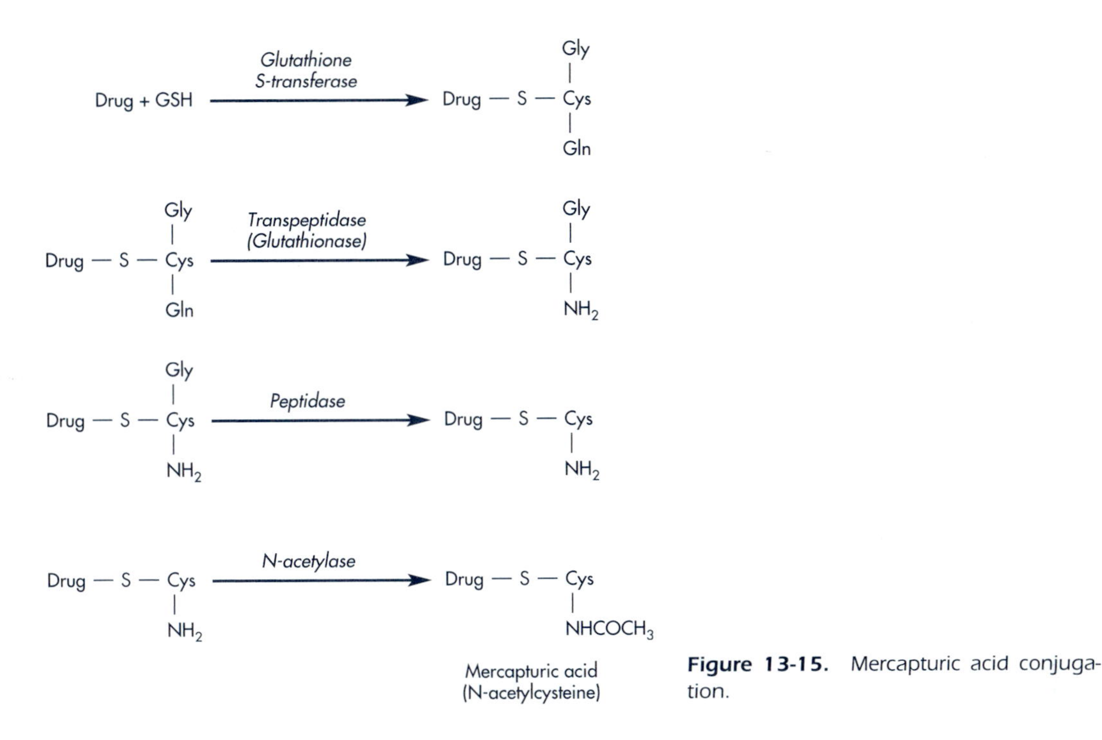

Figure 13-15. Mercapturic acid conjugation.

ent for each stereoisomer. For example, (*S*)-(+)disopyramide is more highly bound in man than (*R*)-(−)disopyramide. Carprofen, a nonsteroidal antiinflammatory drug, also exists in both an *S* and an *R* configuration. The predominate activity lies in the *S* configuration. The clearance of the *S*-carprofen glucuronide through the kidney was faster than that of the *R* form, 36 versus 26 mL/min (Iwakawa et al, 1989). A list of some common drugs with enantiomers is given in Table 13.5). A review (Ariens and Wuis, 1987) shows that out of 475 semisynthetic drugs derived from natural sources, 469 were enantiomers, indicating that the biologic systems are very stereospecific.

The anticonvulsant drug mephenytoin is another example of a drug that exists as the *R* and *S* enantiomer. Both enantiomers are metabolized by hydroxylation in man (Wilkinson et al, 1989). After an oral dose of 300 mg of the racemic or mixed form, the plasma concentration of the *S* form in most subjects was only about 25% of the *R* form. The elimination half-life of the *S* form (2.13 hrs) was much faster than that of the *R* form (76 hr) in these subjects (Fig. 13-16A). The severity of the sedative side effect of this drug was also less in subjects with rapid metabolism. Hydroxylation reduces the lipophilicity of the metabolite and may reduce the par-

TABLE 13.5 Common Drug Enantiomers

Atropine	Brompheniramine	Cocaine
Disopyramide	Doxylamine	Ephedrine
Propranolol	Nadolol	Verapamil
Tocainide	Propoxyphene	Morphine
Warfarin	Thyroxine	Flecainide
Ibuprofen	Atenolol	Subutamol
Metoprolol	Terbutaline	

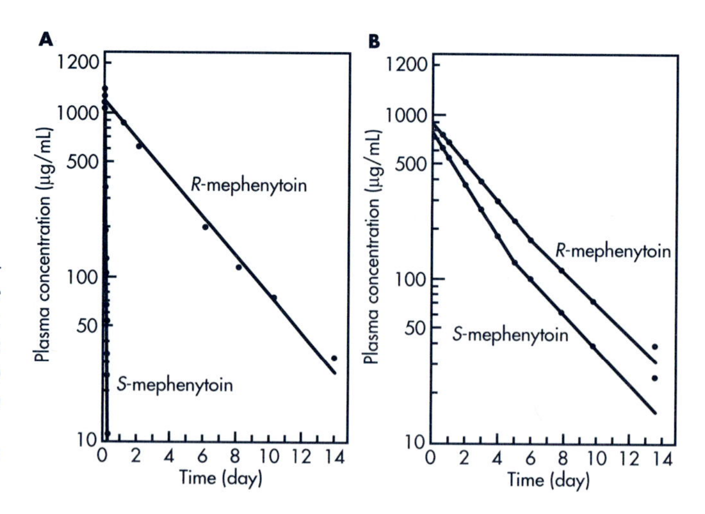

Figure 13-16. Plasma level of mephenytoin after 300 mg oral dose of the racemic drug. **A.** Efficient metabolizer. **B.** Poor metabolizer. The plasma levels of the *R* and *S* form are different due to different rates of metabolism of the two isomers.
(Adapted from Wilkinson et al, 1989, with permission.)

tition of the metabolite into the CNS. Interestingly, some subjects do not metabolize the *S* form of mephenytoin well, and the severity of sedation in these subjects was increased. The plasma level of the *S* form was much higher in these subjects (Fig. 13-16B). The variation in metabolic rate was attributed to genetically controlled enzymatic differences within the population.

Regioselectivity

In addition to stereoselectivity, the biotransformation enzymes may also be regioselective. In this case, the enzymes will catalyze a reaction that is specific for a particular region in the drug molecule. For example, isoproterenol is methylated via catechol-*O*-methyltransferase and *S*-adenosylmethionine primarily in the meta position, resulting in a 3-*O*-methylated metabolite. Very little methylation occurs at the hydroxyl group in the para position.

Species Differences in Hepatic Biotransformation Enzymes

The biotransformation activity of the hepatic enzymes can be affected by a variety of factors (Table 13.6). During the early preclinical phase of drug development, drug metabolism studies attempt to identify the major metabolic pathways of a new drug through the use of animal models. For most drugs, different animal species may have different metabolic pathways. For example, amphetamine is mainly hydroxylated in the rat, whereas in humans and the dog it is largely deaminated. In many cases, the rates of metabolism may differ among different animal species even though the biotransformation pathways are the same. In other cases, a specific pathway may be absent in a particular species. Generally, the researcher tries to find the best animal model that will be predictive of the metabolic profile in humans.

Variation of Biotransformation Enzymes in Humans

In humans, variation in metabolism may be caused by a number of biologic and environmental variables (Table 13.6). Genetic differences in drug elimination has

TABLE 13.6 Sources of Variation in Intrinsic Clearance

Sources of Variation
Genetic Factors
Genetic differences within population
Racial differences among different populations
Environmental Factors and Drug Interactions
Enzyme induction
Enzyme inhibition
Physiologic Conditions
Age
Gender
Diet/nutrition
Pathophysiology
Drug Dosage Regimen
Route of drug administration
Dose dependent (nonlinear) pharmacokinetics

led to the study of *pharmacogenetics.* For example, the *N*-acetylation of isoniazid has been found to be genetically determined with at least two identifiable groups, including rapid and slow acetylators (Evans et al, 1960). The difference is referred to as *genetic polymorphism.* Individuals with slow acetylation are prone to isoniazid-induced neurotoxicity. Procainamide and hydralazine are other drugs that are acetylated and demonstrate genetic polymorphism.

Another example of genetic differences in drug metabolism is glucose-6-phosphate-dehydrogenase deficiency, which is observed in approximately 10% of black Americans. A well-documented example of genetic polymorphism occurred with phenytoin (Wilkinson et al, 1989). Two phenotypes, EM (efficient metabolizer) and PM (poor metabolizer), were identified in the study population. The PM frequency in Caucasians was about 4% and among Japanese about 16%. Variation in metabolic rate was also observed with mephobarbital. The incidence of side effects was higher in Japanese subjects, possibly due to a slower oxidative metabolism. Metabolism difference of propranolol due to genetic difference among Chinese populations was also recently reported (Lai et al, 1995). It is important to note that some variations in metabolism may be also related to geographical difference rather racial differences (Bertilsson, 1995).

Besides genetic influence, the basal level of enzyme activity may be altered by environmental factors and exposure to chemicals. Shorter theophylline elimination half-life due to smoking was observed in smoking subjects. Apparently, the aromatic hydrocarbons, such as benzpyrene, released during smoking stimulate the enzymes involved in theophylline metabolism. Young children are also known to eliminate theophylline faster. The drug phenobarbital is a potent inducer of a wider variety of hepatic enzymes. Polycyclic hydrocarbons such as 3-methylcholanthrene and benzpyrene also induce hepatic enzyme formation. These compounds are carcinogenic.

Hepatic enzyme activity may also be inhibited by a variety of agents including carbon monoxide, heavy metals, and certain imidazole drugs such as cimetidine. Enzyme inhibition by cimetidine may lead to higher plasma levels and longer elimination of coadministered phenytoin or theophylline. The physiologic condition of the host—including age, gender, nutrition, diet, and pathophysiology—also affects the level of hepatic enzyme activities.

Genetic Variation of Cytochrome P-450 (CYP) Isozymes

One of the most important groups of enzymes accounting for variation in phase I metabolism of drugs is the cytochrome P-450 enzyme group, which exists in many forms among individuals because of genetic differences (May, 1994; Tucker, 1994). The genes encoding many of these enzymes have been identified. Multiforms of P-450 are referred to as *isozymes*, which are classified into families (originally denoted by Roman numerals: I, II, III, etc), and subfamilies (denoted by A, B, C, etc) based on the similarity of the amino acid sequences of the isozymes. If an isozyme amino acid sequence is 60% similar or more, it is placed within a family. Within the family, isozymes with amino acid sequences of 70% or more similarity are placed into a subfamily, and an Arabic number follows for further classification.

The substrate specificities of the P-450 enzymes appear to be due to the nature of the amino acid residues, size of the amino acid side chain, polarity and charge of the amino acids (Negishi, 1996). The individual gene is denoted by an Arabic number (last number) after the subfamily. For example, cytochrome P-450IA2 is involved in the oxidation of caffeine and cytochrome, P-450IID6 is involved in the oxidation of drugs, such as codeine, propranolol, and dextromethorphan. The well-known cytochrome P-450IID6 is responsible for debrisoquine metabolism among individuals showing genetic polymorphism. The vinca alkaloids used in cancer treatment have shown great inter- and intraindividual variabilities. P-450IIIA cytochromes are known to be involved in the metabolism of vindesine, vinblastine, and other vinca alkaloids (Rahmani–Zhou, 1993). Failing to recognize variations in drug clearance in cancer chemotherapy may result in greater toxicity or even therapeutic failure.

There are now at least eight families of cytochrome isozymes known in humans and animals. Cytochrome P-450 I–III (CYP 1–3) are best known for metabolizing clinically useful drugs in humans. Variation in isozyme distribution and content in the hepatocytes may affect intrinsic hepatic clearance of a drug. Clinically, it is important to look for evidence of unusual metabolic profiles in patients prior to dosing. Pharmacokinetic experiments using a "marker" drug such as antipyrine, dextromethorphan may be used to determine if the intrinsic hepatic clearance of the patient is significantly different from an average subject.

The nomenclature of the P-450 family of enzymes was reviewed by Nebert et al (1989) and by Hansch and Zhang (1993); new nomenclature starting with "CYP" as the root denoting cytochrome P-450 with an Arabic number replacing the Roman numeral was discussed. See Table 13.7 for comparison. The CYP3A subfamily of an

TABLE 13.7 Comparison of P-450 Nomenclatures Currently in Use

P-450 GENE FAMILY/SUBFAMILY	NEW NOMENCLATURE
P-450I	CYP1
P-450IIA	CYP2A
P-450IIB	CYP2B
P-450IIC	CYP2C
P-450IID	CYP2D
P-450IIE	CYP2E
P-450III	CYP3
P-450IV	CYP4

Sources: Nebert et al (1989) and Hansch and Zhang (1993).

important family, CYP3, appears to be responsible for the metabolism of a large number of structurally diverse endogenous agents (eg, testosterone, cortisol, progesterone, estradiol) and xenobiotics (eg, nifedipine, lovastatin, midazolam, terfenadine, erythromycin).

The metabolism of debrisoquin is polymorphic in the population with some individuals having extensive metabolism (EM) and other individuals having poor metabolism (PM). Those individuals who are PM lack functional CYP2D6 (P-450IID6). In EM individuals, quinidine will block CYP2D6 so that the genotypic EM individuals appear to be phenotypic PM individuals (Caraco et al, 1996). Some drugs which are metabolized by CYP2D6 (P-450IID6) are codeine, flecainide, dextromethorphan, imipramine and other cyclic antidepressants that undergo ring hydroxylation. The inability to metabolize substrates for CYP2D6 results in increased plasma concentrations of the parent drug in PM individuals.

Drug Interactions Involving Drug Metabolism

The enzymes involved in the metabolism of drugs may be altered by diet and the coadministration of other drugs and chemicals. *Enzyme induction* is a drug or chemical-stimulated increase in enzyme activity usually due to an increase in the amount of enzyme present. Enzyme induction usually requires some onset time for the synthesis of enzyme protein. For example, rifampin induction occurs within 2 days, while phenobarbital induction takes about one week to occur. Enzyme induction for carbmazepine begins after 3 to 5 days and is not complete for approximately 1 month or longer. Smoking can change the rate of metabolism of many cyclic antidepressant drugs (CAD) through enzyme induction (Toney, Ereshefsky, 1995). Agents (see also Chapter 17) that induce enzymes include aromatic hydrocarbons (such as benzopyrene found in cigarette smoke), insecticides (such as chlordane), and drugs, such as carbamazepine, rifampin, and phenobarbital. *Enzyme inhibition* may be due to substrate competition or due to direct inhibition of the drug metabolizing enzymes, particularly one of several of the cytochrome P-450 enzymes. Many widely prescribed antidepressants generally known as selective serotonin reuptake inhibitors (SSRI) have been reported to inhibit the P-450IID6 system resulting in significantly elevated plasma concentration of coadministered psychotropic drugs. Fluoxetine (FLX) was found to cause a tenfold decrease in the clearance of imipramine (IMI) and desipramine (DMI) due to its inhibitory effect on hydroxylation (Toney, Ereshefsky, 1995).

A few clinical examples of enzyme inhibitors and inducers are listed in Table 13.8. Diet also affects drug metabolizing enzymes. For example, plasma theophylline concentrations and theophylline clearance in patients on a high protein diet are lower than in subjects whose diets are high in carbohydrates. Sucrose or glucose plus fructose decrease the activity of mixed function oxidase, which is related to a slower metabolism rate and a prolongation in hexobarbital sleeping time in rats. Chronic administration of 5% glucose was suggested to affect sleeping time in subjects receiving barbiturates. A decreased intake of fatty acids may lead to decreased basal MFO activities (Campbell, 1977) and affect the rate of drug metabolism.

The protease inhibitor, saquinavir mesylate (Invirase, Roche Labs), has very low bioavailability—only about 4%. In studies conducted by Hoffmann-La Roche, the AUC of saquinavir was increased to 150% when the volunteers took a 150-mL glass of grapefruit juice with the saquinavir, and then another 150-mL glass an hour later. Concentrated grapefruit juice increased the AUC up to 220%. Naringin, a

TABLE 13.8 Examples of Drug Interactions Affecting Mixed Function Oxidase Enzymes

INHIBITORS OF DRUG METABOLISM	EXAMPLE	RESULT
Acetaminophen	Ethanol	Increased hepatotoxicity in chronic alcoholics
Cimetidine	Warfarin	Prolongation of prothrombin time
Erythromycin	Carbamazepine	Decreased carbazepine clearance
Fluoxetine	Imipramine (IMI)	Decreased clearance of CAD
Fluoxetine	Desipramine (DMI)	Decreased clearance of CAD
INDUCERS OF DRUG METABOLISM	**EXAMPLE**	**RESULT**
Carbamazepine	Acetaminophen	Increased acetaminophen metabolism
Rifampin	Methadone	Increased methadone metabolism, may precipitate opiate withdrawal
Phenobarbital	Dexamethasone	Decreased dexamethasone elimination half-life
Rifampin	Prednisolone	Increased elimination of prednisolone

bioflavonoid in grapefruit juice was found to be at least partially responsible for the inhibition of the enzyme cytochrome P-450IIIA4, (CYP3A4), present in the liver and the intestinal wall, which metabolizes saquinavir resulting in an increase in its AUC. Ketoconazole and ranitidine (Zantac) may also increase the AUC of saquinavir by inhibition of the cytochrome P-450 enzymes. In contrast, rifampin greatly reduces the AUC of saquinavir, apparently due to enzymatic stimulation. Other drugs recently shown to have increased bioavailability when taken with grapefruit juice include several sedatives and the anticoagulant coumarin (Table 13.9). Increases in drug levels may be dangerous and the pharmacokinetics of drugs with potential interaction should be closely monitored.

ROUTE OF DRUG ADMINISTRATION AND EXTRAHEPATIC DRUG METABOLISM

The liver is the main organ involved in drug metabolism. However, other areas associated with portals of drug entry into the body may be involved in drug metabolism. These sites include the lung, skin, gastrointestinal mucosal cells, microbiological flora in the distal portion of the ileum, and large intestine. The kidney may also be involved in certain drug metabolism reactions. For many drugs, the principle site of metabolism is often assumed to take place in the liver. A simple way to assess ex-

TABLE 13.9 Change in Drug Availability Due to Oral Coadministration of Grapefruit Juice

DRUG	STUDY
Triazolam	Hukkinen, 1995
Midazolam	Kupferschmidt, 1995
Cyclosporine	Yee, 1995
Coumarin	Merkel, 1994
Nisoldipine	Bailey DG, 1993
Felodipine	Baily DG, 1993

trahepatic metabolism is to calculate hepatic (metabolic) clearance of the drug. For example, for morphine clearance, Cl_T is 1600 mL/min, and the fraction of drug excreted unchanged in the urine is $f_e = 0.08$. Therefore, metabolic clearance is expressed as $Cl_{nr} = 0.08 \times 1600$ mL/min = 1472 mL/min. Since hepatic blood flow is about 1250 mL/min, the drug appears to be metabolized faster than the rate of blood flow. Thus, at least some of the drug must be metabolized outside the liver. Nitroglycerin is another drug that is metabolized extensively outside the liver.

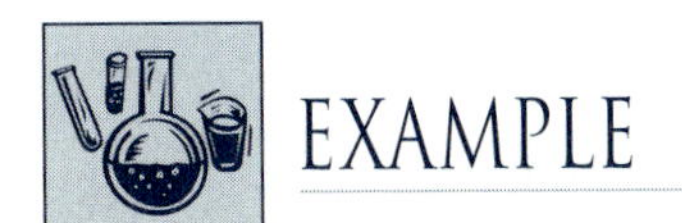

EXAMPLE

Flutamide, (Evlexin, Schering Corp.) used to treat prostate cancer, is rapidly metabolized to an active metabolite, alpha-hydroxyflutamide in humans. The steady-state level is 51 ng/mL (range, 24–78 ng/mL) after oral multiple doses of 250 mg flutamide 3 times daily or every 8 hours (manufacturer-supplied information). Calculate the total body clearance and hepatic clearance assuming that flutamide is 90% metabolized, and is completely (100%) absorbed.

Solution

$$Cl_T = \frac{FD_0}{C_{av}^{\infty}\tau}$$

$$Cl_T = (250 \times 1{,}000{,}000)/(51 \times 8) = 6.127 \times 10^5 \text{ mL/hr} = 10200 \text{ mL/min}$$

$$Cl_{nr} = 10200 \text{ mL/min} \times 0.9 = 9180 \text{ mL/min}.$$

The Cl_{nr} of flutamide is far greater than the rate of hepatic blood flow (about 1500 mL/min), indicating extensive extrahepatic clearance.

Both the nature of the drug and the route of administration may influence the type of drug metabolite formed. For example, isoproterenol given orally forms a sulfate conjugate in the gastrointestinal mucosal cells, whereas, after IV administration, it forms the 3-*O*-methylated metabolite due to *S*-adenosylmethionine and catechol-*O*-methyltransferase. Azo drugs such as sulfasalazine are poorly absorbed after oral administration. However, the azo group of sulfasalazine is cleaved by the intestinal microflora, producing 5-aminosalicylic acid and sulfapyridine, which is absorbed in the lower bowel.

FIRST-PASS EFFECTS

For some drugs, the route of administration affects the metabolic rate of the compound. For example, a drug given parenterally, transdermally, or by inhalation may distribute within the body prior to metabolism by the liver. In contrast, drugs given orally are normally absorbed in the duodenal segment of the small intestine and transported via the mesenteric vessels to the hepatic portal vein and then to the liver prior to the systemic circulation. Drugs that are highly metabolized by the liver or by the intestinal mucosal cells demonstrate poor systemic availability when given orally. This rapid metabolism of an orally administered drug prior to reaching the general circulation is termed *first-pass effects* or *presystemic elimination.*

Evidence of First-Pass Effects

First-pass effects may be suspected when there is a lack of parent (or intact) drug in the systemic circulation after oral administration. In such a case, the AUC for a drug given orally is less than the AUC for the same dose of drug given intravenously. Due to experimental findings in animals, first-pass effects may be assumed if the intact drug appears in a cannulated hepatic portal vein but not in general circulation.

Assuming the drug is chemically stable in the gastrointestinal tract and that drug is administered orally in solution to ensure complete absorption, the area under the plasma drug concentration curve (AUC) should be the same when the *same dose* is administered intravenously. Therefore, the absolute bioavailability (F) may reveal evidence of drug being removed by the liver due to first-pass effects as follows:

$$F = \frac{[\mathrm{AUC}]_0^\infty \ \mathrm{oral}/dose_{\mathrm{oral}}}{[\mathrm{AUC}]_0^\infty \ \mathrm{IV}/dose_{\mathrm{IV}}} \tag{13.32}$$

For drugs that undergo first-pass effects $[\mathrm{AUC}]_0^\infty$ oral is smaller than $[\mathrm{AUC}]_0^\infty$ IV and F is less than 1. A drug like isoproterenol or nitroglycerin would have an F value less than 1 because these drugs undergo significant first-pass effects.

Liver Extraction Ratio

Because there are many other reasons for a drug to have a reduced F value, the extent of first-pass effects is not very precisely measured from the F value. The liver extraction ratio (ER) provides a direct measurement of drug removal from the liver after oral administration of a drug.

$$ER = \frac{C_a - C_v}{C_a} \tag{13.33}$$

where C_a is the drug concentration in the blood entering the liver and C_v is the drug concentration leaving the liver. Because C_a is usually greater than C_v, ER is usually less than 1. For example, for propranolol, ER or (E) is about 0.7—that is, about 70% of the drug is actually removed by the liver before it is available for general distribution to the body. By contrast, if the drug is injected intravenously, most of the drug would be distributed before reaching the liver, and less of the drug would be metabolized.

Relationship Between Absolute Bioavailability and Liver Extraction

Liver ER provides a measurement of liver extraction of a drug orally administered. Unfortunately, the sampling of drug from the hepatic portal vein and artery is difficult. Therefore, most ER measurements for drugs are done in animals. These ER values may be quite different from those in humans. The following relationship between bioavailability and liver extraction enables a rough estimate of the extent of liver extraction.

$$F = 1 - ER - F'' \tag{13.34}$$

where F is the fraction of bioavailable drug, ER is the drug fraction extracted by the liver, and F'' is the fraction of drug removed by nonhepatic process.

If F'' is assumed to be negligible—that is, there is no loss of drug due to chemical degradation, gut metabolism, and incomplete absorption—ER may be estimated from

$$ER = 1 - F \tag{13.35}$$

After substitution of Equation 13.32 into Equation 13.35,

$$ER = 1 - \frac{[\text{AUC}]_0^\infty \text{ oral}/dose_{\text{oral}}}{[\text{AUC}]_0^\infty \text{ IV}/dose_{\text{IV}}} \tag{13.36}$$

It should be noted that the ER is a rough estimation of liver extraction for a drug. Many other factors may alter this estimation: the size of the dose, the formulation of the drug, and the physiologic condition of the patient all may effect the ER value obtained.

Liver ER provides valuable information in determining the oral dose of a drug when the intravenous dose is known. With the drug propranolol, a much higher oral dose is necessary to produce sufficient therapeutic blood levels because of drug extraction by the liver. Because liver extraction is affected by blood flow to the liver, dosing of drug with extensive liver metabolism may produce erratic plasma drug levels. Formulation of this drug into an oral dosage form would require extensive, careful testing.

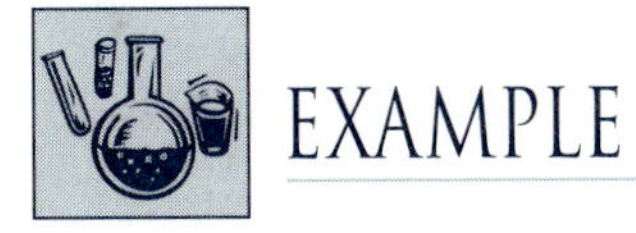

EXAMPLE

A new 5-mg tablet of propranolol was developed and tested in volunteers. The bioavailability of propranolol from the tablet was 70%, relative to an oral solution of propranolol, and 21.6%, relative to an intravenous dose of propranolol (absolute bioavailability). Comment on the feasibility of improving the absolute bioavailability of the propranolol tablet.

Solution

From the table of ER values (Table 13.10), the ER for propranolol is 0.6 to 0.8. If the product is perfectly formulated (ie, the tablet dissolves completely and is all absorbed), the fraction of drug absorbed after deducting for the fraction of drug extracted is calculated below.

$$\begin{aligned} F' &= 1 - ER \\ &= 1 - 0.7 \text{ (mean } ER = 0.7) \\ &= 0.3 \end{aligned}$$

TABLE 13.10 Pharmacokinetic Classification of Drugs Eliminated Primarily by Hepatic Metabolism

DRUG CLASS	EXTRACTION RATIO (APPROX.)	PERCENT BOUND
	Flow-Limited	
Lidocaine	0.83	45–80[a]
Propranolol	0.6–0.8	93
Pethidine (meperidine)	0.60–0.95	60
Pentazocine	0.8	—
Propoxyphene	0.95	—
Nortriptyline	0.5	95
Morphine	0.5–0.75	35
	Capacity-Limited, Binding-Sensitive	
Phenytoin	0.03	90
Diazepam	0.03	98
Tolbutamide	0.02	98
Warfarin	0.003	99
Chlorpromazine	0.22	91–99
Clindamycin	0.23	94
Quinidine	0.27	82
Digitoxin	0.005	97
	Capacity-Limited, Binding-Insensitive	
Theophylline	0.09	59
Hexobarbital	0.16	—
Amobarbital	0.03	61
Antipyrine	0.07	10
Chloramphenicol	0.28	60–80
Thiopental	0.28	72
Acetaminophen	0.43	5[a]

[a]Concentration dependent in part.

From Blaschke (1977), with permission.

A similar calculation using ER of 0.6 and 0.8 would give F′ of 0.4 and 0.2, respectively. Because the drug is 26% available relative to an intravenous dose, the oral tablet is within limits of the absolute bioavailability of this drug—that is, the drug is only 20 to 40% available relative to an intravenous dose even if all the drug is absorbed from the gastrointestinal tract.

It is important to note that the same tablet tested experimentally resulted in a bioavailability of 70% relative to an oral solution. In this case the relative bioavailability is higher because the drug extracted by the liver is not reflected in the relative bioavailability. In measuring the AUC of the oral solution, liver extraction resulted in a smaller AUC in the oral solution as well as in the tablet, therefore canceling out the effect of each other in calculating the relative availability of the tablet.

The following shows a method for calculating the absolute bioavailability from the relative bioavailability providing that the ER is accurately known. Using the above example,

$$\text{Absolute availability of the solution} = 1 - ER = 1 - 0.7 = 0.3 = 30\%$$

$$\text{Relative availability of the solution} = 100\%$$

$$\text{Absolute availability of the solution} = x \text{ percent}$$

$$\text{Relative availability of the tablet} = 70\%$$

$$x = \frac{30 \times 70}{100} = 21\%$$

Therefore, this product has an absolute bioavailability of 21%. The small percent of calculated and actual absolute bioavailability is due largely to liver extraction fluctuation. All calculations are performed with the assumption of linear pharmacokinetics, which is generally a good approximation. When therapeutic drugs are administered, saturation may occur rapidly with some drugs, and ER may deviate significantly with changes in blood flow.

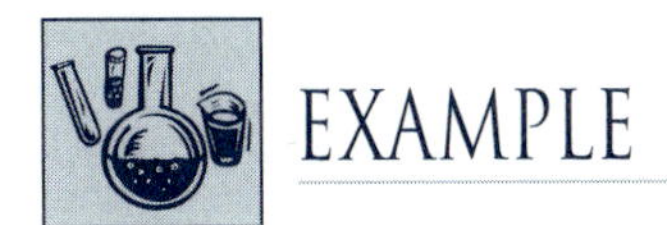

EXAMPLE

Fluvastatin sodium (Lescol, Novartis) is a drug used to lower cholesterol, whose absolute bioavailability after an oral dose is reported to be 19 to 29% after oral administration. The drug is rapidly and completely absorbed (manufacturer's product information). What are the reasons for the low oral bioavailability in spite of reportedly good absorption? What is the extraction ratio of fluvastatin? (The absolute bioavailability was 46%, according to values reported in the literature.)

Solution

Assuming the drug to be completely absorbed as reported, using Equation 13.35

$$ER = 1 - 0.46 = 0.54$$

54% of the drug is lost due to first-pass effect because of a relatively large extraction ratio. Since bioavailability is only 19 to 29%, there is probably some nonhepatic loss (F''), according to Equation 13.34. The drug was reported to be extensively metabolized, with some drug excreted in feces.

Estimation of Reduced Bioavailability Due to Liver Metabolism with Variable Blood Flow to the Liver

Blood flow to the liver plays an important role in the extent of drug metabolized after oral administration. Changes in blood flow to the liver may substantially alter the percent of drug metabolized and therefore alter the percent of bioavailable drug. The relationship between blood flow, hepatic clearance, and percent of drug bioavailable is

$$F' = 1 - \frac{Cl_h}{Q} \qquad (13.37)$$

where Cl_h is the hepatic clearance of the drug and Q is the effective hepatic blood flow. F' is the bioavailability factor obtained from estimates of liver blood flow and hepatic clearance, ER.

The usual effective hepatic blood flow is 1.5 L/min, but it may vary from 1 to 2 L/min depending on diet, food intake, physical activity, or drug intake (Rowland, 1973). This equation provides a reasonable approach for evaluating the reduced bioavailability due to first-pass effect. With the drug propoxyphene hydrochloride

TABLE 13.11 Hepatic and Renal Extraction Ratios of Representative Drugs

EXTRACTION RATIOS		
LOW (<0.3)	**INTERMEDIATE (0.3–0.7)**	**HIGH (>0.7)**
	HEPATIC EXTRACTION[a]	
Amobarbital	Aspirin	Arabinosyl–cytosine
Antipyrine	Quinidine	Encainide
Chloramphenicol	Desipramine	Isoproterenol
Chlordiazepoxide	Nortriptyline	Meperidine
Diazepam		Morphine
Digitoxin		Nitroglycerin
Erythromycin		Pentazocine
Isoniazid		Propoxyphene
Phenobarbital		Propranolol
Phenylbutazone		Salicylamide
Phenytoin		Tocainide
Procainamide		Verapamil
Salicylic acid		
Theophylline		
Tolbutamide		
Warfarin		

From Rowland (1978), with permission and Brouwer et al (1992).

F' has been calculated from hepatic clearance (990 mL/min) and an assumed liver blood flow of 1.53 L/min.

$$F' = 1 - \frac{0.99}{1.53} = 0.35$$

The results show that 35% of the drug is systemically absorbed after liver extraction are reasonable compared with the experimental values for propranolol. Although Equation 13.37 seems to provide a convenient way of estimating the effect of liver blood flow on bioavailability, this estimation is actually more complicated. A change in liver blood flow may alter hepatic clearance and F'. A large blood flow may deliver enough drug to the liver to alter the rate of metabolism. In contrast, a small blood flow may decrease the delivery of drug to the liver and become the rate-limiting step for metabolism. The hepatic clearance of a drug is usually calculated from plasma drug data rather than whole blood data. Significant nonlinearity may be the result of drug equilibration due to partitioning into the red blood cells.

Presystemic elimination or first-pass effects is a very important consideration for drugs that have a high extraction ratio (Table 13.11). Drugs with low extraction ratios, such as theophylline, have very little presystemic elimination, as demonstrated by complete systemic absorption after oral administration. In contrast, drugs with high extraction ratios have poor bioavailability when given orally. Therefore, the oral dose must be higher than the intravenous dose to achieve the same therapeutic response. In some cases, oral administration of a drug with high presystemic elimination, such as nitroglycerin, may be impractical due to very poor oral bioavailability, and, thus, the sublingual, transdermal or nasal routes of administration may be preferred. Furthermore, if an oral drug product has slow dissolution characteristics or release rates, then more of the drug will be subject to first-pass effects compared to the doses of drug given in a more bioavailable form (such as a solution). In addition, drugs with high presystemic elimination tend to demonstrate more variability in drug bioavailability between and within individuals. Finally, the quantity and quality of the metabolites formed may vary according to the route of drug administration, which may be clinically important if one or more of the metabolites has pharmacologic or toxic activity.

To overcome first-pass effects, the route of administration of the drug may be changed. For example, nitroglycerin may be given sublingually or topically and xylocaine may be given parenterally to avoid the first-pass effects. Another way to overcome first-pass effects is to either enlarge the dose or change the drug product to a more rapidly absorbable dosage form. In either case, a large amount of drug is presented rapidly to the liver, and some of the drug will reach the general circulation in the intact state.

HEPATIC CLEARANCE

The clearance concept may be applied to any organ and is used as a measure of elimination of drug by the organ (see also Chapter 12). *Hepatic clearance* may be defined as the volume of blood that perfuses the liver that is cleared of drug per unit of time. Hepatic clearance (Cl_h) is also equal to total body clearance (Cl_T) minus renal clearance (Cl_R) as follows:

$$Cl_h = Cl_T - Cl_R \quad \textbf{(13.38)}$$

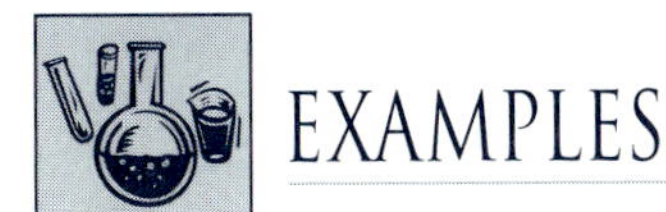

EXAMPLES

1. The total body clearance for a drug is 15 mL/min per kg. Renal clearance accounts for 10 mL/min per kg. What is the hepatic clearance for the drug?

Solution

Hepatic clearance = 15 − 10 = 5 mL/min per kg

Sometimes the renal clearance is not known, in which case, hepatic clearance and renal clearance may be calculated from the percent of intact drug recovered in the urine.

2. The total body clearance of a drug is 10 mL/min per kg. The renal clearance is not known. From a urinary drug excretion study, 60% of the drug is recovered intact and 40% is recovered as metabolites. What is the hepatic clearance for the drug assuming metabolism occurs in the liver?

Solution

$$\begin{aligned}\text{Hepatic clearance} &= \text{body clearance} \times (100 - f_e) \quad \textbf{(13.39)}\\ &= 10 \times (1 - 0.6)\\ &= 4 \text{ mL/min per kg}\end{aligned}$$

where f_e = percent of intact drug recovered in the urine. In this example, the metabolites are recovered completely and hepatic clearance may be obtained as total body clearance times the percent of dose recovered as metabolites. Often, the metabolites are not completely recovered, thus precluding the accuracy of this approach. In this case, hepatic clearance is estimated as the difference between body clearance and the renal clearance.

Relationship Between Blood Flow, Intrinsic Clearance, and Hepatic Clearance

Factors that affect the hepatic clearance of a drug include (1) blood flow to the liver, (2) intrinsic clearance, and (3) the fraction of drug bound to protein.

In experimental animals, the blood flow (Q) to the liver may be measured as well as the concentration of drug in the artery (C_a) and the concentration of drug in the vein (C_v). As the arterial blood containing drug perfuses the liver, a certain portion of the drug is removed by metabolism and/or biliary excretion. Therefore, the drug concentration in the vein is less than the drug concentration in the artery. An *extraction ratio* may be expressed as 100% of the drug entering the liver less the relative concentration (C_v/C_a) of drug that is removed by the liver

$$ER = \frac{C_a - C_v}{C_a} \tag{13.40}$$

The ER may vary from 0 to 1.0. An ER of 0.25 means that 25% of the drug was removed by the liver. If both the ER for the liver and blood flow to the liver are known, then hepatic clearance may be calculated by the following expression.

$$Cl_h = \frac{Q(C_a - C_v)}{C_a} = Q \cdot \mathrm{ER} \tag{13.41}$$

For some drugs (such as isoproterenol, lidocaine, and nitroglycerin), the extraction ratio is high (greater than 0.7), and the drug is removed by the liver almost as rapidly as the organ is perfused by blood in which the drug is contained. For drugs with very high extraction ratios, the rate of drug metabolism is sensitive to changes in hepatic blood flow. Thus, an increase in blood flow to the liver will increase the rate of drug removal by the organ. Propranolol, a β-adrenergic blocking agent, decreases hepatic blood flow by decreasing cardiac output. In such a case, the drug decreases its own clearance through the liver when given orally. Many drugs that demonstrate first-pass effects are drugs that have high extraction ratios with respect to the liver.

Intrinsic clearance (Cl_{int}) is used to describe the total ability of the liver to metabolize a drug in the absence of flow limitations, reflecting the inherent activities of the mixed-function oxidases and all other enzymes. Intrinsic clearance is a distinct characteristic of a particular drug, and, as such, it reflects the inherent ability of the liver to metabolize the drug. Intrinsic clearance may be shown to be analogous to the ratio of V_{max}/K_M for a drug that follows Michaelis–Menten kinetics. Hepatic clearance is a concept for characterizing drug elimination based on both blood flow and the intrinsic clearance of the liver as shown in Equation 13.42.

$$Cl_h = Q\left[\frac{Cl_{int}}{Q + Cl_{int}}\right] \tag{13.42}$$

When the blood flow to the liver is constant, hepatic clearance is equal to the product of blood flow (Q) and the extraction ratio (E). However, the hepatic clear-

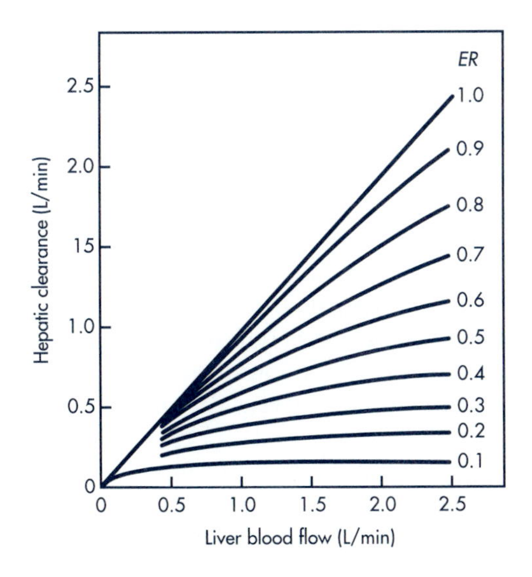

Figure 13-17. The relationship between liver blood flow and total hepatic clearance for drugs with varying extraction rates (*ER*).

ance of a drug is not constant. Hepatic clearance changes with blood flow (Fig. 13-17) and the intrinsic clearance of the drug, as described in Equation 13.42. For drugs with low extraction ratios (eg, theophylline, phenylbutazone, and procainamide), the hepatic clearance is less affected by hepatic blood flow. Instead, these drugs are more affected by the intrinsic activity of the mixed-function oxidases. Describing clearance in terms of all the factors in a physiologic model allow drug clearance to be estimated when physiologic or disease condition causes changes in blood flow or intrinsic enzyme activity. Smoking, for example, can increase the intrinsic clearance for the metabolism of many drugs.

Changes or alterations in mixed-function oxidase activity or biliary secretion can affect the rate of drug removal by the liver. Drugs that show low extraction ratios and are eliminated primarily by metabolism demonstrate marked variation in overall elimination half-lives within a given population. For example, the elimination half-life of theophylline varies from 3 to 9 hours. This variation in $t_{1/2}$ is thought to be due to genetic differences in intrinsic hepatic enzyme activity. Moreover, the elimination half-lives of these same drugs are also affected by enzyme induction, enzyme inhibition, age of the individual, nutritional, and pathologic factors.

Clearance may also be expressed as the rate of drug removal divided by the plasma drug concentration.

$$Cl_{\mathrm{h}} = \frac{\text{rate of drug removed by liver}}{C_{\mathrm{a}}} \quad \textbf{(13.43)}$$

Because the rate of drug removal by the liver is usually the rate of drug metabolism, Equation 13.41 may be expressed in terms of hepatic clearance and drug concentration entering the liver (C_a).

$$\text{Rate of liver drug metabolism} = Cl_{\mathrm{h}}\ C_{\mathrm{a}} \quad \textbf{(13.44)}$$

Hepatic Clearance of a Protein-Bound Drug

It is generally assumed that bound drugs are not easily metabolized (restrictive clearance), while free (unbound) drugs are subject to metabolism. Protein-bound drugs do not diffuse through cell membranes, while free drugs can reach the site of the mixed-function oxidase enzymes easily. Therefore, an increase in the free drug concentration in the blood will make more drug available for hepatic extraction. The concept is discussed under *restrictive* and *nonrestrictive* clearance (JR Gillette, 1973) of protein-bound drugs (See Chapter 11). Most drugs are restrictively cleared, for example, diazepam, quinidine, tolbutamide, and warfarin. The clearance of these drugs is proportional to the fraction of unbound drug (f_u). However, some drugs such as propranolol, morphine, and verapamil are nonrestrictively extracted by the liver regardless of bound to protein or free. Kinetically, a drug is nonrestrictively cleared if its hepatic extraction ratio (ER) is greater than the fraction of free drug (f_u), and the rate of drug clearance is unchanged when the drug is displaced from binding. Mechanistically, when a bound drug (nonrestrictively cleared) approaches an enzyme, it may involve a conformation change in the protein, weakening the process of binding and subjecting the drug to metabolism.

The elimination half-life of a nonrestrictively cleared drug is not significantly affected by a change in the degree of protein binding. The concept of restrictive clearance is also applicable to renal clearance of drugs by active tubular secretion.

For a drug with restrictive clearance, the relationship of blood flow, intrinsic clearance, and protein binding is as follows:

$$Cl_h = Q\left[\frac{f_u Cl'_{int}}{Q + f_u Cl'_{int}}\right] \tag{13.45}$$

where $= f_u$ is the fraction of drug unbound in the blood and Cl'_{int} is the intrinsic clearance of free drug. Equation 13.45 is derived by substituting $= f_u\ Cl'_{int}$ for Cl_{int} in Equation 13.42.

From Equation 13.45, when Cl'_{int} is very small in comparison to hepatic blood flow (ie, $Q > Cl'_{int}$), then Equation 13.46 reduces to Equation 13.47.

$$Cl_h = \frac{Q f_u Cl'_{int}}{Q} \tag{13.46}$$

$$Cl_h = f_u Cl'_{int} \tag{13.47}$$

As shown in Equation 13.47, a change in Cl'_{int} or f_u will cause a proportional change in Cl_h for drugs with protein binding.

In the case where Cl'_{int} for a drug is very large in comparison to flow ($Cl'_{int} \gg Q$), then Equation 13.48 reduces to Equation 13.49.

$$Cl = Q\frac{Cl'_{int} f_u}{Cl'_{int} f_u} \tag{13.48}$$

$$Cl_h \approx Q \tag{13.49}$$

Thus, for drugs with a very high Cl'_{int}, Cl_h is dependent on hepatic blood flow, and independent of protein binding.

Restrictive and Nonrestrictive Clearance From Binding

For some drugs that are highly extracted by the liver, the percent of plasma protein binding does not significantly alter the rate of metabolism, because the drug is removed from the plasma binding sites during circulation through the liver. Many of these drugs may be kinetically classified as nonrestrictively cleared drugs. Propranolol is an example. A similar situation occurs with the renal excretion of some protein-bound cephalosporins and penicillins; some are actively secreted in the renal tubules in spite of plasma protein binding.

For restrictively cleared drugs, change in binding generally alters drug clearance; for a drug with low hepatic extraction ratio and low plasma binding, clearance will increase, but not significantly when the drug is displaced from binding. For a drug highly bound to plasma proteins (more than 90%), a displacement from these binding sites will significantly increase the free concentration of the drug, and clearance (both hepatic and renal clearance) will increase (Chapter 11). There are some drugs that are exceptional and show a paradoxical increase in hepatic clearance despite an increase in protein binding. In one case, increased binding to AAG was found to concentrate drug in the liver, leading to an increased rate of metabolism because the drug was nonrestrictively cleared in the liver.

Effect of Changing Intrinsic Clearance, or Blood Flow on Hepatic Extraction and Elimination Half-Life After IV and Oral Dosing

The effects of altered hepatic intrinsic clearance and liver blood flow on the blood level–time curve have been described by Wilkinson and Shand (1975) after both IV and oral dosing (Figs. 13-18 and 13-19). These illustrations show how changes

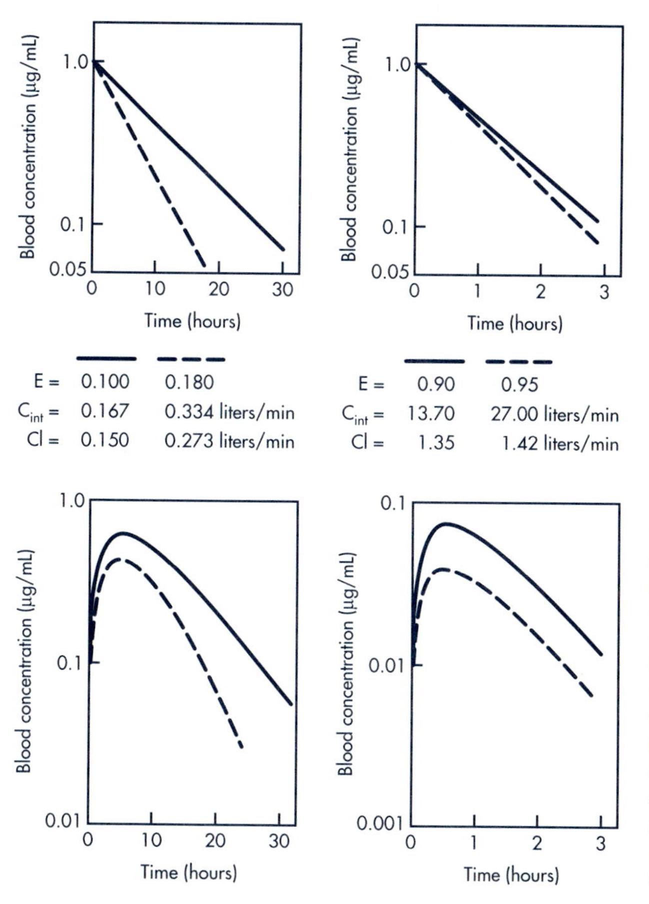

Figure 13-18. The effect of increasing hepatic total intrinsic clearance (Cl_{int}) on the total blood concentration–time curves after intravenous (upper panels) and oral (lower panels) administration of equal doses of two totally metabolized drugs. The left panels refer to a drug with an initial Cl_{int} equivalent to an extraction ratio of 0.1 at a liver blood flow of 1.5 L/min and the right panels to one with an initial extraction ratio of 0.9. The AUCs after oral administration are inversely proportional to Cl_{int}.
(From Wilkinson and Shand, 1975, with permission.)

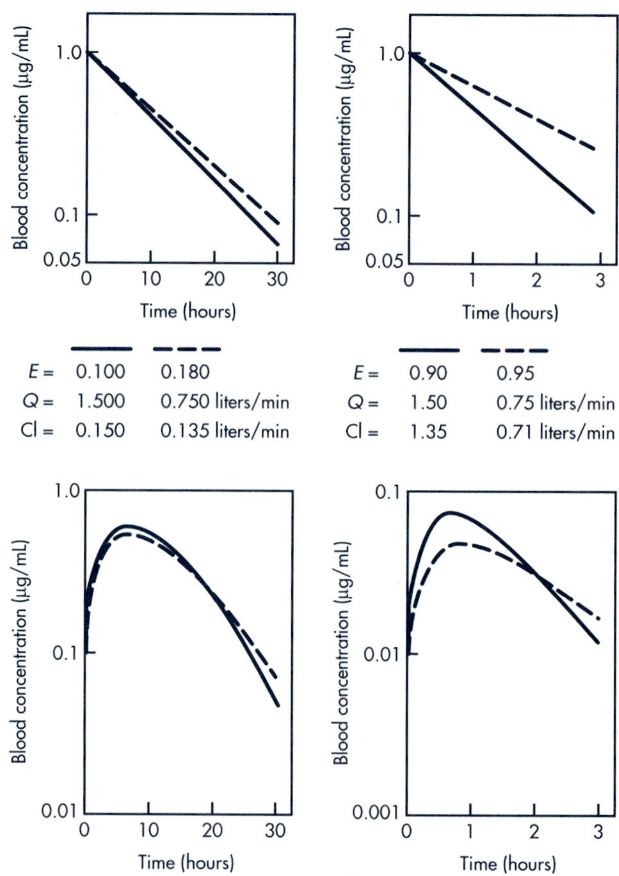

Figure 13-19. Effects of decreasing liver blood flow in the total blood concentration–time curves after intravenous (upper panels) and oral (lower panels) administration of equal doses of two totally metabolized drugs. The left panels refer to a drug with a total intrinsic clearance equivalent to an extraction ratio of 0.1 when blood flow equals 1.5 L/min, and the right panels to a drug with an intrinsic clearance equivalent to an extraction ratio of 0.9.
(From Wilkinson and Shand, 1975, with permission.)

in intrinsic clearance and blood flow affect the elimination half life, first pass effects, and bioavailability of the drug as represented by the area under the curve.

Effect of Changing Intrinsic Clearance

For drugs with low ER, the effect of doubling Cl_{int} (see Fig. 13-18) changing Cl_{int} from 0.167 to 0.334 L/min increases both the extraction ratio (E) and clearance (Cl) of the drug, leading to a steeper slope (dotted line) or shorter $t_{1/2}$. The elimination half-life decreases about 50% due to the increase in intrinsic clearance. Figure 13-18: (bottom left) shows the change in drug concentrations after oral administration, when Cl_{int} doubles. In this case, there is a decrease in both AUC and $t_{1/2}$ (dotted line) due the increase in clearance of the drug.

For drugs with high ER the effect of doubling Cl_{int} (see Fig. 13-18) changing Cl_{int} from 13.70 to 27.00 L/min increases both the extraction ratio and clearance only moderately, leading to a slightly steeper slope. The elimination half-life decreases only marginally. Figure 13-18 (bottom right) shows the change in drug levels after oral administration. Some decrease in AUC is observed and the $t_{1/2}$ is shortened moderately.

The elimination half-life of a drug with a low extraction ratio is decreased significantly by an increase in hepatic enzyme activity. In contrast, the elimination half-life of a drug with a high extraction ratio is not markedly affected by an increase in hepatic enzyme activity because enzyme activity is already quite high. In both cases, an orally administered drug with a higher extraction ratio results in a greater first-pass effect as shown by a reduction in the AUC (Fig. 13-18).

Effect of Changing Blood Flow on Drugs with High or Low Extraction Ratio

Drug clearance and elimination half-life are both affected by changing blood flow to the liver. For drugs with low extraction ($E = 0.1$), a decrease in hepatic blood flow from normal (1.5 L/min) to one half decreases clearance only slightly, and blood level is slightly higher (Fig. 13-19, top left, dotted line). In contrast, for a drug with high extraction ratio ($E = 0.9$), decreasing the blood flow to one half of normal greatly decreases clearance, and the blood level is much higher (Fig. 13-19, top right, dotted line).

Alterations in hepatic blood flow significantly affect the elimination of drugs with high extraction ratios (eg, propranolol) and have very little effect on the elimination of drugs with low extraction ratios (eg, theophylline). For drugs with low extraction ratios, any concentration of drug in the blood that perfuses the liver is more than the liver can eliminate. Consequently, small changes in hepatic blood flow do not affect the removal rate of such drugs. In contrast, drugs with high extraction ratios are removed from the blood as rapidly as they are presented to the liver. If the blood flow to the liver decreases, then the elimination of these drugs are prolonged. Therefore, drugs with high extraction ratios are considered to be *flow dependent.* A number of drugs have been investigated and classified according to their extraction by the liver, as shown in Table 13.10. The relationship between hepatic clearance and blood flow for drugs with different extraction ratio is shown in Figure 13-19.

Effect of Protein Binding on Hepatic Clearance

The effect of protein binding on hepatic clearance is often difficult to quantitate precisely because it is not always known whether the bound drug is restrictively or nonrestrictively cleared. For example, animal tissue levels of imipramine, a nonrestrictively cleared drug, was shown to change as the degree of plasma protein binding changes (see Chapter 11). As discussed, drug protein binding is not a factor in hepatic clearance for drugs that have high extraction ratios. These drugs are considered to be flow limited. In contrast, drugs that have low extraction ratios may be affected by plasma protein binding depending on the fraction of drug bound. For a drug that has a low extraction ratio and is less than 75 to 80% bound, small changes in protein binding would not produce significant changes in hepatic clearance. These drugs are considered *capacity-limited, binding-insensitive drugs* (Blaschke, 1977) and are listed in Table 13.10. Drugs highly bound to plasma protein but with low extraction ratios are considered *capacity limited and binding sensitive* because a small displacement in the protein binding of these drugs will cause a very large increase in the free drug concentration. These drugs are good examples of restrictively cleared drugs. A large increase in free drug concentration will cause an increase in the rate of drug metabolism, resulting in an overall increase in hepatic clearance. Figure 13-20 is a diagram demonstrating the relationship of protein binding, blood flow, and extraction.

SIGNIFICANCE OF DRUG METABOLISM

It is important to consider what fraction of the drug is eliminated by metabolism and what fraction is eliminated by excretion. Drugs that are highly metabolized (such as phenytoin, theophylline, and lidocaine) demonstrate large variations in elimination half-lives in humans. Unlike renal drug excretion, which is highly dependent on the glomerular filtration rate (relatively constant among individuals),

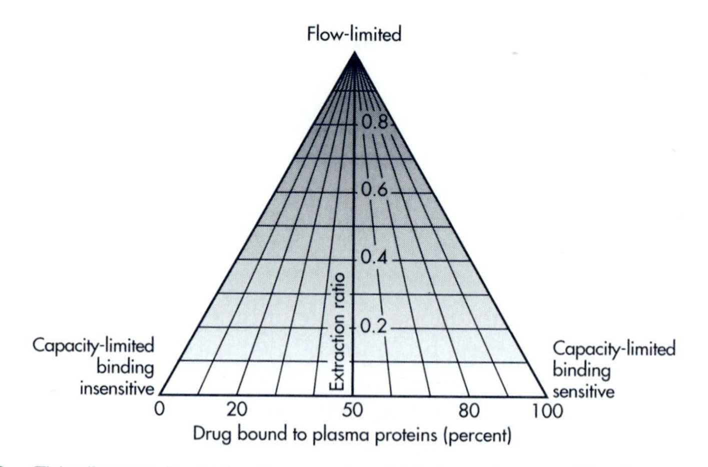

Figure 13-20. This diagram illustrates the way in which two pharmacokinetic parameters (hepatic extraction ratio and percent plasma protein binding) are used to assign a drug into one of three classes of hepatic clearance (flow-limited; capacity-limited, binding sensitive; and capacity-limited, binding insensitive). Any drug metabolized by the liver can be plotted on the triangular graph, but the classification is important only for those eliminated primarily by hepatic processes. The closer a drug falls to a corner of the triangle (shaded areas), the more likely it is to have the characteristic changes in disposition in liver disease as described for the three drug classes in the text.
(From Blaschke, 1977, with permission.)

drug metabolism is dependent on the intrinsic activity of the biotransformation enzymes, which may be altered by genetic and environmental factors.

BILIARY EXCRETION OF DRUGS

The biliary system of the liver is an important system for the secretion of bile and the excretion of drugs. Anatomically, the intrahepatic bile ducts join outside the liver to form the common hepatic duct (Fig. 13-21). The bile that enters the gallbladder becomes highly concentrated. The hepatic duct containing hepatic bile joins the cystic duct that drains the gallbladder to form the common bile duct. The common bile duct then empties into the duodenum. Bile primarily consists of water, bile salts, bile pigments, electrolytes, and, to a lesser extent, cholesterol and fatty

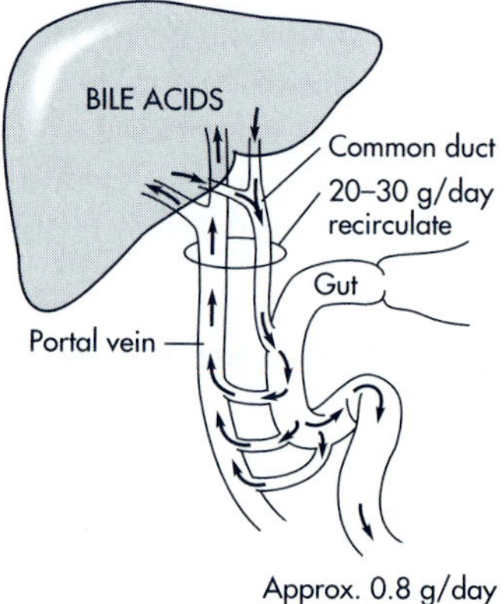

Figure 13-21. Enterohepatic recirculation of bile acids and drug.
(From Dow, 1963.)

TABLE 13.12 Examples of Drugs Undergoing Enterohepatic Circulation and Biliary Excretion

Enterohepatic Circulation	
Imipramine	
Indomethacin	
Morphine	
Pregnenolone	
Biliary Excretion (intact or as metabolites)	
Cefamandole	Fluvastatin
Cefoperazone	Lovastatin
Chloramphenicol	Moxalactam
Diazepam	Practolol
Digoxin	Spironolactone
Doxorubicin	Testosterone
Doxycycline	Tetracycline
Estradiol	Vincristine

acids. The hepatic cells lining the bile canaliculi are responsible for the production of bile. The production of bile appears to be an active secretion process. Separate active biliary secretion processes have been reported for organic anions, organic cations, and for polar, unchanged molecules.

Drugs that are mainly excreted in the bile have molecular weights in excess of 500. Drugs with molecular weights between 300 and 500 are excreted both in urine and in bile. For these drugs, a decrease in one excretory route results in a compensatory increase in excretion via the other route. Compounds with molecular weights of less than 300 are almost exclusively excreted via the kidneys into urine.

In addition to a high molecular weight, drugs excreted into bile usually require a strongly polar group. Many drugs excreted into bile are metabolites, very often glucuronide conjugates. Most metabolites are more polar than the parent drug. In addition, the formation of a glucuronide increases the molecular weight of the compound by nearly 200, as well as increasing the polarity.

Drugs excreted into the bile include the digitalis glycosides, bile salts, cholesterol, steroids, and indomethacin (Table 13.12). Compounds that enhance bile production stimulate the biliary excretion of drugs normally eliminated by this route. Furthermore, phenobarbital, which induces many mixed-function oxidase activities, may stimulate the biliary excretion of drugs by two mechanisms: namely, by an increase in the formation of the glucuronide metabolite and by an increase in bile flow. In contrast, compounds that decrease bile flow or pathophysiologic conditions that cause cholestasis will decrease biliary drug excretion. The route of administration may also influence the amount of the drug excreted into bile. For example, drugs given orally may be extracted by the liver into the bile to a greater extent than if the drugs are given intravenously.

Estimation of Biliary Clearance

The rate of drug elimination may be measured by monitoring the amount of drug secreted into the GI perfusate using a special intubation technique that blocks off a segment of the gut with an inflating balloon. In animals, bile duct cannulation allows both the volume of the bile and the concentration of drug in the bile to be measured directly.

Assuming an average bile flow of 0.5 to 0.8 mL/min in man, biliary clearance can be calculated if the bile concentration, C_{bile} is known.

$$Cl_{biliary} = \frac{\text{bile flow} \times C_{bile}}{C_p} \quad \textbf{(13.50)}$$

Alternatively, using the perfusion technique, the amount of drug eliminated in bile is determined from the GI perfusate, and $Cl_{biliary}$ may be calculated without the bile flow rate, as follows:

$$Cl_{biliary} = \frac{\text{amount of drug secreted from bile per minute}}{C_p} \quad \textbf{(13.51)}$$

To avoid any complication of unabsorbed drug in the feces, the drug should be given by parenteral administration (eg, IV) during biliary determination experiments. The amount of drug in the GI perfusate recovered periodically may then be determined. The extent of biliary elimination of digoxin has been determined in humans using this approach.

Enterohepatic Circulation

A drug or its metabolite is secreted into bile and on contraction of the gallbladder will be excreted into the duodenum via the common bile duct. Subsequently, the drug or its metabolite might be excreted into the feces or the drug may be reabsorbed and become systemically available. The cycle in which the drug is absorbed, excreted into the bile, and reabsorbed is known as *enterohepatic circulation.* Some drugs excreted as a glucuronide conjugate will become hydrolized in the gut back to the parent drug by the action of a β-glucuronidase enzyme present in the intestinal bacteria. In this case, the parent drug becomes available for reabsorption.

Significance of Biliary Excretion

When a drug appears in the feces after oral administration, it is difficult to determine whether this presence of drug is due to biliary excretion or incomplete absorption. If the drug is given parenterally and then observed in the feces, one can assess that some of the drug was excreted in the bile. Because drug secretion into bile is an active process, it is possible to saturate this process with high drug concentrations. Moreover, other drugs may compete for the same carrier system.

Enterohepatic circulation after a single dose of drug is not as important as after multiple doses or a very high dose of drug. With a large dose or multiple doses, a larger amount of drug is secreted in the bile, from which drug is then reabsorbed. This reabsorption process may affect the absorption and elimination rate constants. Furthermore, the biliary secretion process may become saturated, thus altering the plasma level–time curve.

Drugs that undergo enterohepatic circulation sometimes show a small secondary peak in the plasma drug concentration curve. The first peak occurs as the drug in the GI tract is depleted; a small secondary peak then emerges as biliary-excreted drug is reabsorbed. In experimental studies involving animals, bile duct cannulation provides a means of estimating the amount of drug excreted through the bile. In humans, a less accurate estimation of biliary excretion may be made from the recovery of drug excreted through the feces. However, if the drug were given orally, some of the fecal drug excretion could represent unabsorbed drug.

? FREQUENTLY ASKED QUESTIONS

1. Why do we use the term *hepatic drug clearance* to describe drug metabolism in the liver?
2. Please explain why many drugs with significant metabolism often have variable bioavailability.
3. The metabolism of some drugs are affected more than others when there is a change in protein binding. Why?
4. Please give some examples that explain why the metabolic pharmacokinetics of drugs are important in patient care.

LEARNING QUESTIONS

1. A drug fitting a one-compartment model was found to be eliminated from the plasma by the following pathways with the corresponding elimination rate constants.
   - Metabolism $k_m = 0.200\ \text{hr}^{-1}$
   - Kidney excretion $k_e = 0.250\ \text{hr}^{-1}$
   - Biliary excretion $k_b = 0.150\ \text{hr}^{-1}$

   a. What is the elimination half-life of this drug?
   b. What would the half-life of this drug be if biliary secretion were completely blocked?
   c. What would the half-life of this drug be if drug excretion through the kidney were completely impaired?
   d. If drug-metabolizing enzymes were induced so that the rate of metabolism of this drug doubled, what would the new elimination half-life be?
2. A new broad-spectrum antibiotic was administered by rapid intravenous injection to a 50-kg woman at a dose of 3 mg/kg. The apparent volume of distribution of this drug was equivalent to 5% of the body weight. The elimination half-life for this drug is 2 hours.
   a. If 90% of the unchanged drug was recovered in the urine, what is the renal excretion rate constant?
   b. Which is more important for the elimination of the drugs, renal excretion or biotransformation? Why?
3. Explain briefly:
   a. Why does a drug that has a high extraction ratio (eg, propranolol) demonstrate greater differences between individuals after oral administration than after intravenous administration?
   b. Why does a drug with a low hepatic extraction ratio (eg, theophylline) demonstrate greater differences between individuals after hepatic enzyme induction than a drug with a high hepatic extraction ratio?

4. A drug is being screened for antihypertensive activity. After oral administration, the onset time is 0.5 to 1 hours. However, after intravenous administration, the onset time is 6 to 8 hours.
   a. What reasons would you give for the differences in the onset times for oral and intravenous drug administration?
   b. Devise an experiment that would prove the validity of your reasoning.
5. Calculate the hepatic clearance for a drug with an intrinsic clearance of 40 mL/min in a normal adult patient whose hepatic blood flow is 1.5 L/min.
   a. If the patient develops congestive heart failure that reduces hepatic blood flow to 1.0 L/min but does not affect the intrinsic clearance, what is the hepatic drug clearance in this patient?
   b. If the patient is concurrently receiving medication, such as phenobarbital which increases the Cl_{int} to 90 mL/min but does not alter the hepatic blood flow (1.5 L/min), what is the hepatic clearance for the drug in this patient?
6. Calculate the hepatic clearance for a drug with an intrinsic clearance of 12 L/min in a normal adult patient whose hepatic blood flow is 1.5 L/min. If this same patient develops congestive heart failure that reduces his hepatic blood flow to 1.0 L/min but does not affect intrinsic clearance, what is the hepatic drug clearance in this patient?
   a. Calculate the extraction ratio for the liver in this patient before and after congestive heart failure develops.
   b. From the above information, estimate the fraction of bioavailable drug, assuming the drug is given orally and absorption is complete.
7. Why do elimination half-lives of drugs primarily eliminated by hepatic biotransformation demonstrate greater intersubject variability than those drugs eliminated primarily by glomerular filtration?
8. A new drug demonstrates high presystemic elimination when taken orally. From which of the following drug products would the drug be most bioavailable? Why?
   a. Aqueous solution
   b. Suspension
   c. Capsule (hard gelatin)
   d. Tablet
   e. Sustained release
9. For a drug that demonstrated presystemic elimination, would you expect qualitative and/or quantitative differences in the formation of metabolites from this drug given orally compared to intravenous injection? Why?
10. The bioavailability of propranolol is 26%. Propranolol is 87% bound to plasma proteins and has an elimination half-life of 3.9 hr. The apparent volume of distribution of propranolol is 4.3 L/kg. Less than 0.5% of the unchanged drug is excreted in the urine.
    a. Calculate the hepatic clearance for propranolol in an adult male patient (43 yr, 80 kg).
    b. Assuming the hepatic blood flow is 1500 mL/min, estimate the hepatic extraction ratio for propranolol.
    c. Explain why hepatic clearance is more important than renal clearance for the elimination of propranolol.
    d. What would be the effect of hepatic disease such as cirrhosis on the (1) bioavailability of propranolol and (2) hepatic clearance of propranolol?

e. Explain how a change in (1) hepatic blood flow, (2) intrinsic clearance, or (3) plasma protein binding would effect hepatic clearance of propranolol.

f. What is meant by *first-pass effects?* From the data above, why is propranolol a drug with first-pass effects?

11. The following pharmacokinetic information for erythromycin was reported in Gilman et al: *Goodman and Gilman's The Pharmacologic Basis of Therapeutics,* 8th ed. (Pergamon Press, 1990, p 1679).

- Bioavailability (%) 35
- Urinary excretion (%) 12
- Bound in plasma (%) 84
- Volume of distribution (L/kg) 0.78
- Elimination half-life (hr) 1.6

An adult male patient (41 yr, 81 kg) was prescribed 250 mg erythromycin base every 6 hours for 10 days. From the data above, calculate the following:

a. Total body clearance

b. Renal clearance

c. Hepatic clearance

12. Why would you expect hepatic clearance of theophylline in *identical* twins to be less variable compared to hepatic clearance in *fraternal* twins?

13. Which of the following statements describe(s) correctly the properties of a drug that follows nonlinear or capacity-limited pharmacokinetics?

a. The elimination half-life will remain constant when the dose changes.

b. The area under the plasma curve (AUC) will increase proportionately with an increase in dose.

c. The rate of drug elimination = $C_p \times K_M$.

d. At maximum saturation of the enzyme by the substrate, the reaction velocity is at V_{max}.

e. At very low substrate concentrations, the reaction rate approximates a zero-order rate.

14. The V_{max} for metabolizing a drug is 10 μM/hr. The rate of metabolism (v) is 5 μM/hr when drug concentration is 4 μM. Which of the following statements is/are true?

a. K_M is 5 μM for this drug.

b. K_M cannot be determined from the information given.

c. K_M is 4 μM for this drug.

15. Which of the following statements is/are true regarding the pharmacokinetics of diazepam (98% protein bound) and propranolol (87% protein bound)?

a. Diazepam has a long elimination half-life due to its lack of metabolism and its extensive plasma protein binding.

b. Propranolol is a drug with high protein binding but unrestricted (unaffected) metabolic clearance.

c. Diazepam exhibits low hepatic extraction.

16. The hepatic intrinsic clearance of two drugs are as follows:

- Drug *A*: 1300 mL/min
- Drug *B*: 26 mL/min

Which drug is likely to show the greatest increase in hepatic clearance when hepatic blood flow is increased from 1 L/min to 1.5 mL/min? Which drug will likely be blood-flow limited?

REFERENCES

Alvares AP, Pratt WB: Pathways of drug metabolism. In Pratt WB, Taylor P (eds), *Principles of Drug Action*, 3rd ed. New York, Churchill Livingstone, 1990, chap 5

Ariens EJ, Wuis EW: Commentary: Bias in pharmacokinetics and clinical pharmacology. *Clin Pharm Ther* **42:**361–363, 1987

Baily DG, Arnold JMO, Strong HA, Munoz C, Spence JD: Effect of grapefruit juice and naringin on nisoldipine pharmacokinetics. *Clin Pharm Therap* **54:**589–593, 1993

Baily DG, Arnold JMO, Munoz C, Spence JD: Grapefruit juice–felodipine interaction: Mechanism, predictability, and effect of naringin. *Clin Pharm Therap* **53:**637–642, 1993

Bertilsson L: Geographic/interracial differences in polymorphic drug oxidation. *Clin Pharmacokinet* **29**(4):192–209, 1995

Blaschke TF: Protein binding and kinetics of drugs in liver diseases. *Clin Pharmacokinet* **2:**32–44, 1977

Brosen K: Recent developments in hepatic drug oxidation. *Clin Pharmacokinet* **18:**220, 1990

Brouwer KL, Dukes GE, Powell JR: Influence of liver function on drug disposition. Applied pharmacokinetics. In Evans WE et al (eds), *Principles of Therapeutic Drug Monitoring.* Vancouver, WA, Applied Therapeutics, 1992, chap 6

Caldwell J: Conjugation reactions. In Jenner P, Testa B (eds), *Concepts in Drug Metabolism.* New York, Marcel Dekker, 1980, chap 4

Campbell TC: Nutrition and drug-metabolizing enzymes. *Clin Pharm Ther* **22:**699–706, 1977

Caraco Y, Sheller J, Wood AJJ: Pharmacogenetic determination of the effects of codeine and prediction of drug interactions. *J Pharmacol Exp Ther* **278:**1165–1174, 1996

Dow P: *Handbook of Physiology*, vol 2, *Circulation.* Washington, DC, American Physiology Society, 1963, p 1406

Ducharme MP, Warbasse LH, Edwards DJ: Disposition of intravenous and oral cyclosporine after administration with grapefruit juice. *Clin Pharm Therap* **57:**485–491, 1995

Evans DAP: Genetic variations in the acetylation of isoniazid and other drugs. *Ann NY Acad Sci* **151:**723, 1968

Evans DAP, Manley KA, McKusik VC: Genetic control of isoniazid metabolism in man. *Br Med J* **2:**485, 1968

Gilman AG, Rall TW, Nies AS, Taylor (eds): *Goodman and Gilman's The Pharmacological Basis of Therapeutics*, 8th ed. Elmsford, NY, Pergamon Press, 1990

Gray H: *Anatomy of the Human Body*, 30th ed. Philadelphia, Lea & Febiger, 1985, p 1495

Hansch C, Zhang L: Quantitative structure-activity relationships of cytochrome P-450. *Drug Met Rev* **25:**1–48, 1993

Harder S, Baas H, Rietbrock S: Concentration effect relationship of levodopa in patients with Parkinson's disease. *Clin Pharmacok* **29:**243–256, 1995

Hucker HB, Kwan KC, Duggan DE: Pharmacokinetics and metabolism of nonsteroidal antiinflammatory agents. In Bridges JW, Chasseaud LF (eds), *Progress in Drug Research*, vol 5. New York, Wiley, 1980, chap 3

Hukkinen SK, Varhe A, Olkkola KT, Neuvonen PJ: Plasma concentrations of triazolam are increased by concomitant ingestion of grapefruit juice. *Clin Pharm Therap* **58:**127–131, 1995

Iwakawa S, Suganuma T, Lee S, et al: Direct determination of diastereomeric carprofen glucuronides in human plasma and urine and preliminary measurements of stereoselective metabolic and renal elimination after oral administration of carprofen in man. *Drug Metab Disp* **17:**414–419, 1989

Kupferschmidt HH, Ha HR, Ziegler WH, Meier PJ, Krahenbuhl S: Interaction between grapefruit juice and midazolam in humans. *Clin Pharm Therap* **58:**20–28, 1995

Lai ML, Wang SL, Lai MD, Lin ET, Tse M, Huang JD: Propranolol disposition in Chinese subjects of different CYT2D6 genotypes. *Clin Pharm Ther* **58:**264–268, 1995

Levy RH, Boddy AV: Stereoselectivity in pharmacokinetics: A general theory. *Pharm Res* **8:**551–556, 1991

Lanctot KL, Naranjo CA: Comparison of the Bayesian approach and a simple algorithm for assessment of adverse drug events. *Clin Pharm Ther* **58:**692–698, 1995

Merkel U, Sigusch H, Hoffmann A: Grapefruit juice inhibits 7-hydroxylation of coumarin in healthy volunteers. *Eur J Clin Pharm* **46:**175–177, 1994

Nebert DW, et al: The P-450 superfamily: Updated listing of all genes and recommended nomenclature for the chromosomal loci. *DNA* **8:**1, 1989

Negishi M, Tomohide U, Darden TA, Sueyoshi T, Pedersen LG: Structural flexibility and functional versatility of mammalian P-450 enzymes. *FASEB J* **10:**683–689, 1996

Rahmani R, Zhou XJ: Pharmacokinetics and metabolism of vinca alkaloids. *Cancer Surv* **17:**269–281, 1993

Rowland M: Drug administration and regimens. In Melmon K, Morelli HF (eds), *Clinical Pharmacology.* New York, Macmillan, 1978

Rowland M: Effect of some physiologic factors on bioavailability of oral dosage forms. In Swarbrick J (ed), *Current Concepts in the Pharmaceutical Sciences: Dosage Form Design and Bioavailability.* Philadelphia, Lea & Febiger, 1973, chap 6

Toney GB, Ereshefsky L: Cyclic antidepressants. In Schumacher GE, *Therapeutic Drug Monitoring.* Norwalk, CT, Appleton & Lange, 1995, chap 13

Tucker GT, Lennard MS: Enantiomer-specific pharmacokinetics. *Pharmacol Ther* **45:**309–329, 1990

Wilkinson GR, Guengerich FP, Branch RA: Genetic polymorphism of S-mephenytoin hydroxylation. *Pharmacol Ther* **43:**53–76, 1989

Wilkinson GR, Shand DG: A physiological approach to hepatic drug clearance. *Clin Pharmacol Ther* **18:**377–390, 1975

Wolf CR: Distribution and regulation of drug-metabolizing enzymes in mammalian tissues. In Caldwell J, Paulson GD, *Foreign Compound Metabolism.* London, Taylor & Francis, 1984

Yee GC, Stanley DL, Pessa LJ, et al: Effect of grapefruit juice on blood cyclosporin concentration. *Lancet* **345:**955–956, 1995

BIBLIOGRAPHY

Anders MW: *Bioactivation of Foreign Compounds.* New York, Academic Press, 1985

Balant LP, McAinsh JM: Use of metabolite data in the evaluation of pharmacokinetics and drug action. In Jenner P, Testa B (eds), *Concepts in Drug Metabolism.* New York, Marcel Dekker, 1980, chap 7

Benet LZ: Effect of route of administration and distribution on drug action. *J Pharm Biopharm* **6:**559–585, 1978

Blaschke TF: Protein binding and kinetics of drugs in liver diseases. *Clin Pharmacokinet* **2:**32–44, 1977

Brown C (ed): *Chirality in Drug Design and Synthesis: Racemic Therapeutics—Problems All Along the Line* (EJ Ariens), New York, Academic Press, 1990

Geroge CF, Shand DG, Renwick AG (eds): *Presystemic Drug Elimination.* Boston, Butterworth, 1982

Gibaldi M, Perrier D: Route of administration and drug disposition. *Drug Metab Rev* **3:**185–199, 1974

Gibson GG, Skett P: *Introduction to Drug Metabolism,* 2nd ed. New York, Chapman & Hall, 1994

Glocklin VC: General considerations for studies of the metabolism of drugs and other chemicals. *Drug Metab Rev* **13:**929–939, 1982

Gorrod JW, Damani LA: *Biological Oxidation of Nitrogen in Organic Molecules: Chemistry, Toxicology and Pharmacology.* Deerfield Beach, FL, Ellis Horwood, 1985

Hildebrandt A, Estabrook RW: Evidence for the participation of cytochrome b_5 in hepatic microsomal mixed-function oxidation reactions. *Arch Biochem Biophys* **143:**66–79, 1971

Houston JB: Drug metabolite kinetics. *Pharmacol Ther* **15:**521–552, 1982

Jakoby WB: *Enzymatic Basis of Detoxification.* New York, Academic Press, 1980

Jenner P, Testa B: *Concepts in Drug Metabolism.* New York, Marcel Dekker, 1980–1981

Kaplan SA, Jack ML: Physiologic and metabolic variables in bioavailability studies. In Garrett ER, Hirtz JL (eds), *Drug Fate and Metabolism,* vol 3. New York, Marcel Dekker, 1979

LaDu BL, Mandel HG, Way EL: *Fundamentals of Drug Metabolism and Drug Disposition.* Baltimore, Williams & Wilkins, 1971

Levine WG: Biliary excretion of drugs and other xenobiotics. *Prog Drug Res* **25:**361–420, 1981

May GD: Genetic differences in drug disposition. *J Clin Pharmacol* **34:**881–897, 1994

Morris ME, Pang KS: Competition between two enzymes for substrate removal in liver: Modulating effects due to substrate recruitment of hepatocyte activity. *J Pharm Biopharm* **15:**473–496, 1987

Nies AS, Shand DG, Wilkinson GR: Altered hepatic blood flow and drug disposition. *Clin Pharmacokinet* **1:**135–156, 1976

Pang KS, Rowland M: Hepatic clearance of drugs, 1. Theoretical considerations of a "well-stirred" model and a "parallel tube" model. Influence of hepatic blood flow, plasma, and blood cell binding and the hepatocellular enzymatic activity on hepatic drug clearance. *J Pharmacokinet Biopharm* **5:**625, 1977

Perrier D, Gibaldi M: Clearance and biologic half-life as indices of intrinsic hepatic metabolism. *J Pharmacol Exp Ther* **191:**17–24, 1974

Plaa GL: The enterohepatic circulation. In Gillette JR, Mitchell JR (eds), *Concepts in Biochemical Pharmacology.* New York, Springer-Verlag, 1975, chap 63

Pratt WB, Taylor P: *Principles of Drug Action: The Basis of Pharmacology,* 3rd ed. New York, Churchill Livingstone, 1990

Roberts MS, Donaldson JD, Rowland M: Models of hepatic elimination: Comparison of stochastic models to describe residence time distributions and to predict the influence of drug distribution, enzyme heterogeneity, and systemic recycling on hepatic elimination. *J Pharm Biopharm* **16:**41–83, 1988

Routledge PA, Shand DG: Presystemic drug elimination. *Annu Rev Pharmacol Toxicol* **19:**447–468, 1979

Semple HA, Tam YK, Coutts RT: A computer simulation of the food effect: Transient changes in hepatic blood flow and Michaelis–Menten parameters as mediators of hepatic first-pass metabolism and bioavailability of propranolol. *Biopharm Drug Disp* **11:**61–76, 1990

Shand DG, Kornhauser DM, Wilkinson GR: Effects of route administration and blood flow on hepatic drug elimination. *J Pharmacol Exp Ther* **195:**425–432, 1975

Stoltenborg JK, Puglisi CV, Rubio F, Vane FM: High performance liquid chromatographic determination of stereoselective disposition of carprofen in humans. *J Pharm Sci* **70:**1207–1212, 1981

Testa B, Jenner B: *Drug Metabolism: Chemical and Biochemical Aspects.* New York, Marcel Dekker, 1976

Tucker GT: Clinical implications of genetic polymorphism in drug metabolism. *J Pharm Pharmacol* **46**(suppl):417–424, 1994

Venot A, Walter E, Lecourtier Y, et al: Structural identifiability of "first-pass" models. *J Pharm Biopharm* **15:**179–189, 1987

Wilkinson GR: Pharmacodynamics of drug disposition: Hemodynamic considerations. *Annu Rev Pharmacol* **15:**11–27, 1975

Wilkinson GR: Pharmacodynamics in disease states modifying body perfusion. In Benet LZ (ed), *The Effect of Disease States on Drug Pharmacokinetics.* Washington, DC, American Pharmaceutical Association, 1976

Wilkinson GR, Rawlins MD: *Drug Metabolism and Disposition: Considerations in Clinical Pharmacology.* Boston, MTP Press, 1985

Williams RT: Hepatic metabolism of drugs. *Gut* **13:**579–585, 1972

14

INTRAVENOUS INFUSION

Intravenous infusion is a direct method by which the drug is administered systemically into the body. Intravenous (IV) drug solutions may be given either as a bolus dose or infused slowly at a constant or zero-order rate. The main advantage for giving a drug by IV infusion is the precise control of plasma drug concentrations to fit the individual needs of the patient. For drugs with a narrow therapeutic window, IV infusion maintains an effective constant plasma drug concentration by eliminating wide fluctuations between the peak (maximum) and trough (minimum) plasma drug concentration. Moreover, the IV infusion of drugs, such as antibiotics, may be given with IV fluids including electrolytes and nutrients. Furthermore, the duration of drug therapy may be maintained or terminated as needed using IV infusion.

The plasma drug concentration versus time curve of a drug given by constant IV infusion is shown in Figure 14-1. Because no drug was present in the body at zero time, drug level rises from zero drug concentration and gradually becomes constant when a *plateau* or *steady-state* drug concentration is reached. At steady state, the rate of drug leaving the body is equal to the rate of drug (infusion rate) entering the body. Therefore, the rate of change in the plasma drug concentration $dC_p/dt = 0$, and

Rate of drug input = rate of drug output
(infusion rate)   (elimination rate)

Based on this simple mass balance relationship, a pharmacokinetic equation for infusion may be derived depending on whether the drug follows one- or two-compartment kinetics.

ONE-COMPARTMENT MODEL DRUGS

The pharmacokinetics of a drug given by constant IV infusion is a zero-order input process in which the drug is directly infused into the systemic blood circulation. For most drugs, elimination of drug from the plasma is a first-order process. Therefore, in this model, the infused drug follows zero-order input and first-order

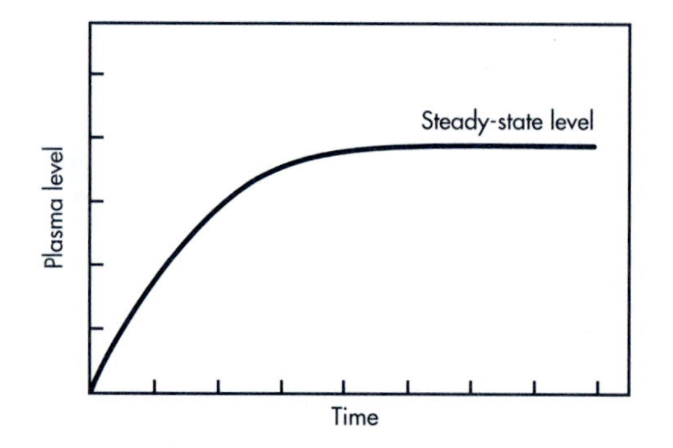

Figure 14-1. Plasma level–time curve for constant IV infusion.

C_{ss}^{∞}

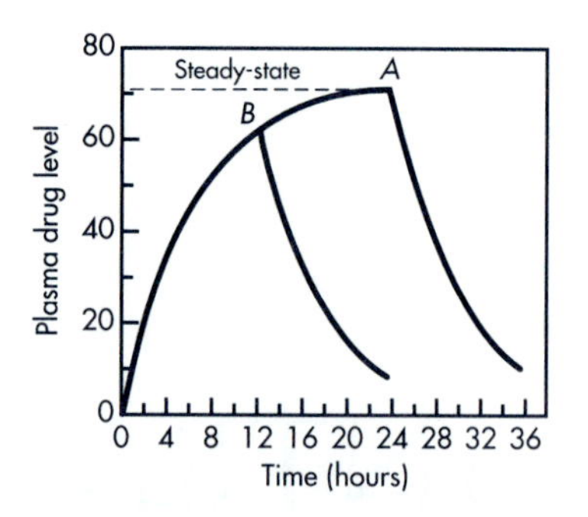

Figure 14-2. Plasma drug concentrations versus time profiles after IV infusion. IV infusion is stopped at steady state **(A)** or prior to steady-state **(B).** In both cases, plasma drug concentrations decline exponentially (first order) according to a similar slope.

output. The change in the amount of drug in the body at any time (dD_B/dt) during the infusion is the rate of input minus the rate of output.

$$\frac{dD_B}{dt} = R - kD_B \tag{14.1}$$

where D_B is the amount of drug in the body, R is the infusion rate (zero order), and k is the elimination rate constant (first order).

Integration of Equation 14.1 and substitution of $D_B = C_p V_D$ gives

$$C_p = \frac{R}{V_D k}(1 - e^{-kt}) \tag{14.2}$$

Equation 14.2 gives the plasma drug concentration at any time during the IV infusion where t is the time for infusion. The graph of Equation 14.2 appears in Figures 14-1 and 14-2. Drug elimination occurs according to first-order elimination rate. Whenever the infusion stops either at steady state, or before steady state is reached, the drug concentration declines according to first-order kinetics with the slope of the elimination curve equal to $-k/2.3$ (Fig. 14-2). If the infusion is stopped before steady state is reached, the slope of the elimination curve remains the same (Fig. 14-2B).

From a mathematical viewpoint, all infusions are stopped before true steady state is reached, because the theoretical steady state is only reached after an infinitely long infusion time. In clinical practice, a plasma drug concentration prior to, but approaching, the theoretical steady state is considered the steady-state plasma drug concentration.

As the drug is infused, the value for time (t) increases in Equation 14.2. At infinite time, $t = \infty$, e^{-kt} approaches zero, and Equation 14.2 reduces to Equation 14.4.

$$C_p = \frac{R}{V_D k}(1 - e^{-\infty}) \tag{14.3}$$

$$C_{ss} = \frac{R}{V_D k} \tag{14.4}$$

$$C_{ss} = \frac{R}{V_D k} = \frac{R}{Cl} \tag{14.5}$$

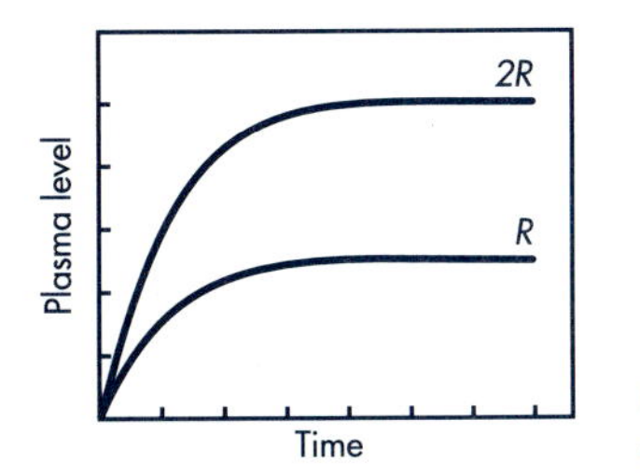

Figure 14-3. Plasma level–time curve for IV infusions given at rates of R and $2R$, respectively.

Steady-State Drug Concentration (C_{ss}) and Time Needed to Reach C_{ss}

The time required to reach the steady-state drug concentration in the plasma is dependent on the elimination rate constant of the drug for a constant volume of distribution. For a zero-order process, if rate of input is greater than rate of elimination, plasma drug concentration will keep increasing and no steady state will be reached. This is a potentially dangerous situation that will occur when saturation of metabolic process occurs.

For most drugs, however, at therapeutic concentrations, drugs are eliminated by a first order process. When infused at a constant rate R, the infusion rate will be fixed while the rate of elimination steadily increases until steady state is reached because rate of elimination is concentration dependent (ie, C_p keeps increasing until steady state is reached).

$$\text{Rate of elimination} = kC_p$$

(See Chapter 2).

For a drug with a small k and a constant (fixed) rate of infusion, a long time is needed for kC_p to reach C_{ss}. In pharmacokinetics, the time to reach steady state is, therefore, inversely related to k or directly related to the elimination half-life of the drug. (See numerical example in Example 2 below.) In theory, an infinite time is needed after the start of the IV infusion for the drug to reach the steady-state drug concentration, because drug elimination is exponential (first order). Thus, the plasma drug concentration becomes asymptotic to the theoretical steady-state plasma drug concentration. The plasma drug concentration at steady state is related to the rate of infusion and inversely related to the body clearance of the drug as shown in Equation 14.5.

In clinical practice, however, the activity of the drug will be observed when the drug concentration is close to the desired plasma drug concentration, which is usually the *target* or steady-state drug concentration. The time to reach 90, 95, and 99% of the steady-state drug concentration may be calculated (Table 14.1). For therapeutic purposes, the time for the plasma drug concentration to reach more than 95% of the steady-state drug concentration in the plasma is often estimated. From Table 14.1, after IV infusion of the drug for 5 half-lives the plasma drug concen-

TABLE 14.1 Number of $t_{1/2}$ to Reach a Fraction of C_{SS}

PERCENT OF C_{SS} REACHED[a]	NUMBER OF HALF-LIVES
90	3.32
95	4.32
99	6.65

[a]C_{ss} is the steady-state drug concentration in plasma.

tration will be between 95% (4.32 $t_{1/2}$) and 99% (6.65 $t_{1/2}$) of the steady-state drug concentration. Thus, the time for a drug whose $t_{1/2}$ is 6 hours to reach >95% of the steady-state plasma drug concentration will be 5 $t_{1/2}$, or 5 × 6 hours = 30 hours.

An increase in the infusion rate will not shorten the time to reach the steady-state drug concentration. If the drug is given at a more rapid infusion rate, a higher steady-state drug level will be obtained, but the time to reach steady state is the same (Fig. 14-3). This equation may also be obtained with the following approach. At steady state, the rate of infusion equals the rate of elimination. Therefore, the rate of change in the plasma drug concentration is equal to zero.

$$\frac{dC_p}{dt} = 0$$

$$\frac{dC_p}{dt} = \frac{R}{V_D} - kC_p = 0$$

$$(\text{Rate in}) - (\text{rate out}) = 0$$

$$\frac{R}{V_D} = kC_p$$

$$C_{ss} = \frac{R}{V_D k} \tag{14.6}$$

Equation 14.6 shows that the steady-state concentration (C_{ss}) is dependent on the volume of distribution, the elimination rate constant, and the infusion rate. Altering any one of these factors can affect steady-state concentration.

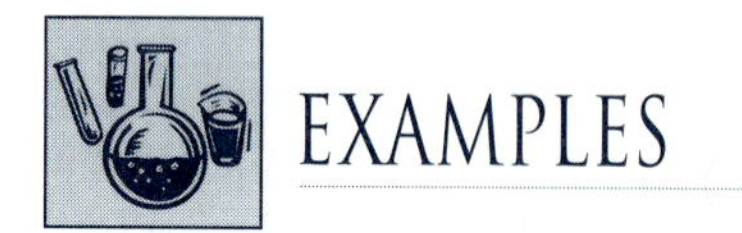

EXAMPLES

1. An antibiotic has a volume of distribution of 10 L and a k of 0.2 hr^{-1}. A steady-state plasma concentration of 10 μg/mL is desired. The infusion rate needed to maintain this concentration can be determined as follows.

Equation 14.6 can be rewritten as

$$\begin{aligned} R &= C_{ss} V_D k \\ &= (10\ \mu\text{g/mL})(10)(1000\ \text{mL})(0.2\ \text{hr}^{-1}) \\ &= 20\ \text{mg/hr} \end{aligned}$$

Assume the patient has a uremic condition and the elimination rate constant has decreased to 0.1 hr^{-1}. To maintain the steady-state concentration of 10 μg/mL, we must determine a new rate of infusion as follows.

$$R = (10\ \mu\text{g/mL})(10)(1000\ \text{mL})(0.1\ \text{hr}^{-1}) = 10\ \text{mg/hr}$$

When the elimination rate constant decreases, then the infusion rate must decrease proportionately to maintain the same C_{ss}. However, because the elimination rate constant is smaller (ie, the elimination $t_{1/2}$ is longer), the time to reach C_{ss} will be longer.

2. An infinitely long period of time is needed to reach steady-state drug levels. However, in practice it is quite acceptable to reach 99% C_{ss} (ie, 99% steady-state level). Using Equation 14.6, we know that the steady-state level is

$$C_{ss} = \frac{R}{V_D k}$$

and 99% steady-state level would be equal to

$$99\% \frac{R}{V_D k}$$

Substituting into Equation 14.2 for C_p, we can find out the time needed to reach steady state by solving for t.

$$99\% \frac{R}{V_D k} = \frac{R}{V_D k}(1 - e^{-kt})$$
$$99\% = 1 - e^{-kt}$$
$$e^{-kt} = 1\%$$

Take the natural logarithm on both sides:

$$-kt = \ln 0.01$$
$$t_{99\%ss} = \frac{\ln 0.01}{-k} = \frac{-4.61}{-k} = \frac{4.61}{k}$$

substituting $(0.693/t_{1/2})$ for k,

$$t_{99\%ss} = \frac{4.61}{(0.693/t_{1/2})} = \frac{4.61}{0.693} t_{1/2}$$
$$t_{99\%ss} = 6.65 t_{1/2}$$

Notice that in the equation directly above, the time needed to reach steady state is not dependent on the rate of infusion, but only on the elimination half-life. Using similar calculations, the time needed to reach any percentage of the steady-state drug concentration may be obtained (Table 14.1).

IV infusion may be used to determine total body clearance if the infusion rate and steady-state level are known, as with Equation 14.6 repeated here:

$$C_{ss} = \frac{R}{V_D k} \quad \textbf{(14.6)}$$
$$V_D k = \frac{R}{C_{ss}}$$

because total body clearance, Cl_T, is equal to $V_D k$,

$$Cl_T = \frac{R}{C_{ss}} \quad \textbf{(14.7)}$$

3. A patient was given an antibiotic ($t_{1/2}$ = 6 hr) by constant IV infusion at a rate of 2 mg/hr. At the end of 2 days, the serum drug concentration was 10 mg/L. Calculate the total body clearance Cl_T for this antibiotic.

Solution

The total body clearance may be estimated from Equation 14.7. The serum sample was taken after 2 days or 48 hours of infusion, which time represents 8 $t_{1/2}$. Therefore, this serum drug concentration approximates the C_{ss}.

$$Cl_T = \frac{R}{C_{ss}} = \frac{2 \text{ mg/hr}}{10 \text{ mg/L}} = 200 \text{ mL/hr}$$

INFUSION METHOD FOR CALCULATING PATIENT ELIMINATION HALF-LIFE

Equation 14.2 may be used to calculate k, or indirectly the elimination half-life of the drug in a patient. Some information about the elimination half-life of the drug in the population must be known, and one or two plasma samples must be taken at a known time after infusion. Knowing the half-life in the general population helps to determine if the sample is taken at steady state in the patient. To simplify calculation, Equation 14.2 is arranged to solve for k,

$$C_p = \frac{R}{V_D k}(1 - e^{-kt}) \qquad \textbf{(14.2)}$$

Since

$$C_{ss} = \frac{R}{V_D k}$$

Substituting into Equation 14.2:

$$C_p = C_{ss}(1 - e^{-kt})$$

Rearranging and taking the log on both sides:

$$\log\left[\frac{C_{ss} - C_p}{C_{ss}}\right] = -\frac{kt}{2.3} \text{ and } k = \frac{-2.3}{t}\log\left[\frac{C_{ss} - C_p}{C_{ss}}\right] \qquad \textbf{(14.8)}$$

C_p is the plasma drug concentration taken at time t; C_{ss} is the approximate steady state plasma drug concentration in the patient.

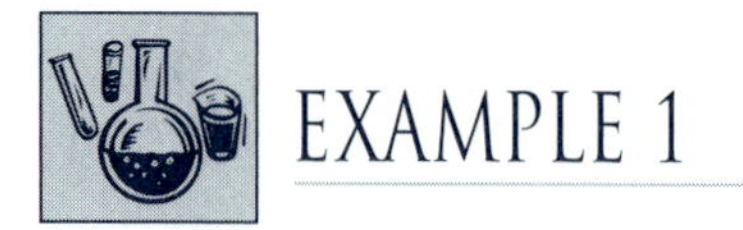

EXAMPLE 1

An antibiotic has an elimination half-life of 3 to 6 hours in the general population. A patient was given an IV infusion of an antibiotic at an infusion rate of 15 mg/hr. Blood samples were taken at 8 and at 24 hours and plasma drug concentrations were 5.5 and 6.5 mg/L, respectively. Estimate the elimination half-life of the drug in this patient.

Solution

Because the second plasma sample was taken at 24 hours, or 24/6 = 4 half-lives after infusion, the plasma drug concentration in this sample is approaching 95% of the true plasma steady-state drug concentration assuming the extreme case of $t_{1/2} = 6$ hours.

By substitution into Equation 14.8:

$$\log\left[\frac{6.5 - 5.5}{6.5}\right] = -\frac{k(8)}{2.3}$$

$$k = 0.234\ \text{hr}^{-1}$$

$$t_{1/2} = 0.693/0.234 = 2.96\ \text{hr}$$

The elimination half-life calculated in this manner is not as accurate as the calculation of $t_{1/2}$ using multiple plasma drug concentration time points after a single IV bolus dose or after stopping the IV infusion. However, this method may be sufficient in clinical practice. As the second blood sample is taken closer to the time for steady state, the accuracy of this method improves. At the 30th hour, for example, the plasma concentration would be 99% of the true steady-state value (corresponding to 30/6 or 5 elimination half-lives), and less error would result in applying Equation 14.8.

When Equation 14.8 was used as in the example above to calculate the drug $t_{1/2}$ of the patient, the second plasma drug concentration was assumed to be the theoretical C_{SS}. As demonstrated below, when $t_{1/2}$ and the corresponding values are substituted,

$$\log\left[\frac{C_{SS} - 5.5}{C_{SS}}\right] = -\frac{(0.231)(8)}{2.3}$$

$$\frac{C_{SS} - 5.5}{C_{SS}} = 0.157$$

$$C_{SS} = 6.5\ \text{mg/L}$$

(Note that C_{SS} is in fact the same as the concentration at 24 hours in the example above.)

In practice, before starting an IV infusion, an appropriate infusion rate (R) is generally calculated from Equation 14.8 using literature values for C_{SS}, k, and V_D or Cl_T. Two plasma samples are taken and the sampling times recorded. The second sample should be taken near the theoretical time for steady state. Equation 14.8 would then be used to calculate a $t_{1/2}$. If the elimination half-life calculated confirms that the second sample was taken at steady state, the plasma concentration is simply assumed as the steady-state concentration and a new infusion rate may be calculated.

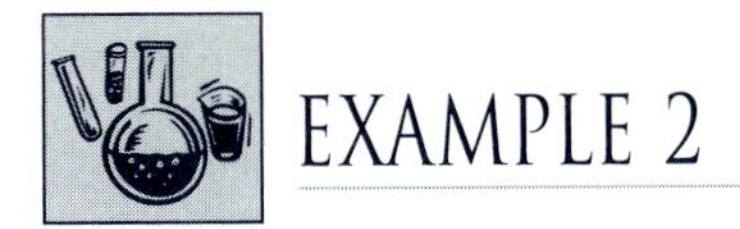

EXAMPLE 2

If the desired therapeutic plasma concentration is 8 mg/L for the above patient (Example 1), what is the suitable infusion rate for the patient?

Solution

From Example 1, the trial infusion rate was 15 mg/hr. Assuming the second blood sample is the steady-state level, 6.5 μg/mL, the clearance of the patient is

$$C_{ss} = R/Cl$$
$$Cl = R/C_{ss} = 15/6.5 = 2.31 \text{ L/hr}$$

The new infusion rate should be

$$R = C_{ss} \times Cl = 8 \times 2.31 = 18.48 \text{ mg/hr}$$

In this example, the $t_{1/2}$ of this patient is a little shorter, about 3 hours compared to 3 to 6 hours reported for the general population. Therefore, the infusion rate should be a little greater in order to maintain the desired steady-state level of 15 mg/L.

Equation 14.7 or the steady-state clearance method has been applied to the clinical infusion of drugs. The method was regarded as simple and accurate compared with other methods, including the two-point method (Hurley and McNeil, 1988).

LOADING DOSE PLUS IV INFUSION

The *loading dose* D_L, or initial bolus dose of a drug, is used to obtain steady-state concentrations as rapidly as possible. The concentration of drug in the body for a one-compartment model after an IV bolus dose is described by

$$C_1 = C_0 e^{-kt} = \frac{D_L}{V_D} e^{-kt} \tag{14.9}$$

and concentration by infusion at the rate R is

$$C_2 = \frac{R}{V_D k}(1 - e^{-kt}) \tag{14.10}$$

Assume that an IV bolus dose D_L of the drug is given and that an IV infusion is started at the same time. The total concentration C_p at t hours after the start of infusion would be equal to $C_1 + C_2$ due to the sum contributions of bolus and infusion, or

$$\begin{aligned} C_p &= C_1 + C_2 \\ &= \frac{D_L}{V_D} e^{-kt} + \frac{R}{V_D k}(1 - e^{-kt}) \\ &= \frac{D_L}{V_D} e^{-kt} + \frac{R}{V_D k} - \frac{R}{V_D k} e^{-kt} \\ &= \frac{R}{V_D k} + \left(\frac{D_L}{V_D} e^{-kt} - \frac{R}{V_D k} e^{-kt}\right) \end{aligned} \tag{14.11}$$

Let the loading dose (D_L) equal the amount of drug in the body at steady state

$$D_L = C_{ss} V_D$$

From Equation 14.4: $C_{ss}V_D = R/k$. Therefore,

$$D_L = R/k \tag{14.12}$$

Substituting $D_L = R/k$ in Equation 14.11 makes the expression in parentheses in Equation 14.12 cancel out. Equation 14.12 reduces to Equation 14.13, which is the same expression for C_{ss} or steady-state plasma concentrations:

$$C_p = \frac{R}{V_D k} \tag{14.13}$$

$$C_{ss} = \frac{R}{V_D k} \tag{14.4}$$

Therefore, if an IV loading dose of R/k is given, followed by an IV infusion, steady-state plasma drug concentrations are obtained immediately and maintained (Fig. 14-4).

The loading dose needed to get immediate steady-state drug levels can also be found by the following approach.

Loading dose equation:

$$C_p = \frac{D_L}{V_D}\, e^{-kt}$$

Infusion equation:

$$C_p = \frac{R}{kV_D}\,(1 - e^{-kt})$$

Adding up the two equations yields Equation 14.14, an equation describing simultaneous infusion after a loading dose.

$$C_p = \frac{D_L}{V_D}\, e^{-kt} + \frac{R}{V_D k}\,(1 - e^{-kt}) \tag{14.14}$$

By differentiating this equation at steady state, we obtain

$$\frac{dC_p}{dt} = 0 = \frac{-D_L k}{V_D}\, e^{-kt} + \frac{Rk}{V_D k}\, e^{-kt} \tag{14.15}$$

$$0 = e^{-kt}\left(\frac{-D_L k}{V_D} + \frac{R}{V_D}\right)$$

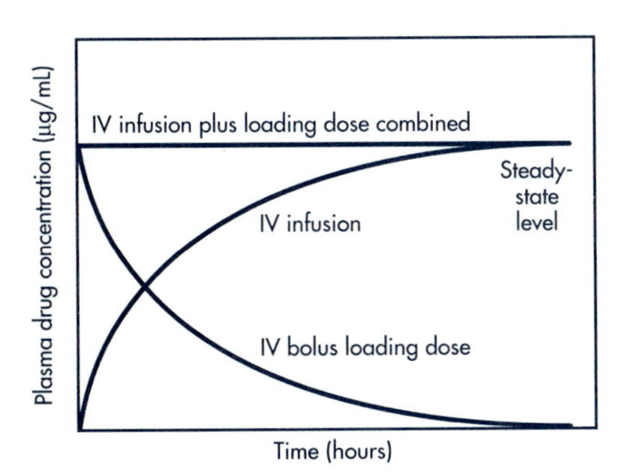

Figure 14-4. IV infusion with loading dose D_L. The loading dose is given by IV bolus injection at the start of the infusion. Plasma drug concentrations decline exponentially after D_L, whereas they increase exponentially during the infusion. The resulting plasma drug concentration versus time curve is a straight line due to the summation of the two curves.

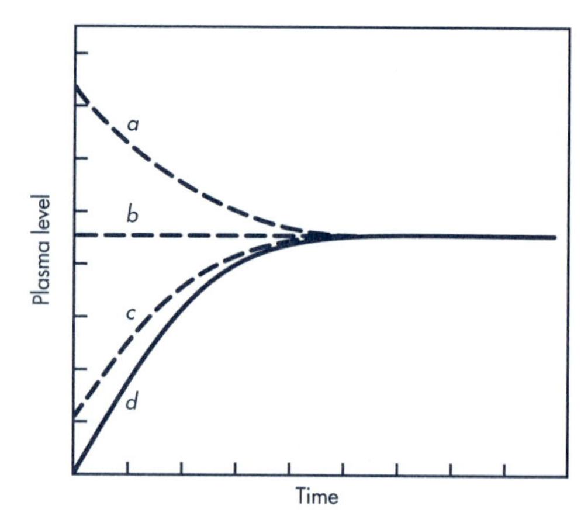

Figure 14-5. Intravenous infusion with loading doses *a*, *b*, and *c*. Curve *d* represents an IV infusion without a loading dose.

$$\frac{D_L k}{V_D} = \frac{R}{V_D} \tag{14.16}$$

$$D_L = \frac{R}{k} = \text{loading dose}$$

In order to maintain instant steady-state level $[(dC_p/dt) = 0]$, the loading dose should be equal to R/k.

In Figure 14-5, curve b shows the blood level after a single loading dose of R/k plus infusion from which the instant steady-state level is obtained. If the loading dose is large, the plasma drug concentration takes longer to decline to steady-state drug levels (curve a). If the loading dose is low, the plasma drug concentrations will increase slowly to steady-state drug levels (curve c), but more quickly than without any loading dose.

Another method for the calculation of loading dose D_L is based on knowledge of the desired steady-state drug concentration C_{ss} and the apparent volume of distribution V_D for the drug, as shown in Equation 14.17.

$$D_L = C_{ss} V_D \tag{14.17}$$

For many drugs, C_{ss} is reported in the literature as the *effective therapeutic drug concentration.* The V_D and the elimination half-life $t_{1/2}$ are also available for these drugs.

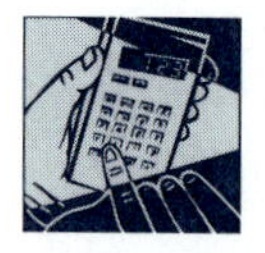

PRACTICE PROBLEMS

1. A physician wants to administer an anesthetic agent at a rate of 2 mg/hr by IV infusion. The elimination rate constant is 0.1 hr^{-1} and the volume of distribution (one compartment) is 10 L. What loading dose should be recommended if the doctor wants the drug level to reach 2 μg/mL immediately?

Solution

$$C_{ss} = \frac{R}{V_D k} = \frac{2000}{(10 \times 10^3)(0.1)} = 2\ \mu\text{g/mL}$$

To reach C_{ss} instantly,

$$D_L = \frac{R}{k} = \frac{2\ \text{mg/hr}}{0.1/\text{hr}} \qquad D_L = 20\ \text{mg}$$

2. What is the concentration of a drug 6 hours after administration of a loading dose of 10 mg and simultaneous infusion at 2 mg/hr (the drug has a $t_{1/2}$ of 3 hr and a volume of distribution of 10 L)?

Solution

$$k = \frac{0.693}{3}\ \text{hr}^{-1}$$

$$C_p = \frac{D_L}{V_D} e^{-kt} + \frac{R}{V_D k}(1 - e^{-kt})$$

$$C_p = \frac{10000}{10000} e^{-(0.693/3)(6)} + \frac{2000}{(10000)(0.693/3)}[1 - e^{-(0.693/3)(6)}]$$

$$C_p = 0.90\ \mu\text{g/mL}$$

3. Calculate the drug concentration in the blood after infusion has been stopped.

Solution

This concentration can be calculated in two parts (see Fig. 14-2**A**). First, calculate the concentration of drug during infusion, and second, calculate the present concentration, C_0. Then use the IV bolus dose equation ($C = C_0 e^{-kt}$) for calculations for any further point in time. For convenience, the two equations can be combined as follows.

$$C_p = \frac{R}{kV_D}(1 - e^{-kb})e^{-k(t - b)} \qquad \textbf{(14.18)}$$

where b = length of time of infusion period, t = total time (infusion and postinfusion), and $t - b$ = length of time after infusion has stopped.

4. A patient was infused for 6 hours with a drug ($k = 0.01\ \text{hr}^{-1}$; $V_D = 10$ L) at a rate of 2 mg/hr. What is the concentration of the drug in the body 2 hours after cessation of the infusion?

Solution

Using Equation 14.18,

$$C_p = \frac{2000}{(0.01)(10000)}(1 - e^{-0.01(6)})e^{-0.01(8 - 6)}$$

$$C_p = 1.14\ \mu\text{g/mL}$$

Alternatively, when infusion stops, C'_p is calculated:

$$C'_p = \frac{R}{kV_D}(1 - e^{-kt})$$

$$C'_p = \frac{2000}{0.01 \times 10000}(1 - e^{-0.01(6)})$$

$$C = C'_p e^{-0.01(2)}$$

$$C = 1.14\ \mu\text{g/mL}$$

The two approaches should give the same answer.

5. An adult male asthmatic patient (78 kg, 48 years old) with a history of heavy smoking was given an IV infusion of aminophylline at a rate of 0.5 mg/kg per hr. A loading dose of 6 mg/kg was given by IV bolus injection just prior to the start of the infusion. At 2 hours after the start of the IV infusion, the plasma theophylline concentration was measured and found to contain 5.8 μg/mL of theophylline. The apparent V_D for theophylline is 0.45 L/kg. Aminophylline is the ethylenediamine salt of theophylline and contains 80% of theophylline base.

Because the patient was responding poorly to the aminophylline therapy, the physician wanted to increase the plasma theophylline concentration in the patient to 10 μg/mL. What dosage recommendation would you give the physician? Would you recommend another loading dose?

Solution

If no loading dose is given and the IV infusion rate is increased, the time to reach steady-state plasma drug concentrations will be about 4 to 5 $t_{1/2}$ to reach 95% of C_{ss}. Therefore, a second loading dose should be recommended to rapidly increase the plasma theophylline concentration to 10 μg/mL. The infusion rate must also be increased to maintain this desired C_{ss}.

The calculation of loading dose D_L must consider the present plasma theophylline concentration.

$$D_L = \frac{V_D(C_{p\ \text{desired}} - C_{p\ \text{present}})}{(S)(F)} \tag{14.19}$$

where S is the salt form of the drug and F is the fraction of drug bioavailable. For aminophylline S is equal to 0.80 and for an IV bolus injection F is equal to 1.

$$D_L = \frac{(0.45\ \text{L/kg})(78\ \text{kg})(10 - 5.8\ \text{mg/L})}{(0.80)(1)}$$

$$D_L = 184\ \text{mg aminophylline}$$

The maintenance IV infusion rate may be calculated after estimation of the patient's clearance, Cl_T. Because a loading dose and an IV infusion of 0.5 mg/hr per kg was given to the patient, the plasma theophylline concentration of 5.8 mg/L is at steady-state C_{ss}. Total clearance may be estimated by

$$Cl_T = \frac{R}{C_{ss\ \text{present}}} = \frac{(0.6\ \text{mg/hr kg})(78\ \text{kg})}{5.8\ \text{mg/L}}$$

$$Cl_T = 8.07\ \text{L/hr or } 1.72\ \text{mL/min kg}$$

The usual Cl_T for adult, nonsmoking patients with uncomplicated asthma is approximately 0.65 mL/min per kg. Heavy smoking is known to increase Cl_T for theophylline.

The new IV infusion rate, R', is calculated by

$$R' = C_{ss\ \text{desired}} Cl_T$$

$$R' = 10\ \text{mg/L} \times 8.07\ \text{L/hr} = 80.7\ \text{mg/hr or } 1.03\ \text{mg/hr per kg}$$

6. An adult male patient (43 yr, 80 kg) is to be given an antibiotic by IV infusion. According to the literature, the antibiotic has an elimination $t_{1/2}$ of 2 hours, V_D of 1.25 L/kg, and is effective at a plasma drug concentration of 14 mg/L. The drug is supplied in 5-mL ampuls containing 150 mg/mL.

a. Recommend a starting infusion rate in milligrams per hour and liters per hour.

Solution

Assume the effective plasma drug concentration is the target drug concentration or C_{SS}.

$$R = C_{SS}kV_D$$
$$= (14 \text{ mg/L})(0.693/2 \text{ hr})(1.5 \text{ L/kg})(80 \text{ kg})$$
$$= 485.1 \text{ mg/hr}$$

Because the drug is supplied at a concentration of 150 mg/mL,

$$(485.1 \text{ mg})(\text{mL}/150 \text{ mg}) = 3.23 \text{ mL}$$

Thus, $R = 3.23$ mL/hr.

b. Blood samples were taken from the patient at 12, 16, and 24 hours after the start of the infusion. Plasma drug concentrations were as shown below:

***t* (hr)**	**C_p (mg/L)**
12	16.1
16	16.3
24	16.5

From this additional data, calculate the total body clearance Cl_T for the drug in this patient.

Solution

Because the plasma drug concentrations at 12, 16, and 24 hours were similar, steady state has essentially been reached. (Note: The continuous increase in plasma drug concentrations could be caused by drug accumulation due to a second tissue compartment, or could be due to variation in the drug assay.) Assuming a C_{SS} of 16.3 mg/mL, Cl_T is calculated.

$$Cl_T = \frac{R}{C_{SS}} = \frac{485.1 \text{ mg/hr}}{16.3 \text{ mg/L}} = 29.8 \text{ L/hr}$$

c. From the above data, estimate the elimination half-life for the antibiotics in this patient.

Solution

Generally, the apparent volume of distribution (V_D) is less variable than $t_{1/2}$. Assuming that the literature value for V_D is 1.25 L/kg, then $t_{1/2}$ may be estimated from the Cl_T.

$$Cl_T = kV_D$$

$$k = \frac{Cl_T}{V_D} = \frac{29.9 \text{ L/hr}}{(1.25 \text{ L/kg})(80 \text{ kg})} = 0.299 \text{ hr}^{-1}$$

$$t_{1/2} = \frac{0.693}{0.299 \text{ hr}^{-1}} = 2.32 \text{ hr}$$

Thus the $t_{1/2}$ for the antibiotic in this patient is 2.32 hours, which is in good agreement with the literature value of 2 hours.

d. After reviewing pharmacokinetics of the antibiotic in this patient, should the infusion rate for the antibiotic be changed?

Solution

To properly decide whether the infusion rate should be changed, the clinical pharmacist must consider the pharmacodynamics and toxicity of the drug. Assuming the drug has a wide therapeutic window and shows no sign of adverse drug toxicity, the infusion rate of 485.1 mg/hr, calculated according to pharmacokinetic literature values for the drug, appears to be correct.

$$C_p = \frac{R}{Cl}\left(1 - e^{-(Cl/V_D)t}\right)$$

ESTIMATION OF DRUG CLEARANCE AND V_D FROM INFUSION DATA

The plasma concentration of a drug during constant infusion was described in terms of volume of distribution and elimination constant k in Equation 14.2. Alternatively, the equation may be described in terms of clearance by substituting for k into Equation 14.2 with $k = Cl/V_D$:

$$C_p = (R/Cl)\left(1 - e^{-(Cl/V_D)t}\right) \qquad \textbf{(14.20)}$$

The drug concentration in this physiologic model is described in terms of volume of distribution of V_D. According to total body clearance (Cl), the independent parameters are clearance and volume of distribution; k is viewed as a dependent variable that depends on Cl and V_D. In this model, the time for steady state and the resulting steady-state concentration will be dependent on both clearance and volume of distribution. When a constant volume of distribution is evident, the time for steady state is then inversely related to clearance. Thus, drugs with small clearance will take a long time to reach steady state. Although this newer approach is preferred by some clinical pharmacists the alternative approach to parameter estimation was known for some time in classical pharmacokinetics. Equation 14.20 has been applied in population pharmacokinetics to estimate both V_D and Cl in individual patients with one or more data points. However, clearance in patients may differ greatly from subjects in the population, especially subjects with different renal functions. Unfortunately, the plasma samples taken at time equivalent to less than one half life after infusion was started may not be very discriminating due to the small change in the drug concentration. Blood samples taken at 3 to 4 half lives later are much more reflective of their difference in clearance.

ESTIMATION OF k AND V_D OF AMINOGLYCOSIDES IN CLINICAL SITUATIONS

Antibiotics are often infused intravenously by multiple doses (see Chapter 15) at fixed dosing interval (τ). It is desirable to adjust dose based on k and V_D. According to Sawchuk and Zaske (1976), individual parameters for aminoglycoside may be determined in a patient by using a limited number of plasma drug samples taken at appropriate time intervals. The equation was simplified by replacing an elaborate model with the one-compartment model to describe drug elimination and appropriately avoiding the distributive phase. The plasma sample should be collected 15 to 30 minutes postinfusion (with infusion lasting about 60 minutes) and in patients with poor renal function, 1 to 2 hours post infusion to allow adequate tissue distribution. The second and third blood sample should be collected about 2 to 3 half-lives later in order to get a good estimation of the slope. The data may be graphically determined or by regression using a scientific calculator or computer program.

$$V_D = \frac{R(1 - e^{-kt_{inf}})}{k[C_{SSmax} - C_{SSmin}\, e^{-kt_{inf}}]} \tag{14.21}$$

C_{SSmax} = steady-state peak plasma drug concentration
C_{SSmin} = steady-state trough plasma drug concentration
t_{inf} = infusion period
τ = dosing interval

The dose of aminoglycoside is generally fixed by the desirable peak and trough plasma concentration. For example, C_{SSmax} for gentamicin may be set at 6 to 10 mcg/mL with the steady-state trough level is generally about 0.5 to 2 mcg/mL, depending on the severity of the infection and renal consideration. The upper range is used only for life-threatening infections. The dose for any desired peak drug concentration may be calculated using Equation 14.22:

$$R = \frac{V_D k\, C_{SSmax}(1 - e^{-k\tau})}{(1 - e^{-kt_{inf}})} \tag{14.22}$$

The dosing interval in between infusion may be adjusted to obtain a desirable concentration. A more detailed discussion of peak and trough drug concentration is available in Chapter 15.

INTRAVENOUS INFUSION OF TWO-COMPARTMENT MODEL DRUGS

Many drugs given by IV infusion follow two-compartment kinetics. For example, the respective distributions of theophylline and lidocaine in humans are described by the two-compartment open model. As with the one-compartment-model drugs, IV infusion requires a distribution and equilibration of the drug before a stable blood level is reached. The time needed to reach a steady-state blood level depends entirely on the half-life of the drug. The equation describing plasma drug concentration as a function of time is as follows:

$$C_p = \frac{R}{V_p k}\left[1 - \left(\frac{k - b}{a - b}\right) e^{-at} - \left(\frac{a - k}{a - b}\right) e^{-bt}\right] \tag{14.23}$$

where a and b are hybrid rate constants and R is the rate of infusion. At steady state (ie, $t = \infty$), Equation 14.23 reduces to

$$C_{ss} = \frac{R}{V_p k} \tag{14.24}$$

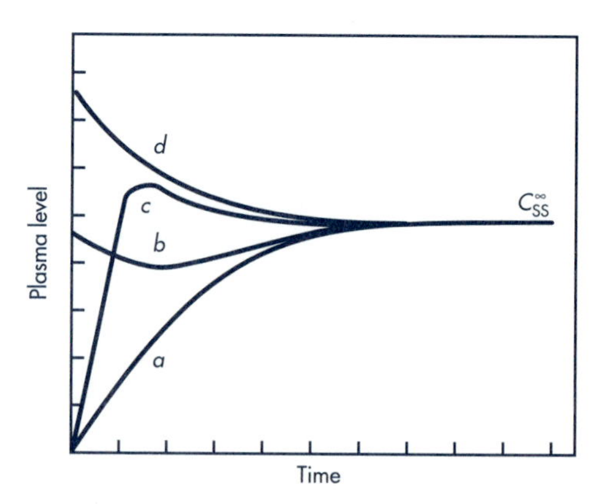

Figure 14-6. Plasma drug level after various loading doses and rates of infusion for a drug that follows a two-compartment model: *a*, no loading dose; *b*, loading dose = *R/k* (rapid infusion); *c*, loading dose = *R/b* (slow infusion); and *d*, loading dose = *R/b* (rapid infusion).

By rearranging this equation, the infusion rate for a desired steady-state plasma drug concentration may be calculated.

$$R = C_{ss} V_p k \tag{14.25}$$

Drugs with long half-lives require a loading dose to rapidly attain steady-state plasma drug levels. The plasma drug concentration of a drug that follows a two-compartment model after various loading doses is shown in Figure 14-6.

It is clinically desirable to achieve rapid therapeutic drug levels by using a loading dose. However, for drugs that follow the two-compartment pharmacokinetic model, the drug distributes slowly into extravascular tissues (compartment 2). Thus, drug equilibrium is not immediate. If a loading dose is given too rapidly, the drug may initially give excessively high concentrations in the plasma (central compartment), which then decreases as drug equilibrium is reached (Fig. 14-6). It is not possible to maintain an instantaneous, stable steady-state blood level for a two-compartment model drug with a zero-order rate of infusion. Therefore, a loading dose produces an initial blood level either slightly higher or lower than the steady-state blood level. To overcome this problem, several IV bolus injections given as short intermittent IV infusions may be used as a method for administering a loading dose to the patient.

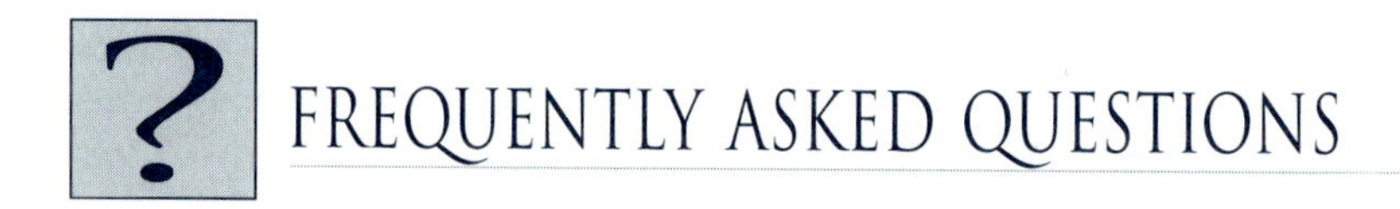

FREQUENTLY ASKED QUESTIONS

1. What is the main reason for giving a drug by slow IV infusion?
2. Why do we use a loading dose to rapidly achieve therapeutic concentration for a drug with a long elimination half-life instead of increasing the rate of drug infusion or increasing the size of the infusion dose?
3. What are some of the complications involved with IV infusion?

LEARNING QUESTIONS

1. A female patient (35 years old, 65 kg) with normal renal function is to be given a drug by IV infusion. According to the literature, the elimination half-life of this drug is 7 hours and the apparent V_D is 23.1% of body weight. The pharmacokinetics of this drug assumes a first-order process. The desired steady-state plasma level for this antibiotic is 10 μg/mL.

a. Assuming no loading dose, how long after the start of the IV infusion would it take to reach 95% of the C_{ss}?

b. What is the proper loading dose for this antibiotic?

c. What is the proper infusion rate for this drug?

d. What is the total body clearance?

e. If the patient suddenly develops partial renal failure, how long would it take for a new steady-state plasma level to be established (assume that 95% of the C_{ss} is a reasonable approximation)?

f. If the total body clearance declined 50% due to partial renal failure, what new infusion rate would you recommend to maintain the desired steady-state plasma level of 10 μg/mL.

2. An anticonvulsant drug was given as (a) a single IV dose and (b) a constant IV infusion. The serum drug concentrations are as presented in Table 14.2.

a. What is the steady-state plasma drug level?

b. What is the time for 95% steady-state plasma drug level?

c. What is the drug clearance?

d. What is the plasma concentration of the drug 4 hours after stopping infusion (infusion was stopped after 24 hours)?

e. What is the infusion rate for a patient weighing 75 kg to maintain a steady-state drug level of 10 μg/mL?

f. What is the plasma drug concentration 4 hours after an IV dose of 1 mg/kg followed by a constant infusion of 0.2 mg/kg per hour?

3. An antibiotic is to be given by IV infusion. How many milliliters per minute should a sterile drug solution containing 25 mg/mL be given to a 75-kg adult male patient to achieve an infusion rate of 1 mg/kg per hour?

4. An antibiotic drug is to be given to an adult male patient (75 kg, 58 years old) by IV infusion. The drug is supplied in sterile vials containing 30 mL of the antibiotic solution at a concentration of 125 mg/mL. What rate in milliliters per hour would you infuse this patient to obtain a steady-state concentration of 20 μg/mL? What loading dose would you suggest? Assume the drug follows the pharmacokinetics of a one-compartment open model. The apparent volume of distribution of this drug is 0.5 L/kg and the elimination half-life is 3 hours.

5. According to the manufacturer, a steady-state serum concentration of 17 μg/mL was measured when the antibiotic, cephradine (Velosef, Bristol-Meyers, Squibb) was given by IV infusion to 9 adult male volunteers (average weight, 71.7 kg) at a rate of 5.3 mg/kg hr for 4 hours.

a. Calculate the total body clearance for this drug.

b. When the IV infusion was discontinued, the cephradine serum concentration

TABLE 14.2 Serum Drug Concentrations for a Hypothetical Anticonvulsant Drug

	CONCENTRATION IN PLASMA (μg/ml)	
Time (hr)	**SINGLE IV DOSE OF 1 mg/kg**	**CONSTANT IV INFUSION OF 0.2 mg/kg per hr**
0	10.0	0
2	6.7	3.3
4	4.5	5.5
6	3.0	7.0
8	2.0	8.0
10	1.35	8.6
12		9.1
18		9.7
24		9.9

decreased exponentially, declining to 1.5 μg/mL at 6.5 hours after the start of the infusion. Calculate the elimination half-life.

c. From the information above, calculate the apparent volume of distribution.

d. Cephradine is completely excreted unchanged in the urine, and studies have shown that probenecid given concurrently causes elevation of the serum cephradine concentration. What is the probable mechanism for this interaction of probenecid with cephradine?

6. Calculate the *excretion rate* at steady state for a drug given by IV infusion at a rate of 30 mg/hr. The C_{ss} is 20 μg/mL. If the rate of infusion were increased to 40 mg/hr, what would be the new steady-state drug concentration, C_{ss}? Would the excretion rate for the drug at the new steady state be the same? Assume first-order elimination kinetics and a one-compartment model.

7. An antibiotic is to be given to an adult male patient (58 yr, 75 kg) by IV infusion. The elimination half-life is 8 hours and the apparent volume of distribution is 1.5 L/kg. The drug is supplied in 60-mL ampules at a drug concentration of 15 mg/mL. The desired steady-state drug concentration is 20 μg/mL.

a. What infusion rate in mL/hr would you recommend for this patient?

b. What loading dose would you recommend for this patient? By what route of administration would you give the loading dose? When?

c. Why should a loading dose be recommended?

d. According to the manufacturer, the recommended starting infusion rate is 15 mL/hr. Do you agree with this recommended infusion rate for your patient? Give a reason for your answer.

e. If you were to monitor the patient's serum drug concentration, when would you request a blood sample? Give a reason for your answer.

f. The observed serum drug concentration is higher than anticipated. Give two possible reasons based on sound pharmacokinetic principles that would account for this observation.

8. Which of the following statements (**a–e**) is/are true regarding the time to reach steady-state for the three drugs below:

	Drug *A*	**Drug *B***	**Drug *C***
rate of infusion (mg/hr)	10	20	15
k (hr^{-1})	0.5	0.1	0.05
Cl (L/hr)	5	20	5

a. Drug A takes the longest time to reach steady-state.
b. Drug B takes the longest time to reach steady-state.
c. Drug C takes the longest time to reach steady-state.
d. Drug A takes 6.9 hours to reach steady-state.
e. None of the above is true.

9. The steady-state drug concentration of a cephalosporin after constant infusion of 250 mg/hr is 45 mcg/mL, what is the drug clearance of this cephalosporin?

REFERENCES

Hurley SF, McNeil JJ: A comparison of the accuracy of a least-squares regression, a Bayesian, Chiou's and the steady-state clearance method of individualizing theophylline dosage. *Clin Pharmacokinet* **14:**311–320, 1988

BIBLIOGRAPHY

Gibaldi M: Estimation of the pharmacokinetic parameters of the two-compartment open model from postinfusion plasma concentration data. *J Pharm Sci* **58:**1133–1135, 1969

Koup J, Greenblatt D, Jusko W, et al: Pharmacokinetics of digoxin in normal subjects after intravenous bolus and infusion dose. *J Pharmacokinet Biopharm* **3:**181–191, 1975

Loo J, Riegelman S: Assessment of pharmacokinetic constants from postinfusion blood curves obtained after IV infusion. *J Pharm Sci* **59:**53–54, 1970

Loughnam PM, Sitar DS, Ogilvie RI, Neims AH: The two-compartment open system kinetic model: A review of its clinical implications and applications. *J Pediatr* **88:**869–873, 1976

Mitenko P, Ogilvie R: Rapidly achieved plasma concentration plateaus, with observations on theophylline kinetics. *Clin Pharmacol Ther* **13:**329–335, 1972

Riegelman JS, Loo JC: Assessment of pharmacokinetic constants from postinfusion blood curves obtained after IV infusion. *J Pharm Sci* **59:**53, 1970

Sawchuk RJ, Zaske DE: Pharmacokinetics of dosing regimens which utilize multiple intravenous infusions: Gentamicin in burn patients. *J Pharmacokinet Biopharm* **4:**183–195, 1976

Wagner J: A safe method for rapidly achieving plasma concentration plateaus. *Clin Pharmacol Ther* **16:**691–700, 1974

15

MULTIPLE-DOSAGE REGIMENS

Many drugs are given in a multiple-dosage regimen for prolonged therapeutic activity. The plasma levels of these drugs must be maintained within narrow limits to achieve maximal clinical effectiveness. Among these drugs are antibacterials, cardiotonics, anticonvulsants, and hormones. Ideally, a dosage regimen is established for each drug to provide the correct plasma level without excessive fluctuation and drug accumulation.

For certain drugs, such as antibiotics, a desirable minimum effective plasma concentration can be determined. Other drugs with narrow therapeutic indices (such as digoxin and phenytoin) require definition of the therapeutic minimum and maximum nontoxic plasma concentrations. In calculating a multiple-dose regimen, the desired or *target* plasma concentration must be related to a therapeutic response. The two main parameters that can be adjusted in developing a dosage regimen are (1) the size of the drug dose and (2) the frequency of drug administration—that is, the time interval between doses.

DRUG ACCUMULATION

Pharmacokinetic parameters are obtained from the plasma level–time curve generated by single dose drug studies to predict the drug plasma levels during a multiple-dosage regimen. With these pharmacokinetic parameters and knowledge of the size of the dose and dosage interval (τ) the complete plasma level–time curve or the plasma level may be predicted at any time after the beginning of the dosage regimen.

To calculate multiple-dosage regimens, it is necessary to decide whether successive doses of drug will have any effect on the previous dose. The principle of *superposition* assumes that early doses of drug do not affect the pharmacokinetics of subsequent doses. Therefore, the blood levels after the second, third, or nth dose will overlay or superimpose the blood level attained after the $(n - 1)$th dose. In addition, the AUC$(\int_0^\infty C_p\, dt)$ following the administration of a single dose equals the AUC $(\int_{t_1}^{t_2} C_p\, dt)$ during a dosing interval at steady state (Fig. 15-1).

The principle of superposition allows one to project the plasma drug concentration–time curve of a drug after several consecutive doses based on the plasma

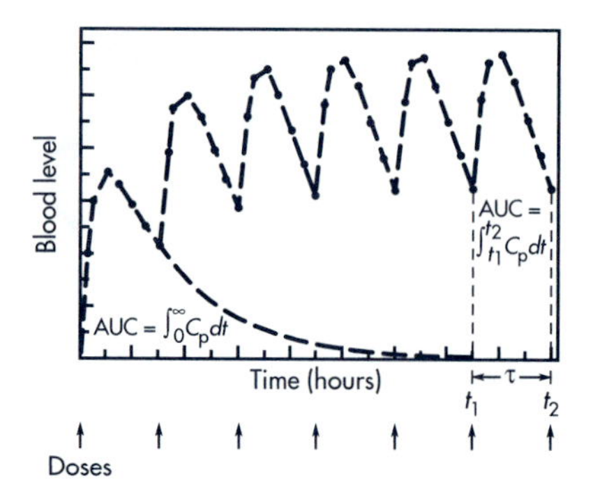

Figure 15-1. Simulated data showing blood levels after administration of multiple doses and accumulation of blood levels when equal doses are given at equal time intervals.

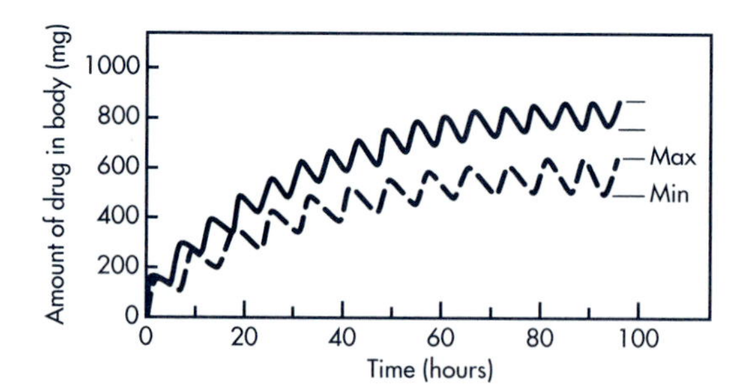

Figure 15-2. Amount of drug in the body as a function of time. Equal doses of drug were given every 6 hours (upper curve) and every 8 hours (lower curve). k_a and k remain constant.

drug concentration-time curve obtained after a single dose. The basic assumptions are that the drug is eliminated by first-order kinetics and that the pharmacokinetics of the drug after a single dose (first dose) are not altered after taking multiple doses.

From the plasma drug concentrations obtained after a single dose, the plasma drug concentrations after multiple doses may be predicted, as shown in Table 15.1. In Table 15.1, the plasma drug concentrations from 0 to 24 hours are measured after a single dose. A constant dose of drug is given every 4 hours and plasma drug concentrations after each dose are generated from the data after the first dose. Thus, the *predicted* plasma drug concentration in the patient would be the total drug concentration obtained by adding the residual drug concentration obtained after each previous dose. The superposition principle may be used to predict drug concentrations after multiple doses of many drugs. Because the superposition principle is an overlay method, it may be used to predict drug concentrations after multiple doses given at *equal* and *unequal* dosage intervals. For example, a drug dose may be given every 8 hours or three times a day before meals at 8 AM, 12 noon, and 6 PM. There are situations, however, for which the superposition principle does not apply. In these cases, the pharmacokinetics of the drug change after multiple dosing due to various factors, including changing pathophysiology in the patient, saturation of a drug carrier system, enzyme induction, and enzyme inhibition. Drugs that follow nonlinear pharmacokinetics (Chapter 16) generally do not have predictable plasma drug concentrations after multiple doses using the superposition principle.

If the drug is administered at a fixed dose and a fixed-dosage interval, the amount of drug in the body will increase and then plateau to a mean plasma level higher than the peak C_p obtained from the initial dose (Figs. 15-1 and 15-2). When the second dose is given after a time interval shorter than the time required to eliminate the previous dose, drug accumulates in the body. However, if the second dose is given after a time interval longer than the time required to eliminate the previous dose, drug will not accumulate (Table 15.1).

As repetitive equal doses are given at a constant frequency, the plasma level–time curve plateaus and a steady state is obtained. At steady state, the plasma drug levels fluctuate between C_{max}^{∞} and C_{min}^{∞}. An average steady state plasma drug concentration (C_{av}^{∞}) is obtained by dividing the AUC for a dosing period (ie, $\int_{t_1}^{t_2} C_p \, dt$) by the dosing interval τ, at steady state. Once steady state is obtained, C_{max}^{∞} and C_{min}^{∞} are constant and remain unchanged from dose to dose. The C_{max}^{∞} is important in determining drug safety. The C_{max}^{∞} should always remain below the minimum toxic concentration. The C_{max}^{∞} is also a good indication of drug accumulation. If a drug produces the same C_{max}^{∞} at steady state, compared with the $(C_{n=1})_{max}$ after the first dose, then there is no drug accumulation. If C_{max}^{∞} is much larger than $(C_{n=1})_{max}$, then there is significant accumulation. Accumulation is affected by the elimination half-life of the drug and the dosing interval. The index for measuring drug accumulation R is as follows:

$$R = \frac{(C^{\infty})_{max}}{(C_{n\,=\,1})_{max}} \tag{15.1}$$

Substituting for C_{max} after the first dose and at steady state yields the following equation:

$$R = \frac{D_0/V_D[1/(1-e^{-k\tau})]}{D_0/V_D} \tag{15.2}$$

$$R = \frac{1}{1-e^{-k\tau}}$$

TABLE 15.1 Predicted Plasma Drug Concentrations for Multiple-Dosage Regimen Using the Superposition Principle[a]

		PLASMA DRUG CONCENTRATION (μg/mL)						
DOSE NUMBER	TIME (HR)	DOSE 1	DOSE 2	DOSE 3	DOSE 4	DOSE 5	DOSE 6	TOTAL
1	0	0						0
	1	21.0						21.0
	2	22.3						22.3
	3	19.8						19.8
2	4	16.9	0					16.9
	5	14.3	21.0					35.3
	6	12.0	22.3					34.3
	7	10.1	19.8					29.9
3	8	8.50	16.9	0				25.4
	9	7.15	14.3	21.0				42.5
	10	6.01	12.0	22.3				40.3
	11	5.06	10.1	19.8				35.0
4	12	4.25	8.50	16.9	0			29.7
	13	3.58	7.15	14.3	21.0			46.0
	14	3.01	6.01	12.0	22.3			43.3
	15	2.53	5.06	10.1	19.8			37.5
5	16	2.13	4.25	8.50	16.9	0		31.8
	17	1.79	3.58	7.15	14.3	21.0		47.8
	18	1.51	3.01	6.01	12.0	22.3		44.8
	19	1.27	2.53	5.06	10.1	19.8		38.8
6	20	1.07	2.13	4.25	8.50	16.9	0	32.9
	21	0.90	1.79	3.58	7.15	14.3	21.0	48.7
	22	0.75	1.51	3.01	6.01	12.0	22.3	45.6
	23	0.63	1.27	2.53	5.06	10.1	19.8	39.4
	24	0.53	1.07	2.13	4.25	8.50	16.9	33.4

[a]A single oral dose of 350 mg was given and the plasma drug concentrations were measured for 0–24 hr. The same plasma drug concentrations are assumed to occur after doses 2–6. The total plasma drug concentration is the sum of the plasma drug concentrations due to each dose. For this example, $V_D = 10$ L, $t_{1/2} = 4$ hr, and $k_a = 1.5$ hr^{-1}. The drug is 100% bioavailable and follows the pharmacokinetics of a one-compartment open model.

Equation 15.2 shows that drug accumulation measured with the R index depends on the elimination constant and the dosing interval and is independent of the dose.

For a drug given in repetitive oral doses, the time required to reach steady state is dependent on the elimination half-life of the drug and is independent of the size of the dose, length of the dosing interval, and number of doses. For example, if the dose or dosage interval of the drug is altered as shown in Figure 15-2, the time required for the drug to reach steady state is the same, but the final steady state plasma level changes proportionately. Furthermore, if the drug is given at the same dosing rate (eg, 25 mg/hr), the average plasma drug concentrations will be the same but the fluctuations between C^{∞}_{max} and C^{∞}_{min} will vary (Fig. 15-3).

An equation for the estimation of the time to reach one-half of the steady-state plasma levels or the accumulation half-life has been described by van Rossum and Tomey (1968).

$$\text{Accumulation } t_{1/2} = t_{1/2}\left(1 + 3.3 \log \frac{k_a}{k_a - k}\right) \tag{15.3}$$

For IV administration, k_a is very rapid; k is very small in comparison to k_a and can be omitted in the denominator of Equation 15.3. Thus, Equation 15.3 reduces to

$$\text{Accumulation } t_{1/2} = t_{1/2}\left(1 + 3.3 \log \frac{k_a}{k_a}\right) \tag{15.4}$$

Because $k_a/k_a = 1$ and $\log 1 = 0$, the accumulation $t_{1/2}$ of a drug administered intravenously is the elimination $t_{1/2}$ of the drug. From this relationship, the time to

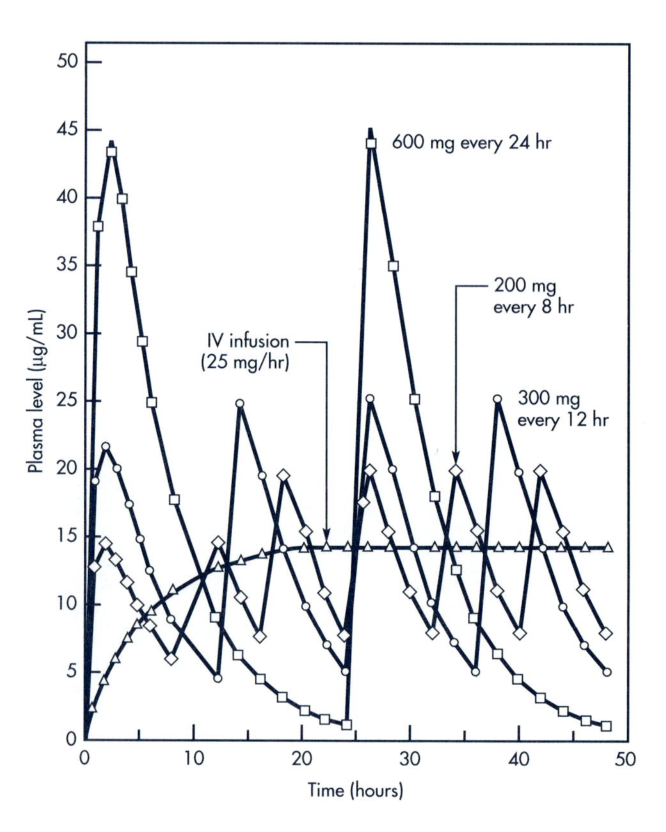

Figure 15-3. Simulated plasma drug concentration versus time curves after IV infusion and oral multiple doses for a drug with an elimination half-life of 4 hours and apparent V_D of 10 L. IV infusion given at a rate of 25 mg/hr, oral multiple doses are 200 mg every 8 hours, 300 mg every 12 hours, and 600 mg every 24 hours.

TABLE 15.2 Effect of Elimination Half-Life and Absorption Rate Constant on Accumulation Half-Life After Oral Administration[a]

ELIMINATION HALF-LIFE (hr)	ELIMINATION RATE CONSTANT (1/hr)	ABSORPTION RATE CONSTANT (1/hr)	ACCUMULATION HALF-LIFE (hr)
4	0.173	1.50	4.70
8	0.0866	1.50	8.67
12	0.0578	1.50	12.8
24	0.0289	1.50	24.7
4	0.173	1.00	5.09
8	0.0866	1.00	8.99
12	0.0578	1.00	13.0
24	0.0289	1.00	25.0

[a]Accumulation half-life is calculated by Equation 15.3, and is the half-time for accumulation of the drug to 90% of the steady-state plasma drug concentration.

reach 50% steady-state drug concentrations is dependent on the elimination $t_{1/2}$ and not on the dose or dosage interval.

As shown in Equation 15.4, the accumulation $t_{1/2}$ is directly proportional to the elimination $t_{1/2}$. Table 15.2 gives the accumulation $t_{1/2}$ of drugs with various elimination half-lives given by multiple oral doses (Table 15.2).

From a clinical viewpoint, the time needed to reach 90% of the steady state plasma concentration is 3.3 times the elimination half-life, whereas the time required to reach 99% of the steady state plasma concentration is 6.6 times the elimination half-life (Table 15.3). It should be noted from Table 15.3 that at a constant dose size, the shorter the dosage interval, the larger the dosing rate (mg/hr), and the higher the steady-state drug level.

The number of doses for a given drug to reach steady state is dependent upon the elimination half-life of the drug and the dosage interval τ (Table 15.3). If the

TABLE 15.3 Interrelation of Elimination Half-Life, Dosage Interval, Maximum Plasma Concentration, and Time to Reach Steady-State Plasma Concentration[a]

ELIMINATION HALF-LIFE (hr)	DOSAGE INTERVAL, τ (hr)	C^{∞}_{max} (μg/mL)	TIME FOR C^{∞}_{av}[b] (hr)	NO. DOSES TO REACH 99% STEADY STATE
0.5	0.5	200	3.3	6.6
0.5	1.0	133	3.3	3.3
1.0	0.5	341	6.6	13.2
1.0	1.0	200	6.6	6.6
1.0	2.0	133	6.6	3.3
1.0	4.0	107	6.6	1.65
1.0	10.0	100[c]	6.6	0.66
2.0	1.0	341	13.2	13.2
2.0	2.0	200	13.2	6.1

[a]A single dose of 1000 mg of three hypothetical drugs with various elimination half-lives but equal volumes of distribution (V_D = 10 L) were given by multiple IV doses at various dosing intervals. All time values are in hours; (C^{∞}_{max}) = maximum steady-state concentration. C^{∞}_{av} = average steady-state plasma concentration. The maximum plasma drug concentration after the first dose of the drug is $(C_{n=1})_{max}$ = 100 μg/mL.

[b]Time to reach 99% of steady-state plasma concentration.

[c]Since the dosage interval, τ, is very large compared to the elimination half-life, no accumulation of drug occurs.

drug is given at a dosage interval equal to the half-life of the drug, then 6.6 doses are required to reach 99% of the theoretical steady-state plasma drug concentration. The number of doses needed to reach steady state is 6.6 $t_{1/2}/\tau$, as calculated in the far right column of Table 15.3. As discussed in Chapter 14, Table 14.1, it takes 4.32 half-lives to reach 95% of steady state.

REPETITIVE INTRAVENOUS INJECTIONS

The maximum amount of drug in the body following a rapid IV injection is equal to the dose of the drug. For a one-compartment open model, the drug will be eliminated according to first-order kinetics.

$$D_B = D_0\, e^{-kt} \tag{15.5}$$

If τ is equal to the dosage interval (ie, the time between the first dose and the next dose), then the amount of drug remaining in the body after several hours can be determined with

$$D_B = D_0 e^{-k\tau} \tag{15.6}$$

The fraction (f) of the dose remaining in the body is related to the elimination constant (k) and the dosage interval (τ) as follows.

$$f = \frac{D_B}{D_0} = e^{-k\tau} \tag{15.7}$$

With any given dose, f depends on k and τ. If τ is large, f will be smaller because D_B (the amount of drug remaining in the body) is smaller.

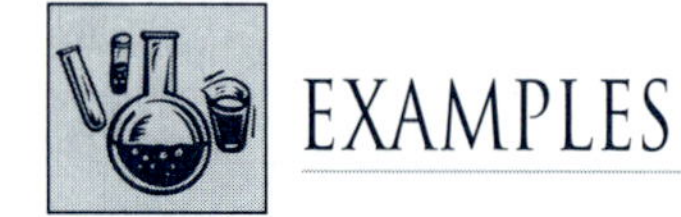

EXAMPLES

1. A patient receives 1000 mg every 6 hours by repetitive IV injection of an antibiotic with an elimination half-life of 3 hours. Assume the drug is distributed according to a one-compartment model and the volume of distribution is 20 L.
a. Find the maximum and minimum amount of drug in the body.
b. Determine the maximum and minimum plasma concentration of the drug.

Solution

a. The fraction of drug remaining in the body is estimated by Equation 15.7. The concentration of the drug declines to one-half after 3 hours ($t_{1/2} = 3$ hrs), after which the amount of drug will again decline by one-half at the end of the next 3 hours. Therefore, at the end of 6 hours only one-quarter, or 0.25, of the original dose remains in the body. Thus f is equal to 0.25.

To use Equation 15.7, we must first find the value of k from the $t_{1/2}$.

$$k = \frac{0.693}{t_{1/2}} = \frac{0.693}{3} = 0.231\ \text{hr}^{-1}$$

The time interval, τ, is equal to 6 hours. From Equation 15.7,

$$f = e^{-(0.231)(6)}$$
$$f = 0.25$$

In this example, 1000 mg of drug is given intravenously so that the amount of drug in the body is immediately increased by 1000 mg. At the end of the dosage interval (ie, before the next dose), the amount of drug remaining in the body is 25% of the amount of drug present just after the previous dose, because $f = 0.25$. Thus, if the value of f is known, a table can be constructed relating the fraction of the dose in the body before and after rapid IV injection (Table 15.4).

From Table 15.4 the maximum amount of drug in the body is 1333 mg, and the minimum amount of drug in the body is 333 mg. The difference between the maximum and minimum values, D_0, will always equal the injected dose.

$$D_{max} - D_{min} = D_0 \tag{15.8}$$

In this example:

$$1333 - 333 = 1000 \text{ mg}$$

D^{∞}_{max} can also be calculated directly by the relationship:

$$D^{\infty}_{max} = \frac{D_0}{1 - f} \tag{15.9}$$

Substituting known data, we obtain the following:

$$D^{\infty}_{max} = \frac{1000}{1 - 0.25} = 1333 \text{ mg}$$

then, from Equation 13.8,

$$D^{\infty}_{min} = 1333 - 1000 = 333 \text{ mg}$$

The average amount of drug in the body at steady state, D^{∞}_{av}, can be found by Equation 15.10 or 15.17. F is the fraction of dose absorbed. For an IV injection, F is equal to 1.0.

$$D^{\infty}_{av} = \frac{FD_0}{k\tau} \tag{15.10}$$

TABLE 15.4 Fraction of the Dose in the Body Before and After Intravenous Injections of a 1000-mg Dose[a]

	AMOUNT OF DRUG IN BODY	
NUMBER OF DOSES	**BEFORE DOSE**	**AFTER DOSE**
1	0	1000
2	250	1250
3	312	1312
4	328	1328
5	332	1332
6	333	1333
7	333	1333
∞	333	1333

[a] $f = 0.25$.

$$D_{av}^{\infty} = \frac{FD_0 1.44 t_{1/2}}{\tau} \tag{15.11}$$

Equations 15.10 and 15.11 can be used for repetitive dosing at constant time intervals and for any route of administration as long as elimination occurs from the central compartment.

Substitution of values from the example into Equation 15.11 gives

$$D_{av}^{\infty} = \frac{(1)(1000)(1.44)(3)}{6} = 720 \text{ mg}$$

Since the drug in the body declines exponentially (ie, first-order drug elimination), the value D_{av}^{∞} is not the arithmetic mean of D_{max}^{∞} and D_{min}^{∞}. The limitation of using D_{av}^{∞} is that the fluctuations of D_{max}^{∞} and D_{min}^{∞} are not known.

b. To determine the concentration of drug in the body after multiple dosing, divide the amount of drug in the body by the volume in which it is dissolved. For a one-compartment model, the maximum, minimum, and steady-state concentrations of drug in the plasma are found by the following equations:

$$C_{max}^{\infty} = \frac{D_{max}^{\infty}}{V_D} \tag{15.12}$$

$$C_{min}^{\infty} = \frac{D_{min}^{\infty}}{V_D} \tag{15.13}$$

$$C_{av}^{\infty} = \frac{D_{av}^{\infty}}{V_D} \tag{15.14}$$

A more direct approach to finding C_{max}^{∞}, C_{min}^{∞}, and C_{av}^{∞} is as follows:

$$C_{max}^{\infty} = \frac{C_p^0}{1 - e^{-k\tau}} \tag{15.15}$$

where C_p^0 is equal to D_0/V_D.

$$C_{min}^{\infty} = \frac{C_p^0 e^{-k\tau}}{1 - e^{-k\tau}} \tag{15.16}$$

$$C_{av}^{\infty} = \frac{FD_0}{V_D k\tau} \tag{15.17}$$

For this example the values for C_{max}^{∞}, C_{min}^{∞}, and C_{av}^{∞} are 66.7, 16.7, and 36.1 μg/mL, respectively.

As mentioned, C_{av}^{∞} is not the arithmetic mean of C_{max}^{∞} and C_{min}^{∞} because plasma drug concentration declines exponentially. The C_{av}^{∞} is equal to the AUC($\int_{t_1}^{t_2} C_p\, dt$) for a dosage interval at steady state divided by the dosage interval τ.

$$C_{av}^{\infty} = \frac{[\text{AUC}]_{t_1}^{t_2}}{\tau} \tag{15.18}$$

The AUC is related to the amount of drug absorbed divided by total body clearance, as shown in the following equation.

$$[\text{AUC}]_{t_1}^{t_2} = \frac{FD_0}{Cl_T} = \frac{FD_0}{kV_D} \tag{15.19}$$

Substitution of FD_0/kV_D for AUC in Equation 15.18 gives Equation 15.17.

Equation 15.17 or 15.18 can be used to obtain C_{av}^{∞} after a multiple-dosage regimen regardless of the route of administration.

It is sometimes desirable to know the plasma drug concentration at any time after the administration of n doses of drug. The general expression for calculating this plasma drug concentration is

$$C_p = \frac{D_0}{V_D}\left(\frac{1 - e^{-nk\tau}}{1 - e^{-k\tau}}\right) e^{-kt} \tag{15.20}$$

where n is the number of doses given and t is the time after the nth dose.

At steady-state $e^{-nk\tau}$ approaches zero and Equation 15.20 reduces to

$$C_p^{\infty} = \frac{D_0}{V_D}\left(\frac{1}{1 - e^{-k\tau}}\right) e^{-kt} \tag{15.21}$$

where C_p^{∞} is the steady state drug concentration at time t after the dose.

2. The patient in the previous example received 1000 mg of an antibiotic every 6 hours by repetitive IV injection. The drug has an apparent volume of distribution of 20 L and elimination half-life of 3 hours. Calculate (a) the plasma drug concentration C_p at 3 hours after the second dose, (b) the steady state plasma drug concentration C_p^{∞} at 3 hours after the last dose, (c) C_{max}^{∞}, (d) C_{min}^{∞}, and (e) C_{ss}.

Solution

a. The C_p at 3 hours after the second dose. Use Equation 15.20 and let $n = 2$, $t = 3$ hours, and make other appropriate substitutions.

$$C_p = \frac{1000}{20}\left(\frac{1 - e^{-(2)(0.231)(6)}}{1 - e^{-(0.231)(6)}}\right) e^{-0.231(3)}$$
$$= 31.3 \text{ mg/L}$$

b. The C_p^{∞} at 3 hours after the last dose. Because steady state is reached, use Equation 13.21 and perform the following calculation.

$$C_p^{\infty} = \frac{1000}{20}\left(\frac{1}{1 - e^{0.231(6)}}\right) e^{-0.231(3)}$$
$$= 33.3 \text{ mg/L}$$

c. The C_{max}^{∞} is calculated from Equation 15.15.

$$C_{max}^{\infty} = \frac{1000/20}{1 - e^{-(0.231)(6)}} = 66.7 \text{ mg/L}$$

d. The C_{min}^{∞} may be estimated as the drug concentration after the dosage interval τ, or just before the next dose:

$$C_{min}^{\infty} = C_{max}^{\infty}\, e^{-kt} = 66.7\, e^{-(0.231)(6)} = 16.7 \text{ mg/L}$$

e. The C_{ss} is estimated by Equation 15.17. Because the drug is given by IV bolus injections, $F = 1$.

$$C_{ss} = \frac{1000}{(0.231)(20)(6)} = 36.1 \text{ mg/L}$$

C_{av}^{∞} is represented as C_{ss} in some references.

Dealing With a Missed Dose

Equation 15.22 describes the plasma drug concentration t hours after the nth dose was administered; the doses are administered at τ hours apart according to a multiple dose regimen:

$$C_p = \frac{D_0}{V_D}\left[\frac{1 - e^{-nk\tau}}{1 - e^{-k\tau}}\right] e^{-kt} \tag{15.22}$$

Concentration contributed by the missing dose is as follows:

$$C'_p = \frac{D_0}{V_D} e^{-kt\text{-}miss} \tag{15.23}$$

in which $t\text{-}miss$ = time elapsed since the scheduled dose was missed. Subtracting Equation 15.23 from Equation 12.20 corrects for the missing dose as shown in Equation 15.24:

$$C_p = \frac{D_0}{V_D}\left[\left(\frac{1 - e^{-nk\tau}}{1 - e^{-kt}}\right) e^{-k\tau} - e^{-kt\text{-}miss}\right] \tag{15.24}$$

NOTE: If steady state is reached (ie, either n = large or after many doses), the equation simplifies to Equation 15.25. Equation 15.25 is useful when steady state is reached.

$$C_p = \frac{D_0}{V_D}\left[\frac{1 - e^{-nk\tau}}{1 - e^{-k\tau}} e^{-kt} - e^{-kt\text{-}miss}\right]$$
$$= \frac{D_0}{V_D}\left[\frac{e^{-k\tau}}{1 - e^{-k\tau}} - e^{-kt\text{-}miss}\right] \tag{15.25}$$

Generally, if the missing dose is recent, it will affect the present drug level more. If the missing dose is several half-lives ago (>5 $t_{1/2}$), it may be omitted because it will be very small. Equation 15.24 accounts for one missing dose, but several can be subtracted in a similar way if necessary.

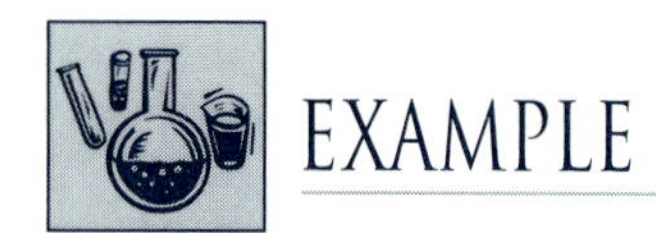

EXAMPLE

A cephalosporin ($k = 0.2$ hr^{-1}, $V_D = 10$ L) was administered by IV multiple dosing, 100 mg was injected every 6 hours for 6 doses. What was the plasma drug concentration 4 hours after the 6th dose (ie, 40 hours later) if: (a) the 5th dose was omitted, (b) the 6th dose was omitted (c) the 4th dose was omitted?

Solution

Substitute $k = 0.2$ hr^{-1}, $V_D = 10$ L, $D = 100$ mg, $n = 6$, $t = 4$ hr and $\tau = 6$ hr into equation 15.20 and evaluate:

$C_p = 6.425$ mg/L

If no dose was omitted, 4 hours after the 6th injection, C_p would be 6.425 mg/L..

(a) Missing the 5th dose, its contribution must be subtracted off, *t-miss* = 6 + 4 = 10 hours (the time elapsed since missing the dose):

$$C'_p = \frac{D_0}{V_D} e^{-kt\text{-}miss} = 100/10\ e^{-(0.2 \times 10)} = 10 \times 0.1353 = 1.353 \text{ mg/L}$$

Drug concentration correcting for the missing dose = 6.425 − 1.353 = 5.072 mg/L.

(b) If the 6th dose is missing, *t-miss* = 4 hr:

$$C_p' = \frac{D_0}{V_D} e^{-kt\text{-}miss} = 100/10\ e^{-(0.2 \times 4)} = 4.493 \text{ mg/L}$$

Drug concentration correcting for the missing dose = 6.425 − 4.493 = 1.932 mg/L.

(c) If the 4th dose is missing, *t-miss* = 12 + 4 = 16 hr:

$$C_p' = \frac{D_0}{V_D} e^{-kt\text{-}miss} = 100/10\ e^{-(0.2 \times 16)} = 0.408 \text{ mg/L}$$

The drug concentration corrected for the missing dose = 6.425 − 0.408 = 6.017 mg/L.

NOTE: The effect of a missing dose becomes less pronounced at a later time. A strict dose regimen compliance is advised for all drugs. With some drugs, missing the dose can have serious effect on therapy. For example, compliance is important for the anti-HIV1 drugs such as the protease inhibitors.

Dealing With an Early or Late Dose Administration During Multiple Dosing

When one of the drug doses is taken earlier or later than scheduled, the resulting plasma drug concentration can still be calculated based on the principle of superposition. The dose could be treated as missing with the late or early dose added back to take into account the actual time of dosing, using Equation 15.26.

$$C_p = \frac{D_0}{V_D}\left[\frac{1 - e^{-nk\tau}}{1 - e^{-k\tau}} e^{-kt} - e^{-kt\text{-}miss} + e^{-kt\text{-}actual}\right] \quad \textbf{(15.26)}$$

in which *t-miss* = time elapsed since the dose (late or early) is scheduled, and *t-actual* = time elapsed since the dose (late or early) is actually taken. Using a similar approach, a second missed dose can be subtracted from Equation 15.20. Similarly, a second late/early dose may be corrected by subtracting the scheduled dose followed by adding the actual dose. Similarly, if a different dose is given, the regular dose may be subtracted and the new dose added back.

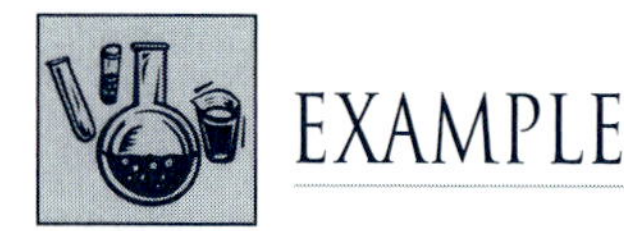

EXAMPLE

Assume the same drug as above (ie, $k = 0.2\ \text{hr}^{-1}$, $V_D = 10$ L) was given by multiple IV bolus injections and that at a dose of 100 mg every 6 hours for 6 doses. What is the plasma drug concentration 4 hours after the 6th dose, if the 5th dose were to be given an hour late? Substitute into Equation 15.26 for all unknowns: $k = 0.2\ \text{hr}^{-1}$, $V_D = 10$ L, $D = 100$ mg, $n = 6$, $t = 4$ hr, $\tau = 6$ hr, *t-miss* = 6 + 4 = 10 hr, *t-actual* = 9 hr (taken 1 hr late—ie, 5 hr before the 6th dose)

$$C_p = \frac{D_0}{V_D}\left[\frac{1 - e^{-nk\tau}}{1 - e^{-k\tau}}e^{-kt} - e^{-kt\text{-}miss} + e^{-kt\text{-}actual}\right]$$

$$= 6.425 - 1.353 + 1.653 = 6.725 \text{ mg/mL}$$

(NOTE: 1.353 was subtracted and + 1.653 added because the 5th dose was not given as planned, but 1 hour later)

INTERMITTENT INTRAVENOUS INFUSION

Intermittent IV infusion is a method of successive short IV drug infusions in which the drug is given by IV infusion for a short period of time followed by a drug elimination period, then followed by another short IV infusion (Fig. 15-4). During the short IV infusions, the drug may not reach steady state. The rational for the intermittent IV infusion is to prevent transient high drug concentrations and accompanying side effects. Many drugs are better tolerated when infused slowly over time compared to IV bolus dosing.

Administering One or More Doses by Constant Infusion: Superposition of Several IV Infusion Doses

For a continuous IV infusion (see Chapter 14):

$$C_p = \frac{R}{Cl}(1 - e^{-kt}) = \frac{R}{kV_D}(1 - e^{-kt}) \quad \textbf{(15.27)}$$

Equation 15.27 may be modified to determine drug concentration after one or more short IV infusions for a specified time period (Eq. 15.28).

$$C_p = \frac{D}{t_{inf}\ V_D k}(1 - e^{-kt}) \quad \textbf{(15.28)}$$

where R = rate of infusion = D/t_{inf}, D = size of infusion dose, t_{inf} = infusion period.

After the infusion is stopped, the drug concentration post-IV infusion is obtained using the first-order equation for drug elimination:

$$C_p = C_{stop}e^{-kt} \quad \textbf{(15.29)}$$

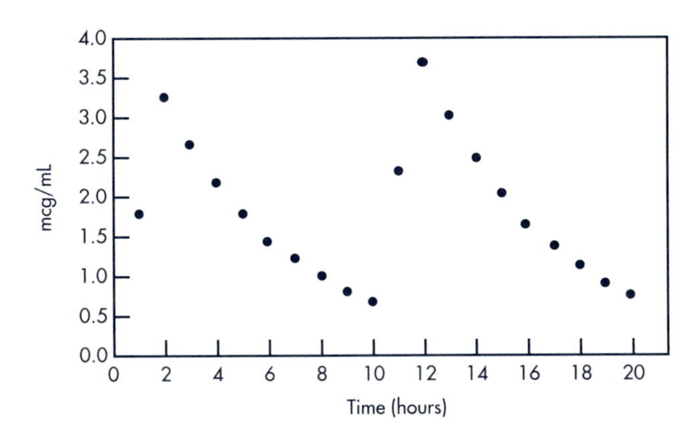

Figure 15-4. Plasma drug concentration after two doses by IV infusion. Data from Table 15.5.

where C_{stop} = concentration when infusion stops, t = time elapsed since infusion stopped.

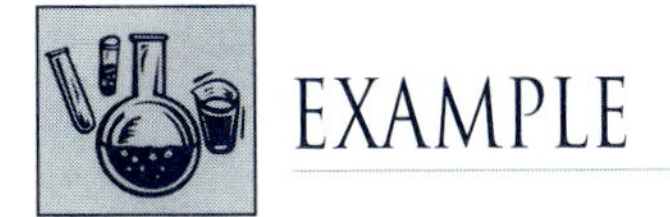

EXAMPLE

An antibiotic was infused with a 40 mg IV dose over 2 hours. Ten hours later, a second dose of 40 mg was infused again over 2 hours. What is the plasma drug concentration after 2 hours? What is the plasma drug concentration 5 hours after the second dose was infused? Assume $k = 0.2\ \text{hr}^{-1}$, $V_{\text{D}} = 10$ L for the antibiotic.

Solution

The predicted plasma drug concentrations after the first and second IV infusions are shown in Table 15.5. Using the principle of superposition, the total plasma drug concentration is the sum of the residual drug concentrations due to the first IV infusion (column 3) and the drug concentrations due to the second IV infusion (column 4). A graphical representation of these data is shown in Figure 15-4.

1. The plasma drug concentration at 2 hours after the first IV infusion starts is calculated from Equation 15.28.

$$C_{\text{p}} = \frac{40/2}{10 \times 0.2}(1 - e^{-0.2 \times 2}) = 3.30\ \text{mg/L}$$

2. From Table 15.5, the plasma drug concentration at 15 hours (ie, 5 hr after the start of the second IV infusion) is 2.06 mcg/mL. At 5 hours after the second IV infusion starts, the plasma drug concentration is the sum of the residual plasma drug concentrations from the first 2-hour infusion according to first-order elimination and the residual plasma drug concentrations from the second 2-hour IV infusion as shown in the following scheme:

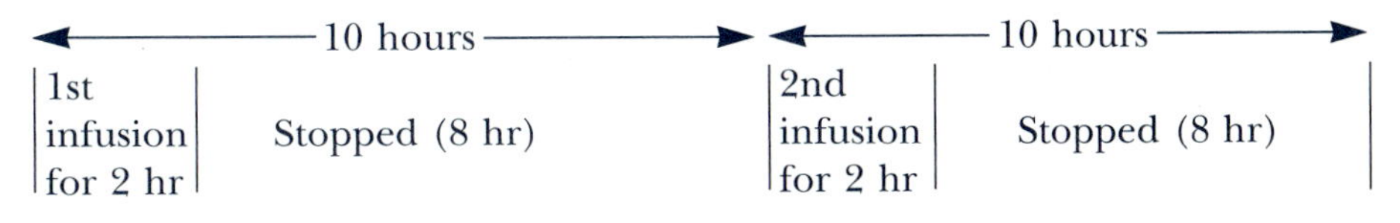

TABLE 15.5 Drug Concentration After Two Intravenous Infusions[a]

	TIME (hr)	PLASMA DRUG CONCENTRATION AFTER INFUSION 1	PLASMA DRUG CONCENTRATION AFTER INFUSION 2	TOTAL PLASMA DRUG CONCENTRATION
Infusion 1 Begins	0	0		0
	1	1.81		1.81
Infusion 1 Stopped	2	3.30		3.30
	3	2.70		2.70
	4	2.21		2.21
	5	1.81		1.81
	6	1.48		1.48
	7	1.21		1.21
	8	0.99		0.99
	9	0.81		0.81
Infusion 2 begins	10	0.67	0	0.67
	11	0.55	1.81	2.36
Infusion 2 Stopped	12	0.45	3.30	3.74
	13	0.37	2.70	3.07
	14	0.30	2.21	2.51
	15	0.25	1.81	2.06

[a]Drug is given by a 2-hr infusion separated by a 10-hr drug elimination interval. All drug concentrations are in mcg/mL. The declining drug concentration after the first infusion dose and the drug concentration after the second infusion dose gives the total plasma drug concentration.

The plasma drug concentration was calculated using the first-order elimination equation, where C_{stop} is the plasma drug concentration at the stop of the 2-hour IV infusion.

The plasma drug concentration after the completion of the first IV infusion, when $t = 13$ hours is as follows:

$$C_p = C_{stop}\, e^{-kt} = 3.30\, e^{-0.2 \times 13} = 0.25 \text{ mg/L}$$

The plasma drug concentration 5 hours after the second IV infusion is shown below:

$$C_p = C_{stop} e^{-kt} = 3.30\, e^{-0.2 \times 3} = 1.81 \text{ mcg/mL}$$

The total plasma drug concentration 5 hours after the start of the second IV infusion

$$= 0.25 \text{ mg/L} + 1.81 \text{ mg/L} = 2.06 \text{ mg/L}.$$

CLINICAL EXAMPLE

Gentamicin sulfate was given to an adult male patient (57 yrs, 70 kg) by intermittent IV infusions. One-hour IV infusions of 90 mg of gentamicin was given at 8-hour intervals. Gentamicin clearance is similar to creatinine clearance and was estimated as 7.2 L/hr with an elimination half-life of 3 hours.

1. What is the plasma drug concentration after the first IV infusion?
2. What is the peak plasma drug concentration, C_{pk} and the trough plasma drug concentration, C_{min} at steady state?

Solution

1. The plasma drug concentration directly after the first infusion is calculated from Equation 15.27, where $R = 90$ mg/hr, $Cl = 7.2$ L/hr and $k = 0.231$ hr^{-1}. The time for infusion, t_{int}, is 1 hour.

$$C_p = \frac{90}{7.2}\left(1 - e^{-(0.231)(1)}\right) = 2.58 \text{ mg/L}$$

2. The C_{pk} at steady state may be obtained from the Equation 15.30:

$$C_{pk} = \frac{R(1 - e^{-kt'})}{Cl} \times \frac{1}{(1 - e^{-k\tau})} \tag{15.30}$$

where C_{pk} is the peak drug concentration following the nth infusion at steady state, t' is the time for infusion and τ is the dosage interval. The term $1/(1 - e^{-k\tau})$ is the accumulation factor for repeated drug administration.

Substitution in Equation 15.30 gives the following:

$$C_{pk} = \frac{90\ (1 - e^{-(0.231)(1)})}{7.2} \times \frac{1}{(1 - e^{-(.231)(8)})} = 3.06 \text{ mg/L}$$

The plasma drug concentration at any time after the last infusion at steady state is obtained by Equation 15.31 and assumes that plasma drug concentrations decline according to first elimination kinetics.

$$C_{pk} = \frac{R\ (1 - e^{-kt\text{-inf}})}{Cl} \times \frac{1}{(1 - e^{-k\tau})} \times e^{-k(t\text{-inf})} \tag{15.31}$$

where t_{inf} is the time for infusion and t is the time after the start of the infusion.

The trough plasma drug concentration, C_{min} at steady state is the drug concentration just before the start of the next IV infusion or after the dosage interval equal to 8 hr after the infusion stopped. Equation 15.31 can be used to determine the plasma drug concentration at anytime after the last infusion is stopped (after steady state has been reached).

$$C_{min} = \frac{90\ (1 - e^{-(0.231)(1)})}{7.2} \times \frac{e^{-(0.231)(9\text{-}1)}}{(1 - e^{-(.231)(8)})} = 0.48 \text{ mg/L}$$

MULTIPLE ORAL DOSE REGIMEN

Figures 15-1 and 15-2 present typical cumulation curves for the concentration of drug in the body after multiple oral doses given at a constant dosage interval. The plasma concentration at any time during a multiple-dose regimen, assuming a one-compartment model and constant doses and dose interval, can be determined as follows:

$$C_p = \frac{Fk_aD_0}{V_D(k - k_a)}\left[\left(\frac{1 - e^{-nk_a\tau}}{1 - e^{-k_a\tau}}\right) e^{-k_at} - \left(\frac{1 - e^{-nk\tau}}{1 - e^{-k\tau}}\right) e^{-kt}\right] \tag{15.32}$$

where n = number of doses; τ = dosage interval; F = fraction of dose absorbed; and t = time after administration of n doses.

The mean plasma level at steady state, C_{av}^{∞}, is determined by a similar method employed for repeat IV injections. Equation 15.17 can be used for finding C_{av}^{∞} for any route of administration.

$$C_{av}^{\infty} = \frac{FD_0}{V_D k\tau} \quad (15.17)$$

Because proper evaluation of F and V_D requires IV data, the AUC of a dosing interval at steady state may be substituted in Equation 15.17 to obtain the following.

$$C_{av}^{\infty} = \frac{\int_0^{\infty} C_p \, dt}{\tau} = \frac{[AUC]_0^{\infty}}{\tau} \quad (15.33)$$

One can see from Equation 15.17 that the magnitude of C_{av}^{∞} is directly proportional to the size of the dose and the extent of drug absorbed. Furthermore, if the dosage interval (τ) is shortened, then the value for C_{av}^{∞} will increase. The C_{av}^{∞} will be predictably higher for drugs distributed in a small V_D (eg, plasma water) or which have long elimination half-lives, than for drugs distributed in a large V_D (eg, total body water) or have very short elimination half-lives. Because body clearance (Cl_T) is equal to kV_D, substitution into Equation 15.17 yields

$$C_{av}^{\infty} = \frac{FD_0}{Cl_T \tau} \quad (15.34)$$

Thus, if Cl_T decreases, C_{av}^{∞} will increase.

The C_{av}^{∞} does not give information concerning the fluctuations in plasma concentration (C_{max}^{∞} and C_{min}^{∞}). In multiple-dosage regimens, C_p at any time can be obtained with Equation 15.32, where n = nth dose. At *steady state*, the *drug* concentration can be determined by letting n equal infinity. Therefore, $e^{-nk\tau}$ becomes approximately equal to zero and Equation 15.22 becomes

$$C_p^{\infty} = \frac{k_a F D_0}{V_D (k_a - k)} \left[\left(\frac{1}{1 - e^{-k\tau}} \right) e^{-kt} - \left(\frac{1}{1 - e^{k_a \tau}} \right) e^{-k_a t} \right] \quad (15.35)$$

The maximum and minimum drug concentrations (C_{max}^{∞} and C_{min}^{∞}) can be obtained with the following equations:

$$C_{max}^{\infty} = \frac{FD_0}{V_D} \left(\frac{1}{1 - e^{-k\tau}} \right) e^{-kt_p} \quad (15.36)$$

$$C_{min}^{\infty} = \frac{k_a F D_0}{V_D (k_a - k)} \left(\frac{1}{1 - e^{-k\tau}} \right) e^{-k\tau} \quad (15.37)$$

The time at which maximum (peak) plasma concentration (or t_{max}) occurs following a single oral dose is as shown:

$$t_{max} = \frac{2.3}{k_a - k} \log \frac{k_a}{k} \quad (15.38)$$

whereas the peak plasma concentration t_p following multiple doses is given by Equation 15.39.

Large fluctuations between C_{max}^{∞} and C_{min}^{∞} can be hazardous, particularly with drugs that have a narrow therapeutic index. The larger the number of divided doses, the smaller the fluctuations in the plasma drug concentrations. For example, a 500-mg dose of drug given every 6 hours will produce the same C_{av}^{∞} value as a 250-mg dose of the same drug given every 3 hours, while the C_{max}^{∞} and C_{min}^{∞} fluctuations for the latter dose will be decreased by one-half (see Figure 15.3). With drugs that have a narrow therapeutic index, the dosage interval should not be longer than the elimination half-life.

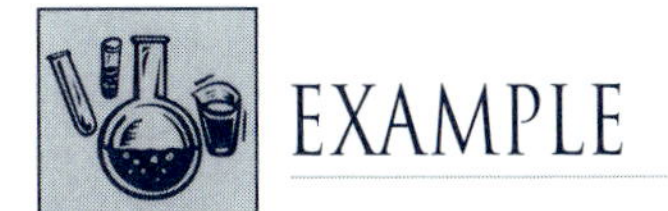

EXAMPLE

An adult male patient (46 years old, 81 kg) was given orally 250 mg of tetracycline hydrochloride every 8 hours for 2 weeks. From the literature, tetracycline hydrochloride is about 75% bioavailable and has an apparent volume of distribution of 1.5 L/kg. The elimination half-life is about 10 hours. The absorption rate constant is 0.9 hr^{-1}. From this information calculate (1) C_{max} after the first dose, (2) C_{min} after the first dose, (3) plasma drug concentration C_p at 4 hours after the seventh dose, (4) maximum plasma drug concentration at steady state C^{∞}_{max}, (5) minimum plasma drug concentration at steady state C^{∞}_{min}, and (6) average plasma drug concentration at steady state C^{∞}_{av}.

Solution

1. C_{max} after the first dose. The C_{max} occurs at t_{max}. Therefore, using Equation 15.38,

$$t_{max} = \frac{2.3}{0.9 - 0.07} \log(0.9/0.07)$$
$$= 3.07 \text{ hr}$$

Then substitute t_{max} into the following equation for a single oral dose (one-compartment model) to obtain C_{max}.

$$C_{max} = \frac{FD_0 k_a}{V_D(k_a - k)}(e^{-kt_{max}} - e^{-k_a t_{max}})$$
$$= \frac{(0.75)(250)(0.9)}{(121.5)(0.9 - 0.07)}(e^{-0.07(3.07)} - e^{-0.9(3.07)})$$
$$= 1.28 \text{ mg/L}$$

2. C_{min} after the first dose. The C_{min} occurs just before the administration of the next dose of drug. Therefore, set $t = 8$ hours and solve for C_{min}.

$$C_{min} = \frac{(0.75)(250)(0.9)}{(121.5)(0.9 - 0.07)}(e^{-0.07(8)} - e^{-0.9(8)})$$
$$= 0.95 \text{ mg/L}$$

3. C_p at 4 hours after the seventh dose. The C_p may be calculated by Equation 15.32, letting $n = 7$, $t = 4$, $\tau = 8$, and making the appropriate substitutions.

$$C_p = \frac{(0.75)(250)(0.9)}{(121.5)(0.07 - 0.9)}$$
$$\times \left[\left(\frac{1 - e^{-(7)(0.9)(8)}}{1 - e^{-0.9(8)}}\right)e^{-0.9(4)} - \left(\frac{1 + e^{-(7)(0.07)(8)}}{1 - e^{-(0.07)(8)}}\right)e^{-0.07(4)}\right]$$
$$= 2.86 \text{ mg/L}$$

4. $C_{\max}^{\infty}$ at steady state. The t_p at steady state is obtained from Equation 15.39.

$$t_p = \frac{1}{k_a - k} \ln \left[\frac{k_a(1 - e^{-k\tau})}{k(1 - e^{-k_a\tau})} \right] \tag{15.39}$$

$$= \frac{1}{0.9 - 0.07} \ln \left[\frac{0.9(1 - e^{-(0.07)(8)})}{0.07(1 - e^{-(0.9)(8)})} \right]$$

$$= 2.05 \text{ hr}$$

Then $C_{\max}^{\infty}$ is obtained using Equation 15.36.

$$C_{\max}^{\infty} = \frac{0.75(250)}{121.5} \left(\frac{1}{1 - e^{-0.07(8)}} \right) e^{-0.07(2.05)}$$

$$= 3.12 \text{ mg/L}$$

5. $C_{\min}^{\infty}$ at steady state. The $C_{\min}^{\infty}$ is calculated from Equation 15.37.

$$C_{\min}^{\infty} = \frac{(0.9)(0.75)(250)}{(121.5)(0.9 - 0.07)} \left(\frac{1}{1 - e^{-0.07(8)}} \right) e^{-(0.07)(8)}$$

$$= 2.23 \text{ mg/L}$$

6. C_{av}^{∞} at steady state. The C_{av}^{∞} is calculated from Equation 15.17.

$$C_{av}^{\infty} = \frac{(0.75)(250)}{(121.5)(0.07)(8)}$$

$$= 2.76 \text{ mg/L}$$

LOADING DOSE

In practice, a loading dose may be given as a bolus dose or a short-term loading IV infusion. As discussed earlier, the time required for the drug to accumulate to a steady-state plasma level is dependent mainly on its elimination half-life. The time needed to reach 90% of C_{av}^{∞} is approximately 3.3 half-lives, and the time required to reach 99% of C_{av}^{∞} is equal to approximately 6.6 half-lives. For a drug with a half-life of 4 hours, it would take approximately 13 and 26 hours to reach 90 and 99% of C_{av}^{∞}, respectively.

To reduce the onset time of the drug—that is, the time it takes to achieve the minimum effective dose (assumed to be equivalent to the C_{av}^{∞})—a loading (priming) or initial dose of drug is given. The main objective of the loading dose is to achieve C_{av}^{∞} as quickly as possible. Thereafter, a maintenance dose is given to maintain C_{av}^{∞} so that the therapeutic effect is also maintained.

For drugs absorbed rapidly in relation to elimination ($k_a \gg k$) and which are distributed rapidly, the loading dose D_L can be calculated as follows:

$$\frac{D_L}{D_0} = \frac{1}{(1 - e^{-k_a\tau})(1 - e^{-k\tau})} \tag{15.40}$$

For extremely rapid absorption, as when the product of $k_a\tau$ is large or in the case of IV infusion, $e^{-k_a\tau}$ becomes approximately zero and Equation 15.40 reduces to

$$\frac{D_L}{D_0} = \frac{1}{1 - e^{-k\tau}} \tag{15.41}$$

The loading dose should approximate the amount of drug contained in the body

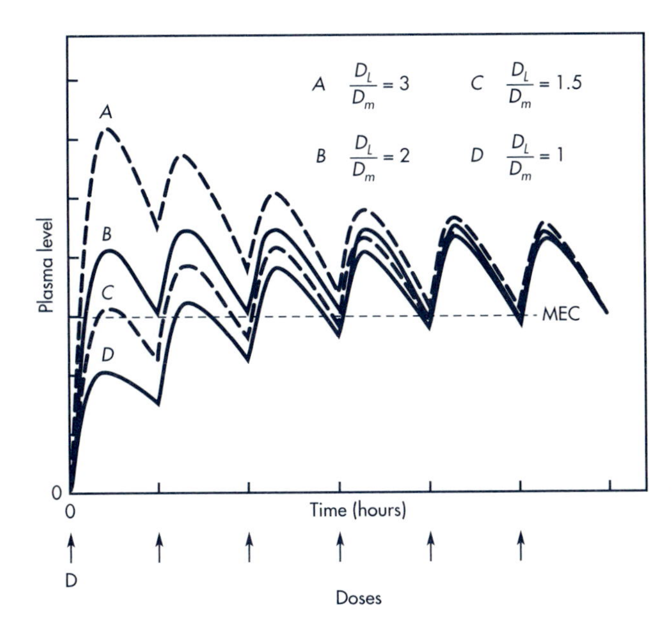

Figure 15-5. Concentration curves for dosage regimens with equal maintenance doses (D) and dosage intervals (τ) and different dose ratios.
(From Kruger-Thiemer (1968), with permission.)

during steady state. The dose ratio is equal to the loading dose divided by the maintenance dose.

$$\text{Dose ratio} = \frac{D_L}{D_0} \tag{15.42}$$

As a general rule, the dose ratio should be equal to 2.0 if the selected dosage interval is equal to the elimination half-life. Figure 15-5 shows the plasma level–time curve for dosage regimens with equal maintenance doses but different loading doses. A rapid approximation of loading dose, D_L, may be estimated from the following equation:

$$D_L = \frac{V_D C_{av}^{\infty}}{(S)(F)} \tag{15.43}$$

where C_{av}^{∞} is the desired plasma drug concentration, S is the salt form of the drug, and F is the fraction of drug bioavailability.

Equation 15.43 assumes very rapid drug absorption from an immediate-release dosage form. The D_L calculated by this method has been used in clinical situations for which only an approximation of the D_L is needed.

These calculations for loading doses are not applicable to drugs that demonstrate multicompartment kinetics. Such drugs distribute slowly into extravascular tissues, and drug equilibration may not take place until after the apparent plateau is reached in the vascular (central) compartment.

DETERMINATION OF BIOAVAILABILITY AND BIOEQUIVALENCE IN A MULTIPLE-DOSE REGIMEN

In evaluating drug bioavailability information, one must consider the experimental design used to obtain the data. Otherwise, differences due to an artifact might be mistaken for real differences in bioavailability. Estimation of the absorption rate constant during multiple dosing is difficult, because the residual drug from the previous dose superimposes on the dose that follows. However, the data obtained in multiple doses are useful in calculating a steady-state plasma level.

Bioavailability may be determined during a multiple-dose regimen only after a steady-state plasma drug level has been reached. As discussed, the time needed to reach the steady-state plasma level is related to the elimination $t_{1/2}$ of the drug. As observed in Table 15.3, it takes approximately 6.6 half-lives to reach 99% of the C_{av}^{∞}.

The parameters for bioavailability of a drug using plasma level data from a multiple-dose regimen are similar to those obtained with a single-dose regimen. In the former case, the first plasma samples are taken just prior to the second dose of the drug. Thereafter, plasma samples are taken periodically after the dose is administered to adequately describe the entire plasma level–time curve (Fig. 15-1). Parameters including AUC, time for peak drug concentration, and peak drug concentration are then used to describe the bioavailability of the drug.

The extent of bioavailability, measured by assuming the $[AUC]_0^{\infty}$, is dependent on clearance:

$$[AUC]_0^{\infty} = \frac{FD_0}{Cl_T} \tag{15.44}$$

Determination of bioavailability using multiple doses reveals changes that are normally not detected in a single-dose study. For example, nonlinear pharmacokinetics may occur after multiple drug doses due to the higher plasma drug concentrations saturating an enzyme system involved in absorption or elimination of the drug. With some drugs a drug-induced malabsorption syndrome can also alter the percentage of drug absorbed. In this case, drug bioavailability may decrease after repeated doses if the fraction of the dose absorbed (F) decreases or if the total body clearance (kV_D) increases.

BIOEQUIVALENCE STUDIES

Most bioequivalence studies use *normal healthy adult subjects.* The Food and Drug Administration, Division of Bioequivalence, Office of Generic Drugs provides a guidance for the determination of bioequivalence for extended-release products which includes the demonstration of *in vivo* bioequivalence using a multiple-dose (steady-state) study (see also Chapter 7). This study is required for oral extended-release (controlled-release) drug products in addition to a single-dose fasting study and a food intervention study.

The multiple-dose study is designed as a steady state, randomized, two-treatment, two-way, crossover study comparing equal doses of the test and reference products in adult, healthy subjects. Each subject receives either the test or reference product separated by a "washout" period, which is the time needed for the drug to be completely eliminated from the body.

To ascertain that the subjects are at steady state, three consecutive trough concentrations (C_{min}) are determined usually on three consecutive days. The last morning dose is given to the subject after an overnight fast with continual fasting for at least 2 hours following dose administration. Blood sampling is then performed similar to the single dose study.

Pharmacokinetic analysis includes calculation for each subject of the steady-state area-under-the-curve (AUC_{0-t}), t_{max}, C_{min}, C_{max}, and the percent fluctuation $[100 \times (C_{max} - C_{min})/C_{min}]$. The data is statistically analyzed using analysis of variance (ANOVA) on the log-transformed AUC and C_{max}. To establish bioequivalence, the AUC and C_{max} parameters for the test (generic) product should be within 80 to 125% of the reference product using the 90% confidence interval.

For some drugs, such as hormone replacement therapy, a bioequivalence study may be performed in *patients* already maintained on the drug. In this case, a washout period would place the patient at substantial risk for being without drug therapy. Therefore, the patient continues on his or her own medication, and blood sampling is performed during a dosage interval (Fig. 15-6, drug product *A*). Once this is accomplished, the patient begins to take equal oral doses of an alternate drug product. Again, time must be allowed for the theoretical attainment of C_{av}^{∞} with the second drug product. When steady state is reached, the plasma level–time curve for a dosage interval with the second drug product is described (Fig. 15-5, drug product *B*). Using the same plasma parameters as before, the bioequivalence or lack of bioequivalence may be determined.

There are a number of advantages to using this method for the determination of bioequivalence: (1) the patient acts as his or her own control, (2) the patient maintains a minimum plasma drug concentration, and (3) the plasma samples after multiple doses contain more drug that can be assayed more accurately. The disadvantages of using this method include the following: (1) the study takes more time to perform, because steady-state conditions must be reached, and (2) sometimes more plasma samples must be obtained from the patient to ascertain that steady state is reached and to describe the plasma level–time curve accurately.

Because the C_{av}^{∞} depends primarily on the dose of the drug and the time interval between doses, the extent of drug systemically available is more important than the rate of drug availability. Small differences in the rate of drug absorption may not be observed with steady-state study comparisons. If there is wide variation in the rate of a drug's availability, then it is possible that initial high blood levels may lead to toxicity.

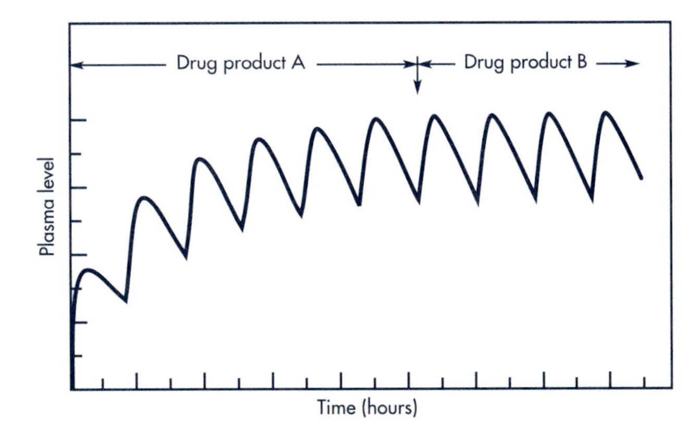

Figure 15-6. Multiple-dose bioequivalency study comparing the bioavailability of drug product *B* to the bioavailability of drug product *A*. Blood levels for such studies must be taken after C_{av}^{∞} is reached. The arrow represents the start of therapy with drug product B.

If the blood level–time curve of the second drug product is comparable to that of the reference drug product, the second product is considered to be bioequivalent. If the second drug has less bioavailability (assuming that only the extent of drug absorption is less than that of the reference drug), the resulting C_{av}^{∞} will be smaller than that obtained with the first drug. Usually the drug manufacturer will perform dissolution and content uniformity tests prior to performing a bioequivalence study. These *in vitro* dissolution tests will help to ensure that the C_{av}^{∞} obtained from each drug product *in vivo* will not be largely different from each other. In contrast, if the extent of drug availability is greater in the second drug product, the C_{av}^{∞} will be higher.

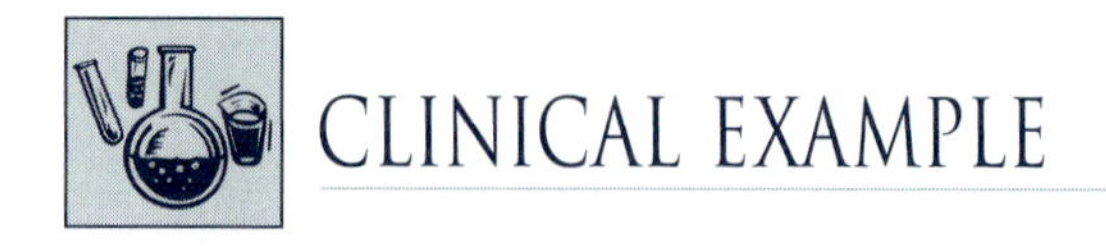

CLINICAL EXAMPLE

The bioequivalence of two synthetic levothyroxine sodium preparations, Levothroid and Synthroid were evaluated in 20 hypothyroid patients (Sista and Albert, 1994). The investigation was designed as a two-way crossover study in which the patients who had been diagnosed as hypothyroid by their primary care physician were given a single 100 μg daily dose of either Levothroid or Synthroid brand levothyroxine sodium tablets for 50 days and then switched over immediately to other treatment for 50 days. Predose blood samples were taken on days 1, 25, 48, 49, and 50 of each phase, and, on day 50, a complete blood sampling was performed. The serum from each blood sample was analyzed for total and free thyroxine (T_4), total and free triiodothyronine (T_3), the major metabolite of T_4, and thyrotropin (TSH).

1. Why were hypothyroid patients used in this study?
2. Why were the subjects dosed for 50 days with each thyroid product?
3. Why were blood samples obtained on days 48, 49, and 50?
4. Why was T_3 measured?
5. Why was TSH measured?

Solution

1. Normal healthy euthyroid subjects would be at risk if they were to take levothyroxine sodium for an extended period of time.
2. The long (50 day) daily dosing for each product was required to obtain steady-state drug levels due to the long elimination half-life of levothyroxine.
3. Serum from blood samples were taken on days 48, 49, and 50 to obtain three consecutive C_{min} drug levels.
4. T_3 is the active metabolite of T_4.
5. The serum TSH concentration is inversely proportional to the free serum T_4 concentrations and gives an indication of the pharmacodynamic activity of the active drug.

DOSAGE REGIMEN SCHEDULES

Predictions of steady-state plasma drug concentrations usually assume the drug is given at a constant dosage interval throughout a 24-hour day. Very often, however, the drug is only given during the waking hours. Niebergall and associates (1974) have discussed the problem of scheduling dosage regimens and have particularly warned against improper timing of the drug dosage. For example, Figure 15-7 shows the plasma levels of theophylline given three times a day. Notice the large fluctuation between the maximum and minimum plasma levels. In comparison, procainamide was given on a 0.5-g, 4-times-a-day maintenance dosage with a 1.0-g loading dose on the first day (Fig. 15-8). However, on the second and third days, plasma levels did not reach the therapeutic range until after the second dose of drug.

Ideally, drug doses should be given at evenly spaced intervals. However, to improve *patient compliance*, dosage regimens may be designed to fit with the life style of the patient. For example, the patient is directed to take a drug such as amoxicillin 4 times a day (QID) before meals and at bedtime for a systemic infection. This dosage regimen will produce *unequal dosage intervals* during the day when the patient takes the drug before breakfast at 0800 hours (8 AM), before lunch at 1200 hours (12 noon), before dinner at 1800 hours (6 PM), and before bedtime at 2300 hours (11 PM). For these drugs, evenly spaced dosage intervals are not that critical to the effectiveness of the antibiotic as long as the plasma drug concentrations are maintained above the minimum inhibitory concentration (MIC) for the microorganism.

Patient compliance to multiple dose regimens may be a problem for the patient in following the prescribed dosage regimen. Occasionally, a patient may miss taking the drug dose at the prescribed dosage interval. For drugs with long elimination half-lives (eg, levothyroxine sodium or oral contraceptives), the consequences of one missed dose is minimal, since only a small fraction of drug is lost between daily dosing intervals. The patient should either take the next drug dose as soon as the patient remembers or continue the dosing schedule starting at the next prescribed dosing period. If it is almost time for the next dose, then the skipped dose is not taken and the regular dosing schedule is maintained. Generally, the patient

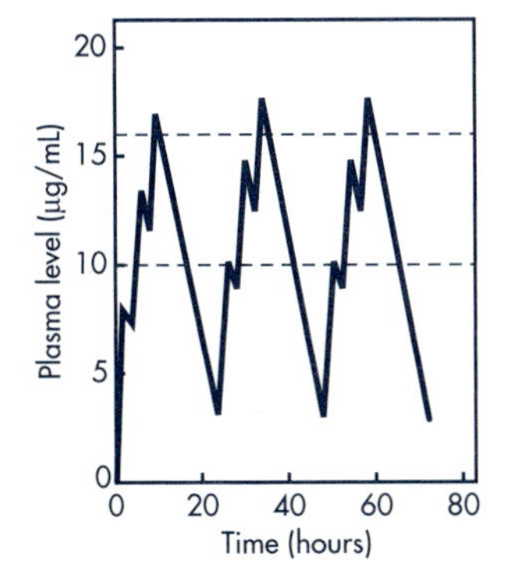

Figure 15-7. Plasma level–time curve for theophylline given in doses of 160 mg 3 times a day. Dashed lines indicate the therapeutic range.
(From Niebergall et al (1974), with permission.)

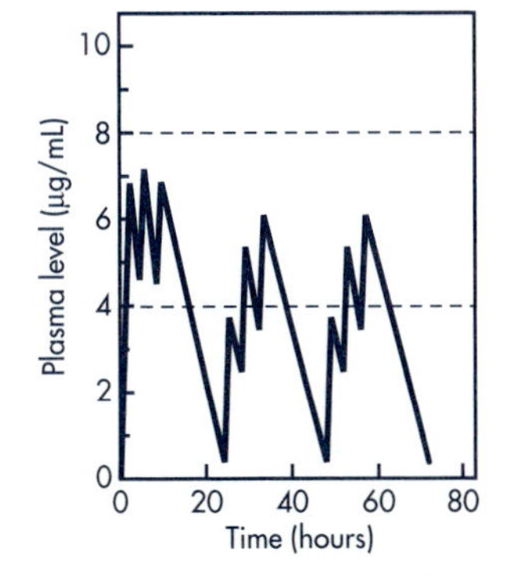

Figure 15-8. Plasma level–time curve for procainamide given in an initial dose of 1.0 g followed by doses of 0.5 g 4 times a day. Dashed lines indicate the therapeutic range.
(From Niebergall et al (1974), with permission.)

should not double the dose of the medication. For specific drug information on missed doses, the USP DI II, *Advice for the Patient* published annually by the United States Pharmacopeia is a good source of information.

The problems of widely fluctuating plasma drug concentrations may be prevented by using a controlled-release formulation of the drug, or a drug in the same therapeutic class that has a long elimination half-life. The use of extended-release dosage forms allows for less frequent dosing and prevents undermedication between the last evening dose and the first morning dose. Extended-release drug products may improve patient compliance by decreasing the number of doses within a 24-hour period which the patient needs to take. Patients generally show better compliance with a twice-a-day (BID) dosage regimen compared to a 3-times-a-day (BID) dosage schedule.

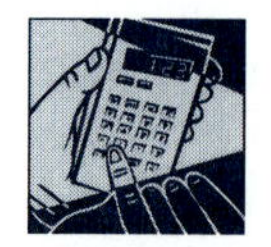

PRACTICE PROBLEMS

1. Patient C.S. is a 35-year-old male weighing 76.6 kg. The patient is to be given multiple IV bolus injections of an antibiotic every 6 hours. The effective concentration of this drug is 15 μg/mL. After the patient is given a single IV dose, the elimination half-life for the drug is determined to be 3.0 hours and the apparent V_D is 196 mL/kg. Determine a multiple IV dose regimen for this drug (assume drug is given every 6 hours).

Solution

$$C_{av}^{\infty} = \frac{FD_0}{V_D k\tau}$$

For IV dose, $F = 1$,

$$D_0 = (15\ \mu\text{g/mL})\left(\frac{0.693}{3\ \text{hr}}\right)(196\ \text{mL/kg})(6\ \text{hr})$$
$$= 4.07\ \text{mg/kg every 6 hr}$$

Since patient C.S. weighs 76.6 kg, the dose should be as shown:

$$D_0 = (4.07\ \text{mg/kg})(76.6\ \text{kg})$$
$$= 312\ \text{mg every 6 hr}$$

After the condition of this patient has stabilized, the patient is to be given the drug orally for convenience of drug administration. The objective is to design an oral dosage regimen that will produce the same steady-state blood level as the multiple IV doses. The drug dose will depend on the bioavailability of the drug from the drug product, the desired therapeutic drug level, and the dosage interval chosen. Assume that the antibiotic is 90% bioavailable and that the physician would like to continue oral medication every 6 hr.

The average or steady-state plasma drug level is given by the following:

$$C_{av}^{\infty} = \frac{FD_0}{V_D k\tau}$$

Because $k = 0.693/t_{1/2}$

$$C_{av}^{\infty} = \frac{FD_0 1.44 t_{1/2}}{V_D \tau}$$

Because the literature may give the total body clearance Cl_τ for the drug, the above equation is equivalent to

$$C_{av}^{\infty} = \frac{FD_0}{Cl_T \tau}$$

Where $Cl_T = kV_D$ for a one-compartment model, or $Cl_T = bV_p$ for a two-compartment model:

$$D_0 = \frac{(15\ \mu g/mL)(196\ mL/kg)(6\ hr)}{(0.9)(1.44)(3\ hr)}$$
$$= 4.54\ mg/kg$$

Because patient C.S. weighs 76.6 kg, he should be given the following dose:

$$D_0 = (4.54\ mg/kg)(76.6\ kg)$$
$$= 348\ mg\ every\ 6\ hr$$

For drugs with equal absorption but slower absorption rates (F is the same but k_a is smaller), the initial dosing period may show a lower blood level; however, the steady-state blood level will be unchanged.

2. In practice, drug products are usually commercially available in certain specified strengths. Using the information provided in the preceding problem, assume that the antibiotic is available in 125-, 250-, and 500-mg tablets. Therefore, the pharmacist or prescriber must now decide which tablets are to be given to the patient. In this case, it may be possible to give the patient 375 mg (eg, one 125-mg tablet and one 250-mg tablet) every 6 hours. However, the C_{av}^{∞} should be calculated to determine if the plasma level is approaching a toxic value. Alternatively, a new dosage interval might be appropriate for the patient. It is very important to design the dosage interval and the dose to be as simple as possible, so that the patient will not be confused and will be able to comply with the medication program properly.

a. What is the new C_{av}^{∞} if the patient is given 375 mg every 6 hours?

Solution

$$C_{av}^{\infty} = \frac{(0.9)(375{,}000)(1.44)(3)}{(196)(76.6)(6)}$$
$$= 16.2\ \mu g/mL$$

Because the therapeutic objective was to achieve a minimum effective concentration (MEC) of 15 μg/mL, a value of 16.2 μg/mL is reasonable.

b. The patient has difficulty in distinguishing tablets of different strengths. Can the patient take a 500-mg dose (eg, two 250-mg tablets)?

Solution

The dosage interval (τ) for the 500-mg tablet would have to be calculated as follows.

$$\tau = \frac{(0.9)(500{,}000)(1.44)(3)}{(196)(76.6)(15)}$$
$$= 8.63\ hr$$

c. A dosage interval of 8.63 hours is difficult to remember. Is a dosage regimen of 500 mg every 8 hours reasonable?

Solution

$$C_{av}^{\infty} = \frac{(0.9)(500{,}000)(1.44)(3)}{(196)(76.6)(8)}$$
$$= 16.2\ \mu g/mL$$

Notice that a larger dose is necessary if the drug is given at longer intervals.

In designing a dosage regimen, one should consider a regimen that is practical and convenient for the patient. For example, the dosage interval should be spaced conveniently for the patient for improved compliance. In addition, one should consider the commercially available dosage strengths of the prescribed drug product.

The use of Equation 15.17 to initially estimate a dosage regimen has wide utility. The C_{av}^{∞} is equal to the dosing rate divided by the total body clearance of the drug in the patient:

$$C_{av}^{\infty} = \frac{FD_0}{\tau}\frac{1}{Cl_T} \tag{15.45}$$

where FD_0/τ is equal to the dosing rate R, and $1/Cl_T$ is equal to $1/kV_D$.

In designing dosage regimens, the dosing rate D_0/τ is adjusted for the patient's drug clearance to obtain the desired C_{av}^{∞}. For an IV infusion, the zero-order rate of infusion (R) is used to obtain the desired steady-state plasma drug concentration C_{ss}. If R is substituted for FD_0/τ in Equation 15.45, then the following equation for estimating C_{ss} after an IV infusion is obtained.

$$C_{ss} = \frac{R}{Cl_T} \tag{15.46}$$

From Equations 15.45 and 15.46, all dosage schedules having the same dosing rate D_0/τ, or R, will have the same C_{av}^{∞} or C_{ss}, whether the drug is given by multiple doses or by IV infusion. For example, dosage schedules of 100 mg every 4 hours, 200 mg every 8 hours, 300 mg every 12 hours, and 600 mg every 24 hours will yield the same C_{av}^{∞} in the patient. An IV infusion rate of 25 mg/hr in the same patient will give a C_{ss} equal to the C_{av}^{∞} obtained with the multiple-dose schedule (Fig. 15-3; Table 15.6).

TABLE 15.6 Effect of Dosing Schedule on Predicted Steady-State Plasma Drug Concentrations[a]

DOSING SCHEDULE			STEADY-STATE DRUG CONCENTRATION (μg/mL)		
DOSE (mg)	τ (hr)	DOSING RATE, D_0/τ (mg/hr)	C_{max}^{∞}	C_{av}^{∞}	C_{min}^{∞}
—	—	25[b]	14.5	14.5	14.5
100	4	25	16.2	14.5	11.6
200	8	25	20.2	14.5	7.81
300	12	25	25.3	14.5	5.03
600	24	25	44.1	14.5	1.12
400	8	50	40.4	28.9	15.6
600	8	75	60.6	43.4	23.4

[a]Drug has an elimination half-life of 4 hr and an apparent V_D of 10 L.

[b]Drug given by IV infusion. The first-order absorption rate constant k_a is 1.2 hr^{-1} and the drug follows a one-compartment open model.

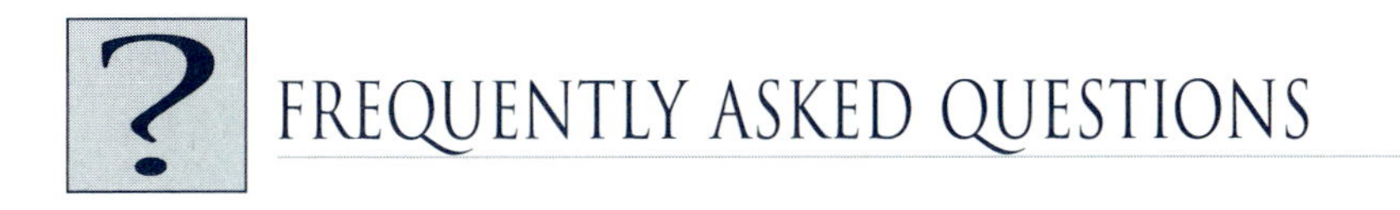

FREQUENTLY ASKED QUESTIONS

1. What are the advantages/disadvantages for giving a drug by a constant IV infusion, intermittent IV infusion, or multiple IV bolus injections? What drugs would most likely be given by each route of administration? Why?
2. Is a loading dose always necessary when placing a patient on a multiple-dose regimen? What are the determining factors?
3. Is the drug accumulation index (R) applicable to any drug given by multiple dose or only to drugs that are eliminated slowly from the body?
4. Does a loading dose significantly affect the steady-state concentration of a drug given by a constant multiple-dose regimen?
5. Give two examples of a drug that requires a loading dose because of its long $t_{1/2}$.
6. Why is the steady-state peak plasma drug concentration often measured sometime after an IV dose is given in a clinical situation?

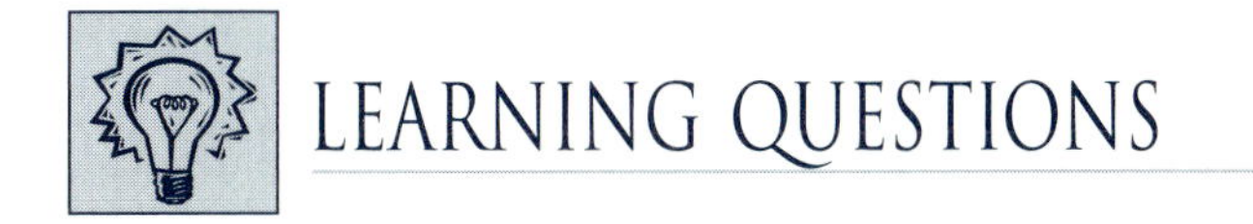

LEARNING QUESTIONS

1. Gentamicin has an average elimination half-life of approximately 2 hours and an apparent volume of distribution of 20% of body weight. It is necessary to give gentamicin, 1 mg/kg every 8 hours by multiple IV injections, to a 50-kg woman with normal renal function. Calculate (a) C_{max}, (b) C_{min}, and (c) C_{av}^{∞}.
2. A physician wants to give theophylline to a young male asthmatic patient (age 29, 80 kg). According to the literature, the elimination half-life for theophylline is 5 hours and the apparent V_D is equal to 50% of body weight. The plasma level of theophylline required to provide adequate airway ventilation is approximately 10 μmg/mL.
   - **a.** The physician wants the patient to take medication every 6 hours around the clock. What dose of theophylline would you recommend (assume theophylline is 100% bioavailable)?
   - **b.** If you were to find that theophylline is available to you only in 225-mg capsules, what dosage regimen would you recommend?
3. What pharmacokinetic parameter is most important in determining the time at which the steady-state plasma drug level (C_{av}^{∞}) is reached?
4. Name two ways in which the fluctuations of plasma concentrations (between C_{max}^{∞} and C_{min}^{∞}) can be minimized for a person on a multiple-dose drug regimen without altering the C_{av}^{∞}.
5. What is the purpose of giving a loading dose?

6. What is the loading dose for an antibiotic ($k = 0.23\ \text{hr}^{-1}$) with a maintenance dose of 200 mg every 3 hours?

7. What is the main advantage of giving a potent drug by IV infusion as opposed to multiple IV injections?

8. A drug has an elimination half-life of 2 hours and a volume of distribution of 40 L. The drug is given at a dose of 200 mg every 4 hours by multiple IV bolus injections. Predict the plasma drug concentration at 1 hour after the third dose.

9. The elimination half-life of an antibiotic is 3 hours and the apparent volume of distribution is 20% of body weight. The therapeutic window for this drug is from 2 to 10 μmg/mL. Adverse toxicity is often observed at drug concentrations above 15 μmg/mL. The drug will be given by multiple IV bolus injections.

a. Calculate the dose for an adult male patient (68 years old, 82 kg) with normal renal function to be given every 8 hours.

b. Calculate the anticipated C_{max}^{∞} and C_{min}^{∞} values.

c. Calculate the C_{av}^{∞} value.

d. Comment on the adequacy of your dosage regimen.

10. Tetracycline hydrochloride (Achromycin V, Lederle) is prescribed for a young adult male patient (28 years old, 78 kg) suffering from gonorrhea. According to the literature, tetracycline HCl is 77% orally absorbed, is 65% bound to plasma proteins, has an apparent volume of distribution of 0.5 L/kg, has an elimination half-life of 10.6 hours, and is 58% excreted unchanged in the urine. The minimum inhibitory drug concentration (MIC) for gonorrhea is 25 to 30 μmg/mL.

a. Calculate an *exact* maintenance dose for this patient to be given every 6 hours around the clock.

b. Achromycin V is available in 250-mg and 500-mg capsules. How many capsules (state dose) should the patient take every 6 hours?

c. What loading dose using the above capsules would you recommend for this patient?

11. The body clearance of sumatriptan (Imitrex) is 250 mL/min. The drug is about 14% bioavailable. What would be the average plasma drug concentration after 5 doses of 100 mg po every 8 hours in a patient. (Assume steady state was reached.)

12. Cefotaxime has a volume of distribution of 0.17L/kg and an elimination half life of 1.5 hours. What is the peak plasma drug concentration in a patient weighing 75 kg after receiving 1 gm IV of the drug 3 times daily for 3 days?

REFERENCES

Kruger-Thiemer E: Pharmacokinetics and dose-concentration relationships. In Ariens EJ (ed), *Physico-Chemical Aspects of Drug Action.* New York, Pergamon Press, 1968, p 97

Niebergall PJ, Sugita ET, Schnaare RC: Potential dangers of common drug dosing regimens. *Am J Hosp Pharm* **31**:53–58, 1974

Sista S, Albert KS: A two-way crossover, multiple dose bioavailability study of levothyroxine sodium tablets in hypothyroid patients. *Pharm Res* Oct 1994 (abstract)

Van Rossum JM, Tomey AHM: Rate of accumulation and plateau concentration of drugs after chronic medication. *J Pharm Pharmacol* **20**:390–392, 1968

BIBLIOGRAPHY

Gibaldi M, Perrier D: *Pharmacokinetics*, 2nd ed. New York, Marcel Dekker, 1962, pp 451–457

Levy G: Kinetics of pharmacologic effect. *Clin Pharmacol Ther* **7:**362, 1966

Van Rossum JM: Pharmacokinetics of accumulation. *J Pharm Sci* **75:**2162–2164, 1968

Wagner JG: Kinetics of pharmacological response, I: Proposed relationship between response and drug concentration in the intact animal and man. *J Theor Biol* **20:**173, 1968

Wagner JG: Relations between drug concentrations and response. *J Mond Pharm* **14:**279–310, 1971

16

NONLINEAR PHARMACOKINETICS

In the previous chapters, linear pharmacokinetic models using simple first-order kinetics were introduced to describe the course of drug action. These linear models assumed that the pharmacokinetic parameters for a drug would not change when different doses or multiple doses of a drug were given. With some drugs, increased doses or chronic medication can cause deviations from the linear pharmacokinetic profile observed with single low doses of the same drug. This nonlinear pharmacokinetic behavior is also termed *dose-dependent pharmacokinetics*.

Many of the processes of drug absorption, distribution, biotransformation, and excretion involve enzymes or carrier-mediated systems. For some drugs given at therapeutic levels, one of these specialized processes may become saturated. As shown in Table 16.1, various causes of nonlinear pharmacokinetic behavior are theoretically possible. Besides saturation of a carrier-mediated system, drugs may demonstrate nonlinear pharmacokinetics due to a pathologic alteration in drug absorption, distribution, and elimination. For example, aminoglycosides may cause renal nephrotoxicity, thereby altering renal drug excretion.

In addition, an obstruction of the bile duct due to the formation of gallstones will alter biliary drug excretion. In most cases, the main pharmacokinetic observation is a change in the apparent elimination rate constant.

A number of drugs for which saturation or capacity-limited metabolism has been demonstrated in humans. These drug processes include glycine conjugation of salicylate, sulfate conjugation of salicylamide, acetylation of *p*-aminobenzoic acid, and the elimination of phenytoin (Tozer et al, 1981). Drugs that demonstrate saturation kinetics usually show the following characteristics.

1. Elimination of drug does not follow simple first-order kinetics—that is, elimination kinetics are nonlinear.
2. The elimination half-life changes as dose is increased. Usually, the elimination half-life increases with increased dose due to saturation of an enzyme system. However, the elimination half-life might decrease due to "self" induction of liver biotransformation enzymes as observed for carbamazepine.
3. The AUC is not proportional to the amount of bioavailable drug.
4. The saturation of capacity-limited processes may be affected by other drugs that require the same enzyme or carrier-mediated system.

TABLE 16.1 Examples of Drugs Showing Nonlinear Kinetics

CAUSE[a]	DRUG
GI Absorption	
Saturable transport in gut wall	Riboflavin, gebapentin, L-dopa, baclofen, ceftibuten
Intestinal metabolism	Salicylamide, propranolol
Drugs with low solubility in GI but relatively high dose	Chorothiazide, griseofulvin, danazol
Saturable gastric or GI decomposition	Penicillin G, omeprazole, saquinavir
Distribution	
Saturable plasma protein binding	Phenylbutazone, lidocaine, salicylic acid, ceftriaxone, diazoxide, phenytoin, warfarin, disopyramide
Cellular uptake	Methicillin (rabbit)
Tissue binding	Imiprimine (rat)
CSF transport	Benzylpenicillins
Saturable transport into or out of tissues	Methotrexate
Renal Elimination	
Active secretion	Mezlocillin, para-aminohippuric acid
Tubular reabsorption	Riboflavin, ascorbic acid, cephapirin
Change in urine pH	Salicylic acid, dextroamphetamine
Metabolism	
Saturable metabolism	Phenytoin, salicyclic acid, theophylline, valproic acid[b]
Cofactor or enzyme limitation	Acetaminophen, alcohol
Enzyme induction	Carbamazepine
Altered hepatic blood flow	Propranolol, verapamil
Metabolite inhibition	Diazepam
Biliary Excretion	
Biliary secretion	Iodipamide, sulfobromophthalein sodium
Enterohepatic recycling	Cimetidine, isotretinoin

[a]Hypothermia, metabolic acidosis, altered cardiovascular function, and coma are additional causes of dose and time dependencies in drug overdose.
[b]In guinea pig and probably in some younger subjects.

Compiled by author and from Evans et al (1992), with permission

5. The composition of the metabolites of a drug may be affected by a change in the dose.

Because these drugs have a changing apparent elimination constant with larger doses, prediction of drug concentration in the blood based on a small dose is difficult. Drug concentration in the blood can increase rapidly once an elimination process is saturated. In general, metabolism (biotransformation) and active tubular secretion of drugs by the kidney are the processes most usually saturated. Figure 16-1 shows plasma level–time curves for a drug that exhibits saturable kinetics. When a large dose is given, a curve is obtained with an initial slow elimination phase followed by a much more rapid elimination at lower blood concentrations

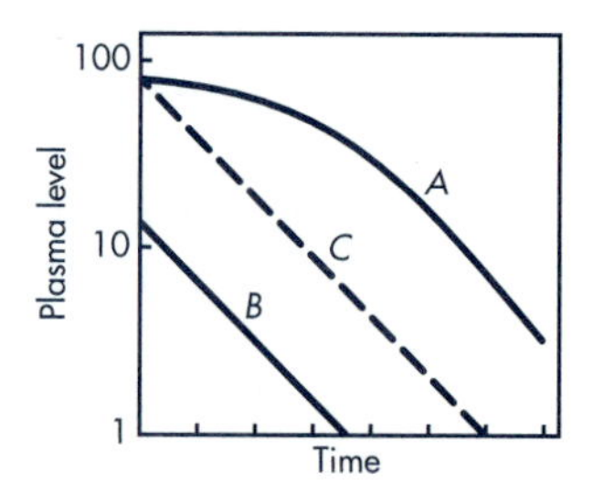

Figure 16-1. Plasma level–time curves for a drug that exhibits a saturable elimination process. Curves *A* and *B* represent high and low doses of drug, respectively, given in a single IV bolus. Curve *C* represents the normal first-order elimination of a different drug.

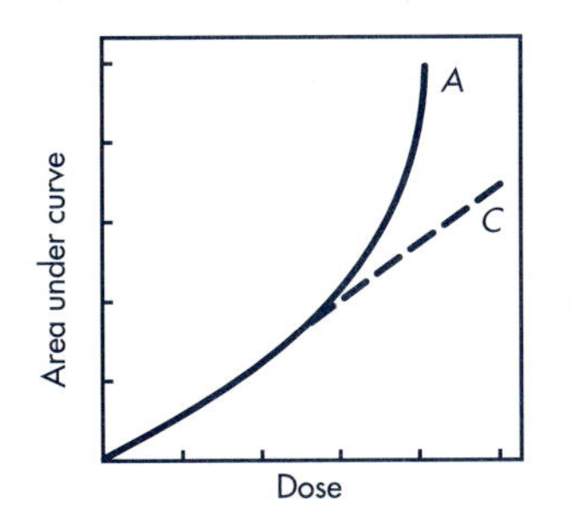

Figure 16-2. Area under the plasma level–time curve versus dose for a drug that exhibits a saturable elimination process. Curve *A* represents dose-dependent or saturable elimination kinetics. Curve *C* represents dose-independent kinetics.

(curve *A*). With a small dose of the drug, apparent first-order kinetics are observed, because no saturation kinetics occur (curve *B*). If the pharmacokinetic data were estimated only from the blood levels described by curve *B*, then a twofold increase in the dose would give the blood profile presented in curve *C*, which considerably underestimates the drug concentration as well as the duration of action. In order to determine whether a drug is following dose-dependent kinetics, the drug is given at various dosage levels and a plasma level–time curve is obtained for each dose. The curves should exhibit parallel slopes if the drug follows dose-independent kinetics. Alternatively, a plot of the areas under the plasma level–time curves at various doses should be linear (Fig. 16-2).

SATURABLE ENZYMATIC ELIMINATION PROCESSES

The elimination of drug by a saturable enzymatic process is described by *Michaelis–Menten* kinetics. If C_p is the concentration of drug in the plasma, then

$$\text{Elimination rate} = \frac{dC_p}{dt} = \frac{V_{max} C_p}{K_M + C_p} \tag{16.1}$$

where V_{max} is the maximum elimination rate and K_M is the Michaelis constant. The values for K_M and V_{max} are dependent on the nature of the drug and the enzymatic process involved.

The elimination rate of a hypothetical drug with a K_M of 0.1 μg/mL and a V_{max} of 0.5 μg/mL per hour is calculated in Table 16.2 by means of Equation 16.1. Because the ratio of elimination rate to drug concentration changes as the drug concentration changes, the rate of drug elimination is not a first-order or linear process. A first-order elimination process would yield a constant elimination rate: drug concentration value known as the rate constant. At drug concentrations of 0.4 to 10 μg/mL, the enzyme system is not saturated and the rate of elimination is a *mixed* or *nonlinear* process. At higher drug concentrations, 11.2 μg/mL and above, the elimination rate approaches the maximum velocity (V_{max}) of approximately 0.5 μg/mL per hour.

Equation 16.1 describes a nonlinear enzyme process that encompasses a broad range of drug concentrations. When the drug concentration C_p is large in relation to K_M, saturation of the enzymes occurs and the rate of elimination proceeds at a fixed or constant rate equal to V_{max}. Thus, elimination of drug becomes a zero-order process.

$$-\frac{dC_p}{dt} = \frac{V_{max}\ C_p}{C_p} = V_{max} \tag{16.2}$$

TABLE 16.2 Effect of Drug Concentration on the Elimination Rate and Rate Constant[a]

DRUG CONCENTRATION (μg/mL)	ELIMINATION RATE (μg/mL per hr)	ELIMINATION RATE/ CONCENTRATION[b] (hr^{-1})
0.4	0.400	1.000
0.8	0.444	0.556
1.2	0.462	0.385
1.6	0.472	0.294
2.0	0.476	0.238
2.4	0.480	0.200
2.8	0.483	0.172
3.2	0.485	0.152
10.0	0.495	0.0495
10.4	0.495	0.0476
10.8	0.495	0.0459
11.2	0.496	0.0442
11.6	0.496	0.0427

[a]K_M = 0.1 μg/mL, V_{max} = 0.5 μg/mL per hr.
[b]The ratio of the elimination rate to the concentration is equal to the rate constant.

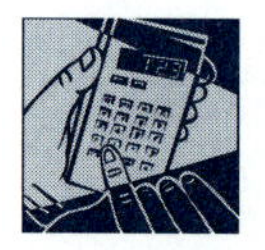

PRACTICE PROBLEM

Using the hypothetical drug considered in Table 16.2 (V_{max} = 0.5 μg/mL per hour, K_M = 0.1 μg/mL), how long would it take for the plasma drug concentration to decrease from 20 to 12 μg/mL?

Solution

Because 20 μg/mL is above the saturable level, as indicated in the table, elimination occurs at a zero-order rate of 0.5 μg/hr.

$$\text{Time needed for the drug to decrease to 12 } \mu\text{g/mL} = \frac{20 - 12\ \mu\text{g}}{0.5\ \mu\text{g/hr}} = 16\ \text{hr}$$

Based on data generated from Equation 16.2, Table 16.3 shows how enzymatic drug elimination can change from a nonlinear to a linear process over a restricted concentration range.

When the drug concentration C_p is small in relation to the K_M ($C_p \leq 0.05$ μg/mL, Table 16.3), the rate of drug elimination becomes a first-order process. This is evident since the rate constant (or elimination rate–drug concentration) values are constant. At drug concentrations below 0.05 μg/mL, the ratio of elimination rate to drug concentration has a constant value of 1.1 hr^{-1}. Mathematically, when C_p is much smaller than K_M, C_p in the denominator is negligible.

$$-\frac{dC_p}{dt} = \frac{V_{max}C_p}{C_p + K_M} = \frac{V_{max}}{K_M}C_p \qquad \textbf{(16.3)}$$

$$-\frac{dC_p}{dt} = k'C_p$$

TABLE 16.3 Effect of Drug Concentration on the Elimination Rate and Rate Constant[a]

DRUG CONCENTRATION (C_P) (μg/mL)	ELIMINATION RATE (μg/mL per hr)	ELIMINATION RATE CONCENTRATION[b] (hr^{-1})
0.01	0.011	1.1
0.02	0.022	1.1
0.03	0.033	1.1
0.04	0.043	1.1
0.05	0.053	1.1
0.06	0.063	1.0
0.07	0.072	1.0
0.08	0.082	1.0
0.09	0.091	1.0

[a] $K_M = 0.8\ \mu g/mL$, $V_{max} = 0.9\ \mu g/mL$ per hr.
[b] The ratio of the elimination rate to the concentration is equal to the rate constant.

The first-order rate constant, k' can be calculated from Equation 16.3:

$$k' = \frac{V_{max}}{K_M} = \frac{0.9}{0.8} = \sim 1.1\ hr^{-1}$$

This calculation confirms the data in Table 16.3, because enzymatic drug elimination at drug concentrations below 0.05 μg/mL is a first-order rate process with a rate constant of 1.1 hr^{-1}. Therefore, the $t_{1/2}$ due to enzymatic elimination can be calculated:

$$t_{1/2} = \frac{0.693}{1.1} = 0.63\ hr$$

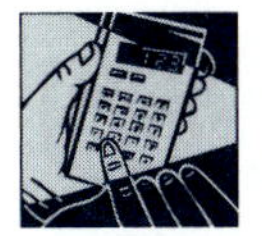

PRACTICE PROBLEM

How long would it take for the plasma concentration of the drug in Table 16.3 to decline from 0.05 to 0.005 μg/mL?

Solution

Because drug elimination is a first-order process for the specified concentrations,

$$C_p = C_p^0 e^{-kt}$$

$$\log C_p = \log C_p^0 - \frac{kt}{2.3}$$

$$t = 2.3\,\frac{\log C_p - \log C_p^0}{k}$$

Because $C_p^0 = 0.05\ \mu g/mL$, $k = 1.1\ hr^{-1}$, and $C_p = 0.005\ \mu g/mL$,

$$t = \frac{2.3(\log 0.05 - \log 0.005)}{1.1} = \frac{2.3(-1.30 + 2.3)}{1.1} = \frac{2.3}{1.1} = 2.09\ hr$$

When given in therapeutic doses, most drugs produce plasma drug concentrations well below K_M for all carrier-mediated enzyme systems affecting the pharmacokinetics of the drug. Therefore, most drugs at normal therapeutic concentrations follow first-order rate processes. Only a few drugs, such as salicylate and phenytoin, tend to saturate the hepatic mixed-function oxidases at higher therapeutic doses. With these drugs, elimination kinetics are first-order with very small doses, *mixed* at higher doses, and may approach zero-order with very high therapeutic doses.

DRUG ELIMINATION BY CAPACITY-LIMITED PHARMACOKINETICS: ONE-COMPARTMENT MODEL, IV BOLUS INJECTION

The rate of elimination of a drug that follows capacity-limited pharmacokinetics is governed by the V_{max} and K_M of the drug. Equation 16.1 describes the elimination of a drug that distributes in the body as a single compartment and is eliminated by Michaelis–Menten or capacity-limited pharmacokinetics. If a single IV bolus injection of drug (D_0) is given at $t = 0$, the drug concentration (C) in the plasma at any time t may be calculated by an integrated form of Equation 16.1 described by

$$\frac{C_0 - C}{t} = V_{max} - \frac{K_M}{t} \ln \frac{C_0}{C} \tag{16.4}$$

Alternatively, the amount of drug in the body after an IV bolus injection may be calculated by the following relationship. Equation 16.5 may be used to simulate the decline of drug in the body after various size doses are given provided the K_M and V_{max} of drug are known.

$$\frac{D_0 - D_t}{t} = V_{max} - \frac{K_M}{t} \ln \frac{D_0}{D_t} \tag{16.5}$$

where D_0 is the amount of drug in the body at $t = 0$. In order to calculate the time for the dose of the drug to decline to a certain amount of drug in the body, Equation 16.5 must be rearranged and solved for time t.

$$t = \frac{1}{V_{max}} \left(D_0 - D_t + K_M \ln \frac{D_0}{D_t} \right) \tag{16.6}$$

The relationship of K_M and V_{max} to the time for an IV bolus injection of drug to decline to a given amount of drug in the body is illustrated in Figures 16-3 and 16-4. Using Equation 16.6, the time for a single 400-mg dose given by IV bolus injection to decline to 20 mg was calculated for a drug with a K_M of 38 mg/L and a V_{max} that is varied from 200 to 100 mg/hr (Table 16.4). With a V_{max} of 200 mg/hr, the time for the 400-mg dose to decline to 20 mg in the body is 2.46 hours, whereas, when the V_{max} is decreased to 100 mg/hr, the time for the 400-mg dose to decrease to 20 mg is increased to 4.93 hours. Thus, there is an inverse relationship between the time for the dose to decline to a certain amount of drug in the body and the V_{max} as shown in Equation 16.6.

Using a similar example, the effect of K_M on the time for a single 400-mg dose given by IV bolus injection to decline to 20-mg in the body is described in Table

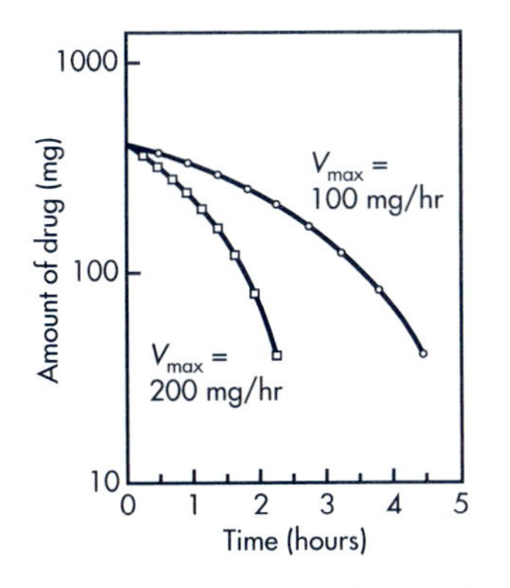

Figure 16-3. Amount of drug in the body versus time for a capacity-limited drug following an IV dose. Data generated using V_{max} of 100 (○) and 200 mg/hr (□). K_M is kept constant.

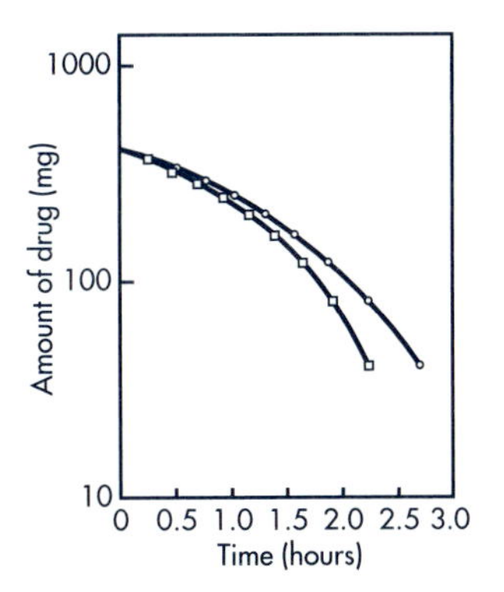

Figure 16-4. Amount of drug in the body versus time for a capacity-limited drug following an IV dose. Data generated using K_M of 38 mg/L (□) and 76 mg/L (○). V_{max} is kept constant.

16.5 and Fig. 16-4. Assuming V_{max} is 200 mg/hr, the time for the drug to decline from 400 to 20 mg is 2.46 hours when K_M is 38 mg/L; whereas, when K_M is 76 mg/L, the time for the drug dose to decline to 20 mg is 3.03 hours. Thus, an increase in K_M (with no change in V_{max}) will increase the time for the drug to be eliminated from the body. It is important to note that K_M is not an elimination

TABLE 16.4 Capacity-Limited Pharmacokinetics: Effect of V_{max} on the Elimination of Drug[a]

AMOUNT OF DRUG IN BODY (mg)	TIME FOR DRUG ELIMINATION (hr)	
	V_{MAX} = 200 mg/hr	V_{MAX} = 100 mg/hr
400	0	0
380	0.109	0.219
360	0.220	0.440
340	0.330	0.661
320	0.442	0.884
300	0.554	1.10
280	0.667	1.33
260	0.781	1.56
240	0.897	1.79
220	1.01	2.02
200	1.13	2.26
180	1.25	2.50
160	1.37	2.74
140	1.49	2.99
120	1.62	3.25
100	1.76	3.52
80	1.90	3.81
60	2.06	4.12
40	2.23	4.47
20	2.46	4.93

[a]A single 400-mg dose is given by IV bolus injection. The drug is distributed into a single compartment and is eliminated by capacity-limited pharmacokinetics. K_M is 38 mg/L. The time for drug to decline from 400 to 20 mg is calculated from Equation 16.6 assuming the drug has V_{max} = 200 mg/hr or V_{max} = 100 mg/hr.

TABLE 16.5 Capacity-Limited Pharmacokinetics: Effects of K_m on the Elimination of Drug[a]

AMOUNT OF DRUG IN BODY (mg)	TIME FOR DRUG ELIMINATION (hr)	
	K_M = 38 mg/L	K_M = 76 mg/L
400	0	0
380	0.109	0.119
360	0.220	0.240
340	0.330	0.361
320	0.442	0.484
300	0.554	0.609
280	0.667	0.735
260	0.781	0.863
240	0.897	0.994
220	1.01	1.12
200	1.13	1.26
180	1.25	1.40
160	1.37	1.54
140	1.49	1.69
120	1.62	1.85
100	1.76	2.02
80	1.90	2.21
60	2.06	2.42
40	2.23	2.67
20	2.46	3.03

[a]A single 400-mg dose is given by IV bolus injection. The drug is distributed into a single compartment and is eliminated by capacity-limited pharmacokinetics. V_{max} is 200 mg/hr. The time for drug to decline from 400 to 20 mg is calculated from Equation 16.6 assuming the drug has K_M = 38 mg/L or K_M = 76 mg/L.

constant, but is actually a hybrid rate constant in enzyme kinetics, representing both the forward and backward reaction rates and equal to the drug concentration or amount of drug in the body at $1/2V_{max}$.

The one-compartment open model with capacity-limited elimination pharmacokinetics adequately describes the plasma drug concentration–time profiles for some drugs. The mathematics needed to describe nonlinear pharmacokinetic behavior of drugs that follow two-compartment models and/or have both combined capacity-limited and first-order kinetic profiles are very complex and have little practical application for dosage calculations and therapeutic drug monitoring.

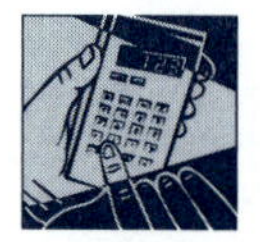

PRACTICE PROBLEMS

1. A drug eliminated from the body by capacity-limited pharmacokinetics has a K_M of 100 mg/L and a V_{max} of 50 mg/hr. If 400 mg of the drug is given to a patient by IV bolus injection, calculate the time for the drug to be 50% eliminated. If 320 mg of the drug is to be given by IV bolus injection, calculate the time for 50% of the dose to be eliminated. Explain why there is a difference in the time for 50% elimination of a 400-mg dose compared to a 320-mg dose.

Solution

Use Equation 16.6 to calculate the time for the dose to decline to a given amount of drug in the body. For this problem, D_t, is equal to 50% of the dose D_0.

If the dose is 400 mg,

$$t = \frac{1}{50}\left(400 - 200 + 100 \ln \frac{400}{200}\right) = 5.39 \text{ hr}$$

If the dose is 320 mg,

$$t = \frac{1}{50}\left(320 - 160 + 100 \ln \frac{320}{160}\right) = 4.59 \text{ hr}$$

For capacity-limited elimination, the elimination half-life is dose dependent, because the drug elimination process is partially saturated. Therefore, small changes in the dose will produce large differences in the time for 50% drug elimination. The parameters K_M and V_{max} determine when the dose is saturated.

2. Using the same drug as in Problem 1, calculate the time for 50% elimination of the dose when the dose is 10 and 5 mg, respectively. Explain why the times for 50% drug elimination are similar even though the dose is reduced by one-half.

Solution

As in Practice Problem 1, use Equation 16.6 to calculate the time for the amount of drug in the body at zero time (D_0) to decline 50%.

If the dose is 10 mg,

$$t = \frac{1}{50}\left(10 - 5 + 100 \ln \frac{10}{5}\right) = 1.49 \text{ hr}$$

If the dose is 5 mg,

$$t = \frac{1}{50}\left(5 - 2.5 + 100 \ln \frac{5}{2.5}\right) = 1.44 \text{ hr}$$

Whether the patient is given a 10- or 5-mg dose by IV bolus injection, the times for the amount of drug to decline 50% are approximately the same. At 10- and 5-mg doses the amount of drug in the body is much less than the K_M of 100 mg. Therefore, the amount of drug in the body is well below saturation of the elimination process and the drug declines at a first-order rate.

Determination of K_M and V_{max}

Equation 16.1 relates the rate of drug biotransformation to the concentration of the drug in the body. The same equation may be applied to determine the rate of enzymatic reaction of a drug in vitro (Eq. 16.7). When an experiment is performed with solutions of various concentration of the drug C, a series of reaction rates (v) may be measured for each concentration. Special plots may then be used to determine K_M and V_{max} (see also Chapter 13).

Equation 16.7 may be rearranged into Equation 16.8.

$$v = \frac{V_{max} C}{K_M + C} \quad \textbf{(16.7)}$$

$$\frac{1}{v} = \frac{K_M}{V_{max}} \frac{1}{C} + \frac{1}{V_{max}} \quad \textbf{(16.8)}$$

TABLE 16.6 Information Necessary for Graphic Determination of V_{max} and K_M

OBSERVATION NUMBER	C (μM/mL)	v (μM/mL per min)	$1/v$ (mL per min/μM)	$1/C$ (mL/μM)
1	1	0.500	2.000	1.000
2	6	1.636	0.611	0.166
3	11	2.062	0.484	0.090
4	16	2.285	0.437	0.062
5	21	2.423	0.412	0.047
6	26	2.516	0.397	0.038
7	31	2.583	0.337	0.032
8	36	2.504	0.379	0.027
9	41	2.673	0.373	0.024
10	46	2.705	0.369	0.021

Equation 16.8 is a linear equation when $1/v$ is plotted against $1/C$. The intercept for the line is $-1/K_M$ and the slope is K_M/V_{max}. An example of a drug reacting enzymatically with rate (v) at various concentrations C is shown in Table 16.6 and Figure 16-5. A plot of $1/v$ versus $1/C$ is shown in Figure 16-6. A plot of $1/v$ versus $1/C$ is linear with an intercept of 0.33 μmol. Therefore,

$$\frac{1}{V_{max}} = 0.33 \text{ min mL}/\mu\text{mol}$$

$$V_{max} = 3\ \mu\text{mol/mL min}$$

because slope = 1.65 = $K_M/V_{max} = K_M/3$ or $K_M = 3 \times 1.65\ \mu$mol/mL = 5 μmol/mL. Alternatively, K_M may be found from the x intercept where $-1/K_M$ is equal to the x intercept. (This may be seen by extending the graph to intercept the x axis at the negative region.)

With this plot (Fig. 16-6) the points are clustered. Other methods are available that may spread the points more evenly. These methods are derived from rearranging Equation 16.8 into Equations 16.9 and 16.10:

$$\frac{C}{v} = \frac{1}{V_{max}}C + \frac{K_M}{V_{max}} \tag{16.9}$$

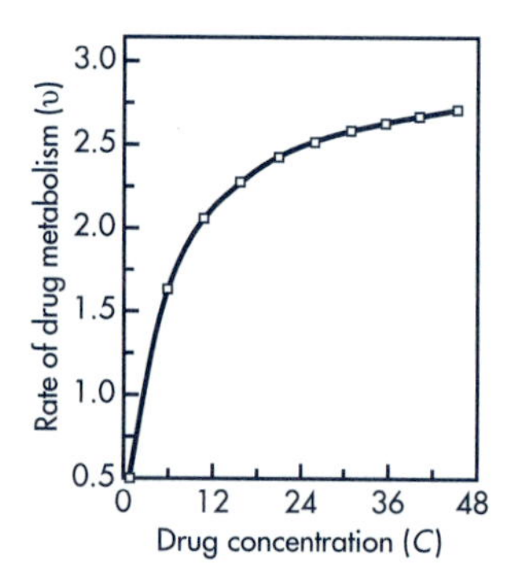

Figure 16-5. Plot of rate of drug metabolism at various drug concentrations. (K_M = 5.0 μmol/mL, V_{max} = 3 μmol/mL per min.)

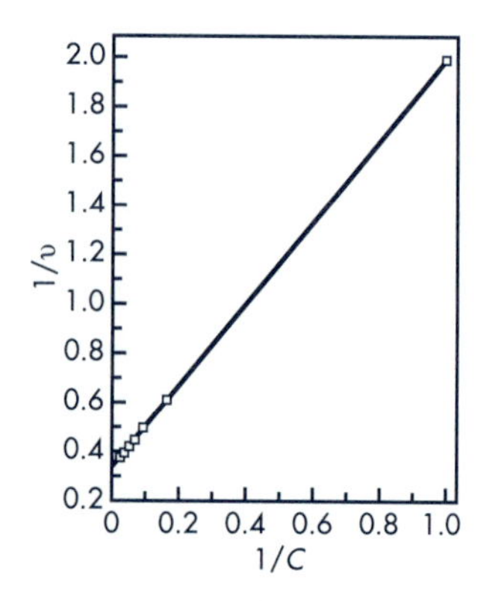

Figure 16-6. Plot of $1/v$ versus $1/C$ for determining K_M and V_{max}.

TABLE 16.7 Calculations Necessary for Graphic Determination of K_M and V_{max}

C (μM/mL)	v (μM/mL per min)	C/v (min)	v/C (1/min)
1	0.500	2.000	0.500
6	1.636	3.666	0.272
11	2.062	5.333	0.187
16	2.285	7.000	0.142
21	2.423	8.666	0.115
26	2.516	10.333	0.096
31	2.583	12.000	0.083
36	2.634	13.666	0.073
41	2.673	15.333	0.065
46	2.705	17.000	0.058

$$v = -K_M \frac{v}{C} + V_{max} \tag{16.10}$$

A plot of C/v versus C would yield a straight line with $1/V_{max}$ as slope and K_M/V_{max} as intercept (Eq. 16.9). A plot of v versus v/C would yield a slope of $-K_M$ and an intercept of V_{max} (Eq. 16.10).

The necessary calculations for making the above plots are shown in Table 16.7. The plots themselves are shown in Figures 16-7 and 16-8. It should be noted that the data are spread out better by the two latter plots. Calculations from the slope show that the same K_M and V_{max} are obtained as in Figure 16-6. When the data are more scattered, one method may be more accurate than the other; a simple approach is to graph the data and examine the linearity of the graphs. The same basic type of plot is used in the clinical literature to determine K_M and V_{max} for individual patients for drugs that undergo capacity-limited kinetics.

Determination of K_M and V_{max} in Patients

Equation 16.7 shows that the rate of drug metabolism (v) is dependent on the concentration of the drug (C). This same basic concept may be applied to the rate of drug metabolism of a capacity-limited drug in the body (Chapter 13). The body may be regarded as a single compartment in which the drug is dissolved. The rate of drug metabolism will vary depending on the concentration of drug C_p as well as on the metabolic rate constants K_M and V_{max} of the drug in each individual.

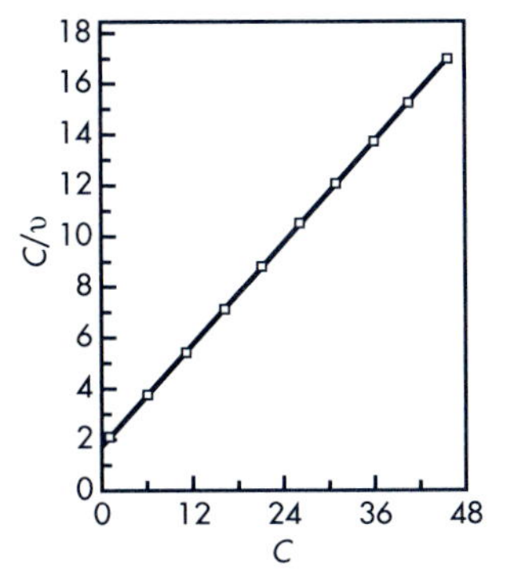

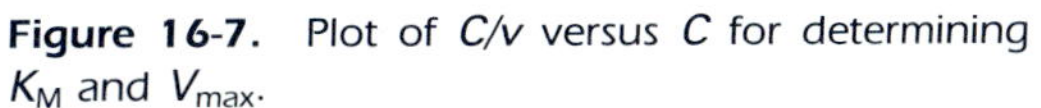
Figure 16-7. Plot of C/v versus C for determining K_M and V_{max}.

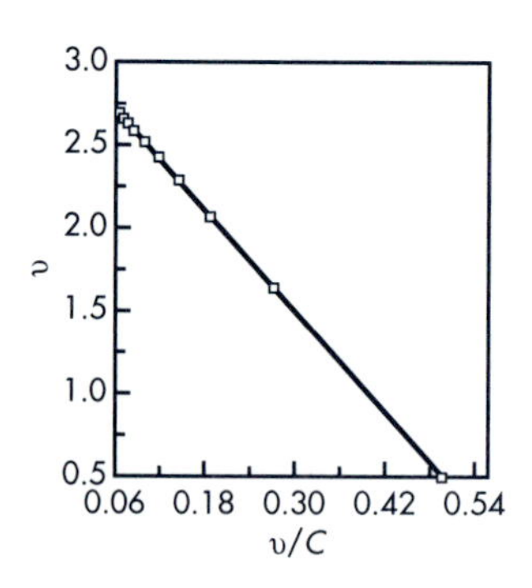

Figure 16-8. Plot of v versus v/C for determining K_M and V_{max}.

An example for the determination of K_M and V_{max} is given for the drug phenytoin. Phenytoin undergoes capacity-limited kinetics at therapeutic drug concentrations in the body. To determine K_M and V_{max}, two different dose regimens are given at different times, until steady state is reached. The steady state drug concentrations are then measured by assay. At steady state, the rate of drug metabolism (v) is assumed to be the same as the rate of drug input R (dose/day). Therefore Equation 16.11 may be written for drug metabolism in the body similar to the way drugs are metabolized *in vitro* (Eq. 16.7).

$$R = \frac{V_{max} C_{ss}}{K_M + C_{ss}} \tag{16.11}$$

where R = dose/day or dosing rate; C_{ss} = steady-state plasma drug concentration, V_{max} = maximum metabolic rate constant in the body, and K_M = Michaelis–Menten constant of the drug in the body.

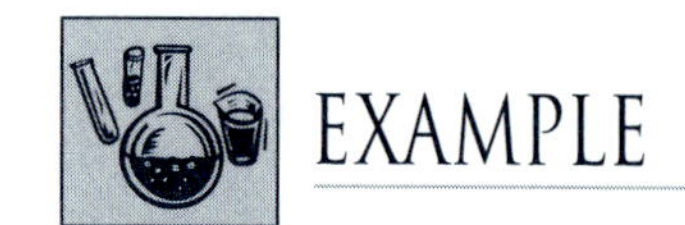

EXAMPLE

Phenytoin was administered to a patient at dosing rates of 150 and 300 mg/day, respectively. The steady-state plasma drug concentrations were 8.6 mg/L and 25.1 mg/L, respectively. Find the K_M and V_{max} of this patient. What dose is needed to achieve a steady-state concentration of 11.3 mg/L?

Solution

There are three methods for solving this problem, all based on the same basic equation (Eq. 16.11).

Method A

Inverting Equation 16.11 on both sides yields:

$$\frac{1}{R} = \frac{K_M}{V_{max}} \frac{1}{C_{ss}} + \frac{1}{V_{max}} \tag{16.12}$$

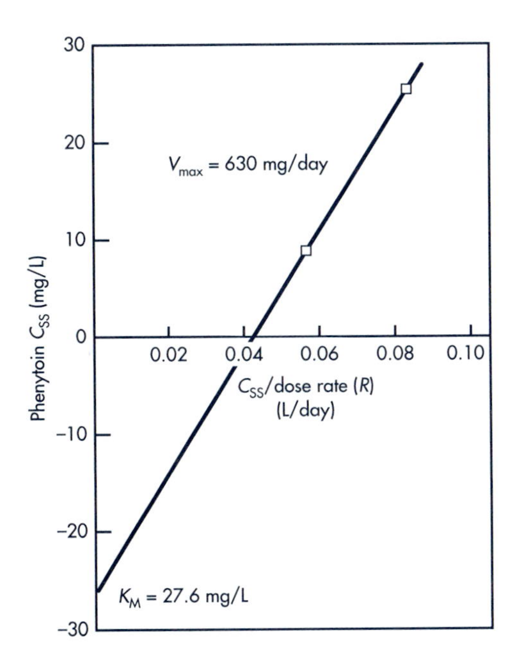

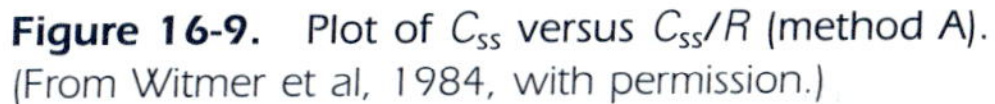
Figure 16-9. Plot of C_{ss} versus C_{ss}/R (method A). (From Witmer et al, 1984, with permission.)

Multiply both sides by $C_{ss}V_{max}$.

$$\frac{V_{max}C_{ss}}{R} = K_M + C_{ss}$$

Rearrange.

$$C_{ss} = \frac{V_{max}C_{ss}}{R} - K_M \tag{16.13}$$

A plot of C_{ss} versus C_{ss}/R is shown in Figure 16-9. V_{max} is equal to the slope, 630 mg/day, and K_M is found from the y-intercept, 27.6 mg/L (note negative intercept).

Method B

From Equation 16.11,

$$RK_M + RC_{ss} = V_{max}C_{ss}$$

Dividing both sides by C_{ss} yields

$$R = V_{max} - \frac{K_M R}{C_{ss}} \tag{16.14}$$

A plot of R versus R/C_{ss} is shown in Figure 16-10. The K_M and V_{max} found are similar to those by the previous method (Fig. 16-9).

Method C

A plot of R versus C_{ss} is shown in Figure 16-11. To determine K_M and V_{max}:

1. Mark points for R of 300 mg/day and C_{ss} of 25.1 mg/L as shown. Connect with a straight line.
2. Mark points for R of 150 mg/day and C_{ss} of 8.6 mg/L as shown. Connect with a straight line.

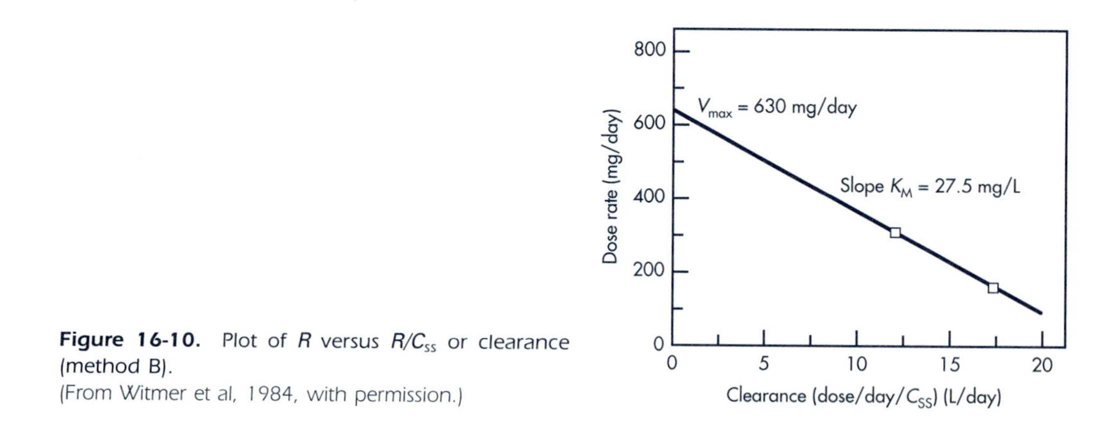

Figure 16-10. Plot of R versus R/C_{ss} or clearance (method B).
(From Witmer et al, 1984, with permission.)

3. Where lines from the first two steps cross is called point A.

4. From point A, read V_{max} on the y axis, and K_M on the x axis. (Again, V_{max} of 630 mg/day and K_M of 27 mg/L are found.)

This V_{max} and K_M can be used in Equation 16.11 to find R. Alternatively, join point A on the graph to meet 11.3 mg/L on the x axis; R can be read where this line meets the y axis (190 mg/day).

To calculate the dose needed to keep steady state phenytoin concentration of 11.3 mg/L in this patient, use Equation 16.7.

$$R = \frac{(630 \text{ mg/day})(11.3 \text{ mg/L})}{27 \text{ mg/L} + 11.3 \text{ mg/L}} = \frac{7119 \text{ mg/day}}{38.3} = 186 \text{ mg/day}$$

This answer compares very closely with the value obtained by the graphic method. All three methods have been used clinically. Vozeh and associates (1981) introduced a method that allows for an estimation of phenytoin dose based on steady-

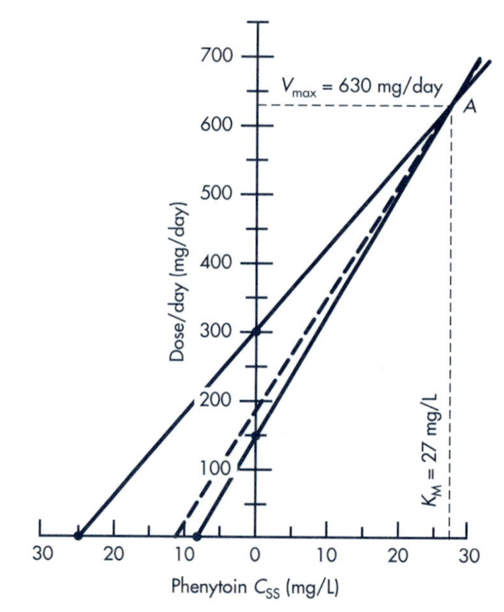

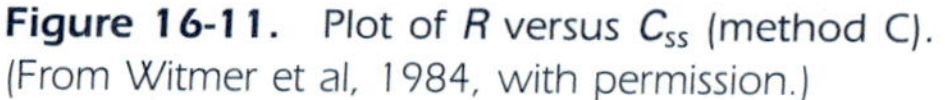

Figure 16-11. Plot of R versus C_{ss} (method C).
(From Witmer et al, 1984, with permission.)

state concentration resulting from one dose. This method is based on a statistically compiled nomogram that makes it possible to project a most likely dose for the patient.

Determination of K_M and V_{max} by Direct Method

When steady-state concentrations of phenytoin are known only at two dose levels, there is no advantage in using the graphic method. K_M and V_{max} may be calculated by solving two simultaneous equations formed by substituting C_{ss} and R (Eq. 16.11) with C_1, R_1, C_2, and R_2. The equations contain two unknowns, K_M and V_{max}, and may be solved easily.

$$R_1 = \frac{V_{max} C_1}{K_M + C_1}$$

$$R_2 = \frac{V_{max} C_2}{K_M + C_2}$$

Combining the two equations yields Equation 16.15.

$$K_M = \frac{R_2 - R_1}{\frac{R_1}{C_1} - \frac{R_2}{C_2}} \tag{16.15}$$

where C_1 is steady-state plasma drug concentration after dose 1, C_2 is steady-state plasma drug concentration after dose 2, R_1 is the first dosing rate, and R_2 is the second dosing rate. To calculate K_M and V_{max}, use Equation 16.15 with the values $C_1 = 8.6$ mg/L, $C_2 = 25.1$ mg/L, $R_1 = 150$ mg/day, and $R_2 = 300$ mg/day. The results are

$$K_M = \frac{300 - 150}{\frac{150}{8.6} - \frac{300}{25.1}} = 27.3 \text{ mg/L}$$

Substitute K_M into either of the two simultaneous equations to solve for V_{max}:

$$150 = \frac{V_{max}(8.6)}{27.3 + 8.6}$$

$$V_{max} = 626 \text{ mg/day}$$

Interpretation of K_M and V_{max}

An understanding of Michaelis–Menten kinetics provides insight into the nonlinear kinetics and helps to avoid dosing a drug at concentration near enzyme saturation. For example, in the above phenytoin dosing example, since K_M occurs at half V_{max}, $K_M = 27.3$ mg/L, the implication is that, at an average plasma concentration of 27.3 mg/L, enzymes responsible for phenytoin metabolism are eliminating the drug at 50% V_{max}, ie, 0.5×626 mg/day or 313 mg/day at steady state. When the subject is receiving 300 mg of phenytoin per day, the plasma drug concentration of phenytoin is 8.6 mg/L, which is considerably below the K_M of 27.3 mg/L. In practice, the K_M in patients can range from 1 to 15 mg/L, V_{max} can range from 100 to 1000 mg/day. Patients with low K_M tend to have problems in adjust-

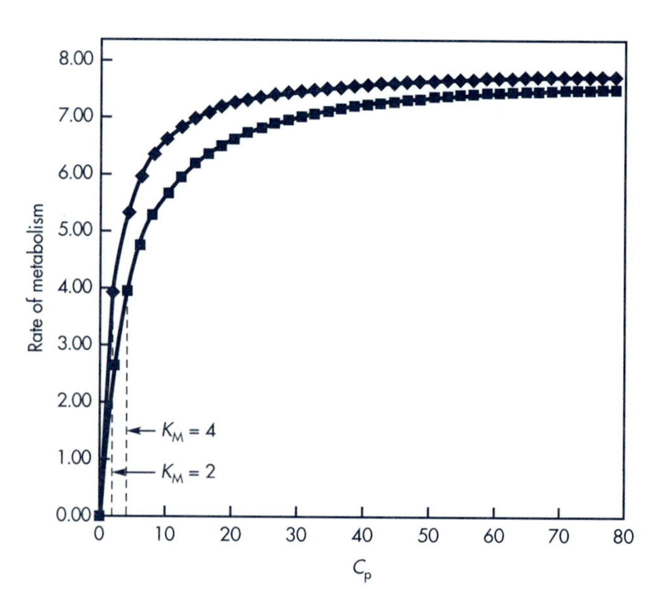

Figure 16-12. Diagram showing the rate of metabolism when V_{max} is constant (8 mcg/mL/hr) and K_M is changed (K_M = 2 mcg/mL for top curve and K_M = 4 mcg/mL for bottom curve). Note the rate of metabolism is faster for the lower K_M, but saturation starts at lower concentration.

ing dosing. Patients with a smaller K_M (same V_{max}) will show a greater change in the rate of elimination when plasma drug concentration changes. A subject with the same V_{max}, but different K_M, is shown in Figure 16-12. (For another example, see the slopes of the two curves generated in Figure 16-4 also.)

Dependence of Elimination Half-Life on Dose

For drugs that follow linear kinetics, the elimination half-life is constant and does not change with dose or drug concentration. For a drug that follows nonlinear kinetics, the elimination half-life and drug clearance both change with dose or drug concentration. Generally, the elimination half-life becomes longer, clearance becomes smaller, and the area under the curve becomes disproportionately larger with increasing dose. The relationship between elimination half-life and drug concentration is shown in Equation 16.16. The elimination half-life is dependent on the Michaelis–Menten parameters and concentration.

$$t_{1/2} = \frac{0.693}{V_{max}}(K_M + C_p) \quad \textbf{(16.16)}$$

Some pharmacokineticists prefer not to calculate the elimination half-life of a nonlinear drug because the elimination half-life is not constant. Clinically, if the half-life is increasing as plasma concentration increases, and there is no apparent change in metabolic or renal function, then there is a good possibility that the drug may be metabolized by nonlinear kinetics.

Dependence of Clearance on Dose

The total body clearance of a drug given by IV bolus injection that follows a one-compartment model with Michaelis–Menten elimination kinetics changes with respect to time and plasma drug concentration. Within a certain drug concentration range, an average or *mean clearance* (Cl_{av}) may be determined for the time of the dose. Because the drug follows Michaelis–Menten kinetics, Cl_{av} is dose dependent.

Cl_{av} may be estimated from the area under the curve and the dose given (Wagner et al, 1985).

According to the Michaelis–Menten equation,

$$\frac{dC_p}{dt} = \frac{V_{max} C_p}{K_M + C_p} \quad (16.17)$$

Inverting Equation 16.17 and rearranging yields:

$$C_p dt = \frac{K_M}{V'_{max}} dC_p - \frac{C_p}{V'_{max}} dC_p \quad (16.18)$$

The area under the curve $[AUC]_0^\infty$ is obtained by integration of Equation 16.18 (ie, $[AUC]_0^\infty = \int_0^\infty C_p dt$).

$$\int_0^\infty C_p dt = \int_{C_p^0}^\infty \frac{K_M}{V'_{max}} dC_p + \int_{C_p^0}^\infty \frac{C_p}{V'_{max}} dC_p \quad (16.19)$$

where V'_{max} is the maximum velocity for metabolism. Units for V'_{max} are mass/compartment volume per unit time. $V'_{max} = \frac{V_{max}}{V_D}$; Wagner and coworkers (1985) used V_{max} in Equation 16.20 as mass/time to be consistent with biochemistry literature, which considers the initial mass of the substrate reacting with the enzyme.

Integration of Equation 16.18 from time 0 to infinity gives Equation 16.20.

$$[AUC]_0^\infty = \frac{C_p^0}{V_{max}/V_D}\left(\frac{C_p^0}{2} + K_M\right) \quad (16.20)$$

where V_D is the apparent volume of distribution.

Because the dose $D_0 = C_p^0 V_D$, Equation 16.20 may be expressed as

$$[AUC]_0^\infty = \frac{D_0}{V_{max}}\left(\frac{C_p^0}{2} + K_M\right) \quad (16.21)$$

To obtain mean body clearance, Cl_{av} is then calculated from the dose and the AUC.

$$Cl_{av} = \frac{D_0}{[AUC]_0^\infty} = \frac{V_{max}}{(C_p^0/2) + K_M} \quad (16.22)$$

$$Cl_{av} = \frac{V_{max}}{\frac{D_0}{2V_D} + K_M} \quad (16.23)$$

Alternatively,

$$Cl = \frac{V_D \frac{dC_p}{dt}}{C_p} = \frac{V_{max}}{K_M + C_p} \quad (16.24)$$

Equation 16.22 or 16.23 calculates the average clearance Cl_{av} for the drug after a single IV bolus dose over the entire time course of the drug in the body. For any time period, clearance may be calculated according to Chapter 12 (Eq. 12.10) as

$$Cl_T = \frac{dD_E/dt}{C_p} \quad (16.25)$$

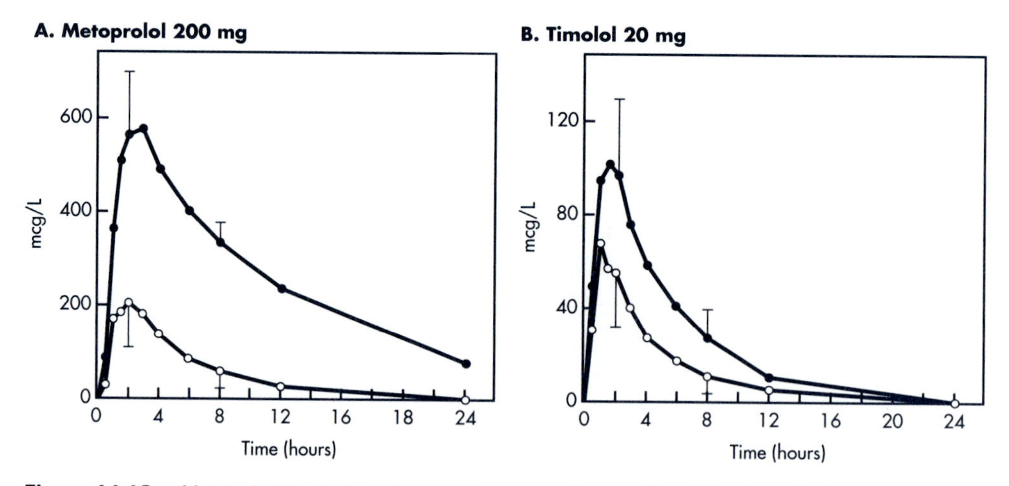

Figure 16-13. Mean plasma drug concentration versus time profiles following administration of single oral doses of (A) metoprolol tartrate 200 mg to 6 extensive metabolizers (EMs) and 6 poor metabolizers (PMs), (B) timolol maleate 20 mg to 6 EMs (○) and 4 PMs (●).
(From Lennard et al, 1986, with permission.)

Dividing Equation 16.17 by C_p gives Equation 16.24, which shows that the clearance of a drug that follows nonlinear pharmacokinetics is dependent upon the plasma drug concentration C_p, K_M, and V_{max}.

In Chapter 13, the physiologic model based on blood flow and intrinsic clearance was used to describe drug metabolism. The extraction ratios of many drugs are listed in the literature. Actually, extraction ratios are dependent on dose, enzymatic system, blood flow, and for practical purposes, they were often assumed to be constant at normal doses.

A paucity of K_M, and V_{max} data is available in the literature defining the nature of nonlinear drug elimination in patients except for phenytoin, however, abundant information is available supporting variable metabolism due to genetic polymorphism. The clearance (apparent) of many of these drugs in slow metabolizers changes with dose, although these drugs may exhibit linear kinetics in normal subjects. Metoprolol and many β-adrenergic antagonists are extensively metabolized. The plasma levels of metoprolol in slow metabolizers (Lennard et al, 1986) were much greater, and the AUC, after equal doses, is several times greater among the slow metabolizers of metoprolol (Fig. 16-13). A similar picture is observed with the other β-adrenergic antagonist, timolol. These drugs will have smaller clearance than normal.

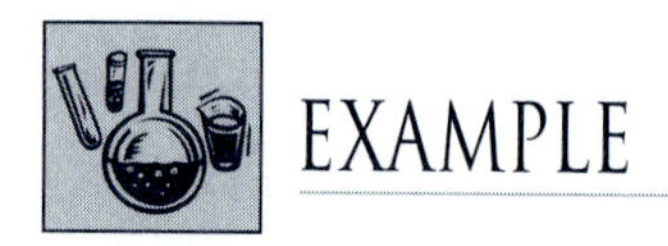

EXAMPLE

The dose-dependent pharmacokinetic of sodium valproate (VPA) was studied in guinea pigs at 20, 200, and 600 mg/kg by rapid intravenous infusion. The area under the plasma concentration-time curve (AUC) increased out of proportion at the 600 mg/kg dose level in all groups (Yu et al, 1987). The total clearance (*Cl*) was significantly decreased and the beta elimination half-life ($t_{1/2}$) was significantly increased at the 600 mg/kg dose level. The dose dependent kinetics of VPA was due to saturation of metabolism. Metabolic capacity was greatly reduced in young guinea pigs and, clinically, it is not uncommon to observe similar enzymatic saturation in infants and in special patient populations, whereas drug metabolism may be linear with dose in normal subjects. These patients have lower V_{max} and longer elimination half-life. Variability in drug metabolism is described in Chapter 13.

EQUATIONS FOR DRUGS DISTRIBUTED AS ONE-COMPARTMENT MODEL AND ELIMINATED BY NONLINEAR PHARMACOKINETICS

The equations presented thus far in this chapter have been for drugs given by IV bolus, distributed as a one-compartment model, and eliminated only by nonlinear pharmacokinetics. The following are useful equations describing other possible routes of drug administration and including mixed drug elimination, by which the drug may be eliminated by both nonlinear (Michaelis–Menten) and linear (first-order) processes.

Mixed Drug Elimination

Drugs may be metabolized by parallel pathways to several different metabolites. At low drug doses corresponding to low drug concentrations at the site of the biotransformation enzymes, the rate of formation of both metabolites is first order. However, with higher doses of drug, or, as more drug is absorbed, higher drug concentrations are presented to the biotransformation enzymes. At the higher drug concentration, the enzyme process for the formation of one of these metabolites may become saturated, and the rate of formation of this metabolite becomes nonlinear and approaches zero order. For example, sodium salicylate is metabolized to both a glucuronide and a glycine conjugate (hippurate). The rate of formation of the glycine conjugate is limited by the amount of glycine available. Thus, the rate of formation of the glucuronide continues as a first-order process; whereas the rate of conjugation with glycine is capacity limited.

The equation that describes a drug that is eliminated by both first-order and Michaelis–Menten kinetics after IV bolus injection is given by

$$-\frac{dC_p}{dt} = kC_p + \frac{V'_{max}C_p}{K_M + C_p} \tag{16.26}$$

where k is the first-order rate constant representing the sum of all first-order elimination processes, while the second term of Equation 16.26, represents the saturable process. V'_{max} is simply V_{max} expressed as concentration by dividing by V_D.

Zero-Order Input and Nonlinear Elimination

The usual example of zero-order input is constant IV infusion. If the drug is given by constant IV infusion and is eliminated only by nonlinear pharmacokinetics, then the following equation describes the rate of change of the plasma drug concentration.

$$\frac{dC_{\mathrm{p}}}{dt} = \frac{k_0}{V_{\mathrm{D}}} - \frac{V'_{\max} C_{\mathrm{p}}}{K_{\mathrm{M}} + C_{\mathrm{p}}} \tag{16.27}$$

where k_0 is the infusion rate and V_{D} is the apparent volume of distribution.

First-Order Absorption and Nonlinear Elimination

The relationship that describes the rate of change in the plasma drug concentration for a drug that is given extravascularly (eg, orally), absorbed by first-order absorption, and eliminated only by nonlinear pharmacokinetics, is given by the following equation. C_{GI} is concentration in the GI tract.

$$\frac{dC_{\mathrm{p}}}{dt} = k_{\mathrm{a}} C_{\mathrm{GI}} e^{-k_{\mathrm{a}} t} - \frac{V'_{\max} C_{\mathrm{p}}}{K_{\mathrm{M}} + C_{\mathrm{p}}} \tag{16.28}$$

where k_{a} is the first-order absorption rate constant.

If the drug is eliminated by parallel pathways consisting of both linear and nonlinear pharmacokinetics, Equation 16.28 may be extended to Equation 16.29.

$$\frac{dC_{\mathrm{p}}}{dt} = k_{\mathrm{a}} C_{\mathrm{GI}} e^{-k_{\mathrm{a}} t} - \frac{V'_{\max} C_{\mathrm{p}}}{K_{\mathrm{M}} + C_{\mathrm{p}}} - kC_{\mathrm{p}} \tag{16.29}$$

where k is the first-order elimination rate constant.

TIME-DEPENDENT PHARMACOKINETICS

Time-dependent pharmacokinetics, unlike dose-dependent pharmacokinetics, involve an alteration in the biochemistry in an organ or physiologic change in the patient (Levy, 1983). One type of time dependency is termed *chronopharmacokinetics,* which describes changes in drug absorption, distribution, and/or elimination due to normal physiologic circadian rhythms. A second type of time dependency leading to nonlinear pharmacokinetics is based on a biochemical change due to *autoinduction* or *autoinhibition* of biotransformation enzymes. For example, Pitlick and Levy (1977) have shown that repeated doses of carbamazepine induce the enzymes responsible for its elimination (ie, autoinduction), thereby increasing the clearance of the drug. Autoinhibition may occur during the course of metabolism of certain drugs (Perrier et al, 1973). In this case, the metabolites formed increase in concentration and further inhibit metabolism of the parent drug. In biochemistry, this phenomenon is known as *product inhibition.* Drugs undergoing time-dependent pharmacokinetic will have variable clearance and elimination half-life. It is important to take that into consideration during drug therapy. The steady-state concentration of a drug that causes autoinduction may be due to in-

TABLE 16.8 Drugs Showing Circadian or Time-Dependent Disposition

Cefodizime	Fluorouracil	Ketoprofen	Theophylline
Cisplatin	Heparin	Mequitazine	

From Reinberg et al, 1991.

creased clearance over time. Some anticancer drugs are better tolerated at certain times of the day; for example, the antimetabolite drug, fluorouracil (FU) was least toxic when given in the morning to rodents (Von Roemeling, 1991). A list is shown in Table 16.8.

BIOAVAILABILITY OF DRUGS THAT FOLLOW NONLINEAR PHARMACOKINETICS

The bioavailability of drugs that follow nonlinear pharmacokinetics is difficult to estimate accurately. As shown in Table 16.1, each process of drug absorption, distribution, and elimination is potentially saturable. Drugs that follow linear pharmacokinetics follow the principle of *superposition* (Chapter 15). The assumption in applying the rule of superposition is that each dose of drug superimposes on the previous dose. Consequently, the bioavailability of subsequent doses is predictable and not affected by the previous dose. In the presence of a saturable pathway in drug absorption, distribution, or elimination, drug bioavailability will change within a single dose or with subsequent (multiple) doses. An example of a drug with dose-dependent absorption is chlorothiazide (Hsu et al, 1987).

The extent of bioavailability is generally estimated by the $[\mathrm{AUC}]_0^\infty$. If drug absorption is saturation limited in the gastrointestinal tract, then a smaller fraction of drug is absorbed systemically when the gastrointestinal drug concentration is high. A drug with a saturable elimination pathway may also have a concentration-dependent AUC affected by the magnitude of K_M and V_{max} of the enzymes involved in drug elimination (Eq. 16.21). At low systemic drug concentrations at the beginning of drug absorption from the gastrointestinal tract, the rate of elimination is first order. As more drug is absorbed, either from a single dose or after multiple doses, systemic drug concentrations increase to levels that saturate the enzymes involved in drug elimination. The body drug clearance changes and the AUC increases disproportionally to the increase in dose (Fig. 16-2).

NONLINEAR PHARMACOKINETICS DUE TO DRUG–PROTEIN BINDING

Protein binding may prolong the elimination half-life of a drug. Drugs that are protein bound must dissociate into the free or nonbound form to be eliminated by glomerular filtration. The nature and extent of drug–protein binding affects the magnitude of the deviation from normal linear or first-order elimination rate process.

For example, consider the plasma level–time curves of two hypothetical drugs given intravenously in equal doses (Figure 16-14). One drug is 90% protein bound, whereas the other drug does not bind plasma protein. Both drugs are eliminated solely by glomerular filtration through the kidney.

The plasma curves in Fig. 16-14 demonstrate that the protein-bound drug is more concentrated in the plasma than a drug that is not protein bound, and the protein-bound drug is eliminated at a slower, nonlinear rate. Because the two drugs are eliminated by identical mechanisms, the characteristically slower elimination

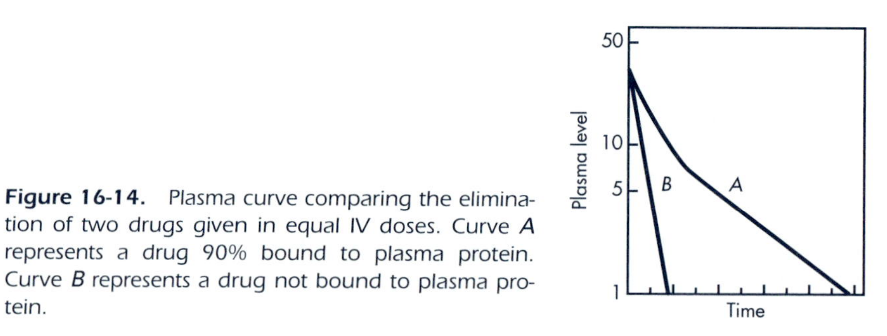

Figure 16-14. Plasma curve comparing the elimination of two drugs given in equal IV doses. Curve *A* represents a drug 90% bound to plasma protein. Curve *B* represents a drug not bound to plasma protein.

rate for the protein-bound drug is due to the fact that less free drug is available for glomerular filtration in the course of renal excretion.

The concentration of free drug, C_f, can be calculated at any time, as follows.

$$C_f = C_p\ (1 - \text{fraction bound}) \tag{16.30}$$

For any protein-bound drug, the free drug concentration (C_f) will always be less than the total drug concentration (C_p).

A careful examination of Figure 16-14 shows that the slope of the bound drug decreases gradually as the drug concentration decreases. This indicates that the percent of drug bound is not constant. *In vivo,* the percent of drug bound usually increases as the plasma drug concentration decreases (see Chapter 11). Since protein binding of drug can cause nonlinear elimination rates, pharmacokinetic fitting of protein-bound drug data to a simple one-compartment model without accounting for binding results in erroneous estimates of the volume of distribution and elimination half-life. Sometimes plasma drug data for drugs that are highly protein bound have been inappropriately fitted to two-compartment models.

One-Compartment Model Drug with Protein Binding

The process of elimination of a drug distributed in a single compartment with protein binding is illustrated in Figure 16-15. The one compartment contains both free drug and bound drug, which are dynamically interconverted with rate constants k_1 and k_2. Elimination of drug occurs only with the free drug at a first-order rate. The bound drug is not eliminated. Assuming a saturable and instantly reversible drug-binding process: P = protein concentration in plasma, C_f = plasma concentration of free drug, $k_d = k_2/k_1$ = dissociation constant of the protein drug complex, C_p = total plasma drug concentration, and C_b = plasma concentration of bound drug.

$$\frac{C_b}{P} = \frac{\dfrac{1}{k_d}C_f}{1 + \left(\dfrac{1}{k_d}\right)C_f} \tag{16.31}$$

This equation can be rearranged as follows:

$$C_b = \frac{PC_f}{k_d + C_f} = C_p - C_f \tag{16.32}$$

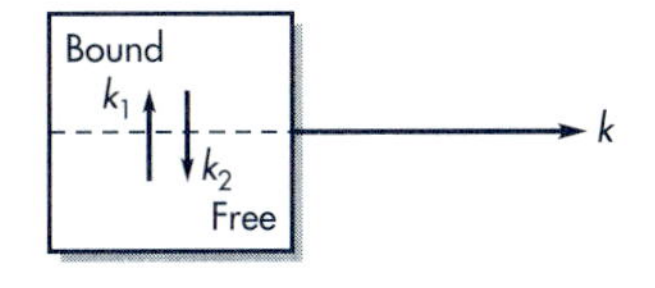

Figure 16-15. One-compartment model with drug–protein binding.

Solving for C_f,

$$C_f = \frac{1}{2}\left[-(P + k_d - C_p) + \sqrt{(P + k_d - C_p)^2 + 4k_d C_p}\,\right] \tag{16.33}$$

Because the rate of drug elimination is dC_p/dt,

$$\frac{dC_p}{dt} = -kC_f \tag{16.34}$$

$$\frac{dC_p}{dt} = -\frac{k}{2}\left[-(P + k_d - C_p) + \sqrt{(P + k_d - C_p)^2 + 4k_d C_p}\,\right]$$

This differential equation describes the relationship of changing plasma drug concentrations during elimination. The equation is not easily integrated but could be solved by means of a numerical method. Figure 16-16 shows the plasma drug concentration curves for a one-compartment protein-bound drug having a volume of distribution of 50 mL/kg and an elimination half-life of 30 minutes. The protein concentration is 4.4% and the molecular weight of the protein is 67,000 d. At various doses, the pharmacokinetics of elimination of the drug, as shown by the plasma curves, range from linear to nonlinear, depending on the total plasma drug concentration.

Nonlinear elimination pharmacokinetics occur more dramatically at higher doses, because more free drug is then available, and initial drug elimination occurs more rapidly. For drugs demonstrating nonlinear pharmacokinetics, the free drug concentration may increase slowly at first, but when the dose of drug is raised beyond the protein-bound saturation point, free plasma drug concentrations may rise abruptly. Therefore, the concentration of free drug should always be calculated to make sure the patient receives a proper dose.

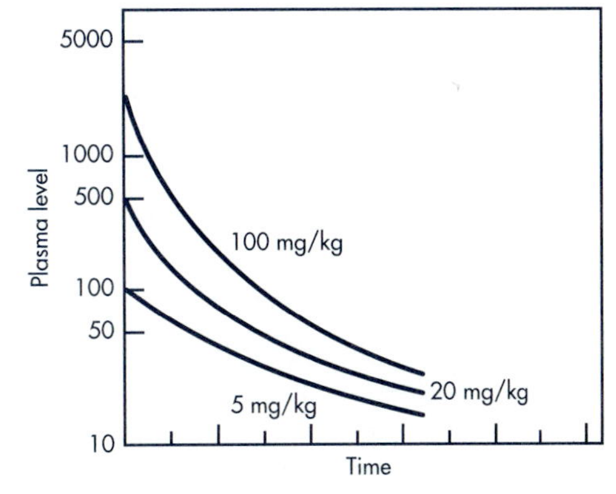

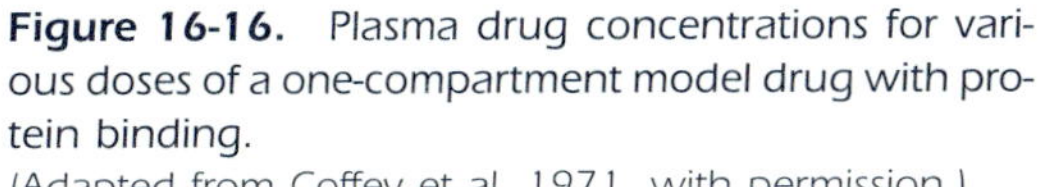

Figure 16-16. Plasma drug concentrations for various doses of a one-compartment model drug with protein binding.
(Adapted from Coffey et al, 1971, with permission.)

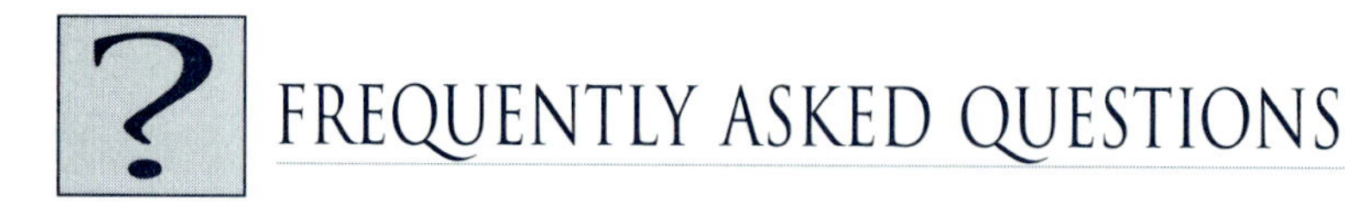

FREQUENTLY ASKED QUESTIONS

1. Most drugs follow linear pharmacokinetics at therapeutic doses. Why is it important to monitor drug level carefully for dose dependency?
2. What are the main differences in pharmacokinetic parameters between a drug that follows linear and a drug that follows nonlinear pharmacokinetic?
3. What are the main differences between a model based on Michaelis–Menten kinetic (V_{max} and K_M) and the physiologic model that describes hepatic metabolism based on clearance?
4. What is the cause of nonlinear pharmacokinetics that is not dose related?

LEARNING QUESTIONS

1. Define *nonlinear pharmacokinetics*. How do drugs that follow nonlinear pharmacokinetics differ from drugs that follow linear pharmacokinetics?
   a. What is the rate of change in the plasma drug concentration with respect to time, dC_p/dt, when $C_p \ll K_M$?
   b. What is the rate of change in the plasma drug concentration with respect to time, dC_p/dt, when $C_p \gg K_M$?
2. What processes of drug absorption, distribution, and elimination may be considered "capacity limited," "saturated," or "dose dependent?"
3. Drugs, such as phenytoin and salicylates, have been reported to follow dose-dependent elimination kinetics. What changes in pharmacokinetic parameters, including $t_{1/2}$, V_D, AUC, and C_p, could be predicted if the amounts of these drugs administered were increased from low pharmacologic doses to high therapeutic doses?
4. A given drug is metabolized by capacity-limited pharmacokinetics. Assume K_M is 50 μg/mL, V_{max} is 20 μg/mL per hr, and the apparent V_D is 20 L/kg.
   a. What is the reaction order for the metabolism of this drug when given in a single intravenous dose of 10 mg/kg?
   b. How much time is necessary for the drug to be 50% metabolized?
5. How would induction or inhibition of the hepatic enzymes involved in drug biotransformation theoretically affect the pharmacokinetics of a drug that demonstrates nonlinear pharmacokinetics due to saturation of its hepatic elimination pathway?
6. Assume that both the active parent drug and its inactive metabolites are excreted by active tubular secretion. What might be the consequences of increasing the dosage of the drug on its elimination half-life?

7. The drug isoniazid was reported to interfere with the metabolism of phenytoin. Patients taking both drugs together would show higher phenytoin levels in the body. Using the basic principles in this chapter, do you expect K_M to increase or decrease in patients taking both drugs? (Hint: see Fig. 16-4.)
8. Explain why K_M is often seen to have units of μM/mL and sometimes mg/L.
9. The V_{max} for metabolizing a drug is 10 μmol/hr. The rate of metabolism (v) is 5 μmol/hr when drug concentration is 4 μmol. Which of the following statements is/are true?
   - **a.** K_M is 5 μmol for this drug
   - **b.** K_M cannot be determined from the information given
   - **c.** K_M is 4 μmol for this drug
10. Which of the following statements is/are true regarding the pharmacokinetics of diazepam (98% protein bound) and propranolol (87% protein bound)?
    - **a.** Diazepam has a long elimination half-life because it is difficult to be metabolized due to extensive plasma–protein binding.
    - **b.** Propranolol is an example of a drug with high protein binding but unrestricted (unaffected) metabolic clearance.
    - **c.** Diazepam is an example of a drug with low hepatic extraction.
    - **d.** All of the above.
    - **e.** a and c
    - **f.** b and c
11. Which of the following statements describe(s) correctly the properties of a drug that follows nonlinear or capacity-limited pharmacokinetics?
    - **a.** The elimination half-life will remain constant when the dose changes.
    - **b.** The area under the plasma curve (AUC) will increase proportionally as dose increases.
    - **c.** The rate of drug elimination = $C_p \times K_M$.
    - **d.** All of the above.
    - **e.** a and b
    - **f.** None of the above.
12. The hepatic intrinsic clearance of two drugs are:
    Drug A: 1300 mL/min
    Drug B: 26 mL/min
    Which drug is likely to show the greatest increase in hepatic clearance when hepatic blood flow is increased from 1 L/min to 1.5 L/min?
    - **a.** Drug A.
    - **b.** Drug B.
    - **c.** No change for both drugs.

REFERENCES

Coffey J, Bullock FJ, Schoenemann PT: Numerical solution of nonlinear pharmacokinetic equations: Effect of plasma protein binding on drug distribution and elimination. *J Pharm Sci* **60:**1623, 1971

Evans WE, Schentag JJ, Jusko WJ: *Applied Pharmacokinetics—Principles of Therapeutic Drug Monitoring*, 3rd ed. Applied Therapeutics, 1992, pp 2–33

Hsu F, Prueksaritanont T, Lee MG, Chiou WL: The phenomenon and cause of the dose-dependent oral absorption of chlorothiazide in rats: Extrapolation to human data based on the body surface area concept. *J Pharmacokinet Biopharm* **15:**369–386, 1987

Lennard MS, Tucker GT, Woods HF: The polymorphic oxidation of beta-adrenoceptor antagonists—Clinical pharmacokinetic considerations. *Clin Pharmacol* **11:**1–17, 1986

Levy RH: Time-dependent pharmacokinetics. *Pharmacol Ther* **17:**383–392, 1983

Perrier D, Ashley JJ, Levy G: Effect of product inhibition in kinetics of drug elimination. *J Pharmacokinet Biopharm* **1:**231, 1973

Pitlick WH, Levy RH: Time-dependent kinetics, I. Exponential autoinduction of carbamazepine in monkeys. *J Pharm Sci* **66:**647, 1977

Reinberg AE: Concepts of circadian chronopharmacology. In Hrushesky WJM, Langer R, Theeuwes F (eds), *Temporal Control of Drug Delivery.* New York, Annals of the Academy of Science, 1991, vol 618, p 102

Tozer TN et al: In Breimer DD, Speiser P (eds), *Topics in Pharmaceutical Sciences.* New York, Elsevier, 1981, p 4

Von Roemeling R: The therapeutic index of cytotoxic chemotherapy depends upon circadian drug timing. In Hrushesky WJM, Langer R, Theeuwes F, (eds), *Temporal Control of Drug Delivery.* New York, Annals of the Academy of Science, 1991, vol 618, pp 292–311

Vozeh S, Muir KT, Sheiner LB: Predicting phenytoin dosage. *J Pharm Biopharm* **9:**131–146, 1981

Wagner JG, Szpunar GJ, Ferry JJ: Michaelis–Menten elimination kinetics: Areas under curves, steady-state concentrations, and clearances for compartment models with different types of input. *Biopharm Drug Disp* **6:**177–200, 1985

Witmer DR, Ritschel WA: Phenytoin isoniazid interaction: A kinetic approach to management. *Drug Intell Clin Pharm* **18:**483–486, 1984

Yu HY, Shen YZ, Sugiyama Y, Hanano M: Dose-dependent pharmacokinetics of valproate in guinea pigs of different ages. *Epilepsia* **28**(6):680–687, 1987

BIBLIOGRAPHY

Amsel LP, Levy G: Drug biotransformation interactions in man, II. A pharmacokinetic study of the simultaneous conjugation of benzoic and salicylic acids with glycine. *J Pharm Sci* **58:**321–326, 1969

Gibaldi M: Pharmacokinetic aspects of drug metabolism. *Ann NY State Acad Sci* **179:**19, 1971

Kruger-Theimer E: Nonlinear dose concentration relationships. *Il Farmaco* **23:**718–756, 1968

Levy G: Pharmacokinetics of salicylate in man. *Drug Metab Rev* **9:**3–19, 1979

Levy G, Tsuchiya T: Salicylate accumulation kinetics in man. *N Engl J Med* **287:**430–432, 1972

Ludden TM: Nonlinear pharmacokinetics. Clinical applications. *Clin Pharmacokinet* **20:**429–446, 1991

Ludden TM, Hawkins DW, Allen JP, Hoffman SF: Optimum phenytoin dosage regimen. *Lancet* **1:**307–308, 1979

Mullen PW: Optimal phenytoin therapy: A new technique for individualizing dosage. *Clin Pharm Ther* **23:**228–232, 1978

Mullen PW, Foster RW: Comparative evaluation of six techniques for determining the Michaelis–Menten parameters relating phenytoin dose and steady state serum concentrations. *J Pharm Pharmacol* **31:**100–104, 1979

Tozer TN, Rubin GM: Saturable kinetics and bioavailability determination. In Welling PG, Tse FLS (eds), *Pharmacokinetics: Regulatory, Industrial, Academic Perspectives.* New York, Marcel Dekker, 1988

Van Rossum JM, van Lingen G, Burgers JPT: Dose-dependent pharmacokinetics. *Pharmacol Ther* **21:**77–99, 1983

Wagner J: Properties of the Michaelis–Menten equation and its integrated form which are useful in pharmacokinetics. *J Pharm Biopharm* **1:**103, 1973

17

APPLICATION OF PHARMACOKINETICS IN CLINICAL SITUATIONS

The success of drug therapy is highly dependent on the dosage regimen design. A properly designed dosage regimen tries to achieve an optimum concentration of the drug at a receptor site to produce an optimal therapeutic response with minimum adverse effects. Individual variation in pharmacokinetics and pharmacodynamics makes the design of dosage regimens difficult. Therefore, the application of pharmacokinetics to dosage regimen design must be coordinated with proper clinical evaluation and monitoring.

INDIVIDUALIZATION OF DRUG DOSAGE REGIMEN

Not all drugs need rigid individualization of the dosage regimen. Many drugs have a large margin of safety (ie, exhibit a wide therapeutic window), and strict individualization of the dose is unnecessary. The United States Food and Drug Administration (FDA) has approved an over-the-counter (OTC) classification for drugs that the public may buy without prescription. In the past few years, many prescription drugs, such as ibuprofen, cimetidine, naproxen, nicotine patches, and others, have been approved by the FDA for OTC status. These OTC drugs and certain prescription drugs when taken as directed are generally safe and effective for the labeled indications without medical supervision. For drugs that are relatively safe and have a broad safety dose range, such as the penicillins, cephalosporins, and tetracyclines, the antibiotic dosage is not dose titrated precisely but rather based on clinical judgment of the physician to maintain an effective plasma antibiotic concentration above a minimum inhibitory concentration.

For drugs with a narrow therapeutic window, such as digoxin, aminoglycosides, antiarrhythmics, anticonvulsants, and some antiasthmatics, such as theophylline, individualization of the dosage regimen is very important. The objective of the dosage regimen design for these drugs is to produce a safe plasma drug concentration that does not exceed the minimum toxic concentration or fall below a critical minimum drug concentration below which the drug is not effective. For this reason, the dose of these drugs is carefully individualized to avoid plasma drug concentration fluctuations due to intersubject variation in drug absorption, distribution, or elimination processes.

For drugs, such as phenytoin, that follow nonlinear pharmacokinetics at therapeutic plasma drug concentrations, a small change in the dose may cause a huge increase in the therapeutic response, leading to possible adverse effects.

The monitoring of plasma drug concentrations is valuable only if there is a relationship between the plasma drug concentration and the desired clinical effect or between the plasma drug concentration and an adverse effect. For those drugs in which plasma drug concentration and clinical effect are not related, other pharmacodynamic parameters may be monitored. For example, the clotting time may be measured directly in patients on warfarin anticoagulant therapy. For asthmatic patients, the bronchodilator albuterol is given by inhalation via a metered dose inhaler and the patient's FEV_1 is a measurement of drug efficacy. In cancer chemotherapy, dose adjustment for individual patients may depend upon the severity of side effects and the patient's ability to tolerate the drug. For some drugs that have large inter- and intra-subject variability, clinical judgment and experience with the drug is needed to properly dose the patient.

THERAPEUTIC DRUG MONITORING

The therapeutic range for a drug is an approximation of the average plasma drug concentrations that are safe and efficacious in most patients. When using published therapeutic drug concentration ranges, such as those in Table 17.1, the prescriber must realize that the therapeutic range is more a probability concept and should never be considered as absolute values (Evans, 1992; Schumacher, 1995). For example, the accepted therapeutic range for theophylline is 10 to 20 μg/mL. Some patients may exhibit signs of theophylline intoxication such as central nervous system excitation and insomnia at serum drug concentrations below 20 μg/mL (Fig. 17.2,

TABLE 17.1 Therapeutic Range for Commonly Monitored Drugs

Drug	Therapeutic Range
Amikacin	20–30 mcg/mL
Carbamazepine	4–12 mcg/mL
Digoxin	1–2 ng/mL
Gentamicin	5–10 mcg/mL
Lidocaine	1–5 mcg/mL
Lithium	0.6–1.2 mEq/L
Phenytoin	10–20 mcg/mL
Procainamide	4–10 mcg/mL
Quinidine	1–4 mcg/mL
Theophylline	10–20 mcg/mL
Tobramycin	5–10 mcg/mL
Valproic acid	50–100 mcg/mL
Vancomycin	20–40 mcg/mL

From Schumacher GE: Therapeutic Drug Monitoring, Appleton & Lange, Norwalk (1995), with permission p 512), whereas other patients may show drug efficacy at serum drug concentrations below 10 $\mu g/mL$.

In administering potent drugs to patients, the physician must maintain the plasma drug level within a narrow range of therapeutic concentrations (Table 17.1). Various pharmacokinetic methods may be used to calculate the initial dose or dosage regimen. Usually, the initial dosage regimen is calculated based on body weight or body surface after a careful consideration of the known pharmacokinetics of the drug, the pathophysiologic condition of the patient, and the patient's drug history.

Due to interpatient variability in drug absorption, distribution, and elimination as well as changing pathophysiologic conditions in the patient, *therapeutic drug-monitoring* (TDM) or clinical pharmacokinetic (laboratory) services (CPKS) have been established in many hospitals to evaluate the response of the patient to the recommended dosage regimen. The improvement in the clinical effectiveness of the drug by therapeutic drug monitoring may decrease the cost of medical care by preventing untoward adverse drug effects. The functions of a TDM service are listed below.

- Select drug
- Design dosage regimen
- Evaluate patient response
- Determine need for measuring serum drug concentrations
- Assay for drug
- Perform pharmacokinetic evaluation of drug levels
- Readjust dosage regimen
- Monitor serum drug concentrations
- Recommend special requirements

Drug Selection

The choice of drug and drug therapy is usually made by the physician. However, many practitioners consult with the clinical pharmacist in drug product selection and dosage regimen design. Increasingly, clinical pharmacists in hospitals and nursing care facilities are closely involved in prescribing, monitoring, and substitution of medications. Drugs are selected not only on the basis of therapeutic consideration, but also based on cost and therapeutic equivalency. Pharmacokinetics and pharmacodynamics are part of the overall considerations in the selection of a drug for inclusion into the Drug Formulary (DF). New pharmacokinetic and pharmacodynamic data are periodically reviewed and updated by the Institutional Pharmacy and Therapeutic Committees (IPTC).

Drugs with similar therapeutic indications may differ in dose and pharmacokinetics. The pharmacist may choose one drug over another based on cost, therapeutic and pharmacokinetic considerations. Other factors include patient specific information such as medical history, pathophysiologic states, concurrent drug therapy, known allergies, drug sensitivity, and drug interactions; all are important considerations in drug selection (Table 17.2).

Dosage Regimen Design

Once the proper drug is selected for the patient, a number of factors must be considered when designing a therapeutic dosage regimen. First, the usual pharmacokinetics of the drug—including its absorption, distribution, and elimination profile—are considered in the patient. Some patients have unusual first-pass metabolism and bioavailability may be reduced. Second, the physiology of the patient, the

TABLE 17.2 Factors Producing Variability in Drug Response

PATENT FACTORS	DRUG FACTORS
Age	Bioavailability and biopharmaceutics
Weight	Pharmacokinetics (including absorption, distribution and elimination)
Pathophysiology	Drug interactions
Nutritional status	Receptor sensitivity
Genetic variability	Rapid or slow metabolism
Gender	

age, weight, gender, and nutritional status will impact on the disposition of the drug and should be considered. Third, any pathophysiologic conditions, such as renal dysfunction, hepatic disease, and congestive heart failure, may change the normal pharmacokinetic profile of the drug, and the dose must be carefully adjusted. For some patients, the hidden effect of exposure to long-term medication or drug abuse are important. Personal life style factors, such as cigarette smoking and ethanol abuses, are known to alter the pharmacokinetics of drugs.

The overall objective of dosage regimen design is to achieve a *target drug concentration* at the receptor site. Careful assessment of the patient including changes in the drug's pharmacokinetics, drug tolerance, cross sensitivity, or history of unusual reactions to related drugs should alert a pharmacist to change the dosage or consider the selection of another medication with the same therapeutic objective. Several mathematical approaches to dosage regimen design are given in the later sections of this chapter and in Chapter 18. Optimal dosing design can greatly improve the safety and efficacy of the drug including reduced side effects and a decrease in frequency of *therapeutic drug monitoring* (*TDM*) and its associated costs. However, the pharmacists must develop competency and experience in clinical pharmacology and therapeutics in addition to the necessary pharmacokinetic skills. For some drugs, TDM will be necessary due to the unpredictable nature of their pharmacodynamics and pharmacokinetics.

Pharmacokinetics of the Drug

Various popular drug references list pharmacokinetic parameters such as clearance, bioavailability, and elimination half-life. The values for these pharmacokinetic parameters are often obtained from small clinical studies. Therefore, it is difficult to determine if these reported pharmacokinetic parameters are reflected in the general population. Differences in study design, patient population, and data analysis may lead to conflicting values for the same pharmacokinetic parameters. For example, values for the apparent volume of distribution and clearance can be estimated by different methods, as discussed in previous chapters. Ideally, the *target drug concentration* and the *therapeutic window* for the drug should be obtained, if available. In using the target drug concentration in the development of a dosage regimen, the clinical pharmacist should know whether the reported target (effective) drug concentration represents an average steady-state drug concentration, a peak drug concentration, or a trough concentration.

Drug Dosage Form

The drug dosage form will affect the bioavailability of the drug and thus the subsequent pharmacodynamics of the drug in the patient. These biopharmaceutic factors have been discussed in Chapter 6. The route of drug administration and the desired onset and duration of the clinical response will affect the choice of the drug dosage form.

Patient Compliance

Institutionalized patients may have very little choice as to the prescribed drug and drug dosage form. Moreover, patient compliance is dictated by the fact that medication is provided by the medical personnel. Ambulatory patients must remember to take the medication as prescribed to obtain the optimum clinical effect of the drug. Factors that may effect patient compliance include cost of the medication, complicated instructions, multiple daily doses, difficulty in swallowing, and adverse drug reactions. Therefore, it is very important that the clinician or clinical pharmacist consider the patient's life-style and needs when developing a drug dosage regimen.

Evaluation of Patient's Response

After a drug product is chosen and the patient receives the initial dosage regimen, the practitioner should clinically evaluate the patient's response. If the patient is not responding to drug therapy as expected, then the drug and dosage regimen should be reviewed. The dosage regimen should be reviewed for adequacy, accuracy, and patient compliance to the drug therapy. In many situations, sound clinical judgment may preclude the need for measuring serum drug concentrations.

Measurement of Serum Drug Concentrations

Before blood samples are taken from the patient, the practitioner needs to determine whether serum drug concentrations should be measured in the patient. In some cases, the patient's response may not be related to the serum drug concentration. For example, allergy or mild nausea may not be dose related. In other cases, the response of a drug may be related to its chronopharmacology (see examples in Chapter 16).

A major assumption made by the practitioner is that serum drug concentrations relate to the therapeutic and/or toxic effects of the drug. For many drugs, clinical studies have demonstrated a therapeutically effective range of serum concentrations. Knowledge of the serum drug concentration may clarify why a patient is not responding to the drug therapy or why the drug is having an adverse effect. In addition, the practitioner may want to verify the accuracy of the dosage regimen.

When ordering serum drug concentrations to be measured, a single serum drug concentration may not yield useful information unless other factors are considered. For example, the dosage regimen of the drug should be known, including the size of the dose and dosage interval, the route of drug administration, the time of sampling (peak, trough, or steady-state), and the type of drug product (eg, immediate release or extended release).

In many cases, a single blood sample gives insufficient information and several blood samples are needed to clarify the adequacy of the dosage regimen. In practice, trough serum concentrations are easier to obtain than peak or C_{av}^{∞} samples during a multiple-dose regimen. In addition, there may be limitations in terms of the number of blood samples that may be taken, total volume of blood needed for the assay, and time to perform the drug analysis. Schumacher (1985) has suggested that blood sampling times for therapeutic drug monitoring be taken during the postdistributive phase for loading and maintenance doses and at steady-state for maintenance doses. After distribution equilibrium has been achieved, the plasma drug concentration during the postdistributive phase is better correlated with the tissue concentration and, presumably, the drug concentration at the site of action. In some cases, the clinical pharmacist might want an early time sample that approximates the peak drug level, whereas a blood sample taken at 3 to 4 half-lives of the drug would approximate the steady-state drug concentration. The practitioner who orders the measurement of serum concentrations should also consider the cost of the assays, the risks and discomfort for the patient, and the utility of the information gained.

Assay for Drug

Drug analyses are usually performed by either a clinical chemistry laboratory or a clinical pharmacokinetics laboratory. A variety of analytic techniques are available for drug measurement, including high-pressure liquid chromatography, gas chromatography, spectrophotometry, fluorometry, immunoassay, and radioisotopic methods. The methods used by the analytic laboratory may depend on such factors as the physicochemical characteristics of the drug, target concentration for measurement, amount and nature of the biological specimen (serum, urine), available instrumentation, cost for each assay, and analytical skills of the laboratory personnel. The laboratory should have a standard operating procedure for each drug analysis technique and follow good laboratory practices. Moreover, analytic method used for the assay of drugs in serum should be validated with respect to specificity, linearity, sensitivity, precision, accuracy, stability, and ruggedness. Due to cost and equipment constraint, most *Clinical Pharmacokinetic Services*, or CPKD, routinely analyze drugs by immunoassay. The Abbott TDx system is a fluorescence polarization immunoassay (FPI), which measures most of the antiarrhythmics and aminoglycosides and other drugs of abuse (Table 17.3). TDxFLx is a newer equipment that allows flexible handling of samples. Other dedicated systems routinely used in hospitals include the Autocarousel (Syva Corp.) which markets many EMIT test kits for many drugs. Other makers of instruments or kits for drug testing include Syntex, Eastman Kodak, Hoffman-LaRoche, and Miles Laboratories.

Specificity

Specificity should be established by the demonstration of chromatographic evidence that the method is specific for the drug. The method should demonstrate that there is no interference between the drug metabolites of the drug, and endogenous or exogenous substances. In addition, the internal standard should be resolved completely and also demonstrate no interference with other compounds. Immunoassays are dependent upon an antibody and antigen (usually the drug to be measured) reaction. The antibody may not be specific for the drug analyte, but may also cross-react with drugs that have similar structures, including related compounds (endogenous or exogenous chemicals) and metabolites of the drug. Colorimetric and spectrophotometric assays are usually less specific. Interference from other materials may erroneously inflate the results.

Sensitivity

Sensitivity is the minimum detectable level or concentration of drug in serum that may be approximated as that lowest drug concentration that is 2 to 3 times the

TABLE 17.3 Common Drugs Monitored in Hospitals

ANTIARRHYTHMICS	ANTIBIOTICS	ANTICONVULSANTS
Disopyramide	Amikacin	Carbamazepine, free carbamazepine
Flecainide	Gentamicin	Valproic acid, free valproic acid
Lidocaine	Netilmicin	Ethosuximide
N-acetylprocainamide	Tobramycin	Phenobarbital
Procainamide	Vancomycin	Phenytoin, free phenytoin
Quinidine		Primidone
OTHERS	**TOXICOLOGY ASSAYS**	**DRUG SCREENING ASSAYS**
Digoxin	Acetaminophen	Amphetamine
Digitoxin	Ethanol	Barbiturates
Methotrexate	Salicylate	Salicylate
Benzodiazepines	Tricyclic antidepressants	Cannabinoids
Theophylline		Cocaine
		Methadone
		Opiates
		Phencyclidine
		Propoxyphene

background noise. A *minimum quantifiable level* (MQL) is a statistical method for the determination of the precision of the lower level.

Linearity and Dynamic Range

Dynamic range refers to the relationship between the drug concentration and the instrument response (or signal) used to measure the drug. Many assays show a linear drug concentration versus instrument response relationship. Immunoassays generally have a nonlinear dynamic range. High serum drug concentrations above the dynamic range of the instrument response must be diluted prior to assay. The dynamic range is determined by using serum samples that have known (standard) drug concentrations (including a blank serum sample or zero drug concentration). Extrapolation of the assay results above or below the measured standard drug concentrations may be inaccurate since the relationship between instrument response and extrapolated drug concentration is unknown.

Precision

Precision is a measurement of the variability or reproducibility of the data. Precision measurements are obtained by replication of various drug concentrations and by replication of standard concentration curves prepared separately on different days. A suitable statistical measurement of the dispersion of the data, such as standard deviation or coefficient of variation, is then performed.

Accuracy

Accuracy refers to the difference between the average assay values and the true or known drug concentrations. Control (known) drug serum concentrations should be prepared by an independent technician using such techniques to minimize any error in their preparation. These samples, including a "zero" drug concentration, are assayed by the technician assigned to the study along with a suitable standard drug concentration curve.

Stability

Standard drug concentrations should be maintained under the same storage conditions as the unknown serum samples and assayed periodically. The stability study should continue for at least the same length of time as that for which the patient samples are to be stored. Freeze-thaw stability studies are performed to determine the effect of thawing and refreezing on the stability of the drug in the sample. On occasion, a previously frozen biological sample must be thawed and reassayed if the first assay result is uncertain.

Serum samples obtained from subjects on a drug study are usually assayed along with a minimum of three standard processed serum samples containing known standard drug concentrations and a minimum of three control serum samples whose concentrations are unknown to the analyst. These control serum samples are randomly distributed in each day's run. Control samples are replicated in duplicate to evaluate within day precision and between day precision. The concentration of drug in each serum sample is based on each day's processed standard curve.

Ruggedness

Ruggedness is the degree of reproducibility of the test results obtained by the analysis of the same samples by different analytical laboratories. The determination of ruggedness measures the reproducibility of the results under normal operational conditions from laboratory to laboratory and analyst to analyst.

Because each method for drug assay may have differences in sensitivity, precision, and specificity, the pharmacokineticist should be aware of which drug assay method the laboratory used.

Pharmacokinetic Evaluation

After the serum drug concentrations are measured, the pharmacokineticist must properly evaluate the data. Most laboratories report total drug (free plus bound drug) concentrations in the serum. The pharmacokineticist should be aware of the usual therapeutic range of serum concentrations from the literature. However, the literature may not indicate if the reported values were trough or peak serum levels. Moreover, the assay used in reporting the methodology may be different in terms of specificity and precision.

The assay results from the laboratory may show that the patient's serum drug levels are higher, lower, or similar to the expected serum levels. The pharmacokineticist should evaluate these results while considering the patient and the patient's pathophysiologic condition. Table 17.4 gives a number of factors for the pharmacokineticist to consider when interpreting the drug serum concentration. Often, other data, such as a high serum creatinine and high blood urea nitrogen (BUN), may help verify that an observed high serum drug concentration in a patient is due to slow renal drug clearance because of compromised kidney function. In another case, a complaint by the patient of overstimulation and insomnia might collaborate the laboratory's finding of higher than anticipated serum concentrations of theophylline. Therefore, the clinician or pharmacokineticist should evaluate the data using sound medical judgment and observation. The therapeutic decision should not be based solely on serum drug concentrations.

TABLE 17.4 Pharmacokinetic Evaluation of Serum Drug Concentrations

Serum Concentrations Lower than Anticipated
Patient compliance
Error in dosage regimen
Wrong drug product (controlled-release instead of immediate-release)
Poor bioavailability
Rapid elimination (efficient metabolizer)
Reduced plasma protein binding
Enlarged apparent volume of distribution
Steady state not reached
Timing of blood sample
Improving renal/hepatic function
Drug interaction due to stimulation of elimination enzyme autoinduction
Changing hepatic blood flow
Serum Concentrations Higher than Anticipated
Patient compliance
Error in dosage regimen
Wrong drug product (immediate release instead of controlled release)
Rapid bioavailability
Smaller than anticipated apparent volume of distribution
Slow elimination (poor metabolizer)
Increased plasma protein binding
Deteriorating renal/hepatic function
Drug interaction due to inhibition of elimination
Serum Concentration Correct but Patient Does not Respond to Therapy
Altered receptor sensitivity (eg, tolerance)
Drug interaction at receptor site
Changing hepatic blood flow

Dosage Adjustment

From the serum drug concentration data and patient observations, the clinician or pharmacokineticist may recommend an adjustment in the dosage regimen. Ideally, the new dosage regimen should be calculated using the pharmacokinetic parameters derived from the patient's serum drug concentrations. Although there may not be enough data for a complete pharmacokinetic profile, the pharmacokineticist should still be able to derive a new dosage regimen based on the available data and the pharmacokinetic parameters in the literature that are based on average population data.

Monitoring Serum Drug Concentrations

In many cases, the patient's pathophysiology may be unstable, either improving or further deteriorating. For example, proper therapy for congestive heart failure will improve cardiac output and renal perfusion, thereby increasing renal drug clearance. Therefore, continuous monitoring of serum drug concentrations is necessary to ensure proper drug therapy for the patient. For some drugs, an acute pharmacologic response can be monitored in lieu of actual serum drug concentration. For example, prothrombin clotting time might be useful for monitoring anticoagulant therapy and blood pressure monitoring for hypotensive agents.

Special Recommendations

At times, the patient may not be responding to drug therapy due to other factors. For example, the patient may not be following instructions for taking the medication (patient noncompliance), may be taking the drug after a meal instead of before, or may not be adhering to a special diet (eg, low salt). Therefore, the patient may need special instructions that are simple and easy to follow.

DESIGN OF DOSAGE REGIMENS

Several methods may be used to design a dosage regimen. Generally, the initial dosage of the drug is estimated using average population pharmacokinetic parameters as obtained from the literature. The patient is then monitored for the therapeutic response by physical diagnosis and, if necessary, by measurement of serum drug levels. After evaluation of the patient, a readjustment of the dosage regimen may be indicated, with further therapeutic drug monitoring.

Many versions of clinical pharmacokinetic software are available for dose calculations of drugs with narrow therapeutic index (eg, DataKinetics (ASHSP), and Abbottbase pharmacokinetic system). The dosing strategies are based generally on basic pharmacokinetic principles that have been estimated manually. Computer automation and pharmacokinetic software packages improve the accuracy of the calculation, make the calculations "easier" and have an added advantage in maintaining proper documentation.

Individualized Dosage Regimens

The most accurate approach to dosage regimen design would be the calculation of the dose based on the pharmacokinetics of the drug in the patient. This approach is not feasible for the calculation of the initial dose. However, once the patient has been medicated, the readjustment of the dose may be calculated using pharmacokinetic parameters derived from measurement of the serum drug levels from the patient after the initial dose. Most dosing programs record the patient's age and weight and calculate the individual dose based on creatinine clearance and lean body weight.

Dosage Regimens Based on Population Averages

The method most often used to calculate a dosage regimen is based on average pharmacokinetic parameters obtained from clinical studies published in the drug literature. This method may be based on a fixed or adaptive model (Greenblatt, 1979; Mawer, 1976).

The *fixed model* assumes that the population average pharmacokinetic parameters may be used directly to calculate a dosage regimen for the patient without any alteration. Usually, pharmacokinetic parameters, such as absorption rate constant k_a, bioavailability factor F, apparent volume of distribution V_D, and elimination rate constant k, are assumed to remain constant. Most often the drug is assumed to follow the pharmacokinetics of a one-compartment model. When a multiple-dose regimen is designed, then the multiple-dosage equations based on principle of superposition (Chapter 15) are used to evaluate the dose. The practitioner may use the usual dosage suggested by the literature and also make a small adjustment of the dosage based on the patient's weight and/or age.

The *adaptive model* for the dosage regimen calculation uses patient variables such as weight, age, sex, body surface area, and known patient pathophysiology, such as renal disease, as well as the known population average pharmacokinetic parameters of the drug. In this case, the calculation of dosage regimen takes into consideration any changing pathophysiology of the patient and attempts to adapt or modify the dosage regimen according to the needs of the patient. The adaptive model generally assumes that pharmacokinetic parameters, such as drug clearance, does not change from one dose to the next. However, some adaptive models allow for continuously adaptive change with time in order to simulate more closely the changing process of drug disposition in the patient, especially during a disease state (Whiting et al, 1991).

Dosage Regimens Based on Partial Pharmacokinetic Parameters

For many drugs, the entire pharmacokinetic profile for the drug is unknown or unavailable. Therefore, the pharmacokineticist needs to make some assumptions to calculate the dosage regimen. For example, a common assumption is to let the bioavailability factor F equal 1 or 100%. Thus, if the drug is less than fully absorbed systemically, the patient would be undermedicated rather than overmedicated. Some of these assumptions will be dependent on the safety, efficacy, and therapeutic range of the drug.

The use of *population pharmacokinetics* (discussed later in this chapter) uses average patient population characteristics and only a few serum drug concentrations from the patient. Population pharmacokinetic approaches to therapeutic drug monitoring have increased with the increased availability of computerized databases and the development of statistical tools for the analysis of observational data (Schumacher, 1993).

Empirical Dosage Regimens

In many cases, the physician selects a dosage regimen for the patient without using any pharmacokinetic variables. In such a situation, the physician makes the decision based on empirical clinical data, personal experience, and observations. The physician characterizes the patient as representative of a similar well-studied clinical population that has used the drug successfully.

CONVERSION FROM INTRAVENOUS INFUSION TO ORAL DOSING

After the patient's condition is controlled by intravenous infusion, it is often desirable to continue to medicate the patient with the same drug using the oral route of administration. When the intravenous infusion is stopped, then the serum drug concentration decreases according to first-order elimination kinetics (Chapter 14). For most oral drug products, the time to reach steady state is dependent on the first-order elimination rate constant for the drug. Therefore, if the patient starts the dosage regimen with the oral drug product at the same time when the intravenous infusion is stopped, then the exponential decline of serum levels from the intravenous infusion should be matched by the exponential increase in serum drug levels from the oral drug product.

The conversion from intravenous infusion to a controlled release oral medication given once or twice daily has become more common with the availability of controlled release-drug products, such as theophylline (Stein et al, 1982) and quinidine. Computer simulation for the conversion of intravenous theophylline (aminophylline) therapy to oral controlled release theophylline demonstrated that oral therapy should be started at the same time as intravenous infusion is stopped (Iafrate et al, 1982). With this method, minimal fluctuations are observed between the peak and trough serum theophylline levels. Moreover, giving the first oral dose may make it easier for the nursing staff or patient to comply with the dosage regimen.

The following methods may be used to calculate an appropriate oral dosage regimen for a patient whose condition has been stabilized by an intravenous drug infusion. Both methods assume that the patient's plasma drug concentration is at steady state.

Method 1

This method assumes that the steady-state plasma drug concentration C_{ss}, after IV infusion is identical to the desired C_{av}^{∞} after multiple oral doses of the drug. Therefore, the following equation may be used:

$$C_{av}^{\infty} = \frac{SFD_0}{kV_D\tau} \quad \textbf{(17.1)}$$

$$\frac{D_0}{\tau} = \frac{C_{av}^{\infty} kV_D}{SF} \quad \textbf{(17.2)}$$

where S is the salt form of the drug.

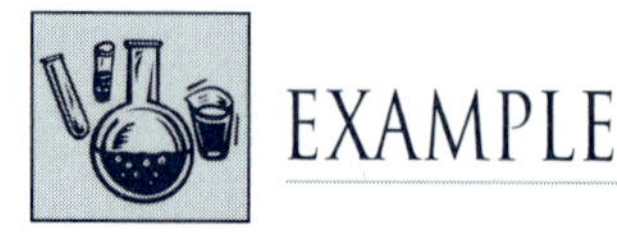

EXAMPLE

An adult male asthmatic patient (age 55, 78 kg) has been maintained on an intravenous infusion of aminophylline at a rate of 34 mg/hr. The steady-state theophylline drug concentration was 12 μg/mL and total body clearance was calculated as 3.0 L/hr. Calculate an appropriate oral dosage regimen of theophylline for this patient.

Solution

Aminophylline is a soluble salt of theophylline and contains 85% of theophylline ($S = 0.85$). Theophylline is 100% bioavailable ($F = 1$) after an oral dose. Because total body clearance $Cl_T = kV_D$, Equation 17.2 may be expressed as

$$\frac{D_0}{\tau} = \frac{C_{av}^{\infty} Cl_T}{SF} \quad \textbf{(17.3)}$$

The dose rate D_0/τ (34 mg/hr) was calculated on the basis of aminophylline. The patient, however, will be given theophylline orally. To convert to oral theophylline, S and F should be considered.

$$\text{Theophylline dose rate} = \frac{SFD_0}{\tau} = \frac{(0.85)(1)(34)}{1} = 28.9 \text{ mg/hr}$$

The theophylline dose rate of 28.9 mg/hr must be converted to a reasonable schedule for the patient with a consideration of the various commercially available theophylline drug products. Therefore, the total daily dose is 28.9 mg/hr × 24 hr or 693.6 mg/day. Possible theophylline dosage schedules could be 700 mg/day, 350 mg every 12 hours, or 175 mg every 6 hours. Each of these dosage regimens would achieve the same C_{av}^{∞} but different C_{max}^{∞} and C_{min}^{∞}, which should be calculated. The dose of 350 mg every 12 hours could be given in sustained-release form to avoid any excessive high drug concentration in the body.

Method 2

This method assumes that the rate of intravenous infusion (mg/hr) is the same desired rate of oral dosage.

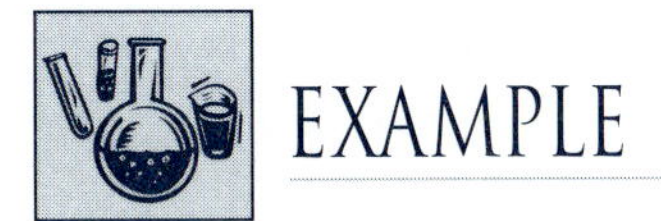

EXAMPLE

Using the example in method 1, the following calculations may be used.

Solution

The aminophylline is given by IV infusion at a rate of 34 mg/hr. The total daily dose of aminophylline would be 34 mg/hr × 24 hr = 816 mg. The equivalent daily dose in terms of theophylline would be 816 × 0.85 = 693.6 mg. Thus, the patient should receive approximately 700 mg of theophylline per day or 350 mg controlled-release theophylline every 12 hours.

DETERMINATION OF DOSE

The drug dose is estimated to deliver a desirable (target) therapeutic level of the drug to the body. The dose of a drug is estimated with the objective of delivering a desirable therapeutic level of the drug to the body. For many drugs, the desirable therapeutic drug levels and pharmacokinetic parameters are available in the clinical literature. However, the literature in some cases may not yield complete drug information, or the information available may be partly equivocal. Therefore, the pharmacokineticist must make certain necessary assumptions in accordance with the best pharmacokinetic information available.

For a drug that is given in multiple doses for an extended period of time, the dosage regimen is usually calculated so that the average steady-state blood level is within the therapeutic range. The dose can be calculated with Equation 17.4, which expresses the C_{av}^{∞} in terms of dose (D_0), dosing interval (τ), volume of distribution

(V_D), and the elimination half-life of the drug. F is the fraction of drug absorbed and is equal to 1 for drugs administered intravenously.

$$C_{av}^{\infty} = \frac{1.44 D_0 t_{1/2} F}{V_D \tau} \qquad \textbf{(17.4)}$$

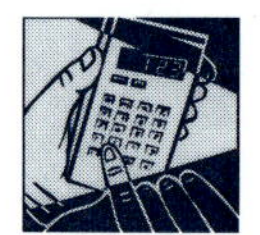

PRACTICE PROBLEMS

1. The pharmacokinetic data of clindamycin were reported by DeHann et al (1972) as follows:

$$k = 0.247\ \text{hr}^{-1}$$
$$t_{1/2} = 2.81\ \text{hr}$$
$$V_D = 43.9\ \text{L}/1.73\ \text{m}^2$$

What is the steady-state concentration of the drug after 150 mg of the drug was given orally every 6 hours for a week (assume the drug is 100% absorbed)?

Solution

$$C_{av}^{\infty} = \frac{1.44 D_0 t_{1/2} F}{V_D \tau}$$
$$= \frac{1.44 \times 150{,}000 \times 2.81 \times 1}{43{,}900 \times 6}\ \mu\text{g/mL}$$
$$= 2.3\ \mu\text{g/mL}$$

2. The elimination half-life of tobramycin was reported by Regamey and associates (1973) to be 2.15 hours; the volume of distribution was reported to be 33.5% of body weight.

a. What is the dose for an 80-kg individual if a steady-state level of 2.5 μg/mL is desired? Assume that the drug is given intravenously every 8 hours.

Solution

Assuming the drug is 100% bioavailable due to IV injection,

$$C_{av}^{\infty} = \frac{1.44 D_0 t_{1/2} F}{V_D \tau}$$
$$2.5 = \frac{1.44 \times 2.15 \times 1 \times D_0}{80 \times 0.335 \times 1000 \times 8}$$
$$D_0 = \frac{2.5 \times 80 \times 0.335 \times 1000 \times 8}{1.44 \times 2.15}\ \mu\text{g}$$
$$= 173\ \text{mg}$$

The dose should be 173 mg every 8 hours.

b. The manufacturer has suggested that in normal cases tobramycin should be given at a rate of 1 mg/kg every 8 hours. With this dosage regimen, what would the average steady-state level be?

Solution

$$C_{av}^{\infty} = \frac{1.44 \times 1 \times 1000 \times 2.15}{0.335 \times 1000 \times 8}$$
$$= 1.16\ \mu g/mL$$

Because the bacteriocidal concentration of an antibiotic varies with the organism involved in the infection, the dose prescribed may change. The average plasma drug concentration is used to indicate whether optimum drug levels have been reached. With certain antibiotics, the steady-state peak and trough levels are sometimes used as therapeutic indicators. (See Chapter 19 for discussion of time above MIC.) For example, the effective concentration of tobramycin was reported to be around 4 to 5 μg/mL for peak level and around 2 μg/mL for trough level when given intramuscularly every 12 hours. Although peak and trough levels are frequently reported in clinical journals, these drug levels are only transitory in the body. Peak and trough drug levels are less useful pharmacokinetically because peak and trough levels fluctuate more and are usually reported less accurately than average plasma drug concentrations. When the average plasma drug concentration is used as a therapeutic indicator, an optimum dosing interval must be chosen. The dosing interval is usually set at approximately 1 to 2 elimination half-lives of the drug, unless the drug has a very narrow therapeutic index. In this case the drug must be given in small doses more frequently or by IV infusion.

EFFECT OF CHANGING DOSE AND DOSING INTERVAL ON C_{max}^{∞}, C_{min}^{∞}, AND C_{av}^{∞}

The C_{av}^{∞} is used most often in dosage calculation. However, when monitoring serum drug concentrations, C_{av}^{∞} cannot be measured directly but may be obtained by the AUC/τ during multiple-dosage regimens. As discussed in Chapter 15, the C_{av}^{∞} is not the arithmetic average of C_{max}^{∞} and C_{min}^{∞} because serum concentrations decline exponentially. In contrast, C_{ss} may be used to monitor the steady-state serum concentrations after intravenous infusion. When considering therapeutic drug monitoring of serum concentrations after the initiation of a multiple-dosage regimen, the trough serum drug concentrations or C_{min}^{∞} may be used to validate the dosage regimen. The blood sample withdrawn just prior to the administration of the next dose represents C_{min}^{∞}. To obtain C_{max}^{∞}, the blood sample must be withdrawn exactly at the time for peak absorption, or closely spaced blood samples must be taken and the plasma drug concentrations graphed. In practice, an approximate time for maximum drug absorption is estimated and a blood sample is withdrawn. Due to differences in rates of drug absorption, C_{max}^{∞} measured in this manner is only an approximation of the true C_{max}^{∞}.

The advantage of using C_{av}^{∞} as an indicator for deciding therapeutic blood level is that C_{av}^{∞} is determined on a set of points and is generally less fluctuating than either C_{max}^{∞} or C_{min}^{∞}. Moreover, when the dosing interval is changed, the dose may be proportionally increased to keep C_{av}^{∞} constant. This approach works well for some drugs. For example, if the drug diazepam is given either 10 mg tid (three times a day) or 15 mg bid (twice daily), the same C_{av}^{∞} is obtained as shown by Equation 17.1. In fact, if the daily dose is the same, the C_{av}^{∞} should be the same.

The dosing interval must be set with the elimination half-life of the drug; otherwise, the patient may suffer either toxic effect of a high C_{max}^{∞} even if the C_{av}^{∞} is kept constant. For example, using the same example of diazepam, the same C_{av}^{∞} is achieved at 10 mg tid or 60 mg every other day. Obviously, the C_{max}^{∞} of the latter dose regimen would produce a C_{max}^{∞} several times larger than that achieved with 10 mg tid dose regimen. In general, if a drug has a relatively wide therapeutic index and a relatively long elimination half-life, then there is good flexibility in changing the dose or dosing interval using C_{av}^{∞} as an indicator. When the drug has a narrow therapeutic index, C_{max}^{∞} and C_{min}^{∞} must be monitored to ensure safety and efficacy.

As the size of the dose or dosage intervals change proportionately, the C_{av}^{∞} may be the same but the steady-state peak, C_{max}^{∞}, and trough, C_{min}^{∞}, drug levels will change. C_{max}^{∞} is influenced by the size of the dose and dosage interval. An increase in the size of the dose given at a longer dosage interval will cause an increase in C_{max}^{∞} and a decrease in C_{min}^{∞}. In this case C_{max}^{∞} may be very close or above the minimum toxic drug concentration (MTC). However, the C_{min}^{∞} may be lower than the minimum effective drug concentration (MEC). In this latter case the low C_{min}^{∞} may be subtherapeutic and dangerous for the patient depending on the nature of the drug.

DETERMINATION OF FREQUENCY OF DRUG ADMINISTRATION

The size of a drug dose is often related to the frequency of drug administration. The more frequently a drug is administered, the smaller the dose must be to obtain the same C_{av}^{∞}. Thus, a dose of 250 mg every 3 hours could be changed to 500 mg every 6 hours without affecting the average steady-state plasma concentration of the drug. However, as the dosing intervals get longer, the size of the dose required to maintain the average plasma drug concentration gets correspondingly larger. When an excessively long dosing interval is chosen, the large dose may result in peak plasma levels that are above toxic drug concentration, although the C_{av}^{∞} will remain the same. In general, the dosing interval for most drugs is determined by the elimination half-life. Drugs like penicillins, which have relatively low toxicity, may be given at intervals much longer than their elimination half-lives without any toxicity problems. Drugs having a narrow therapeutic index, such as digoxin and phenytoin, must be given relatively frequently to minimize excessive "peak and trough" fluctuations in blood levels. For example, the common maintenance schedule for digoxin is 0.25 mg/day and the elimination half-life of digoxin is 1.7 days. In contrast, penicillin G is given at 250 mg every 6 hours, while the elimination half-life of penicillin G is 0.75 hours. Penicillin is given at a dosage interval equal to 8 times its elimination half-life, whereas digoxin is given at a dosing interval only 0.59 times its elimination half-life. The toxic plasma concentration of penicillin G is over 100 times greater than its effective concentration, whereas digoxin has an effective concentration of 1 to 2 ng/mL and a toxicity level of 3 ng/mL. The toxic concentration of digoxin is only 1.5 times the effective concentration. Therefore, a drug with a large therapeutic index (ie, a large margin of safety) can be given in large doses and at relatively long dosing intervals.

DETERMINATION OF BOTH DOSE AND DOSAGE INTERVAL

Both the dose and dosage interval should be considered in the dosage regimen calculations. Ideally, the calculated dosage regimen should maintain the serum drug concentrations between C_{max}^{∞} and C_{min}^{∞}. For intravenous multiple-dosage regimens the ratio of $C_{max}^{\infty}/C_{min}^{\infty}$ may be expressed by

$$\frac{C_{max}^{\infty}}{C_{min}^{\infty}} = \frac{C_p^0/(1 - e^{-k\tau})}{C_p^0 e^{-k\tau}/(1 - e^{-k\tau})} \quad (17.5)$$

which can be simplified to

$$\frac{C_{max}^{\infty}}{C_{min}^{\infty}} = \frac{1}{e^{-k\tau}} \quad (17.6)$$

From Equation 17.6 a maximum dosage interval, τ, may be calculated that will maintain the serum concentration between C_{min}^{∞} and C_{max}^{∞}. After the dosage interval is calculated, then a dose may be calculated.

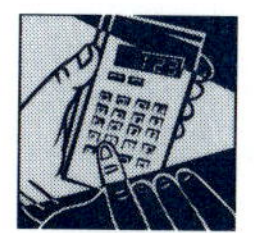

PRACTICE PROBLEM

1. The elimination half-life of an antibiotic is 3 hours with an apparent volume of distribution equivalent to 20% of body weight. The usual therapeutic range for this antibiotic is between 5 and 15 μg/mL. Adverse toxicity for this drug is often observed at serum concentrations greater than 20 μg/mL. Calculate a dosage regimen (multiple IV doses) that will just maintain the serum drug concentrations between 5 and 15 μg/mL.

Solution

From Equation 17.6 determine the dosage interval τ.

$$\frac{15}{5} = \frac{1}{e^{-(0.693/3)\tau}}$$

$$e^{-0.231\tau} = 0.333$$

Take the natural logarithm (ln) on both sides of the equation.

$$-0.231\tau = -1.10$$

$$\tau = 4.76 \text{ hr}$$

Then determine the dose from Equation 17.7 after substitution of $C_p^0 = D_0/V_D$:

$$C_{max}^{\infty} = \frac{D_0/V_D}{1 - e^{-k\tau}} \quad (17.7)$$

Solve for dose D_0, letting V_D = 200 mL/kg (20% body weight).

$$15 = \frac{D_0/200}{1 - e^{-(0.231)(4.76)}}$$

$$D_0 = 2 \text{ mg/kg}$$

To check this dose for therapeutic effectiveness, calculate $C_{\min}^{\infty}$ and C_{av}^{∞}.

$$C_{\min}^{\infty} = \frac{(D_0/V_D)\,e^{-k\tau}}{1 - e^{-k\tau}} = \frac{(2000/200)\,e^{-0.231(4.76)}}{1 - e^{(-0.231)(4.76)}}$$

$$C_{\min}^{\infty} = 4.99\ \mu\text{g/mL}$$

As a further check on the dosage regimen, C_{av}^{∞} is calculated:

$$C_{\text{av}}^{\infty} = \frac{D_0}{V_D k\tau} = \frac{2000}{(200)(0.231)(4.76)}$$

$$C_{\text{av}}^{\infty} = 9.09\ \mu\text{g/mL}$$

By calculation, the dose of this antibiotic should be 2 mg/kg every 4.76 hours to maintain the serum drug concentrations between 5 and 15 μg/mL.

In practice, rather than a dosage interval of 4.76 hours, the dosage regimen and the dosage interval should be made as convenient as possible for the patient and the size of the dose should take into account the commercially available drug formulation. Therefore, the dosage regimen should be recalculated to have a convenient value (4 to 6 hours) and the size of the dose adjusted accordingly.

NOMOGRAMS AND TABULATIONS IN DESIGNING DOSAGE REGIMENS

For ease of calculation of dosage regimens, many clinicians rely on nomograms to calculate the proper dosage regimen for their patients. The use of a nomogram may give a quick dosage regimen adjustment for patients with characteristics requiring adjustments, such as age, body weight, and physiologic state. In general, the nomogram of a drug is based on population pharmacokinetic data collected and analyzed using a specific pharmacokinetic model. In order to keep the dosage regimen calculation simple, complicated equations are often solved and the result displayed diagrammatically on special scaled axes to produce a simple dose recommendation based on patient information. Some nomograms make use of certain physiologic parameters, such as serum creatinine concentration, to help modify the dosage regimen according to renal function (Chapter 18).

For marketed drugs, the manufacturer often provides tabulated general guidelines for use in establishing a dosage regimen for patients, including loading and maintenance doses. For example, the initial doses and subsequent serum moni-

TABLE 17.5 Maintenance Dose of Theophylline When the Serum Concentration Is Not Measured[a]

AGE	DOSE	DOSE PER 12 HOURS
6–9 yrs	24 mg/kg/day	12.0 mg/kg
9–12 yrs	20 mg/kg/day	10.0 mg/kg
12–16 yrs	18 mg/kg/day	9.0 mg/kg
Over 16 yrs	13 mg/kg/day or 900 mg: WHICHEVER IS LESS	6.5 mg/kg

[a]WARNING: DO NOT ATTEMPT TO MAINTAIN A DOSE THAT IS NOT TOLERATED.

Adapted from product information for Theo-Dur Sprinkle (Theophylline Anhydrous Sustained Action Capsules, 1993, and Facts and Comparisons, 1991).

TABLE 17.6 Dosage Guidelines for Rapid Theophyllinization[a]

PATIENT GROUP	MAINTENANCE DOSE
Children 1 to 9 yrs	4 mg/kg every 6 hr
Children 9 to 16 and young adult smokers	3 mg/kg every 6 hr
Otherwise healthy nonsmoking adults	3 mg/kg every 8 hr
Older patients and patients with cor pulmonale	2 mg/kg every 8 hr
Patients with congestive heart failure	1–2 mg/kg every 8 hr

[a]In patients not receiving theophylline. The recommended loading dose for each patient group is 5 mg/kg.

Adapted from Facts and Comparisons, 1991, with permission.

toring of theophylline anhydrous sustained action capsules (Theo-Dur Sprinkle) and theophylline extended release tablets (Theo-Dur Tablets) are shown in Tables 17.5 and 17.6, respectively.

For narrow therapeutic index drugs, such as theophylline, a guide for monitoring serum drug concentrations is given. Another example is the aminoglycoside antibiotic, tobramycin sulfate, USP (Nebcin, Eli Lilly), which is eliminated primarily by renal clearance. Thus, the dosage of tobramycin sulfate should be reduced in direct proportion to a reduction in creatinine clearance (see Chapter 18). The manufacturer provides a nomogram for estimating the percent of the normal dose of tobramycin sulfate assuming the serum creatinine (mg/100 mL) has been obtained.

DETERMINATION OF ROUTE OF ADMINISTRATION

The selection of the proper route of administration is an important consideration in drug therapy. The rate of drug absorption and the duration of action are influenced by the route of drug administration. Moreover, the use of certain routes of administration are precluded due to physiologic and safety considerations. For example intra-arterial and intrathecal drug injections are less safe than other routes of drug administration and are only used when absolutely necessary. Drugs that are unstable in the gastrointestinal tract or drugs that undergo extensive first-pass effect are not suitable for oral administration. For example, insulin is a protein that is degraded in the gastrointestinal tract by proteolytic enzymes. Drugs like xylocaine and nitroglycerin are not suitable for oral administration because of first-pass effect. These drugs, therefore, must be given by an alternate route of administration.

Certain drugs are not suitable for administration intramuscularly due to erratic drug release, pain, or local irritation. Even though the drug is injected into the muscle mass, the drug must reach the circulatory system or other body fluid to become bioavailable. The anatomic site of the intramuscular injection will affect the rate of drug absorption. A drug injected into the deltoid muscle is more rapidly absorbed than a drug similarly injected into the gluteus maximus due to better blood flow in the former. In general, the method of drug administration that provides the most consistent and greatest bioavailability should be used to ensure maximum therapeutic effect. The various routes of drug administration can be classified as either extravascular or intravascular (Table 17.7).

Intravenous administration is the fastest and most reliable way of delivering the drug into the circulatory system. Drugs administered intravenously are removed

TABLE 17.7 Common Routes of Drug Administration

Parenteral	Extravascular
Intravascular	Enteral
Intravenous injection (IV bolus)	Buccal
Intravenous infusion (IV drip)	Sublingual
Intra-arterial injection	Oral
Intramuscular injection	Rectal
Intradermal injection	Inhalation
Subcutaneous injection	Transdermal
Intradermal injection	
Intrathecal injection	

more rapidly because the entire dose is subject to elimination immediately. Consequently, more frequent drug administration is required. Drugs administered extravascularly must be absorbed into the bloodstream, and the total absorbed dose is eliminated more slowly. The frequency of administration can be lessened by using routes of administration that give a sustained rate of drug absorption. Intramuscular injection generally provides more rapid absorption than does oral administration of preparations that are not very soluble. However, precipitation of the drug at the injection site may result in slower absorption and a delayed response. For example, a dose of 50 mg of chlordiazepoxide (Librium) is more quickly absorbed after oral administration than after intramuscular injection. Some drugs, such as haloperidol decanoate, are very oil-soluble products that release very slowly after intramuscular injection (Chapter 6).

DOSING OF DRUGS IN INFANTS AND CHILDREN

Infants and children have different dosing requirements than adults. Dosing of drugs in this population requires a thorough consideration of the differences in the pharmacokinetics and pharmacology of a specific drug in the newborn (birth

TABLE 17.8 Comparison of Newborn and Adult Renal Clearances[a]

	AVERAGE INFANT	AVERAGE ADULT
Body weight (kg)	3.5	70
Body water		
(%)	77	58
(L)	2.7	41
Inulin clearance		
(mL/min)	Approx 3	130
k (min^{-1})	3/2700 = 0.0011	130/41,000 = 0.0032
$t_{1/2}$ (min)	630	220
PAH clearance		
(mL/min)	Approx 12	650
k (min^{-1})	12/2800 = 0.0043	650/41,000 = 0.016
$t_{1/2}$ (min)	160	43

[a]Computations are for a drug distributed in the whole body water, but any other V_D would give the same relative values.

Data for average infant from West et al (1948), with permission from Charles C Thomas and Cambridge University Press.

TABLE 17.9 Elimination Half-Lives of Drugs in Infants and Adults

DRUG	HALF-LIFE IN NEONATES[a] (hr)	HALF-LIFE IN ADULTS (hr)
Penicillin G	3.2	0.5
Ampicillin	4	1–1.5
Methicillin	3.3/1.3	0.5
Carbenicillin	5–6	1–1.5
Kanamycin	5–5.7	3–5
Gentamicin	5	2–3

[a]0–7 days old.

to 1 month), infant (1 to 24 months), young child (1 to 5 yrs), older child (6 to 12 yrs), adolescent (13 to 18 yrs), and the adult. Unfortunately, the pharmacokinetics and pharmacodynamics of most drugs are not well known in children under age 12 years of age. The variation in body composition and the maturity of liver and kidney function are potential sources of differences in pharmacokinetics with respect to age. For convenience, "infants" are here arbitrarily defined as children 0 to 2 years of age. However, within this group, special consideration is necessary for infants less than 4 weeks (1 month) old, because their ability to handle drugs often differs from more mature infants.

In general, complete hepatic function is not attained until the third week of life. Oxidative processes are fairly well developed in infants, but there is a deficiency of conjugative enzymes. In addition, many drugs exhibit reduced binding to plasma albumin in infants.

Newborns show only 30 to 50% the renal activity of adults on the basis of activity per unit of body weight (Table 17.8). Drugs that are heavily dependent on renal excretion will have a sharply increased elimination half-life. For example, the penicillins are excreted for the most part through the kidney. The elimination half-lives of such drugs are much reduced in infants, as shown in Table 17.9.

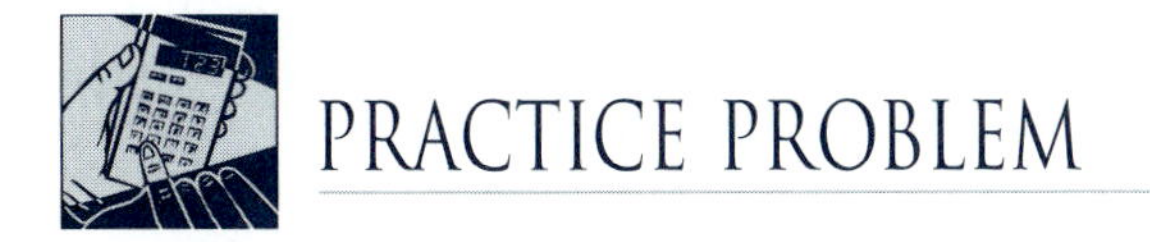

PRACTICE PROBLEM

The elimination half-life of penicillin G is 0.5 hours in adults and 3.2 hours in neonates (0 to 7 days old). Assuming that the normal adult dose of penicillin G is 4 mg/kg every 4 hours, calculate the dose of penicillin G for an 11-pound infant.

Solution

$$\frac{\tau_1}{\tau_2} = \frac{(t_{1/2})_1}{(t_{1/2})_2}$$

$$t_{1/2} = 0.5 \text{ hr}$$

$$\tau_2 = \frac{4 \times 3.2}{0.5} = 25.6 \text{ hr}$$

Therefore, this infant may be given the following dose:

$$\text{Dose} = 4 \text{ mg/kg} \times \frac{11 \text{ lb}}{2.2 \text{ lb/kg}} = 20 \text{ mg every 24 hr}$$

Alternatively, 10 mg every 12 hr would achieve the same C_{av}^{∞}.

Various methods have been used in the past for the estimation of a dose for a child. Methods such as Young's rule or Clark's rule for dose adjustment are at best crude approximations in that they take into account only body age and size change attributable to growth and do not consider the rate of drug elimination. Another dose adjustment method is based on *body surface area.* This approach has the advantage of avoiding bias due to obesity or unusual body weight because the height and weight of the patient are both considered. Again, the body surface area method gives only a rough estimation of the proper dose, because the pharmacokinetic differences of specific drugs are not considered.

DOSING OF DRUGS IN THE ELDERLY

Physiologic and cognitive functions tend to change with the aging process and can affect the therapeutic safety and efficacy of the prescribed drug. Since the elderly tend to be on multiple drug therapy, decreased cognitive function in geriatric patients may result in poor compliance with the desired dosage schedules, in turn resulting in lack of drug efficacy and possible drug interactions and drug intoxication.

Several vital physiologic functions measured by markers show that renal plasma flow, glomerular filtration, cardiac output, and breathing capacity can drop from 10 to 30% in the elderly subjects relative to those at age 30. The physiologic changes due to aging may necessitate special considerations in administering drugs in the elderly. For some drugs, an age-dependent increase in adverse drug reactions or toxicity may be observed in the elderly patient. This apparent increased drug sensitivity in the elderly may be due to pharmacodynamic and/or pharmacokinetic changes (Schmucker, 1985).

The pharmacodynamic hypothesis assumes that age causes alterations in the quantity and quality of the target drug receptors, leading to an enhanced drug response. Quantitatively, the number of drug receptors may decline with age, whereas, qualitatively, a change in the affinity for the drug may occur. Alternatively, the pharmacokinetic hypothesis assumes that age-dependent increases in adverse drug reactions are due to physiologic changes in drug absorption, distribution, and elimination including renal excretion and hepatic clearance.

In the elderly, age-dependent alterations in drug absorption may include a decline in the splanchnic blood flow, altered gastrointestinal motility, increase in gastric pH, and alteration in the gastrointestinal absorptive surface. From a distribution consideration, drug protein binding in the plasma may decrease due to a decrease in the albumin concentration, and the apparent volume of distribution may change due to a decrease in muscle mass and an increase in body fat. Renal drug excretion generally declines with age due to decrease in the glomerular filtration rate and/or active tubular secretion. Moreover, the activity of the enzymes responsible for drug biotransformation may decrease with age, leading to a decline in hepatic drug clearance.

The elderly may have several different pathophysiologic conditions that require multiple drug therapy and, therefore, increasing the likelihood for a drug interaction. Moreover, increased adverse drug reactions and toxicity may result from poor patient compliance. Both penicillin and kanamycin show prolonged $t_{1/2}$ in the aged patient, as a consequence of age related gradual reduction in the kidney size and function. The Gault and Cockroft rule for calculating creatinine clearance clearly quantitate a reduction in clearance when the age is increased (Chapter 18). Age-related changes in plasma albumin and α_1 acid glycoprotein may also be a factor in the binding of drugs in the body.

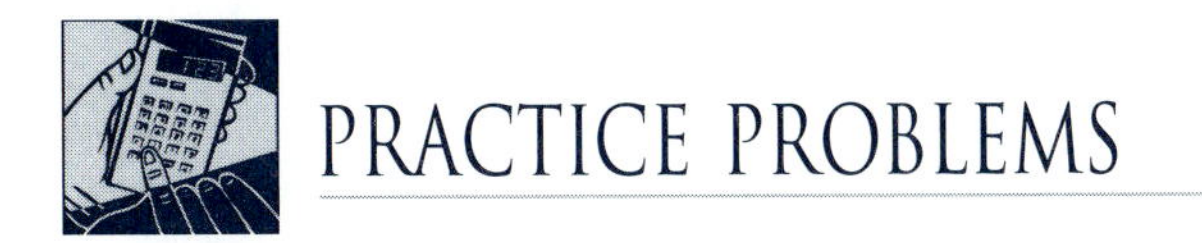

PRACTICE PROBLEMS

1. An aminoglycoside has a normal elimination half-life of 107 minutes in young adults. In patients 70 to 90 years old, the elimination half-life of the aminoglycoside is 282 minutes. The normal dose of the aminoglycoside is 15 mg/kg per day divided into two doses. What is the dose for a 75-year-old patient, assuming that the volume of distribution per body weight is not changed by the patient's age?

Solution

The longer elimination half-life of the aminoglycoside in the elderly is due to a decrease in renal function. A good inverse correlation has been obtained of elimination half-life to the aminoglycoside and creatinine clearance. To maintain the same average concentration of the aminoglycoside in the elderly as in young adults, the dose may be reduced.

$$C_{av}^{\infty} = \frac{1.44D_N(t_{1/2})_N}{\tau_N V_N} = \frac{1.44D_0(t_{1/2})_0}{\tau_0 V_0}$$

$$\frac{D_N(t_{1/2})_N}{\tau_N} = \frac{D_0(t_{1/2})_0}{\tau_0}$$

Keeping the dose constant,

$$D_N = D_0$$

where D_N is the new dose, and D_0 is the old dose.

$$\frac{\tau_0}{\tau_N} = \frac{(t_{1/2})_0}{(t_{1/2})_N}$$

$$\tau_0 = 12 \times \frac{282}{107} = 31.6 \text{ hr}$$

Therefore, the same dose of the aminoglycoside may be administered every 32 hours without affecting the average steady-state level of the aminoglycoside.

2. The clearance of lithium was determined to be 41.5 mL/min in a group of patients with an average age of 25 years. In a group of elderly patients with an average age of 63 years, the clearance of lithium was 7.7 mL/min. What percentage of the normal dose of lithium should be given to a 65-year-old patient?

Solution

The dose should be proportional to clearance; therefore,

$$\text{Dose reductions (\%)} = \frac{7.7 \times 100}{41.5} = 18.5\%$$

The dose of lithium may be reduced to about 20% of the regular dose in the 65-year-old patient without affecting the steady-state blood level.

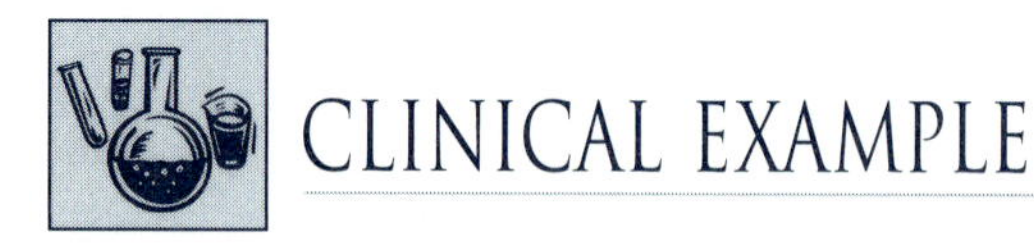

CLINICAL EXAMPLE

Hypertension is common in elderly patients. The pharmacokinetics of felodipine (Plendil), a calcium channel antagonist for hypertension was studied in young and elderly subjects. After a dose of 5 mg oral felodipine, the AUC and C_{max} in the elderly patients (67–79 yrs of age, mean wt = 71 kg) were found to be 3 times that of the young subjects (20–34 years of age, mean wt = 75 kg) as shown in Figure 17-1. Side effects of felodipine in the elderly patients, such as flushing, were reported in 9/11 subjects and palpitation in 3/11 subjects, whereas, only 1/12 of the young subjects reported side effects. Systemic clearance in the elderly was 248 ± 108 L/hr compared to 619 ± 214 L/hr in the young subjects. The bioavailability of felodipine was reported to be about 15.5% in the elderly and 15.3% in the young subjects. (Concomitant medications included a diuretic and beta-blocker.)

1. What is the main cause for the difference in the observed AUC between the elderly and young subjects?
2. What would be the steady-state level of felodipine in the elderly if dose and dosing interval are unchanged?
3. Can felodipine be given safely to elderly patients?

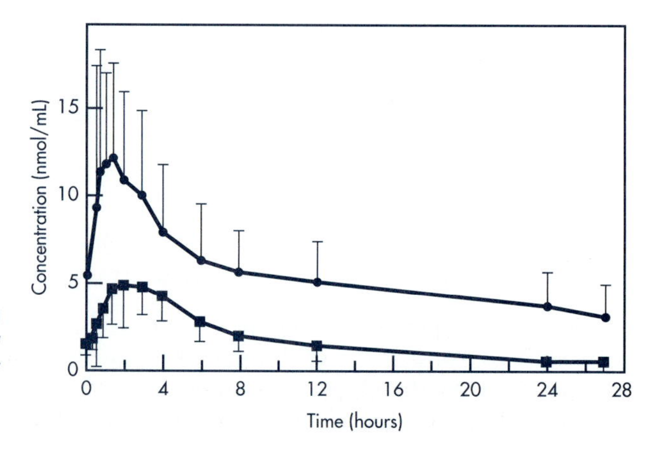

Figure 17-1. Plasma concentrations (mean ± SD) of felodipine after an oral dose during steady-state treatment with 5 mg twice daily in healthy subjects (n = 12) [■] and elderly hypertensive patients (n = 1) [●].
From Landahl et al, 1988, with permission.

Solution

1. The higher AUC in the elderly compared to young adults is due to the decreased drug clearance in the older subjects.
2. The elderly have more side effects with felodipine compared to young adults. Factors that may have increased side effects in the elderly could be due to (a) reduced hepatic blood flow, (b) potassium depletion in the body, (c) increased bioavailability or (d) reduced clearance.
3.

$$C_{av}^{\infty} = \frac{FD}{Cl_T} \tag{17.8}$$

If D, F, and T are the same, the steady-state drug concentration C_{av}^{∞} would be inversely proportional to clearance:

$$\frac{C_{av\ elderly}^{\infty}}{C_{av\ young}^{\infty}} = \frac{Cl_{young}}{Cl_{elderly}}$$

$$\frac{C_{av\ elderly}^{\infty}}{C_{av\ young}^{\infty}} = \frac{619}{248} = 2.5$$

(Note: Cl is in the denominator in Equation 17.8 and is inversely related to concentration.) The steady concentration of felodipine would be 250% or 2.5× that in the young subjects.

Changes in Renal Function with Age

Many studies have shown a general decline in glomerular filtration rate (GFR) with age (Lindeman, 1992). Lindeman (1992) reports that the GFR as measured by creatinine clearance (see Chapter 18) decreases at a mean rate of 1% per year after 40 years of age. However, there is considerable variation in this rate of decline in normal healthy aging adults. In one study by Lindeman et al (1985), approximately two-thirds of the subjects (162 of 254) had declining creatinine clearances, whereas, about one-third of the subjects (92 of 254) had no decrease in creatinine clearance. Since muscle mass and urinary creatinine excretion decrease at nearly the same rate in the elderly, mean serum concentrations may stay relatively constant. Creatinine clearance measured by serum creatinine concentrations only (see Chapter 18) may yield inaccurate GFR function if the urinary creatinine excretion is not measured.

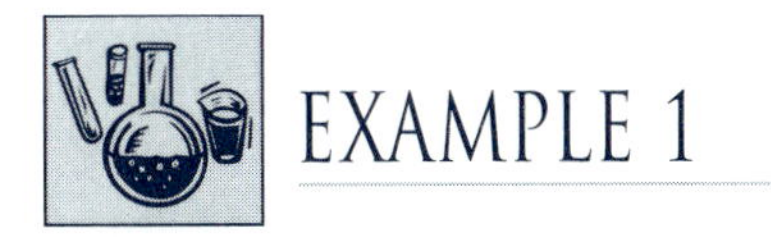

EXAMPLE 1

An elderly 85-yr-old adult patient with congestive heart failure has a serum creatinine of 1.0 mg/dL. The 24-hour urinary creatinine excretion was 0.7 gm. Based on the serum creatinine only, this patient has normal renal function, whereas, based on both serum creatinine concentration and total 24-hour urinary creatinine excretion, the patient has a GFR of less than 50 mL/min. In practice, serum creatinine clearance is often estimated from serum creatinine concentration alone for dose adjustment. In elderly subjects, the clinician should carefully assess the patient, since substantial deviation from the true clearance may occur in some elderly subjects.

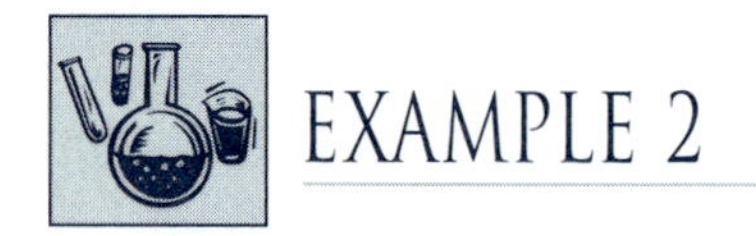

EXAMPLE 2

Diflunisal pharmacokinetics were studied in healthy young and old subjects. After a single dose of diflunisal, the terminal plasma half-life, mean residence time and apparent volume of distribution were higher in elderly subjects than in young adults (Erikson, 1989). This study shows that renal function in old subjects is generally reduced somewhat compared to younger patients due to diminished rate of glomerular filtration.

DOSING OF DRUGS IN THE OBESE PATIENT

The obese patient has a greater accumulation of fat tissue than necessary for normal body functions. The patient is considered obese if the actual body weight exceeds the ideal or desirable body weight by 20%, according to the Metropolitan Life Insurance data (latest published tables). In contrast, athletes who have a greater body weight due to greater muscle mass are not considered obese. Obesity sometimes is defined by *body mass index* (BMI), a value that normalizes body weight based on height. Adipose (fat) tissue has a smaller proportion of water compared to muscle tissue. Thus, the obese patient has a smaller proportion of total body water to total body weight compared to the patient with ideal body weight, which could affect the apparent volume of distribution of the drug. For example, Abernethy et al (1982) showed a significant difference in the apparent volume of distribution of antipyrine in obese patients (0.46 L/kg) compared to the ideal body weight patient (0.62 L/kg) based on actual total body weight. The *ideal body weight* (IBW) is a term that refers to the appropriate or normal weight for a male or female based on age, height, weight, and frame size; ideal body weights are generally obtained from the latest table of desirable weights for men and women compiled by the Metropolitan Life Insurance Company.

In addition to the differences in total body water per kilogram body weight in the obese patient, the greatest proportion of body fat in this patient could lead to distributional changes in the drug's pharmacokinetics due to partitioning of the drug between lipid and aqueous environments. Drugs such as digoxin and gentamicin are very polar and tend to distribute into water rather than into fat tissue. Other pharmacokinetic parameters may be altered in the obese patient due to possible physiologic alterations, such as fatty infiltration of the liver affecting biotransformation and cardiovascular changes that may affect renal blood flow and renal excretion (Abernethy and Greenblatt, 1982).

Dosing by actual body weight may result in overdose for drugs such as the aminoglycosides (eg, gentamicin) that are very polar and are distributed in extracellular fluids. Dosing for these drugs is based on ideal body weight. *Lean body weight* has been estimated by several empirical equations based on the patient's height and actual (total) body weight. The following equations have been used for estimating lean body weight, particularly for adjustment of dosage in renally impaired patients.

$$\text{LBW (males)} = 50\text{ kg} + 2.3\text{ kg for each inch over 5 ft} \quad \textbf{(17.9)}$$

$$\text{LBW (females)} = 45.5\text{ kg} + 2.3\text{ kg for each inch over 5 ft} \quad \textbf{(17.10)}$$

where LBW is lean body weight.

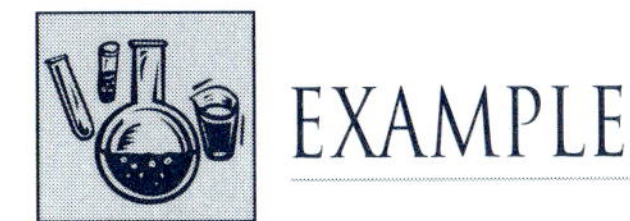

EXAMPLE

Calculate the lean body weight for an adult male patient who is 5 ft 9 in (175.3 cm) tall and weighs 264 lb (120 kg).

Solution

Using Equation 17.8:

$$\text{LBW} = 50 + (2.3 \times 9) = 70.7\text{ kg}$$

PHARMACOKINETICS OF DRUG INTERACTIONS

A *drug interaction* generally refers to a modification of the expected drug response in the patient, due to exposure of the patient to another drug or substance. Some unintentional drug interactions produce adverse reactions in the patient, whereas some drug interactions may be intentional to provide an improved therapeutic response or to decrease adverse drug effects. Drug interactions may include *drug–drug interactions, food–drug interactions* or *chemical–drug interactions*, such as the interaction of a drug with alcohol or tobacco. A listing of food interactions is given in Chapter 5. A *drug–laboratory* test interaction pertains to an alteration in a diagnostic laboratory test results due to the drug.

The risk of a drug interaction increases with multiple drug therapy, multiple prescribers, poor patient compliance, and patient risk factors, such as a predisposing illness (diabetes, hypertension, etc), or advancing age. Use of multiple drugs for therapy are routine in most acute and chronic care settings. Elderly patients and patients with various predisposing illnesses tend to be a population using multiple drug therapy. A recent student survey found an average of 8 to 12 drugs per patient used in a group of hospital patients.

Screening for drug interactions should be performed whenever multiple drug uses are involved. Many computer programs will "flag" a potential drug interaction.

However, the pharmacist needs to determine the clinical significance of the interaction. The determination of the clinical significance of a potential drug interaction should be documented in the literature. The likelihood of a drug interaction may be classified as an established drug interaction, probable drug interaction, possible drug interaction, or unlikely drug interaction. The size of the dose and the duration of therapy, the onset (rapid, delayed), and severity (major, minor) of the potential interaction, and the extrapolation to related drugs should also be considered.

Preferably, drugs that interact should be avoided or given sufficiently far apart so that the interaction is minimized. In situations involving two drugs of choice that may interact, dose adjustment based on pharmacokinetic and therapeutic considerations of one or both of the drugs in question may be necessary. Dose adjustment may be based on clearance or elimination half-life of the drug. Assessment of the patient's renal function, such as serum creatinine concentration, and liver function indicators, such as alkaline phosphatase, alanine aminotransferase (ALT), aspartate aminotransferase (AST) or other markers of hepatic metabolism (Chapter 18) should be undertaken. In general, if the therapeutic response is predictable from serum drug concentration, dosing at regular intervals may be based on a steady-state concentration equation such as Equation 17.1. When the elimination half-life is changed due to drug interaction, the dosing interval may be extended or the dose reduced according to Equation 17.4. Some examples of pharmacokinetic drug interactions are listed in Table 17.10. A more complete discussion of pharmacologic and therapeutic drug interactions of drugs is available in standard textbooks on clinical pharmacology.

Some examples of pharmacokinetic drug interactions are discussed in more detail below. Many side effects occur as a result of impaired drug metabolism. The changes in pharmacokinetics due to impaired drug metabolism should be evalu-

TABLE 17.10 Pharmacokinetic Drug Interactions

DRUG INTERACTION	EXAMPLES (PRECIPITANT DRUGS)	EFFECT (OBJECT DRUGS)
Bioavailability		
Complexation/chelation	Calcium, magnesium or aluminum and iron salts	Tetracycline complexes with divalent cations, causing a decreased bioavailability
Adsorption binding/ionic interaction	Cholestyramine resin (anion exchange resin binding)	Decreased bioavailability of Thyroxine, and digoxin; binds anionic drugs and reduces absorption
Adsorption	Antacids (adsorption)	Decreased bioavailability of antibiotics
	Charcoal, Antidiarrheals	Decreased bioavailability of many drugs
Increased GI motility	Laxatives, cathartics	Increases GI motility, decreases bioavailability for drugs which are absorbed slowly; may also affect the bioavailability of drugs from controlled release products
Decreased GI motility	Anticholinergic agents	Propantheline decreases the gastric emptying of acetaminophen (APAP) delaying APAP absorption from the small intestine
Alteration of gastric pH	H-2 blockers, antacids	Both H-2 blockers and antacids increase gastric pH; the dissolution of ketoconazole is reduced causing decreased drug absorption

TABLE 17.10 Pharmacokinetic Drug Interactions (continued)

DRUG INTERACTION	EXAMPLES (PRECIPITANT DRUGS)	EFFECT (OBJECT DRUGS)
Alteration of intestinal flora	Antibiotics (eg, tetracyclines, penicillin)	Digoxin has better bioavailability after erythromycin; erythromycin administration reduces bacterial inactivation of digoxin.
Inhibition of drug metabolism in intestinal cells	Monoamine oxidase inhibitors (MAO-I) (eg tranylcypromine, phenelzine)	Hypertensive crisis may occur in patients treated with MAO-I and foods containing tyramine
Distribution		
Protein binding	Warfarin–phenylbutazone	Displacement of warfarin from binding
	Phenytoin–valproic acid	Displacement of phenytoin from binding
Hepatic Elimination		
Enzyme induction	Smoking (polycyclic aromatic hydrocarbons)	Smoking increase theophylline clearance
	Barbiturates	Phenobarbital increases the metabolism of warfarin
Enzyme inhibition Mixed-function oxidase	Cimetidine	Decreased theophylline, diazepam metabolism
	Fluvoxamine	Diazepam $t_{1/2}$ longer
	Quinidine	Decreased nifedipine metabolism
	Fluconazole	Increased levels of phenytoin, warfarin
Other enzymes	Monoamine oxidase inhibitors, MAO-I (eg, pargyline, tranylcypromine)	Serious hypertensive crisis may occur following ingestion of foods with a high content of tyramine or other pressor substances (eg, cheddar cheese, red wines)
Inhibition of biliary secretion	Verapamil	Decreased biliary secretion of digoxin causing increased digoxin levels
Renal Clearance		
Glomerular filtration rate (GFR) and renal blood flow	Methylxanthines (eg, caffeine, theobromine)	Increased renal blood flow and GFR will decrease time for reabsorption of various drugs leading to more rapid urinary drug excretion
Active tubular secretion	Probenecid	Probenecid blocks the active tubular secretion of penicillin and some cephalosporin antibiotics
Tubular reabsorption and urine pH	Antacids, sodium bicarbonate	Alkalinization of the urine increases the reabsorption of amphetamine and decreases its clearance Alkalinization of urine pH increases the ionization of salicylates, decreases reabsorption and increases its clearance.
Diet		
Charcoal hamburgers	Theophylline	Elimination half-life of theophylline decreases due to increased metabolism
Grapefruit	Terfenadine, cyclosporin	Blood levels of terfenadine and cyclosporine increase due to decreased metabolism
Virus Drug Interactions		
Reye's syndrome	Aspirin	Aspirin in children exposed to certain viral infections such as influenza B virus leads to Reye's syndrome

ated quantitatively. For example, acetaminophen is an OTC drug safely used for decades, but incidences of severe hepatic toxicity leading to coma have occurred in some subjects with impaired liver function due to chronic alcohol use. Drugs that have reactive intermediates, active metabolites, and or metabolites with longer half-life than the parent drug need to be considered carefully if there is a potential for a drug interaction. A polar metabolite may also distribute to a smaller fluid volume, leading to high concentration in some tissues. Many drugs share common metabolic pathways for the same liver enzyme so that the administration of one drug affects the rate of metabolism of the other drug. Drug interactions involving metabolism may be *temporal*, observed as a delayed effect. Temporal drug interactions are more difficult to detect in a clinical situation.

INHIBITION OF DRUG METABOLISM

Numerous clinical instances of severe adverse reactions as a result of drug interaction involving a change in the rate of drug metabolism have been reported. Knowledge of pharmacokinetics allows the clinical pharmacist to evaluate the clinical significance of the drug interaction. Pharmacokinetic models help to determine the need for dose reduction or discontinuing a drug. In assessing the situation, the pathophysiology of the patient and the effect of chronic therapy on drug disposition in the patient must be considered. A severe drug reaction in a patient with liver impairment has resulted in near fatal reaction in subjects taking otherwise safe doses of acetaminophen. In some patients with injury or severe cardiovascular disease, blood flow may be impaired resulting in delayed drug absorption and distribution. Many incidences of serious toxicity or accidents are caused by the premature administration of a "booster dose" when the expected response is not immediately observed. Potent drugs such as morphine, midazolam, lidocaine, pentothal, and fentenyl can result in serious adverse reactions if the kinetics of multiple dosing is not carefully assessed.

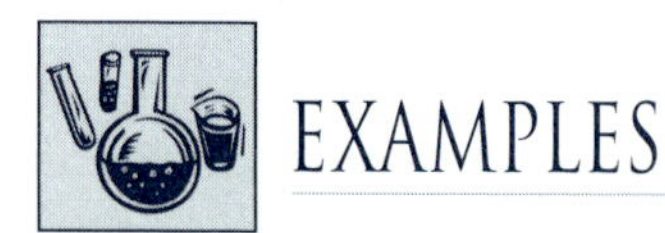

EXAMPLES

Inhibition of Drug Metabolism

1. Fluvoxamine Doubles the Half-Life of Diazepam
The effect of fluvoxamine on the pharmacokinetics of diazepam was investigated in healthy volunteers. Concurrent fluvoxamine intake increased mean peak plasma diazepam concentrations from 108 to 143 ng/mL, oral diazepam clearance was reduced from 0.40 to 0.14 mL/min/kg. The half-life of diazepam increased from 51 to 118 hours. The area under the plasma concentration time curve values for the diazepam metabolite, *N*-desmethyldiazepam were also significantly increased during fluvoxamine treatment. These data suggest that fluvoxamine inhibits the biotransformation of diazepam and its active *N*-demethylated metabolite (Perucca et al, 1994).

In this example, the dosing interval, τ may be increased to twofold to account for the doubling of elimination half-life to keep average steady-state concentration unchanged based on Equation 17.4. The rationale for this recommendation may be demonstrated by sketching a diagram showing how the steady-state plasma drug level of diazepam differs after taking 10 mg orally twice a day with or without taking fluvoxamine for a week.

$$C_{\mathrm{av}}^{\infty} = \frac{1.44 D_0 t_{1/2} F}{V_{\mathrm{D}} \tau}$$

2. Quinidine Inhibits the Metabolism of Nifedipine and Other Calcium Channel Blocking Agents

Quinidine coadministration significantly inhibited the aromatization of nifedipine to its major first-pass pyridine metabolite and prolonged the elimination half-life by about 40%. The interaction between quinidine and nifedipine supports the involvement of a common cytochrome P450 (P450IIIA4) in the metabolism of the two drugs (Schellens et al, 1991). Other calcium channel antagonists may also be affected by a similar interaction.

What other drugs are metabolized by CYP3A4? (See Chapter 13.) What could be a potential problem if two drugs metabolized by the same isozyme are coadministered?

3. Theophylline Clearance Decreased by Cimetidine

Controlled studies have shown that cimetidine can decrease theophylline plasma clearance by 20 to 40% (apparently by inhibiting demethylation). Prolongation of half-life by as much as 70% was found in some patients. Elevated theophylline plasma concentrations with toxicity may lead to nausea, vomiting, cardiovascular instability, and even seizure.

What could happen to an asthmatic patient whose meals are high in protein and low in carbohydrate, and who takes Tagamet 400 mg bid? (Hint: check the effect of food on theophylline below.)

4. Beta-Interferon Reduces Metabolism of Theophylline

Theophylline pharmacokinetics were also examined before and after interferon treatment. Interferon beta treatment reduced the activities of both O-dealkylases by 47%. The total body clearance of theophylline was also decreased (from 0.76 to 0.56 mL/kg/min) and its elimination half-life was increased (from 8.4 to 11.7 hr; $P < 0.05$). This study provides the first direct evidence that interferon beta can depress the activity of drug-metabolizing enzymes in the human liver (Okuno et al, 1993).

What percent of steady-state theophylline plasma concentration would be changed due to the interaction? (Use Equation 17.8.)

5. Erythromycin and Terfenadine (Seldane) Interaction

Erythromycin can reduce hepatic metabolism of terfenadine leading to fatal cardiac toxicity in some subjects due to high levels of terfenadine. The active metabolite of terfenadine is not cardiac toxic and is now marked as fexofenadine (Allegra), a nonsedative antihistamine.

6. Cimetidine and Diazepam Interaction

The administration of 800 mg of cimetidine daily for 1 week increased the steady-state plasma diazepam and nordiazepam concentrations due to a cimetidine-induced impairment in microsomal oxidation of diazepam and nordiazepam. The concurrent administration of cimetidine caused a decrease in total metabolic clearance of diazepam and its metabolite, nordiazepam (Lima et al, 1991).

How would the following pharmacokinetic parameters of diazepam be affected due to coadministration of cimetidine?

a. Areas under the curve in the dose intervals (AUC_{0-24h})
b. Maximum plasma concentrations (C_{max})
c. Time to peak concentrations ($t_{1/2}$)
d. Elimination rate constant (k)
e. Total body clearance, Cl

INHIBITION OF BILIARY EXCRETION

The interaction between digoxin and verapamil (Hedman et al, 1991) was studied in six patients (mean age: 61 ± 5 years) with chronic atrial fibrillation. The effects of adding verapamil (240 mg/day) on steady-state plasma concentrations of digoxin were studied. Verapamil induced a 44% increase in steady-state plasma concentrations of digoxin. The biliary clearance of digoxin was determined by a duodenal perfusion technique. The biliary clearance of digoxin decreased by 43%, from 187 ± 89 to 101 ± 55 mL/min, whereas the renal clearance was not significantly different (153 ± 31 versus 173 ± 51 mL/min).

INDUCTION OF DRUG METABOLISM

Cytochrome P450 isozymes are often involved in the metabolic oxidation of many drugs (Chapter 13). Many drugs can stimulate the production of hepatic enzymes. Therapeutic dose of phenobarbital and other barbiturates accelerate the metabolism of coumarin anticoagulants such as warfarin and substantially reduce the hypoprothrombinemic effect. Fatal hemorrhagic episodes can result when phenobarbital is withdrawn and warfarin dosage maintained at its previous level. Other drugs known to stimulate drug metabolism include carbamazepine, rifampin, valproic acid and phenytoin. Enzymatic stimulation can shorten the elimination half life of the affected. For example, phenobarbital can result in lower level of dexamethasone in asthmatic patients taking both drugs.

ALTERED RENAL REABSORPTION DUE TO CHANGING URINARY PH

The normal adult urinary pH ranges from 4.8 to 7.5 but can increase due to chronic antacids. This change in urinary pH affects the ionization and reabsorption of weak electrolyte drugs (Chapter 12). An increased ionization of salicylate due to an increase in urine pH reduces salicylate reabsorption in the renal tubule resulting in an increased renal excretion. Magnesium aluminum hydroxide gel (Maalox) 120 mL/day for 6 days decreased serum salicylate levels from 19.8 mg/dL to 15.8 mg/dL in six subjects who had achieved a control serum salicylate level of >10 mg/dL with the equivalent of 3.76 g/day aspirin (Hansten et al, 1980). Single doses of magnesium aluminum hydroxide gel did not alter urine pH significantly. Five mL Titralac (calcium carbonate with glycine) 4 times a day or magnesium hydroxide for 7 days also increased urinary pH. In general, drugs with pKa values within the urinary pH range are affected the most. Basic drugs tend to have longer half-lives when urinary pH is increased, especially near its pKa.

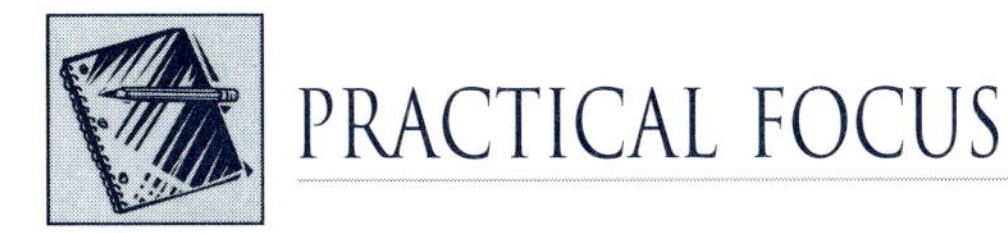

PRACTICAL FOCUS

Which of the following treatments would be most likely to decrease the $t_{1/2}$ of aspirin?

1. calcium carbonate PO

2. sodium carbonate PO

3. IV sodium bicarbonate

(Hint: Which drug can be absorbed and change urinary pH and the reabsorption of aspirin?)

INHIBITION OF DRUG ABSORPTION

Various drugs and dietary supplements can decrease the absorption of drugs from the gastrointestinal tract. Antacids containing magnesium and aluminum hydroxide often interfere with absorption of many drugs. Coadministration of magnesium and aluminum hydroxide caused a decrease of plasma levels of perfloxacin. The drug interaction is caused by the formation of chelate complexes and is possibly also due to adsorption of the quinolone to aluminum hydroxide gel. Perfloxacin should be given at least 2 hours before the antacid to ensure sufficient therapeutic efficacy of the quinolone.

Sucralfate is an aluminum glycopyranoside complex that is not absorbed but retards the oral absorption of ciprofloxacin. Sucralfate is used in the local treatment of ulcers. Cholestyramine is an anion exchange resin that binds bile acid and many drugs in the GI tract. Cholestyramine can bind digitoxin in the gastrointestinal tract and shorten the elimination half-life of digitoxin by approximately 30 to 40%. Absorption of thyroxine may be reduced by 50% when administered closely with cholestyramine.

EFFECT OF FOOD ON DRUG DISPOSITION

1. Diet Theophylline Interaction

Theophylline disposition is influenced by diet. A protein-rich diet will increase theophylline clearance. Average theophylline half-lives in subjects on a low carbohydrate-high protein diet increased from 5.2 to 7.6 hours when subjects were changed to a high carbohydrate-low protein diet. A diet of charcoal-broiled beef which contains polycyclic aromatic hydrocarbons from the charcoal resulted in a decrease in theophylline half-life of up to 42% when compared to a control non-charcoal-broiled beef diet. Irregular intake of vitamin K may modify the anticoagulant effect of warfarin. Many foods, especially green, leafy vegetables, such as broccoli and spinach, contain high concentrations of vitamin K. In one study, warfarin therapy was interfered with in patients receiving vitamin K, broccoli, or spinach daily for 1 week (Pedersen et al, 1991).

2. Grapefruit Drug Interactions

Recent investigations have shown that the ingredients in a common food product, grapefruit juice, taken in usual dietary quantities can significantly inhibit the metabolism of gut wall cytochrome P450 3A4 (CYP3A4) (Spence, 1997). For example, grapefruit juice increases average felodipine levels about 3-fold, increases cyclosporine levels and increases the levels of terfenadine, a common antihistamine. In the case of terfenadine, Spence (1997) reported a death of a 29-year-old male who had been taking terfenadine and drinking grapefruit juice 2 to 3 times per week. Death was attributed to terfenadine toxicity.

ADVERSE VIRAL DRUG INTERACTIONS

Recent findings have suggested that some interactions of viruses and drugs may predispose individuals to specific disease outcomes (Haverkos et al, 1991). For example, Reye's syndrome has been observed in children who have been taking aspirin and were concurrently exposed to certain viruses, including influenza B virus and varicella-zoster virus. The mechanism by which salicylates and certain viruses interact is not clear. However, the publication of this interaction has led to the prevention of morbidity and mortality due to this complex interaction (Haverkos et al, 1991).

POPULATION PHARMACOKINETICS

Introduction to Bayesian Theory

Bayesian theory was originally developed to improve forecast accuracy by combining subjective prediction with improvement from newly collected data. In the diagnosis of disease, the physician may make a preliminary diagnosis based on symptoms and physical examination. Later, the results of the laboratory tests are received. The clinician then makes a new diagnostic forecast based on both sets of information. Bayesian theory provides a method to weigh the prior information (eg, physical diagnosis) and new information (eg, results from laboratory tests) to estimate a new probability for predicting the disease.

In developing a drug dosage regimen, we assess the patient's medical history and then use average pharmacokinetic parameters appropriate for the patient's condition to calculate the initial dose. After the initial dose, plasma or serum drug concentrations are obtained from the patient providing new information to assess the adequacy of the dosage. The dosing approach of combining old information with new involves a "feedback" process and is, in some degree, inherent in many dosing methods involving some parameter readjustment when new serum drug concentrations become known. The advantage of the Bayesian approach is the improvement in estimating the patient's pharmacokinetic parameter based on Bayesian probability versus an ordinary least-squares-based program. An example comparing the Bayesian method with an alternative method for parameter estimation from some simulated theophylline data will be shown in the next section. The method is particularly useful when only a few blood samples are available.

Due to inter- and intrasubject variability, the pharmacokinetic parameters of an individual patient must be estimated from limited data in the presence of unknown random error (assays, etc), known covariates and variables such as clearance, weight, and disease factor, etc, and possible structural (kinetic model) error. From knowledge of the mean population pharmacokinetic parameters and their variability, the Bayesian methods often employ a special *weighted least-squares* (WLS) approach and allow an improved estimation of the patient pharmacokinetic parameter when there is a lot of variation in data. The methodology is discussed in more detail under the Bayes estimator in the next section and also under pharmacokinetic analysis.

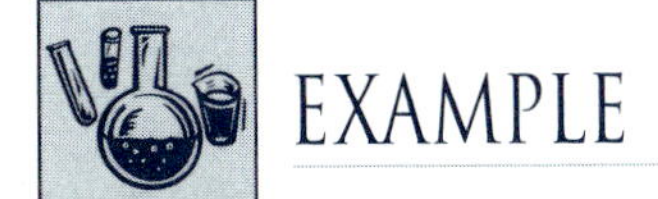

EXAMPLE

After diagnosing a patient, the physician gave the patient a probability of 0.4 for having a disease. The physician then ordered a clinical laboratory test. A positive laboratory test value has a probability of 0.8 of positively identifying the disease in patients with the disease (*true positive*) and a probability of 0.1 of positive identification of the disease in subjects without the disease (*false positive*). From the prior information (physician's diagnosis) and current patient-specific data (laboratory test), what is the *posterior probability* of the patient having the disease using the Bayesian method?

Solution

Prior probability of having the disease = 0.4
Prior probability of not having the disease = 1 − 0.4 = 0.6

Ratio of disease positive/disease negative = 0.4/0.6 = 2/3, or, the physician's evaluation shows a 2/3 chance for the presence and absence of the disease.

The probabilities for a positive laboratory test of 0.8 and 0.1 for the detection of disease in positive patients (with disease) and negative patient (without disease) are equal to a ratio of 0.8/0.1 or 8/1. This ratio is known as the *likelihood ratio.* Combining the prior probability, the posterior probability ratio is

Posterior probability ratio = (2/3)(8/1) = 16/3
Posterior probability = 16/(16 + 3) = 84.2%

Thus, the laboratory test that estimates the likelihood ratio and the preliminary diagnostic evaluation are both used in determining the posterior probability. The results of this calculation show that with a positive diagnosis by the physician *and* a positive value for the laboratory test, the probability that the patient actually has the disease is 84.2%.

The Bayes probability theory when applied to dosing of a drug involves a given pharmacokinetic parameter (P) and plasma or serum drug concentration (C), which is shown in Equation 17–11.

The probability of the patient with a given pharmacokinetic parameter P taking into account the measured concentration is Prob $(P|C)$:

$$\text{Prob }(P|C) = \frac{\text{Prob }(P)^{\circ}\text{ Prob }(C|P)}{\text{Prob }(C)} \qquad \textbf{(17.11)}$$

Prob (P) = the probability of the patient's parameter within the assumed population distribution, Prob $(C|P)$ = the probability of measured concentration within the population, Prob (C) = the unconditional probability of the observed concentration.

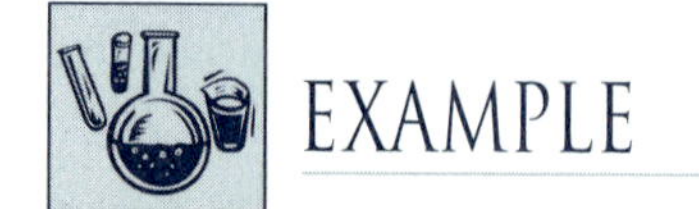

EXAMPLE

Theophylline has a therapeutic window of 10 to 20 μg/mL. Serum theophylline concentrations above 20 μg/mL produces mild side effects, such as nausea and insomnia; more serious side effects, such as sinus tachycardia, may occur at drug concentrations above 40 μg/mL; at serum concentration above 45 μg/mL, cardiac arrhythmia and seizure may occur (Figure 17-2). However, the probability of some side effect occurring is by no means certain. Side effects are not solely determined by plasma concentration as other known or unknown variables (called covariates) may affect the side effect outcome. Some patients have initial side effects of nausea and restlessness (even at very low drug concentrations) that later disappear when therapy is continued. The clinician would therefore assess the probability of side effects in the patient, order a blood sample for serum theophylline determination and then estimate a combined (or posterior) probability for side effects in the patient.

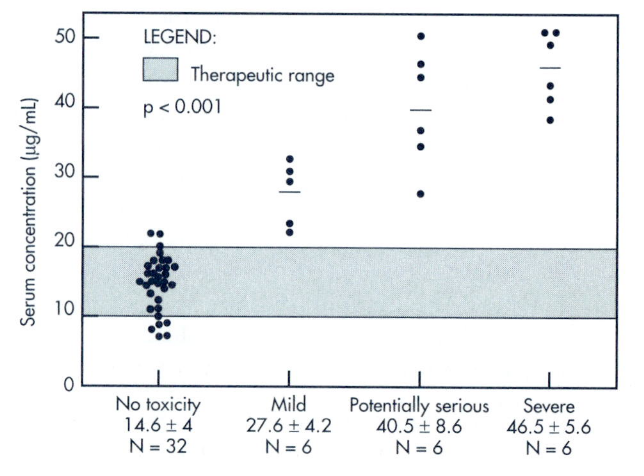

Figure 17-2. Correlation between the frequency and severity of adverse effects and plasma concentration of theophylline (mean ± SD) in 50 adult patients. Mild symptoms of toxicity included nausea, vomiting, headache, and insomnia: a potentially serious effect was sinus tachycardia, and severe toxicity was defined as the occurrence of life-threatening cardiac arrhythmias and seizures. Adapted from Hendeles and Weinberger, 1980, with permission.

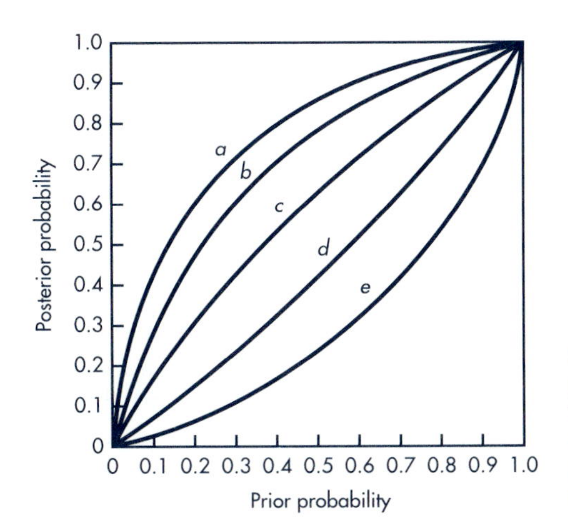

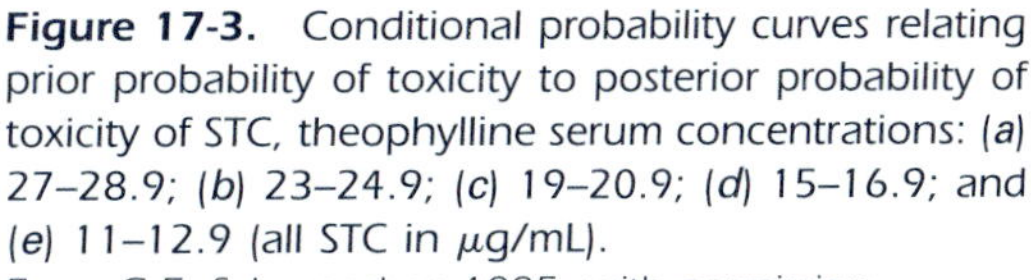

Figure 17-3. Conditional probability curves relating prior probability of toxicity to posterior probability of toxicity of STC, theophylline serum concentrations: (*a*) 27–28.9; (*b*) 23–24.9; (*c*) 19–20.9; (*d*) 15–16.9; and (*e*) 11–12.9 (all STC in μg/mL).
From G.E. Schumacher, 1995, with permission.

The decision process is illustrated graphically in Figure 17-3. The probability of initial (prior) estimation of side effects is plotted on the *x*-axis, and the final (posterior) probability of side effects is on the *y*-axis for various serum theophylline concentrations. For example, a patient was placed on theophylline, and the physician estimated the chance of side effects to be 40%, but TDM shows a theophylline level of 27 μg/mL. A vertical line of prior probability at 0.4 intersects curve A at about 0.78 or 78%. Hence, the Bayesian probability of having side effects is 78% by taking both the laboratory and physician assessments into consideration. The curves (*a* to *e* in Fig. 17-3) for various theophylline concentrations are called conditional probability curves. Bayesian theory does not replace clinical judgment but gives a quantitative tool for incorporating subjective judgment (human) with objective (laboratory assay) in making risk decisions. When complex decisions involving several variables are involved, this objective tool can be very useful.

Bayesian probability is used to improve forecasting in medicine. One example is its use in the diagnosis of healed myocardial infarction (HMI) from a 12-lead electrocardiogram (ECG) by artificial neural networks using the Bayesian concept. Bayesian results were comparable to those of the experienced electrocardiographer (Heden et al, 1996). In pharmacokinetics, Bayesian theory is applied to "feed forward neural networks" for gentamicin concentration predictions (Smith, Brier, 1996). A brief literature search of Bayesian applications revealed over 400 therapeutic applications between 1992 to 1996. Bayesian parameter estimations were most frequently used for drugs with narrow therapeutic ranges such as the aminoglycosides, cyclosporin, digoxin, anticonvulsants (especially phenytoin), lithium, and theophylline. The technique has now been extended to cytotoxic drugs, factor VIII and warfarin. Bayesian methods have also been used to limit the number of samples required in more conventional pharmacokinetic studies with new drugs (Thomson and Whiting, 1992). The main disadvantage of Bayesian methods is the subjective selection of prior probability. Therefore, it is not considered to be unbiased by many statisticians for drug approval purposes.

Adaptive Method or Dosing with Feedback

In dosing drugs with narrow therapeutic ratios, an initial dose is calculated based on mean population pharmacokinetic parameters. After dosing, plasma drug concentrations are obtained from the patient. As more blood samples are drawn from the patient, the calculated individualized patient pharmacokinetic parameters will become increasingly more reliable. This type of approach has been referred to as adaptive, or *Bayesian adaptive method* with feedback when a spacial extended least-squares algorithm is used. Many ordinary least-squares computer software packages are available in clinical practice for parameter and dosage calculation. Some software packages record medical history and provide adjustments for weight, age, and in some cases, disease factors. A common approach is to estimate the clearance and volume of distribution from intermittent infusion (see Chapter 14). Abbottbase Pharmacokinetic Systems (1986 and 1988) is an example of a patient-oriented software that records patient information and dosing history based on 24-hour clock time. An adaptive-type algorithm is used to estimate pharmacokinetic parameters. The average population clearance and volume of distribution of drugs are used for initial estimates and the program computes patient-specific Cl and V_D as serum drug concentrations are entered. The program accounts for renal dysfunction based on creatinine clearance which is estimated from serum creatinine concentration using the Cockroft-Gault equation (see Chapter 18). The software package allows specific parameter estimation for digoxin, theophylline, and aminoglycosides, although other drugs can also be manually analyzed.

Many least-squares (LS) and weighted-least-squares (WLS) algorithms are available for estimating patient pharmacokinetic parameters. Their common objective involves estimating the parameters with minimum bias and good prediction, often as evaluated by mean predictive error. The advantage of the Bayesian method is the ability to input known information into the program, so that the search for the real pharmacokinetic parameter is more efficient and, perhaps, more precise.

For example, a drug is administered by intravenous infusion at a rate, R to a patient. The drug is infused over t hours (t may be 0.5 to 2 hours for a typical infusion). The patient's clearance, *Cl*, may be estimated from a plasma drug concentration taken at known time later according to a one-compartment model equation. Sheiner and Beal (1982) simulated a set of theophylline data and estimated pa-rameters from the data using one- and two-serum concentrations, assuming different variability. These investigators tested the method with a Bayesian approach and with an *ordinary least-squares method*, OBJ_{OLS}.

$$C_i = f(P, t_i) + \epsilon_i \tag{17.12}$$

$$OBJ_{OLS} = \sum_{i=1}^{n} (C_i - \hat{C}_i)^2/\sigma_i^2 \tag{17.13}$$

The Bayes Estimator

When the pharmacokinetic parameter P is estimated from a set of plasma drug concentration data (C_i) having several potential sources of error with different variance, the ordinary least-squares (OLS) method for parameter estimation is no longer adequate (yield trivial estimates). The intersubject variation, intrasubject variance and random error must be minimized properly to allow a condition for efficient parameter estimation. The weighted least-squares function in Equation 17.14 was suggested by Sheiner and Beal (1982). The equation represents the least-squares estimation of the concentration by minimizing deviation squares (first summation term of Eq. 17.14), and deviation of population parameter squares (second summation term). Equation 17.14 is termed the *Bayes estimator.* This approach is frequently referred to as extended least-squares (ELS).

$$\text{Intrasubject} \quad C_i = f(P, X_i) + \epsilon_i$$
$$\text{Intersubject} \quad P_k = \hat{P}_k + \eta_k$$
$$\text{OBJ}_{\text{BAYES}} = \sum_{i=1}^{n} (C_i - \hat{C}_i)^2/\sigma_i^2 + \sum_{k=1}^{s} (P_k - \hat{P}_k)^2/\omega_k^2 \qquad \textbf{(17.14)}$$

For n number of drug plasma concentration data, i is an index to refer to each data item, C_i is the ith concentration, $\hat{C}_i$ is the ith model-estimated concentration, and σ^2 is the variance of random error, ϵ_i (assays errors, random intrasubject variation, etc). There is a series of population parameters in the model for the kth population parameter, P_k, $\hat{P}_k$ is the estimated population parameter and η_k is the kth parameter random error with variance of ω_k^2.

To compare the performance of the Bayesian method versus other methods in drug dosing, Sheiner and Beal (1982) generated some theophylline plasma drug concentrations based on known clearance. They added various error levels to the data and divided the patients into groups with one and two plasma drug samples. The two pharmacokinetic parameters used were based on population pharmacokinetics for theophylline derived from the literature: (1) for P_1, a V_D of 0.5 L/kg and coefficient of variation of 32%; and (2) for P_2, clearance of 0.052 L/kg/hr and coefficient of variation of 44%.

The data were then analyzed using the Bayesian method and a second (alternative) approach in determining the pharmacokinetic parameter (Cl). In the presence of various levels of error, the Bayesian approach was robust and resulted in better estimation of clearance in both the one- and two-sample group (Fig. 17-4 and Table 17.11). The success of the Bayesian approach is due to the ability of the

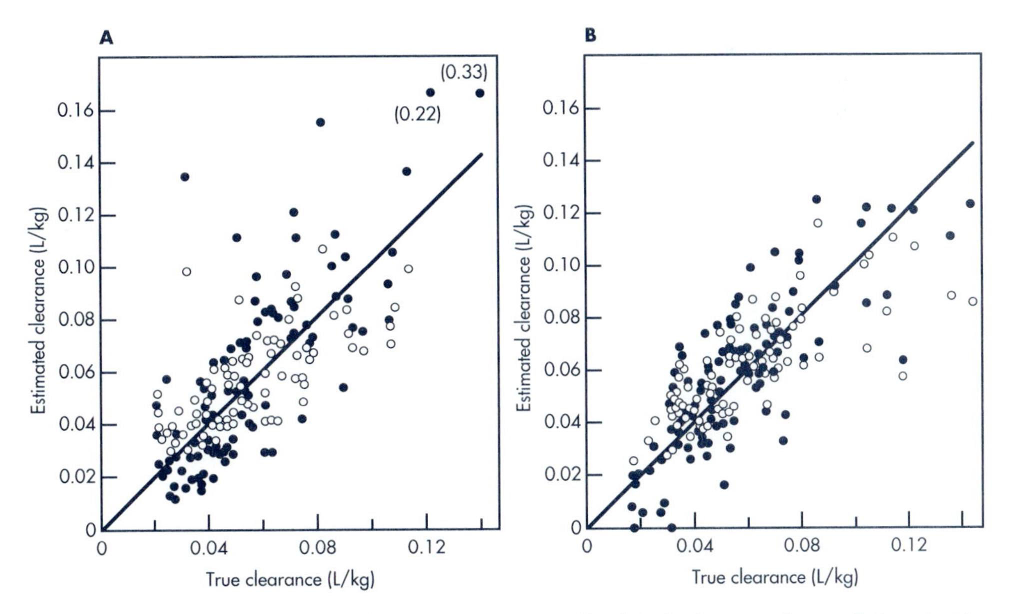

Figure 17-4. Plots of predicted clearance versus true (simulated) clearance for predictions by the Bayesian (○) and alternative (●) methods. The diagonal line on each graph is the line of identity. **A** shows results for one-sample group; **B** shows results for two-sample group.
(From Sheiner and Beal, 1982, with permission.)

TABLE 17.11 Performance of Clearance Estimation Methods

METHOD	$\frac{\omega_{Cl}{}^{a}}{\sigma}$	$\frac{\omega_{V_D}{}^{a}}{\sigma}$	MEAN CLEARANCE ERROR (±SEM) AS PERCENT OF MEAN CLEARANCE: ERROR, Example 1	ERROR, Example 2	ABSOLUTE ERROR, Example 1	ABSOLUTE ERROR, Example 2
Alternative	—	—	−5.77(5.8)	−2.82(3.3)	37.1(4.5)	26.4(2.1)
Bayesian	1	1	−1.02(3.0)	−1.08(3.1)	22.2(2.0)[b]	21.7(2.2)[b]
	3/2	1	−4.94(3.4)	−3.77(3.0)	25.6(2.3)[b]	23.1(2.1)[b]
	2/3	1	5.02(3.2)	2.52(3.4)	23.7(2.2)[b]	23.5(2.4)
	1	3/2	0.44(3.0)	−0.26(3.1)	22.5(2.1)[b]	21.4(2.2)[b]
	1	2/3	−0.76(3.0)	−1.56(3.1)	22.5(1.9)[b]	21.7(2.2)

[a]Ratio of standard deviation of clearance (or V_D) to σ used in the Bayesian method. All ratios are divided by the correct ratio so that a value of unity signifies that the correct ratio itself was used.
[b]Mean absolute error of Bayesian method less than that of alternative ($P < .05$).

From Sheiner and Beal (1982), with permission.

algorithm to minimize the total mean square terms of errors. A more precise clearance estimation would lead to more accurate dose estimation in the patient.

The implementation of the Bayesian (ELS) approach uses the NONMEM computer software, facilitated by a response criteria defined through a first-order (FO) Taylor series expansion. Among other computer software packages available, the NPME2 (USC*PACK) is a nonparametric maximum expectation maximization method that makes no parametric assumptions about the mean and standard deviation of the distribution. The program can also discover unrecognized subpopulations. The new NONMEM also features FOEM, a first-order expectation maximization method. Generally, finding a set of best parameter estimates to describe the data involves minimizing the error terms; alternatively, another paradigm that maximizes the probability of the parameter estimates in the distribution serves the same purpose equally well or better. Thus, the first-order expectation maximization (FOEM) paradigm is also available in the present NONMEM and in other programs, such as the P-PHARM (Mentre and Gomeni, 1995).

Comparison of Bayes, Least-Squares, Steady-State, and Chiou Methods

For theophylline dosing, the Bayes method and others, including the conventional steady-state method, were compared by Hurley and McNeil (1988). The Bayes method compared favorably with other methods (Table 17.12 and 17.13). The steady-state method was also useful, but none of the methods was sufficiently accurate, probably due to other variables, such as saturation kinetics or use of an inappropriate compartment model.

Model fitting in pharmacokinetics often involves the search for a set of parameters that fits the data, a situation analogous to finding a point within a large geometrical space. The ordinary least-squares (OLS) approach of iteratively minimizing the error terms may not be adequate when data are sparse, but are fine when sufficient data and good initial estimates are available. The Bayesian approach uses prior information, and, in essence, guides the search pointer to a proximity in the geometric space where the estimates are more likely to be found (reducing vari-

TABLE 17.12 Pharmacokinetic Parameter Estimates (Mean ± SD)

METHOD	Cl[a] (L/h/kg IBW)	k[b] (h^{-1})	V_D (L/kg IBW)
Least-Squares			
Day 1	0.0383 ± 0.0129	0.105 ± 0.014	0.519 ± 0.291
Final	0.0391 ± 0.0117	0.095 ± 0.064	0.511 ± 0.239
Chiou			
1	0.0399 ± 0.0306		
2	0.0437 ± 0.0193		
3	0.0438 ± 0.0212		
Steady-State Clearance			
	0.0408 ± 0.0174		
Bayesian			
1	0.0421 ± 0.0143	0.081 ± 0.030	0.534 ± 0.0745
2	0.0424 ± 0.0158	0.082 ± 0.035	0.532 ± 0.0802
3	0.0408 ± 0.0182	0.078 ± 0.037	0.531 ± 0.0820
4	0.0403 ± 0.0147	0.077 ± 0.027	0.530 ± 0.0787
Final	0.0372 ± 0.0113	0.070 ± 0.026	0.536 ± 0.0741

Cl = total body clearance, k = elimination rate constant, V_D = volume of distribution, IBW = ideal body weight.
[a]Calculated from least-squares estimates.
[b]Calculated by Bayesian estimates.

From Hurley and McNeil (1988), with permission.

ability but increasing subjectivity). Many algorithms use some form of gradient- or derivative-based method; other algorithms use variable sequential simplex method. A discussion of the pharmacokinetic estimation methods was given by D'Argenio et al (1979). Some common pharmacokinetic algorithms for parameter estimation are: (1) Newton-Raphson with first and second derivative, (2) Gauss-Newton method, (3) Levenberg-Marquardt method, and (4) Nelder-Mead simplex method. The Gauss-Newton method was used in the early versions of NONLIN. As discussed in the mixed-effect models in later sections, assuming a relationship such as Cl_R proportional to Cl_{cr} (technically called linearization) reduces the minimum number of data necessary for parameter estimation.

TABLE 17.13 Predictive Accuracy at the End of Infusion 1[a]

METHOD	MEAN PREDICTION ERROR (mg/L)	MEAN PERCENT ABSOLUTE PREDICTION ERROR (%)
Least-Squares		
Day 1	−0.06 (−1.1, 0.95)	17.6 (13.4, 21.7)
Chiou		
1	0.96 (−1.7, 3.60)	36.8 (27.3, 46.3)
2	−1.7 (−3.3, −0.08)	20.8 (14.1, 27.5)
3	−1.5 (−3.7, 0.80)	27.7 (17.8, 37.5)
Bayesian		
1	−0.61 (−1.7, 0.50)	18.8 (14.1, 23.6)
2	−0.65 (−2.0, 0.69)	22.7 (16.3, 29.2)
3	0.16 (−1.1, 1.40)	21.7 (16.1, 27.2)
4	−0.15 (−1.2, 0.96)	19.8 (15.6, 24.1)

[a]Figures in parentheses are 95% confidence intervals.

From Hurley and McNeil (1988), with permission.

Analysis of Population Pharmacokinetic Data

Traditional pharmacokinetic study involves taking multiple blood samples periodically over time in a few individual patients, and characterizing basic pharmacokinetic parameters such as K, V_D and Cl; because the studies are generally well designed, there are fewer parameters than data points (ie, that provide sufficient degree of freedom to reflect lack of fit of model), and the parameters are efficiently estimated from the model with most least-squares programs. Traditional pharmacokinetic parameter estimation is very accurate, providing, however, that enough samples can be taken for the individual patient to be dosed. The disadvantage is that only a few relatively homogeneous healthy subjects are included in pharmacokinetic studies from which dosing in different patients must be projected.

In the clinical setting, patients are usually not very homogeneous; patients vary in sex, age, body weight; they may have concomitant disease and may be receiving multiple drug treatment. Even the diet, life style, ethnic, and geographical location can differ from a selected group of "normal" subjects. Further, it is often not possible to take multiple samples in the same subject, and, therefore, no data is available to reflect intrasubject difference, so that iterative procedure for finding the maximum likelihood estimate can be complex and unpredictable due to incomplete or missing data. However, the vital information needed about the pharmacokinetics of drugs in patients at different stages of their disease with various therapies can only be obtained from the same population, or from a collection of pooled blood samples. The advantages of population pharmacokinetic analysis using pooled data were reviewed by Sheiner and Ludden (1992) that included a summary of population pharmacokinetics for dozens of drugs. Pharmacokinetic analysis of pooled data of plasma drug concentration from a large group of subjects may reveal much information about the disposition of a drug in a population. Unlike data from an individual subject collected over time, inter- and intrasubject variations must be considered. Both kinetic and nonkinetic related factors, such as age, weight, sex, and creatinine concentration should be examined in the model to determine the relevance to the estimation of pharmacokinetic parameters.

Nonlinear mixed effect model (or *NONMEM*) is so called because the model uses both fixed and random factors to describe data. Fixed factors such as patient weight, age, gender, and creatinine concentration are assumed to have no error; whereas random factors include inter- and intraindividual differences. NONMEM is a statistical program written in Fortran (see Appendix B) that allows Bayesian pharmacokinetic parameters to be estimated using an efficient algorithm called the first-order (FO) method. The parameters may now be estimated also with a first-order conditional estimate (FOCE) algorithm. In addition, to pharmacokinetic parameters, many examples of population plasma data have been analyzed to determine population factors. Multiplicative coefficients or parameters for patient factors may also be estimated.

NONMEM fits plasma drug concentration data for all subjects in the groups simultaneously and estimates the population parameter and its variance. The parameter may be clearance and/or V_D. The model may also test for other fixed effects on the drug due to factors such as age, weight, and creatinine concentration.

The model describes the observed plasma drug concentration (C_i) in terms of a model with:

1. P_k = fixed effect parameters, which include pharmacokinetic parameters or patient factor parameters. For example, P_1 is Cl, P_2 is the multiplicative coefficient including creatinine factor, and P_3 is the multiplicative coefficient for weight.

2. Random effect parameters, including (a) the variance of the structural (kinetic) parameter P_k or intersubject variability within the population ω_k^2; and (b) the residual intrasubject variance or variance due to measurement errors, fluctuations in individual parameter values, and all other errors not accounted for by the other parameters.

There are generally two reliable and practical approaches for population pharmacokinetic data analysis. One approach is the *standard two-stage method* (STS), which estimates parameters from the plasma drug concentration data for an individual subject during the first stage. The estimates from all subjects are then combined to obtain an estimate of the parameters for the population. The method is useful because unknown factors that affect the response in one patient would not carry over and bias parameter estimates of the others. The method works well when sufficient drug concentration–time data are available.

A second approach, the *first-order method* (FO), is also used but is perhaps less well understood. The estimation procedure is based on minimization of an extended least-squares criterion, which was defined through a first-order Taylor series expansion of the response vector about the fixed effects and which utilized a Newton-Raphson-like algorithm (Beal and Sheiner, 1980). This method attempts to fit the data and partition the unpredictable differences between theoretical and observed values into random error terms. When this model includes concomitant effects, it is called a *mixed-effect statistical model* (Beal and Sheiner, 1985). The advantage of the first-order model is that it is applicable even when the amount of time concentration data obtained from each individual is small, provided that the total number of individuals is sufficiently large. For example, in the example cited (Beal and Sheiner, 1985), 116 plasma concentrations were collected from 39 patients with various weight, age, gender, serum creatinine, and congestive heart failure conditions. The two-stage method was not suitable, but the FO method was useful for this set of data analysis. With a large number of factors and only limited data, and with hidden factors possibly affecting the pharmacokinetics of the drug, the analysis may sometimes be misleading. Beal and Sheiner (1985) suggested that the main concomitant factor should be measured whenever possible. Several examples of population pharmacokinetic data analysis using clinical data are listed below. Typically, a computer method is used in the data analysis based on a statistical model using either the weighted least-squares (WLS) or the extended least-squares (ELS) method in estimating the parameters. In the last few years, NONMEM has been continuously updated and improved. Many drugs were analyzed with population pharmacokinetics to yield information not obtainable within the traditional two-stage method (Sheiner and Ludden, 1992). An added feature is the development of a population model involving both pharmacokinetics and pharmacodynamics, the so-called population *PK/PD* models.

One example involving analysis of population plasma concentration data involved the drug procainamide. The drug clearance of an individual in a group may be assumed to be affected by several factors (Whiting et al, 1986). These factors include body weight, creatinine clearance, and a clearance factor P_1 described in the following equation.

$$Cl_{\text{drug j}} = P_1 + P_2(C_{\text{creatinine j}}) + P_3(\text{weight}_j) + \eta_{\text{Cl j}} \tag{17.15}$$

η_{Cl_j} is the intersubject error of clearance and its variance is $\omega^2{}_{Cl_j}$.

In another mixed effect model involving the analysis of lidocaine and maxiletine (Fig. 17-5), Vozeh and associates (1984) tested age, sex, time on drug therapy,

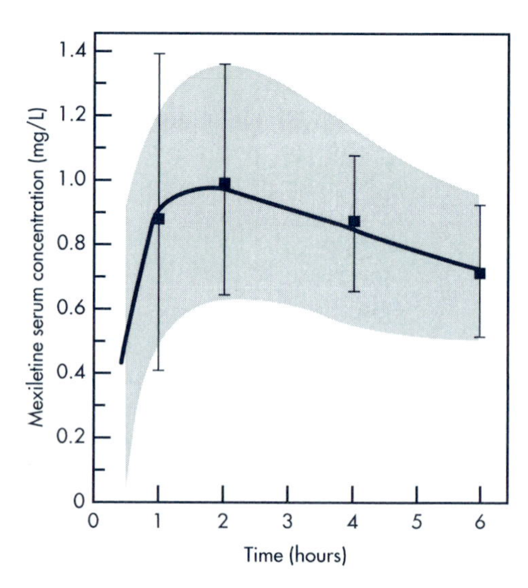

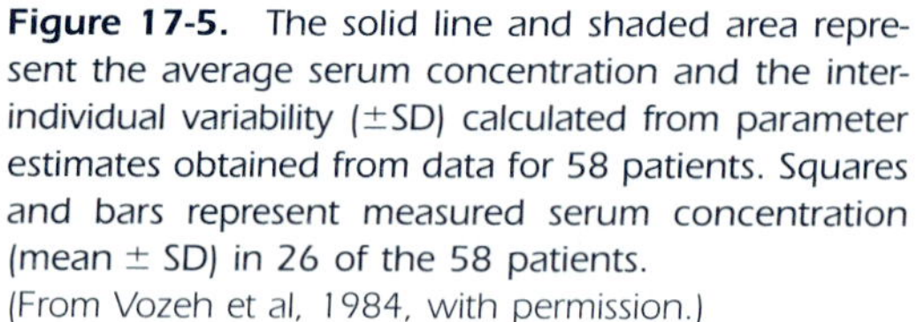
Figure 17-5. The solid line and shaded area represent the average serum concentration and the interindividual variability (±SD) calculated from parameter estimates obtained from data for 58 patients. Squares and bars represent measured serum concentration (mean ± SD) in 26 of the 58 patients.
(From Vozeh et al, 1984, with permission.)

and congestive heart failure (CHF) for effects on drug clearance. The effects of CHF and weight on V_D were also examined. The test statistic, ΔELS, or difference extended least-squares, was significant for CHF and moderately significant for weight on lidocaine clearance (Table 17.14).

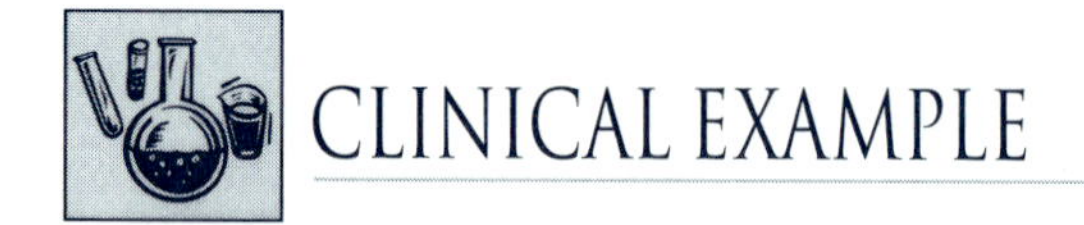

CLINICAL EXAMPLE

Fitting Warfarin Population Data

Population pharmacokinetics may be analyzed from various clinical sites. The population pharmacokinetics of racemic warfarin was evaluated using 613 measured warfarin plasma concentrations from 32 adult hospitalized patients and 131 adult outpatients (Mungall et al, 1985). Warfarin concentrations were measured in duplicate using a high-performance liquid chromatographic procedure. The pharmacokinetic model used was a one-compartment open model with first-order absorption and first-order elimination. The extent of availability was assumed to be

TABLE 17.14 Testing for Factors Affecting Lidocaine Pharmacokinetics

HYPOTHESIS	ΔELS[a]
Cl influenced by:	
Age	0.1
Sex	2.4
Time on therapy	1.0
CHF $[Cl_{CHF} = Cl_{no}(1 - \theta_5)]$	52.7
V_1 influenced by CHF $[V_{1CHF} = V_{1no}(1 - \theta_6)]$	9.0
Cl and V_1 normalized for body weight	13.4

[a]ΔELS = change in extended least-squares.

From Vozeh et al (1984).

one. A linear regression model was used to evaluate the influence of various disease and demographic factors (Table 17.15) on warfarin drug clearance. Age appeared to be an important determinant of warfarin clearance in this adult population. There was about a 1% per year decrease in oral clearance over the age range of 20 to 70 years. Smoking appeared to result in a 10% increase in warfarin clearance, while coadministration of the inducers phenytoin or phenobarbital yielded about a 30% increase in clearance. Other factors such as race, gender, and hospital site did not significantly affect *Cl* based on this model. This study has yielded a predictive model that, when combined with appropriate pharmacological response data, may be useful in the design and adjustment of warfarin regimens.

$$\text{SIZEVD} = \text{TBW}/70$$
$$\text{VD} = \text{SIZEVD (P1)}$$
$$\text{SIZECL} = (\text{TBW}/70)^{\text{P2}}$$

$$Cl = \text{SIZECL (P3 + P4 CHF + P5 VAH + P6 AGE + P7 GEN + P8 SKG + P9 ANG + P10 BLK + P11 INH + P12 IND + P13 DIS)}$$

The patient variables are the following: 1 = present 0 = absent; CHF = congestive heart failure; VAH = VA hospital site; Age = age in year; GEN = 1 for male and 0 for female; SKG = smoker; ANG = 1 if Caucasian; BLK = 1 if Black; INH = 1 if taking an inhibitor drug; IND = 1 if taking an inducer drug; DIS = 1 if taking a displacer (protein binding) drug.

Thus, the information content is better when sampling is strategically designed. Proper sampling can yield valuable information about the distribution of pharmacokinetic parameters in a population. Pooled clinical drug concentrations taken from hospital patients are generally not well controlled and are much harder to analyze. This example shows that a mixed-effect model can yield valuable information about various demographic and pathophysiologic factors that may influence drug disposition in the patient population.

TABLE 17.15 Population Pharmacokinetics of Warfarin Regression

PARAMETER	REGRESSION VALUE	EXPLANATION
P1	7.85 L/70 kg	Factor relating TBW to V_D
P2	0.460	exponential factor relating TBW to SIZECL
P3	3.31 L/day	Factor relating SIZECL to *Cl*
P4	0	Factors relating CHF to *Cl*
P5	0	Factor relating VAH-site to *Cl*
P6	−0.0214 L/day/year of age	Factor relating age to *Cl*
P7	0	Factor relating gender to *Cl*
P8	0.367 L/day	Factor relating smoking to *Cl*
P9	0	Factor relating Caucasian vs Latin difference to *Cl*
P10	0	Factor relating Black vs Latin difference to *Cl*
P11	0	Factor relating drug inhibitor to *Cl*
P12	1.16 L/day	Factor relating drug inducer to *Cl*
P13	0	Factor relating drug displacer to *Cl*

From Mungall et al, 1985.

Model Selection Criteria

Data analysis in pharmacokinetics frequently selects either a monoexponential or polyexponential that will better describe the concentration–time relationship. The selection criteria for the better model is determined by the goodness-of-fit, taking into account the number of parameters involved. Three common model selection criteria are: (1) the *Akaike Information Criterion* (AIC), (2) the *Schwarz Criterion* (SC), and (3) the F test (alpha = 0.05). The performance characteristics of these criteria were examined by Ludden et al (1994) using Monte Carlo (random or stochastic) simulations. The precision and bias of the estimated parameters were considered. The Akaike Information Criterion and the Schwarz Criterion lead to selection of the correct model more often than does the F test, which tends to choose the simpler model even when the more complex model is correct. The F test is also more sensitive to deficient sampling designs. Clearance was quite robust among the different methods and generally well estimated. Other pharmacokinetic parameters are more sensitive to model choice, particularly the apparent elimination rate constant. Prediction of concentrations is generally more precise when the correct model is chosen.

Decision Analysis Involving Diagnostic Tests

Diagnostic tests may be performed to determine the presence or absence of a disease. A scheme for the predictability of a disease by a diagnostic test is shown in Table 17.16. A *true positive*, represented by "*a*" indicates that the laboratory test correctly predicted the disease, whereas a *false positive*, represented by "*b*," shows that the laboratory test incorrectly predicted that the patient had the disease when, in fact, the patient did not have the disease. In contrast, a *true negative*, represented by "*d*" correctly gives a negative test in patients without the disease, whereas a *false negative*, represented by "*c*" incorrectly gives a negative test when, in fact, the patient does have the disease.

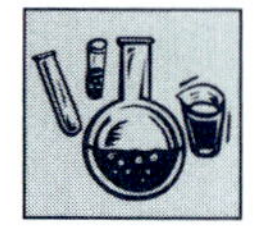

CLINICAL EXAMPLE

A new diagnostic test for HIV^+/AIDS was developed and tested in 5772 intravenous drug users. The results of this study are tabulated in Table 17.17.

From the results in Table 17.17, a total of 2863 subjects had a positive diagnostic test for HIV^+/AIDS and 2909 subjects had a negative diagnostic test for

TABLE 17.16 Errors in Decision Predictability

DECISION	DIAGNOSTIC TEST RESULT		TOTALS
	DISEASE PRESENT	DISEASE ABSENT	
Accept disease Present	Test positive (*True positive*) *a*	Test positive (*False positive*) *b*	*a* + *b*
Reject disease Present	Test negative (*False negative*) *c*	Test negative (*True negative*) *d*	*c* + *d*
Totals	*a* + *c*	*b* + *d*	*a* + *b* + *c* + *d*

TABLE 17.17 Results of HIV^+/AIDS Test

	DIAGNOSTIC TEST RESULT		
DECISION	DISEASE PRESENT	DISEASE ABSENT	TOTALS
Accept HIV^+/AIDS Present	2756	107	2863
Reject HIV^+/AIDS Present	211	2698	2909
Totals	2967	2805	5772

HIV^+/AIDS. Further tests on these subjects showed that 2967 subjects actually had HIV^+/AIDS, although 211 of these subjects had negative diagnostic test results. Moreover, 107 subjects who had a positive diagnostic test result did not, in fact, have HIV^+/AIDS after further tests were made.

1. The *positive predictability* of the test or the likelihood that the test will correctly predict the disease if the test is positive is estimated as shown:

$$\text{Positive predictability} = \frac{a}{a+b} = 2756/2863 = 0.963\ (96.3\%)$$

2. The *negative predictability* of the test is the likelihood that the patient will not have the disease if the test is negative is estimated as shown:

$$\text{Negative predictability} = \frac{d}{c+d} = 2698/2909 = 0.927\ (92.7\%)$$

3. The *total predictability* of the test is the likelihood that the patient will be predicted correctly is estimated as shown:

$$\text{Total predictability} = \frac{a+d}{a+b+c+d} = (2756 + 2698)/5772 = 0.945\ (94.5\%)$$

4. The *sensitivity* of the test is the likelihood that a test result will be positive in a patient with the disease is estimated as shown:

$$\text{Sensitivity} = a/(a+c) = 2756/2967 = 0.929\ (92.9\%)$$

5. The *specificity* of a test is the likelihood that a test result will be negative in a patient without the disease is estimated as shown:

$$\text{Specificity} = d/(b+d) = 2698/2805 = 0.962\ (96.2\%)$$

Analysis of the results in Table 17.17 shows that a positive result from the new test for HIV^+/AIDS will only predict the disease correctly 94.5%. Therefore, the clinician must use other measures for predicting whether the patient does or does not have the disease. These other measures may include physical diagnosis of the patient, other laboratory tests, normal incidence of the disease in the patient population (in this case, intravenous drug users), and the experience of the clinician. Each test has different predictive values.

Regional Pharmacokinetics

Pharmacokinetics is the study of the time course of drug concentrations in the body. Pharmacokinetics is based generally on the time course of drug concentrations in systemic blood sampled from either the vein or the artery. This general approach is useful as long as the drug concentrations in the tissues of the body are well reflected by drug concentrations in the blood. Clinically, the blood drug concentration may not be proportional to the drug concentration in tissues. For example, after IV bolus administration, the distributive phase is attributed to temporally different changes in mixing and redistribution of drug in organs such as the lung, heart, and kidney (Upton, 1990). The time course for the pharmacodynamics of the drug may have no relationship to the time course for the drug concentrations in the blood. The pharmacodynamics of the drug may be related to local tissue drug levels and the status of homeostatic physiologic functions. After an IV bolus dose, Upton (1990) reported that lignocaine (lidocaine) rapidly accumulates in the spleen and kidney but is slowly sequestered into fat. More than 30 minutes were needed before the target site (heart and brain) drug levels established equilibrium with drug concentrations in the blood. These regional equilibrium factors are often masked in conventional pharmacokinetic models that assume rapid drug equilibrium.

Regional pharmacokinetics is the study of pharmacokinetics within a given tissue region. The tissue region is defined as an anatomic area of the body between specified afferent and efferent blood vessels. For example, the myocardium includes the region perfused by the coronary arterial (afferent) and the coronary sinus (efferent) blood vessels. The selection of a region bounded by its network of blood vessel is based on the movement of drug between the blood vessels and the interstitial and intracellular spaces of the region. The conventional pharmacokinetic approach for calculating systemic clearance and volume of distribution tends to average various drug distributions together, such that the local perturbations are neglected. Regional pharmacokinetics supplement systemic pharmacokinetics when inadequate information is provided by conventional pharmacokinetics.

Various homeostatic physiologic functions may be responsible for the nonequilibrium of drug concentrations between local tissue regions and the blood. For example, most cells have an electrochemical difference across the cell membrane consisting of a membrane potential of negative 70 mV inside the membrane relative to the outside. Moreover, regional differences in pH normally exist within a cell. For example, the pH within the lysosome is between 4 and 5, which could allow a basic drug to accumulate within the lysosome with a concentration gradient of 400-fold to 160,000-fold over the blood. Other explanations for regional drug concentration differences have been reviewed by Upton (1990), who also considers that dynamic processes may be more important than equilibrium processes in affecting dynamic response. Thus, regional pharmacokinetics is another approach in applying pharmacokinetics to pharmacodynamics and clinical effect.

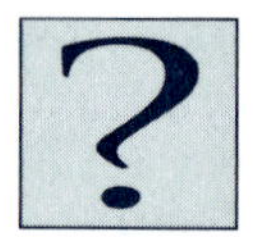

FREQUENTLY ASKED QUESTIONS

1. Can therapeutic drug monitoring be performed without taking blood samples?
2. What is meant by "population" pharmacokinetics? What advantages does population pharmacokinetics have over classical pharmacokinetics?
3. What are the major considerations in therapeutic drug monitoring?

4. Why is it possible to estimate individual pharmacokinetic parameters with just a few data points using the Bayesian method?
5. Why is pharmacokinetics important in studying drug interactions?

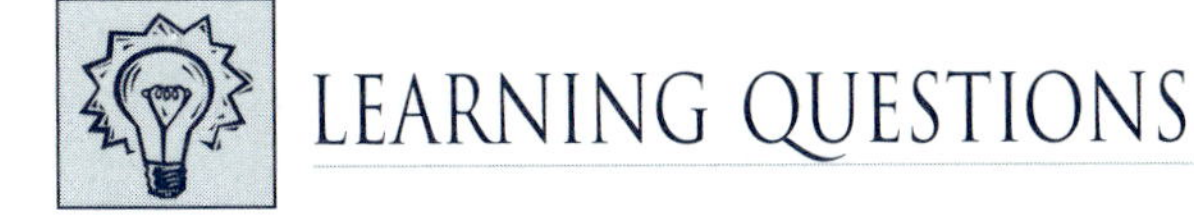

LEARNING QUESTIONS

1. Why is it harder to titrate patients with a drug whose elimination half-life is 36 hours compared to a drug whose elimination is 6 hours?
2. Penicillin G has a volume of distribution of 42 L/1.73 m^2 and an elimination rate constant of 1.034 hr^{-1}. Calculate the maximum peak concentration that would be produced if the drug were given intravenously at a rate of 250 mg every 6 hours for a week.
3. Dicloxacillin has an elimination half-life of 42 minutes and a volume of distribution of 20 L. Dicloxacillin is 97% protein bound. What would be the steady-state free concentration of dicloxacillin if the drug were given intravenously at a rate of 250 mg every 6 hours?
4. The normal elimination half-life of cefamandole is 1.49 hours and the apparent volume of distribution (V_D) is 39.2% of body weight. The elimination half-life for a patient with a creatinine clearance of 15 mL/min was reported by Czerwinski and Pederson (1979) to be 6.03 hours, and cefamandole's V_D is 23.75% of body weight. What doses of cefamandole should be given the normal and the uremic patient (respectively) if the drug is administered intravenously every 6 hours and the desired objective is to maintain an average steady concentration of 2 μg/mL?
5. The maintenance dose of digoxin was reported to be 0.5 mg/day for a 60-kg patient with normal renal function. The half-life of digoxin is 0.95 days and the volume of distribution is 306 L. The bioavailability of the digoxin tablet is 0.56.
   a. Calculate the steady-state concentration of digoxin.
   b. Determine whether the patient is adequately dosed (effective serum digoxin concentration is 1–2 ng/mL).
   c. What is the steady-state concentration if the patient is dosed with the elixir instead of the tablet? (Assume the elixir to be 100% bioavailable.)
6. An antibiotic has an elimination half-life of 2 hours and an apparent volume of distribution of 200 mL/kg. The minimum effective serum concentration is 2 μg/mL and the minimum toxic serum concentration is 16 μg/mL. A physician ordered a dosage regimen of this antibiotic to be given at 250 mg every 8 hours by repetitive intravenous bolus injections.
   a. Comment on the appropriateness of this dosage regimen for an adult male patient (23 years, 80 kg) whose creatinine clearance is 122 mL/min.
   b. Would you suggest an alternate dosage regimen for this patient? Give your reasons and suggest an alternative dosage regimen.
7. Gentamycin (Garamycin, Schering) is a highly water-soluble drug. The dosage

of this drug in obese patients should be based on an estimate of the lean body mass or "ideal body weight." *Why?*

8. Why is the calculation for the loading dose (D_L) for a drug based on the apparent volume of distribution, whereas the calculation of the maintenance dose is based on the elimination rate constant?

9. A potent drug with a narrow therapeutic index is ordered for a patient. After making rounds, the attending physician observes that the patient is not responding to drug therapy and orders a single plasma level measurement. Comment briefly on the value of measuring the drug concentration in a single blood sample and on the usefulness of the information that may be gained.

10. Calculate an oral dosage regimen for a cardiotonic drug for an adult male (63 years old, 68 kg) with normal renal function. The elimination half-life for this drug is 30 hours and its apparent volume of distribution is 4 L/kg. The drug is 80% bioavailable when given orally, and the suggested therapeutic serum concentrations for this drug range from 0.001 to 0.002 μg/mL.

a. This cardiotonic drug is commercially supplied as 0.075 mg, 0.15 mg, and 0.30 mg white, scored, compressed tablets. Using these readily available tablets, what dose would you now recommend for this patient?

b. Are there any advantages for this patient to give smaller doses more frequently compared to a higher dosage less frequently? Any disadvantages?

c. Would you suggest a loading dose for this drug? Why? What loading dose would you recommend?

d. Is there a rationale for preparing a controlled-release product of this drug?

11. The dose of sulfisoxazole (Gantrisin, Roche Labs) recommended for an adult female patient (age 26, 63 kg) with a urinary tract infection was 1.5 g every 4 hours. The drug is 85% bound to serum proteins. The elimination half-life of this drug is 6 hours and the apparent volume of distribution is 1.3 L/kg. Sulfisoxazole is 100% bioavailable.

a. Calculate the steady-state plasma concentration of sulfisoxazole in this patient.

b. Calculate an appropriate loading dose of sulfisoxazole for this patient.

c. Gantrisin (sulfisoxazole) is supplied in tablets containing 0.5 g of drug. How many tablets would you recommend for the loading dose?

d. If no loading dose were given, how long would it take to achieve 95 to 99% of steady state?

12. The desired plasma level for an antiarrhythmic agent is 5 μg/mL. The drug has an apparent volume of distribution of 173 mL/kg and an elimination half-life of 2.0 hours. The kinetics of the drug follow the kinetics of a one-compartment open model.

a. An adult male patient (75 kg, 56 years of age) is to be given an IV injection of this drug. What loading dose (D_L) and infusion rate (R) would you suggest?

b. The patient did not respond very well to drug therapy. Plasma levels of drug were measured and found to be 2 μg/mL. How would you readjust the infusion rate to increase the plasma drug level to the desired 5 μg/mL?

c. How long would it take to achieve 95% of steady-state plasma drug levels in this patient assuming no loading dose was given and the apparent V_D was unaltered?

13. An antibiotic is to be given to an adult male patient (75 kg, 58 years of age) by intravenous infusion. The elimination half-life for this drug is 8 hours and the apparent volume of distribution is 1.5 L/kg. The drug is supplied in 30-mL ampules at a concentration of 15 mg/mL. The desired steady-state serum concentration for this antibiotic is 20 μg/mL.

a. What infusion rate (R) would you suggest for this patient?
b. What loading dose would you suggest for this patient?
c. If the manufacturer suggests a starting infusion rate of 0.2 mL/hr per kg body weight, what is the expected steady-state serum concentration in this patient?
d. You would like to verify that this patient received the proper infusion rate. At what time after the start of the IV infusion would you take a blood sample to monitor the serum antibiotic concentration? Why?
e. Assume that the serum antibiotic concentration was measured and found to be higher than anticipated. What reasons, based on sound pharmacokinetic principles, would account for this situation?

14. Nomograms are frequently used in lieu of pharmacokinetic calculations to determine an appropriate drug dosage regimen for a patient. Discuss the advantages and disadvantages for using nomograms to calculate a drug dosage regimen.

15. Based on the following pharmacokinetic data for Drug *A*, Drug *B*, and Drug *C*: (a) Which drug takes the longest time to reach steady state? (b) Which drug would achieve the highest steady-state drug concentration? (c) Which drug has the largest apparent volume of distribution?

	Drug A	**Drug B**	**Drug C**
Rate of infusion (mg/hr)	10	20	15
k (hr^{-1})	0.5	0.1	0.05
Cl (L/hr)	5	20	5

16. The effect of repetitive administration of phenytoin (PHT) on the single-dose pharmacokinetics of primidone (PRM) was investigated by Sato et al (1992) in 3 healthy male subjects. The peak concentration of unchanged PRM was achieved at 12 and 8 hours after the administration of PRM in the absence and the presence of PHT, respectively. The elimination half-life of PRM was decreased from 19.4 ± 2.2 (mean ± S.E.) to 10.2 ± 5.1 h ($p < .05$) and the total body clearance was increased from 24.6 ± 3.1 to 45.1 ± 5.1 mL/h/kg ($p < .01$) in the presence of PHT. No significant change was observed for the apparent volume of distribution between the two treatments. Based on pharmacokinetics of the two drugs, what are the possible reasons for phenytoin to reduce primidone elimination half-life and increase its renal clearance?

17. Traconazole (Sporanox, Janssen) is a lipophilic drug with extensive lipid distribution. The drug levels in fatty tissue and organs contains 2 to 20 times the drug levels in the plasma. Little or no drug was found in the saliva and in the cerebrospinal fluid and the half-life is 64 ± 32 hours. The drug is 99.8% bound. How does (a) plasma drug protein binding, (b) tissue drug distribution and (c) lipid tissue partitioning contribute to the long elimination half-life for traconazole?

18. JL (29-year-old male, 180 kg) received oral ofloxacin 400 mg twice a day for presumed bronchitis due to *S. pneumoniae*. His other medications were the following: 400 mg cimetidine, orally, three times a day; 400 mg metronidazole, as directed. JL was still having a fever of 100.1°C a day after taking the quinolone antibiotic. Comment on any appropriate action.

19. CK (70-year-old male, 177 lbs). Scr = 0.9 mg/dL Allergy: PCN. Claudication, rhinitis: URI infection. His medication includes: Ilosone: 250 qid × 1wk; Trental: 200 mg tid; Colace: 100 mg bid; Seldane: one tid prn. Which of the following should the pharmacist conclude from this information?

a. There is an interaction between colace and seldane.

b. The dose of Trental is too high for this patient based on his renal function.

c. Seldane should be substituted with a therapeutic alternative due to an interaction.

REFERENCES

Abernethy DR, Greenblatt DJ: Pharmacokinetics of drugs in obesity. *Clin Pharmacokinet* **7:**108–124, 1982

Abernethy DR, Greenblatt DJ, Divoll M, et al: Alterations in drug distribution and clearance due to obesity. *J Pharmacol Exp Ther* **217:**681–685, 1981

Beal SL: *NONMEM Users Guide VII: Conditional Estimation Methods.* San Francisco, NONMEM Project Group, University of California, San Francisco, 1992

Beal SL, Sheiner LB: Methodology of population pharmacokinetics. In Garrett ER, Hirtz JL (eds), *Drug Fate and Metabolism: Methods and Techniques,* vol 5. New York, Marcel Dekker, 1985

Beal SL, Sheiner LB: The NONMEM system, AM. *Statistics* **34:**118–119, 1980

Czerwinski AW, Pederson JA: Pharmacokinetics of cefamandole in patients with renal impairment. *Antimicrob Agents Chemother* **15:**161–164, 1979

D'Argenio DZ, Schumitzky A: A program package for simulation and parameter estimation in pharmacokinetic systems, *Computer Prog Biomed* **9:**115–134, 1979

DeHaan RM, Metzler CM, Schellenberg D, et al: Pharmacokinetic study of clindamycin hydrochloride in humans. *Int J Clin Pharmacol Biopharm* **6:**105–119, 1972

Erikson LO, Wahlin Boll-E, Odar Cederlof I, Lindholm L, Melander A: Influence of renal failure, rheumatoid arthritis and old age on the pharmacokinetics of diflunisal. *Eur J Clin Pharmaco* **36**(2):165–74, 1989

Evans WE, Schentag JJ, Jusko WJ: *Applied Pharmacokinetics. Principles of Therapeutic Drug Monitoring.* San Francisco, Applied Therapeutics, 1992

Gomeni R, Pineau G, Mentre F: Population kinetics and conditional assessment of the optimal dosage regimen using the P-pharm software package. *Cancer Res* **14:**2321–2326, 1994

Greenblatt DJ: Predicting steady state serum concentration of drugs. *Annu Rev Pharmacol Toxicol* **19:**347–356, 1979

Haverkos HW, Amsel Z, Drotman DP: Adverse virus-drug interactions. *Rev Infect Dis* **13:**697–704, 1991

Heden B, et al: Agreement between artificial neural networks and experienced electrocardiographer on electrocardiographic diagnosis of healed myocardial infarction. *J Am Coll Cardiol* **28**(4):1012–1016, 1996

Hedman A, Angelin B, Arvidsson A, Beck O, Dahlqvist R, Nilsson B, Olsson M, Schenck-Gustafsson K: Digoxin-verapamil interaction: Reduction of biliary but not renal digoxin clearance in humans. *Clin Pharmacol Ther* **49**(3):256–262, 1991

Hendeles L, Weinberger M: Avoidance of adverse effects during chronic therapy with theophylline. *Drug Intell Clin Pharm* **14:**523, 1980

Hurley SF, McNeil JF: A comparison of the accuracy of a least-squares regression, a Bayesian, Chiou's and the steady state clearance method of individualizing theophylline dosage. *Clin Pharmacokinet* **14:**311–320, 1988

Iafrate RP, Glotz VP, Robinson JD, Lupkiewicz SM: Computer simulated conversion from intravenous to sustained-release oral theophylline drug. *Intel Clin Phar* **16:**19–25, 1982

Jaehde U, Sorgel F, Stephan U, Schunack W: Effect of an antacid containing magnesium and aluminum on absorption, metabolism, and mechanism of renal elimination of pefloxacin in humans. *Antimicrob Agents Chemother* **38**(5):1129–33, 1994

Kaminori GH, et al: The effects of obesity and exercise on the pharmacokinetics of caffeine in lean and obese volunteers. *Eur J Clin Pharmacol* **31:**595–600, 1987

Landahl S, et al: Pharmacokinetics and blood pressure effects of felodipine in elderly hypertensive patients—A comparison with the young healthy subjects. *Clin Pharmacokinet* **14:**374–383, 1988

Lima DR, Santos RM, Werneck E, Andrade GN: Effect of orally administered misoprostol and cimetidine on the steady-state pharmacokinetics of diazepam and nordiazepam in human volunteers. *Eur J Drug Metab Pharmacokinet* **16**(3):61–70, 1991

Lindeman RD, Tobin J, Shock NW: Longitudinal studies on the rate of decline in renal function with age. *J Am Geriatr Soc* 33:278–285, 1985

Ludden TM, Beal SL, Sheiner LB: Comparison of the Akaike Information Criterion, the Schwarz criterion and the F test as guides to model selection. *J Pharmacokinet Biopharm* **22**(5):431–445, 1994

Mawer GE: Computer assisted prescribing of drugs. *Clin Pharmacokinet* **1**:67–78, 1976

Mentre F, Gomeni R: A two-step iterative algorithm for estimation in nonlinear mixed-effect models with an evaluation in population pharmacokinetics. *J Biopharm Stat* **5**(2):141–158, 1995

Mentre F, Pineau, Gomeni R: Population kinetics and conditional assessment of the optimal dosage regimen using the P-Pharm software package. *Anticancer Res* **14**:2321–2326, 1994

Mungall DR, Ludden TM, Marsh II J, Hawkin DW, Talbert RL, Crawford MH: Population pharmacokinetics of racemic warfarin in adult patients. *J Pharmacokinet Biopharm* **13**(3):213–227, 1985

Okuno H, Takasu M, Kano H, Seki T, Shiozaki Y, Inoue K: Depression of drug metabolizing activity in the human liver by interferon-beta. *Hepatology* **17**(1):65–69, 1993

Perucca E, Gatti G, Cipolla G, Spina E, Barel S, Soback S, Gips M, Bialer M: Inhibition of diazepam metabolism by fluvoxamine: A pharmacokinetic study in normal volunteers. *Clin Pharmacol Ther* **56**(5):471–476, 1994

Regamey C, Gordon RC, Kirby WMM: Comparative pharmacokinetics of tobramycin and gentamicin. *Clin Pharmacol Ther* **14**:396–403, 1973

Sato J, Sekizawa Y, Yoshida A, Owada E, Sakuta N, Yoshihara M, Goto T, Kobayashi Y, Ito K: Single-dose kinetics of primidone in human subjects: effect of phenytoin on formation and elimination of active metabolites of primidone, phenobarbital and phenylethylmalonamide. *J Pharmacobiodyn* **15**(9):467–472, 1992

Schellens JH, Ghabrial H, van-der-Wart HH, Bakker EN, Wilkinson GR, Breimer DD: Differential effects of quinidine on the disposition of nifedipine, sparteine, and mephenytoin in humans. *Clin Pharmacol Ther 50*(5 Pt 1):520–528, 1991

Schumacher GE: Choosing optimal sampling times for therapeutic drug monitoring. *Clin Pharm* **4**:84–92, 1985

Schumacher GE, Barr JT: Applying decision analysis in therapeutic drug monitoring: Using decision trees to interpret serum theophylline concentrations. *Clin Pharm* 5:325–333, 1986

Schumacker GE: *Therapeutic Drug Monitoring*, Chapter 7, p 152, Appleton & Lange, Norwalk, CT 1995

Schumucker DL: Aging and drug disposition: An update: *Pharmacol Rev* **37**:133–148, 1985

Sheiner LB, Beal SL: Bayesian individualization of pharmacokinetics. Simple implementation and comparison with nonBayesian methods. *J Pharm Sci* **71**:1344–1348, 1982

Sheiner LB, Ludden TM: Population pharmacokinetics/dynamics. *Ann Rev Pharmacol Toxicol* **32**:185–209, 1992

Smith BP, Brier ME: Statistical approach to neural network model building for gentamicin peak predictions *J Pharm Sci* **85**(1):65–69, 1996

Spence JD: Drug interactions with grapefruit: Whose responsibility is it to warn the public? *Clin Pharmacol Therap* **61**:395–400, 1997

Stein GE, Haughey DB, Ross RJ, Vakoutis J: Conversion from intravenous to oral dosing using sustained release theophylline tablets. *Clin Pharm* **1**:772–773, 1982

Thomson AH: Bayesian feedback methods for optimizing therapy. *Clin Neuropharmacol* **15**(suppl 1, part A):245A–246A, 1992

Thomson AH, Whiting B: Bayesian parameter estimation and population pharmacokinetics. *Clin Pharmacokinet* **22**(6):447–467, 1992

Upton RN: Regional Pharmacokinetics, I. Physiological and physicochemical basis. *Biopharm Drug Disp* **11**:647–662, 1990

Vonesh EF, Carter RL: Mixed-effects nonlinear regression for unbalanced repeated measures. *Biometrics* **48**:1–17, 1992

Vozeh S, Wenk M, Follath F: Experience with NONMEM: Analysis of serum concentration data in patients treated with mexiletine and lidocaine. *Drug Metab Rev* **15**:305–315, 1984

West JR, Smith HW, Chasis H: Glomerular filtration rate, effective blood flow and maximal tubular excretory capacity in infancy. *J Pediatr* **32**:10, 1948

Whiting B, Kelman AW, Grevel J: Population pharmacokinetics: Theory and clinical application. *Clin Pharmacokin* **11**:387–401, 1986

BIBLIOGRAPHY

Abernethy DR, Azarnoff DL: Pharmacokinetic investigations in elderly patients. Clinical and ethical considerations. *Clin Pharmacokinet* **19:**89–93, 1990

Anderson KE: Influences of diet and nutrition on clinical pharmacokinetics. *Clin Pharmacokinet* **14:**325–346, 1988

Aranda JV, Stern L: Clinical aspects of developmental pharmacology and toxicology. *Pharmacol Ther* **20:**1–51, 1983

Benet LZ (ed): *The Effect of Disease States on Drug Pharmacokinetics.* Washington, DC, American Pharmaceutical Association, 1976

Benowitz NL, Meister W: Pharmacokinetics in patients with cardiac failure. *Clin Pharmacokinet* **1:**389–405, 1976

Besunder JB, Reed MD, Blumer JL: Principles of drug biodisposition in the neonate: A critical evaluation of the pharmacokinetic—Pharmacodynamic interface, Part I. *Clin Pharmacokinet* **14:**189–216, 1988

Chiou WL, Gadalla MAF, Pang GW: Method for the rapid estimation of total body clearance and adjustment of dosage regimens in patients during a constant-rate infusion. *J Pharmacokinet Biopharm* **6:**135–151, 1978

Chrystyn H, Ellis JW, Mulley BA, Peak MD: The accuracy and stability of Bayesian theophylline predictions. *Ther Drug Monit* **10:**299–303, 1988

Clinical symposium on drugs and the unborn child. *Clin Pharmacol Ther* **14:**621–770, 1973

Crooks J, O'Malley K, Stevenson IH: Pharmacokinetics in the elderly. *Clin Pharmacokinet* **1:**280–296, 1976

Crouthamel WG: The effect of congestive heart failure on quinidine pharmacokinetics. *Am Heart J* **90:**335, 1975

DeVane CL, Jusko WJ: Dosage regimen design. *Pharmacol Ther* **17:**143–163, 1982

Dimascio A, Shader RI: Drug administration schedules, *Am J Psychiatry* **126:**6, 1969

Friis-Hansen B: Body-water compartments in children: Changes during growth and related changes in body composition. *Pediatrics* **28:**169–181, 1961

Giacoia GP, Gorodisher R: Pharmacologic principles in neonatal drug therapy. *Clin Perinatol* **2:**125–138, 1975

Gillis AM, Kates R: Clinical pharmacokinetics of the newer antiarrhythmic agents. *Clin Pharmacokinet* **9:**375–403, 1984

Godley PJ, Black JT, Frohna PA, Garrelts JC: Comparison of a Bayesian program with three microcomputer programs for predicting gentamicin concentrations. *Ther Drug Monit* **10:**287–291, 1988

Grasela TH, Sheiner LB: Population pharmacokinetics of procainamide from routine clinical data. *Clin Pharmacokinet* **9:**545, 1984

Gross G, Perrier CV: Intrahepatic portasystemic shunting in cirrhotic patients. *N Engl J Med* **293:**1046, 1975

Harnes HT, Shiu G, Shah VP: Validation of bioanalytical methods. *Pharm Res* **8:**421–426, 1991

Holloway DA: Drug problems in the geriatric patient. *Drug Intell Clin Pharm* **8:**632–642, 1974

Jensen EH: Current concepts for the validation of compendial assays. *Pharmacopoeial Forum* March–April:1241–1245, 1986

Jusko WJ: Pharmacokinetic principles in pediatric pharmacology. *Pediatr Clin North Am* **19:**81–100, 1972

Klotz U, Avant GR, Hoyumpa A, et al: The effects of age and liver disease on the disposition and elimination of diazepam in adult man. *J Clin Invest* **55:**347, 1975

Krasner J, Giacoia GP, Yaffe SJ: Drug–protein binding in the newborn infant. *Ann NY State Acad Sci* **226:**102–114, 1973

Kristensen M, Hansen JM, Kampmann J, et al: Drug elimination and renal function. *Int J Clin Pharmacol Biopharm* **14:**307–308, 1974

Latini R, Bonati M, Tognoni G: Clinical role of blood levels. *Ther Drug Monit* **2:**3–9, 1980

Latini R, Maggioni AP, Cavalli A: Therapeutic drug monitoring of antiarrhythmic drugs. Rationale and current status. *Clin Pharmacokinet* **18:**91–103, 1990

Lehmann K, Merten K: Die Elimination von Lithium in Abhangigkeit vom Lebensalten bei Gesunden und Niereninsuffizienten. *Int J Clin Pharmacol Biopharm* **10:**292–298, 1974

Levy G (ed): *Clinical Pharmacokinetics: A Symposium.* Washington, DC, American Pharmaceutical Association, 1974

Lindeman RD: Changes in renal function with aging. Implications for treatment. *Drugs Aging* **2:**423–431, 1992

Ludden TM: Population pharmacokinetics. *J Clin Pharmacol* **28:**1059–1063, 1988

Matzke GR, St Peter WL: Clinical pharmacokinetics 1990. *Clin Pharmacokinet* **18:**1–19, 1990

Maxwell GM: Paediatric drug dosing. Body weight versus surface area. *Drugs* **37:**113–115, 1989

Meister W, Benowitz NL, Melmon KL, Benet LZ: Influence of cardiac failure on the pharmacokinetics of digoxin. *Clin Pharmacol Ther* **23:**122, 1978

Morley PC, Strand LM: Critical reflections on therapeutic drug monitoring. *J Pharm Pract* **2:**327–334, 1989

Morselli PL: Clinical pharmacokinetics in neonates. *Clin Pharmacokinet* **1:**81–98, 1976

Mungall DR: *Applied Clinical Pharmacokinetics.* New York, Raven, 1983

Neal EA, Meffin PJ, Gregory PB, Blaschke TF: Enhanced bioavailability and decreased clearance of analgesics in patients with cirrhosis. *Gastroenterology* **77:**96, 1979

Niebergall PJ, Sugita ET, Schnaare RL: Potential dangers of common drug dosing regimens. *Am J Hosp Pharm* **31:**53–58, 1974

Rane A, Sjoquist F: Drug metabolism in the human fetus and newborn infant. *Pediatr Clin North Am* **19:**37–49, 1972

Rane A, Wilson JT: Clinical pharmacokinetics in infants and children. *Clin Pharmacokinet* **1:**2–24, 1976

Richey DP, Bender DA: Pharmacokinetic consequences of aging. *Annu Rev Pharmacol Toxicol* **17:**49–65, 1977

Roberts J, Tumer N: Age and diet effects on drug action. *Pharmacol Ther* **37:**111–149, 1988

Rowland M, Tozer TN: *Clinical Pharmacokinetics Concepts and Applications.* Philadelphia, Lea & Febiger, 1980

Schumacher GE, Barr JT: Making serum drug levels more meaningful. *Ther Drug Monit* **11:**580–584, 1989

Schumacher GE, Barr JT: Pharmacokinetics in drug therapy. Bayesian approaches in pharmacokinetic decision making. *Clin Pharm* **3:**525–530, 1984

Schumacher GE, Griener JC: Using Pharmacokinetics in drug therapy II. Rapid estimates of dosage regimens and blood levels without knowledge of pharmacokinetic variables. *Am J Hosp Pharm* **35:**454–459, 1978

Sheiner LB, Benet LZ: Premarketing observational studies of population pharmacokinetics of new drugs. *Clin Pharmacol Ther* **38:**481–487, 1985

Sheiner LB, Rosenberg B, Marathe V: Estimation of population characteristics of pharmacokinetic parameters from routine clinical data. *J Pharmacokinet Biopharm* **9:**445–479, 1977

Shirkey HC: Dosage (Dosology). In Shirkey HC (ed), *Pediatric Therapy.* St. Louis, Mosby, 1975, pp 19–33

Spector R, Park GD, Johnson GF, Vessell ES: Therapeutic drug monitoring. *Clin Pharmacol Ther* **43:**345–353, 1988

Thompson PD, Melmon KL, Richardson JA, et al: Lidocaine pharmacokinetics in advanced heart failure, liver disease, and renal failure in humans. *Ann Intern Med* **78:**499–508, 1973

Uematsu T, Hirayama H, Nagashima S, et al: Prediction of individual dosage requirements for lignocaine. A validation study for Bayesian forecasting in Japanese patients. *Ther Drug Monit* **11:**25–31, 1989

Vestel RE: Drug use in the elderly: A review of problems and special considerations. *Drugs* **16:**358–382, 1978

Whiting B, Niven AA, Kelman AW, Thomson AH: A Bayesian kinetic control strategy for cyclosporin in renal transplantation. In D'Argenio DZ, (ed), *Advanced Methods of Pharmacokinetic and Pharmacodynamic Systems Analysis.* New York, Plenum Press, 1991

Williams RW, Benet LZ: Drug pharmacokinetics in cardiac and hepatic disease. *Annu Rev Pharmacol Toxicol* **20:**289, 1980

Winter ME: *Basic Clinical Pharmacokinetics.* San Francisco, Applied Therapeutics, 1980

Yuen GJ, Beal SL, Peck CC: Predicting phenytoin dosages using Bayesian feedback. A comparison with other methods. *Ther Drug Monit* **5:**437–441, 1983

18

DOSAGE ADJUSTMENT IN RENAL AND HEPATIC DISEASE

The kidney is an important organ in regulating body fluid levels, electrolyte balance, and metabolic waste and drug removal from the body. Impairment or degeneration of the kidney function will have an impact on the pharmacokinetics of drugs. Some of the more common causes of kidney failure include disease, injury, and drug intoxication. Table 18.1 lists some of the conditions that may lead to chronic or acute renal failure. The condition in which glomerular filtration is impaired or reduced, leading to accumulation of excessive fluid and blood nitrogenous products in the body, is commonly described as *uremia.* Uremia can also be caused by acute diseases or trauma to the kidney. However, the influence of uremia on drug elimination is pharmacokinetically the same, generally producing a reduction of glomerular filtration and/or active secretion, which leads to a longer elimination half-life of the administered drug.

Declining renal function leads not only to disturbances in electrolyte and fluid balance, but also causes physiologic and metabolic changes that may alter the pharmacokinetics and pharmacodynamics of a drug. Pharmacokinetic processes such as drug distribution (including both the volume of distribution and protein binding) and elimination (including both biotransformation and renal excretion) may be altered by renal impairment. Both therapeutic and toxic responses may be altered due to changes in drug sensitivity at the receptor site.

PHARMACOKINETIC CONSIDERATIONS

The oral bioavailability of a drug in severe uremia may be decreased due to disease-related changes in gastrointestinal motility and pH caused by nausea, vomiting, and diarrhea. Mesenteric blood flow may also be changed. However, the oral bioavailability of a drug such as propranolol (with a high first-pass effect) may be

TABLE 18.1 Common Causes of Kidney Failure

Pyelonephritis	Inflammation and deterioration of the pyelonephrons due to infection, antigens, or other idiopathic causes.
Hypertension	Chronic overloading of the kidney with fluid and electrolytes may lead to kidney insufficiency.
Diabetes mellitus	The disturbance of sugar metabolism and acid-base balance may lead to or predispose a patient to degenerative renal disease.
Nephrotoxic drugs/metals	Certain drugs taken chronically may cause irreversible kidney damage—eg, the aminoglycosides, phenacetin, and heavy metals, such as mercury and lead.
Hypovolemia	Any condition that causes a reduction in renal blood flow will eventually lead to renal ischemia and damage.
Neophroallergens	Certain compounds may produce an immune type of sensitivity reaction with nephritic syndrome—eg, quartan malaria nephrotoxic serum.

increased in patients with renal impairment due to a decrease in first-pass hepatic metabolism (Bianchetti et al, 1978).

The apparent volume of distribution depends largely upon drug protein binding in plasma or tissues and the total body water. Renal impairment may alter the distribution of the drug due to changes in fluid balance, drug protein binding or other factors causing changes in the apparent volume of distribution (Chapter 11). The plasma protein binding of weak acidic drugs in uremic patients is decreased, whereas the protein binding of weak basic drugs is less affected. The decrease in drug protein binding results in a larger fraction of free drug and an increase in the volume of distribution. However, the net elimination half-life is generally increased due to the dominant effect of reduced glomerular filtration. Protein binding of the drug may be further compromised due to the accumulation of metabolites of the drug and accumulation of various biochemical metabolites, such as free fatty acids and urea, that may compete for the protein binding sites for the active drug.

Total body clearance of drugs in uremic patients is also reduced by either a decrease in the glomerular filtration rate and possibly active tubular secretion or reduced hepatic clearance due to a decrease in intrinsic hepatic clearance.

In clinical practice, the estimation of the appropriate drug dosage regimen in patients with impaired renal function is based on an estimate of the remaining renal function of the patient and a prediction of the total body clearance. A complete pharmacokinetic analysis of the drug in the uremic patient is not possible. Moreover, the patient's uremic condition may not be stable and may be changing too rapidly for pharmacokinetic analysis. Each of the approaches for the calculation of a dosage regimen have certain assumptions and limitations that must be carefully assessed by the clinician before any approach is taken. Dosing guidelines for individual drugs in patients with renal impairment may be found in the various reference books, such as the *Physicians' Desk Reference* and the medical literature (Bennett 1988, 1990; St Peter et al, 1992).

GENERAL APPROACHES FOR DOSE ADJUSTMENT IN RENAL DISEASE

Several approaches are available for estimating the appropriate dosage regimen for a patient with renal impairment. Each of these approaches has similar assumptions, including: (1) no change in the desired or target plasma drug concentration, (2) diminished renal clearance but unchanged nonrenal clearance, (3) unaltered drug protein binding and volume of distribution in the renally impaired patient, and (4) unchanged drug absorption from the gastrointestinal tract.

Most of these methods assume that the required therapeutic plasma drug concentration in uremic patients is similar to that required in patients with normal renal function. Uremic patients are maintained on the same C_{av}^{∞} after multiple oral doses or multiple IV bolus injections. For IV infusions, the same C_{ss} is maintained. (C_{ss} is the same as C_{av}^{∞} after the plasma drug concentration reaches steady state.)

The design of dosage regimens for the uremic patient is based on the pharmacokinetic changes that have occurred due to the uremic condition. Generally, drugs in patients with uremia or kidney impairment have prolonged elimination half-lives and a change in the apparent volume of distribution. In less severe uremic conditions there may not be edema nor a significant change in the apparent volume of distribution. Consequently, the methods for dose adjustment in uremic patients are based on an accurate estimation of the drug clearance in these patients.

Several specific clinical approaches for the calculation of drug clearance based on monitoring kidney function are presented later in this chapter. Two general pharmacokinetic approaches for dose adjustment include methods based on drug clearance and methods based on the elimination half-life.

DOSE ADJUSTMENT BASED ON DRUG CLEARANCE

This method tries to maintain the desired C_{av}^{∞} after multiple oral doses of multiple IV bolus injections as total body clearance, Cl_T changes. The calculation for C_{av}^{∞} is

$$C_{av}^{\infty} = \frac{FD_0}{Cl_T \tau} \tag{18.1}$$

For patients with a uremic condition or renal impairment, total body clearance will change to a new value, Cl_T^u. Therefore, to maintain the same desired C_{av}^{∞}, the dose must change to D_0^u or the dosage interval must change to τ^u, as shown in the following equation:

$$C_{av}^{\infty} = \underset{\text{(normal)}}{\frac{D_0^N}{Cl_T^N \tau^N}} = \underset{\text{(uremic)}}{\frac{D_0^u}{Cl_T^u \tau^u}} \tag{18.2}$$

where the superscripts N and u represent normal and uremic conditions, respectively.

Rearranging Equation 18.2 and solving for D_0^u

$$D_0^u = \frac{D_0^N Cl_T^u \tau^u}{Cl_T^N \tau} \tag{18.3}$$

If the dosage interval τ is kept constant, then the uremic dose D_0^u is equal to a fraction (Cl_T^u / Cl_T^N) of the normal dose, as shown in the equation:

$$D_0^u = \frac{D_0^N Cl_T^u}{Cl_T^N} \tag{18.4}$$

For IV infusions the same desired C_{ss} is maintained both for patients with normal renal function and for patients with renal impairment. Therefore, the rate of infusion, R must be changed to a new value of R^{u} for the uremic patient, as described by the equation:

$$C_{ss} = \underset{\text{(normal)}}{\frac{R}{Cl_T^N}} = \underset{\text{(uremic)}}{\frac{R^u}{Cl_T^u}} \tag{18.5}$$

METHOD BASED ON CHANGES IN THE ELIMINATION RATE CONSTANT

The overall elimination rate constant for many drugs is reduced in the uremic patient. A dosage regimen may be designed for the uremic patient either by reducing the normal dose of the drug and keeping the frequency of dosing (dosage interval) constant or by decreasing the frequency of dosing (prolong the dosage interval) and keeping the dose constant. Doses of drugs with a narrow therapeutic window should be reduced—particularly if the drug has accumulated in the patient prior to deterioration of kidney function.

The usual approach to estimating a multiple-dosage regimen in the normal patient is to maintain a desired C_{av}^{∞}, as shown in Equation 18.1. Assuming the V_D is the same in both normal and uremic patients and τ is constant, then the uremic dose D_0^u is a fraction (k^u/k^N) of the normal dose:

$$D_0^u = \frac{D_0^N\, k^u}{k^N} \tag{18.6}$$

When the elimination rate constant for a drug in the uremic patient cannot be determined directly, indirect methods are available to calculate the predicted elimination rate constant based on the renal function of the patient. The assumption on which these dosage regimens are calculated include the following:

1. The renal elimination rate constant (k_R) decreases proportionately as renal function decreases.
2. The nonrenal routes of elimination (primarily, the rate constant for metabolism) remains unchanged.
3. Changes in the renal clearance of the drug are reflected by changes in the creatinine clearance.

The overall elimination rate constant is the sum total of all the routes of elimination in the body including the renal rate and the nonrenal rate constants.

$$k^u = k_{nr} + k_R^u \tag{18.7}$$

where k_{nr} is the nonrenal elimination rate constant, and k_R is the renal excretion rate constant.

Renal clearance is the product of the apparent volume of distribution and the rate constant for renal excretion.

$$Cl_R^u = k_R^u\, V_D^u \tag{18.8}$$

Rearrangement of Equation 18.8 gives

$$k_R^u = \frac{1}{V_D^u}\, Cl_R^u \tag{18.9}$$

Assuming that the apparent volume of distribution and nonrenal routes of elimination do not change in uremia, the $k^{u}_{nr} = k^{N}_{nr}$ and $V^{u}_{D} = V^{N}_{D}$.

Substitution of Equation 18.9 into Equation 18.7 gives

$$k^{u} = k_{nr} + \frac{1}{V_D} Cl^{u}_{R} \quad \textbf{(18.10)}$$

From Equation 18.10, a change in the renal clearance Cl^{u}_{R} due to renal impairment will be reflected by a change in the overall elimination rate constant k^{u}. Because changes in the renal drug clearance cannot be assessed directly in the uremic patient, Cl^{u}_{R} is usually related to a measurement of kidney function as the glomerular filtration rate (GFR), which in turn is estimated by changes in the patient's creatinine clearance.

MEASUREMENT OF GLOMERULAR FILTRATION RATE

Several drugs and endogenous substances have been used as markers to measure GFR. These markers are carried to the kidney by the blood via the renal artery and are filtered at the glomerulus.

Several criteria are necessary for using a drug to measure GFR:

1. The drug must be freely filtered at the glomerulus.
2. The drug must not be reabsorbed nor actively secreted by the renal tubules.
3. The drug should not be metabolized.
4. The drug should not bind significantly to plasma proteins.
5. The drug should not have an effect on the filtration rate nor alter renal function.
6. The drug should be nontoxic.
7. The drug may be infused in a sufficient dose which permits simple and accurate quantitation in plasma and in urine.

Therefore, the rate at which these drug markers are filtered from the blood into the urine per unit of time reflects the glomerular filtration rate of the kidney. Changes in GFR reflect changes in kidney function that may be diminished in uremic conditions.

Inulin, a fructose polysaccharide, fulfills most of the criteria listed above and is therefore used as a standard reference for the measurement of GFR. In practice, however, the use of inulin involves a time-consuming procedure in which inulin is given by intravenous infusion until a constant steady-state plasma level is obtained. Clearance of inulin may then be measured by the rate of infusion divided by the steady-state plasma inulin concentration. Although this procedure gives an accurate value for GFR, inulin clearance is not used frequently in clinical practice.

The clearance of creatinine is used most extensively as a measurement of GFR. *Creatinine* is an endogenous substance formed during muscle metabolism from creatine phosphate. Creatinine production varies with the age, weight, and sex of the individual. In humans, creatinine is mainly filtered at the glomerulus with no reabsorption. However, a small amount of creatinine may be actively secreted by the renal tubules, and the values for GFR obtained by the creatinine clearance tend to be higher than GFR measured by inulin clearance. Creatinine clearance tends to decrease in the elderly patient. As mentioned in Chapter 17, the physiologic changes due to aging may necessitate special considerations in administering drugs in the elderly.

Blood urea nitrogen (BUN) is a commonly used clinical diagnostic laboratory test for renal disease. Urea is the end-product of protein catabolism and is excreted through the kidney. Normal BUN levels range from 10 to 20 mg/dL. Higher BUN levels generally indicate the presence of renal disease. However, other factors, such as excessive protein intake, reduced renal blood flow, hemorrhagic shock, and gastric bleeding may affect increased BUN levels. The renal clearance of urea is by glomerular filtration and partial reabsorption in the renal tubules. Therefore, the renal clearance of urea is less than creatinine or inulin clearance and does not give a quantitative measure of kidney function.

SERUM CREATININE CONCENTRATION AND CREATININE CLEARANCE

Under normal circumstances, creatinine production is roughly equal to creatinine excretion, so that the serum creatinine level remains constant. In a patient with reduced glomerular filtration, serum creatinine will accumulate in accordance with the degree of loss of glomerular filtration in the kidney. The serum creatinine concentration alone is frequently used to determine creatinine clearance, Cl_{Cr}. Creatinine clearance from the serum creatinine concentration is a rapid and convenient way to monitor kidney function.

Creatinine clearance may be defined as the rate of urinary excretion of creatinine/serum creatinine. Creatinine clearance can be calculated directly by determining the patient's serum creatinine concentration and the rate of urinary excretion of creatinine. The approach is similar to that used in the determination of drug clearance. In practice, the rate of urinary excretion of creatinine is measured for the entire day to obtain a reliable excretion rate. The serum creatinine concentration is determined at the midpoint of the urinary collection period. Creatinine clearance is clinically expressed in mL/min and serum creatinine concentration in mg/dL or mg%.

Creatinine clearance may be estimated from the 24-hour urinary creatinine excretion or from the serum creatinine concentration. Other Cl_{Cr} methods based solely on serum creatinine are generally compared to the creatinine clearance obtained from the 24-hour urinary creatinine excretion.

The following equation is used to calculate creatinine clearance in mL/min when the serum creatinine concentration is known:

$$Cl_{Cr} = \frac{\text{rate of urinary excretion of creatinine}}{\text{serum concentration of creatinine}} \quad \textbf{(18.11)}$$

$$Cl_{Cr} = \frac{C_u V 100}{C_{Cr} 1440}$$

where C_{Cr} = creatinine concentration (mg/dL) of the serum taken at the 12th hour or at the midpoint of the urine collection period, V = volume of urine excreted (mL) in 24 hours, C_u = concentration of creatinine in urine (mg/mL), and Cl_{Cr} = creatinine clearance in mL/min.

Creatinine is primarily eliminated by glomerular filtration. A small fraction of creatinine also is eliminated by active secretion and some nonrenal elimination. Therefore, the Cl_{Cr} value obtained from creatinine measurements overestimate the actual glomerular filtration rate (GFR).

Creatinine clearance has been normalized both to body surface area using 1.73 m^2 as the average and to body weight for a 70-kg adult male. Creatinine distributes into total body water, and when clearance is normalized to a standard V_D, similar drug half-lives in adults and children correspond with identical clearances.

Creatinine clearance values must be considered carefully in special populations such as the elderly, obese, and emaciated patients. In elderly and emaciated patients, muscle mass may have declined thus lowering the production of creatinine. However, serum creatinine concentration values may appear to be in the normal range due to lower renal creatinine excretion. Thus, the calculation of creatinine clearance from serum creatinine may give an inaccurate estimation of the renal function. For the obese patient, generally defined as having greater than 20% of ideal body weight (IBW), creatinine clearance should be based on ideal body weight. Estimation of creatinine clearance based on total body weight, TBW would exaggerate the Cl_{Cr} values in the obese patient. Women with normal kidney function have smaller creatinine clearance values, approximately 80 to 85% of that in men with normal kidney function.

Several empirical equations have been used to estimate lean body weight (LBW) based on the patient's height and actual (total) body weight (see Chapter 17). The following equations have been used for the estimate of LBW in renally impaired patients.

LBW (males) = 50 kg + 2.3 kg for each inch over 5 ft
LBW (females) = 45.5 kg + 2.3 kg for each inch over 5 ft

For the purpose of dose adjustment in renal patients, normal creatinine clearance has generally been assumed to be between 100 to 125 mL/min per 1.73 M^2 for an ideal body weight subject. For a female adult, $Cl_{Cr} = 108.8 \pm 13.5$ mL/173 M^2, and for an average adult male, $Cl_{Cr} = 124.5 \pm 9.7$ mL/173 sq M (*Scientific Table*, 1973). Creatinine clearance is affected by diet and salt intakes. As a convenient approximation, the normal clearance has often been assumed to be approximately 100 mL/min by many clinicians.

Calculation of Creatinine Clearance from Serum Creatinine Concentration

The problems of obtaining a complete 24-hour urine collection from a patient, the time necessary for urine collection, and the analysis time preclude a direct estimation of creatinine clearance. *Serum creatinine concentration* C_{Cr} is related to creatinine clearance and C_{Cr} is measured routinely in the clinical laboratory. Therefore, creatinine clearance, Cl_{Cr} is most often estimated from the patient's C_{Cr}.

Several methods are available for the calculation of creatinine clearance from the serum creatinine concentration. The more accurate methods are based on the patient's age, height, weight, and gender. These methods should only be used in patients with intact liver function and no abnormal muscle disease, such as hypertrophy or dystrophy. Moreover, most of the methods assume a stable creatinine clearance. Creatinine clearance in obese patients is generally based on lean body weight or actual body weight of the patient using the lower of the two values.

Adults

The following method by Jellife (1973) takes into account the patient's age and is generally applicable for adult patients age 20 to 80 years. With this method, the older the patient, the smaller is the creatinine clearance for the same serum creatinine concentration.

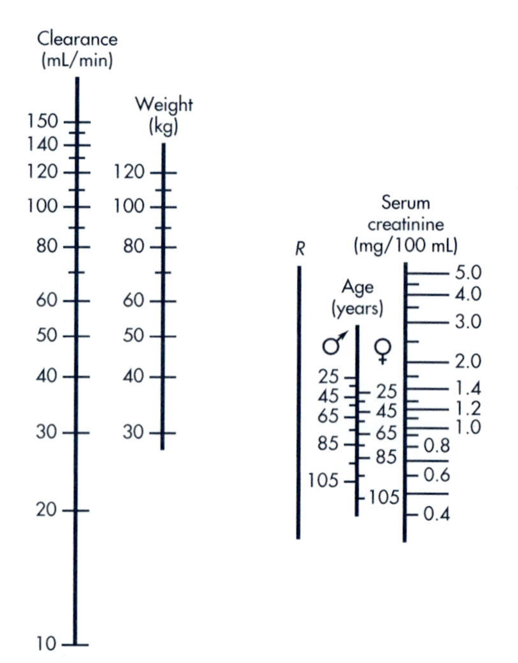

Figure 18-1. Nomogram for evaluation of endogenous creatinine clearance. To use the nomogram, connect the patient's weight on the second line from the left with the patient's age on the fourth line with a ruler. Note the point of intersection on *R* and keep the ruler there. Turn the right part of the ruler to the appropriate serum creatinine value and the left side will indicate the clearance in mL/min.
(From Kampmann and Siersback-Nielsen, 1974, with permission.)

The *Jellife method* for males is shown in Equation 18.4. For female patients one uses 90% of the Cl_{Cr} obtained for males to make the calculation shown in Equation 18.12.

$$Cl_{Cr} = \frac{98 - 0.8\ (\text{age} - 20)}{C_{Cr}} \tag{18.12}$$

The method by *Crockcroft and Gault* (1976) shown in Equation 18.13 is also used to estimate creatinine clearance from serum creatinine concentration. This method does include both age and weight of the patient.

Males:

$$Cl_{Cr} = \frac{[140 - \text{age (yr)}] \times \text{body weight (kg)}}{72(C_{Cr})} \tag{18.13}$$

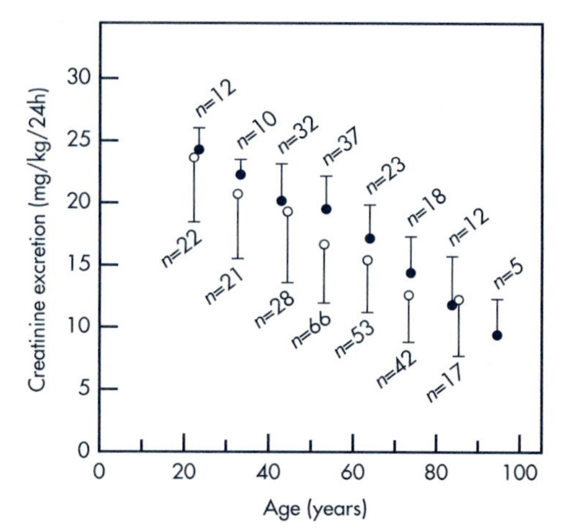

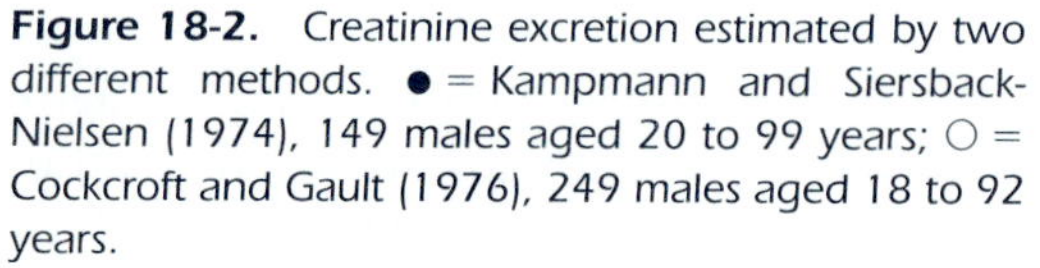

Figure 18-2. Creatinine excretion estimated by two different methods. ● = Kampmann and Siersback-Nielsen (1974), 149 males aged 20 to 99 years; ○ = Cockcroft and Gault (1976), 249 males aged 18 to 92 years.
(From Cockcroft and Gault, 1976, with permission.)

Females:

For female patients, use 85% of the Cl_{Cr} value obtained in males.

The *nomogram method* estimates creatinine clearance on the basis of age, weight, and serum creatinine concentration, as shown in Figure 18-1.

Cockcroft and Gault (1976) compared their method with the nomogram method of Siersback-Nielsen et al (1971) in adult males of various ages. Creatinine clearance estimated by both methods were comparable. Both methods also demonstrated an age-related linear decline in creatinine excretion (Fig. 18-2), which may be due to a decrease muscle mass with age.

Children

There are a number of methods for calculation of creatinine clearance in children based on body length and serum creatinine concentration. Equation 18.14 is a method by Schwartz and associates (1976).

$$Cl_{Cr} = \frac{0.55 \text{ body length (cm)}}{C_{Cr}} \tag{18.14}$$

where Cl_{Cr} is given in mL/min 1.73 m^2.

Another method for the calculation of creatinine clearance in children uses the nomogram by Traub and Johnson (1980) shown in Figure 18-3. This nomogram was based on observations of 81 children aged 6 to 12 years and requires the patient's height and serum creatinine concentration.

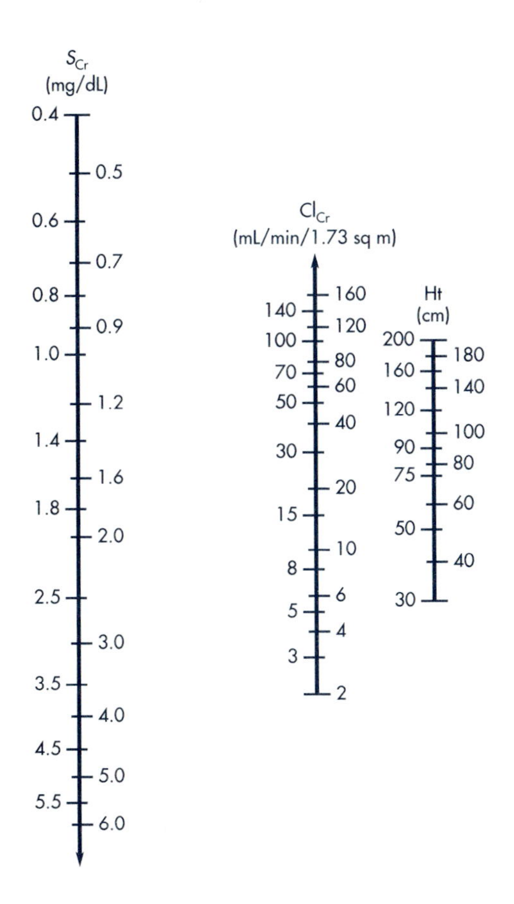

Figure 18-3. Nomogram for rapid evaluation of endogenous creatinine clearance (Cl_{Cr}) in pediatric patients (aged 6–12 yr). To predict Cl_{Cr}, connect the child's S_{Cr} (serum creatinine) and Ht (height) with a ruler and read the Cl_{Cr} where the ruler intersects the center line.
(From Taub and Johnson, 1980, with permission.)

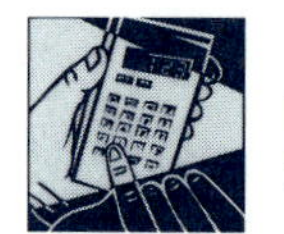

PRACTICE PROBLEMS

1. What is the creatinine clearance for a 25-year-old male patient with a C_{Cr} of 1 mg/dL and a body weight of 80 kg?

Solution

Using the Jellife equation (Eq. 18.12),

$$Cl_{Cr} = \frac{98 - 0.8(25 - 20)}{1\%} = 94 \text{ mL/min } 1.73 \text{ m}^2$$

2. Using the nomogram (Fig. 18-1), join the points at 25 years (male) and 80 kg with a ruler—let the line intersect line *R*. Connect the intersection point at line *R* with the creatinine concentration point of 1 mg/dL—extend the line to intersect the "clearance line." The extended line will intersect the clearance line at 110 mL/min, giving the creatinine clearance for the patient.

3. What is the creatinine clearance for a 25-year-old male patient with a C_{Cr} of 1 mg/dL? The patient is 5 ft, 4 in in height and weighs 103 kg.

Solution

The patient is obese and the Cl_{Cr} calculation should be based on ideal body weight.

LBW (males) = 50 kg + 2.3 (4) kg = 59.2 kg

Using the Cockcroft and Gault method (Eq. 18.13), the Cl_{Cr} can be calculated.

$$Cl_{Cr} = \frac{(140 - 25)(59.2 \text{ kg})}{72(1)} = 94.6 \text{ mL/min}$$

The practice problems show that, depending on the formula used, the calculated Cl_{Cr} can vary considerably. Consequently, unless a significant change in the creatinine clearance occurs, use of these methods will result in a rather large margin of error. According to St Peter et al, 1992, dosage adjustment of many antibiotic drugs is only necessary when the glomerular filtration rate as measured by Cl_{Cr} is less than 50 mL/min. For the aminoglycoside antibiotics and vancomycin, dosage adjustment is individualized according to the wide range of Cl_{Cr}. Therefore, dosage adjustment for all drugs on the basis of these Cl_{Cr} methods alone is not justified.

The serum creatinine methods for the estimation of the creatinine clearance assume stabilized kidney function and a steady-state serum creatinine concentration. In acute renal failure and in other situations in which kidney function is changing, the serum creatinine may not represent steady-state conditions. If C_{Cr} is measured daily and the C_{Cr} value is constant, then the serum creatinine concentration is probably at steady state. If the C_{Cr} values are changing daily, then kidney function is changing and the serum creatinine is not at steady state.

DOSAGE ADJUSTMENT FOR UREMIC PATIENTS

Dosage adjustment for drugs in uremic or renally impaired patients should be made in accordance with changes in pharmacodynamics and pharmacokinetics of the drug in the individual patient. Active metabolites of the drug may also be formed and must be considered for additional pharmacologic effects.

The following methods may be used to estimate an initial and maintenance dose regimen. After initiating the dose, the clinician should continue to monitor the pharmacodynamics and pharmacokinetics of the drug. He or she should also evaluate the patient's renal function, which may be changing.

Basis of Dosage Adjustment in Uremia

The loading drug dose is based on the apparent volume of distribution of the patient. It is generally assumed that the apparent volume of distribution is not altered significantly, and, therefore, that the loading dose of the drug is the same in the uremic patient as in subjects with normal renal function.

The maintenance dose is based on clearance of the drug in the patient. In the uremic patient, the rate of renal drug excretion has decreased, leading to a decrease in total body clearance. Most methods for dosage adjustment assumes nonrenal drug clearance to be unchanged. The fraction of normal renal function remaining in the uremic patient is estimated from creatinine clearance.

After the remaining total body clearance in the uremic patient is estimated, a dosage regimen may be developed by (1) decreasing the maintenance dose, (2) increasing the dosage interval, or (3) changing both maintenance dose and dosage interval.

Although total body clearance is a more accurate index of drug dosing, the elimination half-life of the drug is used more commonly for dose adjustment due to its convenience. Clearance allows for the prediction of steady-state drug concentrations, while elimination half-life yields information on the time it takes to reach steady-state concentration.

Nomograms

Nomograms are charts available for use in estimating dosage regimens in uremic patients (Bjornsson, 1986; Chennavasin and Craig Brater, 1981; Tozer, 1974). The nomograms may be based on serum creatinine concentrations, patient data (height, weight, age, gender), and the pharmacokinetics of the drug. As discussed by Chennavasin and Craig Brater (1981), each nomogram has errors in its assumptions and drug data base.

Most methods for dose adjustment in renal disease assume that nonrenal elimination of the drug is not affected by renal impairment and that the remaining renal excretion rate constant in the uremic patient is proportional to the product of a constant and the creatinine clearance, Cl_{Cr}.

$$k_u = k_{nr} + \alpha\, Cl_{Cr} \qquad \textbf{(18.15)}$$

where k_{nr} is the nonrenal elimination rate constant and α is a constant.

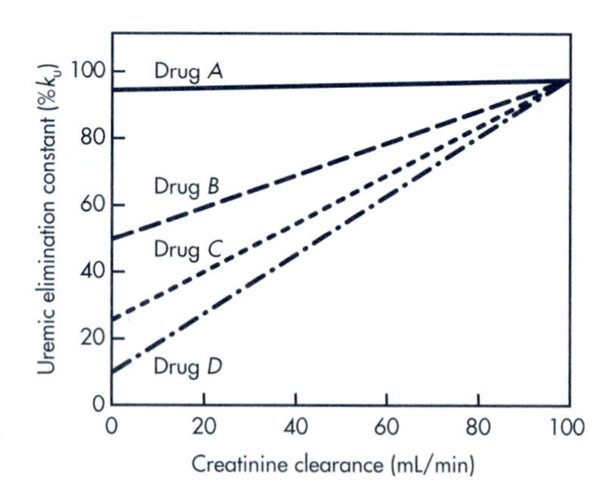

Figure 18-4. Relationship between creatinine clearance and the drug elimination rate constant.

Equation 18.15 is similar to Equation 18.10, where $\alpha = 1/V_D$, and can be used for the construction of a nomogram. Figure 18-4 shows a graphical representation of Equation 18.15 for four different drugs, each with a different renal excretion rate constant. The fraction of drug excreted in the urine unchanged *fe* for drugs *A*, *B*, *C*, and *D* is 5, 50, 75, and 90%, respectively. A creatinine clearance of ≥100 mL/min is considered an adequate glomerular filtration rate in subjects with normal renal function. The uremic elimination rate constant (k_u) is expressed as a percent and is equal to the sum of the nonrenal and renal elimination rate constants. If the patient has complete renal shutdown (ie, creatinine clearance = 0 mL/min), then the intersect on the *y*-axis, represents the percent of drug elimination due to nonrenal drug elimination routes. Thus, drug *D*, which is excreted 90% unchanged in the urine, has the steepest slope (equivalent to α in Eq. 18.15) and is most affected by small changes in creatinine clearance. In contrast, drug *A*, which is excreted only 5% unchanged in the urine (ie, 95% eliminated by nonrenal routes), is least affected by a decrease in creatinine clearance.

The nomogram method of Welling and Craig (1976) provides an estimation of the ratio of the uremic elimination rate constant (k_u) to the normal elimination rate constant (k_N) on the basis of creatinine clearance (Fig. 18-5). For this method, Welling and Craig (1976) provided a list of drugs grouped according to the amount of drug excreted unchanged in the urine (Table 18.2). From the k_u/k_N ratio, the uremic dose could be estimated according to Equation 18.16.

$$\text{Uremic dose} = \frac{k_u}{k_N} \times \text{normal dose} \quad \textbf{(18.16)}$$

When the dosage interval τ is kept constant, the uremic dose is always a smaller fraction of the normal dose. Instead of reducing the dose for the uremic patient, the usual dose is kept constant and the dosage interval τ is prolonged according to the following equation.

$$\text{Dosage interval in uremia, } \tau_u = \frac{k_N}{k_u} \times \tau_N \quad \textbf{(18.17)}$$

where τ_u is the dosage interval for the dose in the uremic patient and τ_N is the dosage interval for the dose in patients with normal renal function.

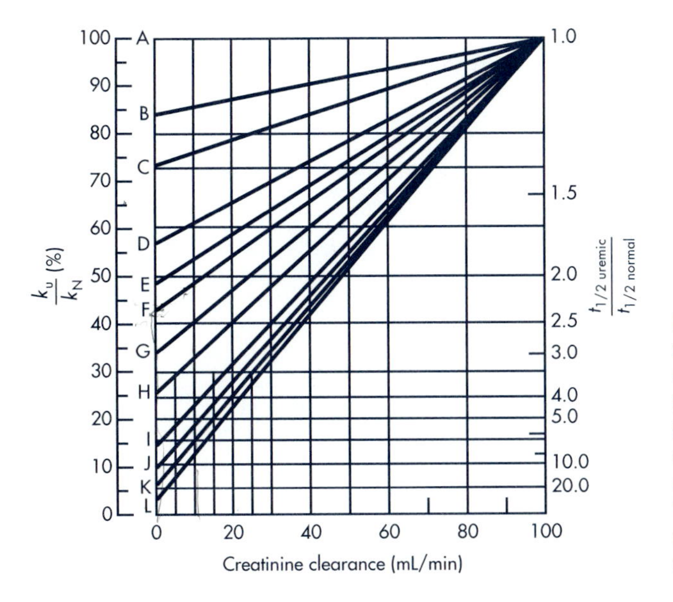

Figure 18-5. This nomograph describes the changes in the percentage of normal elimination rate constant (left ordinate) and the consequent geometric increase in elimination half-life (right ordinate) as a function of creatinine clearance. The drugs associated with the individual slopes are given in Table 18.2.
(From Welling and Craig, 1976, with permission.)

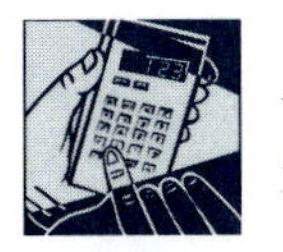

PRACTICE PROBLEM

Lincomycin is given at 500 mg every 6 hours to a 75-kg normal patient. What doses would be used (a) in complete renal shutdown ($Cl_{Cr} = 0$) and (b) when $Cl_{Cr} = 10$ mL/min?

Solution

To use the nomogram method, follow the steps below:

1. Locate the group to which the drug belongs in Table 18.2.

2. Find k_u/k_N at the point corresponding to the Cl_{Cr} of the patient (Fig. 18-5).

3. Determine k_u for the patient.

4. Make the dose adjustment in accordance with pharmacokinetic principles.

a. When $Cl_{Cr} = 0$,

$$k_u = k_{nr} + k_r$$

In complete renal shutdown ($k_r = 0$),

$$k_u = k_{nr} = 0.06 \text{ hr}^{-1} \text{ (Table 18.2, group F)}$$

or find k_u/k_N in Figure 18-5, group F, at $Cl_{Cr} = 0$ mL/min:

$$\frac{k_u}{k_N} = 0.425$$

$$k_u = 0.425(0.15) = 0.0638 \text{ hr}^{-1}$$

$$\text{Uremic dose} = 500 \text{ mg} \times \frac{0.0638}{0.15} = 212 \text{ mg every 6 hr}$$

b. At $Cl_{Cr} = 10$ mL

$$\frac{k_u}{k_N} = 0.48$$

$$k_N = 0.15\ \text{hr}^{-1}$$
$$k_u = (0.48)(0.15) = 0.072\ \text{hr}^{-1}$$
$$\text{Dose} = \frac{0.072}{0.15} \times 500\ \text{mg} = 240\ \text{mg}$$

Alternatively,

$$\text{Dose} = (0.48)(500) = 240\ \text{mg}$$

TABLE 18.2 Elimination Rate Constants for Various Drugs[a]

GROUP	DRUG	k_N (hr^{-1})	k_{nr} (hr^{-1})	k_{nr}/k_N%
A	Minocycline	0.04	0.04	100.0
	Rifampicin	0.25	0.25	100.0
	Lidocaine	0.39	0.36	92.3
	Digitoxin	0.114	0.10	87.7
B	Doxycycline	0.037	0.031	83.8
	Chlortetracycline	0.12	0.095	79.2
C	Clindamycin	0.16	0.12	75.0
	Chloramphenicol	0.26	0.19	73.1
	Propranolol	0.22	0.16	72.8
	Erythromycin	0.39	0.28	71.8
D	Trimethoprim	0.054	0.031	57.4
	Isoniazid (fast)	0.53	0.30	56.6
	Isoniazid (slow)	0.23	0.13	56.5
E	Dicloxacillin	1.20	0.60	50.0
	Sulfadiazine	0.069	0.032	46.4
	Sulfamethoxazole	0.084	0.037	44.0
F	Nafcillin	1.26	0.54	42.8
	Chlorpropamide	0.020	0.008	40.0
	Lincomycin	0.15	0.06	40.0
G	Colistimethate	0.154	0.054	35.1
	Oxacillin	1.73	0.58	33.6
	Digoxin	0.021	0.007	33.3
H	Tetracycline	0.120	0.033	27.5
	Cloxacillin	1.21	0.31	25.6
	Oxytetracycline	0.075	0.014	18.7
I	Amoxicillin	0.70	0.10	14.3
	Methicillin	1.40	0.19	13.6
J	Ticarcillin	0.58	0.066	11.4
	Penicillin G	1.24	0.13	10.5
	Ampicillin	0.53	0.05	9.4
	Carbenicillin	0.55	0.05	9.1
K	Cefazolin	0.32	0.02	6.2
	Cephaloridine	0.51	0.03	5.9
	Cephalothin	1.20	0.06	5.0
	Gentamicin	0.30	0.015	5.0
L	Flucytosine	0.18	0.007	3.9
	Kanamycin	0.28	0.01	3.6
	Vancomycin	0.12	0.004	3.3
	Tobramycin	0.32	0.010	3.1
	Cephalexin	1.54	0.032	2.1

[a]k_N is for patients with normal renal function, k_{nr} is for patients with severe renal impairment, and k_{nr}/k_N% = percent of normal elimination in severe renal impairment.

From Welling and Craig (1976), with permission.

Fraction of Drug Excreted Unchanged *fe* Methods

For many drugs, the fraction of drug excreted unchanged (*fe*) is available in the literature. Table 18.3 lists various drugs with their *fe* value and elimination half-life. The *fe* method for estimation of a dosage regimen in the uremic patient is a general method that may be applied to any drug whose *fe* is known.

TABLE 18.3 Fraction of Drug Excreted Unchanged (*fe*) and Elimination Half-Life Values

DRUG	*fe*	$t_{1/2}$ normal (hr)[a]	DRUG	*fe*	$t_{1/2}$ normal (hr)[a]
Acebutolol	0.44 ± 0.11	2.7 ± 0.4	Erythromycin	0.15	1.1–3.5
Acetaminophen	0.03 ± 0.01	2.0 ± 0.4	Ethambutol	0.79 ± 0.03	3.1 ± 0.4
Acetohexamide	0.4	1.3	Ethosuximide	0.19	33 ± 6
Allopurinol	0.1	2–8	Flucytosine	0.63–0.84	5.3 ± 0.7
Active metabolite		16–30	Flunitrazepam	0.01	15 ± 5
Alprenolol	0.005	3.1 ± 1.2	Furosemide	0.74 ± 0.07	0.85 ± 0.17
Amantadine	0.85	10	Gentamicin	0.98	2–3
Amikacin	0.98	2.3 ± 0.4	Griseofulvin	0	15
Amiloride	0.5	8 ± 2	Hydralazine	0.12–0.14	2.2–2.6
Amoxicillin	0.52 ± 0.15	1.0 ± 0.1	Hydrochlorothiazide	0.95	2.5 ± 0.2
Amphetamine	0.4–0.45	12	Indomethacin	0.15 ± 0.08	2.6–11.2
Amphotericin B	0.03	360	Isoniazid		
Ampicillin	0.90 ± 0.08	1.3 ± 0.2	Rapid acetylators	0.07 ± 0.02	1.1 ± 0.2
Atenolol	0.85	6.3 ± 1.8	Slow acetylators	0.29 ± 0.05	3.0 ± 0.8
Azlocillin	0.6	1.0	Isosorbide dinitrate	0.05	0.5
Bacampicillin	0.88	0.9	Kanamycin	0.9	2.1 ± 0.2
Baclofen	0.75	3–4	Lidocaine	0.02 ± 0.01	1.8 ± 0.4
Bleomycin	0.55	1.5–8.9	Lincomycin	0.6	5
Bretylium	0.8 ± 0.1	4–17	Lithium	0.95 ± 0.15	22 ± 8
Bumetanide	0.33	3.5	Lorazepam	0.01	14 ± 5
Carbenicillin	0.82 ± 0.09	1.1 ± 0.2	Meperidine	0.04–0.22	3.2 ± 0.8
Cefalothin	0.52	0.6 ± 0.3	Methadone	0.2	22
Cefamandole	0.96 ± 0.03	0.77	Methicillin	0.88 ± 0.17	0.85 ± 0.23
Cefazolin	0.80 ± 0.13	1.8 ± 0.4	Methotrexate	0.94	8.4
Cefoperazone	0.2–0.3	2.0	Methyldopa	0.63 ± 0.10	1.8 ± 0.2
Cefotaxime	0.5–0.6	1–1.5	Metronidazole	0.25	8.2
Cefoxitin	0.88 ± 0.08	0.7 ± 0.13	Mexiletine	0.1	12
Cefuroxime	0.92	1.1	Mezlocillin	0.75	0.8
Cephalexin	0.96	0.9 ± 0.18	Minocycline	0.1 ± 0.02	18 ± 4
Chloramphenicol	0.05	2.7 ± 0.8	Minoxidil	0.1	4
Chlorphentermine	0.2	120	Moxalactam	0.82–0.96	2.5–3.0
Chlorpropamide	0.2	36	Nadolol	0.73 ± 0.04	16 ± 2
Chlorthalidone	0.65 ± 0.09	44 ± 10	Nafcillin	0.27 ± 0.05	0.9–1.0
Cimetidine	0.77 ± 0.06	2.1 ± 1.1	Nalidixic acid	0.2	1.0
Clindamycin	0.09–0.14	2.7 ± 0.4	Netilmicin	0.98	2.2
Clofibrate	0.11–0.32	13 ± 3	Neostigmine	0.67	1.3 ± 0.8
Clonidine	0.62 ± 0.11	8.5 ± 2.0	Nitrazepam	0.01	29 ± 7
Colistin	0.9	3	Nitrofurantoin	0.5	0.3
Cytarabine	0.1	2	Nomifensine	0.15–0.22	3.0 ± 1.0
Cyclophosphamide	0.3	5	Oxacillin	0.75	0.5
Dapsone	0.1	20	Oxprenolol	0.05	1.5
Dicloxacillin	0.60 ± 0.07	0.7 ± 0.07	Pancuronium	0.5	3.0
Digitoxin	0.33 ± 0.15	166 ± 65	Pentazocine	0.2	2.5
Digoxin	0.72 ± 0.09	42 ± 19	Phenobarbital	0.2 ± 0.05	86 ± 7
Disopyramide	0.55 ± 0.06	7.8 ± 1.6	Pindolol	0.41	3.4 ± 0.2
Doxycycline	0.40 ± 0.04	20 ± 4	Pivampicillin	0.9	0.9

(Continued)

TABLE 18.3 Fraction of Drug Excreted Unchanged (*fe*) and Elimination Half-Life Values (continued)

DRUG	*fe*	$t_{1/2}$ normal (hr)[a]	DRUG	*fe*	$t_{1/2}$ normal (hr)[a]
Polymyxin B	0.88	4.5	Thiazinamium	0.41	
Prazosin	0.01	2.9 ± 0.8	Theophylline	0.08	9 ± 2.1
Primidone	0.42 ± 0.15	8.0 ± 4.8	Ticarcillin	0.86	1.2
Procainamide	0.67 ± 0.08	2.9 ± 0.6	Timolol	0.2	3–5
Propranolol	0.005	3.9 ± 0.4	Tobramycin	0.98	2.2 ± 0.1
Quinidine	0.18 ± 0.05	6.2 ± 1.8	Tocainide	0.20–0.70 (0.40 mean)	1.6–3
Rifampin	0.16 ± 0.04	2.1 ± 0.3			
Salicylic acid	0.2	3	Tolbutamide	0	5.9 ± 1.4
Sisomicin	0.98	2.8	Triamterene	0.04 ± 0.01	2.8 ± 0.9
Sotalol	0.6	6.5–13	Trimethoprim	0.53 ± 0.02	11 ± 1.4
Streptomycin	0.96	2.8	Tubocurarine	0.43 ± 0.08	2 ± 1.1
Sulfisoxazole	0.53 ± 0.09	5.9 ± 0.9	Valproic acid	0.02 ± 0.02	16 ± 3
Sulfinpyrazone	0.45	2.3	Vancomycin	0.97	5–6
Tetracycline	0.48	9.9 ± 1.5	Warfarin	0	37 ± 15
Thiamphenicol	0.9	3			

[a]Half-life is a derived parameter that changes as a function of both clearance and volume of distribution. It is independent of body size, because it is a function of these two parameters (Cl, V_D), each of which is proportional to body size. It is important to consider that half-life is the time to eliminate 50% of the "drug" from the body (plasma), not the time in which 50% of the effect is lost.

From Benet et al (1984), with permission.

The Giusti–Hayton Method

This method assumes that the effect of reduced kidney function on the renal portion of the elimination constant can be estimated from the ratio of the uremic creatinine clearance (Cl^{u}_{Cr}) to the normal creatinine clearance (Cl^{N}_{Cr}).

$$\frac{k^{u}_{r}}{k^{N}_{r}} = \frac{Cl^{u}_{Cr}}{Cl^{N}_{Cr}} \tag{18.18}$$

where k^{u}_{r} is the uremic renal excretion rate constant and k^{N}_{r} is the normal renal excretion rate constant.

$$k^{u}_{r} = k^{N}_{r}\frac{Cl^{u}_{Cr}}{Cl^{N}_{Cr}} \tag{18.19}$$

Because the overall uremic elimination rate constant k_u is the sum of renal and nonrenal factors,

$$k_u = k^{u}_{nr} + k^{u}_{r} \tag{18.20}$$

$$k_u = k^{u}_{nr} + k^{N}_{r}\left(\frac{Cl^{u}_{Cr}}{Cl^{N}_{Cr}}\right)$$

Dividing Equation 18.20 by k_N on both sides yields:

$$\frac{k_u}{k_N} = \frac{k^{u}_{nr}}{k_N} + \frac{k^{N}_{r}}{k_N}\left(\frac{Cl^{u}_{Cr}}{Cl^{N}_{Cr}}\right) \tag{18.21}$$

Let $fe = k^{N}_{r}/k_N$ = fraction of drug excreted unchanged in the urine and $1 - fe =$

k_{nr}^{u}/k_N = fraction of drug excreted by nonrenal routes. Substitution into Equation 18.21 yields

$$\frac{k_u}{k_N} = (1 - fe) + fe\left(\frac{Cl_{Cr}^{u}}{Cl_{Cr}^{N}}\right)$$

or

$$\frac{k_u}{k_N} = 1 - fe\left(1 - \frac{Cl_{Cr}^{u}}{Cl_{Cr}^{N}}\right) = G \quad \textbf{(18.22)}$$

where the G factor is a ratio that can be obtained from the fraction of drug excreted by the kidney and the creatinine clearance of the uremic patient. Equation 18.22 is known as the *Giusti–Hayton equation* (Giusti and Hayton, 1973).

The Giusti–Hayton equation is useful for most drugs in the literature for which the fraction of drug excreted by renal routes has been reported.

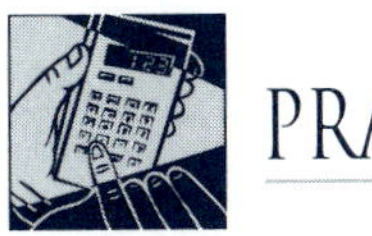

PRACTICE PROBLEM

The maintenance dose of gentamicin is 80 mg every 6 hours for a patient with normal renal function. Calculate the maintenance dose for a uremic patient with creatinine clearance of 20 mL/min?

Solution

From the literature, gentamicin was reported to be 100% excreted by the kidney (ie, $fe = 1$). Using Equation 18.22 and assuming a normal creatinine clearance of 100 mL/min,

$$G = 1 - 1\left(1 - \frac{20}{100}\right) = 0.2$$

Because

$$\frac{D_u}{D_N} = \frac{k_u}{k_N} = G \quad \textbf{(18.23)}$$

where D_u = uremic dose, D_N = normal dose.

$$D_u = D_N \times \frac{k_u}{k_N} = 80 \text{ mg} \times 0.2 = 16 \text{ mg}$$

The maintenance dose would be 16 mg every 6 hours. Alternatively, the dosing interval can be adjusted without changing the dose.

$$\frac{\tau_u}{\tau_N} = \frac{k_N}{k_u}$$

$$\tau_u = \tau_N \frac{k_N}{k_u} = 6 \text{ hr} \times \frac{1}{0.2} = 30 \text{ hr}$$

where τ_u and τ_N are dosing intervals for uremic and normal patients, respectively. The patient may be given 80 mg every 30 hours.

The approach developed by Giusti and Hayton (1973) was followed by Tozer (1974) and Bjornsson (1986). Their approach uses the following equation:

$$Q = 1 - fe(1 - kf) \tag{18.24}$$

where Q is the dosage adjustment factor, which is the same as G in the Giusti–Hayton Equation (18.22); $kf = Cl^{u}_{Cr}/Cl^{N}_{Cr}$, and fe is the fraction of unchanged drug excreted renally.

Equation 18.24 is used in the same way as Equation 18.23 to estimate the initial maintenance dose in the uremic patient.

All the methods discussed earlier assumed that nonrenal elimination, k_{nr}, is unchanged, thereby ignoring potential side effects resulting from an increase in the half-life for metabolism of the parent drug and/or an accumulation of active metabolites of the drug.

Bodenham and associates (1988) have shown that although lorazepam pharmacokinetics were not significantly altered in patients with chronic renal failure, the clearance of lorazepam glucuronide, a major metabolite, was reduced significantly. Therefore, there are potential sedative side effects in the renally impaired patient due to a longer metabolite half-life. Bodenham and coworkers (1988) also cited literature references to potentiation of sedative and analgesic drug effects in renal, liver, and other multisystem disease states.

In addition to pharmacokinetic changes, possible changes in pharmacodynamic effects in patients with renal and other diseases must be considered. Neuromuscular blocking drugs may be potentiated or antagonized by changes in potassium, phosphate, and hydrogen ion concentration brought about by uremic states. Morphine potentiation has been reported in hypocalcemic states. These authors also cautioned that, in many patients, plasma creatinine concentration may not rise for some time until creatinine clearance has fallen significantly, thereby adding to the uncertainty of any method that depends on plasma C_{Cr} for dose adjustment.

Comparison of the Various Methods for Dose Adjustment in Uremic Patients

All of the methods mentioned previously have the common limitations that the drug must follow dose-independent kinetics and that the volume of distribution of the drug must remain relatively constant in the uremic patient. As mentioned, it is usually assumed that the nonrenal routes of elimination, such as hepatic clearance, do not change. Because no correction for metabolites is made, any drug having an active pharmacologic metabolite must be additionally modified. Another assumption in the use of these methods is that pharmacologic response is unchanged in the uremic patient. This assumption may be unrealistic with drugs that act differently in the disease state. For example, the pharmacologic response with digoxin is dependent on the potassium level in the body, and the potassium level in the uremic patient may be rather different from that of the normal individual. In a patient undergoing dialysis, loss of potassium may increase the potential of toxic effect of the drug digoxin. With many drugs, studies have shown that the incidence of adverse effects was increased in uremic patients. It is often impossible to distinguish whether the increase in adverse effect is due to a pharmacokinetic change or to a pharmacodynamic change in the receptor sensitivity to the drug. In any event, these observations point out the fact that dose adjustment must be regarded as a preliminary estimation to be followed with further adjustments in accordance with the observed clinical response.

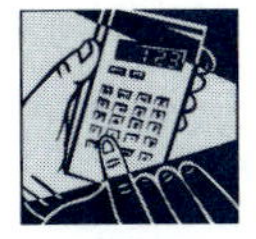

PRACTICE PROBLEMS

1. An adult male patient (52 yr, 75 kg) whose serum creatinine is 2.4 mg/dL is to be given gentamicin sulfate for a confirmed Gram-negative infection. The usual dose of gentamicin in adult patients with normal renal function is 1 mg/kg every 8 hours by multiple IV bolus injections. Gentamicin sulfate (Garamycin) is available in 2-mL vials containing 40 mg gentamicin sulfate per mL. Calculate (a) the creatinine clearance in this patient by the Cockcroft and Gault method and (b) the appropriate dosage regimen of gentamicin sulfate for this patient in mg and mL.

Solution

a. The creatinine clearance is calculated by the Cockcroft and Gault method using Equation 18.13.

$$Cl_{Cr} = \frac{(140 - 52)(75)}{72(2.4)} = 38.19 \text{ mL/min}$$

b. The initial dose of gentamicin sulfate in this patient may be estimated using Equation 18.22 or 18.24. Normal creatinine clearance is assumed to equal 100 mL/min. The fraction of dose excreted unchanged in the urine $fe = 0.98$ for gentamicin sulfate (Table 18.3).

$$\frac{k_u}{k_N} = Q = 1 - 0.98\left(1 - \frac{38.19}{100}\right) = 0.39$$

The usual dose of gentamicin sulfate = 1 mg/kg every 8 hours. Therefore, for a 75-kg adult, the usual dose is 75 mg every 8 hours. The dose may be estimated by:

(1) Reducing the maintenance dose and keeping the dosing interval constant:

$$\text{Uremic dose} = \frac{k_u}{k_N} \times \text{normal dose}$$

$$\text{Uremic dose} = 0.39 \times 75 = 29.25 \text{ mg}$$

Give 29.25 mg (about 30 mg) every 8 hours. Because the concentration of gentamicin sulfate solution is 40 mg/mL, then 30 mg gentamicin sulfate is equivalent to 0.75 mL.

(2) Increasing the dosing interval and keeping the maintenance dose constant:

$$\text{Dosage interval in uremia, } \tau_u = \frac{k_N}{k_u} \times \tau_N$$

$$\tau_u = 2.564 \times 8 = 20.5 \text{ hr (2.564 is the reciprocal of 0.39)}$$

Give 75 mg every 20.5 hours.

(3) Change both the maintenance dose and dosing interval. Using the dosing rate $D_\tau = 29.25$ mg/8 hr = 3.66 mg/hr, then a dose of 21.9 mg every 6 hours or 43.9 mg every 12 hours will produce the same average steady-state plasma drug concentration.

Although each estimated dosage regimen shown above produces the same average steady-state plasma drug concentration, the peak drug concentration, trough drug concentration, and duration of time in which the drug concentration will be above or below the minimum effective plasma drug concentration will be different. The choice of the appropriate dosage regimen requires consideration of these issues, the patient, and the safety and efficacy of the drug.

2. Using the Giusti–Hayton equation (Eq. 18.22) calculate the dose adjustment needed for uremic patients with (a) 75% of normal kidney function (ie, $Cl^{u}_{Cr}/Cl^{N}_{Cr} = 75\%$); (b) 50% of normal kidney function; and (c) 25% of normal kidney function. Make calculations for (a) a drug that is 50% excreted by the kidney, and (b) a drug that is 75% excreted by the kidney.

Solution

The values for percent of normal creatinine clearance in uremic patients with various renal functions are listed in Table 18.4.

The percent of dose adjustment in a given uremic state is obtained using the procedure detailed below. The important facts to remember are (1) although the elimination rate constant is usually composed of two components, only the renal component is reduced in a uremic patient, and (2) the kidney function of the uremic patient may be expressed as a percent of uremic Cl^{u}_{Cr}/normal Cl^{N}_{Cr}. The reduction in the renal elimination rate constant can be estimated from the percent of kidney function remaining in the patient. The steps involved in making the calculations are as follows:

a. Determine *fe*, or the fraction of drug excreted by the kidney.

b. Express the Cl^{u}_{Cr} of the uremic patient as a percent of the Cl^{N}_{Cr} of a normal patient—that is, $Cl^{u}_{Cr}/100$.

c. Multiply $fe(Cl^{u}_{Cr}/100)$ to obtain the uremic renal elimination constant.

d. Adding the uremic renal elimination constant to $1 - fe$, the nonrenal elimination constant, will give the new overall elimination rate constant as a percent of the normal elimination constant. This also gives the fraction of normal dose required for a uremic patient.

3. What is the dose for a drug that is 75% excreted through the kidney in a uremic patient with a creatinine clearance of 10 mL/min?

Solution

$fe = 75\%$

$$\text{Renal function of uremic patient} = \frac{10}{100} = 10\% \text{ normal}$$

$$\text{Uremic patient's renal elimination constant} = 75\% \times 10\% = 7.5\% \text{ normal}$$

$$\text{Uremic patient's overall elimination constant} = 7.5\% + (1 - 75\%)$$

$$= 7.5\% + 25\% = 32.5\%$$

Alternatively, using the Giusti–Hayton equation,

$$G = 1 - 0.75\left(1 - \frac{10}{100}\right) = 0.325$$

Therefore, the uremic patient's dose should be 32.5% of that of normal patient. It should be noted that the first method described is actually the same as the

Giusti–Hayton method. The intuitive approach, however, may be useful if the practitioner is unfamiliar with the Giusti–Hayton equation. Table 18.4 provides some of the calculated dosage adjustments for drugs eliminated to various degrees by renal excretion in different stages of renal failure.

General Clearance Method

The general clearance method is based on the methods discussed above. This method is popular in many clinical settings due to its simplicity. The method assumes that creatinine clearance, Cl_{Cr}, is a good indicator of renal function and that the renal clearance of a drug, Cl_r is proportional to Cl_{Cr}. Therefore, renal drug clearance, Cl_r^u, in the uremic patient is as shown below:

$$Cl_r^u = \frac{Cl_{Cr}^u}{Cl_{Cr}^N} \times Cl_r \tag{18.25}$$

$$Cl_u = Cl_{nr} + Cl_r \frac{Cl_{Cr}^u}{Cl_{Cr}^N} \tag{18.26}$$

where Cl_u is the total body clearance in the uremic patient.

If the ratio of Cl_{Cr}^u/Cl_{Cr}^N, Cl_{nr} and Cl_r are known, the total body clearance in the uremic patient may be estimated using Equation 18.26. Alternatively, if the normal total body clearance Cl and fe are known, Equation 18.27 may be obtained by substitution of Equation 18.26:

$$Cl_u = Cl\,(1 - fe) + fe\;Cl \frac{Cl_{Cr}^u}{Cl_{Cr}^N} \tag{18.27}$$

Equation 18.27 provides a simple calculation for drug clearance in the uremic patient that requires knowing the fraction of drug excreted unchanged (fe); total body clearance of the drug (Cl) in the normal subject, and the ratio of creatinine clearance of the uremic to normal patient.

Dividing Equation 18.27 on both sides yields by Cl the ratio, Cl_u/Cl, reflecting the ratio of the uremic/normal drug dose.

$$\frac{Cl_u}{Cl} = (1 - fe) + fe \frac{Cl_{Cr}^u}{Cl_{Cr}^N} \tag{18.28}$$

TABLE 18.4 Dosage Adjustment in Uremic Patients

FRACTION OF DRUG EXCRETED UNCHANGED (k_r/k_N)	PERCENT OF NORMAL DOSE			
	50% NORMAL Cl_{Cr}	25% NORMAL Cl_{Cr}	10% NORMAL Cl_{Cr}	0% NORMAL Cl_{CR}
0.25	87	81	77	75
0.50	75	62	55	50
0.75	62	44	32	25
0.90	55	32	19	10

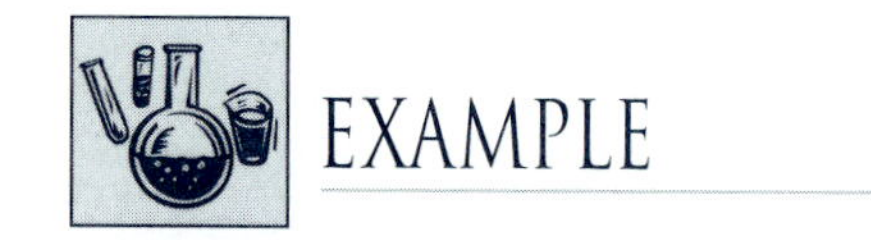

M.S., a 34-year-old, 110 lb female patient, is to be given tobramycin for sepsis. The usual dose of tobramycin is 150 mg twice a day by intravenous injection. The creatinine clearance in this patient was decreased to a stable level of 50 mL/min. Calculate the appropriate dose of tobramycin for this patient.

Solution

Obtain $fe = 0.9$ from literature (Appendix E) and apply Equation 18.29,

$$\frac{Cl_u}{Cl} = (1 - fe) + fe\frac{Cl^u_{Cr}}{Cl^N_{Cr}} \tag{18.29}$$

$$= 1 - 0.9 + 0.9\ (50/100) = 0.55$$

Therefore, the dose for the uremic patient = 150 mg × 0.55 = 82.5 mg (given twice a day).

Equation (18.29) may be derived by simplifying Equation 18.22, the Giusti–Hayton equation. The right side of Equation 18.28 is equal to the G factor in the Giusti–Hayton equation as shown below. Assuming the volume of distribution, V_D is unchanged in renal disease, multiplication of k_u/k_N of Equation 18.22 with V_D/V_D yields the left side of Equation 18.28. The right side of Equation 18.22 is identical to the right side of Equation 18.28. In both equations, fe refers to the fraction of drug excreted unchanged.

$$\frac{k_u}{k_N} = 1 - fe\left(1 - \frac{Cl^u_{Cr}}{Cl^N_{Cr}}\right) = G \tag{18.22}$$

$$= 1 - fe + fe\frac{Cl^u_{Cr}}{Cl^N_{Cr}} = G \tag{18.29}$$

The Giusti-Hayton method assumes that the elimination rate constant ratio is reflected by the creatinine clearance ratio of the uremic patient to that of the normal, whereas the clearance method assumes that the drug clearance ratio, Cl_u/Cl_N is reflected by the relative ratio of the creatinine clearances in the uremic and normal patient.

The Wagner Method

The methods for renal dose adjustment discussed in the previous sections all assumed that the volume of distribution and fraction of drug excreted by nonrenal routes are unchanged. These assumptions are convenient and hold true for many drugs. However, in the absence of reliable information assuring the validity of these assumptions, the equations should be demonstrated as statistically reliable in prac-

TABLE 18.5 Adjustment of Drug Dosage in Patients with Impaired Renal Function, Based on Endogenous Creatinine Clearance

DRUG	PATIENT $k_{\%} = a + b \times Cl_{Cr}$ (%/hr) a	b	NORMAL $k_{\%}$ (%/hr)	NORMAL $t_{1/2}$ (hr)
α-Acetyldigoxin	1.0	0.02	3.0	23.0
Ampicillin	11.0	0.59	70.0	1.0
Carbenicillin	6.0	0.54	60.0	1.2
Cephalexin	3.0	0.67	70.0	1.0
Cephaloridine	3.0	0.37	40.0	1.7
Cephalothin	6.0	1.34	140.0	0.5
Chloramphenicol	20.0	0.10	30.0	2.3
Chlortetracycline	8.0	0.04	12.0	5.8
Colistin	8.0	0.23	31.0	2.2
Digitoxin	0.3	0.001	0.4	173.0
Digoxin	0.8	0.009	1.7	41.0
Doxycycline	3.0	0.0	3.0	23.0
Erythromycin	13.0	0.37	50.0	1.4
5-Fluorocytosine	0.7	0.243	25.0	2.8
Gentamicin	2.0	0.28	30.0	2.3
Isoniazid—fast inactivators	34.0	0.19	53.0	1.3
Isoniazid—slow inactivators	12.0	0.11	23.0	3.0
Kanamycin	1.0	0.24	25.0	2.75
Methicillin	17.0	1.23	140.0	0.5
Methyldigoxin	0.7	0.009	1.6	43.0
Oxacillin	35.0	1.05	140.0	0.5
Penicillin G	3.0	1.37	140.0	0.5
Polymyxin B	2.0	0.14	16.0	4.3
Rolitetracycline	2.0	0.04	6.0	11.6
Streptomycin	1.0	0.26	27.0	2.6
Strophanthin G	1.2	0.038	5.0	14.0
Strophanthin K	1.0	0.03	4.0	17.0
Sulfadiazine	3.0	0.05	8.0	8.7
Sulfamethoxazole	7.0	0.0	7.0	9.9
Sulfasomidine (children)	1.0	0.14	15.0	4.6
Tetracycline	0.8	0.072	8.0	8.7
Thiamphenicol	2.0	0.24	26.0	2.7
Trimethoprim	2.0	0.04	6.0	12.0
Vancomycin	0.3	0.117	12.0	5.8

From Wagner, 1975, with permission.

tice. A statistical approach was used by Wagner (1975) who established a linear relationship between creatinine concentration and the first-order elimination constant of the drug in patients (Table 18.5). The regression parameters are listed for different drugs.

This method takes advantage of the fact that the elimination constant for a patient can be obtained from the creatinine clearance, as follows:

$$k\% = a + bCl_{Cr} \quad \textbf{(18.30)}$$

The values of a and b are statistically determined for each drug from the pooled data on uremic patients. The method is simple to use and should provide accurate determination of elimination constants for patients when a good linear relationship exists between elimination constant and creatinine concentration. The theoretical derivation of this approach is as follows:

$k\%$ = total elimination rate constant
k_{nr} = nonrenal elimination rate constant (%)
k_r = renal excretion rate constant

$$R = \frac{Cl_d}{Cl_{Cr}} = \frac{\text{drug clearance}}{\text{creatinine clearance}} \tag{18.31}$$

$$Cl_d = RCl_{Cr}$$

$$k_r = \frac{R}{V_D} Cl_{Cr}$$

$$k = k_{nr} + \frac{R}{V_D} Cl_{Cr}$$

$$100k = 100k_{nr} + \frac{100R}{V_D} Cl_{Cr}$$

$$k\% = a + bCl_{Cr} \tag{18.32}$$

Equation 18.32 can also be used with drugs that follow the two-compartment model. In such cases the terminal half-life is used and b would be substituted for k. Since the equation assumes a constant nonrenal elimination constant (k_{nr}) and volume of distribution, any changes in these two parameters will result in error in the estimated elimination constant.

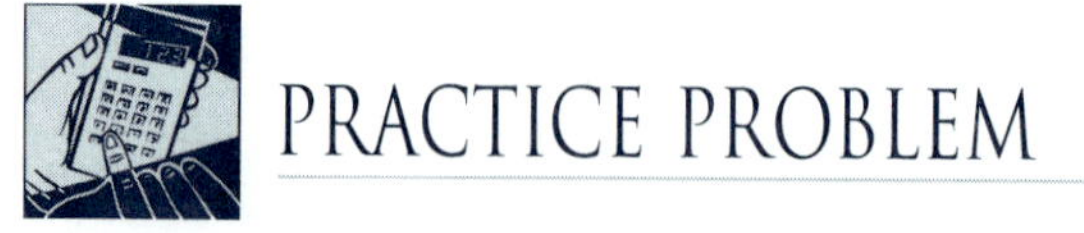

PRACTICE PROBLEM

A patient normally takes 500 mg ampicillin every 6 hours. What would the dose be for a patient with a Cl_{Cr} of 80 mL/min?

Solution

From Table 18-5 the following information on ampicillin is obtained: $a = 11$, $b = 0.59$, and normal $k\% = 70$. Using Equation 18.32, $k\%$ for the uremic patient is obtained:

$$k\% = a + bCl_{Cr} = 11 + 0.59 \times 80 = 58.2\%$$

$$\text{Uremic patient's dose} = \text{normal dose} \times \frac{\text{patient's } k\%}{\text{normal } k\%}$$

$$\text{Dose of ampicillin} = 500 \times \frac{58.2}{70} = 416 \text{ mg (every 6 hr)}$$

EXTRACORPOREAL REMOVAL OF DRUGS

Patients with *end-stage renal disease* (ESRD) and patients who have become intoxicated with a drug due to drug overdose require supportive treatment to remove the accumulated drug and its metabolites. Several methods for the extracorporeal removal of drugs are available. These methods include hemodialysis, peritoneal dialysis, hemoperfusion, and hemofiltration. The objective of these methods is to rapidly remove the undesirable drugs and metabolites from the body without disturbing the fluid and electrolyte balance in the patient.

Patients with impaired renal function may be taking other medication concurrently. For these patients, dosage adjustment may be needed to replace drug loss during extracorporeal drug removal.

DIALYSIS

Dialysis is an artificial process in which the accumulation of drugs or waste metabolites is removed by diffusion from the body into the dialysis fluid. Two common dialysis treatments are *peritoneal dialysis* and *hemodialysis.* Both processes work on the principle that as the uremic blood or fluid is equilibrated with the dialysis fluid, waste metabolites diffuse through a membrane into the dialysis fluid and are removed. The dialysate contains water, dextrose, electrolytes (eg, potassium, sodium, chloride, bicarbonate, acetate, calcium, etc), and other elements similar to normal body fluids without the toxins.

Peritoneal Dialysis

Peritoneal dialysis uses the peritoneal membrane in the abdomen as the filter. The peritoneum consists of visceral and parietal components. The peritoneum membrane provides a large natural surface area for diffusion of approximately 1 to 2 square meters in adults; the membrane is permeable to solutes of molecular weights ≤30,000 daltons (Merck Manual, 1997). Total splanchnic flow is 1200 mL/min at rest, but only a small portion, approximately 70 mL/min, comes in contact with the peritoneum. Placement of a peritoneal catheter is surgically more simple than hemodialysis and does not require vascular surgery and heparinization. The dialysis fluid is pumped into the peritoneal cavity, where waste metabolites in the body fluid are discharged rapidly. The dialysate is periodically drained and fresh dialysate is reinstilled and then drained. Peritoneal dialysis is also more amenable to self-treatment. However, slower drug clearance rates are obtained with peritoneal dialysis compared to hemodialysis and thus requires longer dialysis time.

Continuous Ambulatory Peritoneal Dialysis (CAPD) is the most common form of peritoneal dialysis. Many diabetic patients become uremic due to lack of control of their diabetes. About 2 L of dialysis fluid is instilled into the peritoneal cavity of the patient through a surgically placed resident catheter. The objective is to remove accumulated urea and other metabolic waste in the body. The catheter is sealed and the patient is able to continue in an ambulatory mode. Every 4 to 6 hours, the fluid is emptied from the peritoneal cavity and replaced with fresh dialysis fluid. The technique uses about 2 L of dialysis fluid; it does not require dialysis machine and can be performed at home.

Hemodialysis

Hemodialysis uses a dialysis machine and filters blood through an artificial membrane. Hemodialysis requires access to the blood vessels to allow the blood to flow to the dialysis machine and back to the body. For temporary access, a shunt is created in the arm with one tube inserted into an artery and another tube inserted in a vein. The tubes are joined above the skin. For permanent access to the blood vessels, an *arteriovenous fistula* or graft is created by a surgical procedure to allow access to the artery and vein. Patients who are on chronic hemodialysis treatment need to be aware of the need for infection control of the surgical site of the fistula. At the start of the hemodialysis procedure, an arterial needle allows the blood to flow to the dialysis machine, and blood is returned to the patient to the venous side. Heparin is used to prevent blood clotting during the dialysis period.

During hemodialysis, the blood flows through the dialysis machine, where the waste material is removed from the blood by diffusion through an artificial membrane before the blood is returned to the body. Hemodialysis is a much more effective method of drug removal and is preferred in situations where rapid removal of the drug from the body is important, as in overdose or poisoning. In practice, hemodialysis is most often applied to patients with end-stage renal failure. Early dialysis is appropriate with patients with acute renal failure in whom resumption of renal function can be expected and in patients who are to be renally transplanted. Other patients may be placed on dialysis according to clinical judgement concerning the patient's quality of life and risk/benefit ratio (Carpenter and Lazarus, 1994).

Dialysis may be required from once every 2 days to 3 times a week, with each treatment period lasting 2 to 4 hours. The time required for dialysis depends upon the amount of residual renal function in the patient, any complicating illness (eg, diabetes mellitus), the size and weight of the patient, including muscle mass, and the efficiency of the dialysis process. Dosing of drugs in patients receiving hemodialysis is affected greatly by the frequency and type of dialysis machine used and by the physicochemical and pharmacokinetic properties of the drug. Factors that affect drug removal in hemodialysis are listed in Table 18.6. These factors are carefully considered before hemodialysis is used for drug removal.

In hemodialysis, blood is pumped to the dialyzer by a roller pump at a rate of 300 to 450 mL/min. The drug and metabolites diffuse from the blood through the semipermeable membrane. In addition, hydrostatic pressure also forces the drug molecules into the dialysate by ultrafiltration. The composition of the dialysate is similar to plasma but may be altered according to the needs of the patient. Many

TABLE 18.6 Factors Affecting Dialyzability of Drugs

PHYSICOCHEMICAL AND PHARMACOKINETIC PROPERTIES OF THE DRUG	
Water solubility	Insoluble or fat-soluble drugs are not dialyzed—eg, glutethimide, which is very water insoluble.
Protein binding	Tightly bound drugs are not dialyzed because dialysis is a passive process of diffusion—eg, propranolol is 94% bound.
Molecular weight	Only molecules with molecular weights of less than 500 are easily dialyzed—eg, vancomycin is poorly dialyzed and has a molecular weight of 1800.
Drugs with large volumes of distribution	Drugs widely distributed are dialyzed more slowly because the rate-limiting factor is the volume of blood entering the machine—eg, for digoxin, $V_D = 250 - 300$ L. Drugs concentrated in the tissues are usually difficult to remove by dialysis.
CHARACTERISTICS OF THE DIALYSIS MACHINE	
Blood flow rate	Higher blood flows give higher clearance rates.
Dialysate	Composition of the dialysate and flow rate.
Dialysis membrane	Permeability characteristics and surface area.
Transmembrane pressure	Ultrafiltration increases with increase in transmembrane pressure.
Duration and frequency of dialysis	

dialysis machines use a hollow fiber or capillary dialyzer in which the semipermeable membrane is made into fine capillaries, of which thousands are packed into bundles with blood flowing through the capillaries and the dialysate is circulated outside the capillaries. The permeability characteristics of the membrane and the membrane surface area are determinants of drug diffusion and ultrafiltration.

The effect of newer hemodialysis membranes for the removal of vancomycin by hemodialysis has been reviewed by DeHart, 1996. Vancomycin is an antibiotic effective against most Gram-positive organisms such as *Staphylococcus aureus* which may be responsible for vascular access infections in patients undergoing dialysis. In this study, vancomycin hemodialysis in patients was compared using a cuprophan membrane or a cellulose acetate and polyacrylonitrile membrane. The cellulose acetate and polyacrylonitrile membrane is considered a "high flux" filter. Serum vancomycin concentrations decreased only 6.3% after dialysis when using the cuprophan membrane, whereas the serum drug concentration decreased 13.6 to 19.4% after dialysis with the cellulose acetate and polyacrylonitrile membrane (De Hart, 1996).

In dialysis involving uremic patients receiving drugs for therapy, the rate at which a given drug is removed depends on the flow rate of blood to the dialysis machine and the performance of the dialysis machine. The term *dialysance* is used to describe the process of drug removal from the dialysis machine. Dialysance is a clearance term similar in meaning to renal clearance, and it describes the amount of blood completely cleared of drugs (in mL/min). Dialysance is defined by the equation:

$$Cl_D = \frac{Q(C_a - C_v)}{C_a} \qquad \textbf{(18.33)}$$

where C_a = drug concentrations in arterial blood (blood entering kidney machine), C_v = drug concentration in venous blood (blood leaving kidney machine), Q = rate of blood flow to the kidney machine, and Cl_D = dialysance. Dialysance is sometimes referred to as *dialysis clearance.*

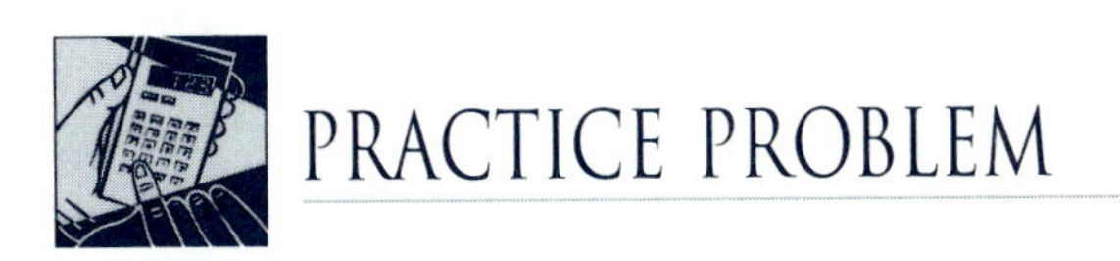

PRACTICE PROBLEM

Assume the flow rate of blood to the dialysis machine is 350 mL/min. By chemical analysis, the concentrations of drug entering and leaving the machine are 30 and 12 μg/mL, respectively. What is the dialysis clearance?

Solution

The rate of drug removal is equal to the volume of blood passed through the machine divided by the arterial difference in blood drug concentrations before and after dialysis. Thus,

$$\text{Rate of drug removal} = 350 \text{ mL/min} \times (30 - 12)\ \mu\text{g/mL} = 6300\ \mu\text{g/min}$$

Since clearance is equal to the rate of drug removal divided by the arterial concentration of drug,

$$Cl_D = \frac{6300\ \mu\text{g/min}}{30\ \mu\text{g/mL}} = 210 \text{ mL/min}$$

Alternatively, using Equation 18.33,

$$Cl_D = 350 \text{ mL/min} \times \frac{(30 - 12)}{30} = 210 \text{ mL/min}$$

These calculations show that the two terms are the same. In practice, dialysance has to be measured experimentally by determining C_a, C_v, and Q. In dosing drugs involving dialysis, the average plasma drug concentration of a patient is given by the equation:

$$C_{av}^{\infty} = \frac{FD_0}{(Cl_T + Cl_D)\tau} \tag{18.34}$$

where F represents fraction of dose absorbed, Cl_T is total body drug clearance of the patient, C_{av}^{∞} is average steady-state plasma drug concentration, and τ is the dosing interval.

In practice, if Cl_D is 30% or more of Cl_T, adjustment is usually made for the amount of drug lost in dialysis.

The elimination half-life $t_{1/2}$ for the drug in the patient off dialysis is related to the remaining total body clearance Cl_T and the volume of distribution V_D, as shown below.

$$t_{1/2} = \frac{0.693\ V_D}{Cl_T} \tag{18.35}$$

Drugs that are easily dialyzed will have a high dialysis clearance Cl_D, and the elimination half-life $t_{1/2}$ will be shorter in the patient on dialysis.

$$t_{1/2} = \frac{0.693\ V_D}{Cl_T + Cl_D} \tag{18.36}$$

$$k_{ON} = \frac{Cl_T + Cl_D}{V_D} \tag{18.37}$$

where k_{ON} is the first-order elimination half-life of the drug in the patient on dialysis.

The *fraction of drug lost* due to elimination and dialysis may be estimated from Equation 18.38. Equation 18.38 is based on first-order drug elimination and the substitution of t hours for the dialysis period.

$$\text{Fraction drug lost} = 1 - e^{-(Cl_T + Cl_D)t/V_D} \tag{18.38}$$

Several hypothetical examples illustrating the use of Equation 18.38 have been developed by Gambertoglio (1984). These are given in Table 18.7.

Equation 18.38 shows that as the V_D increases, the fraction of drug lost decreases. The fraction of drug lost during a 4-hour dialysis period for phenobarbital and salicylic acid was 0.30 to 0.50, respectively, whereas, for digoxin and phenytoin, the fraction of drug lost was only 0.07 and 0.04, respectively. Both phenobarbital and salicylic acid are easily dialyzed due to their smaller volumes of distribution, small molecular weights, and aqueous solubility. In contrast, digoxin has a large volume of distribution and phenytoin is highly bound to plasma proteins, making these drugs difficult to dialyze. Thus, dialysis is not very useful for treating digoxin intoxication, but is useful for salicylate overdosage.

TABLE 18.7 Predicted Effects of Hemodialysis on Drug Half-Life and Removal in the Overdose Setting

DRUG	V_D (L)	*Cl* (mL/min)	Cl_D (mL/min)	$t_{1/2\ off}$ (hr)	$t_{1/2\ on}$ (hr)	*FL*[a]
Digoxin[b]	560	150	20	43	38	0.07
Digoxin[c]	300	40	20	86	58	0.05
Ethchlorvynol	300	35	60	99	36	0.07
Phenobarbital	50	5	70	115	8	0.30
Phenytoin	100	5	10	231	77	0.04
Salicylic acid	40	20	100	23	4	0.51

[a]*FL* = fraction lost during a dialysis period of 4 hours.
[b]Parameters for a patient with normal renal function.
[c]Parameters for a patient with no renal function.

From Gambertoglio (1984), with permission.

An example of the effect of hemodialysis on drug elimination is shown in Figure 18-6. During the interdialysis period, the patient's total body clearance is very low and the drug concentration declines slowly. In this example, the drug has an elimination $t_{1/2}$ of 48 hours during the interdialysis period. When the patient is placed on dialysis, the drug clearance (sum of the total body clearance and the dialysis clearance) removes the drug more rapidly.

CLINICAL EXAMPLE

The aminoglycoside antibiotics, such as gentamicin and tobramycin, are eliminated primarily by the renal route. Dosing of these aminoglycosides are adjusted according to the residual renal function in the patient as estimated by creatinine clearance. During hemodialysis or peritoneal dialysis, the elimination half-lives for these antibiotics are significantly decreased as shown in Table 18.8. After dialysis, the aminoglycoside concentrations are below the therapeutic range, and the patient needs to be given another dose of the aminoglycoside antibiotic. The data in Table 18.8 also shows that hemodialysis is more efficient in removing the aminoglycoside antibiotic as shown by a smaller half-life during the dialysis period compared to peritoneal dialysis.

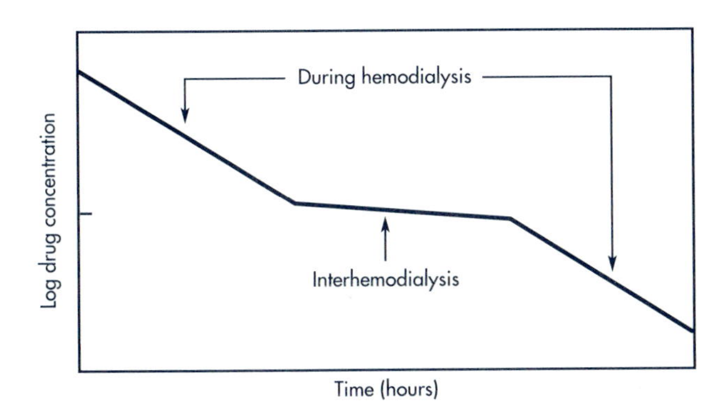

Figure 18-6. Effect of dialysis on drug elimination.

TABLE 18.8 Range of Aminoglycoside Half-Lives (Hours) During Dialysis[a]

AMINOGLYCOSIDE	INTERDIALYSIS[b]	HEMODIALYSIS	PERITONEAL DIALYSIS
Kanamycin	40–96	5	12
Gentamicin	21–59	6–11	5–29
Tobramycin	27–70	3–10	10–37
Amikacin	28–87	4–7	18–29
Netlimicin	24–52	5	—

[a]Patient renal function creatinine clearance ≤5 mL/min.
[b]Interdialysis, period in between dialysis treatment.

From *Facts and Comparisons*, 1992, with permission

CLINICAL EXAMPLE

An adult male (73 yr, 65 kg) with diabetes mellitus is placed on hemodialysis. His residual creatinine clearance is <5 mL/min. The patient is given the aminoglycoside antibiotic, tobramycin, at a dose of 1 mg/kg by IV bolus injection. Tobramycin is 90% excreted unchanged in the urine, is less than 10% bound to plasma proteins and has an elimination half-life of approximately 2.2 hours in patients with normal renal function. In this patient, tobramycin has an elimination $t_{1/2}$ of 50 hours during the interdialysis period and an elimination $t_{1/2}$ of 8 hours during hemodialysis. The apparent volume of distribution for tobramycin is about 0.33 L/kg. For this patient, calculate (1) the initial plasma antibiotic concentration after the first dose of tobramycin; (2) the plasma drug concentration just prior to the start of hemodialysis (48 hours after the initial tobramycin dose); (3) the plasma drug concentration at the end of 4 hours hemodialysis; (4) the amount of drug lost from the body after dialysis, (5) the tobramycin dose (replenishment dose) needed to be given to the patient after hemodialysis.

Solution

1. The initial plasma antibiotic concentration after the first dose of tobramycin:

$$\textit{Patient dose} = \frac{1\text{ mg}}{\text{kg}} \times 65\text{ kg} = 65\text{ mg}$$

$$V_{\text{d}} = \frac{0.33\text{ L}}{\text{kg}} \times 65\text{ kg} = 21.45\text{ L}$$

$$\text{Plasma drug concentration, } C_{\text{p}}^{0} = \frac{D_0}{V_{\text{D}}} = 65\text{ mg}/21.45\text{ L} = 3.03\text{ mg/L}$$

2. The plasma drug concentration just prior to the start of hemodialysis (48 hours after the initial tobramycin dose):

After 48 hours, the plasma drug concentration declines according to first-order kinetics:

$$C_{\text{p}} = 3.03\ e^{-(0.693/50)(48)} = 1.58\text{ mg/L}$$

3. The plasma drug concentration at the end of a 4-hour hemodialysis:

$$C_{\text{p}} = 1.58\ e^{-(0.693/8)(4)} = 0.547\text{ mg/L}$$

4. The amount of drug lost from the body after dialysis:

$$\begin{matrix}\textit{The amount of} & & \textit{The amount of} & & \textit{The amount of} & \\ \textit{drug lost} & = & \textit{drug in the body} & - & \textit{drug in the body} & = \\ \textit{after dialysis} & & \textit{before dialysis} & & \textit{after dialysis} & \end{matrix}$$

$$(1.58 \text{ mg/L})(21.45 \text{ L}) - (0.547 \text{ mg/L})(21.45 \text{ L}) = 22.16 \text{ mg}$$

5. The tobramycin dose (replenishment dose) needed to be given to the patient after hemodialysis:

The recommended range of peak and trough concentrations of tobramycin (Mathews, 1995) is 5–10 mg/L (peak) and 0.5–<2 mg/L (trough). The usual replenishment dose of tobramycin after hemodialysis is 1–1.5 mg/kg.

If a replenishment dose of 65 mg (ie, 1 mg/kg) is given to the patient, then the estimated plasma drug concentration is estimated as:

$$\begin{matrix}\textit{Plasma drug concentration} & \\ \textit{after 65 mg given by bolus} & = 65 \text{ mg}/21.45 \text{ L} + 0.547 \text{ mg/L} = 3.58 \text{ mg/L} \\ \textit{IV injection after hemodialysis} & \end{matrix}$$

The patient is given tobramycin, 65 mg by IV bolus injection after completion of hemodialysis to produce a tobramycin plasma concentration of 3.58 mg/L.

HEMOPERFUSION

Hemoperfusion is the process of removing drug by passing the blood from the patient through an adsorbent material and back to the patient. Hemoperfusion is a useful procedure for rapid drug removal in accidental poisoning and drug overdosage. Because the drug molecules in the blood are in direct contact with the adsorbent material, any molecule that has great affinity for the adsorbent material will be removed. The two main adsorbents used in hemoperfusion include (1) activated charcoal, which adsorbs both polar and nonpolar drugs, and (2) Amberlite resins. Amberlite resins, such as Amberlite XAD-2 and Amberlite XAD-4, are available as insoluble, polymeric beads, each bead containing an agglomerate of cross-linked polystyrene microspheres. The Amberlite resins have a greater affinity for nonpolar organic molecules than does activated charcoal. The factors important for the drug removal by hemoperfusion include affinity of the drug for the adsorbent, surface area of the adsorbent, absorptive capacity of the adsorbent, rate of blood flow through the adsorbent, and the equilibration rate of the drug from the peripheral tissue into the blood.

HEMOFILTRATION

An alternative to hemodialysis and peritoneal dialysis is hemofiltration. Hemofiltration is a process by which fluids, electrolytes, and small-molecular-weight substances are removed from the blood by means of low-pressure flow through hollow artificial fibers or flat plate membranes (Bickley, 1988). Hemofiltration is a slow, continuous filtration process that removes nonprotein bound, small molecules (<10,000 d) from the blood by convective mass transport. The clearance of the drug depends upon the sieving coefficient and ultrafiltration rate. Hemofiltration provides a creatinine clearance of approximately 10 mL/min (Bickley, 1988) and may have limited use for such drugs as aminoglycosides, cephalosporins, and acyclovir. A major problem with this method is the formation of blood clots within the hollow filter fibers.

EFFECT OF HEPATIC DISEASE ON PHARMACOKINETICS

The major difficulty in estimating hepatic clearance in patients with hepatic disease is the complexity and stratification of the liver enzyme systems. Several physiologic and pharmacokinetic factors are relevant in considering dosing a drug in patients with hepatic disease. Drugs are often metabolized by one or more enzymes that are located in cellular membranes in different parts of the liver. Chronic disease or tissue injury may change the accessibility of some enzymes due to redirection or detour of hepatic blood circulation. Liver disease affects the quantitative and qualitative synthesis of albumin, globulins, and other circulating plasma proteins that will subsequently affect drug plasma protein binding and distribution (Chapter 11). Liver function tests, such as alanine aminotransferase (ALT) and aspartate aminotransferase (AST), only indicate that the liver has been damaged, but they do not assess the function of the Cytochrome P-450 enzymes or intrinsic clearance by the liver.

Fraction of Drug Metabolized

Drug elimination in the body may be divided into: (1) fraction of drug excretion unchanged fe, and (2) fraction of drug metabolized. The latter is usually estimated from $1 - fe$; alternatively, the fraction of drug metabolized may be estimated from the ratio of Cl_h/Cl, where Cl_h is hepatic clearance and Cl is total body clearance. Knowing the fraction of drug eliminated from the liver allows an estimation of total body clearance when hepatic clearance is reduced. Drugs with low fe values (or conversely, drugs with a higher fraction of metabolized drug) are more affected by a change in liver function due to hepatic disease.

$$Cl_h = Cl\,(1 - fe) \tag{18.39}$$

Equation 18.39 assumes that all metabolism occurs in the liver, and all the unchanged drug is excreted in the urine. Assuming linear kinetics are applicable (after determining that there is no enzyme saturation), dosing adjustment may be based on residual hepatic function in patients with hepatic disease as shown in the following example.

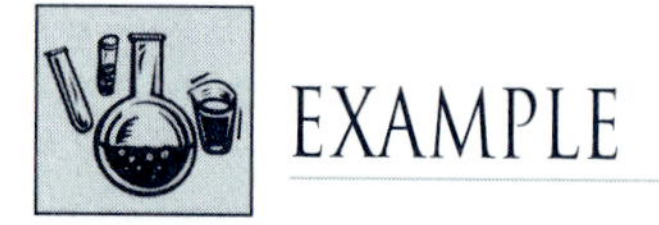

EXAMPLE

The hepatic clearance of a drug in a patient is reduced by 50% due to chronic viral hepatitis. How is the total body clearance of the drug affected? What should be the new dose of the drug in the patient? Assume that renal drug clearance (fe = 0.4) and plasma drug protein binding are not altered.

Solution

RL = *residual liver function*, estimated by $\dfrac{[Cl_h]_{hepatitis}}{[Cl_h]_{normal}}$

$[Cl_h]_{normal}$ = hepatic clearance of drug in normal subject
$[Cl_h]_{hepatitis}$ = hepatic clearance of drug in patient with hepatitis
Cl_{normal} = total clearance of drug in normal subject
$Cl_{hepatitis}$ = total clearance of drug in patient with hepatitis
fe = fraction of drug excreted unchanged
$1 - fe$ = fraction of drug metabolized
$[Cl_h]_{hepatitis} = RL\ [Cl_h]_{normal}$

Substituting for $[Cl_h]_{normal}$ with $Cl_{normal}\ (1 - fe)$,

$$[Cl_h]_{hepatitis} = RL\ Cl_{normal}\ (1 - fe) \qquad \textbf{(18.40)}$$

Assuming no renal clearance deterioration due to hepatitis,

$$Cl_{hepatitis} = [Cl_h]_{hepatitis} + [Cl_R]_{normal} \qquad \textbf{(18.41)}$$

Combine Equation 18.40 with Equation 18.41 and let $[Cl_R]_{normal} - Cl_{normal}\ fe$ will yield Equation 18.42:

$$Cl_{hepatitis} = RL\ Cl_{normal}\ (1 - fe) + Cl_{normal}\ fe \qquad \textbf{(18.42)}$$

$$= Cl_{normal}\ [RL\ (1 - fe) + fe] \qquad \textbf{(18.43)}$$

$$\frac{D_{hepatitis}}{D_{normal}} = \frac{Cl_{hepatitis}}{Cl_{normal}} = \frac{RL\ (1 - fe) + fe}{1} \qquad \textbf{(18.44)}$$

Substituting Equation 18.44 with $RL = 0.5$ and $fe = 0.4$:

$$\frac{D_{hepatitis}}{D_{normal}} = 0.5\ (1 - 0.4) + 0.4 = 0.3 + 0.4 = 0.7 \text{ (or 70\%)}$$

The adjusted dose of the drug in the hepatic patient would be 70% of the normal subject due to a 50% decrease in hepatic function in the above case ($fe = 0.4$). An example of a correlation established between actual residual liver function (measured by marker) and hepatic clearance was reported for cefoperazone (Hu et al, 1995) and other drugs in patients with cirrhosis. The method should be applied only to drugs that have low protein binding or are nonrestrictively bound. For drugs with restrictive binding, the fraction of free drug must be used to correct the change in free drug concentration and the change in free drug clearance. In some cases, the increase in free drug is partly offset by a larger volume of distribution resulted from the decrease in protein binding. There are many variables that can complicate dose correction when binding profoundly affects distribution, elimination and penetration of the drug to the active site. In general, the approach is limited only to drugs with hepatic metabolism approximated by linear kinetics.

Active Drug and the Metabolite

For many drugs, both the drug and the metabolite contribute to the overall response of the drug. The concentration of both the drug and the metabolite in the body should be known. When the pharmacokinetic parameters of the metabolite and the drug are similar, the overall activities of the drug can become more or less potent due to a change in liver function; that is, (1) when the drug is more potent

TABLE 18.9 Pugh's Modification of Child's Classification[a]

	1 POINT	2 POINTS	3 POINTS
Encephalopathy (grade)	None	1 or 2	3 or 4
Ascites	Absent	Slight	Moderate
Bilirubin (mg/dL)	1–2	2–3	>3
Albumin (gm/dL)	>3.5	2.8–3.5	<2.8
Prothrombin time (sec > control)	1–4	4–10	>10

[a]Total points: 5–6 = mild dysfunction; 7–9 = moderate dysfunction; >9 = severe dysfunction.

From Brouwer et al, 1992

than the metabolite, the overall pharmacologic activity will increase in the hepatic-impaired patient since the parent drug concentration will be higher; (2) when the drug is less potent than the metabolite, the overall pharmacologic activity in the hepatic patient will decrease since less of the active metabolite is formed. Changes in pharmacologic activity due to hepatic disease (Table 18.9) may be much more complex when both the pharmacokinetic parameters as well as the pharmacodynamics of the drug change due to the disease process. In such cases, the overall pharmacodynamic response may be greatly modified, making it necessary to monitor the response change with the aid of a pharmacodynamic model (see Chapter 19).

Hepatic Blood Flow and Intrinsic Clearance

Blood flow changes can occur in patients with chronic liver disease (often due to viral hepatitis or chronic alcohol use). In some patients with severe liver cirrhosis, fibrosis of liver tissue may occur resulting in intra- or extrahepatic shunt. Hepatic arterial-venous shunts may lead to reduced drug fraction of drug extracted (see Chapter 13) and an increase in the bioavailability of drug. In other patients, resistance to blood flow may be increased due to tissue damage and fibrosis, causing a reduction in intrinsic hepatic clearance.

The following equation may be applied to estimate hepatic clearance of a drug after assessing changes in blood flow and intrinsic clearance:

$$Cl_h = \frac{Q\,Cl_{int}}{Q + Cl_{int}}$$

Alternatively, when both Q and ER are known in the patient, Cl may also be estimated:

$$Cl = Q\,(ER)$$

Unlike changes in renal disease where serum creatinine concentration may be consistently used to monitor changes in renal function such as glomerular filtration (GFR), the physiologic model equation developed may not be adequate to account for all the factors necessary for accurate prediction of changes in hepatic clearance. Calculations based on model equations must be corroborated with clinical assessment.

Pathophysiologic Assessment

In practice, patient information about changes in hepatic blood flow may not be available since special electromagnetic (Nuxmalo et al, 1978) or ultrasound techniques that are not routinely available are required for measuring blood flow. The clinician/pharmacist may have to make an empirical estimate of the blood flow

TABLE 18.10 Severity Classification Schemes for Liver Disease

	CHILD-TURCOTTE CLASSIFICATION		
	GRADE A	**GRADE B**	**GRADE C**
Bilirubin (mg/dL)	<2.0	2.0–3.0	>3.0
Albumin (gm/dL)	>3.5	3.0–3.5	<3.0
Ascites	None	Easily controlled	Poorly controlled
Neurological disorder	None	Minimal	Advanced
Nutrition	Excellent	Good	Poor

From Brouwer et al, 1992

change after examining the patient and reviewing the available liver function tests (Table 18.10). While chronic hepatic disease is more likely to change the metabolism of a drug (Howden et al, 1989), acute hepatitis due to hepatoxin or viral inflammation is often associated with marginal or less severe changes in metabolic drug clearance (Farrel et al, 1978). The clinician may make an assessment based on an acceptable risk criteria on a case by case basis. Brouwer et al listed a set of useful endpoints for assessing hepatic dysfunction (Table 18.9). A practical method for dosing hepatic-impaired patients is still in its early stages of development. While the hepatic blood flow model is useful in simulating the effect of blood flow, pitfalls result from treating the liver as a single perfusion organ where entering blood Q_a is extracted of drug and exiting blood with Q_v. Global changes in distribution may occur outside the liver. Extrahepatic metabolism and other hemodynamic changes may be accounted for more completely by monitoring total body clearance of the drug using basic pharmacokinetics. For example, lack of local change in hepatic drug clearance should not be prematurely interpreted as "no change" in overall drug clearance. Reduced albumin and AAG, for example, may change the volume of distribution of the drug and therefore alter total body clearance on a global basis. In general, basic pharmacokinetics treats the body globally and more readily applies to dosing. However, drug clearance based on individual eliminating organs is more informative and provides more insight into the pharmacokinetic changes in the disease process.

Hormonal or Immunomodular Influence

In hyperthyroid patients, the rate of metabolism of many drugs is increased, as for example, are the rates for theophylline, digoxin, and propranolol. In hypothyroid disease, the rate of metabolism of these drugs may be decreased. (See Table 18.11).

TABLE 18.11 Drugs with Significantly Decreased Metabolism in Chronic Liver Disease

Antipyrine	Caffeine
Cefoperazone	Chlordiazepoxide
Chloramphenicol	Diazepam
Erythromycin	Hexobarbital
Metronidazole	Lidocaine
Meperidine	Metoprolol
Pentazocine	Propranolol
Tocainide	Theophylline
Verapamil	Promazine

From Howden et al (1989), Williams (1983), Hu et al (1995).

In children with HGH deficiency, administration of HGH decreases the half-life of theophylline.

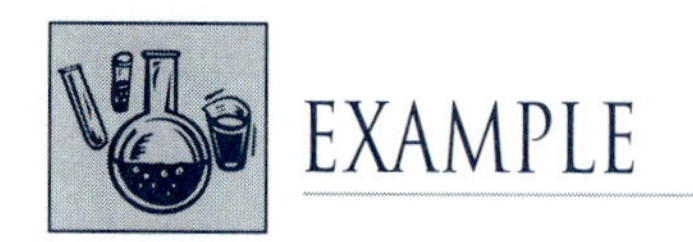

EXAMPLE

After IV bolus administration of 1 gm of cefoperazone to normal and chronic hepatitis patients, urinary excretion of cefoperazone was significantly increased in cirrhosis patients, from 23.95 ± 5.06% for normal patients to 51.09 ± 11.50% in cirrhosis patients (Hu et al, 1995). Explain (1) why there is a change in the percent of unchanged cefoperazone excreted in the urine of patients with cirrhosis, and (2) suggest a quantitative test to monitor the hepatic elimination of cefoperazone. (Hint: consult Hu et al 1994.)

Liver Function Tests and Hepatic Metabolic Markers

Drug markers used to measure residual hepatic function may correlate well with hepatic clearance of one drug but correlate poorly with substrate metabolized by a different enzyme within the same cytochrome P450 superfamily. Some useful marker compounds used are as listed below:

1. Antipyrine
   The pharmacokinetic properties of antipyrine makes the drug useful for reflecting changes in liver disease. Antipyrine is a drug that is well absorbed, almost completely biotransformed by the liver. Antipyrine is not appreciably bound to plasma proteins and distributes mostly in total body water. Antipyrine has a low extraction ratio that allows the drug to be used to measure hepatic drug metabolism independent of blood flow.
2. Indocyanine Green (ICG)
   This drug marker is a tricarbocyanine dye and is 97% cleared through the bile without reabsorption. ICG has an extraction ratio of 0.7–0.9, and its clearance changes with hepatic blood flow. The biliary excretion of ICG has been correlated with the severity of chronic liver disease and other indicators such as bilirubin concentration and prothrombin time (Brouwer et al, 1992).
3. Galactose Blood Concentration
   A simple, clinically useful quantitative liver function test, called the single point GSP method was developed to assess residual liver function by measuring galactose blood concentration 1 hour after galactose (0.5 g/kg) was administered (Hu et al, 1995). A newly developed galactose single point (GSP) was successfully correlated with promazine elimination half-life, total plasma clearance of free promazine. GSP may be a convenient index for promazine dosage adjustment in patients with liver cirrhosis.
4. Erythromycin Breath Test
   The erythromycin breath test is an *in vivo* test to measure CYP3A activity (Watkins et al, 1990). The test consists of giving subjects a small amount of radioactive erythromycin, (^{14}C-*N*-methyl)-erythromycin, as an IV injection. Erythromycin is

enzymatically demethylated and the resulting ^{14}C-methyl group initially forms ^{14}C-formaldehyde and then $^{14}CO_2$ which is measured in the expired air. The cytochrome P-450 (CYP) enzymes are expressed both in the liver and in the intestine. This test has been mainly used in clinical research investigations.

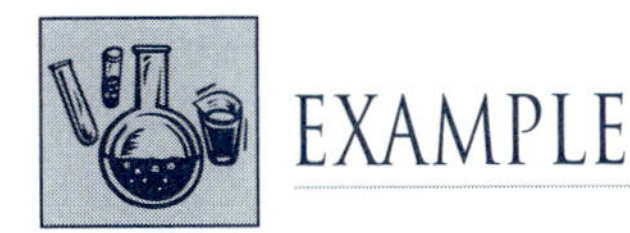

EXAMPLE

Paclitaxel, an anticancer agent for solid tumors and leukemia has extensive tissue distribution, high plasma protein binding (approximately 90 to 95%), and variable systemic clearance. Average paclitaxel clearance ranges from 87 to 503 mL/min/m^2 (5.2–30.2 L/h/m2) with minimal renal excretion of parent drug $<10\%$ (Sonnichsen; Relling, 1994). Paclitaxel is extensively metabolized by the liver to 3 primary metabolites. Cytochrome P450 enzymes of the CYP3A and CYP2C subfamilies appear to be involved in hepatic metabolism of paclitaxel. What are the precautions in administering paclitaxel to patients with liver disease?

Solution

Although paclitaxel has first-order pharmacokinetics at normal dose, its elimination may be saturable in some patients with genetically reduced intrinsic clearance due to CYP3A or CYP2C. The clinical importance of saturable elimination would be greatest when large dosages are infused over a shorter period of time. In these situations, achievable plasma concentrations are likely to cause saturation of binding. Thus, small changes in dosage or infusion duration may result in disproportionately large alterations in paclitaxel systemic exposure, potentially influencing patient response and toxicity.

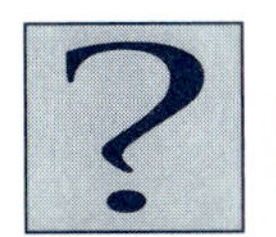

FREQUENTLY ASKED QUESTIONS

1. What are the main factors that influence drug dosing in renal disease?
2. Name and contrast the two methods for adjusting drug dose in renal disease.
3. What are the pharmacokinetic considerations in designing a dosing regimen? Why is dosing once a day for aminoglycosides recommended by many clinicians?
4. Protein binding of drugs is often affected by renal and hepatic disease. How are those changes accounted for in dose adjustment?
5. Drug clearance is often decreased 20 to 50% in many patients with congestive heart failure (CHF)? Explain how it may affect drug disposition.

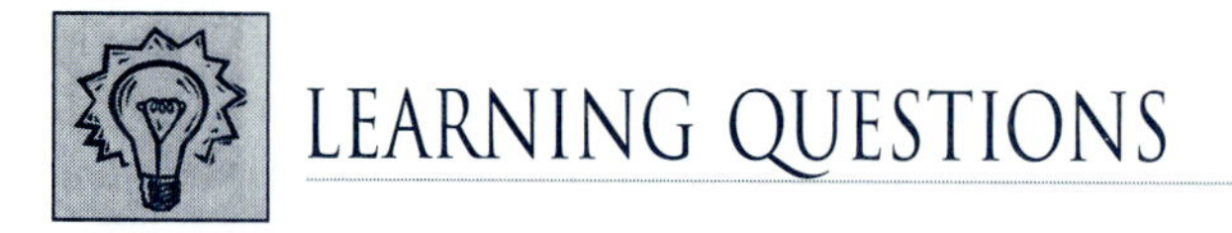

LEARNING QUESTIONS

1. The normal dosing schedule for a patient on tetracycline is 250 mg PO (peroral) every 6 hours. Suggest a dosage regimen for this patient when laboratory analysis shows his renal function to have deteriorated from a Cl_{Cr} of 90 to 20 mL/min.
2. A patient receiving antibiotic treatment is on dialysis. The flow rate of serum into the kidney machine is 50 mL/min. Assays show that the concentration of drug entering the machine is 5 μg/mL and the concentration of drug in the serum leaving the machine is 2.4 μg/mL. The drug clearance for this patient is 10 mL/min. To what extent should the dose be increased if the average concentration of the antibiotic is to be maintained?
3. Glomerular filtration rate (GFR) may be measured by either insulin clearance or creatinine clearance.
   a. Why is creatinine or insulin clearance used to measure GFR?
   b. Which clearance method, insulin or creatinine, gives a more accurate estimate of GFR? Why?
4. A uremic patient has a urine output of 1.8 L/24 hr and an average creatinine concentration of 2.2 mg/dL. What is the creatinine clearance? How would you adjust the dose of a drug normally given at 20 mg/kg every 6 hours in this patient (assume the urine creatinine concentration is 0.1 mg/mL and creatinine clearance is 100 mL/min)?
5. A patient on lincomycin at 600 mg every 12 hours intramuscular was found to have a creatinine clearance of 5 mL/min. Should the dose be adjusted? If so, **(a)** adjust the dose by keeping the dosing interval constant; **(b)** adjust the dosing interval and give the same dose; and **(c)** adjust both dosing interval and dose. What are the significant differences in the adjustment methods?
6. Using the method of *Cockcroft and Gault,* calculate the creatinine clearance for a woman (38 years old, 62 kg) whose serum creatinine is 1.8 mg/dL.
7. Would you adjust the dose of cephamandole, an antibiotic which is 98% excreted unchanged in the urine, for the patient in question 6? *Why?*
8. What assumptions are usually made when adjusting a dosage regimen according to the creatinine clearance in a patient with renal failure?
9. The usual dose of gentamicin in patients with normal renal function is 1.0 mg/kg every 8 hours by multiple IV bolus injections. Using the nomogram method (Fig. 18-5), what dose of gentamicin would you recommend for a 55-year-old male patient weighing 72 kg with a creatinine clearance of 20 mL/min?
10. A single intravenous bolus injection (1 g) of an antibiotic was given to a male anephric patient (age 68, 75 kg). During the next 48 hours, the elimination half-life of the antibiotic was 16 hours. The patient was then placed on hemodialysis for 8 hours and the elimination half-life was reduced to 4 hours.
    a. How much drug was eliminated by the end of the dialysis period?
    b. Assuming the apparent volume of distribution of this antibiotic is 0.5 L/kg, what was the plasma drug concentration just prior to and after dialysis?

11. There are several pharmacokinetic methods for the adjustment of a drug dosage regimen for patients with uremic disease based on the serum creatinine concentration in that patient. From your knowledge of clinical pharmacokinetics, discuss the following questions:

a. What is the basis of these methods for the calculation of drug dosage regimens in uremic patients?

b. What is the validity of the assumptions upon which these calculations are made?

12. After assessment of the uremic condition of the patient, the drug dosage regimen may be adjusted by one of two methods: (a) by keeping the dose constant and prolonging the dosage interval, τ, or (b) by decreasing the dose and maintaining the dosage interval constant. Discuss the advantages and disadvantages of adjusting the dosage regimen using either method.

REFERENCES

Benet LZ, Massoud N, Gambertoglio JG (eds): *Pharmacokinetic Basis for Drug Treatment.* New York, Raven, 1984

Bennett WM: Guide to Drug Dosage in Renal Failure. *Clinical Pharmacokinetics Drug Data Handbook.* New York, Adis Press, 1990

Bennett WM: Guide to Drug Dosage in Renal Failure. *Clin Pharmacokinet* 15:326–354, 1988

Bianchetti G, Graziani G, Brancaccio D, et al: Pharmacokinetics and effects of propranolol in terminal uraemic patients and in patients undergoing regular dialysis treatment. *Clin Pharmacokinet* 1:373–384, 1978

Bickley SK: Drug dosing during continuous arteriovenous hemofiltration. *Clin Pharm* **7:**198–206, 1988

Bjornsson TD: Nomogram for drug dosage adjustment in patients with renal failure. *Clin Pharmacokinet* **11:**164–170, 1986

Bodenham A, Shelly MP, Park GR: The altered pharmacokinetics and pharmacodynamics of drugs commonly used in critically ill patients. *Clin Pharmacokinet* **14:**347–373, 1988

Brouwer KBR, Dukes GE, Powell JR: Influence of liver function on drug disposition, *Applied Pharmacokinetics—Principles of Therapeutic Drug Monitoring.* In Evans WE et al (eds): Vancouver, WA, Applied Therapeutics, Inc, 1992, chap 6

Carpenter CB, Lazarus JM: Dialysis and transplantation in the treatment of renal failure. In Isselbacher KJ et al (ed): *Harrison's Principles of Internal Medicine.* New York, McGraw-Hill, 1994, chap 238

Chennavasin P, Craig Brater D: Nomograms for drug use in renal disease. *Clin Pharmacokinet* **6:**193–215, 1981

Cockcroft DW, Gault MH: Prediction of creatinine clearance from serum creatinine. *Nephron* **16:**31–41, 1976

De Hart RM: Vancomycin removal via newer hemodialysis membranes, *Hosp Pharm* **31:**1467–1477, 1996

Farrel GC et al: Drug metabolism in liver disease. Identification of patients with impaired hepatic drug metabolism. *Gastroenterology* **75:**580, 1978

Gambertoglio JG: Effects of renal disease: Altered pharmacokinetics. In Benet LZ, Massoud N, Gambertoglio JG (eds): *Pharmacokinetic Basis of Drug Treatment.* New York, Raven, 1984

Giusti DL, Hayton WL: Dosage regimen adjustments in renal impairment. *Drug Intell Clin Pharm* **7:**382–387, 1973

Hallynck TH, Soeph HH, Thomis VA, et al: Should clearance be normalized to body surface or lean body mass? *Br J Clin Pharm* **11:**523–526, 1981

Howden CW et al: Drug metabolism in liver disease. *Pharmacol Ther* **40:**439, 1989

Hu OY, Tang HS, Chang CL: The influence of chronic lobular hepatitis on pharmacokinetics of cefoperazone—A novel galactose single-point method as a measure of residual liver function. *Biopharm Drug Dispos* **15**(7):563–576, 1994

Hu OY, Tang HS, Chang CL: Novel galactose single point method as a measure of residual liver function: Example of cefoperazone kinetics in patients with liver cirrhosis. *J Clin Pharmacol* **35**(3):250–258, 1995

Jellife RW: Creatinine clearance: Bedside estimate. *Ann Int Med* **79:**604–605, 1973

Mathews SJ: Aminoglycosides, In Schumacher GE (ed), *Therapeutic Drug Monitoring*. Norwalk, CT, Appleton & Lange, 1995, chap 9

Merck Manual. Whitehouse Station, NJ, Merck & Co, 1996–1997

Nuxmalo JL, et al: Hepatic blood flow measurement. *Arch Surg* **113:**169, 1978

Physicians' Desk Reference, Montvale, NJ, Medical Economics Co. Inc, (published annually)

St Peter WL, Redic-Kill KA, Halstenson CE: Clinical pharmacokinetics of antibiotics in patients with impaired renal function, *Clin Pharmacokinet* **22:**169–210, 1992

Schwartz GV, Haycock GB, Edelmann CM, Spitzer A: A simple estimate of glomerular filtration rate in children derived from body length and plasma creatinine. *Pediatrics* **58:**259–263, 1976

Scientific Table, 7th ed. Ciba Geigy, 1973

Siersback-Nielson K, Hansen JM, Kampmann J, Kirstensen M: Rapid evaluation of creatinine clearance. *Lancet* **i:**1133–1134, 1971

Sonnichsen DS, Relling MV: Clinical pharmacokinetics of paclitaxel. *Clin Pharmacokinet* **27**(4):256–269, 1994

Tozer TN: Nomogram for modification of dosage regimen in patients with chronic renal function impairment. *J Pharmacokinet Biopharm* **2:**13–28, 1974

Traub SL, Johnson CE: Comparison methods of estimating creatinine clearance in children. *Am J Hosp Pharm* **37:**195–201, 1980

Wagner JG: *Fundamentals of Clinical Pharmacokinetics*. Hamilton, IL, Drug Intelligence Publ, 1975, p 161

Watkins PB, Hamilton TA, Annesley TM, Ellis CN, Kolars JC, Voorhees JJ: The erythromycin breath test as a predictor of cyclosporine blood levels, *Clin Pharmacol Ther* **48:**120–129, 1990

Welling PG, Craig WA: Pharmacokinetics in disease states modifying renal function. In Benet LZ (ed): *The Effects of Disease States on Drug Pharmacokinetics*. Washington, DC, American Pharmaceutical Assoc, 1976

Williams RL: Drug administration in hepatic disease. *N Engl J Med* 309:1616, 1983

BIBLIOGRAPHY

Benet L: *The Effect of Disease States on Drug Pharmacokinetics*. Washington, DC, American Pharmaceutical Association, 1976

Bennett WM, Singer I: Drug prescribing in renal failure: Dosing guidelines for adults—An update. *Am J Kidney Dis* **3:**155–193, 1983

Bjornsson TD: Use of serum creatinine concentration to determine renal function. *Clin Pharmacokinet* **4:**200–222, 1979

Bjornsson TD, Cocchetto DM, McGowan FX, et al: Nomogram for estimating creatinine clearance. *Clin Pharmacokinet* **8:**365–399, 1983

Brater DC: *Drug Use in Renal Disease*. Boston, AIDS Health Science Press, 1983

Brater DC: Treatment of renal disorders and the influence of renal function on drug disposition. In Melmon KL, Morrelli HF, Hoffman BB, Nierenberg DW (eds): *Clinical Pharmacology—Basic Principles in Therapeutics*, 3rd ed. New York, McGraw-Hill, 1992, chap 11

Chennavasin P, Brater DC: Nomograms for drug use in renal disease. *Clin Pharmacokinet* **6:**193–214, 1981

Craig Brater D, Chennavasin P: Effects of renal disease: Pharmacokinetic considerations. In Benet LZ et al (eds): *Pharmacokinetic Basis of Drug Treatment*. New York, Raven, 1984

Cutler RE, Forland SC, St. John PG, et al: Extracorporeal removal of drugs and poisons by hemodialysis and hemoperfusion. *Annu Rev Pharmacol Toxicol* **27:**169–191, 1987

Dettli L: Elimination kinetics and dosage adjustment of drugs in patients with kidney disease. In Grobecker H et al (eds): *Progress in Pharmacology*, vol 1. New York, Gustav Fischer Verlag, 1977

Fabre J, Balant L: Renal failure, drug pharmacokinetics and drug action. *Clin Pharmacokinet* **1:**99–120, 1976

Gibaldi M: Drug distribution in renal failure. *Am J Med* **62:**471–474, 1977

Gibson TP, Nelson HA: Drug kinetics and artificial kidneys. *Clin Pharmacokinet* **2:**403–426, 1977

Giusti DL, Hayton WL: Dosage regimen adjustments in renal impairment. *Drug Intell Clin Pharm* **7:**382–387, 1973

Jellife RW: Estimation of creatinine clearance when urine cannot be collected. *Lancet* **1:**975–976, 1971

Jellife RW, Jellife SM: A computer program for estimation of creatinine clearance from unstable serum creatinine concentration. *Math Biosci* **14:**17–24, 1972

Kampmann JP, Hansen JM: Glomerular filtration rate and creatinine clearance. *Br J Clin Pharmacol* **12:**7–14, 1981

Lee CC, Marbury TC: Drug therapy in patients undergoing haemodialysis. Clinical pharmacokinetic considerations. *Clin Pharmacokinet* **9:**42–66, 1984

LeSher DA: Considerations in the use of drugs in patients with renal failure. *J Clin Pharmacol* **16:**570, 1976

Levy G: Pharmacokinetics in renal disease. *Am J Med* **62:**461–465, 1977

Lott RS, Hayton WL: Estimation of creatinine clearance from serum creatinine concentration—A review. *Drug Intell Clin Pharm* **12:**140–150, 1978

Maher JF: Principle of dialysis and dialysis of drugs. *Am J Med* **62:**475–481, 1977

Parker PR, Parker WA: Pharmacokinetic considerations in the haemodialysis of drugs. *J Clin Hosp Pharm* **7:**87–99, 1982

Paton TW, Cornish WR, Manuel MA, Hardy BG: Drug therapy in patients undergoing peritoneal dialysis. Clinical pharmacokinetic considerations. *Clin Pharmacokinet* **10:**404–426, 1985

Rhodes PJ, Rhodes RS, McClelland GH, et al: Evaluation of eight methods for estimating creatinine clearance in man. *Clin Pharm* **6:**399–406, 1987

Rosenberg J, Benowitz NL, Pond S: Pharmacokinetics of drug overdosage. *Clin Pharmacokinet* **6:**161–192, 1981

Schumacher GE: Practical pharmacokinetic techniques for drug consultation and evaluation, II: A perspective on the renal impaired patient. *Am J Hosp Pharm* **30:**824–830, 1973

Traub SL: Creatinine and creatinine clearance. *Hosp Pharm* **13:**715–722, 1978

Watanabe AS: Pharmacokinetic aspects of the dialysis of drugs. *Drug Intell Clin Pharm* **11:**407–416, 1977

19

RELATIONSHIP BETWEEN PHARMACOKINETICS AND PHARMACODYNAMICS

PHARMACODYNAMICS AND PHARMACOKINETICS

The interaction of a drug molecule with a receptor causes the initiation of a sequence of molecular events resulting in a pharmacologic response. The term *pharmacodynamics* refers to the relationship between drug concentrations at the site of action (receptor) and pharmacologic response, including biochemical and physiologic effects that influence the interaction of drug with the receptor. Early pharmacologic research demonstrated that the pharmacodynamic response produced by the drug was dependent upon the chemical structure of the drug molecule. Receptors interacted only with drugs of specific chemical structure and receptors were classified according to the type of pharmacodynamic response induced.

Because most pharmacologic responses are the result of noncovalent interaction between the drug and the receptor, the nature of the interaction is generally assumed to be reversible and conforms to the *law of mass action*. One or several drug molecules may interact simultaneously with the receptor to produce a pharmacologic response. Typically, a single drug molecule interacts with a receptor with a single binding site to produce a pharmacologic response, as illustrated below.

$$[\text{Drug}] + [\text{receptor}] \longleftrightarrow [\text{Drug–receptor complex}] \rightarrow \text{Response}$$

where the brackets [ ] denote molar concentrations.

The scheme above illustrates the *occupation theory* and the interaction of a drug molecule with a receptor molecule. The following assumptions were made in this model:

1. The drug molecule combines with the receptor molecule as a bimolecular association and the resulting drug–receptor complex disassociates as a unimolecular entity.

2. The binding of drug with the receptor is fully reversible.
3. A single type of binding site with one site per molecule is assumed in the basic model. It is also assumed that a receptor with multiple sites may be modeled after this (Taylor and Insel, 1990).

The occupancy of the drug molecule at one receptor site does not change the affinity of other drug molecules to complex at other binding sites (the model may not be suitable for drugs with allosteric type of binding to the receptor). As more receptors are occupied by drug molecules, a greater pharmacologic response is obtained until a maximum response is reached.

The receptor occupancy concept was further applied to show how an agent might elicit a pharmacologic response (an agonist), or produce an opposing pharmacologic response as an antagonist through receptor interaction. Basically, three types of related responses may occur at the receptor: (1) a drug molecule that interacts with the receptor and elicits a maximal pharmacologic response is referred to as an *agonist;* (2) a drug that elicits a partial (below maximal) response is termed a *partial agonist;* and (3) an agent that elicits no response from the receptor, but inhibits the receptor interaction of a second agent, is termed an *antagonist.* An antagonist may prevent the action of an agonist by competitive (reversible) or noncompetitive (irreversible) inhibition. *Spare receptors* are assumed to be present at the site of action, because a maximal pharmacologic response may be obtained when only a small fraction of the receptors are occupied by drug molecules. Equimolar concentrations of different drug molecules that bind to the same receptor may give different pharmacologic responses. The term *intrinsic activity* is used to distinguish the resulting pharmacologic response from different drug molecules that bind to the same receptor. The *potency* of a drug is the concentration of drug needed to obtain a specific pharmacologic effect, such as the EC_{50} (see E_{max} model).

The receptor occupation theory, however, was not consistent with all kinetic observations, and the alternative *rate theory* was proposed. This hypothesis essentially states that the pharmacologic response is not dependent on drug–receptor complex concentration but rather depends on the rate of association of the drug and the receptor. Each time a drug molecule "hits" a receptor, a response is produced, similar to a ball bouncing back and forth from the receptor site. The rate theory predicted that an agonist would associate rapidly to form a receptor complex, which dissociates rapidly to produce a response. An antagonist associates rapidly to form a receptor drug complex and dissociates slowly to maintain the antagonist response. Both theories are consistent with the saturation (sigmoidal) drug dose responses observed, but neither theory is sufficiently advanced to give a detailed description of the "*lock-key*" or the more recent "*induced-fit*" type of interactions with enzymatic receptors. Newer theories of drug action are based on *in vitro* studies on isolated tissue receptors and on observation of the conformational and binding changes with different drug substrates. These *in vitro* studies show that other types of interactions between the drug molecule and the receptor are possible. However, the results from the *in vitro* studies are difficult to extrapolate to *in vivo* conditions. The pharmacologic response in drug therapy is often a product of physiologic adaptation to a drug response. Many drugs trigger the pharmacologic response through a cascade of enzymatic events highly regulated by the body.

The complexity of the molecular events triggering a pharmacologic response is less difficult to describe using a pharmacokinetic approach. Pharmacokinetic models allow very complex processes to be simplified. The process of pharmacokinetic modeling continues until a model is found that quantitatively describes the real process. The understanding of drug response is greatly enhanced when pharmacokinetic modeling techniques are combined with clinical pharmacology, resulting in the development of *pharmacokinetic–pharmacodynamic models*. The pharmacokinetic–pharmacodynamic model uses data derived from the plasma drug concentration versus time profile and from the time course of the pharmacologic effect to predict the pharmacodynamics of the drug. Pharmacokinetic–pharmacodynamic models have been reported for antipsychotic medications, anticoagulants, neuromuscular blockers, antihypertensives, anesthetics, and many antiarrhythmic drugs (the pharmacologic response of these drugs are well studied because of easy monitoring).

RELATION OF DOSE TO PHARMACOLOGIC EFFECT

The onset, intensity, and duration of the pharmacologic effect are dependent upon the dose and the pharmacokinetics of the drug. As the dose increases, the drug concentration at the receptor site increases, and the pharmacologic response (effect) increases up to a maximum effect. The relationship between dose and pharmacologic effect is shown in Figure 19-1 and the same curve is shown after log is transformed in Figure 19-2. A plot of the pharmacologic effect to dose on a linear scale generally results in a hyperbolic curve with maximum effect at the plateau (Fig. 19-1). The same data may be compressed and plotted on a log–linear scale that results in a sigmoid curve (Fig. 19-2).

For many drugs, the graph of log dose versus response curve shows a linear relationship at a dose range between 20 and 80% of the maximum response, which typically includes the therapeutic dose range for many drugs. For a drug that follows one-compartment pharmacokinetics, the volume of distribution is constant; therefore the pharmacologic response is also proportional to the log plasma drug concentration within a therapeutic range, as shown in Figure 19-3.

Mathematically, the relationship in Figure 19-3 may be expressed by the following equation, where m is the slope, e is an extrapolated intercept, and E is the drug effect at drug concentration, C.

$$E = m \log C + e \tag{19.1}$$

Solving for log C yields the expression

$$\log C = \frac{E - e}{m} \tag{19.2}$$

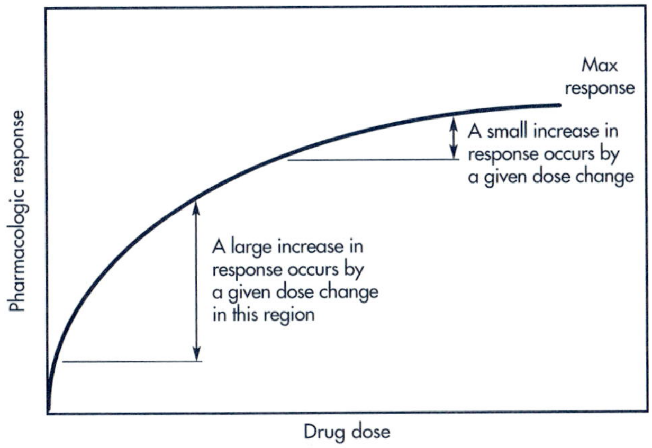

Figure 19-1. Plot of pharmacologic response versus dose on a linear scale.

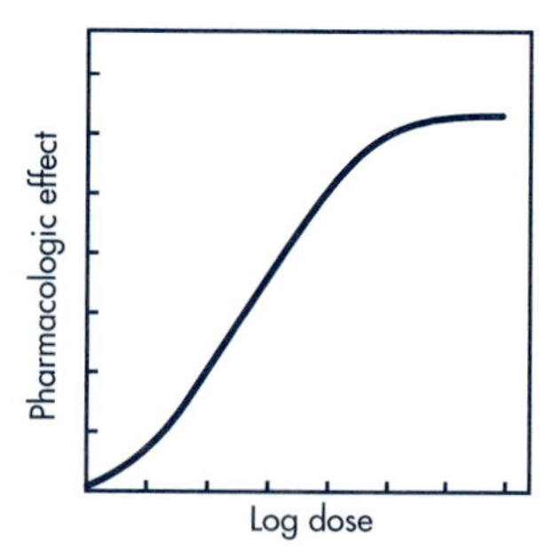

Figure 19-2. Typical log dose versus pharmacologic response curve.

However, after an intravenous dose, the concentration of a drug in the body in a one-compartment open model is described as follows:

$$\log C = \log C_0 - \frac{kt}{2.3} \quad \textbf{(19.3)}$$

By substituting Equation 19.2 into Equation 19.3, we get Equation 19.4, where E_0 = effect at concentration C_0.

$$\frac{E - e}{m} = \frac{E_0 - e}{m} - \frac{kt}{2.3} \quad \textbf{(19.4)}$$

$$E = E_0 - \frac{kmt}{2.3}$$

The pharmacologic response at any time after an intravenous dose of a drug may be calculated theoretically with Equation 19.4. From this equation, the pharmacologic effect declines with a slope of $km/2.3$. The decrease in pharmacologic effect is affected by both the elimination constant k and the slope m. For a drug with a large m, the pharmacologic response declines rapidly and requires that multiple doses be given at small intervals to maintain the pharmacologic effect. Furthermore, Equation 19.4 predicts that the pharmacologic effect will decline linearly with respect to time for a drug that follows a one-compartment model with a linear log dose–pharmacologic response.

The relationship between pharmacokinetics and pharmacologic response can be demonstrated by observing the percent depression of muscular activity after an IV dose of (+)-tubocurarine. The decline of pharmacologic effect is linear as a function of time (Fig. 19-4). For each pharmacologic response, the slope of each curve is the same. Because the values for each slope, which include km (Eq. 19.4), are the same, it is assumed that the sensitivity of the receptors for (+)-tubocurarine is the same at each site of action. Note that a plot of the log concentration of drug versus time yields a straight line.

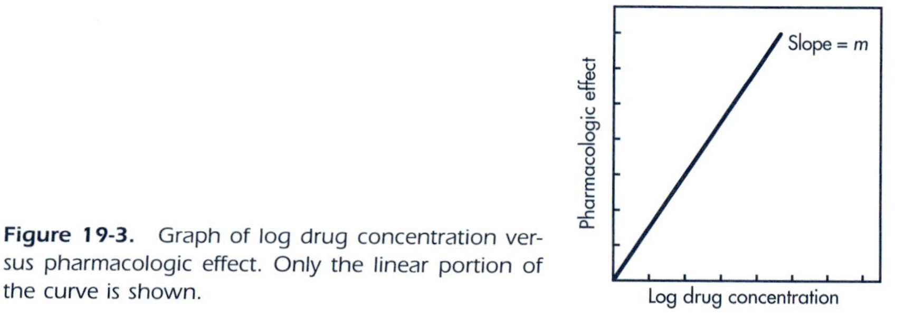

Figure 19-3. Graph of log drug concentration versus pharmacologic effect. Only the linear portion of the curve is shown.

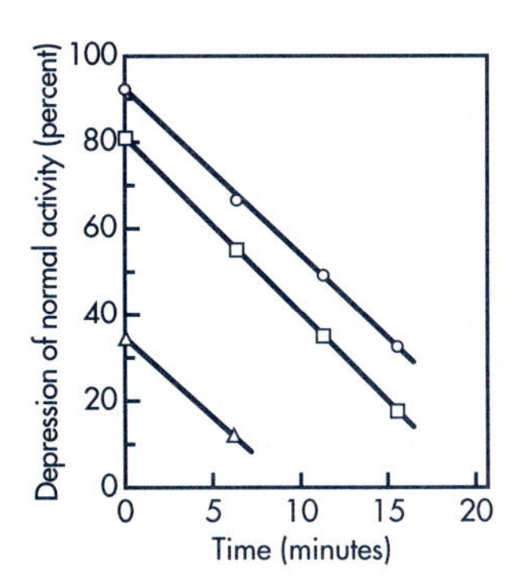

Figure 19-4. Depression of normal muscle activity as a function of time after IV administration of 0.1–0.2 mg (+)-tubocurarine per kilogram to unanesthetized volunteers, presenting mean values of 6 experiments on 5 subjects. Circles represent head lift; squares, hand grip; and triangles, inspiratory flow.
(Adapted from Johansen et al, 1964, with permission.)

A second example of the pharmacologic effect declining linearly with time was observed with lysergic acid diethylamide, or LSD (Fig. 19-5). After an IV dose of the drug, log concentrations of drug decreased linearly with time except for a brief distribution period. Furthermore, the pharmacologic effect, as measured by the performance score of each subject, also declined linearly with time. Because the slope is governed in part by the elimination rate constant, the pharmacologic effect declines much more rapidly when the elimination rate constant is increased due to increased metabolism or renal excretion. Conversely, an increased pharmacologic response is experienced among patients with longer drug half-lives.

RELATIONSHIP BETWEEN DOSE AND DURATION OF ACTIVITY (t_{eff}), SINGLE IV BOLUS INJECTION

The relationship between the duration of the pharmacologic effect and the dose can be inferred from Equation 19.3. After an intravenous dose, assuming a one-compartment model, the time needed for any drug to decline to a concentration C is given by the following equation, assuming the drug takes effect immediately:

$$t = \frac{2.3(\log C_0 - \log C)}{k} \tag{19.5}$$

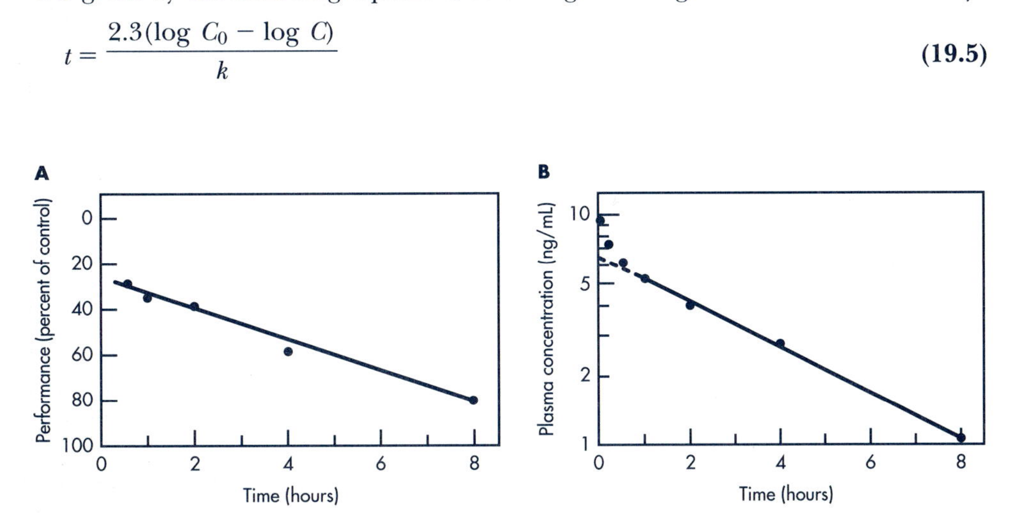

Figure 19-5. Mean plasma concentrations of LSD and performance test scores as a function of time after IV administration of 2 μg LSD per kilogram to 5 normal human subjects.
(Adapted from Aghajanian and Bing, 1964, with permission.)

Using C_{eff} to represent the minimum effective drug concentration, the duration of drug action can be obtained as follows.

$$t_{\text{eff}} = \frac{2.3\left(\log \dfrac{D_0}{V_D} - \log C_{\text{eff}}\right)}{k} \tag{19.6}$$

Some practical applications are suggested by this equation. For example, a doubling of the dose will not result in a doubling of the effective duration of pharmacologic action. On the other hand, a doubling of $t_{1/2}$ or a corresponding decrease in k will result in a proportional decrease in duration of action. A clinical situation is often encountered in the treatment of infections where C_{eff} is the bacteriocidal concentration of the drug, and, in order to double the duration of the antibiotic, a considerably greater increase than simply doubling the dose is necessary.

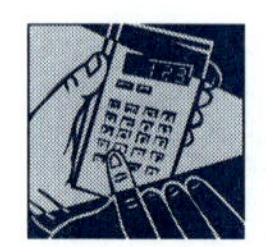

PRACTICE PROBLEM

The MEC in plasma for a certain antibiotic is 0.1 μg/mL. The drug follows a one-compartment open model and has an apparent volume of distribution (V_D) of 10 L and a first-order elimination rate constant of 1.0 hr^{-1}.

1. What is the t_{eff} for a single 100 mg IV dose of this antibiotic?
2. What is the new t_{eff} or t'_{eff} for this drug if the dose were increased 10-fold to 1000 mg?

Solution

1. The t_{eff} for a 100 mg dose is calculated as follows:

   Because $V_D = 10{,}000$ mL, then:

   $$C_0 = \frac{100 \text{ mg}}{10{,}000 \text{ mL}} = 10\ \mu\text{g/mL}$$

   For a one-compartment model IV dose, $C = C_0 e^{-kt}$. Thus

   $$0.1 = 10e^{-(1.0)t_{\text{eff}}}$$
   $$t_{\text{eff}} = 4.61 \text{ hr}$$

2. The t'_{eff} for a 1000-mg dose is calculated as follows (prime refers to a new dose):

   Because $V_D = 10{,}000$ mL, then:

   $$C'_0 = \frac{1000 \text{ mg}}{10{,}000 \text{ mL}} = 100\ \mu\text{g/mL}$$

   and

   $$C'_{\text{eff}} = C'_0 e^{-Kt'_{\text{eff}}}$$
   $$0.1 = 100e^{-(1.0)t'_{\text{eff}}}$$
   $$t'_{\text{eff}} = 6.91 \text{ hr}$$

The percent increase in t_{eff} is therefore found by the following:

$$\text{Percent increase in } t_{eff} = \frac{t'_{eff} - t_{eff}}{t_{eff}} \times 100$$

$$= \frac{6.91 - 4.61}{4.61} \times 100$$

$$\text{Percent increase in } t_{eff} = 50\%$$

This example shows that a 10-fold increase in the dose increases the duration of action of a drug (t_{eff}) by only 50%.

EFFECT OF BOTH DOSE AND ELIMINATION HALF-LIFE ON THE DURATION OF ACTIVITY

A single equation can be derived to describe the relationship of dose (D_0) and the elimination half-life ($t_{1/2}$) on the effective time for therapeutic activity (t_{eff}). This expression is derived below:

$$\ln C_{eff} = \ln C_0 - kt_{eff}$$

Because $C_0 = D_0/V_D$,

$$\ln C_{eff} = \ln\left(\frac{D_0}{V_D}\right) - kt_{eff} \tag{19.7}$$

$$kt_{eff} = \ln\left(\frac{D_0}{V_D}\right) - \ln C_{eff}$$

$$t_{eff} = \frac{1}{k} \ln\left(\frac{D_0/V_D}{C_{eff}}\right)$$

Substitute $0.693/t_{1/2}$ for k:

$$t_{eff} = 1.44t_{1/2} \ln\left(\frac{D_0}{V_D C_{eff}}\right) \tag{19.8}$$

From Equation 19.8 an increase in $t_{1/2}$ will increase the t_{eff} in direct proportion. However, an increase in the dose D_0 does not increase the t_{eff} in direct proportion. The effect of an increase in V_D or C_{eff} could be seen by using generated data. Only the positive solutions for Equation 19.8 are valid, although mathematically t_{eff} can be obtained by increasing C_{eff} or V_D. The effect of changing dose on t_{eff} is shown in Figure 19-6 using data generated with Equation 19.8. The nonlinear increase in t_{eff} is observed as dose increases.

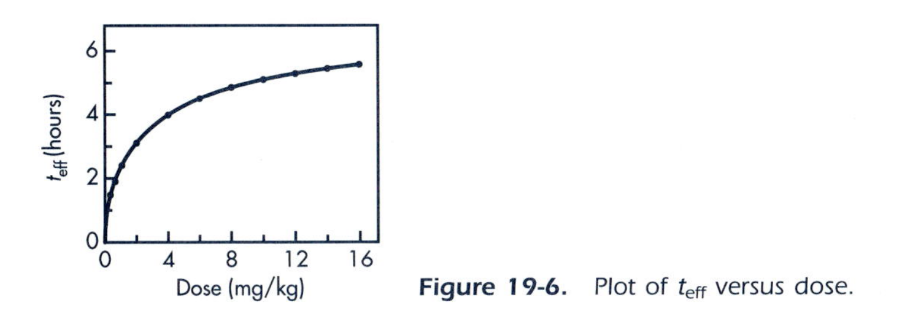

Figure 19-6. Plot of t_{eff} versus dose.

EFFECT OF ELIMINATION HALF-LIFE ON DURATION OF ACTIVITY

Because elimination of drugs is due to the processes of excretion and metabolism, an alteration of any of these elimination processes will effect the $t_{1/2}$ of the drug. In certain disease states, pathophysiologic changes in hepatic or renal function will decrease the elimination of a drug observed by a prolonged $t_{1/2}$. This prolonged $t_{1/2}$ will lead to retention of the drug in the body, thereby increasing the duration of activity of the drug (t_{eff}) as well as increasing the possibility of drug toxicity.

To improve antibiotic therapy with the penicillin and cephalosporin antibiotics, clinicians have intentionally prolonged the elimination of these drugs by giving a second drug, probenecid, which competitively inhibits renal excretion of the antibiotic. This approach to prolong the duration of activity of antibiotics that are rapidly excreted through the kidney has been used successfully for a number of years. The data in Table 19.1 illustrate how a change in the elimination $t_{1/2}$ will affect the t_{eff} for a drug. For all doses, a 100% increase in the $t_{1/2}$ will result in a 100% increase in the t_{eff}. For example, for a drug whose $t_{1/2}$ is 0.75 hours and is given at a dose of 2 mg/kg, the t_{eff} is 3.24 hours. If the $t_{1/2}$ is increased to 1.5 hours, the t_{eff} is increased to 6.48 hours, an increase of 100%. However, the effect of doubling the dose from 2 to 4 mg/kg (no change in elimination processes) will only increase the t_{eff} to 3.98 hours, an increase of 22.8%. The effect of prolonging the elimination half-life has an extremely important effect on the treatment of infections, particularly in patients with high metabolism, or clearance, of the antibiotic. Therefore, antibiotics must be dosed with full consideration of the effect of alteration of the $t_{1/2}$ on the t_{eff}. Consequently, a simple proportional increase in dose will leave the patient's blood concentration below the effective antibiotic level most of the time during drug therapy.

TABLE 19.1 The Relationship Between Elimination Half-Life and the Duration of Activity

DOSE (mg/kg)	$t_{1/2}$ = 0.75 hr t_{eff} (hr)	$t_{1/2}$ = 1.5 hr t_{eff} (hr)
2.0	3.24	6.48
3.0	3.67	7.35
4.0	3.98	7.97
5.0	4.22	8.45
6.0	4.42	8.84
7.0	4.59	9.18
8.0	4.73	9.47
9.0	4.86	9.72
10	4.97	9.95
11	5.08	10.2
12	5.17	10.3
13	5.26	10.5
14	5.34	10.7
15	5.41	10.8
16	5.48	11.0
17	5.55	11.1
18	5.61	11.2
19	5.67	11.3
20	5.72	11.4

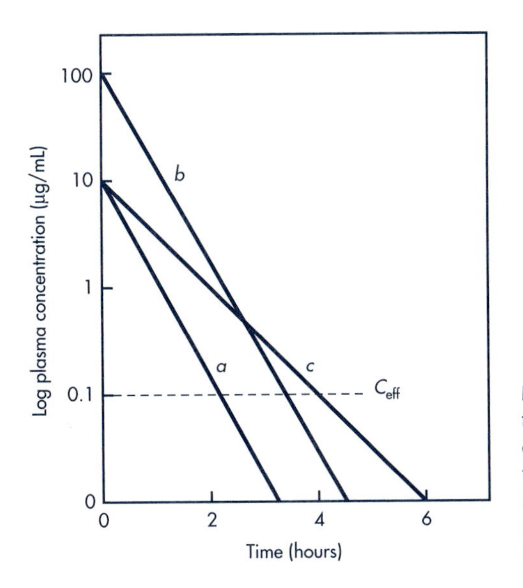

Figure 19-7. Plasma level–time curves describing the relationship of both dose and elimination half-life on duration of drug action. C_{eff} = effective concentration. Curve a = single 100 mg IV injection of drug; $k = 1.0\ hr^{-1}$. Curve b = single 1000-mg IV injection; $k = 1.0\ hr^{-1}$. Curve c = single 100-mg IV injection; $k = 0.5\ hr^{-1}$. V_D is 10 L.

Changes in elimination half-life will proportionately change the t_{eff}. It is interesting to note that, indeed, clinicians have long observed the therapeutic usefulness of combining probenecid with penicillin. The effect of a prolonged t_{eff} is shown in lines a and c in Figure 19-7, and the disproportionate increase in t_{eff} as the dose is increased 10-fold is shown in lines a and b.

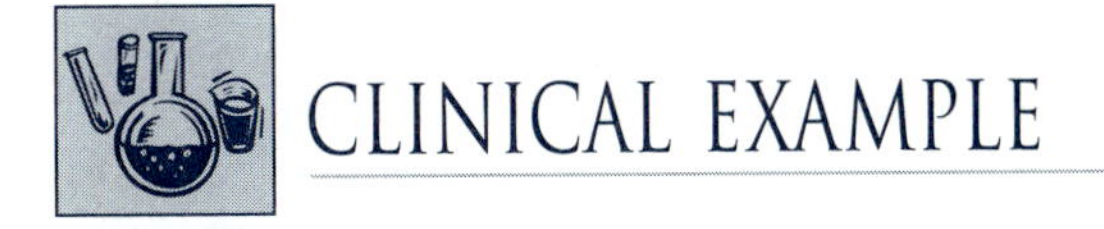

CLINICAL EXAMPLE

Pharmacokinetic/Pharmacodynamic Relationships and Efficacy of Antibiotics

In the previous section, the time above the effective concentration, t_{eff} was shown to be important in optimizing the therapeutic response of many drugs. This concept has been applied to the antibiotic drugs (Drusano, 1988; Craig, 1995; Craig and Andes, 1996; Scaglione, 1997). For example, Craig and Andes (1996) have discussed the antibacterial treatment of otitis media. Using the *minimum inhibitory antibiotic concentration* (MIC) for the microorganism in serum, the percent time for the antibiotic drug concentration to be above the MIC was calculated for several antibacterial classes including cephalosporins, macrolides, and trimethoprim-sulfamethoxazole (TMP/SMX) combination. The percent time above MIC of the dosing interval during therapy correlated well to the percent of bacteriologic cure (Figure 19-8). When the percent of time above MIC falls below a critical value, bacteria will regrow, thereby prolonging the time for eradication of the infection. Although the drug concentration in the middle ear fluid (MEF) is important, once the ratio (MEF/serum) is known, the serum drug level may be used to project MEF drug levels. Craig and Andes (1996) tested the antibiotics listed in Table 19.2.

An almost 100% cure was shown in Figure 19-8 by maintaining 60 to 70% of the

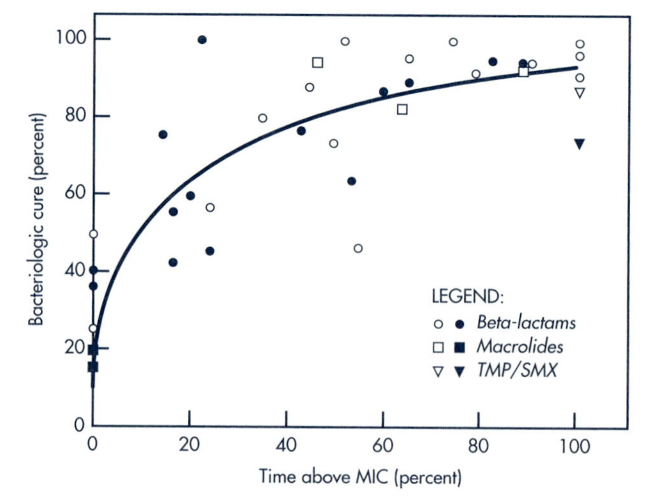

Figure 19-8. Relationship between the percent time above MIC_{90} of the dosing interval during therapy and percent of bacteriologic cure in otitis media caused by *S. pneumoniae* (open symbols) and beta lactamase positive and negative *H. influenzae* (closed symbols). (Circles, closed and open = beta-lactams; squares, closed and open = macrolides; triangles, closed and open = TMP/SMX.

From Craig and Andres, 1995, with permission.

dosing interval with the drug concentration above the MIC; an 80 to 85% cure was achieved with 40 to 50% time above MIC. These results show the importance of pharmacokinetics in optimizing drug therapy. The pharmacokinetic model was further supported by experiments from a mouse infectious model in which an infection in the thigh due to *P. aeruginosa* was treated with ticarcillin and tobramycin.

In another study, Craig (1995) compared the AUC/MIC, the time above MIC, and drug peak concentration over MIC and found that the best fit was obtained when CFU was plotted versus time above MIC for cefotaxime in a mouse infection model (Fig. 19-9).

Both Drusano (1988) and Craig (1995) have reviewed the relationship of pharmacokinetics and pharmacodynamics in the therapeutic efficacy of antibiotics. For some antibiotics, such as the aminoglycosides and fluoroquinolones, both the drug concentration and the dosing interval have an influence on the antibacterial effect. For some antibiotics, such as the beta-lactams, vancomycin, and the macrolides, the duration of exposure (time dependent killing) or the time the drug levels are maintained above the MIC is most important for efficacy. For many antibiotics (eg, fluoroquinolones), there is a defined period of bacterial growth suppression after short exposures to the antibiotic. This phenomenon is known as the *postantibiotic effect* (PAE). Other influences on antibiotic activity include the presence of active metabolite(s), plasma drug protein binding, and the penetration of the antibiotic into the tissues. Finally, the MIC for the antibiotic depends upon the infectious microorganism and the resistance of the microorganism to the antibiotic. In the case

TABLE 19.2 Middle-Ear Fluid to Serum Ratios for Common Antibiotics

ANTIBIOTIC	MIDDLE EAR FLUID (MEF)/SERUM RATIO
Cephalosporins	
Cefaclor	0.18–0.28
Cefuroxime	0.22
Macrolide antibiotic	
Erythromycin	0.49
Sulfa drug	
Sulfisoxazole	0.20

From Craig and Andes (1996).

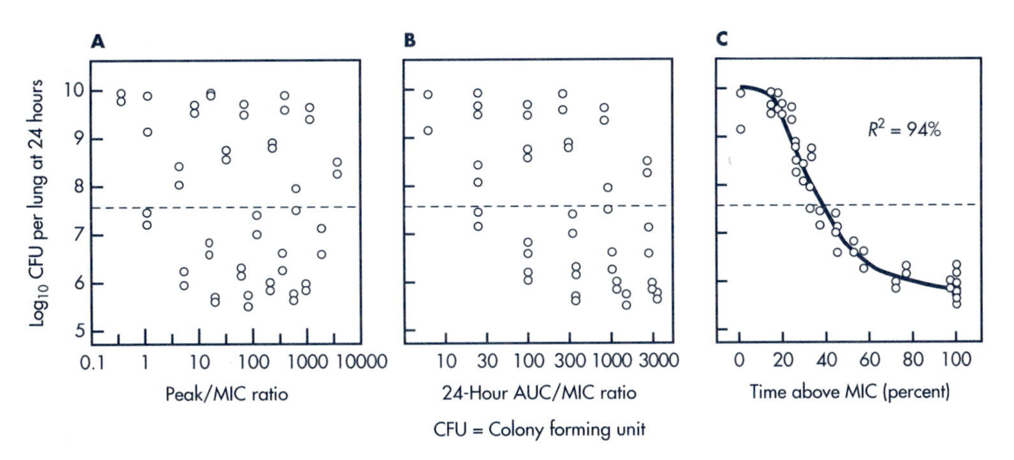

Figure 19-9. Relationship between three pharmacodynamic parameters and the number of *Klebsiella pneumonia* in the lungs of neurotroponic mice after 24-hr therapy with cefotaxime. Each point represents one mouse.
From Craig WA, 1995, with permission.

of ciprofloxacin, a quinolone, the percent of cure of infection at various doses was better related to AUIC, which is the product of area under the curve and the reciprocal of minimum inhibition concentration, MIC (Forrest et al, 1993). Interestingly, quinolones inhibit bacterial DNA gyrase, quite different from the beta-lactam antibiotics, which involve damage to bacterial cell walls.

Relationship Between Systemic Exposure and Response-Anticancer Drugs

For some drugs, the plasma drug concentrations are very scattered even after intravenous infusion due to variable drug clearance in individual patients (Rodman and Evans, 1991). No clear recognizable relationship is apparent between the therapeutic response and the drug dose. An example is the steady-state drug concentration of the anticancer drug teniposide given at three different doses (Figure 19-9A). In some patients, single point drug concentrations were variable and are even higher with lower doses. Careful pharmacokinetic–pharmacodynamic analy-

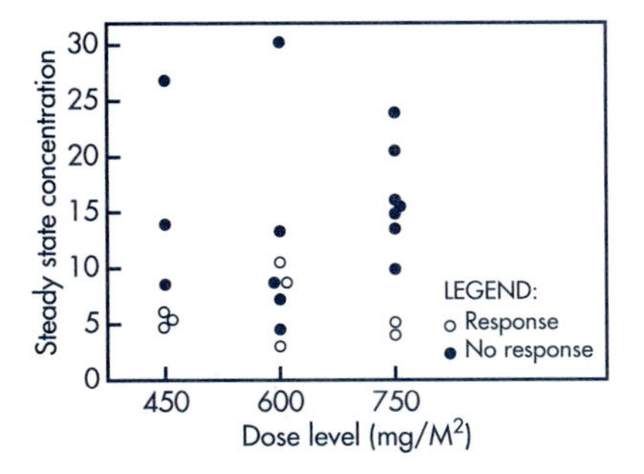

Figure 19-10. Steady-state concentration and response after three levels of teniposide administered by intravenous infusion.
From Rodman and Evans, 1991, with permission.

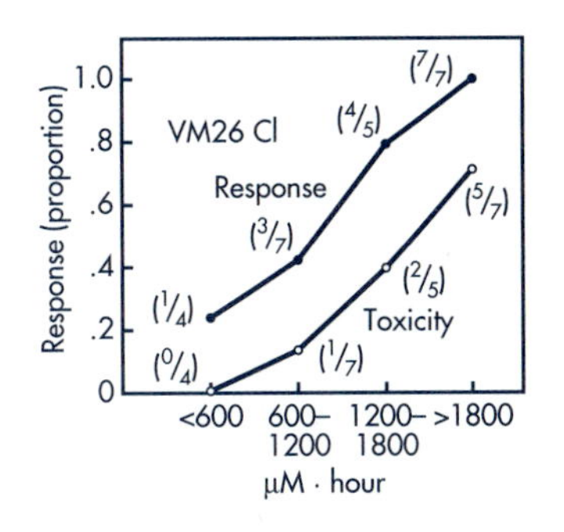

Figure 19-11. Relationship between systemic exposure for teniposide and toxicity and efficacy—shown as proportions of patients.
From Rodman and Evans, 1991, with permission.

sis showed that a graded response curve may be obtained when responses are plotted versus systemic exposure as measured by "concentration × time" (Figure 19-11). This example is one of many showing that anticancer responses may be better correlated to total area under the drug concentration curve (AUC), even when no apparent dose response relationship is observed. Undoubtedly, the cytotoxic effect of the drug involves killing cancer-cells with multiple-resistance thresholds that require different time exposures to the drug. The objective of applying PK/PD principles is to achieve therapeutic efficacy without triggering drug toxicity. This relationship is illustrated by the sigmoid curve for response and toxicity (Fig. 19-11), both of which lie close to each other and intensify as concentration increases.

RATE OF DRUG ABSORPTION AND PHARMACODYNAMIC RESPONSE

The rate of drug absorption influences the rate in which the drug gets to the receptor and the subsequent pharmacologic effect. For drugs that exert an acute pharmacologic effect, usually a direct acting drug agonist, extremely rapid drug absorption may have an intense and possibly detrimental effect. For example, niacin (nicotinic acid) is a vitamin given in large doses to decrease elevated plasma cholesterol and triglycerides. Large doses of niacin will also cause vasodilation, leading to flushing and postural hypertension when given in an immediate-release niacin tablet. Sustained-release niacin products are preferred because the more slowly absorbed niacin allows the baroreceptors to adjust to the hypotensive effect of the drug. Phenylpropanolamine is commonly used as a nasal decongestant in cough and cold products or as an anorectant in weight-loss products. Phenylpropanolamine acts as a pressor increasing the blood pressure much more intensely when given as an immediate-release product compared to a controlled-release product.

Equilibration Pharmacodynamic Half-Life

For some drugs, the half-time for drug equilibration has been estimated by observing the onset of response. A list of drugs reported by Lalonde (1992) are shown in Table 19.3. The factors that affect this parameter include perfusion of the effect compartment, blood-tissue partitioning, drug diffusion from capillaries to the effect compartment, protein binding, and elimination of the drug from the effect compartment.

Substance Abuse Liability

The rate of drug absorption has been associated with the potential for substance abuse. Drugs taken by the oral route have the lowest abuse potential. For example, cocoa leaves containing cocaine alkaloid have been chewed by South American Indians for centuries (Johanson and Fischman, 1989). Cocaine abuse has become a current problem due to the availability of the cocaine alkaloid ("crack" cocaine) and because of the use of other routes of drug administration (intravenous, intranasal delivery, or smoking) that allow a very rapid rate of drug absorption and onset of action (Cone, 1996). Studies on diazepam (de Wit et al, 1993) and nicotine (Henningfield and Keenan, 1993) have shown that the rate of drug delivery correlates with the abuse liability of such drugs. Thus, the rate of drug absorption

TABLE 19.3 Equilibration Half-Times Determined Using the Effect Compartment Method

DRUG	EQUILIBRATION $t_{1/2}$ (min)	PHARMACOLOGIC RESPONSE
d-Tubocurarine	4	Muscle paralysis
Disopyramide	2	QT prolongation
Quinidine	8	QT prolongation
Digoxin	214	LVET shortening
Terbutaline	7.5	FEV-1
Terbutaline	11.5	Hypokalemia
Theophylline	11	FEV-1
Verapamil	2	PR prolongation
Nizatidine	83	Gastric pH
Thiopental	1.2	Spectral edge
Fentanyl	6.4	Spectral edge
Alfentanil	1.1	Spectral edge
Ergotamine	595	Vasoconstriction
Vercuronium	4	Muscle paralysis
N-Acetylprocainamide	6.4	QT prolongation

From Lalonde, 1992, with permission.

influences the abuse potential of these drugs, and the route of drug administration that provides faster absorption and more rapid onset leads to greater abuse.

DRUG TOLERANCE AND PHYSICAL DEPENDENCY

The study of drug tolerance and physical dependency is of particular interest in understanding the actions of abused drug substances, such as opiates and cocaine. Drug *tolerance* is a quantitative change in the sensitivity of the drug and is demonstrated by a decrease in pharmacodynamic effect after repeated exposure to the same drug. The degree of tolerance may vary greatly (Cox, 1990). Drug tolerance has been well described for organic nitrates, opioids, and other drugs. For example, the nitrates relax vascular smooth muscle and have been used for both acute angina (eg, nitroglycerin sublingual spray or transmucosal tablet) or angina prophylaxis (eg, nitroglycerin transdermal, oral controlled-release isosorbide dinitrate). Well-controlled clinical studies have shown that tolerance to the vascular and antianginal effects of nitrates may develop. For nitrate therapy, the use of a low nitrate or nitrate-free periods has been advocated as part of the therapeutic approach. The magnitude of drug tolerance is a function of both the dosage and the frequency of drug administration. *Cross tolerance* can occur for similar drugs that act on the same receptors. Tolerance does not develop uniformly to all the pharmacologic or toxic actions of the drug. For example, patients showing tolerance to the depressant activity of high doses of opiates will still exhibit "pinpoint" pupils and constipation.

The mechanism of drug tolerance may be due to (1) disposition or pharmacokinetic tolerance or (2) pharmacodynamic tolerance. *Pharmacokinetic tolerance* is often due to enzyme induction (discussed in earlier chapters) in which the hepatic drug clearance increases with repeated drug exposure. *Pharmacodynamic tolerance* is due to a cellular or receptor alteration in which the drug response is less than what is predicted in the patient given subsequent drug doses. Measurement of serum drug concentrations may differentiate between pharmacokinetic tolerance and pharmacodynamic tolerance. Acute tolerance, or *tachyphylaxis,* which is the rapid development of tolerance, may occur due to a change in the sensitivity of the receptor or depletion of a cofactor after only a single or a few doses of the drug. Drugs that work indirectly by releasing norepinephrine may show tachyphylaxis. Drug tolerance should be differentiated from genetic factors which account for normal variability in the drug response.

Physical dependency is demonstrated by the appearance of withdrawal symptoms after cessation of the drug. Workers exposed to volatile organic nitrates in the work place may initially develop headaches and dizziness followed by tolerance with continuous exposure. However, after leaving the workplace for a few days, the workers may demonstrate nitrate withdrawal symptoms. Factors that may affect drug dependency may include the dose or amount of drug used (intensity of drug effect), the duration of drug use (months, years, and peak use) and the total dose (amount of drug × duration). The appearance of withdrawal symptoms may be abruptly precipitated in opiate-dependent subjects by the administration of naloxone (Narcan), an opioid antagonist that has no agonist properties.

HYPERSENSITIVITY AND ADVERSE RESPONSE

Many drug responses such as hypersensitivity and allergic response are not fully explained by pharmacodynamics and pharmacokinetics. Allergic responses generally are not dose related, although some penicillin-sensitive patients may respond to threshold skin concentrations, but, otherwise, no dose response relationship has been established. Skin eruption is a common symptom of drug allergy. Allergic reactions can occur at extremely low drug concentrations. Some urticaria episodes in patients have been traced to penicillin contamination in food or due to penicillin contamination during dispensing or manufacturing. Allergic reactions are important data that must be recorded in the patient's profile along with other adverse reactions. Penicillin-allergic reaction in the population is often detected by skin test with a PPL mixture. The incidence of penicillin-allergic reaction occurs in about 1 to 10% of the patients. The majority of these reactions are minor cutaneous reactions such as urticaria, angioedema, and pruritus. Serious allergic reactions, such as anaphylaxis, are rare, with an incidence of 0.021% to 0.106% for penicillins (Lin, 1992). For cephalosporins, the incidence of anaphylactic reaction is less than 0.02%. Anaphylactic reaction for cefaclor was reported to be 0.001% in a postmarketing survey. There are emerging trends showing that there may be a difference between the original and the new generations of cephalosporins (Reisman and Reisman, 1995). Cross sensitivity to similar chemical classes of drugs can occur.

Allergic reactions may be immediate or delayed and have been related to IgE mechanisms. In beta-lactam (penicillin) drug allergy, immediate reactions occur in about 30 to 60 minutes, but delayed reaction, or accelerated reaction, may occur from 1 to 72 hours after administration. Anaphylactic reaction may occur in both groups. Although some early evidences of cross hypersensitivity between penicillin and cephalosporin were observed, the incidence in patients sensitive to penicillin show only a two-fold increase in sensitivity to cephalosporin compared with that of the general population. The report rationalized that it is safe to administer cephalosporin to penicillin-sensitive patients and that the penicillin skin test is not useful in identifying patients allergic to cephalosporin due to the low incidence of cross reactivity (Reisman and Reisman, 1995). In practice, the clinician should evaluate the risk of the drug allergy against the choice of alternative medication. Some earlier reports showed that cross sensitivity between penicillin and cephalosporin was due to the presence of trace penicillin present in those products.

DRUG DISTRIBUTION AND PHARMACOLOGIC RESPONSE

After systemic absorption, the drug is carried throughout the body by the general circulation. Most of the drug dose will reach unintended target tissues, in which the drug may be passively stored, produce an adverse effect, or be eliminated. A fraction of the dose will reach the target site and establish equilibrium there. The receptor site is unknown most of the time, but, kinetically, it is known as the *effect compartment.* The time course of drug delivery to the effect compartment will determine whether the onset of pharmacologic response is immediate or delayed. The delivery of drug to the effect compartment is affected by the rate of blood flow, diffusion, and partition properties of the drug and the receptor molecules.

At the receptor site, the onset, duration, and intensity of the pharmacologic response are controlled by receptor concentration and the concentration of the drug and/or its active metabolites. The ultimate pharmacologic response (effect) may largely depend upon the stereospecific nature of the interaction of the drug with the receptor and the rates of association and dissociation of the drug receptor complex. Depending on their location and topography, not all receptor molecules are occupied by drug molecules when a maximum pharmacologic response is produced. Other variables such as age, sex, genetics, nutrition, and tolerance may also modify the pharmacologic response, making it difficult to relate the pharmacologic response to plasma drug concentration. To control data fluctuation and simplify pharmacodynamic fitting, the pharmacologic response is often expressed as a percent of response above a baseline or percent of maximum response. By combining pharmacokinetics and pharmacodynamics, some drugs with relatively complex pharmacologic responses have been described by pharmacodynamic models accounting for their onset, intensity, and duration of action.

After the pharmacodynamics of a drug are characterized, the time course of pharmacologic response may be predicted after drug administration. Also, from these data, it would be possible to determine from the pharmacokinetic parameters whether an observed change in pharmacologic response is due to pharmacodynamic factors, such as tachyphylaxis or tolerance, or due to pharmacokinetic factors, such as a change in drug absorption, elimination or distribution.

Drug–Receptor Theory Relating Pharmacologic Effect and Dose

The relationship between pharmacologic effect and dose was advanced by Wagner (1968), who derived a kinetic expression that relates drug concentration to pharmacologic effect. This theoretical development transformed the semiempirical dose–effect relationship (the hyperbolic or log sigmoid profile) into a theoretical equation that relates pharmacologic effect to pharmacokinetics (ie, a pharmacokinetics/pharmacodynamic, PK/PD model). Because the equation was developed for a drug receptor with either single or multiple drug binding, many drugs with a sigmoid concentration effect profile may be described by this model. The slope of the profile also provides some insight into the drug–receptor interaction.

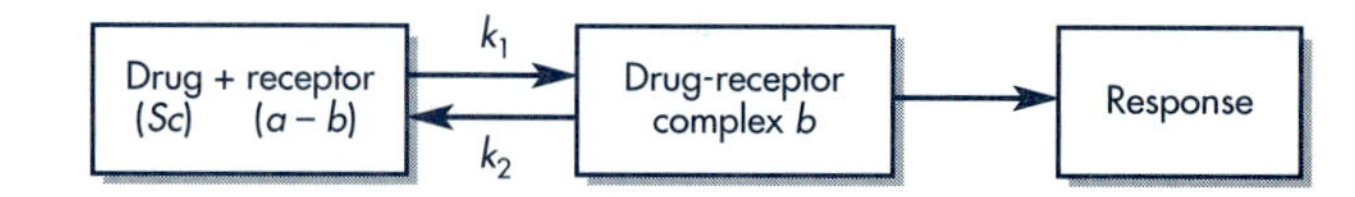

Figure 19-12. Model of the drug–receptor theory: a = total number of drug receptors, c = concentration of drug, S = number of moles of drug that combine with one receptor (constant for each drug), and b = number of drug–receptor complexes.

The basic equation mimics somewhat the kinetic equation for protein drug binding (Chapter 11). One or more drug molecules may interact with a receptor to form a complex that in turn elicits a pharmacokinetic response, as illustrated in Figure 19-12. The rate of change in the number of drug–receptor complexes is expressed as db/dt. From Figure 19-12, a differential equation is obtained as shown:

$$db/dt = k_1 C^s(a - b) - bk_2 \tag{19.9}$$

where $k_1 C^S(a - b)$ = rate of receptor complex formation and bk_2 = rate of dissociation of the receptor complex.

At steady state, $db/dt = 0$ and Equation 19.9 reduces to:

$$k_1 c^s a - k_1 c^s b - bk_2 = 0 \tag{19.10}$$

$$\frac{b}{a} = \frac{k_1 c^s}{k_1 c^s + k_2} = \frac{1}{1 + \left(\dfrac{k_2}{k_1 c^s}\right)}$$

For many drugs, the pharmacologic response (R) is proportio+nal to the number of receptors occupied:

$$R \propto \frac{b}{a} \tag{19.11}$$

The pharmacologic response (R) is related to the maximum pharmacologic response (R_{max}), concentration of drug, and rate of change in the number of drug receptor complexes occupied:

$$R = \frac{R_{max}}{1 + \left(\dfrac{k_2}{k_1 c^s}\right)} \tag{19.12}$$

A graph of Equation 19.12 constructed from the percent pharmacologic response, $(R/R_{max}) \times 100$, versus the concentration of drug gives the response–concentration curve (Fig. 19-13). This type of theoretical development explains that the pharmacologic response versus dose curve is not completely linear over the entire dosage range, as is frequently observed.

The total pharmacologic response elicited by a drug is difficult to quantitate in terms of the intensity and the duration of the drug response. The *integrated phar-*

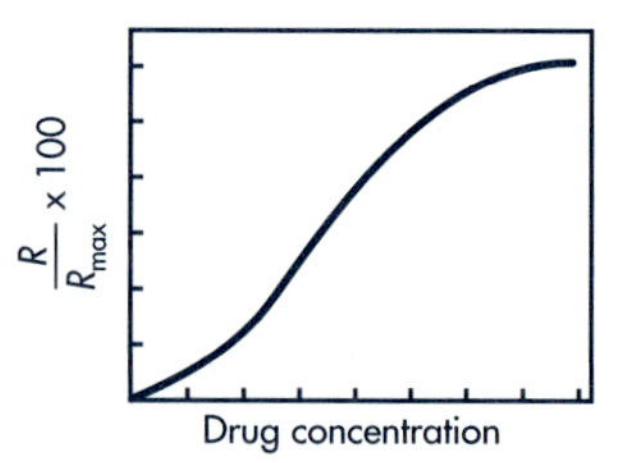

Figure 19-13. Graph of drug concentration versus pharmacologic response.

TABLE 19.4 Hypothetical Drug Given Intravenously in Single and Divided Doses[a]

DOSE NUMBER	SINGLE DOSE	DOSE GIVEN INITIALLY AND AT 12TH hr	DOSE GIVEN AT 0, 6, 12, 18 hr	DOSE GIVEN AT 0, 3, 6, 9, 12, 15, 18, 21 hr
1	422	272	139.4	62.53
2		276	148.2	71.46
3			148.5	74.41
4			149.0	75.61
5				76.27
6				76.44
7				76.71
8				76.81
Total response	422	548	585.1	590.2
% Response	100	130	138.7	138.9

[a]The drug follows a one-compartment open model. Each value represents a unit of integrated pharmacologic response.

Adapted with permission from Wagner (1968).

macologic response is a measure of the total pharmacologic response and is mathematically expressed as the product of these two factors (ie, duration and intensity of drug action) summed up over a period of time. Using Equation 19.12, an integrated pharmacologic response is generated if the drug plasma concentration–time curve can be adequately described by a pharmacokinetic model.

Table 19.4 is based on a hypothetical drug that follows a one-compartment open model. The drug is given intravenously in divided doses. With this drug, the total integrated response increases considerably when the total dose is given in a greater number of divided doses. By giving the drug in a single dose, two doses, four doses, and eight doses, an integrated response was obtained that ranged from 100 to 138.9%, using the single-dose response as a 100% reference. It should be pointed out that when the bolus dose is broken into a smaller number of doses, the largest percent increase in the integrated response occurs when the bolus dose is divided into two doses. Further division will cause less of an increase, proportionally. The actual percent increase in integrated response depends on the $t_{1/2}$ of the drug as well as the dosing interval.

The values in Table 19.2 were theoretically generated. However, these data illustrate that the pharmacologic response is dependent on the dosing schedule. A large total dose given in divided doses may produce a pharmacologic response quite different from that obtained by administration of the drug in a single dose.

The correlation of pharmacologic response to pharmacokinetics is not always possible with all drugs. Sometimes intermediate steps are involved in the mechanism of drug action of the drug that are more complex than is assumed in the model. For example, warfarin (an anticoagulant) produces a delayed response and there is no direct correlation of the anticoagulant activity to the plasma drug concentration. The plasma warfarin level is correlated with the inhibition of the prothrombin complex production rate. However, many of the correlations of pharmacologic effect and plasma drug concentration are performed by proposing models that may be discarded after more data is collected. The process of pharmacokinetic modeling can greatly enhance our understanding of the way drugs act in a quantitative manner.

PHARMACODYNAMIC MODELS

No unified general pharmacodynamic model relating pharmacologic response to pharmacokinetics is available based on detailed drug receptor theory. Most of the drug receptor based models are descriptive and lack quantitative details. Successful modeling of pharmacologic response has been achieved with semiempirically based assumptions and usually with some oversimplification of the real process. The successful modeling of the degree of muscle paralysis of *d*-tubocurarine to plasma concentrations is an interesting example in which the exact mechanism of the drug–receptor interaction was not considered. Many of the classic pharmacodynamic models were developed without detailed knowledge of the drug–receptor interaction. One of the few pharmacodynamic models that take into account the interaction between the receptor and the drug molecule leading to a pharmacologic effect was described by Boudinot and associates (1986) using the drug prednisolone as an example. Prednisolone is a corticosteroid that binds to cytosolic receptors within the cell (Fig. 19-14). The bound steroid receptor complex is activated and translocated into the nucleus of the cell. Within the cell, the drug receptor complex associates with specific DNA sequences and modulates the transcription of RNA, which ultimately initiates protein synthesis (Boudinot et al, 1986). *Tyrosine amino transferase* (TAT) is an enzyme protein that is increased (induced) due to the action of prednisolone. In the liver cell, the prednisolone concentration, drug receptor concentration, and TAT enzyme were measured with respect to time. The

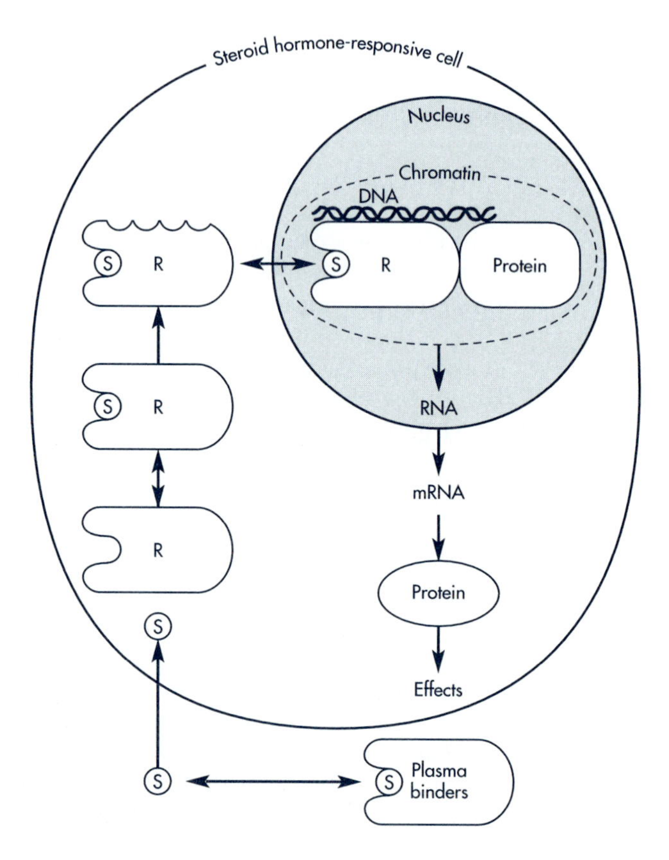

Figure 19-14. Receptor-mediated (R) mechanism of action of corticosteroid (S) hormones.
(From Baxter and Funder, 1979, with permission.)

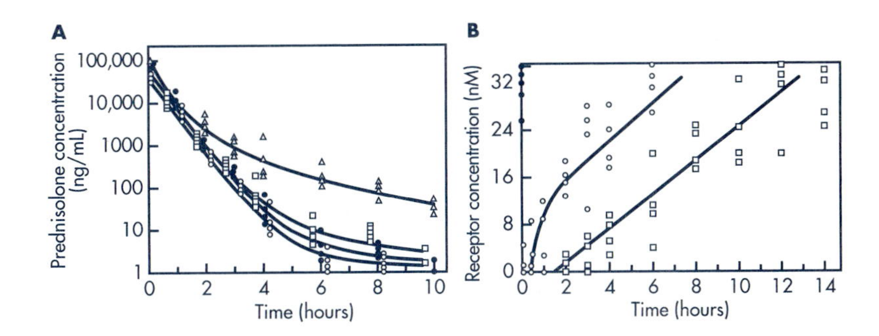

Figure 19-15. **A.** Prednisolone levels in plasma (□) and liver (△) fall exponentially after 50 mg/kg of drug IV during the first 10 hours, as described by a pharmacokinetic model. **B.** Free cytosolic glucocorticoid receptor (CGR) concentration fell from control level (●) after 5 (○) and 50 mg/kg (□) IV dose of prednisolone. Free CGR fell as prednisolone interacted with receptor to form receptor complex. The free CGR returned to baseline level after about 10 hours.
(From Boudinot et al, 1986, with permission.)

pharmacodynamic model accounted for the delayed response of prednisolone, a characteristic of corticosteroid response. In this model, prednisolone is bound to plasma protein, and free drug must leave the plasma compartment and enter the cell to form a drug–receptor complex; creation of this complex then triggers the pharmacologic events leading to an increase in intracellular TAT concentration. The model was able to account for a delay in response. A decrease in free receptor or an increase in bound receptor complexes after drug administration was observed. Plasma prednisolone concentrations were described by a triexponential equation and a time lag was built into the model to account for the delay between TAT increase and the drug–receptor–DNA complex formation (Figs. 19-15 and 19-16).

The Maximum Effect (E_{max}) Model

The *maximum effect model* (E_{max}) is an empirical model that relates pharmacologic response to drug concentrations. This model incorporates the observation known as the *law of diminishing return,* which shows that an increase in drug concentration near the maximum pharmacologic response produces a disproportionately smaller increase in the pharmacologic response (Fig. 19-17). The E_{max} model describes drug action in terms of maximum effect (E_{max}) and EC_{50}.

$$E = \frac{E_{max} C}{EC_{50} + C} \tag{19.13}$$

where C is the plasma drug concentration and E is the pharmacologic effect.

Equation 19.13 is a saturable process resembling Michaelis–Menton enzyme kinetics. As the plasma drug concentration C increases, the pharmacologic effect E approaches E_{max} asymptotically. A double reciprocal plot of Equation 19.13 may be used to linearize the relationship similar to a Lineweaver–Burke equation.

E_{max} is the maximum pharmacologic effect that may be obtained by the drug, and EC_{50} is the drug concentration that produces one-half (50%) of the maximum pharmacologic response. In this model, both E_{max} and EC_{50} can be measured.

For example, the bronchodilator activity of theophylline may be monitored by measuring FEV_1 (forced expiratory volume) at various plasma drug concentrations

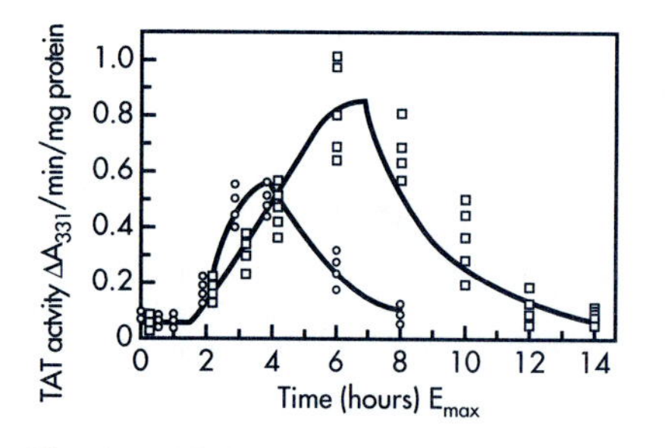

Figure 19-16. Tyrosine aminotransferase (TAT) activity in liver was described by a pharmacodynamic model (solid line) after 5 (○) and 50 mg/kg (□) IV prednisolone. The pharmacodynamic model accounts for the delay of TAT activity. (From Boudinot et al, 1986, with permission.)

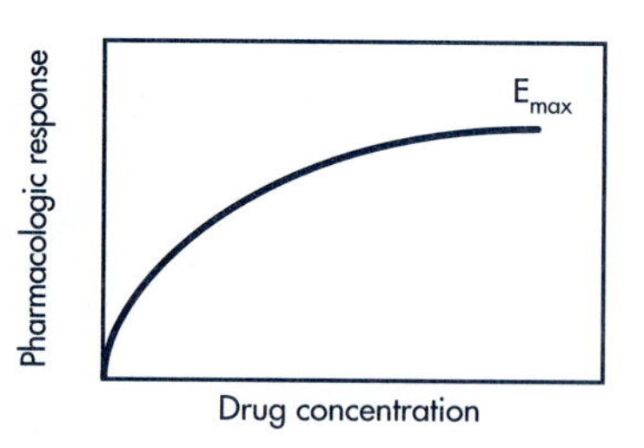

Figure 19-17. Plot of pharmacologic response versus plasma drug concentration in a hyperbolic model.

(Fig. 19-18). For theophylline, a small gradual increase in FEV_1 is obtained as the plasma drug concentrations are increased higher than 10 mg/L. Only a 17% increase in FEV_1 is observed when the plasma theophylline concentration is doubled from 10 to 20 mg/L. The EC_{50} for theophylline is 10 mg/L. The E_{max} is equivalent to 63% of normal FEV_1. A further increase in the plasma theophylline concentration will not obtain an improvement in the FEV_1 beyond E_{max}. Either drug saturation of the receptors or other limiting factors prevent further improvement in the pharmacologic response.

The E_{max} model describes two key features of the pharmacologic response: (1) the model mimics the hyperbolic shape of the pharmacologic response versus drug concentration, and (2) there is a maximum pharmacologic response (E_{max}) induced by a certain drug concentration beyond which no further increases in pharmacologic response is obtained (Fig. 19-17). The drug concentration that produces a 50% maximum pharmacologic response (EC_{50}) is useful as a guide for achieving drug concentration that lies within the therapeutic range.

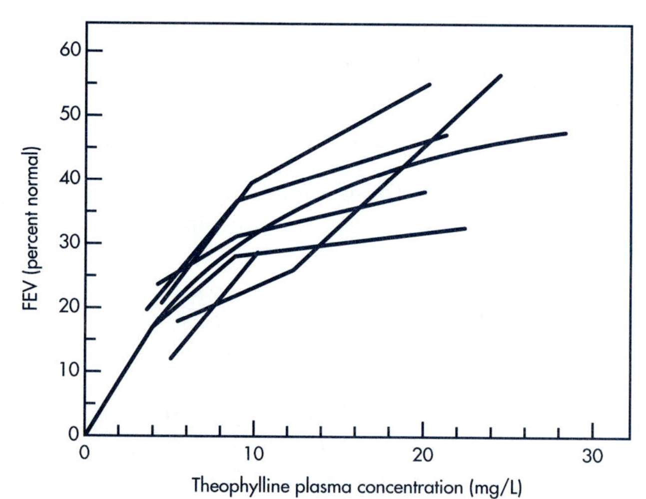

Figure 19-18. Use of E_{max} model to describe the effects of theophylline on change in normalized forced expiratory volume (FEV_1); E_{max} = 63%, EC_{50} = 10 mg/L. (From Mitenko and Ogilvie, 1973, and Holford and Sheiner, 1981, with permission.)

In many cases, the measured pharmacologic effect has some value when drug is absent (eg, blood pressure, heart rate, respiration rate). E_0 is the measured pharmacologic effect (baseline activity) at zero drug concentration in the body. The measurement for E_0 may be variable due to intra- and intersubject differences. Using E_0 as a baseline constant effect term, Equation 19.13 may be modified as follows:

$$E + E_0 + \frac{E_{\max} C}{EC_{50} + C} \tag{19.14}$$

The Sigmoid $E_{\max}$ Model

The *sigmoid $E_{\max}$ model* describes the pharmacologic response versus drug concentration curve for many drugs that appear to be S-shaped (ie, sigmoidal) rather than hyperbolic as described by the more simple $E_{\max}$ model. The model was first used by Hill (1910) to describe the association of oxygen with hemoglobin, in which the association with one oxygen molecule influences the association of the hemoglobin with the next oxygen molecule. The equation for the sigmoid $E_{\max}$ model is an extension of the $E_{\max}$ model:

$$E = \frac{E_{\max} C^n}{EC_{50} + C^n} \tag{19.15}$$

where n is an exponent describing the number of drug molecules that combine with each receptor molecule.

When n is equal to unity ($n = 1$), the sigmoidal $E_{\max}$ model reduces to the $E_{\max}$ model. A value of $n > 1$ influences the slope of the curve and the model fit.

The sigmoidal $E_{\max}$ model has been used to describe the effect of tocainamide on the suppression of ventricular extrasystoles (Winkle et al, 1976). As shown in Figure 19-19, the very steep slope of the tocainamide concentration versus response curve required that $n = 20$ in order to fit the model. Although this model is developed empirically, the mathematical equation describing the model is similar to the one elaborated by Wagner (1968) and discussed earlier in this chapter.

In the sigmoid $E_{\max}$ model, the slope is influenced by the number of drug molecules, bound to the receptor. Moreover, a very large n value may indicate *allosteric* or *cooperative effects* in the interaction of the drug molecules with the receptor.

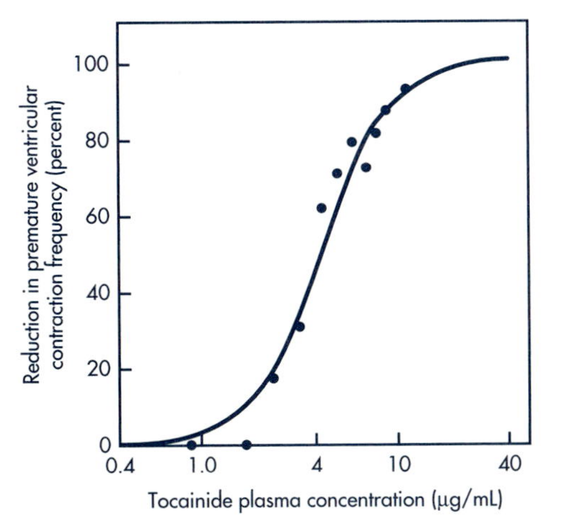

Figure 19-19. Steep concentration response curve for tocainide requiring use of the sigmoid $E_{\max}$ model. (From Winkle et al, 1976, with permission.)

Pharmacokinetic Pharmacodynamic Models with an Effect Compartment

Many pharmacokinetic models describe the time course for drug and metabolite concentrations in the body. Using either the sigmoid E_{max} or one of the other pharmacodynamic models described earlier, the pharmacologic response may be obtained at various time periods. This simple approach has worked for some neuromuscular blockers and anesthetic agents, whose activity is related to plasma drug concentrations.

For some drugs, the time course for the pharmacologic response may not directly parallel the time course of the plasma drug concentration. The maximum pharmacologic response produced by the drug may be observed before or after the plasma drug concentration has peaked. Moreover, other drugs may produce a delayed pharmacologic response unrelated to the plasma drug concentration.

A pharmacokinetic/pharmacodynamic model with an effect compartment is used to describe the pharmacokinetics of the drug in the plasma and the time course of a pharmacologic effect of a drug in the site of action. To account for the pharmacodynamics of an indirect or delayed drug response, a hypothetical effect compartment has been postulated (Fig. 19-20). This *effect compartment* is not part of the pharmacokinetic model but is a hypothetical pharmacodynamic compartment that links the plasma compartment containing drug. Drug transfers from the plasma compartment to the effect compartment, but no significant amount of drug moves from the effect compartment to the plasma compartment. Only free drug will diffuse into the effect compartment, and the transfer rate constants are usually first order. The pharmacologic response is determined from the rate constant, k_{e0} and the drug concentration in the effect compartment (Fig. 19-20).

The amount of drug in the hypothetical effect compartment after a bolus IV dose may be obtained by writing a differential describing the rate of change in drug amounts in each compartment:

$$\frac{dD_e}{dt} = k_{1e}D_1 - k_{e0}D_e \tag{19.16}$$

where D_e is the amount of drug in the effect compartment, D_1 is the amount of drug in the central compartment, k_{1e} is the transfer rate constant for drug movement from the central compartment into the effect compartment, and k_{e0} is the transfer rate constant out of the effect compartment.

Integrating Equation 19.16 yields the amount of drug in the effect compartment D_e.

$$D_e = \frac{D_0 k_{1e}}{(k_{e0} - k)}\left(e^{-kt} - e^{-k_{e0}t}\right) \tag{19.17}$$

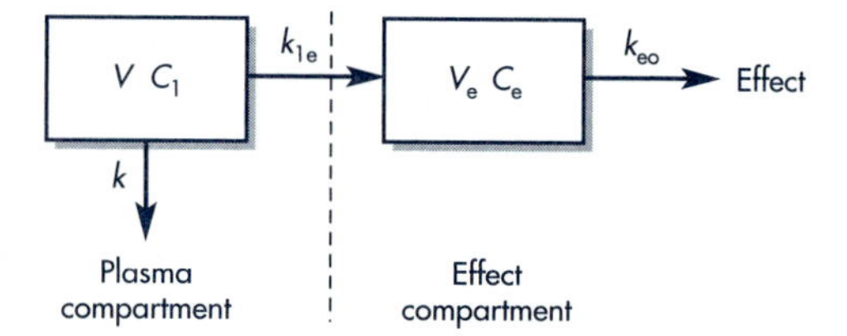

Figure 19-20. Pharmacokinetic–pharmacodynamic model with an effect compartment.

Dividing Equation 19.17 by V_e, the volume of the effect compartment, yields the concentration C_e of the effect compartment.

$$C_e = \frac{D_0 k_{1e}}{V_e(k_{e0} - k)} (e^{-kt} - e^{-k_{e0}t}) \tag{19.18}$$

where D_0 is the dose, V_e is the volume of the effect compartment and k is the elimination rate constant from the central compartment. Equation 19.18 is not very useful because the parameters V_e and k_{1e} are both unknown and are not obtainable from plasma drug concentration data. Several assumptions were made to simplify this equation.

The pharmacodynamic model assumes that even though an effect compartment is present in addition to the plasma compartment, this hypothetical effect compartment takes up only a negligible amount of the drug dose, so that plasma drug level still follows a one-compartment equation. After an IV bolus dose, the rate of drug entering and leaving the effect compartment is controlled by the incoming rate constant k_{1e} and the elimination rate constant k_{e0}. (There is no diffusion of drug from the effect compartment into the plasma compartment.) At steady state, both the input and output rates are equal,

$$k_{1e} D_1 = D_e k_{e0} \tag{19.19}$$

Rearranging,

$$D_1 = \frac{k_{e0} D_e}{k_{1e}} \tag{19.20}$$

Dividing by V_D yields the steady state plasma drug concentration C_1.

$$C_1 = \frac{k_{e0} D_e}{k_{1e} V_D} \tag{19.21}$$

$$D_e = \frac{D_0 k_{1e}}{(k_{e0} - k)} (e^{-kt} - e^{-k_{e0}t}) \tag{19.22}$$

Substituting for D_e into Equation 19.21 yields

$$C_1 = \frac{k_{e0} D_0 k_{1e}}{k_{1e} V_D (k_{e0} - k)} (e^{-kt} - e^{-k_{e0}t}) \tag{19.23}$$

Cancelling the common term k_{1e},

$$C_1 = \frac{k_{e0} D_0}{V_D (k_{e0} - k)} (e^{-kt} - e^{-k_{e0}t}) \tag{19.24}$$

At steady state, C_1 is unaffected by k_{1e} and is only controlled by the elimination constant k and k_{e0}. C_1 is called C_{pss}, or steady-state concentration, and has been used successfully to relate the pharmacodynamics of many drugs including some with delayed equilibration between the plasma and effect compartment. Thus k and k_{e0} jointly determine the pharmacodynamic profile of a drug. In fitting the pharmacokinetic–pharmacodynamic model, the IV bolus equation is fitted to the plasma drug concentration versus time data to obtain k and V_D, while C_{pss}, or C_1 from Equation 19.24, is used to substitute into the concentration in Equation 19.15 to fit the pharmacologic response.

Many drug examples have been described by this type of pharmacokinetic–pharmacodynamic model. The key feature of this model is its dynamic flexibility and adaptability to pharmacokinetic models that account for drug distribution and pharmacologic response. The aggregate effects of drug elimination, binding, partitioning, and distribution in the body are accommodated by the model. The basic assumptions are practical and pragmatic, although some critics of the model (Colburn, 1987) believe the hypothetical effect compartment may oversimplify more complex drug receptor events. On the positive side, the model represents elegantly an *in vivo* pharmacologic event relating to the plasma drug concentrations that a clinician can monitor and adjust.

Until more information is known about the effect compartment, a pharmacokinetic–pharmacodynamic model is proposed to describe these kinetic processes combining some of the variables. A good fit of the data to the model is useful but does not necessarily describe the actual pharmacodynamic process. The process of model development evolves until a better model replaces an inadequate one. Several examples of drugs incorporating the effect compartment concept cited in the next section support the versatility of this model. The model accommodates some difficult drug response–concentration profiles, such as the puzzling hysteresis profile of some drug responses (eg, responses to cocaine and ajmaline).

Pharmacodynamic Models Using an Effect Compartment

The antiarrhythmic drug ajmaline slows the heart rate by delaying the depolarization of the heart muscle in the atrium and the ventricle. The pharmacologic effect of the drug is observed in the ECG by measuring the prolongation of the PQ and QRS interval after an IV infusion of ajmaline. A two-compartment model with binding described the pharmacokinetics of the drug, and a pharmacodynamic model with an effect compartment was linked to the central compartment in which free drug may diffuse into the effect compartment. The effect compartment was necessary because the plasma ajmaline concentration did not correlate well with change in recorded ECG events. When the effect compartment drug concentration was used instead, drug activity was well described by the model (Figs. 19-21 and 19-22).

Hysteresis of Pharmacologic Response

Many pharmacologic responses are complex and do not show a direct relationship between pharmacologic effect and plasma drug concentration. Some drugs have a plasma drug concentration versus pharmacologic response resembling a hysteresis

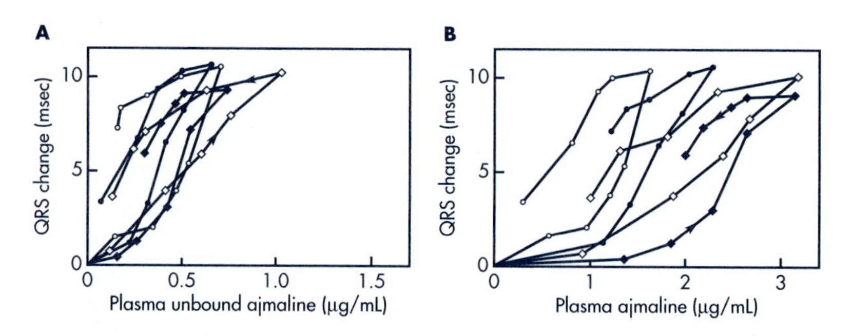

Figure 19-21. Plot of ajmaline concentration versus change in QRS interval for four dogs: (◆) 1, (◇) 2, (●) 3, (○) 4. **A.** Unbound plasma ajmaline versus response. **B.** Plasma ajmaline versus response. (From Yasuhara et al, 1987, with permission.)

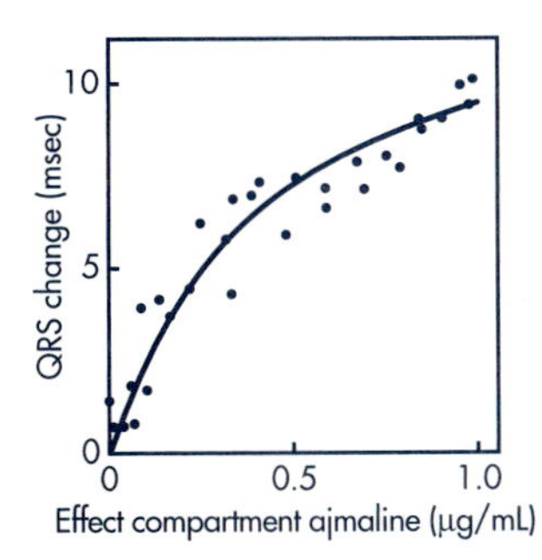

Figure 19-22. Plot of change in QRS interval versus ajmaline concentration in the effect compartment in dog 2. The lines were generated based on the effect compartment model.
(From Yasuhara et al, 1987, with permission.)

loop (Fig. 19-23). For these drugs, an identical plasma concentration can result in significantly different pharmacologic responses, depending on whether the plasma drug concentration is on the ascending or descending phase of the loop. The time-dependent nature of a pharmacologic response may be due to tolerance, induced metabolite deactivation, reduced response, or translocation of receptors at the site of action. This type of time-dependent pharmacologic response is characterized by a *clockwise* profile when pharmacologic response is plotted versus plasma drug concentrations over time (Fig. 19-23).

For example, fentanyl (a lipid-soluble, narcotic anesthetic) and alfentanil (a closely related drug) display a clockwise hysteresis, apparently due to rapid lipid partition. β-adrenoreceptors, such as isoproterenol, apparently have no direct relationship between response and plasma drug concentration and show hysteresis features. The diminished pharmacologic response was speculated to be a result of cellular response and physiologic adaptation to intense stimulation of the drug. A decrease in the number of receptors as well as translocation of receptors was proposed as the explanation for the observation. The euphoria produced by cocaine also displays a clockwise profile when responses were plotted versus plasma cocaine concentration (Fig. 19-24).

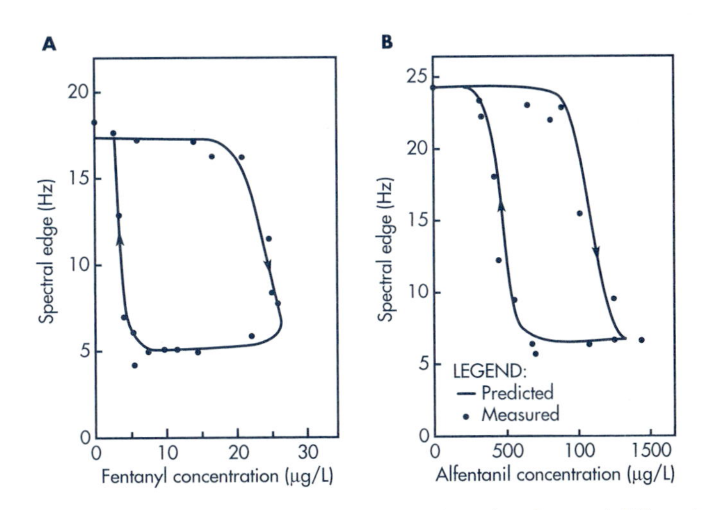

Figure 19-23. Response of the EEG spectral edge to changing fentanyl **(A)** and alfentanil **(B)** serum concentrations. Plots are data from single patients after rapid drug infusion. Time is indicated by arrows. The clockwise hysteresis indicates a significant time lag between blood and effect site.
(From Scott and Stanski, 1985, with permission.)

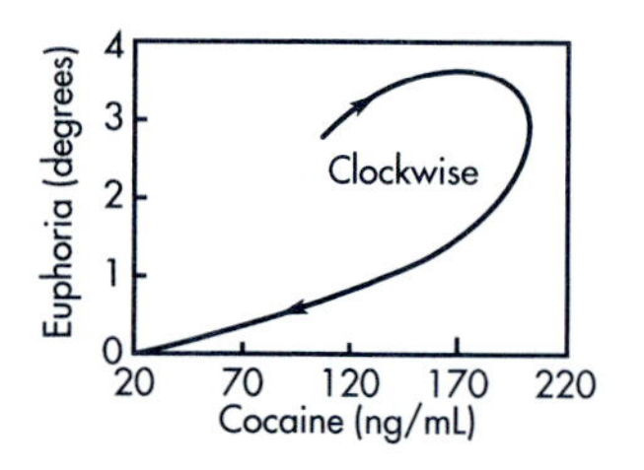

Figure 19-24. Clockwise hysteresis loop typical of tolerance is seen after intranasal administration of cocaine when related to degree of euphoria experienced in volunteers.
(From van Dyke et al, 1978.)

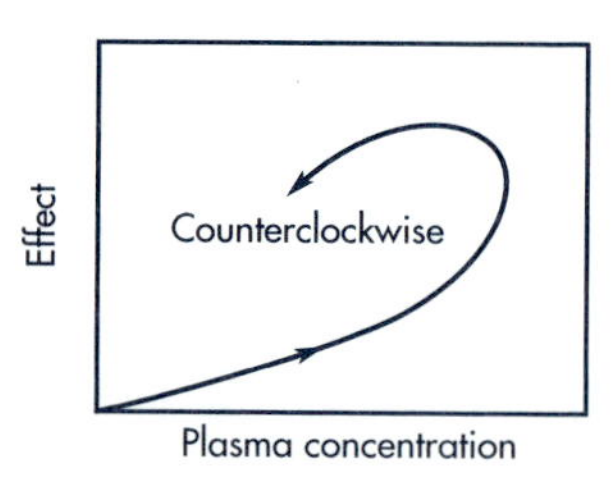

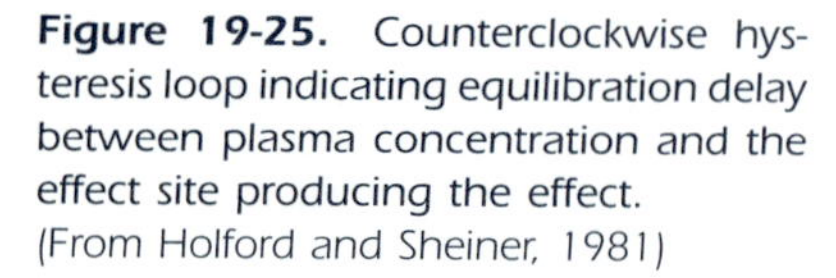

Figure 19-25. Counterclockwise hysteresis loop indicating equilibration delay between plasma concentration and the effect site producing the effect.
(From Holford and Sheiner, 1981)

A second type of pharmacologic response shows a *counterclockwise* hysteresis profile (Fig. 19-25). The pharmacologic response is increased with time as the pharmacologic response is plotted versus plasma drug concentrations. An example of a counterclockwise hysteresis loop is the antiarrhythmic drug ajmaline. When the QRS interval changes in dogs were plotted versus plasma ajmaline concentration in each dog, an interesting counterclockwise hysteresis loop was seen (Fig. 19-21) (Yasuhara et al, 1987). Yasuhara and coworkers (1987) developed a pharmacodynamic model to analyze the molecular events between drug concentration and change in ECG parameters such as QRS. A relationship was established between pharmacologic response and drug concentration in the effect compartment drug level (Fig. 19-22). The hysteresis profile (Fig. 19-21) is the result of the drug being highly bound to the plasma protein (α_1 − acid glycoprotein), and of a slow initial diffusion of drug into the effect compartment.

To predict the time course of drug response using a pharmacodynamic model, a mathematical expression is developed to describe the drug concentration time profile of the drug at the receptor site. This equation is then used to relate drug concentrations to the time course and intensity of the pharmacologic response. Most pharmacodynamic models assume that pharmacologic action is due to a drug–receptor interaction, and the magnitude of the response is quantitatively related to the drug concentration in the receptor compartment. In the simplest case, the drug receptor lies in the plasma compartment and pharmacologic response is established through a one-compartment model with drug response proportional to log drug concentration (Eq. 19.1). A more complicated model involving a receptor compartment that lies outside the central compartment was proposed by Sheiner and associates (1979). This latter model locates the receptor in an effect compartment in which a drug equilibrates from the central compartment by a first-order rate constant k_{1e}. There is no back diffusion of drug away from the effect compartment, thereby simplifying the complexity of the equations. This model was successfully applied to monitor the pharmacologic effects of the drug trimazosin (Meredith et al, 1983).

The pharmacokinetics of trimazosin are described as a two-compartment open model with conversion to a metabolite by a first-order rate constant k_{1m}. The pharmacokinetics of the metabolite are described by a one-compartment model with a first-order elimination constant k_{mo}. The drug effect may be described by two pharmacodynamic models, either model *A* or *B*. Model *A* assumes that the drug effect

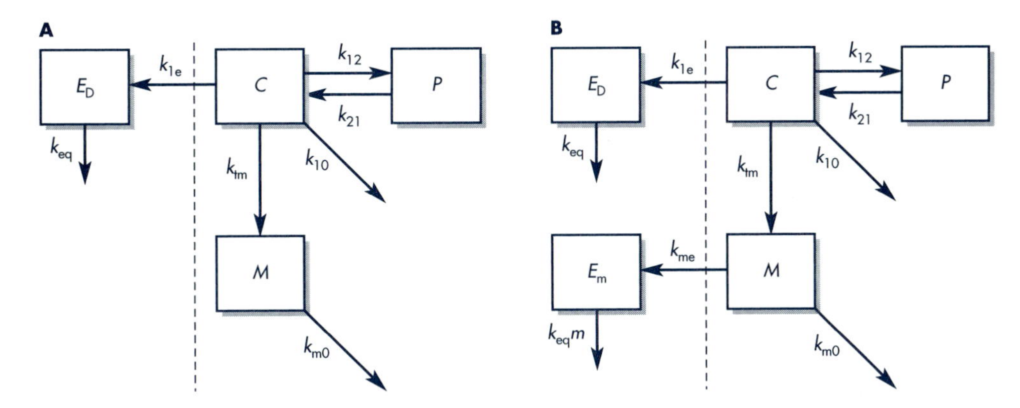

Figure 19-26. Two proposed pharmacodynamic models for describing the hypotensive effect of trimazosin. *A* assumes an effect compartment (left of dotted line) for the drug. *B* assumes an effect compartment for the drug as well as the metabolite.
(From Meredith et al, 1983, with permission.)

in the effect compartment is produced by the drug only. Model *B* assumes that both the drug and a metabolite produce drug effect (Fig. 19-26).

The following equation describes the pharmacokinetics and pharmacodynamics of the drug:

$$C_p = Ae^{-at} + Be^{-bt} \tag{19.25}$$

where C_p is concentration of the drug in the central compartment.

$$C_m = \frac{V_1 k_{1m}}{V_m}\left[\frac{A}{(k_{mo} - a)}(e^{at} - e^{-k_{mo}t}) + \frac{B}{(k_{mo} - b)}(e^{-bt} - e^{-k_{mo}t})\right] \tag{19.26}$$

where C_m is concentration of the metabolite in the body, V_m is volume of distribution of the metabolite, V_1 is the volume of central compartment of the body, k_{1m} is the first-order constant for converting drug to metabolite, k_{mo} is the elimination rate constant of the metabolite, A and B are two-compartment model coefficients for the drug (see Chapter 4), and k_{10} is elimination rate constant of the drug.

The drug concentration in the effect compartment is calculated by assuming that at equilibrium the concentration of the drug in the effect compartment and the central compartment are equal,

$$k_{1e} V_1 = k_{eq} V_e \tag{19.27}$$

where V_e is volume of the effect compartment. Therefore, the drug concentration in effect compartment $C(e,d)$ is calculated as

$$C(e, d) = \frac{Ak_{eq}}{(k_{eq} - a)}(e^{-at} - e^{-k_{eq}t}) + \frac{Bk_{eq}}{(k_{eq} - b)}(e^{-bt} - e^{-k_{eq}t}) \tag{19.28}$$

The effect due to drug is assumed to be linear.

$$E = M_d C(e, d) + i \tag{19.29}$$

where M_d is the sensitivity slope to the drug (ie, effect per unit of drug concentration in the effect compartment). The parameters M_d, i, and k_{eq} are determined by least-squares fitting of the data. For the metabolite, the concentration of metabolite in the effect compartment is $C(e, m)$.

$$\begin{aligned} C(e,m) = {} & \frac{AV_1 k_{1m} k_{eq} m}{V_m} \\ & \times \left[\frac{e^{-at}}{(a - k_{mo})(a - k_{eq} m)} + \frac{e^{-k_{mo} t}}{(a - k_{mo})(k_{eq} m - k_{mo})} \right. \\ & - \frac{e^{-k_{eq} mt}}{(a - k_{eq} m)(k_{eq} m - k_{mo})} \\ & + \frac{BV_1 k_{im} k_{eq} m}{V_m} \frac{e^{-bt}}{(b - k_{mo})(b - k_{eq} m)} \\ & \left. + \frac{e^{-k_{mo} t}}{(b - k_{mo})(k_{eq} m - k_{mo})} - \frac{e^{-k_{eq} mt}}{(b - k_{eq} m)(k_{eq} m - k_{mo})} \right] \end{aligned} \tag{19.30}$$

The concentration of the metabolite in the effect compartment is in turn related to drug effect as for the parent drug. The total effect produced is

$$E_t = M_d C(e,d) + M_m C(e,m) + \mathrm{I} \tag{19.31}$$

From Equation 19.20, the five parameters M_d, M_m, i, k_{eq}, k_{eq}m may be estimated. Figure 19-27 shows the observed decline in systolic blood pressure compared with the theoretical decline in blood pressure predicted by the model. An excellent fit of the data was obtained by assuming that both drug and metabolite are active.

This example illustrates that, for a dose of a drug, the drug concentration in the effect compartment and others may be described by a mathematical model. These equations were further developed to describe the time course of a pharmacologic event. In this case, Meredith and associates (1983) demonstrated that both the drug

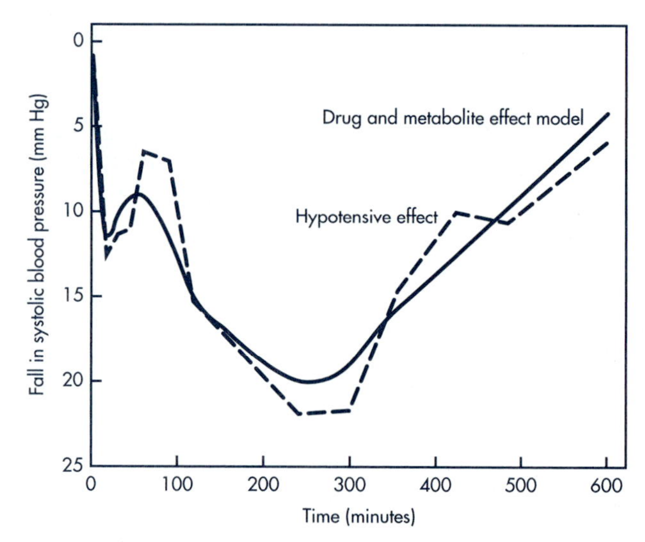

Figure 19-27. Diagram showing the agreement between recorded hypotensive effect (solid line) and hypotensive effect as projected by model B (broken line).
(From Meredith et al, 1983, with permission.)

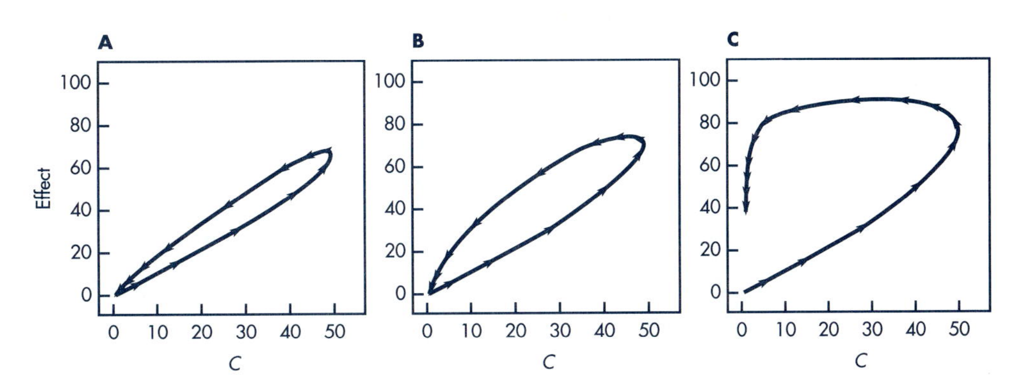

Figure 19-28. Simulated in *in vitro* pharmacodynamic response versus concentration (*C*) contributed by a drug and a metabolite. Potency of parent drug and metabolite are equal, but (*A*) k_{mo} = large (*B*) k_{mo} = medium (*C*) k_{mo} = small.
From Gupta et al, 1993, with permission.

and the metabolite formed in the body may affect the time course of the pharmacologic action of the drug in the body.

Simulation of *In Vitro* Pharmacodynamic Effect Involving Hysteresis

An *in vitro* model simulation of the sum of pharmacologic effect contributed by a drug and its active metabolite may explain the observation of the hysteresis response curve in vivo. Gupta et al (1993) have discussed the factors that impact the shape of the response curve. In the simplest case, pharmacokinetic equations are developed to calculate C_p, the drug concentration and C_m, the metabolite concentration. To estimate the pharmacologic effect due to both the drug and active metabolite, the potency for the drug is defined as P, the potency of the metabolite is P_m, and the sum of the pharmacologic effect is as shown below. (Gupta et al assume that the effect is linearly related to drug and metabolite concentrations in their first simulation.)

$$E = P\,C_p + P_m\,C_m \qquad \textbf{(19.32)}$$

The shape of hysteresis simulated is very dependent on P_m and k_{mo}, the rate constant of metabolite elimination. If k_{mo} is given a high, medium, or low value, the effect on the shape of the hysteresis loop is changed dramatically as is shown in Figure 19-28. A temporal effect causes a counterclockwise loop. In the case of a metabolite that acts as an antagonist, the hysteresis loop is clockwise. The more elaborate features of an E_{max} model were simulated by Gupta et al (1993) in their paper.

CLINICAL EXAMPLE

Lorazepam Pharmacodynamics—Example of an *In Vivo* Hysteresis Loop

Many drugs acting on the central nervous systems (CNS) involve a lag time before the tissues and the plasma are equilibrated with drug. The site at which the pharmacodynamic effect takes place is referred to as the effect compartment. The onset time of the drug is affected by the *equilibration time* of the drug. The pharmacokinetics of lorazepam after oral absorption was fitted to a two-compartment model

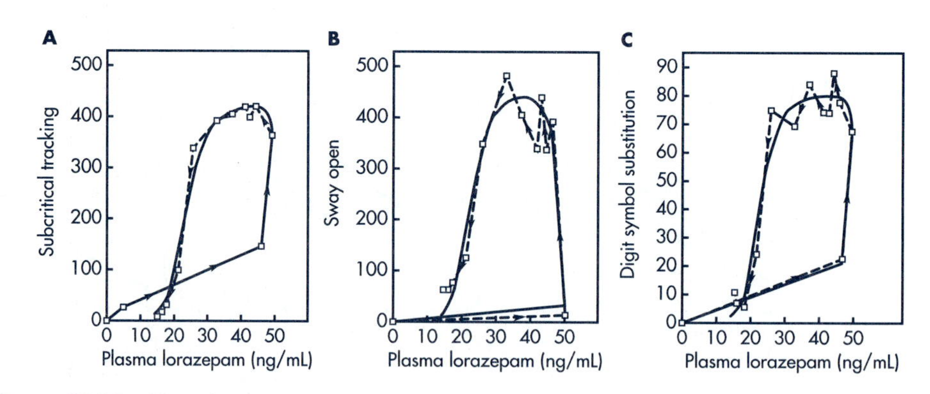

Figure 19-29. Plot of responses of lorazepam versus plasma drug concentration showing counterclockwise hysteresis.
From Gupta et al, 1990, with permission.

with lag time. Lorazepam was studied because the drug accounts for all the activity, such that the counterclockwise response profile may be attributed to equilibration rather than to metabolism (Gupta, et al, 1990).

The description of the plasma drug concentrations, C_p is obtained by conventional pharmacokinetic equations; whereas, the pharmacodynamic effect E is described by a sigmoid-E_{max} model similar to Equation 19.15, except that the baseline effect is also included. Gupta et al (1990) monitored three pharmacodynamic effects due to lorazepam. The monitored pharmacodynamic effects were mental impairment processes evaluated by the cognitive and psychomotor performance of the subjects, including (*A*) subcritical tracking, (*B*) sway open (a measurement of gross body movements), and (*C*) digital symbol substitution. When the time course of each effect is plotted versus plasma drug concentration, a counterclockwise loop is observed (Fig. 19-29). When the same pharmacodynamic responses are plotted versus lorazepam concentration in the effect compartment accounting for the equilibration lag, a classical sigmoid relation is observed (Fig. 19-30). The observations show that the temporal response of many drugs may be the result of pharmacodynamic and distributional factors interacting together. Thus, a model with an effect compartment can more fully help to understand the time course of the drug response.

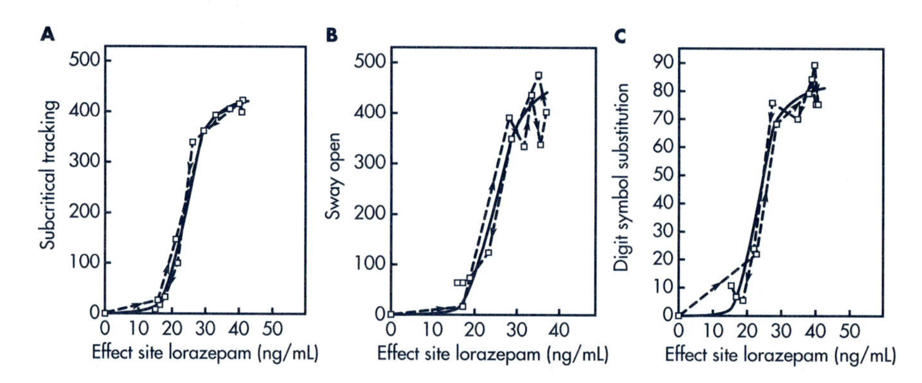

Figure 19-30. Plot of responses to lorazepam versus effect compartment concentration showing sigmoid relationship between effect and concentration without hysteresis.
From Gupta et al, 1990, with permission.

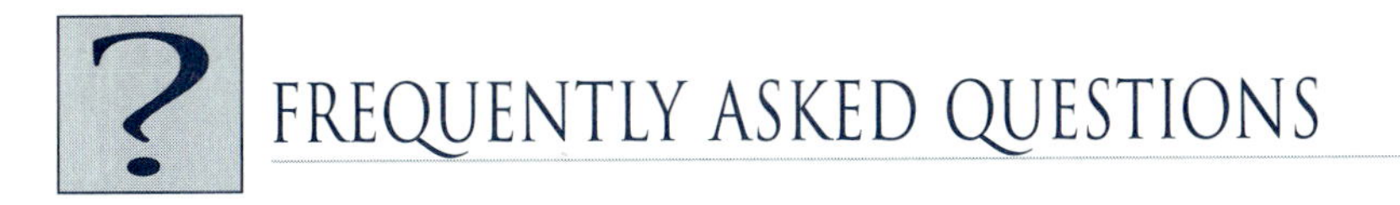

FREQUENTLY ASKED QUESTIONS

1. Explain why doubling the dose of a drug does not double the pharmacodynamic effects of the drug.
2. What is meant by a hysteresis loop? Who do some drugs follow a *clockwise* hysteresis loop and other drugs follow a *counterclockwise* hysteresis loop?
3. What is meant by an *effect compartment*? How does the effect compartment differ from pharmacokinetic compartments, such as the central compartment and the tissue compartment?

LEARNING QUESTIONS

1. On the basis of the graph in Figure 19-31, answer "true" or "false" to statements (a) to (e) and state the reason for each answer.
   a. The plasma drug concentration is more related to the pharmacodynamic effect of the drug compared to the dose of the drug.
   b. The pharmacologic response is directly proportional to the log plasma drug concentration.
   c. The volume of distribution is not changed by uremia.
   d. The drug is exclusively eliminated by hepatic biotransformation.
   e. The receptor sensitivity is unchanged in the uremic patient.
2. What do clavulanate, sublactam, and tazobactam have in common? Why are they used together with antibiotics?
3. Explain why subsequent equal doses of a drug do not produce the same pharmacodynamic effect as the first dose of drug.
   a. Provide an explanation based on *pharmacokinetic* considerations.
   b. Provide an explanation based on *pharmacodynamic* considerations.
4. How are the parameters, AUC and t_{eff} used in pharmacodynamic models?
5. What class of drug tends to have a lag time between the plasma and the effect compartment?

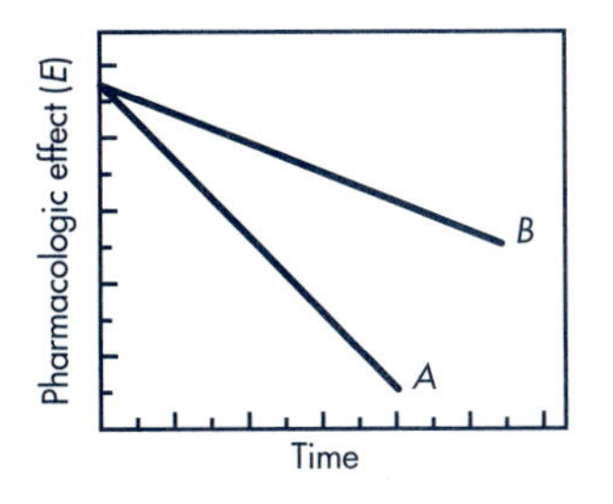

Figure 19-31. Graph of pharmacologic response *E* as a function of time for the same drug in patients with normal (*A*) and uremic (*B*) kidney function, respectively.

6. Name an example of a pharmacodynamic response that does not follow a drug dose response profile?
7. When an antibiotic concentration falls below the MIC, there is a short time period in which bacteria fail to regrow because of postantibiotic effect (PAE). This time period is referred to as PAT. What is PAT?
8. What is AUIC with regard to an antibiotic?

REFERENCES

Aghajanian OK, Bing OHL: Persistence of lysergic acid diethylamide in the plasma of human subjects. *Clin Pharmacol Ther* **5:**611–614, 1964

Baxter JD, Funder JW: Hormone receptors. *N Engl J Med* **301:**1149–1161, 1979

Boudinot FD, D'Ambrosio R, Jusko WJ: Receptor-mediated pharmacodynamics of prednisolone in the rat. *J Pharmacokinet Biopharm* **14:**469–493, 1986

Colburn WA: Perspectives in pharmacokinetics: Pharmacokinetic/pharmacodynamic modeling: What is it! *J Pharmacokinet Biopharm* **15:**545–553, 1987

Cone EJ: Pharmacokinetics and pharmacodynamics of cocaine. *J Anal Toxicol* **19:**459–478, 1995

Cox, BM: Drug tolerance and physical dependence. In WB Pratt, P Taylor (ed), *Principles of Drug Action. The Basis of Pharmacology.* New York, Churchill Livingstone, 1990, chap 10

Craig, WA: Interrelationship between pharmacokinetics and pharmacodynamics in determining dosage regimens for broad-spectrum cephalosporins. *Diag Microbiol Infect Dis* **22:**89–96, 1995

Craig WA, Andes D: Pharmacokinetics and pharmacodynamics of antibiotics in otitis media. *J Pediatr Infect Dis* **15:**255–259, 1996

deWit H, Dudish S, Ambre J: Subjective behavioral effects of diazepam depend upon its rate of onset. *Psychopharmacol* **112:**324–330, 1993

Drusano GL: Minireview: Role of pharmacokinetics in the outcome of infections. *Antimicrob Agents Chemother* March: 289–297, 1988

Drusano GL: Human pharmacodynamics of beta-lactams, aminoglycosides and their combination. *Scand J Infec Dis* **74**(suppl):235–248, 1991

Drusano GL, Craig WA: Relevance of pharmacokinetics and pharmacodynamics in the selection of antibiotics for respiratory tract infections. *J Chemother* **9**(suppl 3):38–44, 1997

Forrest A, Nix DE, Ballow CH, Goss TF, Birmingham MC, Schentag JJ: Pharmacodynamics of intravenous ciprofloxacin in seriously ill patients. *Antimicrob Agents Chemother* **37**(5):1073–1081, 1993

Gupta SK, Ellinwood EH, Nikaido AM, Heatherly DG: Simultaneous modeling of the pharmacokinetic and pharmacodynamic properties of benzodiazepines I: Lorazepam. *J Pharmacokin Biopharm* **18:**89–102, 1990

Gupta SK, Hwang SS, Benet LZ, Gumbleton M: Interpretation and utilization of effect and concentration data collected in an in vivo pharmacokinetic and in vitro pharmacodynamic study. *Pharm Res* **10:**889–894, 1993

Henningfield JE, Keenan RM: Nicotine delivery kinetics and abuse liability. *J Consulting Clin Pharmacol* **61:**743–750, 1993

Hill AV: The possible effects of the aggregation of the molecules of haemoglobin on its dissociation curves. *J Physiol* **40:**4–7, 1910

Holford NHG, Sheiner LB: Kinetics of pharmacologic response. *Pharm Ther* **16:**143–166, 1982

Holford NHG, Sheiner LB: Understanding the dose–effect relationship. Clinical application of pharmacokinetic–pharmacodynamic models. *Clin Pharmacokinet* **6:**429–453, 1981

Johanson C-E, Fischman MW: The pharmacology of cocaine related to its abuse. *Pharmacol Rev* **41:**3–52, 1989

Johansen SH, Jorgensen M, Molbech S: Effect of tubocurarine on respiratory and nonrespiratory muscle power in man. *J Appl Physiol* **19:**990–991, 1964

Lalonde RL: Pharmacodynamics. In Evans WE et al. (eds), *Applied Pharmacokinetics,* 3rd ed. Vancouver, WA, Applied Therapeutics Inc, 1992, chap 4

Lin RY: A perspective on penicillin allergy. *Arch Intern Med* **152:**930–937, 1992

Meredith PA, Kelman AW, Eliott HL, Reid JL: Pharmacokinetic and pharmacodynamic modeling of trimazosin and its major metabolite. *J Pharmacokinet Biopharm* **11:**323–334, 1983

Mitenko PA, Ogilvie RI: Rational intravenous doses of theophylline. *N Engl J Med* **289:**600–603, 1973

Reisman AS, Reisman RE: Risk of administering cephalosporin antibiotics to patients with histories of penicillin allergy. *Ann Aller Asthma Immunol* **74:**167–170, 1995

Rodman JH, Evans WE: Targeted systemic exposure for pediatric cancer therapy. In D'Argenio (ed), *Advanced Methods of Pharmacokinetic and Pharmacodynamic Systems Analysis.* New York, Plenum Press, 1991, p 177–183

Scaglione F: Predicting the clinical efficacy of antibiotics: Toward definitive criteria. *Pediatr Infect Dis J* **3:**S56–S59, 1997

Scott JC, Stanski DR: Decreased fentanyl/alfentanil dose requirement with increasing age: A pharmacodynamic basis. *Anesthesiology* **63:**A374, 1985

Sheiner LB, Stanski DR, Vozeh S, et al: Simultaneous modeling of pharmacokinetics and pharmacodynamics: Application to *d*-tubocurarine. *Clin Pharmacol Ther* **25:**358–370, 1979

Suresh A, Reisman RE: Risk of administering cephalosporin antibiotics to patients with histories of penicillin allergy. *Ann Allergy Asthma Immunol* **74:**167–170, 1995

Van Dyke C, Jatlow P, Ungerer J, et al: Oral cocaine: Plasma concentration and central effects. *Science* **200:**211–213, 1978

Wagner JG: Kinetics of pharmacologic response: 1. Proposed relationship between response and drug concentration in the intact animal and man. *J Theor Biol* **20:**173–201, 1968

Winkle RA, Meffin PJ, Fitzgerald JW, Harrison DC: Clinical efficacy and pharmacokinetics of a new orally effective antiarrhythmic tocainide. *Circulation* **54:**884–889, 1976

Yasuhara M, Hashimoto Y, Okumura K, et al: Kinetics of ajmaline disposition and pharmacologic response in beagle dogs. *J Pharmacokinet Biopharm* **15:**39–56, 1987

BIBLIOGRAPHY

Galeazzi RL, Benet LZ, Sheiner LB: Relationship between the pharmacokinetics and pharmacodynamics of procainamide. *Clin Pharmacol Ther* **20:**278–289, 1976

Gibaldi M, Levy G, Weintraub H: Drug distribution and pharmacologic effects. *Clin Pharmacol Ther* **12:**734, 1971

Harron DWG: Digoxin pharmacokinetic modeling—10 years later. *Int J Pharm* **53:**181–188, 1989

Holford NHG: Clinical pharmacokinetics and pharmacodynamics of warfarin. Understanding the dose–effect relationship. *Clin Pharmacokinet* **11:**583–604, 1986

Jusko WJ: Pharmacodynamics of chemotherapeutic effects: Dose–time–response relationship for phase-nonspecific agents. *J Pharm Sci* **60:**892, 1971

Levy G: Kinetics of pharmacologic effects. *Clin Pharmacol Ther* **1:**362, 1966

Meffin PJ, Winkle RA, Blaschke RF, et al: Response optimization of drug dosage: Antiarrhythmic studies with tocainide. *Clin Pharmacol Ther* **22:**42–57, 1977

Packer M, Carver JR, Rodeheffer RJ, et al: Effect of oral milrinone on mortality in severe chronic heart failure. *N Engl J Med* **21:**1468, 1991

Schwinghammer TL, Kroboth PD: Basic concepts in pharmacodynamic modeling. *J Clin Pharmacol* **28:**388–394, 1988

Seeman P, Lee T, Chau-Wong M, Wong K: Antipsychotic drug doses and neuroleptic/dopamine receptors. *Nature* **261:**717–719, 1976

Sheiner LB: Commentary to pharmacokinetic/pharmacodynamic modeling: What it is! *J Pharmacokinet Biopharm* **15:**553–555, 1987

Swerdlow BN, Holley FO: Intravenous anaesthetic agents. Pharmacokinetic/pharmacodynamic relationships. *Clin Pharmacokinet* **12:**79–110, 1987

Taylor P, Insel PA: Molecular basis of pharmacologic selectivity. In Pratt WB, Taylor P (eds), *Principles of Drug Action. The Basis of Pharmacology*, 3rd ed. New York, Churchill Livingstone, 1990

Verrijk R, Vleeming W, Hans H, et al: Plasma elimination of milrinone in rats in relation to its hemodynamic effects. *J Pharm Sci* **79:**P236–P239, 1990

Whiting B, Holford NHG, Sheiner LB: Quantitative analysis of the disopyramide concentration–effect relationship. *Br J Clin Pharmacol* **9:**67–75, 1980

20

PHYSIOLOGIC PHARMACOKINETIC MODELS, MEAN RESIDENCE TIME, AND STATISTICAL MOMENT THEORY

The study of pharmacokinetics quantitatively describes the absorption, distribution, and elimination of the active drug and metabolites (Chapter 2). Ideally, a pharmacokinetic model uses the observed time course for drug concentration in the body and obtains various pharmacokinetic parameters predictive of the pharmacodynamics and toxicity of the drug.

In developing a model, the pharmacokineticist makes certain underlying assumptions as to the type of pharmacokinetic model, the order of the rate process, the blood flow to a tissue, the method for the estimation of volume, and other factors. Even with the model-independent approach, first-order drug elimination is assumed in the calculation of AUC_0^∞. In addition, the pharmacokineticist may use more than one method of modeling depending upon the available data, the goodness-of-fit to the model, and the desired pharmacokinetic parameters. Each estimated pharmacokinetic parameter has an inherent variability due to the variability of the biologic system and of the observed data. Moreover, because pharmacokinetic studies are performed on a limited number of subjects, the estimated pharmacokinetic parameters may not be representative of the entire population.

In spite of difficulties in the construction of these pharmacokinetic models, such models have been extremely useful in describing the time course of drug action, improving drug therapy and efficacy, minimizing toxicity and adverse reactions, and developing new drug delivery systems.

The human body is composed of organ systems containing living cells bathed

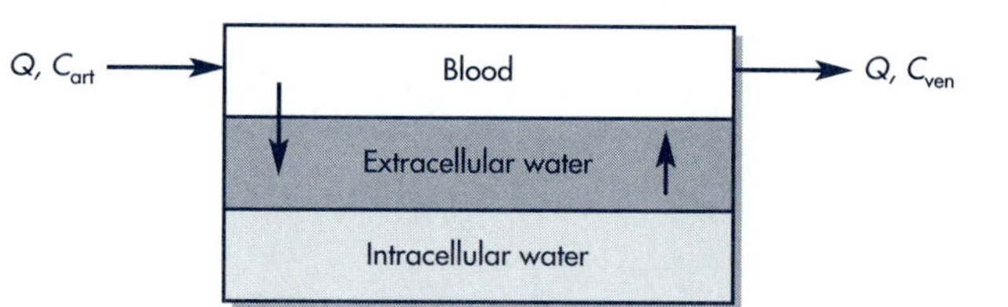

Figure 20-1. The physiologic pharmacokinetic model divides a body organ into three parts in describing drug transfer: capillary vessels, extracellular space, and intracellular space.

in an extracellular aqueous fluid (Chapter 11). Both drugs and endogenous substances, such as hormones, nutrients, and oxygen, are transported to the organs by the same network of blood vessels (arteries). The drug concentration within a target organ depends upon the rate of blood flow to an organ and the rate of uptake of drug. Physiologically, uptake (accumulation) of drug by organ tissues occurs in the extracellular fluid, which equilibrates rapidly with the capillary blood in the organ. Some drugs cross the cell membrane into the interior fluid (intracellular water) of the cell (Fig. 20-1).

In addition to drug accumulation, some organs of the body are involved in drug elimination either by excretion (eg, kidney) or by metabolism (eg, liver). The elimination of drug by an organ may be described by drug clearance in the organ (Chapters 12 and 13). The liver is an example of an organ with drug metabolism and drug uptake (accumulation). Physiologic pharmacokinetic models consider all processes of drug uptake and elimination.

PHYSIOLOGIC PHARMACOKINETIC MODELS

Physiologic pharmacokinetic models are mathematical models describing drug movement and disposition in the body based on blood flow and the organ spaces penetrated by the drug. In its simplest form, a physiologic pharmacokinetic model considers the drug to be blood-flow limited. Drugs are carried from the administration (input) site by blood flow to various body organs, where the drug rapidly equilibrates with the interstitial water in the organ. In such a model, transmembrane movement of drug is rapid, and the cell membrane does not offer any resistance to drug permeation. Drugs are carried to organs by arterial blood and leave organs by venous blood (Fig. 20-2). Uptake of drug into the tissues is rapid, and a constant ratio of drug concentrations between the organ and the venous blood is quickly established. This ratio is the *tissue/blood partition coefficient* (shown below).

$$P_{\text{tissue}} = C_{\text{tissue}}/C_{\text{blood}} \qquad \textbf{(20.1)}$$

where P is the partition coefficient.

The magnitude of the partition coefficient can vary depending upon the drug and on the type of tissue. Adipose tissue, for example, has a high partition for lipophilic drugs. The rate of drug carried to a tissue organ and tissue drug uptake are dependent on the rate of blood flow to the organ and on the tissue/blood partition coefficient, respectively.

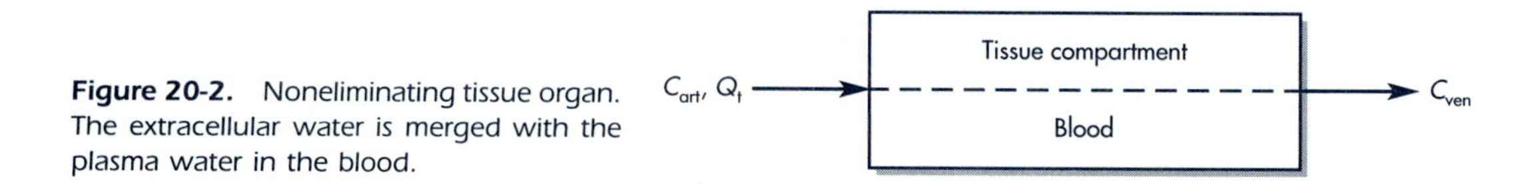

Figure 20-2. Noneliminating tissue organ. The extracellular water is merged with the plasma water in the blood.

The rate of blood flow to the tissue is expressed as Q_t (mL/min), and the rate of change in the drug concentration with respect to time within a given tissue organ is expressed as:

$$d(V_{tissue}C_{tissue})/dt = Q_t(C_{in} - C_{out}) \quad \textbf{(20.2)}$$
$$d(V_{tissue}C_{tissue})/dt = Q_t(C_{art} - C_{ven}) \quad \textbf{(20.3)}$$

where C_{art} is the arterial blood drug concentration and C_{ven} is the venous blood drug concentration.

Q_t represents the volume of blood flowing through a typical tissue organ per unit of time. If drug uptake occurs in the tissue, the incoming concentration C_{art} would be higher than the venous concentration C_{ven}. The rate of drug concentration change in the tissue is equal to the rate of blood flow multiplied by the difference between the blood concentration entering and leaving the tissue organ. In the *blood-flow-limited model*, drug concentration in the blood leaving the tissue and the drug concentration within the tissue are in equilibrium, and C_{ven} may be estimated from the tissue/blood partition coefficient in Equation 20.1. Substituting for Equation 20.3 with $C_{ven} = C_{tissue}/P_{tissue}$ yields

$$d(V_{tissue}C_{tissue})/dt = Q_t(C_{art} - C_{tissue}/P_{tissue}) \quad \textbf{(20.4)}$$

Equation 20.4 describes drug distribution in a noneliminating organ or tissue group. For example, drug distribution to muscle, adipose tissue, and skin is represented in a similar manner by Equations 20.5, 20.6, and 20.7, respectively. For tissue organs in which drug is eliminated (Fig. 20-3), parameters representing drug elimination from the liver (k_{LIV}) and kidney (k_{KID}) are added to account for drug removal through metabolism or excretion. Equations 20.8 and 20.9 are derived similarly to those for the noneliminating organs above.

Removal of drug from any organ is described by drug clearance (Cl) from the organ. The rate of drug elimination is the product of the drug concentration in the organ and the organ clearance.

$$\text{Rate of drug elimination} = V_{tiss}dC_{tiss} - dt = C_{tiss} \times Cl_{tiss}$$

The rate of drug elimination may be described for each organ or tissue (Fig. 20-4).

Muscle: $d(V_{MUS}C_{MUS})/dt = Q_{MUS}(C_{MUS} - C_{MUS}/P_{MUS})$ **(20.5)**

Adipose tissue: $d(V_{FAT}C_{FAT})/dt = Q_{FAT}(C_{FAT} - C_{FAT}/P_{FAT})$ **(20.6)**

Skin: $d(V_{SKIN}C_{SKIN})/dt = Q_{SKIN}(C_{SKIN} - C_{SKIN}/P_{SKIN})$ **(20.7)**

Liver: $d(V_{LIV}C_{LIV})/dt = C_{LIV}(Q_{LIV} - Q_{GI} - Q_{SP}) + Q_{GI}(C_{GI}/P_{GI}) + Q_{SP}(C_{SP}/P_{SP}) - Q_{LIV}C_{LIV}/P_{LIV} - C_{LIV}Cl_{int}/P_{LIV}$ **(20.8)**

Kidney: $d(V_{KID}C_{KID}/dt = Q_{KID}(C_{KID} - C_{KID}/P_{KID}) - C_{KID}Cl_{KID}/P_{KID}$ **(20.9)**

Lung: $d(V_{LU}C_{LU})/dt = Q_{LU}(C_{LU}/P_{LU})$ **(20.10)**

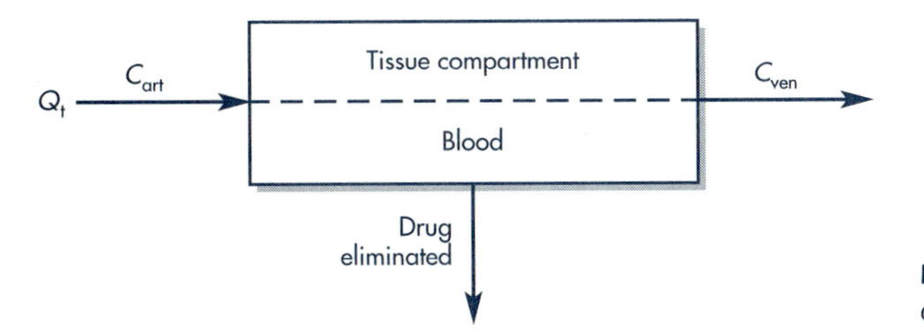

Figure 20-3. A typical eliminating tissue organ.

where LIV = liver, SP = spleen, GI = GI tract, KID = kidney, LU = lung, FAT = adipose, SKIN = skin, and MUS = muscle.

The mass balance for the rate of change in drug concentration in the blood pool is as follows:

$$d(V_b C_b)/dt = \underbrace{Q_{MUS}C_{MUS}/P_{MUS}}_{\{muscle\}} + \underbrace{Q_{LIV}C_{LIV}/P_{LIV}}_{\{liver\}} + \underbrace{Q_{KID}C_{KID}/P_{KID}}_{\{kidney\}} \quad \textbf{(20.11)}$$

$$+ \underbrace{Q_{SKIN}C_{SKIN}/P_{SKIN}}_{\{skin\}} + \underbrace{Q_{FAT}C_{FAT}/P_{FAT}}_{\{adipose\}} + \underbrace{Q_{LU}C_{LU}/P_{LU}}_{\{lung\}} - \underbrace{Q_b C_b}_{\{blood\}}$$

Lung perfusion is unique because the pulmonary artery returns venous blood flow to the lung where carbon dioxide is exchanged for oxygen and the blood becomes oxygenated. The blood from the lungs flows back to the heart (into the left atrium) through the pulmonary vein, and the quantity of blood that perfuses the pulmonary system ultimately passes through the remainder of the body. In describing drug clearance through the lung, perfusion from the heart (right ventricle) to the lung is considered as venous blood (Fig. 20-4). Therefore, the terms in Equation 20.11 describing lung perfusion are reversed compared to those for the perfusion of other tissues. After intravenous drug administration, drug uptake in the lungs may be very significant if the drug has high affinity for lung tissue. If actual drug clear-

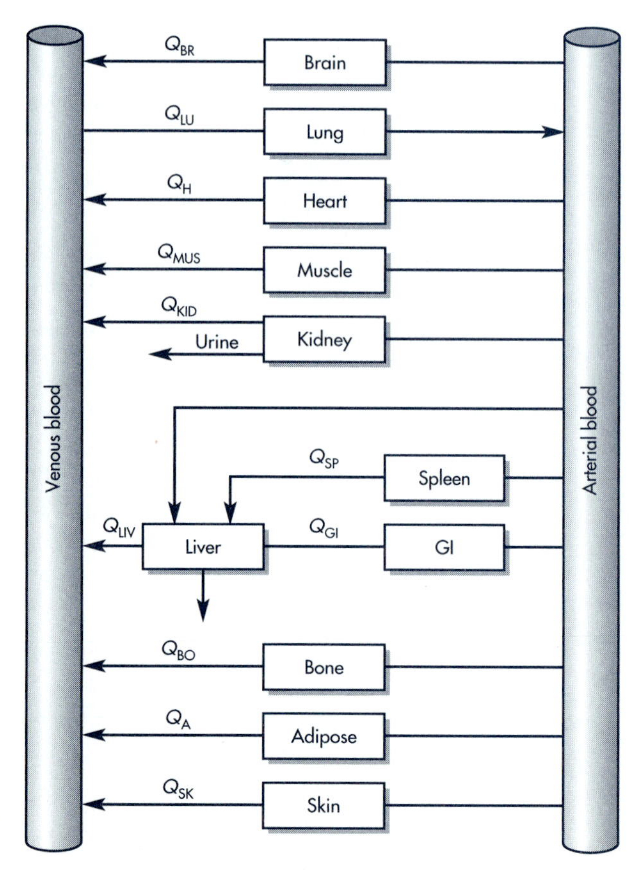

Figure 20-4. Example of blood flow to organs in a physiologic pharmacokinetic model.

ance is at a much higher rate than the drug clearance accounted for by renal and hepatic clearance, then lung clearance of the drug should be suspected, and a lung clearance term should be included in the equation in addition to lung tissue distribution.

The system of differential equations used to describe the blood-flow-limited model is usually solved through computer programs. The *Runge–Kutta* method is often used in computer methods for series of differential equations. Because of the large number of parameters involved in the mass balance, more than one set of parameters may fit the experimental data. This is especially true with human data, in which many of the organ tissue data items are not available. The lack of sufficient tissue data sometimes leads to unconstrained models. As additional data become available, new or refined models are adopted. For example, methotrexate was initially described by a flow-limited model, and later work refined this to a diffusion-limited model.

Using experimental pharmacokinetic data in animals, physiologic pharmacokinetic models may yield more reliable information, because invasive methods are available in animals such that tissue/blood ratios or partition coefficients can be accurately determined by direct measurement.

Physiologic Pharmacokinetic Model with Binding

The physiologic pharmacokinetic model assumes flow-limited drug distribution without drug binding to either plasma or tissues. In reality, many drugs are bound to a variable extent in either plasma or tissues. With most physiologic models, drug binding is assumed to be linear (not saturable or concentration dependent). Moreover, bound and free drug in both tissue and plasma are in equilibrium. Further, the free drug in the plasma and in the tissue equilibrates rapidly. Therefore, the free drug concentration in the tissue and the free drug concentration in the emerging blood are equal.

$$[C_b]_f = [C_t]_f \tag{20.12}$$
$$[C_b]_f = f_b[C_b] \tag{20.13}$$
$$[C_t]_f = f_t[C_t] \tag{20.14}$$

where f_b is the blood free drug fraction, f_t is the tissue free drug fraction, C_t is the total drug concentration in tissue, and C_b is the total drug concentration in blood.

Therefore, the partition ratio P_t of the tissue drug concentration to that of the plasma drug concentration is

$$f_b/f_t = [C_t]/[C_b] = P_t \tag{20.15}$$

By assuming linear drug binding and rapid drug equilibration, the free drug fraction in tissue and blood may be incorporated into the partition ratio and the differential equations. These equations are similar to those above except that free drug concentrations are substituted for C_b. Drug clearance in the liver was assumed to occur only with the free drug. The inherent capacity for drug metabolism (and elimination) is described by the term Cl_{int} (Chapter 13). General mass balance of various tissues is described by Equation 20.16:

$$\begin{aligned} d(V_{tissue}C_{tissue})/dt &= Q_t(C_{art} - C_{ven}) \\ &= Q_t(C_{art} - C_t/P_t) \\ \text{or } &= Q_t(C_{art} - C_t f_t/f_b) \end{aligned} \tag{20.16}$$

For liver metabolism,

$$d(V_{LIV}C_{LIV})/dt = C_b(Q_{LIV} - Q_{GI} - Q_{SP}) - \underset{\{\text{hepatic drug elimination}\}}{Q_{LIV}C_{LIV}/P_{LIV}} + Q_{GI}(C_{GI}/P_{GI}) + Q_{SP}(C_{SP}/P_{SP}) \tag{20.17}$$

The mass balance for the drug in blood pool is

$$d(V_bC_b)/dt = \underset{\{\text{muscle}\}}{Q_{MUS}C_{MUS}} + \underset{\{\text{liver}\}}{Q_{LIV}C_{LIV}/P_{LIV}} + \underset{\{\text{kidney}\}}{Q_{KID}C_{KID}/P_{KID}} + \underset{\{\text{skin}\}}{Q_{SKIN}C_{SKIN}/P_{SKIN}} + \underset{\{\text{adipose}\}}{Q_{FAT}C_{FAT}/P_{FAT}} + \underset{\{\text{lung}\}}{Q_{LU}C_{LU}/P_{LU}} - \underset{\{\text{blood}\}}{Q_bC_b} \tag{20.18}$$

The influence of binding on drug distribution is an important factor in interspecies difference in pharmacokinetics. In some instances, animal data may predict drug distribution in humans by taking into account the difference in drug binding. For the most part, extrapolations from animals to humans or between species are rough estimates only, and there are many instances where species differences are not entirely attributable to drug binding and metabolism.

Blood-Flow-Limited Versus Diffusion-Limited Model

Most physiologic pharmacokinetic models assume rapid drug distribution between tissue and venous blood. Rapid drug equilibrium assumes that drug diffusion is extremely fast and that the cell membrane offers no barrier to drug permeation. If no drug binding is involved, the tissue drug concentration is the same as that of the venous blood leaving the tissue. This assumption greatly simplifies the mathematics involved. Table 20.1 lists some of the drugs that have been described by a flow-limited model. This model is also referred to as *perfusion model.* A more complex type of physiologic pharmacokinetic model is called the *diffusion-limited model* or the *membrane-limited model.* In the diffusion-limited model, the cell membrane acts as a barrier for the drug, which gradually permeates by diffusion. Because blood flow is very rapid and drug permeation is slow, a drug concentration gradient is established between the tissue and the venous blood (Lutz and Dedrick, 1985). The rate-limiting step of drug diffusion into the tissue is dependent on the cell membrane rather than blood flow. Because of the time lag in equilibration between blood and tissue, the pharmacokinetic equation for the diffusion-limited model is very complicated.

TABLE 20.1 Drugs Described by Physiologic Pharmacokinetic Model

DRUG	CATEGORY	COMMENT	REFERENCE
Thiopental	Anesthetic	Blood, flow limited	Chen and Andrade (1976)
BSP	Diagnostic	Plasma, flow limited	Luecke and Thomason (1980)
Nicotine	Stimulant	Blood, flow limited	Gabrielsson and Bondesson (1987)
Lidocaine	Antiarrhythmic	Blood, flow limited	Benowitz et al (1974)
Methotrexate	Antineoplastic	Plasma, flow limited	Bischoff et al (1970)
Biperiden	Anticholinergic	Blood, flow limited	Nakashima and Benet (1988)
Cisplatin	Antineoplastic	Plasma, multiple metabolite, binding	King et al (1986)

Application and Limitations of Physiologic Pharmacokinetic Models

The physiologic pharmacokinetic model is related to drug concentration and tissue distribution using physiologic and anatomical information. For example, the effect of a change in blood flow on the drug concentration in a given tissue may be estimated once the model is characterized. Similarly, the effect of a change in mass size of different tissue organs on the redistribution of drug may also be evaluated using the system of physiologic model differential equations generated. When several species are involved, the physiologic model may predict the pharmacokinetics of a drug in humans when only animal data are available. Changes in drug–protein binding, tissue organ drug partition ratios, and intrinsic hepatic clearance may be inserted into the physiologic pharmacokinetic model.

Interspecies Scaling

Various approaches have been used to compare the toxicity and pharmacokinetics of a drug among different species. *Interspecies scaling* is a method used in *toxicokinetics* (the application of pharmacokinetics to toxicology) for interpolation and extrapolation based on anatomic, physiologic, and biochemical similarities (Mordenti and Chappell, 1989).

The basic assumption in interspecies scaling is that physiologic variables, such as clearance, heart rate, organ weight, and biochemical processes, are related to the weight or body surface area of the animal species (including humans). The physiologic variable y is graphed against body weight of the species on log–log axes to transform the data into a linear relationship (Fig. 20-5). The general allometric equation obtained by this method is the following:

$$y = bW^{a} \tag{20.19}$$

where y is the pharmacokinetic or physiologic property of interest, b is an allometric coefficient, W is the weight or surface area of the animal species, and a is the allometric exponent. *Allometry* is the study of size.

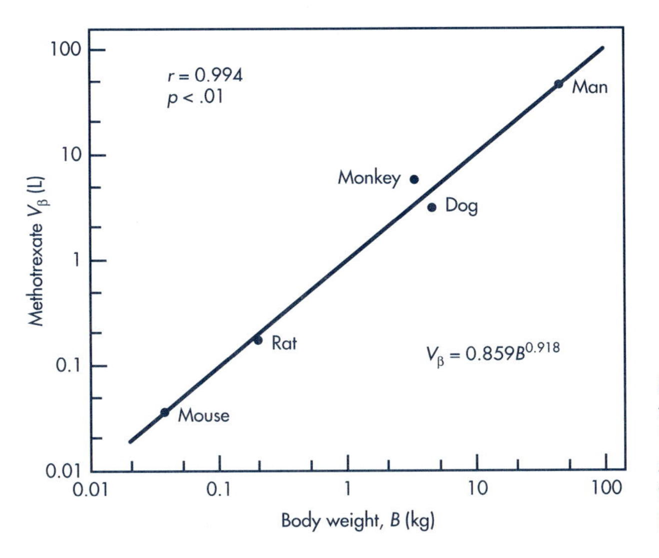

Figure 20-5. Interspecies correlation between methotrexate volume of distribution V_β and body weight. Linear regression analysis was performed on logarithmically transformed data.
(From Boxenbaum, 1982, with permission.)

TABLE 20.2 Examples of Allometric Relationship for Interspecies Parameters

PHYSIOLOGIC OR PHARMACOKINETIC PROPERTY	ALLOMETRIC EXPONENT *a*	ALLOMETRIC COEFFICIENT *b*
Basal O_2 consumption (mL/hr)	0.734	3.8
Endogenous N output (g/hr)	0.72	0.000042
O_2 consumption by liver slices (mL/hr)	0.77	3.3
Clearance		
Creatinine (mL/hr)	0.69	8.72
Inulin (mL/hr)	0.77	5.36
PAH (mL/hr)	0.80	22.6
Antipyrine (mL/hr)	0.89	8.16
Methotrexate (mL/hr)	0.69	10.9
Phenytoin (mL/hr)	0.92	47.1
Aztreonam (mL/hr)	0.66	4.45
Ara-C and Ara-U (mL/hr)	0.79	3.93
Volume of distribution (V_D)		
Methotrexate (L/kg)	0.92	0.859
Cyclophosphamide (L/kg)	0.99	0.883
Antipyrine (L/kg)	0.96	0.756
Aztreonam (L/kg)	0.91	0.234
Kidney weight (g)	0.85	0.0212
Liver weight (g)	0.87	0.082
Heart weight (g)	0.98	0.0066
Stomach and intestines weight (g)	0.94	0.112
Blood weight (g)	0.99	0.055
Tidal volume (mL)	1.01	0.0062
Elimination half-life:		
Methotrexate (min)	0.23	54.6
Cyclophosphamide (min)	0.24	36.6
Digoxin (min)	0.23	98.3
Hexobarbital (min)	0.35	80.0
Antipyrine (min)	0.07	74.5
Turnover times:		
Serum albumin (1/day)	0.30	5.68
Total body water (1/day)	0.16	6.01
RBC (1/day)	0.10	68.4
Cardiac circulation (min)	0.21	0.44

From Ritschel and Banerjee, 1986, with permission.

Both *a* and *b* vary with the drug. Examples of various pharmacokinetic or physiologic properties that demonstrate allometric relationships are listed in Table 20.2.

In the example shown in Figure 20-5, methotrexate volume of distribution is related to body weight *B* of 5 animal species by the equation $V_\beta = 0.859\text{B}^{0.918}$.

The allometric method gives an empirical relationship that allows for approximate interspecies scaling based on the size of the species. Not considered in the method are certain specific interspecies differences such as gender, nutrition, pathophysiology, route of drug administration, and polymorphism. Some of these more specific cases, such as the pathophysiologic condition of the animal or human, may preclude pharmacokinetic or allometric predictions.

Interspecies scaling has been refined by considering the aging rate and life span of the species. In terms of physiologic time, each species has a characteristic life span, its *maximum life span potential* (MLP), which is controlled genetically

(Boxenbaum, 1982). Because many energy-consuming biochemical processes, including drug metabolism, vary inversely with the aging rate or life span of the animal, the allometric approach has been used for drugs that are mainly eliminated by hepatic intrinsic clearance.

Through the study of various species in handling several drugs that are predominantly metabolized by the liver, some empirical relationships regarding drug clearance of several drugs have been related mathematically in a single equation. For example, drug hepatic intrinsic clearance of biperiden in rat, rabbit, and dog was extrapolated to humans (Nakashima et al, 1987). Equation 20.20 describes the relationship between biperiden intrinsic clearance with body weight and MLP:

$$Cl_{\text{int}} \times \text{MLP} = 1.36 \times 10^7 \times B^{0.892} \tag{20.20}$$

where MLP is the maximum life span potential of the species, B is the body weight of the species, and Cl_{int} is the hepatic intrinsic clearance of the free drug. Although further model improvements are needed before accurate prediction of pharmacokinetic parameters can be made from animal data, some interesting results were obtained by Sawada et al (1985) on 9 acid and 6 basic drugs. When interspecies difference in protein–drug binding is properly considered, the volume of distribution of many drugs may be predicted with 50% deviation from experimental values (Table 20.3).

The application of MLP to pharmacokinetics has been described by Boxenbaum (1982). Initially, hepatic intrinsic clearance was considered to be related to the volume or body weight. However, a plot of the log drug clearance versus body weight for various animal species resulted in an approximately linear correlation (ie, a straight line). After correcting intrinsic clearance by MLP, an improved log linear relationship was achieved between free drug Cl_{int} and body weight for many drugs. A possible explanation for this relationship is that the biochemical processes, including Cl_{int}, in each animal species are related to the animal's normal life expectancy (estimated by MLP) through the evolutionary process. Animals with a shorter MLP have higher basal metabolic rates and would tend to have higher intrinsic hepatic clearance and would thus metabolize drugs faster. Boxenbaum (1982, 1983) postulated a constant "life stuff" in each species, such that the faster the life stuff is consumed, the more quickly the life stuff is used up. In the fourth-dimension scale (after correcting for MLP), all species share the same intrinsic clearance for the free drug.

$$(\text{MLP})(Cl_{\text{int}})/B = \text{constant} \tag{20.21}$$

$$Cl_{\text{int}} = aB^{*} \tag{20.22}$$

Recently, extensive work with caffeine in 5 species (mouse, rat, rabbit, monkey, and humans) by Bonati and associates (1985) verified this approach. Caffeine is a drug predominantly metabolized by the liver.

For caffeine,

$$Q = 0.0554 \times B^{0.894}$$
$$L = 0.0370 \times B^{0.849}$$

where B is body weight, L is liver weight; and Q is blood flow.

Hepatic clearance for the unbound drug did not show a direct correlation among the 5 species (Fig. 20-6). After intrinsic clearance was corrected for MLP (calculation based on brain weight), an excellent relationship was obtained among the 5 species (Fig. 20-7).

TABLE 20.3 Relationship Between Predicted and Observed Values of Various Pharmacokinetic Parameters in Humans for 15 Drugs

	V (L/kg)			Cl_m (mL/min PER kg)			$t_{1/2,z}$ (min)		
DRUG	OBSERVED	PREDICTED	PERCENT[a]	OBSERVED	PREDICTED	PERCENT[a]	OBSERVED	PREDICTED	PERCENT[a]
Phenytoin	0.640	0.573	10.5	0.574	0.483	15.9	792	822	3.79
Quinidine	3.20	3.69	22.2	2.91	3.25	11.7	470	785	67.0
Hexobarbital	1.27	0.735	42.1	3.57	4.25	19.0	261	120	54.0
Pentobarbital	0.999	1.57	57.2	0.524	0.964	84.0	1340	1126	16.0
Phenylbutazone	0.122[b]	0.0839[c]	31.2	0.0205	0.0162	21.0	4110	3590	12.7
Warfarin	0.108	0.109	0.926	0.0367	0.0165	55.0	2040	4560	124
Tolbutamide	0.112	0.116	3.57	0.180	0.0589	67.3	434	1360	214
Chlorpromazine	11.2[b]	9.05[c]	19.2	4.29	4.63	7.93	1810	1350	25.2
Propranolol	3.62	3.77	4.14	11.2	15.56	38.9	167	135	19.2
Pentazocine	5.56	7.19	29.3	18.3	11.6	36.6	203	408	101
Valproate	0.151	0.482	219	0.110	0.159	44.5	954	2110	121
Diazepam	0.950	1.44	51.6	0.350	2.13	509	1970	469	76.2
Antipyrine	0.869	0.878	1.04	0.662	0.664	3.02	654	917	40.2
Phenobarbital	0.649	0.817	25.9	0.0530	0.0825	55.7	6600	5870	11.0
Amobarbital	1.04	1.21	16.3	0.556	1.01	81.7	1360	827	39.2

[a]Absolute percent of error.
[b]The value of V_{ss}.
[c]Predicted from the value of V_{ss} in the rat.

From Sawada et al, 1985, with permission.

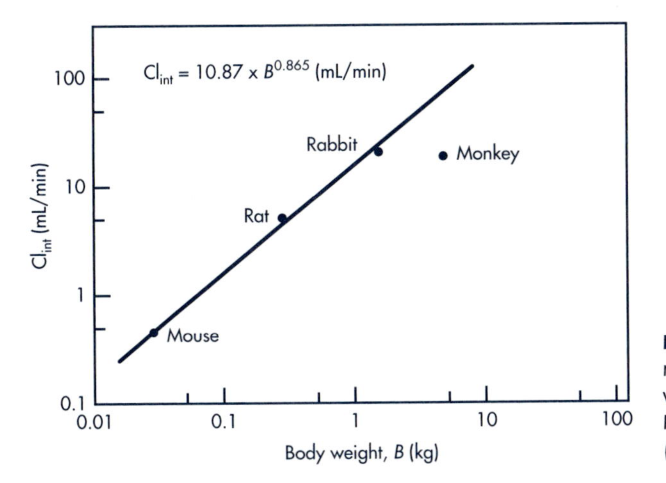

Figure 20-6. Caffeine Cl_{int} (free drug) in mammalian species as a function of body weight. Line does not utilize man and monkey points.
(From Bonati et al, 1985, with permission.)

Physiologic Versus Compartment Approach

Compartmental models represent a simplified kinetic approach to describe drug absorption, distribution, and elimination (Chapters 3 and 4). The major advantage of compartment models is that the time course of drug in the body may be monitored quantitatively with a limited amount of data. Generally, only plasma drug concentrations and limited urinary drug excretion data are available. Compartmental models have been successfully applied to the prediction of the pharmacokinetics of the drug and the development of dosage regimens. Moreover, compartmental models are very useful in relating plasma drug levels to pharmacodynamic and toxic effects in the body.

The simplicity and flexibility of the compartment model is the principal reason for its wide application. For many applications, the compartmental model may be used to extract some information about the underlying physiologic mechanism through model testing of the data. Thus, compartment analysis may lead to a more accurate description of the underlying physiologic processes and the kinetics involved. In this regard, compartmental models are sometimes misunderstood, overstretched, and even abused. For example, the tissue drug levels predicted by a

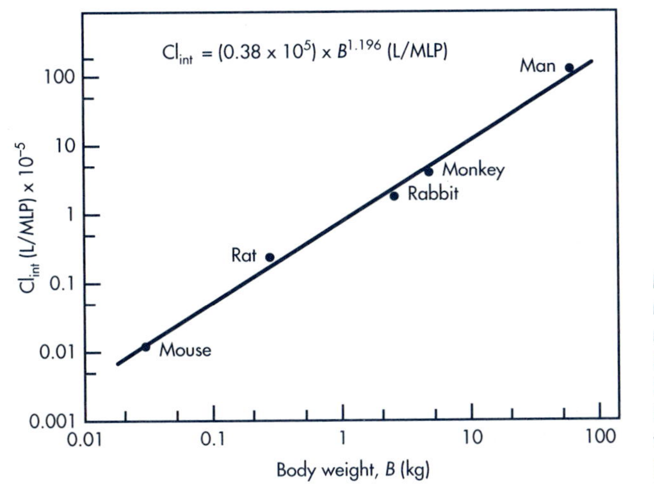

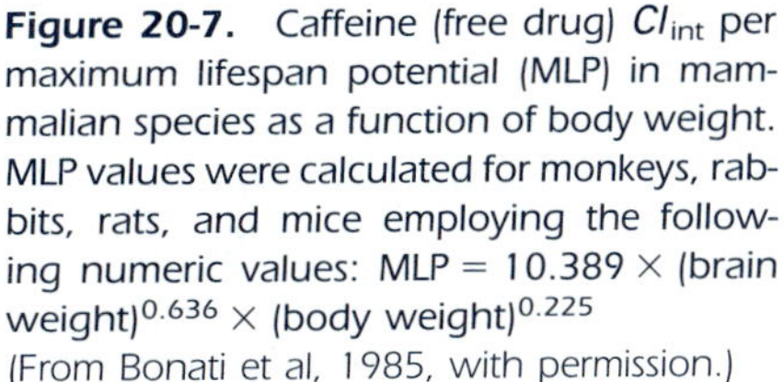
Figure 20-7. Caffeine (free drug) Cl_{int} per maximum lifespan potential (MLP) in mammalian species as a function of body weight. MLP values were calculated for monkeys, rabbits, rats, and mice employing the following numeric values: MLP = 10.389 × (brain weight)$^{0.636}$ × (body weight)$^{0.225}$
(From Bonati et al, 1985, with permission.)

compartment model represent only a composite pool for drug equilibration between all tissues and the circulatory system (plasma compartment). Naturally, any extrapolation to a specific tissue drug concentration is inaccurate and analogous to making predictions without any experimental data. Although specific tissue drug concentration data are missing, many investigators may make predictions about tissue drug levels.

Fundamentally, the principal use of the compartment model is to account accurately for the mass balance of the drug in the plasma, the drug in the tissue pool, and the amount of drug eliminated after dosage administration. The compartment model is particularly useful when several therapeutic agents are compared. In the clinical pharmacokinetic literature, drug data comparisons are based on compartment models, even though alternative pharmacokinetic models have been available for approximately 20 years. The simplicity of the compartment model allows easy tabulation of parameters such as $V_{D_{ss}}$, alpha $t_{1/2}$ and beta $t_{1/2}$. The alternative pharmacokinetic models, including the physiologic and statistical moment approach (mean residence time), are much less frequently used, even though a substantial body of data has been generated using both of these models.

In spite of these advantages, the compartmental model is generally regarded as somewhat empirical and lacking physiologic relevance. Many disease-related changes in pharmacokinetics are the result of physiologic changes, such as impairment of blood flow or a change in organ mass. These pathophysiologic changes are better evaluated using a physiologic-based pharmacokinetic model.

In this regard, the compartment model, owing to its simplicity, often serves as a "first model" that requires further refinement in order to accurately describe the physiologic and drug distribution processes in the body. The physiologic pharmacokinetic model—which accounts for processes of drug distribution, drug binding, metabolism, and drug flow to the body organs—is much more realistic. Disease-related changes in physiologic processes are more readily related to changes in the pharmacokinetics of the drug. Furthermore, organ mass, volumes, and blood perfusion rates are often scalable, based on size, among different individuals and even among different species. This allows a perturbation in one parameter and the prediction of changing physiology on drug distribution and elimination.

The physiologic pharmacokinetic model may also be modified to include the specific feature of a drug. For example, for an antitumor agent that penetrates the inside of a cell, both the drug level in the interstitial water and the intracellular water may be considered in the model. Blood flow and tumor size may even be included in the model to study any change in the drug uptake at that site.

The physiologic pharmacokinetic model can calculate the amount of drug in the blood and in any tissues for any time period if the initial amount of drug in the blood is known and the dose is given IV bolus. In contrast, the tissue compartment in the compartmental model is not related to any actual anatomical tissue groups. The tissue compartment is needed when the plasma drug concentration data are fitted to a multicompartment model. In theory, when tissue drug concentration data are available, the multiple compartment models may be used to fit both tissue and plasma drug data together, including the drug concentration in a specific tissue. In such a case, the compartment model would mimic the system of equations used in the physiologic model, except that in place of blood flows, transfer constants would be used to describe the mass transfer in the model. The latter approach would probably, at best, yield less useful information than that obtained from the physiologic model.

MEAN RESIDENCE TIME (MRT)

After an intravenous bolus drug dose (D_0), the drug molecules distribute throughout the body. These molecules will stay (reside) in the body for various time periods. Some drug molecules will leave the body almost immediately after entering, whereas other drug molecules will leave the body at later time periods. The term *mean residence time* (MRT) describes the average time for *all* the drug molecules to reside in the body. MRT may be considered also as the mean transit time or mean sojourn time.

The residence time for the drug molecules in the dose may be sorted into groups i ($i = 1, 2, 3 \ldots m$) according to their residing time. The total residence time is the summation of the number of molecules in each group i multiplied by the residence time t_i for each group. The summation of n_i (number of molecules in each group) is the total number of molecules N. Thus, MRT is the total residence time for all molecules in the body divided by the total number of molecules in the body, as shown in Equation 20.23.

$$\text{MRT} = \frac{\text{total residence time for all drug molecules in body}}{\text{total number of drug molecules}} \quad \textbf{(20.23)}$$

$$\text{MRT} = \frac{\sum_{i=1}^{m} n_i t_i}{N}$$

where n_i is the number of molecules and t_i is the residence time of the ith group of molecules.

The drug dose (mg) may be converted to the number of molecules by dividing the dose (mg) by 1000 and the molecular weight of the drug to obtain the number of moles of drug, and then multiplying the number of moles of drug by 6.023×10^{23} (Avogadro's number) to obtain the number of drug molecules. For convenience, Equation 20.23 may be written in terms of mg (instead of molecules) by substitution of n_i with $De_i \times f$, where De_i is the number of drug molecules (as mg) leaving the body with residence time $t_i (i = 1, 2, 3 \ldots m)$. The f is simply a conversion factor, the number of molecules/mg of drug that cancels out in Equation 20.24, showing that MRT is independent of mass unit used.

$$\text{MRT} = \frac{\sum_{i=1}^{m} De_i f\, t_i}{\sum_{i=1}^{m} De_i f} = \frac{\sum_{i=1}^{m} De_i\, t_i}{\sum_{i=1}^{m} De_i} \quad \textbf{(20.24)}$$

where $De_i (i = 1\ 2, 3 \ldots m)$ is the amount of drug (mg) in the ith group with residence time t_i.

Drug molecules may have a residence time ranging from values near zero (eg, 0.1, 0.2) to very large values (100, 1000, 10000). The number of i groups may be large and the summation approach to calculate MRT will only be an approximation. Also, for the summation process to be accurate, data must be collected continuously in order not to miss any groups. Integration is an accurate method that replaces summation when the data or function needs to be continuously summed over time.

Mean Residence Time—IV Bolus Dose

The drug concentration in the body after an IV bolus injection for a drug that follows the pharmacokinetics of the one-compartment model is given by the following equation:

$$C_p = (D_0/V_D)e^{-kt} \quad (20.25)$$

$$D_p = D_0 e^{-kt} \quad (20.26)$$

where V_D is the apparent volume of distribution, k is the first-order elimination rate constant, and t is the time after the injection of the drug. The drug exit rate was generated in Table 20.4 with a numerical example until most drug was eliminated.

The rate of change in the amount of drug in the body with respect to time (dD_p/dt) reflects the rate at which the drug molecules leave the body at any time t. Although all drug molecules enter the body at the same time, the exit time, or the residing time, for each molecule is different. Equation 20.27 is obtained by taking the derivative of Equation 20.26, with all the drug molecules exiting the body from $t = 0$ to ∞ (Table 20.4).

$$dD_p/dt = -kD_0 e^{-kt} \quad (20.27)$$

Alternatively, the rate of drug molecules exiting at any time t is given by the following:

$$dDe/dt = -dD_p/dt = kD_0 e^{-kt} \quad (20.28)$$

TABLE 20.4 Simulated Plasma Data After an IV Bolus Dose Illustrating Calculation of MRT[a]

TIME (hr)	RATE ELIMINATED dDe/dt (mg/hr)	RATE ELIMINATED time (t) × dt (mg − hr)	C_P (mg/L)
0	231.000	0	100
1	183.354	183.354	79.374
2	145.535	291.07	63.002
3	115.517	346.551	50.007
4	91.690	366.762	39.693
5	72.778	363.891	31.506
6	57.767	346.602	25.007
7	45.852	320.964	19.849
8	36.395	291.156	15.755
9	28.888	259.990	12.506
10	22.929	229.293	9.926
42	0.014	0.593	0.006
43	0.011	0.482	0.005
44	0.009	0.392	0.004
45	0.007	0.318	0.003
46	0.006	0.258	0.002
47	0.004	0.209	0.002
48	0.004	0.170	0.002
49	0.003	0.137	0.001
Total drug exited = 1004.43[b]		Total drug residence time = 4310[c]	

[a]Drug exiting (first-order rate) tank or body compartment after IV bolus injection. Data generated with Equation 20.25. Dose = 1000 mg, volume = 10 L, $k = 0.231\ \text{hr}^{-1}$.

[b]Total drug exited = average rate × dt and sum total.

[c]Total drug-residence time (expressed as mg − hr) = rate × t × dt and sum total.

Rearranging yields

$$dDe = kD_0e^{-kt}\,dt \tag{20.29}$$

At any time t, dDe molecules exit. Therefore, multiplying Equation 20.29 by t on both sides yields the residence for each molecule exiting with a residence time t. Summation of the residence time for each drug molecule, and division by the total number of molecules, estimates the mean residence time (Eq. 20.30).

$$\frac{\int_0^\infty dD_0e\;t}{D_0} = \frac{\int_0^\infty kD_0e^{-kt}t\,dt}{D_0} \tag{20.30}$$

$$\text{MRT} = \int_0^\infty ke^{-kt}t\,dt \tag{20.31}$$

As shown in Equation 20.30, the MRT is related to the product of the elimination rate constant k and the function describing drug elimination in the body. MRT is the integrated normalized form of the differential function representing drug amount (or concentration) in the body. The term “differential probability” is given to reflect that the function is a *probability density function* (PDF), which represents the residence time probability of a molecule in the population. The mean residence time is the normalized (divided by D_0) differential of the function governing drug elimination in the body. When a function is normalized, it becomes dimensionless without regard to unit.

Equation 20.30 was derived in terms of amount of drug. Because $D_0 = C^0{}_\mathrm{p}V_\mathrm{D}$, substituting for D_0 with $C^0{}_\mathrm{p}V_\mathrm{D}$ into the right side of Equation 20.30 yields:

$$\frac{\int_0^\infty dDe\;t}{D_0} = \frac{\int_0^\infty kC_\mathrm{p}^0e^{-kt}\,t\,dt}{C_\mathrm{p}^0} \tag{20.32}$$

Equation 20.32 may be used to determine MRT directly or may be rearranged to Equation 20.33 by dividing the numerator and denominator by k to yield a moment equation.

$$\text{MRT} = \frac{\int_0^\infty dDe\;t}{D_0} = \frac{\int_0^\infty C_\mathrm{p}^0e^{-kt}t\,dt}{C_\mathrm{p}^0/k} \tag{20.33}$$

The plasma concentration equation (function $f(t)$) multiplied by time and integrated from 0 to ∞ gives a term called the *first moment* of the plasma drug curve. The denominator is the area under the curve, AUC_0^∞. The AUC_0^∞ is equal to $\int_0^\infty C_\mathrm{p}dt$ or $D_0/V_\mathrm{D}k$. Because $C_\mathrm{p}^0 = D_0/V_\mathrm{D}$, the denominator of Equation 20.33 is the $[\text{AUC}]_0^\infty$ of the time concentration curve ($[\text{AUC}]_0^\infty = D_0/(kV_D)$; see Chapter 12). Equation 20.33 is used in pharmacokinetics to determine MRT; the equation is abbreviated as shown in Equation 20.34 in the literature:

$$\text{MRT} = \frac{\text{AUMC}}{\text{AUC}} \tag{20.34}$$

where AUMC is the area under the (first) moment versus time curve from $t = 0$ to infinity. AUC is the area under plasma time versus concentration curve from $t = 0$ to infinity. AUC is also known as the *zero moment curve.* Table 20.5 shows how summation may be used to calculate MRT from generated data when the function is known.

TABLE 20.5 Equations and Parameters Used in Generating Data for Figure 20-8. Summation Method Was Used to Mimic Actual Calculation of MRT by the Moment Method[a]

Parameters	
$i = 0 \ldots 50$	Number of groups summed
$t_i = 1 \times i$	Residence time t_i
$k = 0.231$	
Dose = 1000 mg	
Volume = 10 L	
$Db_i = 1000 \times \exp[-kt_i]$	Equation showing drug in body at t_i
$De_i = 1000\ k \times \exp[-kt_i]$	Equation showing drug exiting at t_i
$rt_i = De_i \times t_i$	
$\sum_i rt_i = 4.31 \times 10^3$	Total residence time found by summation, $\text{MRT} = \dfrac{4310}{1004.43} = 4.29$ hr
$\dfrac{1}{0.231} = 4.329$	MRT by calculation from $1/k$

[a]Mathcad was used for calculation. Complete data generated are listed in Table 20.4.

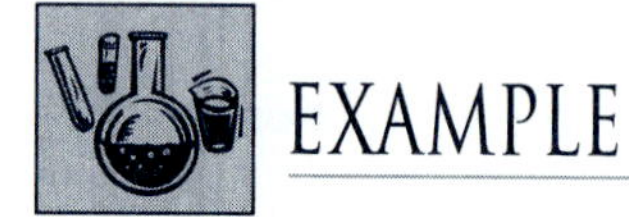

EXAMPLE

A drug that follows the kinetics of a one-compartment model is given by IV bolus injection at a dose of 1000 mg. The drug has an elimination rate constant of 0.231 hr^{-1} and a volume of distribution of 10 L. The body is considered as a single compartment with no drug permanently bound in the body. (Use Table 20.4 for this problem; 50 data points were generated with Equation 20.25 for C_p and Equation 20.28 for dDe/dt.)

1. Calculate the MRT of the drug molecules in the body using the moment method. Assume AUC is 432.9 (mg/L) hr and AUMC is 1865.465 (mg/L) h^2.
2. Calculate MRT using the total residence times of all molecules exited and divide by the total dose. Compare the answer to 1, above.

Solution

1. Using the equation: MRT = AUMC/AUC,

$$\text{MRT} = \frac{1865.465\ (\text{mg/L})\ \text{hr}^2}{432.9\ (\text{mg/L})\ \text{hr}} = 4.309\ \text{hr}$$

2. The residence time for most of the drug molecules exiting from the body ($t =$ 0 to ∞) is approximated by the first 50 points (only few drug molecules remained in the body after 50 hours). Total residence time is the sum of the number of molecules at each exit time point multiplied by the time. The mean residence time is the sum of all the residence times for all drug molecules divided by the total number of molecules (Eq. 20.23). Multiplying columns 1 and 2 yields column 3:

$$\text{Total drug molecule residence time} = 4310\ \text{mg} - \text{hr}$$
$$\text{Sum of drug exited} = 1004.43\ \text{mg}$$

(The sum of drug exited was obtained by averaging the rate of drug exited for each time point and multiplied by the time interval, 1 hour in this case; then sum up to obtain the total drug excreted. See Table 20.4.)

$$\text{MRT} = 4310/1004.43 \text{ hr}$$
$$= 4.29 \text{ hr}$$

The example is basically a verification of Equation 20.30. The approximation shows that when the function is not known, MRT may be estimated from the rate of drug excreted or from the plasma drug concentration versus time curve. In practice, unless the entire dose is known, there is no assurance that all drug molecules are excreted through the plasma compartment if multicompartments are involved.

MRT may also be calculated using the compartmental approach by considering the MRT for a drug after IV bolus injection as the reciprocal of the elimination rate constant k. In this case, MRT is inversely related to the elimination constant, and MRT $= 1/k$. Therefore, MRT $= 1/0.231\ \text{hr}^{-1} = 4.329$ hours.

MRT was estimated as 4.309 hours earlier using the moment method. The slightly smaller value for the MRT is due to approximation in the summation of the moment area and AUC.

Using the method of MRT = AUMC/AUC, MRT may be estimated using the AUC calculated from the C_p versus t curve (Table 20.4). Alternatively, the MRT can be estimated accurately using integration when the function that describes plasma drug concentrations is known (Table 20.5). A plot of De and C_p versus time, and the moment curve $De \times t$ versus t are shown in Figure 20-8. For drugs that follow the kinetics of a one-compartment model with drug elimination only from the plasma, MRT may be calculated by either the area method or from the first moment curve. In data analysis, the function that governs drug disposition is generally not known, and the MRT is generally calculated from the plasma drug concentration versus time curve.

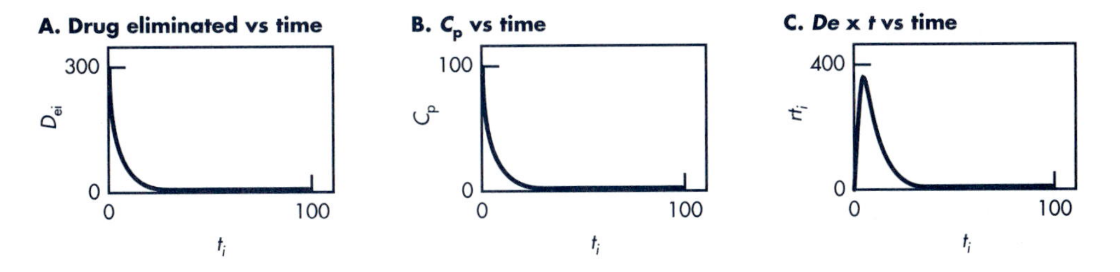

Figure 20-8. Plot of **(A)** drug eliminated versus time; **(B)** C_p versus time; and **(C)** De versus time. The data generated for these plots are tabulated at Table 20.4. The actual equations and parameters used are listed in Table 20.5.

Parameters:

	$t = 0 \ldots 50$	Variable of time from 0 to 50 hr
	$k = 0.231$	Elimination constant k
A	$f(t) = 100\exp(-kt)$	Equation showing first-order exit of tracer
B	$g(t) = \exp(-kt)$	Equation after $f(t)$ divided by C_0, or 100, thus normalizing the function
C	$h(t) = k\exp(-kt)$	Multiplying $g(t)$ with k converts it to a PDF

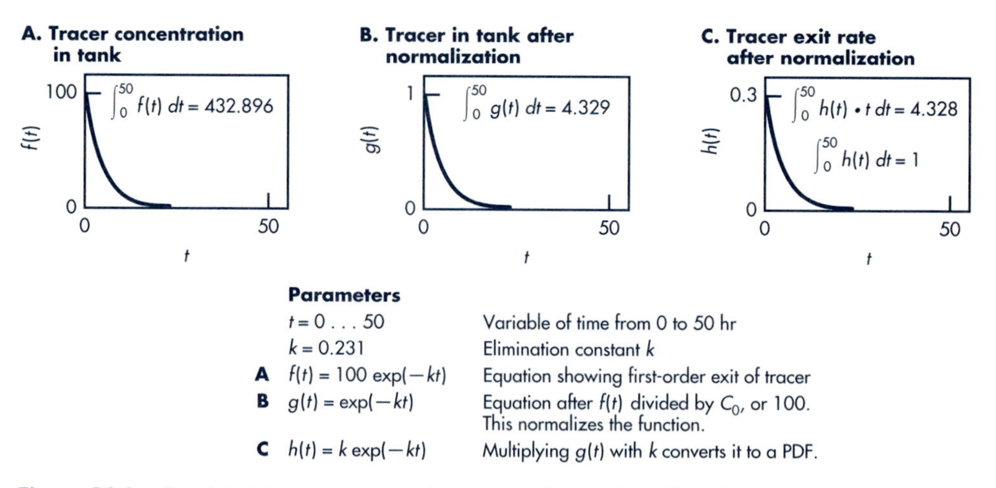

Figure 20-9. Simulated tracer concentration in a tank over time. The three plots were generated by MathCAD. The AUC under each curve is evaluated by integration. In **C**, the tracer concentration exit rate plot is a PDF and the AUC is 1. The mean of this function is simply the first moment and equal to the mean residence time of 4.328.

STATISTICAL MOMENT THEORY

Statistical moment theory provides a unique way to study time-related changes in macroscopic events. A macroscopic event is considered as the overall event brought about by the constitutive elements involved. For example, in chemical processing, a dose of tracer molecules may be injected into a reactor tank to track the transit time (residence time) of materials staying in the tank. The constitutive elements in this example are the tracer molecules, and the macroscopic events are the residence times shared by groups of tracer molecules. Each tracer molecule is well mixed and distributes noninteractively and randomly in the tank. In the case of all the molecules ($\int_0^{D_0} dDe = D_0$) that exit from the tank, the rate of exit of tracer molecules ($-dDe/dt$) divided by D_0 yields the probability of a molecule having a given residence time t (Fig. 20-9C). A mathematical formula describing the probability of a tracer molecule exited at any time is a *probability density function* (PDF). MRT is merely the expected value or mean of the distribution.

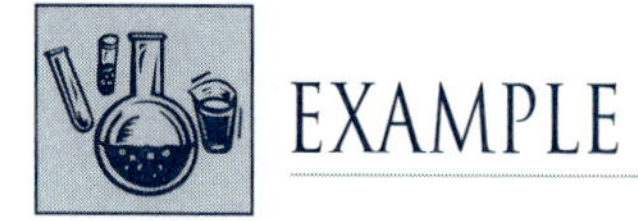

EXAMPLE

Assume the tracer molecules are eliminated according to a kinetic function, $f(t) = C_0e^{-kt}$. The tank volume V_D and k are similar to the previous one compartment model example ($k = 0.231$ hr^{-1}, $D_0 = 1000$ mg, $V_D = 10$). What is the MRT? What is the PDF?

Because $f(t)$ describes drug elimination in terms of concentration unit, it was divided by C_0 to normalize it (Fig. 20-9B). The function was then differentiated to obtain $h(t)$. Next, $h(t) = ke^{-kt}$ was plotted in Figure 20-9C. This is the PDF, also obtained by kC. Integration of $h(t)t\,dt$ yields MRT (4.329 hours) directly. All integrations in Figure 20-9 were computed using Math CAD software. Integration of $f(t)$ yields the AUC of 432.896 (mg/L) hr.

In the one-compartment model, AUC divided by C_0 also yields MRT (432.896/100 = 4.33 hr). This example is another way to calculate MRT, as will be demonstrated later. MRT may also be computed by integrating $f(t)/C_0$ (Fig. 20-9B). However, if $f(t)$ represents a two- or multicompartment function, the computed MRT using this method is only for the central compartment, whereas using the AUMC/AUC approach leads to an MRT for the body (a larger value). The latter method treats the molecules as a single population within the body, tracking them only as they exit and without supposition of any knowledge of molecular exchanges between the plasma and tissue compartments.

In the previous discussion, Equation 20.34 was derived to estimate MRT without applying the PPD concept. However, the equation may be rearranged in the form of a probability density function, as in Equation 20.31. This was plotted in Figure 20-9C for comparison. The moment theory facilitates calculation of MRT and related parameters from the kinetic function, as discussed below.

A probability density function $f(t)$ multiplied by t^m and integrated over time yields the moment curve (Eq. 20.35). The moment curve shows the characteristics of the distribution.

$$\mu_m \text{ or } m\text{th moment} = \int_0^\infty t^m f(t)\, dt \qquad \textbf{(20.35)}$$

where $f(t)$ is the probability density function, t is time, and m is mth moment.

For example, when $m = 0$, substituting for $m = 0$, Equation 20.36 is called the *zero moment.*

$$\mu_0 \text{ or zero moment} = \int_0^\infty f(t)\, dt \qquad \textbf{(20.36)}$$

The area under the zero moment curve is 1, if the distribution is a true probability function.

Substituting into Equation 20.35 with $m = 1$, Equation 20.37 is obtained. The area under the curve $f(t)$ times t is called the AUMC, or the *area under the first moment curve.* The *first moment* defines the *mean* of the distribution.

$$\mu_1 \text{ or first moment} = \int_0^\infty t^1 f(t)\, dt \qquad \textbf{(20.37)}$$

Similarly, when $m = 2$, Equation 20.35 becomes the *second moment:*

$$\mu_2 \text{ or second moment} = \int_0^\infty t^2 f(t)\, dt \qquad \textbf{(20.38)}$$

where μ_2 defines the *variance* of the distribution. Higher moments, such as μ_3 or μ_4, represent skewness and kurtosis of the distribution. Equation 20.35 is therefore useful in characterizing family of moment curves of a distribution.

The principal use of the moment curve is the calculation of the MRT of a drug in the body. The elements of the distribution curve describe the distribution of drug molecules after administration and the residence time of the drug molecules in the body.

In Equation 20.31, the plasma equation $f(t) = C_p^0 e^{-kt}$ was converted to a PDF (ie, $f(t) = ke^{-kt}$). It can be shown that μ_0 for this function = 1 (total probability adds up to 1 by summing zero moment), and the mean of the function is the area under the first moment curve (the mean is the MRT).

By comparison, Equation 20.25 is not a true PDF, because its mean is not given by the AUMC, and its AUC is not 1. Nonetheless, Equation 20.34 may be used to calculate MRT independent of the PDF concept, although some confusion over its application appears in the literature.

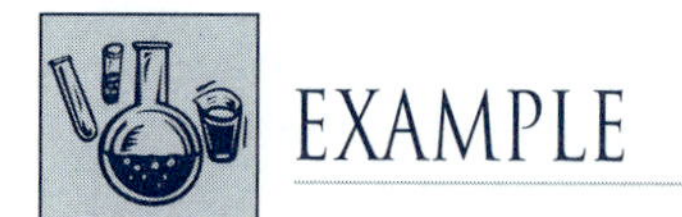

EXAMPLE

An antibiotic was given to two subjects by an IV bolus dose of 1000 mg. The drug has a volume of distribution of 10 L and follows a one-compartment model with an elimination constant of (1) 0.1 hr^{-1} and (2) 0.2 hr^{-1} in two subjects. Determine the MRT from each C_p versus time curve (Table 20.6) and compare your values with the MRT determined by taking the reciprocal of k.

Solution

Noncompartmental Approach (MRT = AUMC/AUC)

1. From Table 20.6, multiply each time point with the corresponding plasma C_p to obtain points for the moment curve. Use the trapezoidal rule and sum the area to obtain area under the moment curve ($AUMC_1$) for subject 1. Also, determine the area under the plasma curve using the trapezoidal rule. The steps are as follows.
   a. Multiply each C_p with t as in column 5 of Table 20.6.
   b. Sum all $C_p \times t$ values, and find area under the moment curve (AUMC)—that is, 9986.45 (μg/mL) hr^2.
   c. Estimate tail area of moment curve (beyond last data point) using the equation

   $$\text{AUMC} = C_p t/k + C_p/k^2 \qquad \textbf{(20.39)}$$

   Substituting the last data point C_p = 0.00454 μg/mL, last time point = 100 hr, and the last moment curve point is 0.454 (μ/mL) hr^2.

   $$\text{Tail AUMC} = 0.454/0.1 + 0.00454/0.1^2 = 4.99\ (\mu\text{g/mL})\ \text{hr}^2$$
   $$\text{Total AUMC} = 9986.46 + 4.99 = 9991.45\ (\mu\text{g/mL})\ \text{hr}^2$$

   Note: k is determined from the slope to be 0.1 hr^{-1}.
   d. Estimate AUC using the trapezoidal rule from columns 1 and 2 (found to be 1000.79 μg/mL/hr).
   e. $$\text{MRT} = \text{AUMC/AUC} = \frac{9991.45\ (\mu\text{g/mL})\ \text{hr}^2}{1000.79\ (\mu\text{g/mL})\ \text{hr}} = 9.98\ \text{hr}$$

   When the data are available for a long period, 6 to 7 half-lives and beyond, the last C_p will be very small and no extrapolation will be needed. If a model-independent approach is needed, no extrapolation beyond the data should be used (in this example, extrapolation was used only for illustration). Instead,

TABLE 20.6 Simulated Data for a Drug Administered by IV Bolus[a]

				SUBJECTS 1 AND 2	
	C_p1	C_p2	t	AUMC1	AUMC2
0	100.000	100.000	0	0.000	0.000
1	90.484	81.873	1	90.484	81.873
2	81.873	67.032	2	163.746	134.064
3	74.082	54.881	3	222.245	164.643
4	67.032	44.933	4	268.128	179.732
5	60.653	36.788	5	303.265	183.940
6	54.881	30.119	6	329.287	180.717
7	49.659	24.660	7	347.610	172.618
8	44.933	20.190	8	359.463	161.517
9	40.657	16.530	9	365.913	148.769
10	36.788	13.534	10	367.879	135.335
11	33.287	11.080	11	366.158	121.883
12	30.119	9.072	12	361.433	108.862
13	27.253	7.427	13	354.291	96.556
14	24.660	6.081	14	345.236	85.134
15	22.313	4.979	15	334.695	74.681
16	20.190	4.076	16	323.034	65.220
17	18.268	3.337	17	310.562	56.735
18	16.530	2.732	18	297.538	49.183
19	14.957	2.237	19	284.180	42.504
20	13.534	1.832	20	270.671	36.631
21	12.246	1.500	21	257.158	31.491
22	11.080	1.228	22	243.767	27.010
23	10.026	1.005	23	230.595	23.119
24	9.072	0.823	24	217.723	19.751
25	8.208	0.674	25	205.212	16.845
26	7.427	0.552	26	193.111	14.343
27	6.721	0.452	27	181.455	12.195
28	6.081	0.370	28	170.268	10.354
29	5.502	0.303	29	159.567	8.780
30	4.979	0.248	30	149.361	7.436
91	0.011167	0.00000125	91	1.0162	0.0001135
92	0.010104	0.00000102	92	0.9296	0.0000939
93	0.009142	0.00000084	93	0.8502	0.0000777
94	0.008272	0.00000068	94	0.7776	0.0000643
95	0.007485	0.00000056	95	0.7111	0.0000532
96	0.006773	0.00000046	96	0.6502	0.0000440
97	0.006128	0.00000038	97	0.5944	0.0000364
98	0.005545	0.00000031	98	0.5434	0.0000301
99	0.005017	0.00000025	99	0.4967	0.0000249
100	0.004540	0.00000021	100	0.4540	0.0000206

[a](1) $k = 0.1\ \text{hr}^{-1}$, (2) $k = 0.2\ \text{hr}^{-1}$
Note the corresponding AUMC for the two subjects in the last two columns.

additional data should be collected, or the assay sensitivity improved so that more data at later time periods may be obtained. All data extrapolation, linear or log linear, will be subject to error, because the real rate process is determined from the experimental data and not assumed.

Note that without the extrapolation to infinity, MRT = 9986.45/1000.79 = 9.978 hr, because extensive plasma drug concentration data are available. This value is fairly close to the value of 9.98 hours when the plasma drug concentration data is extrapolated to infinity.

2. From the tabulated results, summing up column 6, AUMC2 = 2491.68 μg/mL hr^2. AUC for patient 2 = 500 μg/mL·hr (calculated from the trapezoidal rule using the time plasma concentration data of subject 2).

Note: In this case, the AUMC tail area was not extrapolated because the drug concentration was already very low at the last data point.

$$\text{MRT} = \frac{2491.68\ (\mu\text{g/mL})\ \text{hr}^2}{500\ (\mu\text{g/mL})\ \text{hr}}$$
$$= 4.98\ \text{hr}$$

Compartment Approach

1. If a one-compartment model is assumed and k is determined from the slope, MRT is simply $1/k = 1/0.1 = 10$ hr.

2. As determined from the slope of a C_p versus t curve, $k = 0.2\ \text{hr}^{-1}$, and MRT = $1/0.2 = 5$ hr.

In a one-compartment model IV bolus, MRT is inversely proportional to the elimination constant and directly proportional to the half-life of the drug in the patient. The elimination half-lives of the drug in the two patients are 6.93 and 3.47 hours, respectively.

The plasma drug concentration versus time curves for the two cases above were plotted with the moment curves. The use of moment ($C_p \times t$) changes the typical monoexponential plasma time curve into a profile very similar to that of a non-symmetric bell-shaped curve (Fig. 20-10) similar to a statistical distribution (Appendix A). Furthermore, in the one-compartment IV bolus case, the mean of

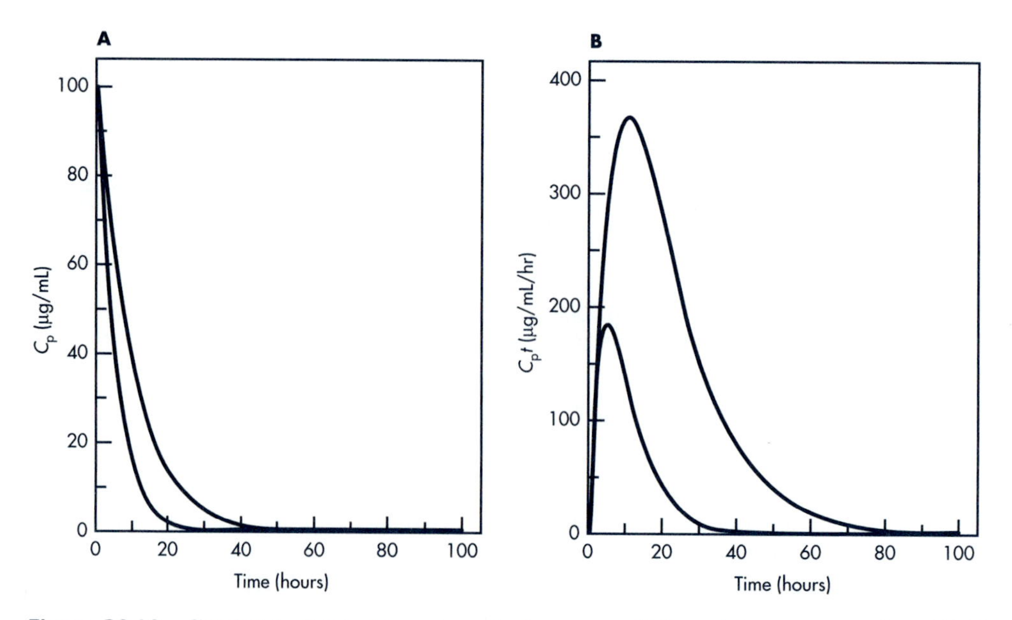

Figure 20-10. Simulated plasma drug concentration curves (left) and the corresponding AUMC curves (right). Dose = 1000 mg, V_D = 10 L, k = 0.1 and 0.2 hr^{-1}, respectively, by IV bolus administration.

the distribution may be seen as 10 and 5 hours, respectively, from the curve. A smaller k widens the distribution and increases the total residing times of all the drug molecules staying in the body. The shape of the moment curve depends on the function describing the plasma drug concentration, and may be skewed.

MRT for Multicompartment Model with Elimination from the Central Compartment

The moment theory provides a means for calculating MRT for the body from plasma drug concentration data obtained for drugs that follow one-compartment models. In this section, the MRT is determined for a drug that has a plasma (central) compartment and one or more tissue or peripheral compartments. The assumptions are (1) that the drug is eliminated only from the central compartment and (2) that all drug is eliminated by a linear process (constant clearance). The MRT for a multicompartment model drug is the summation of the residence time of the drug in each compartment.

$$\text{MRT}_{\text{body}} = \text{MRT}_{\text{c}} + \text{MRT}_{\text{p1}} + \text{MRT}_{\text{p2}} + \ldots + \text{MRT}_{\text{p}n} \quad \textbf{(20.40)}$$

where $\text{MRT}_{\text{p}i}$ represents MRT in the peripheral or tissue compartments and MRT_{c} = MRT for the central compartment.

MRT for the body may be calculated from the plasma concentration curve using AUMC/AUC as discussed earlier, because the body (including all compartments) may be treated as a single compartment similar to that of the single compartment.

MRT_{c} is known as the *mean residence time* or *mean transit time* for the central compartment. This is calculated by AUC/C_{p}^0, where AUC is the area under plasma drug concentration curve and C_{p}^0 is the initial plasma drug concentration curve.

Derivation of MRT_c

Let De = the amount of drug eliminated at time t.

D = dose or drug at time zero.
D_{p} = the amount of drug in plasma compartment from which drug is eliminated at time t.
C_{p} = drug concentration in the plasma compartment (volume V_{D}).

At time t, dDe units of drug are eliminated, the residence time is $t\,dDe$, and integrating from 0 to D_e^∞ will yield the total residence times (see numerator of Eq. 20.41). Integrating De will yield the total units of drug eliminated (see denominator of Eq. 20.41), and MRT is obtained by dividing the total residence time by the total unit of drugs. If elimination occurs only from the central compartment, at any instant dt, $dDe = -dD_{\text{p}}$.

$$\text{MRT}_{\text{c}} = \frac{\int_0^{D_e^\infty} t\,dDe}{\int_0^{D_e^\infty} dDe} = \frac{\int_0^{D_0} t\,dD_{\text{p}}}{\int_0^{D_0} dD_{\text{p}}} \quad \textbf{(20.41)}$$

$$\frac{\int_0^{C_{\text{p}}^0} t\,V_{\text{D}}\,dC_{\text{p}}}{\int_0^{C_{\text{p}}^0} V_{\text{D}}\,dC_{\text{p}}} = \frac{\int_0^{C_{\text{p}}^0} t\,dC_{\text{p}}}{\int_0^{C_{\text{p}}^0} dC_{\text{p}}} \quad \textbf{(20.42)}$$

Since

$$t\,dC_p = -C_p\,dt \text{ and } \int_0^{C_p^0} dC_p = -C_p^0.$$

$$\text{MRT}_c = \frac{\int_0^\infty C_p\,dt}{C_p^0} = \frac{\text{AUC}_0^\infty}{C_p^0} \quad \textbf{(20.43)}$$

When a drug is distributed between a central and one or more peripheral compartments, the peripheral compartment is not available for sampling. Therefore, both the drug and tissue MRT have to be determined from the plasma data. If a two-compartment model is involved, the peripheral MRT is given by the following:

$$\text{MRT}_p = \text{AUMC/AUC} - \text{AUC}/C_p^0 \quad \textbf{(20.44)}$$

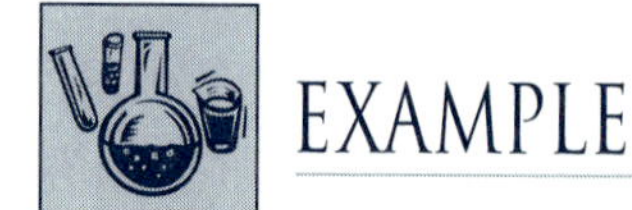

EXAMPLE

The plasma drug concentrations of a drug that follows a two-compartment model after IV bolus were simulated with the following parameters (Nagashima and Benet, 1988) and the plasma concentration equation for the two-compartment model. Determine MRT for the plasma and tissue compartments and verify Equation 20.43.

Use these parameters: $a = 2.2346$, $b = 0.4654$, $k = 0.946$ (overall elimination constant from the central compartment), $k_{12} = 0.655$, $k_{21} = 1.1$ (all rate constant in hr^{-1}). Also, $V_p = 10$ L, $D_0 = 1000$ mg, $C_0 = 100$ μg/mL.

TABLE 20.7 Simulated Data Showing How to Calculate MRT from AUMC/AUC 50 Points Were Generated Using Two-Compartment Equation After IV Bolus

t	C_P	AUC	$C_p t$	AUMC
0	100	21.076	0	2.144
0.25	68.611	14.752	17.153	5.232
0.5	49.404	10.838	24.702	6.585
0.75	37.302	8.336	27.976	7.17
1	29.386	6.67	29.386	7.419
1.25	23.974	5.508	29.968	7.513
1.5	20.092	4.658	30.138	7.523
1.75	17.17	4.006	30.048	7.475
2	14.876	3.485	29.752	7.377
10	0.342	0.081	3.416	0.817
10.25	0.304	0.072	3.117	0.745
10.5	0.271	0.064	2.842	0.679
10.75	0.241	0.057	2.59	0.619
11	0.214	0.051	2.359	0.563
11.25	0.191	0.045	2.148	0.513
11.5	0.17	0.04	1.954	0.467
11.75	0.151	0.036	1.778	0.424
12	0.135	0.032	1.616	0.386
12.25	0.12	0.028	1.469	0.35
Total sum of column		106.6		177.915

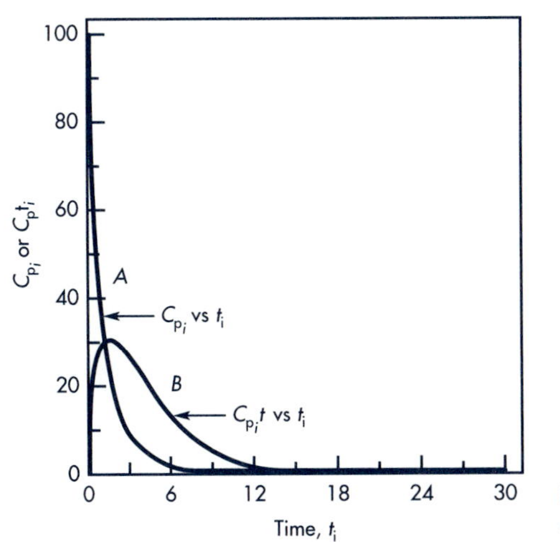

Figure 20-11. Plot of **(A)** C_p and **(B)** C_p versus time $C_p \cdot dt$ after a bolus dose IV.

Using the above parameters, the plasma drug concentrations, C_p, at any point is given by Equation 20.45 (Table 20.7) and plotted in Figure 20-11.

$$C_p = 100\left[\frac{k_{21} - a}{b - a}e^{-at} + \frac{k_{21} - b}{a - b}e^{-bt}\right] \tag{20.45}$$

The AUMC is found by determining the $C_p \times t$ at each point and summed up for the entire curve (Table 20.7). The AUMC = 177.915, and the AUC = 106.6. The MRT of the drug in the body is 1.67 hours. MRT of the drug in the plasma is AUC/C_0 = 106.6/100 = 1.066 hr. The MRT for the tissue compartment is 1.67 − 1.066 = 0.604 hr.

From statistical moment theory, MRT is the mean of the statistical distribution $k \times C_p \times dt$, where k is the elimination constant and each C_p has been normalized by dividing with C_0 (to give a PDF). MRT for the body is then simply the first moment of the distribution as shown below:

$$\text{MRT} = \int_0^{\infty} \frac{100}{C_0}\left[\frac{k_{21} - a}{b - a}e^{-at} + \frac{k_{21} - b}{a - b}e^{-kt}\right]k\,dt$$

$$\text{MRT} = 1.687 \text{ hr} \tag{20.46}$$

The answer should agree with that given above, by AUMC/AUC. The second method illustrates the relationship of the plasma concentration data with the PDF. Because k (elimination constant from the central compartment) is not known from plasma data, the second approach is not applied directly. The PDF approach may also be used to determine the MRT_c, or mean residence from the central compartment. Taking the derivative of the two-compartment equation for plasma drug concentration yields a PDF; this function may be calculated directly using software such as Mathcad. Integration of the result yields MRT = 1.066 hours (the mean of the PDF), the same as that calculated using AUC/C_p^0. AUMC/AUC of the differential function also yields an MRT of 1.066 hours.

In contrast, when AUMC/AUC is applied to the plasma drug concentration equation directly, AUC/C_p^0 yields 1.066 hours, while AUMC/AUC yields 1.687 hours.

The latter approach has caused some controversy in the literature because two different definitions were independently derived that apply independently during calculation. When the PDF approach is applied, this confusion is avoided. When the PDF is applied to the equation describing the drug in the body, an MRT of 1.687 hours is obtained, which is the sum of MRT in tissue and plasma compartment. In each case, MRT is simply the mean of the distribution that has a definite variance. The MRT may still be calculated without any knowledge of the distribution function, in which case the MRT is the ratio of two area-under-the-curve terms used in calculating V_{ss} or Cl. The two approaches are contrasted below.

Analysis Based on $f(t)$, the Function Describing Plasma Drug Concentration

$$f(t) = (k_{21} - a) \times \frac{e^{-at}}{b - a} + (k_{21} - b) \times \frac{e^{-bt}}{a - b}$$

$$\int_0^{50} f(t)\ dt = \text{AUC}_0^\infty = 1.058$$

$$\int_0^{50} f(t) \times t\ dt = \text{AUMC}_0^\infty = 1.784$$

$$\frac{\text{AUMC}}{\text{AUC}} = \frac{1.784}{1.058} = 1.688$$

$$\text{MRT} = \frac{\text{AUC}}{C_\text{p}^0} = \frac{1.058}{1} = 1.058$$

Analysis Based on Differential Function, $f'(t)$, the Derivative of $f(t)$

$$g(t) = (k_{21} - a) \times \frac{e^{-at}}{b - a} \times a + (k_{21} - b) \times \frac{e^{-bt}}{a - b} \times b$$

$$\int_0^{50} g(t) \times t\ dt = \text{AUMC}_0^\infty = 1.058 \qquad \text{(MRT from PDF)}$$

$$\int_0^{50} g(t)\, dt = \text{AUC}_0^\infty = 1$$

$$\frac{\text{AUMC}}{\text{AUC}} = \frac{1.058}{1} = 1.058 \qquad \left(\text{MRT using } \frac{\text{AUMC}}{\text{AUC}}\right)$$

The first approach depends on C_p^0 evaluation. The second approach allows two ways to evaluate MRT. The two approaches agree with each other.

The Model-Independent and Model-Dependent Nature of MRT

MRT evaluated from AUMC/AUC assumes that most drugs are excreted through the central compartment or that they are metabolized in highly vascular tissues that kinetically are considered part of the central compartment. For drugs eliminated through tissues that are not part of the central compartment, the MRT calculated by AUMC/AUC is smaller than that calculated by considering both peripheral and central compartment elimination. Compare models *A* and *B* generated by Nakashima and Benet (1988) in Figure 20-12 and Table 20.8. Both models *A* and *B* have identical rate constants except that model *B* has an elimination rate con-

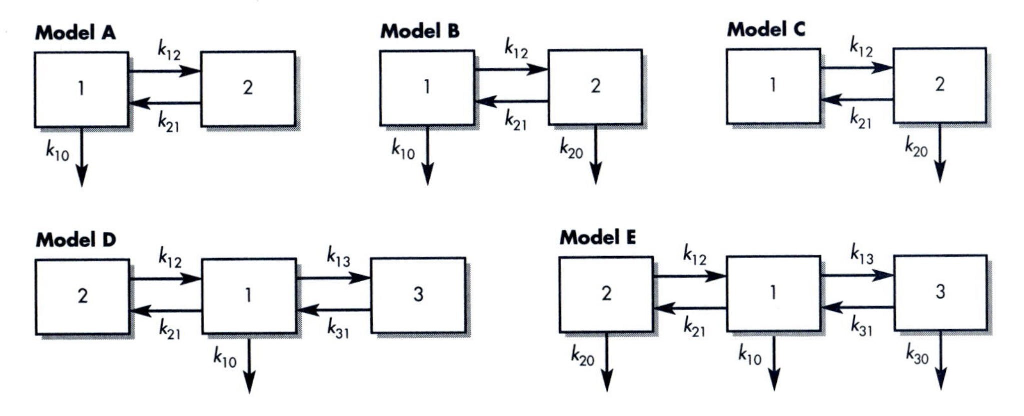

Figure 20-12. The three possible linear two-compartment open models and two possible three-compartment models. In each case, the concentration in compartment 1 (the central compartment) represents the measurable concentration of drug.
(From Nagashima and Benet, 1988, with permission.)

TABLE 20.8 Parameter Values for Models Depicted in Figure 20-12 Consistent with the Following Equations: $C_p = 64.131\ e^{-2.2346t} + 35.869\ e^{-0.4654t}$ for Models *A*, *B*, and *C*; and $C_p = 53.55\ e^{-0.1212t} + 18.4\ e^{-0.0361t} + 28.013\ e^{-0.01049t}$ for Models *D* and *E*

	TWO-COMPARTMENT MODELS			THREE-COMPARTMENT MODELS	
PARAMETER	MODEL A	MODEL B	MODEL C	MODEL D	MODEL E
Dose (D_0)	1000	1000	1000	1000	1000
V_1	10	10	10	10	10
V_{ss}	15.95	20.91	24.55	20.73	25.83
V_{area}	20.32	28.91	35.21	26.31	34.80
Cl	9.455	9.455	9.455	0.276	0.276
k_{12}	0.655	1.2	1.6	0.0323	0.0379
k_{21}	1.1	0.6	0.45	0.0693	0.0593
k_{10}	0.946	0.4	0	0.0276	0.0118
k_{20}	0	0.5	0.65	0	0.01
k_{13}	—	—	—	0.0146	0.0249
k_{31}	—	—	—	0.024	0.0141
k_{30}	—	—	—	0	0.01
f_1	1.0	0.423	0	1.0	0.4265
f_2	0	0.577	1	0	0.1983
f_3	—	—	—	0	0.3752
MRTC	1.058	1.058	1.058	36.23	36.23
$MRTP_2$	0.629	1.154	1.538	16.89	19.83
$MRTP_3$	—	—	—	22.07	37.52
MRT from Eq. 20.48	1.687	2.212	2.596	75.19	93.57
AUMC	178.4	178.4	178.4	272335	272335
AUC	105.8	105.8	105.8	3622	3622
AUMC/AUC	1.687	1.687	1.687	75.19	75.19
MRT from urine	1.687	1.687	ND[a]	75.19	75.19

[a]Intact drug will not be measured in urine.

From Nakashima & Benet (1988), with permission.

stant k_{20} from the peripheral compartment. MRT calculated using the new approach, referred to as MRT (new), is 1.687 hours for model *A* and 2.212 hours for model *B*. The new equation for MRT (new) of model *B* is as shown:

$$\text{MRT (new)} = \text{AUMC/AUC} + (k_{20}/E_2)(V_2/Cl) \quad \textbf{(20.47)}$$

where k_{20} = elimination rate for drug eliminated in the compartment 2; V_2 = the distribution volume of compartment 2; E_2 = the sum of rate constants exiting from compartment 2 (in model *B*, $E_2 = k_{20} + k_{21}$); Cl = total body clearance; MRT_c = MRT from the central compartment; MRT_p = MRT from the peripheral or tissue compartment, also referred to as MRT_t; MRT = AUMC/AUC; and MRT (new) = MRT as calculated with correction for peripheral elimination.

The equation also applies for other multicompartment models. For a three-compartment model, Figure 20-12 (model *E*), a third term is added to Equation 20.47 to reflect drug exiting in compartment 3, as in Equation 20.48.

$$\text{MRT (new)} = \frac{\text{AUMC}}{\text{AUC}} + \frac{k_{20}\ V_2}{E_2\ Cl} + \frac{k_{30}\ V_3}{E_3\ Cl} \quad \textbf{(20.48)}$$

From Table 20.8, MRT (new) calculated using Equations 20.47 and 20.48 is model dependent. The original MRT calculated using AUMC/AUC yields the same MRT value of 1.687 hours for models *A*, *B*, and *C*. The original method, frequently quoted as a model-independent method for calculating MRT from plasma data, in effect, treats the body as a single unit from which drugs are eliminated from the plasma pool regardless of the true nature of the model. Unfortunately, from plasma data alone, it is not possible to know whether drug elimination occurs in the peripheral compartment. Therefore, it is not possible to unambiguously interpret MRT parameters calculated without making some assumptions. Benet and Galeazzi (1979) and Nakashima and Benet (1988) showed MRT is related to V_{ss} and clearance (Eq. 20.49), as illustrated in Table 20.8. The clearances among models *A*, *B*, and *C* are identical, showing that clearance is site independent and may be calculated through MRT. However, the three-compartment model clearances were clearly different.

$$\text{MRT} = Cl/V_{ss} \quad \textbf{(20.49)}$$

MRT is useful in calculating the steady-state volume of distribution and additional parameters in compartmental and other models. In the compartmental models, MRT may give some idea of how long the drug molecules stay in the peripheral

TABLE 20.9 Mean Residence Time for Different Pharmacokinetic Models

MODEL	MRT
One-compartment bolus IV	$1/k$
One-compartment oral bolus	$1/k_a + 1/k$
Two-compartment bolus IV	$(k_{12} + k_{21})/kk_{21}$[a]
Two-compartment oral bolus	$1/k_a + (k_{12} + k_{21})/kk_{21}$
One-compartment infusion (for τ period)	$1/k + \tau/2$
Two-compartment IV bolus	$\text{AUMC} = A_1/a^2 + A_2/b^2$

[a]Alternatively, this may be calculated as $1/a + 1/b - 1/k_{21}$.

Compiled from Riegelman and Collier (1980) and Yamoaka et al (1978).

compartment. For example, for the drug digoxin, MRT for the body is 49.5 hours; for the central and peripheral compartments, MRT is 3.68 hours and 45.8 hours as calculated (Veng-Pedersen, 1989). The peripheral MRT is the mean total time the drug molecules spend in the peripheral tissue, considering the first entry as well as possibly subsequent entries into the peripheral tissue from the central, general systemic circulation. An overview of MRT values for various pharmacokinetic models is shown in Table 20.9.

MEAN ABSORPTION TIME (MAT) AND MEAN DISSOLUTION TIME (MDT)

After IV bolus injection, the rate of systemic drug absorption is zero, because the drug is placed directly into the bloodstream. The MRT calculated for a drug after IV bolus injection basically reflects the elimination rate processes in the body. After oral drug administration, the MRT is the result of both drug absorption and elimination. The relationship between the *mean absorption time* (MAT) and MRT is given by the following equations:

$$\mathrm{MRT_{oral}} = \mathrm{MAT} + \mathrm{MRT_{iv}} \qquad \textbf{(20.50)}$$

$$\mathrm{MAT} = \mathrm{MRT_{oral}} - \mathrm{MRT_{iv}} \qquad \textbf{(20.51)}$$

For a one-compartment model, $\mathrm{MRT_{iv}} = 1/\mathrm{k}$.

$$\mathrm{MAT} = \mathrm{MRT_{oral}} - 1/k$$

In some cases, IV data are not available and an MRT for a solution may be calculated. The *mean dissolution time* (MDT) or *in vivo* mean dissolution time for a solid drug product is

$$\mathrm{MDT_{solid}} = \mathrm{MRT_{solid}} - \mathrm{MRT_{solution}} \qquad \textbf{(20.52)}$$

MDT reflects the time for the drug to dissolve in vivo. Equation 20.52 calculates the in vivo dissolution time for a solid drug product (tablet, capsule) given orally. MDT has been evaluated for a number of drug products. MDT is most readily estimated for the drugs that follow the kinetics of a one-compartment model. MDT is considered model independent because MRT is model independent. MDT has been used to compare the *in vitro* dissolution versus *in vivo* bioavailability for immediate release and extended release-drug products (Chapters 6 and 7). Even with complete experimental data, the parameters obtained are quite dependent on the method of computation method employed.

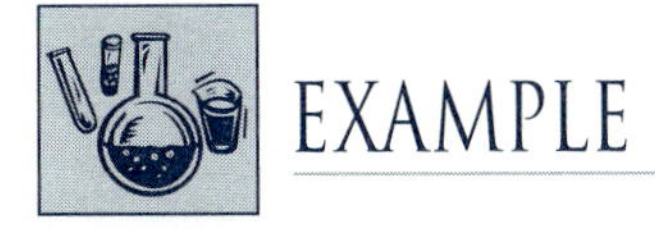

EXAMPLE

Data for ibuprofen (Gillespie et al, 1982) are shown in Table 20.10. Serum concentrations for ibuprofen after a capsule and a solution are tabulated as a function of time in Tables 20.10 and 20.11.

TABLE 20.10 Serum Concentrations for Capsule Ibuprofen

TIME (hr)	C_p	$C_p t$	$tC_p \Delta t$
0	0	0	
0.167	0.06	0.01002	0.000836
0.333	3.59	1.195	0.1000
0.50	7.79	3.895	0.425
1	13.3	13.300	4.298
1.5	14.5	21.750	8.762
2	16.9	33.80	63.887
3	16.6	49.80	41.80
4	11.9	47.60	48.70
6	6.31	37.86	85.46
8	3.54	28.32	66.18
10	1.36	13.60	41.92
12	0.63	7.56	21.16
			Total AUMC = 382.695

$k = 0.347 \text{ hr}^{-1}$, $\text{AUC}_0^\infty = 91.5$

AUMC of tail piece (extrapolation to ∞) $= \frac{C_p' t}{k} + \frac{C_p}{k^2} = \frac{(0.63)(12)}{0.347} + \frac{0.63}{0.347^2}$

$= 21.79 + 5.23 = 27.02$

$\text{AUMC}_0^\infty = 382.695 + 27.02 = 409.72$

$\text{MRT}_{\text{product}} = \frac{409.72}{91.5} = 4.48 \text{ hr}$

Data adapted from Gillespie et al (1982), with permission.

TABLE 20.11 Serum Concentrations for Solution Ibuprofen

TIME (hr)	C_p	$C_p t$	$tC_p \Delta t$
0	0	0	
0.167	17.8	2.973	0.248
0.333	29.0	9.657	1.048
0.5	29.7	14.85	2.046
1	25.7	25.7	10.14
1.5	19.7	29.55	13.81
2	17.0	34.0	15.88
3	11.0	33.0	33.50
4	7.1	28.4	30.70
6	3.82	22.92	51.33
8	1.44	11.52	34.45
10	0.57	5.70	17.22
12	0.38	4.56	10.26
			Total AUMC = 220.64

$k = 0.455 \text{ hr}^{-1}$, $\text{AUC}_0^\infty = 88.5$

AUMC (tailpiece, extrapolation to ∞) $= \frac{C_p t}{k} = \frac{C_p}{k^2} = \frac{(0.38)(12)}{0.455} + \frac{0.38}{0.455^2}$

$= 10.02 + 1.84 = 11.86$

$\text{AUMC}_0^\infty = 220.64 + 11.86 = 232.50 \ (\mu\text{g/mL}) \text{ hr}^2$

$\text{MRT}_{\text{solution}} = \frac{232.50}{88.5} = 2.63 \text{ hr}$

Data adapted from Gillespie et al (1982), with permission.

TABLE 20.12 Parameters for Capsule and Solution Ibuprofen

PARAMETER	UNITS	CAPSULE	SOLUTION
AUC	(μg/mL) hr	92.55	85.50
AUMC	(μg/mL) hr^2	396.1	210.5
k_a	hr^{-1}	0.46	4.90
k	hr^{-1}	0.47	0.437
MRT	hr	4.28	2.49

Parameters were calculated from data of Gillespie et al (1982).

The MRT was determined using the trapezoidal method and Equation 20.43. The MRT for the solution was 2.63 hours and for the product was 4.48 hours. Therefore, MDT for the product is 4.48 − 2.63 = 1.85 hours.

$$\begin{aligned} MAT_{solution} &= MRT_{solution} - 1/k = 2.63 - 1/0.455 = 2.2 \text{ hr} \\ MAT_{product} &= MRT_{product} - 1/k = 4.48 - 1/0.347 \\ &= 4.48 - 2.88 = 1.6 \text{ hr} \end{aligned}$$

Applying Equation 20.52 directly (Riegelman and Collier, 1980),

$$MDT = 4.48 - 2.63 = 1.85 \text{ hr}$$

Alternatively,

$$MDT = MAT_{product} - MAT_{solution} = 2.69 - 2.2 = 0.49 \text{ hr}$$

The MDT obtained for the product differs according to the method of calculation. Therefore, the errors in calculating the elimination constant k may greatly affect the value for MAT and MDT, Equation 20.52 is recommended since it is less affected by k.

When the above data are fitted to an oral one-compartment model and the AUMC and AUC are calculated using Equation 20.34, the results in Table 20.12 are obtained.

SELECTION OF PHARMACOKINETIC MODELS

Several objectives should be considered when using mathematical models to study rate processes such as the pharmacokinetics of a drug. The primary objective in developing a model is to conceptualize the kinetic process in a quantitative manner that can be tested experimentally. A model that cannot be tested is weak and will not improve or yield new knowledge about the process. In contrast, a wrong model may be justified if the hypotheses and its subsequent rejection lead to the correct model. To be statistically vigorous, a hypothesis or model is tested with the null hypothesis (H_0) (Appendix A). Only after rejection of the null hypothesis (tested beyond chance probability) is the hypothesis accepted. When the null hypothesis is rejected, the probability (eg, $p < .05$) means that the chance of error is less than 5% and the hypothesis or model is accepted. In fitting data using linear regression, the correlation of coefficient, r^2, is calculated, where r^2 is an indication of how well the data are predicted by the model. For example, $r = 0.9$ or $r^2 = 0.81$ would indicate 81% of the data agrees with model. The r^2 is not always a very

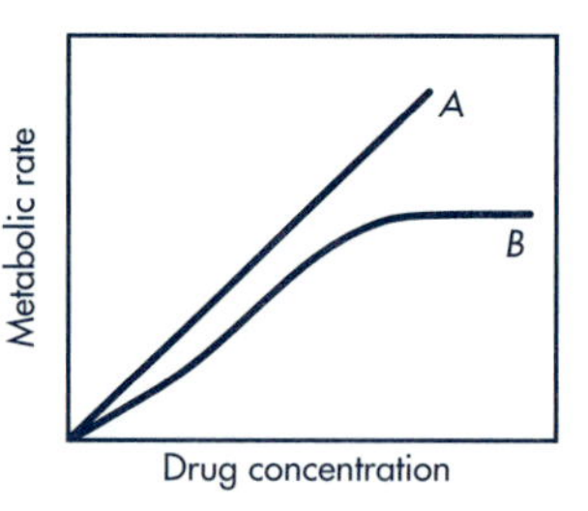

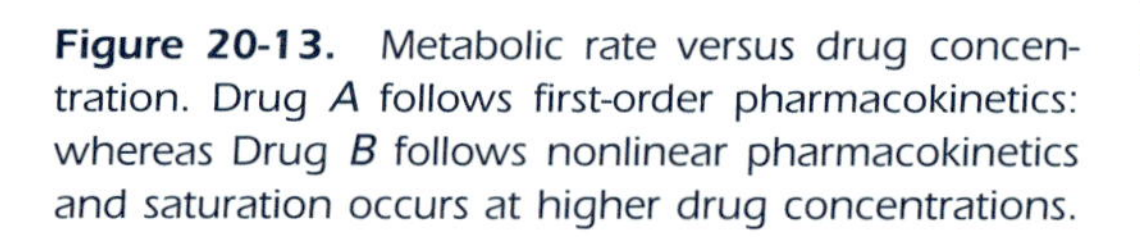

Figure 20-13. Metabolic rate versus drug concentration. Drug *A* follows first-order pharmacokinetics: whereas Drug *B* follows nonlinear pharmacokinetics and saturation occurs at higher drug concentrations.

good criterion; the sums of squared difference (between the observed and predicted data) is a better criterion.

Adequate experimental design and the availability of valid data are important considerations in model selection and testing. For example, the experimental design should determine whether a drug is being eliminated by saturable (dose-dependent) or simple linear kinetics. A plot of metabolic rate versus drug concentration can be done, as in Figure 20-13. Metabolic rate can be measured at various drug concentrations using an *in vitro* system (Chapter 13). In curve B, Figure 20-13, saturation occurs at higher drug concentration.

For illustration, consider the drug concentration versus time profile for a drug given by IV bolus. The combined metabolic and distribution processes may result in profiles like those in Figure 20-14. Curve *A* represents a slow initial decline due to saturation and a faster terminal decline as drug concentration decreases. Curve *C* represents a dominating distributive phase masking the effect of nonlinear metabolism. Finally, a combined process of *A* and *C* may approximate a rough overall linear decline (curve *B*). Notice that the drug concentration versus time profile is shared by many different processes and that the goodness-of-fit is not an adequate criterion for adopting a model. For example, concluding linear metabolism based only on curve *B* would be incorrect. Contrary to common belief, complex models tend to mask opposing variables that must be isolated and tested through better experimental designs. In this case, a constant infusion experiment until steady state would yield information on saturation without the influence of initial drug distribution.

The use of pharmacokinetic models has been critically reviewed by Rescigno and Beck (1987) and Riggs (1963). These authors emphasize the difference between model building and simulation. A model is a secondary system designed to test the primary system (real and unknown). The assumptions in a model must be realistic and consistent with physical observations. On the other hand, a simulation may emulate the phenomenon without resembling the true physical process. A simulation without identifiable support of the physical system does little to aid understanding the basic mechanism. The computation has only hypothetical meaning.

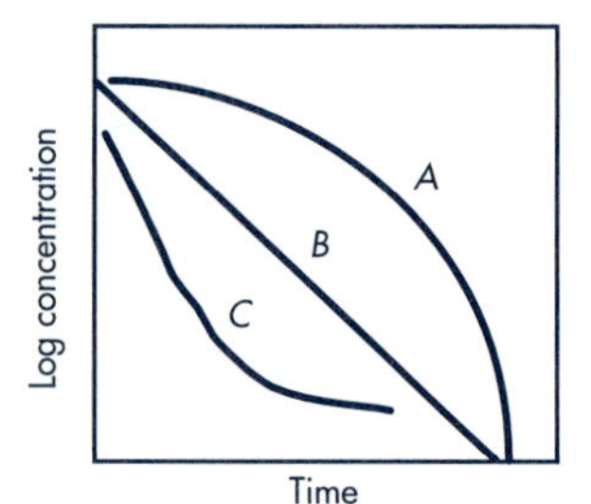

Figure 20-14. Plasma drug concentration profiles due to distribution and metabolic process. (See text for description of *A*, *B*, and *C*.)

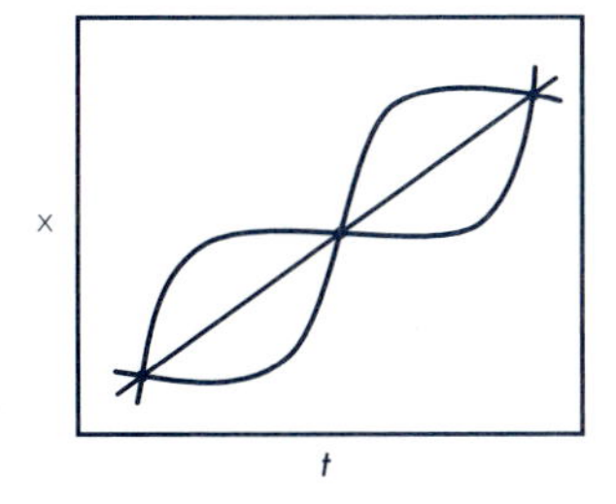

Figure 20-15. Data described by a straight line, a hyperbola, and an equation with trigonometric functions.
(From Roscigno and Beck, 1987, with permission.)

For example, the data in Figure 20-15 may be described by three different equations: a straight line, a hyperbola, and an equation with trigonometric functions. Without physical support, the model gives little understanding of the mechanisms involved. Regression or data fitting (computation of parameters of a given equation so that divergence of the data from the equation is minimized) is considered to be *modulation.* All forms of modulation represent data manipulation and, as such, would decrease information. Information comes from observations and observations only. If more points were available in this example, we could distinguish if the data represent a straight line. Simulations within the realm of data allow for the determination of a quantitative relationship that is useful but does not actually increase understanding of the underlying physiologic processes governing the sojourn of the drug in the body.

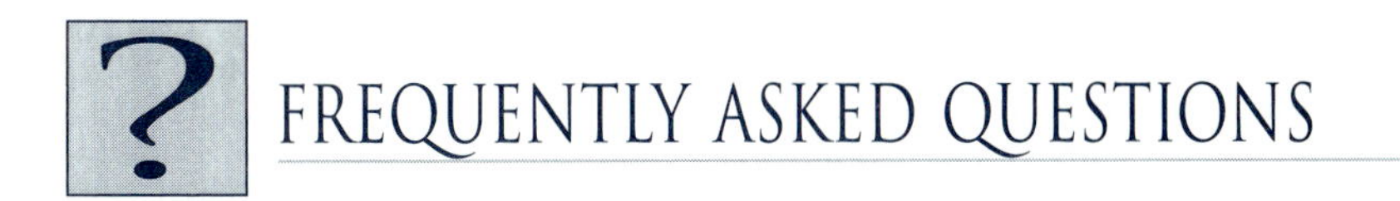

FREQUENTLY ASKED QUESTIONS

1. Why are differential equations used to describe physiologic models?
2. Why do we assume that drug concentrations in venous and arterial blood are the same in pharmacokinetics?
3. Why is statistical moment used in pharmacokinetics?
4. Why is MRT used in pharmacokinetics?

LEARNING QUESTIONS

1. After an intravenous dose (500 mg) of an antibiotic, plasma–time concentration data were collected and the area under the curve was computed to be 20 mg/L·hr. The $AUMC_0^\infty$ area was found to be 100 mg/L·hr^2.
   a. What is the mean residence time of this drug?
   b. What is the clearance of this drug?
   c. What is the steady state volume of distribution of this drug?

2. Why is MRT calculated from moment and AUC curves (ie, $[AUMC]_0^\infty/[AUC]_0^\infty$) rather than $[AUC]_0^\infty/C_0$ directly, as the term was defined in Equation 20.43?
3. If the data in problem 1 are fit to a one-compartment model with an elimination k found to be 0.25 hr, MRT may be calculated simply as $1/k$. What different assumptions are used in problem 3 versus problem 1?
4. What are the principal considerations in interspecies scaling?
5. What are the key considerations in fitting plasma drug data to a pharmacokinetic model?

REFERENCES

Benet LZ, Galeazzi RL: Noncompartmental determination of the steady-state volume of distribution. *J Pharm Sci* **68:**1071–1073, 1979

Benowitz N, Forsyth RP, Melmon KL, Rowland M: Lidocaine disposition kinetics in monkey and man, 1. Prediction by a perfusion model. *Clin Pharmacol Ther* **16:**87–98, 1974

Bischoff KB, Dedrick RL, Zaharko DS: Preliminary model for methotrexate pharmacokinetics. *J Pharm Sci* **59:**149–154, 1970

Bonati M, Latini R, Tognoni G et al: Interspecies comparison of in vivo caffeine pharmacokinetics in man, monkey, rabbit, rat, and mouse. *Drug Metab Rev* **15:**1355–1383, 1985

Boxenbaum H: Evolution biology, animal behavior, fourth-dimensional space, and the raison d'etre of drug metabolism and pharmacokinetics. *Drug Metab Rev* **14:**1057–1097, 1983

Boxenbaum H: Interspecies scaling, allometry, physiological time, and the ground plan of pharmacokinetics. *J Pharmacokinet Biopharm* **10:**201–227, 1982

Chen CN, Andrade JD: Pharmacokinetic model for simultaneous determination of drug levels in organs and tissues. *J Pharm Sci* **65:**717–724, 1976

Gabrielsson J, Bondesson U: Constant-rate infusion of nicotine and cotinine, I. A physiological pharmacokinetic analysis of the cotinine disposition, and effects on clearance and distribution in the rat. *J Pharmacokinet Biopharm* **15:**583–599, 1987

Gillespie WR, Disanto AR, Monovich RE, Albert DS: Relative bioavailability of commercially available ibuprofen oral dosage forms in humans. *J Pharm Sci* **71:**1034–1038, 1982

King FG, Dedrick RL, Farris FF: Physiological pharmacokinetic modeling of *cis*-dichlorodiammineplatinum(II) (DDP) in several species. *J Pharmacokinet Biopharm* **14:**131–157, 1986

Luecke RH, Thomason LE: Physiological flow model for drug elimination interactions in the rat. *Computer Prog Biomed* **11:**88–89, 1980

Lutz RJ, Dedrick RL: Physiological pharmacokinetics: Relevance to human risk assessment. In Li AP (ed), *New Approaches in Toxicity Testing and Their Application in Human Risk Assessment.* New York, Raven, 1985, pp 129–149

Mordenti J, Chappell W: The use of interspecies scaling in toxicology. In Yacobi A, Skelly JP, Batra VK, (eds), *Toxicokinetic and Drug Development.* New York, Pergamon, 1989

Nakashima E, Benet LZ: General treatment of mean residence time, clearance, and volume parameters in linear mammillary models with elimination from any compartment. *J Pharmacokinet Biopharm* **16:**475–492, 1988

Nakashima E, Yokogawa K, Ichimura F et al: A physiologically based pharmacokinetic model for biperiden in animals and its extrapolation to humans. *Chem Pharm Bull* **35:**718–725, 1987

Rescigno A, Beck JS: Perspective in pharmacokinetics and the use and abuses of models. *J Pharmacokinet Biopharm* **15:**327–344, 1987

Riegelman S, Collier P: The application of statistical moment theory to the evaluation of in vivo dissolution time and absorption. *J Pharmacokinet Bipoharm* **8:**509–534, 1980

Riggs DS: *A Mathematical Approach to Physiological Problems.* Baltimore, Williams & Wilkins, 1963

Ritschel WA, Banerjee PS: Physiological pharmacokinetic models: Principles, applications, limitations and outlook. *Meth Find Exp Clin Pharmacol* **8:**603–614, 1986

Sawada Y, Hanano M, Sugiyama Y, Iga T: Prediction of the disposition of nine weakly acidic and six weakly basic drugs in humans from pharmacokinetic parameters in rats. *J Pharmacokinet Biopharm* **13:**477–492, 1985

Veng-Pedersen P: Mean time parameters in pharmacokinetics: Definition, computation and clinical implications, I. *Clin Pharmacol* **17:**345–366, 1989

Yamaoka K, Nakagawa T, Uno T: Statistical moments in pharmacokinetics. *J Pharmacokinet Biopharm* **6:**547–558, 1978

BIBLIOGRAPHY

Banakar UV, Block LH: Beyond bioavailability testing. *Pharm Technol* **7:**107–117, 1983

Benet LZ: Mean residence time in the body versus mean residence time in the central compartment. *J Pharmacokinet Biopharm* **13:**555–558, 1985

Bischoff KB, Dedrick RL, Zaharko DS, Longstreth JA: Methotrexate pharmacokinetics. *J Pharm Sci* **60:**1128–1133, 1971

Boxenbaum H, D'Souza RW: Interspecies pharmacokinetics scaling, biological design and neoteny. In Testa B, D'Souza WD (eds), *Advances in Drug Research.* New York, Academic Press, 1990, vol 19, pp 139–196

Chanter DO: The determination of mean residence time using statistical moments: Is it correct? *J Pharmacokinet Biopharm* **13:**93–100, 1985

Coburn WA, Sheiner LB: Perspective in pharmacokinetics: Pharmacokinetic/pharmacodynamic model: What is it! *J Pharmacokinet Biopharm* **15:**545–555, 1987

Himmelstein KJ, Lutz RJ: A review of the applications of physiologically based pharmacokinetic modeling. *J Pharmacokinet Biopharm* **7:**127–145, 1979

Kasuya Y, Hirayama H, Kubota N, Pang KS: Interpretation and estimation of mean residence time with statistical moment theory. *Biopharm Drug Disposit* **8:**223–234, 1987

Sawada Y, Hanano M, Sugiyama Y, Iga T: Prediction of the disposition of nine weakly acidic and six weakly basic drugs in humans from pharmacokinetic parameters in rats. *J Pharmacokinet Biopharm* **13:**477–492, 1985

Veng-Pedersen P, Gillespie W: The mean residence time of drugs in the systemic circulation. *J Pharm Sci* **74:**791–792, 1985

Wagner JG: Do you need a pharmacokinetic model, and, if so, which one? *J Pharmacokinet Biopharm* **3:**457–478, 1975

Wagner JG: Types of mean residence times. *Biopharm Drug Disp* **9:**41–57, 1988

Wagner JG: Dosage intervals based on mean residence times. *J Pharm Sci* **76:**35–38, 1987

APPENDIX A

STATISTICS

EXPERIMENTAL DESIGN AND COLLECTION OF DATA

All scientific studies must be designed properly to obtain valid conclusions that may be applied to the general population. The experimental design of a study includes the following:

1. A clearly stated hypothesis for the study
2. Assurance that the samples have been randomly selected
3. Control of all experimental variables
4. Collection of adequate data to allow experimental testing of the hypothesis

For example, we want to test the hypothesis that the average weight of young males is greater than that for females in the United States. First, young male and female subjects aged 18 to 24 are selected. The subjects are randomly selected from a pool of subjects who are not interrelated in a way that may affect their weights. A sufficient number of subjects must be selected (sampled) so that the entire population in the country is represented. The need for randomization is easily understood, but poorly met. If all the female subjects in this example were randomly recruited from one health club, the samples would still not be typical of the female population even though the subjects were randomly picked, because many of the subjects exercise at the health club to lose weight. A true sample is one selected randomly from the population of the entire country without connection by any variable that affects their weights. The identification of all covariates in a study is generally difficult and requires thorough consideration. The subject of sample size, inclusion, and exclusion criteria are major considerations in experimental design, which, in its own right, is a very important area in the field of statistics.

Age, gender, genetic background, and health of the subjects are important variables in clinical drug testing. The statistical design of a study is based on the study objectives. Each study should have clearly stated objectives and an appropriate study design indicating how the study is to be performed. Often, the population may be subdivided according to the objectives of the study. For example, a new drug for the treatment of Alzheimer's disease in the elderly might initially be tested in male subjects aged 55 and above. Later clinical studies might test the drug in other patient populations. Many different statistical designs are possible. Some of these designs control experimental variables better than other designs. Specific statistical designs are given in other chapters and in standard statistical texts.

The quality of the data is very important and may be controlled by the researcher and the method of measurement. For example, if the weights of the young males and females in the example above are obtained by using different scales, the investigator must ascertain that each scale weighs the subject accurately. *Accuracy* refers to the closeness of the observation (eg, observed weight) to the actual or true value. *Reproducibility* or *precision* refers to the closeness of repeated measurements.

ANALYSIS AND INTERPRETATION OF DATA

The objective of data analysis is to obtain as much information about the population as possible based on the sample data collected. A common method for analyzing data of a sample population is to classify the data and then plot the frequency of occurrence of all the samples. For example, the frequency of weight distribution of a class of students may be plotted in the form of a histogram, frequency versus weight (Fig. A-1).

An important observation in this example is that the weight of most students lies in the middle of the weight distribution. There is a common tendency for most sample values to occur around the mean. This is described in the *central limit theorem,* which states that the frequency of the values of measurements drawn randomly from a population tends to approximate a bell-shaped curve or normal distribution. Extensive data collection is needed to determine the distributional nature of a sample population. Once the parameters of a distribution are determined, the probability of a given sample's occurring in the population may be calculated.

DESCRIPTIVE TERMS

Descriptive terms are used in statistics to generalize the nature of the data and provide a measure of central tendency. The *mean* or *average* is the sum of the observations divided by the number, *n*, of observations (Table A.1). The *median* is the middle value of the observation between the highest and lowest value. The *mode* is the most frequently occurring value. The term *range* is used to describe the dispersion of the observations and is the difference between the highest and lowest value. For data that are distributed as a normal distribution (discussed below), the mean, median, and mode have the same value.

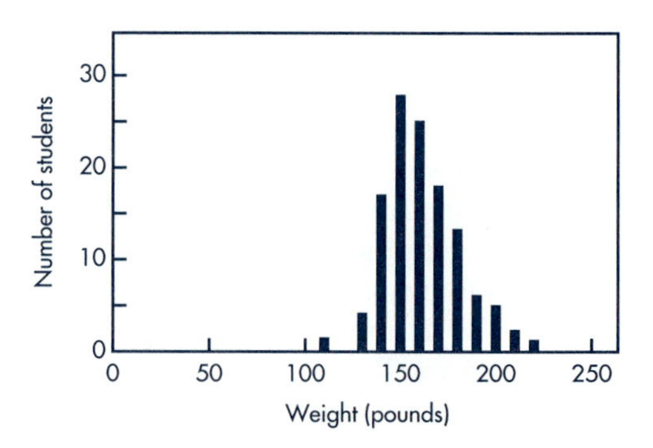

Figure A-1. Weight distribution of 120 students.

TABLE A.1 Descriptive Statistics for a Set of Data[a]

DATA		DESCRIPTIVE TERMS
21	63	Sum = 1274
25	67	Mean = 57.9
29	67	Mode = 67
35	67	Median = 62
37	67	$n = 22$
42	67	Range = 21–91
45	72	SD = 20.3
49	73	RSD = 35.1%
56	75	
57	88	
61	91	

[a]The data represent a set of measurements (observations) in study. The descriptive terms are often used to describe the data. Each term is defined in the text.
SD, standard deviation; RSD, relative standard deviation.

THE NORMAL DISTRIBUTION

If data are plotted according to the frequency of occurrence, a pattern for the distribution of the data is observed. Most data approximate a normal or *Gaussian* distribution. The *normal distribution* is a bell-shaped curve symmetric on both sides of the mean. Statistical tests that assume the data follow normal distribution patterns are known as *parametric tests. Nonparametric tests* do not make any assumption about the central tendency of the data and may be used to analyze data without assuming normal distribution. The shape of the normal distribution is determined by only two parameters, the population mean and the variance, both of which may be estimated from samples. The *variance* is a measure of the spread or variability of the sample. Many biologic and physical random variables are described by the normal distribution (or may be transformed to a normal distribution). These include the weight and height of humans and animal species, the elimination half-lives of many drugs in a population of patients, the duration of a telephone call, and numerous other variables. The item investigated is termed the *random variable* in statistics. For convenience, the standardized normal distribution is introduced to allow easy probability calculation when the standard deviation is known (Fig. A-2). The probability of a sample value occurring from 1 standard deviation above and below the mean is 68% (z of -1 to $+1$). This value is calculated by finding the probability corresponding to $z = -1$ and $z = 1$ from curve B in Figure A-2 as follows:

- Probability between z of -4 to -1 is 0.16.
- Probability between z of -4 to $+1$ is 0.84.
- Therefore, the probability between z of -1 to $+1$ is $0.84 - 0.16 = 0.68$ or 68%.

The area representing probability between any two points on the normal distribution is calculated from this graph. In practice, a cumulative standardized normal distribution table is used to allow better accuracy.

Standard deviation (SD) is a term introduced to measure the variability of a group of data. SD for n number of measurements is calculated according to the following equation:

$$\mathrm{SD} = \sqrt{\frac{(x - \overline{x})^2}{n - 1}} \tag{A.1}$$

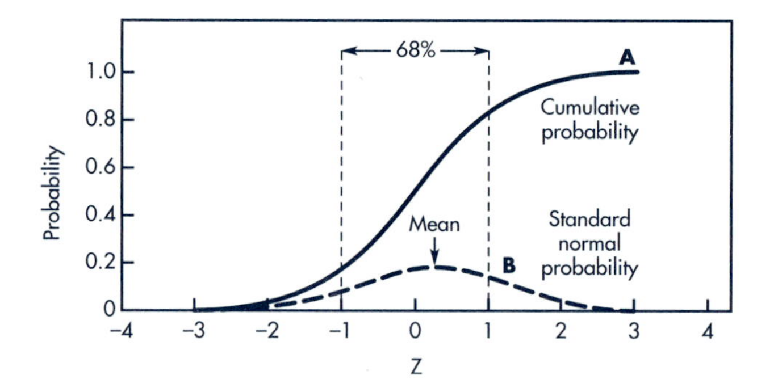

Figure A-2. Probability of a normal distribution. (A = cumulative probability, B = standard normal probability.)

where $\bar{x}$ is the mean, x is the observed value, and n is the number of observations (data). The standard deviation is often calculated by computer or calculator and gives an indication of the spread of data (Fig. A-2). A larger standard deviation indicates that the spread of data about the mean is larger compared to data with the same mean but with a smaller standard deviation.

Relative standard deviation or *coefficient of variation* allows the comparison of variance of measurements. The standard deviation is divided by the mean to give the relative standard deviation (RSD) or coefficient of variation (CV).

$$\text{RSD} = \text{SD}/\bar{x} \tag{A.2}$$

The RSD may be expressed as a percent or %CV by multiplying the RSD by 100. This is commonly known as *percent standard deviation* or percent variation.

The difference between the mean, $\bar{x}$, and each observed datum, x, is the deviation from the mean. Because the deviation from the mean can be either negative or positive, the deviations are squared and summed to give an estimation of the total spread or deviation of the data from the mean. The term $\sum_{i=1}^{n}(x - \bar{x})^2$ is the *sum of the squares.* This term incorporates measurement error as well as inherent variance of the samples. If a single sample is measured several times, the sum of the squares should be very small if the method of measurement is reproducible. The concept of least squares for minimizing error due to model fitting is fundamental in many statistical methods.

CONFIDENCE LIMIT

If normal distribution of the data is assumed, the probability of a random variable within the population can be calculated. For example, data that fall within 1 standard deviation above and below the mean ($\bar{x} \pm 1$ SD) represent approximately 68% of the data, whereas data that fall within 2 standard deviations above and below the mean ($\bar{x} \pm 2$ SD) represent approximately 95% of the data. In the examples below, the random variable in which we are interested is the diameters of drug particles measured from a powdered drug sample lot.

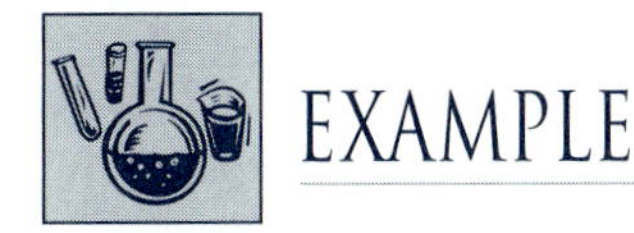

EXAMPLE

The particle size of a powdered drug sample was measured. The average (mean) particle size was 130 μm (microns) with a standard deviation of 20 μm.

1. Determine the range of particle sizes which represent the middle 68% of the powdered drug.

Solution

From a normal distribution table or Figure A-2, 68% of the middle particles represent 34% above and below the mean, corresponding to the mean ±1 SD.

Small particle size = mean − SD = 130 − 20 = 110 μm
Large particle size = mean + SD = 130 + 20 = 150 μm

Therefore, 68% of the particles would have a particle size ranging from 110 to 150 μm.

2. Determine the range of particle sizes that would represent the middle 95% of the powdered drug.

Solution

95%/2 or 47.5% on each side of the mean, corresponding to ±2 SD (Fig. A-2).

Smallest particle size = 130 − (2 × 20) = 90 μm
Largest particle size = 130 + (2 × 20) = 170 μm

Therefore, 95% of the particles would have a particle size ranging from 90 to 170 μm.

In the above example, the calculation shows that most of the particles in the population lie around the mean: to be 95% certain, simply extend from the mean ±2 SD. This approach estimates the *95% confidence limit.* A 95% confidence limit implies that if an experiment is performed 100 times, 95% of the data will be in this range above and below the mean.

The example shows how to reconstruct the population based on the two parameters *mean* and *variance* (approximated by the SD). A more common application is the estimation of experimental data such as assay measurements. Such 95% confidence limits are often calculated from the SD to estimate the reliability of the assay measurement.

In the example given above, the mean for the particle size was 130 μm and the SD is 20 μm. Therefore, from equation A.2, the RSD = 20/130 or 0.15. The RSD may be expressed as a percent or %CV by multiplying the RSD by 100.

As mentioned, *accuracy* refers to the agreement with the observed value or measurement in a group of data and the actual or true value of the population.

Unfortunately, the true value is unknown for many studies. The term *precision* refers to the reproducibility of the data or the variation within a set of measurements. Data that are less precise demonstrate a larger variance or a larger relative standard deviation compared to more precise data, which have a smaller variance.

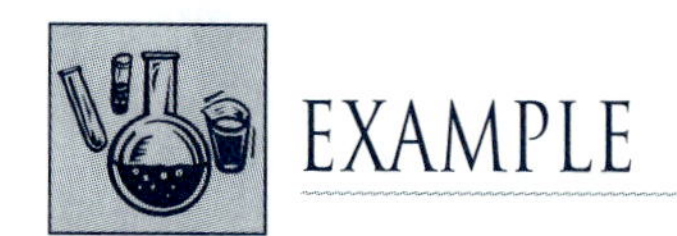

EXAMPLE

A lot of 10 mg tablets was assayed five times by three students (Fig. A-3). Which student most accurately assayed the tablets?

	WEIGHT OF TABLETS (MG)		
ASSAY	STUDENT A	STUDENT B	STUDENT C
1	9.8	13	14
2	10.3	13	14.1
3	10.4	9.9	13.9
4	9.9	7	14
5	10	9.5	14.2
Mean	10.08	9.68	14.04
SD	0.26	4.08	0.11
%SD	2.6	42.1	0.78

Solution

The mean and SD of assays for each student were determined. Because the same lot was assayed, the difference in SD among the students is attributed to assay variations. Student A is closest to the target—that is, the labeled claimed dose, LCD of 10 mg. Student C is most precise (with the smallest %SD) but consistently off target.

The data obtained by student *C* is considered *biased* since all the observed data is above 10 mg. Data is also considered biased if all the observed data were below the true value of 10 mg.

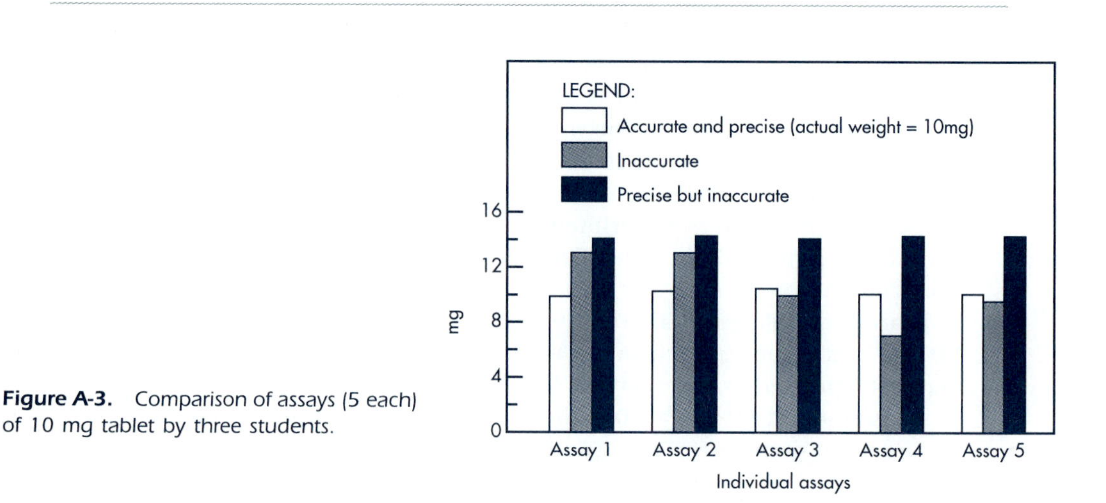

Figure A-3. Comparison of assays (5 each) of 10 mg tablet by three students.

The term *bias* refers to a systematic error when the measurement is consistently not on target. Repeated measurements may be very reproducible (precise) but miss the target. In the example above, student C was most precise, but student A was most accurate. In determining accuracy and precision, a standard (known sample) is usually prepared and assayed several times to determine the variation due to assay errors. In the example above, we assumed that the students used *known* 10 mg standard tablets. If the tablet is an unknown sample, it would not be possible to conclude which student is more accurate, because the true value is unknown. In practice, assay methods are validated for precision and accuracy based on known standards before unknown samples (eg, plasma samples) are assayed.

In the analysis and interpretation of data, statistics makes inferences about a population using experimental data gathered in a sample. After analysis of data, the statistician calculates the likelihood or probability that a given result would happen. *Probability* (P) is the fraction of the population indicating that a given result or event would occur by random sampling or chance. For example, if $P < 0.05$, then the likelihood that a result occurs by random sampling is 5/100, 1/20, or 5%. By convention, if the statistical inference produces a P value of 0.05 or less, it is considered atypical or uncommon of the population. As shown in Figure A-1, the probability of finding a student weighing above 250 lb is small ($P < 0.05$), and we may conclude (somewhat erroneously) that a student who weighs >250 lb is *significantly* different from the rest. This concept for determining the probability of how typical a given sample value occurs in a population may be extended to hypothesis testing. *Hypothesis testing* estimates the probability of whether a given value is typical of the control group or of the treated group.

STATISTICAL DISTRIBUTIONS

The frequency distribution of some data do not appear to be symmetrically shaped. The term *skewness* relates to the assymetry of the data. The data distribution may be skewed to the left or right of the mean. In many pharmacological studies, the sample size in the study is small, and the investigator cannot always be certain that the data obtained from the study are normally distributed. An incorrect assumption of a normal distribution may lead to a biased conclusion. In such cases, a nonparametric test may be used since it does not make any assumption about the underlying test except that it be continuous.

During data analysis, a value or observation may be observed that is several standard deviations above or below the mean; such a value is considered an *outlier.* A value that is an outlier is difficult to use statistically. In general, outlier values should not be excluded from the statistical analysis. Some investigators use *log transformation* of the data to make the distribution of the data appear to be more normally distributed. A *geometric mean* is then obtained after log transformation of the data. In some cases, with sufficient data collection, a *bimodal distribution* may be observed. For example, the acetylation of isoniazide in humans follows a bimodal distribution indicating two populations consisting of fast acetylators and slow acetylators, respectively. In this study, if the data were obtained from subjects of whom all but one subject were fast acetylators, then the single data for the slow acetylator might be considered an outlier (and possibly be discarded from the data analysis).

HYPOTHESIS TESTING

Hypothesis testing is an objective way of analyzing the data and determining whether the data support or reject the hypothesis postulated. For example, we may want to test the hypothesis that a given steroid causes a weight increase. We may want to test this hypothesis using two groups of healthy volunteers, one group (treated) who took the given steroid and the other (control) who took no drug. The two hypotheses generated are as follows:

- H_0: There is no difference in weight between the treated and control group (*null hypothesis*).
- H_1: There is a difference in weight between the treated and control groups (*alternative hypothesis*).

The data will either reject or fail to reject (accept) the null hypothesis. If the null hypothesis is rejected, then the alternative hypothesis is accepted, as there are only two possibilities. A simple hypothesis testing data from two groups is the two-sample *Student t-test* involving a control group and a treated group (the t distribution approximates the normal distribution and is commonly used). The data for the study (simulated) are shown in Figure A-4 using 120 students in the control and treated groups. The mean weight of the treated group is about 175 lb, whereas the mean weight for the control group is about 155 lb. There is a shift to the right in the weight distribution of the treated group. However, a considerable overlapping (shaded area) in weights is observed, making it difficult to reject the null hypothesis. In practice, H_0 is rejected at a known level of uncertainty called *level of significance.* A level of 5% (α = 0.05) is considered statistically significant, and a level of 1% (α = 0.01) is considered highly significant. Commonly, this level of significance is reported as $P < 0.05$ or $P < 0.01$ to indicate the different levels of significance. Because uncertainty is involved, whenever the null hypothesis is rejected or accepted, the level of significance is stated. A significance level of 25% ($P < 0.25$) in the above example suggests that there is a 25% probability that the weight change is not due to drug treatment. A 25% probability is a level far too large to reject the H_0 with certainty. The level of significance is therefore related to the probability of incorrectly rejecting H_0 when it should have been accepted. This level of error is called *Type I error.* Whenever a decision is made, there is the possibility of making the wrong decision. Four possible decisions for a statistical test may be made (Table A.2). A Type II error is committed when H_0 is accepted as being true when it should have been rejected. In contrast, a *Type I error* is committed when H_0 is rejected when it should have been accepted.

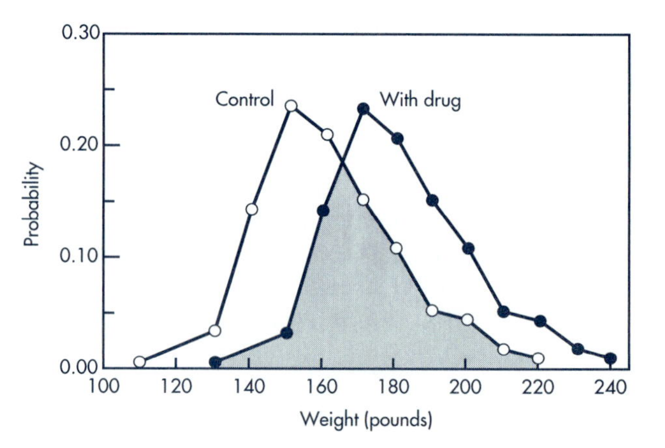

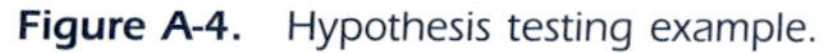
Figure A-4. Hypothesis testing example.

TABLE A.2. Decisions Based on a Statistical Test

	ACCEPT NULL HYPOTHESIS (H_0)	REJECT NULL HYPOTHESIS (H_0)
H_0 true	Correct decision	Type I error
H_1 true	Type II error	Correct decision

The probability of committing a Type I error is defined as the significance level of the statistical test, and is denoted as P or α (alpha). The probability of a Type II error, denoted as β (beta), can also be computed.

The *power test* determines the probability that the statistical test results in the rejection of the null hypothesis if H_0 is really false. The larger the power, the more sensitive the tests. Because power is defined as $1 - \beta$, the larger the β error (Type II error), the weaker the power. The power of the test would equal $1 - \beta$ for a particular power.

To reduce Type I or Type II errors, the sample size needs to be increased or the assay method improved. Because time, expense, and ethical concerns for performing a study may be important issues, the investigator generally tries to keep the sample size (usually the number of subjects in a clinical study) to a minimum. The variability within the samples, number of samples (sample size), and desired level of significance will affect the power of the statistical test. Usually, the greater the variability within the samples, the larger the sample size needed to obtain sufficient power.

ANALYSIS OF VARIANCE (ONE-WAY)

When more than two data sets are compared, ANOVA or analysis of variance is used to determine the probability of the data sets being identical or different among groups. One-way analysis of variance (ANOVA) is a method for testing the differences between the population means of k treatment groups, where each group $i(i = 1, 2, \ldots k)$ consists of n_i observations X_{ij} $(j = 1, 2, \ldots n_i)$. For example, we may want to test if there is a difference in the peak plasma level of a drug resulting from the administration of three different dosage forms—solution, capsule, and tablet. If we decide to have 3 groups of 20 patients per group, $i = 1, 2, 3, j = 1, 2, \ldots 20$, and the observation in each group would be X_{ij}. The formulas for calculation are as follows:

$$\text{Sum of observation in group } i = \sum_{j=1}^{nj} X_{ij}$$

$$\text{Total sum of squares SS} = \sum_{i=1}^{k}\sum_{j=1}^{ni} X_{ij}^2 - \frac{\left(\sum_{i=1}^{k}\sum_{j=1}^{ni} X_{ij}\right)^2}{\sum_{i=1}^{k} n_i}$$

$$\text{Treatment sum of squares TSS} = \sum_{i=1}^{k} \frac{\left(\sum_{j=1}^{ni} X_{ij}\right)^2}{n_i} - \frac{\left(\sum_{i=1}^{k}\sum_{j=1}^{ni} X_{ij}\right)^2}{\sum_{i=1}^{k} n_i}$$

$$\text{Error sum of squares} = \text{ESS} = \text{SS} - \text{TSS}$$

The value of the F statistic is

$$F = \frac{DF_2 \times TSS}{DF_1 \times FSS}$$

$$\text{Treatment degree of freedom } DF_1 = k - 1$$

$$\text{Error degrees of freedom } DF_2 = \sum_{j=1}^{k} n_i - k$$

The ANOVA employed depends upon the objectives and design of the study. ANOVA methods can estimate the variance between different subjects (intersubject variability), groups, or treatments. Using the ANOVA, the statistician determines whether to accept or reject the null hypothesis (H_0), deciding whether there is no significant difference (accept H_0) or there is a significant difference (reject H_0) between the data groups.

After completion of the study and statistical analysis of the data, the investigator must decide whether any statistically significant differences in the data groups have clinical relevance. For example, it may be possible to demonstrate that a new antihypertensive agent lowers the systolic blood pressure in patients by 10 mm Hg and that this effect is statistically significant ($P < 0.05$) using the appropriate statistical test. From these results and statistical treatment of the data, the principal investigator must decide whether the study is clinically relevant and whether the drug will be efficacious for its intended use. An example of ANOVA appears in Chapter 10, Table 10.5.

APPENDIX B

APPLICATION OF COMPUTERS IN PHARMACOKINETICS

The availability of computers has greatly accelerated the development of pharmacokinetics. The main contributions of computer technology have been the easy solution of complicated pharmacokinetic equations and the ability to rapidly model pharmacokinetic processes. Computers automate many mundane tasks and allow more time for experimental work. Other pharmacokinetic computer applications include the development of experimental study designs, statistical data treatment, data manipulation, graphical representation of data, pharmacokinetic model simulation, and projection or prediction of drug action. Furthermore, computers are used frequently for written reports and documentation.

The classification of the computers used in pharmacokinetics is difficult. Generally, computers are divided into three major groups: mainframe computers, minicomputers, and microcomputers. Microcomputers are also known as personal computers (PCs). Minicomputers have intermediate computing power while mainframe computers generally have a large central processing unit (CPU). Both mainframe computers and minicomputers can be shared to perform multiple tasks simultaneously. Increasingly, many PCs are linked together into local networks (LAN) that share many application software packages.

Each type of computer runs under an operating systems (OS), which is a collection of programs that allocate resources and enable algorithms (well-defined rules or processes for solving a problem in a finite number of steps) to be processed. UNIX and WINDOWS are examples of commonly used operating systems. The first generation of PCs used a disk operating system (DOS) which tracks operations for many small personal computers. Most PCs now have Windows 98, 95, or Windows 3.x.

Windows NT is used mostly in network systems that link many PCs. Most PCs today are equipped with a modem to allow access to remote information. Netscape and Microsoft Internet Explorer are browsers that allow PCs to access remote information at various sites in the Internet referred to as Websites. Much information and many applications are now available specifically for pharmacists and pharmacokineticists. Some examples are listed below. Many programs are now also designed to run with a minimum of programming knowledge.

A program of instructions known as a computer package or software is written in a computer language. This software is needed to run the computer. The computer operating system must support the computer language of the software. Common computer languages supported by many computers include Fortran, BASIC, Pascal, and C. BASIC, because of its easy programming of many computations, is particularly suited for beginners. Fortran is somewhat harder to use because of its often strict syntax and format. Pascal is easy to learn and powerful for both number crunching (data manipulation) and string manipulations. The language C is generally reserved for software or system development. With the great number of computer programs available. However, very little computer programming is required for many applications in pharmacokinetics.

PHARMACOKINETIC SOFTWARE

Pharmacokinetic software consists of computer programs designed for computation and easy solution of pharmacokinetic problems. Not all computer programs satisfy the user's full requirements, but many provide the following:

1. Fitting drug concentration versus time data to a series of pharmacokinetic models, and choosing the one that best describes the data statistically.

   Typically, a least-squares program is employed, in which the sum of squared differences between observed data points and theoretic prediction is minimized. Usually, a mathematical procedure is used *iteratively* (repetitively) to achieve a minimum in the sum of squares (convergence). Some data may allow easier convergence with one procedure rather than another. The mathematical method employed should be reviewed prior to use.
2. Fitting data into a pharmacokinetic or pharmacodynamic model defined by the user.

   This method is by far the most useful, because any list of prepared models is often limited. The flexibility of user-defined models allows continuous refinement of the model as new experimental information become available. Some software merely provides a utility program for fitting the data to a series of polynomials. This utility program provides a simple, quantitative way of relating the variables, but offers little insight into the underlying pharmacokinetic processes.
3. Simulation.

   Some software programs generate data based on a model with parameter input by the user. When the parameters are varied, new data are generated based on the model chosen. The user is able to observe how the simulated model data matches the experimental observed data. Because pharmacokinetic processes are conveniently described by systems of differential equations, the simulation process involves a numerical solution of the equation with predefined precision.
4. Experimental design.

   To estimate the parameters of any model, the experimental design of the study must be sufficient for the collected data to have points appropriately spaced to allow curve description and modeling. Although statisticians greatly stress the need for proper experimental design, little information is generally available for experimental design in pharmacokinetics when a study is performed for the first time. For the first pharmacokinetic study, an empirical or a statistical experiment design are both necessarily based on assumptions that may later prove to be wrong.

5. Clinical Pharmacokinetic applications.

   Some software programs are available for the clinical monitoring of narrow therapeutic index drugs (ie, critical dose drugs) such as the aminoglycosides, other antibiotics, theophylline, antiarrythmics, etc. These programs may include calculations for creatinine clearance using Cockcroft and Gault equation (see Chapter 18), dosage estimation, pharmacokinetic parameter estimation for the individual patient and pharmacokinetic simulations.

VALIDATION OF SOFTWARE PACKAGES

Software used for data analysis such as statistical and pharmacokinetic calculations should be validated with respect to the accuracy, quality, integrity, and security of the data. One approach for determining the accuracy of the data analysis is to compare the results obtained from two different software packages using the same set of data (Heatherington et al, 1998). Due to different functionalities of the software packages, different results (eg, pharmacokinetic parameter estimates) may be obtained.

PERSONAL COMPUTERS (PCs)

Two major types of personal computers are currently used including (1) the IBM or IBM-compatible PC and (2) the Apple or Macintosh PC. Many of the IBM-compatible PCs are supported by the DOS or Windows operating system by Microsoft. The CPU (central processing unit) of a PC is a computer chip (8086 chip for the old IBM-XTs, 80286 for IBM-ATs, or 80386 or 80486, and the new Pentium PCs). PCs are also equipped with one or more floppy disk drives that magnetically record information onto floppy disks for storage. Most computers also have a hard disk drive, which records information on a different type of disk and is usually permanently installed in the computer. The hard disk starts at 10 or 20 megabytes, and now up to 8 gigabytes (1000 mega) of information in some of the new PCs. (A double-spaced typed page takes up about 2 kilobytes). Floppy disks store from 180 kilobytes to 1.4 megabytes of information depending on the type of disk and disk drives. Older floppy drives that used 5.25-inch disks have been replaced mostly by the more compact 3.5-inch disk drives. All disks must be formatted before use in the computer. Floppy disk drives are usually named "a:" and "b:" while the hard drive is commonly named the "c:" drive. Additional drives are alphabetically designated. For example, a CD-ROM drive may be labeled "d:" drive.

Older PCs have comparatively little random access memory (RAM) and limited space on the hard disk and do not meet the memory and speed requirements for current software packages. New PCs may contain more than 32 megabytes of RAM depending on the system requirements. Most PCs that features multimedia require a lot of RAM. The software is generally installed on the hard disk, while the floppy drive(s) for data input and transfer. Some software requires special co-processor. Newer versions of operating systems are continuously being developed, and software based on newer versions of DOS may not run on older versions. Windows 95, Windows 98, and Windows NT (Microsoft) are examples of newer operating systems. Windows operating system allows programs to be installed and run easily by "pointing to and clicking menus" on screen using a mouse. Actions are performed when the user simply clicks the mouse after selecting a command.

The Apple PC series includes the Macintosh Apple PCs and iMac, which have their own operating systems. Software written for IBM systems do not run on most of these PCs, although the Power Mac runs some DOS based programs. In general, MAC computers are easier to use. There is always a menu of instructions for the MAC user, although the differences between the two types of PCs are diminishing.

Software Descriptions

Some of the commercially available computer software programs are listed below. The descriptions may not represent the latest versions. New features are often added or old features improved. The user should contact the program vendors directly for more information. See below for information about Internet resources, including user evaluations of software packages.

- PCNonlin
  Scientific Consulting, Inc.
  5625 Dillard Rd. Suite 215
  Cary, NC 27511
  http://www.sciconsulting.com
  PCNonlin is a powerful least-squares program for parameter estimation. Both a user-defined model and a library of over 20 compartmental models are available. The program accepts both differential and regular (analytical) equations. Users may select the Hartley-modified or Levenberg-type Gauss–Newton algorithm or the (Nelder and Mead) simplex algorithm for minimizing the sum of squared residuals. Some training is needed. Prior to commercial release, Nonlin was mostly installed on mainframe computers. PCNonlin includes additional features and was designed to run on PCs. PCGRAPH (Version 4) was bundled to improve the quality of the plots from previous versions of Nonlin. Compartmental models, curve fitting, and simulations are specially designed for pharmacokinetics.

  WinNonlin is a new version with an improved user interface that makes it easier to use and to interface with other Windows applications. WinNonlin is relatively easy to use for modeling or noncompartmental analysis of data files. WinNonlin handles large numbers of subjects or profiles. WinNonlin's input and output data are managed via Excel (Microsoft) compatible spreadsheet files. While WinNonlin will run on a Windows system with at least 4 megabytes RAM, 8 megabytes RAM are recommended. The Noncompartmental Analysis module computes derived PK parameters (eg, AUC_0^t, AUC_0^∞, C_{max}, cumulative excretion, etc). PCNonlin's extensive libraries of models for nonlinear regression and parameter estimation are present in this software. Standard descriptive statistics and confidence intervals are determined from datasets.
- SAS
  SAS Institute, Inc.
  Cary, NC 27511
  (919) 677-8000
  www.sas.com
  An all-purpose data analysis system with a flexible application-development language, SAS graph allows for multidimension plots, for bar, pie, and contour charts, and for all sorts of graphs. Over 5000 SAS products are reported to be

available. Various "procs" (subroutines) are available for statistics as well as general linear and nonlinear regression models. There are over 80 procedures for univariate descriptive statistics; *t*-test, chi square, correlation, autoregression, multidimensional scaling, nonparametric test, factor analysis, and discriminant and stepwise analysis. SAS runs in many user environments including PCSAS for personal computers. A special startup interface, ASSIST will facilitate beginners who are unfamiliar with the default batch data entry.

- RSTRIP
  MicroMath
  PO Box 21550
  Salt Lake City, UT 84121
  RSTRIP is menu driven and very suitable for student use; it fits data to models, mono-, bi-, and tri-exponentials based on model selection criteria (Akaike Information Criteria). A good statistics menu is available for AUC, C_{max}, T_{max}, and MRT. The program gives initial parameter estimates and final parameters after iteration. The program does not handle differential equations or user-defined models. Plot outputs are available, as are pharmacokinetic curve stripping, and least-squares parameter optimization. IBM PC-XT or PC-compatibles with math chip.
- PKAnalyst for Windows
  This program is a bundled pharmacokinetic software incorporating many features of RSTRIP but with more statistics and mathematical functions. The program uses Windows and is generally easier to use. The software is available from MicroMath Scientific Software. This program is very user friendly for routine data analysis in pharmacokinetics.
- DIFFEQ and DIFFEQ Pharmacokinetics Library
  MicroMath Scientific Software
  PO Box 21550
  Salt Lake City, UT 84121
  DIFFEQ is a nonlinear least-squares program for PCs. Model entry uses a generic language with syntax similar to BASIC; it may be used with DIFFEQ Pharmacokinetic Library, which includes many models used in pharmacokinetics.
- P-STAT
  P-Stat Inc.
  Princeton, NJ 08540
  (609) 924-9100
  This program supplies statistical data handling for mainframe computers.
- STELLA
  High Performance Systems
  Lyme, NH 03755
  (603) 643-9636
  STELLA is a structural thinking experimental learning laboratory with animation available for Windows-based PCs. The program was developed on the MAC. STELLA solves differential equations, simulates pharmacokinetic model and other physiologic systems. The software is particularly suitable for teaching because of its animation and learning simulation by drawing the model.
- NONMEM
  NONMEM Project Group, C255
  University of California
  San Francisco, CA 94143
  NONMEM (Nonlinear Mixed Effects Model) developed by S.L. Beal and L.B.

Sheiner is a statistical program used for fitting parameters in population pharmacokinetics. The NONMEM program first appeared in 1979. It is useful in evaluating relationships between pharmacokinetic parameters and demographic data such as age, weight, and disease state. Average population parameters and intersubject variance are estimated. The program fits the data of all the subjects simultaneously and estimates the parameters and their variances. The parameters are useful in estimating doses for individuals based on population pharmacokinetics with calculated risks. A regression program is written in ANSI (American National Standards Institute) Fortran 77 for mainframe computers.

The current version of NONMEM (Version IV) consists of several parts. The NONMEM program itself is a general (noninteractive) regression program which can be used to fit many different types of data. PREDPP consists of subroutines that can be used by NONMEM to compute predictions for population pharmacokinetics. NM-TRAN is a preprocessor, allowing control and other needed inputs and error messages to NONMEM/PREDPP.

- P-PHARM
  Simed
  Creteil, France
  http://www.simed@bioscience.com
  P-PHARM is a population pharmacokinetic-pharmacodynamic data modeling program using a two stage procedure (rich data) and/or EM-type algorithm (sparse data).
- MKMODEL
  Biosoft
  PO Box 10398
  Ferguson, MO
  MKMODEL, by N. Holford, is a pharmacokinetic program from the National Institutes of Health-supported PROPHET system. The program, available for the PC, performs nonlinear least-squares regression and includes both pharmacokinetic and pharmacodynamic models (effect compartment).
- ADAPT II
  D.Z. D'Argenio and A. Schumitzky
  Biomedical Simulation Resource
  University of Southern California
  Los Angeles, CA
  Supplied as FORTRAN code for various operating systems, this program performs simulations, nonlinear regression, and optimal sampling, and includes extended least squares and Bayesian optimization. Models can be expressed as integrated or differential equations.
- USC*PACK PC PROGRAMS
  USC Laboratory of Applied Pharmacokinetics
  2250 Alcazar St, (CSC 134B), Los Angeles, CA 90033.
  http://www.usc.edu/hsc/lab_apk
  The software package consists of various pharmacokinetic programs bundled for clinical pharmacokinetic applications and model parameter estimation. The NPEM2 program (Version 3) is an improved version of the nonparametric expectation maximization algorithm well adapted for population pharmacokinetics. The program is now available for a three-compartment model with various routes of dosing. Lahey Fortran F77EM32 and its associated package is used in this program.

  Clinical programs include related routines in which past therapy data of indi-

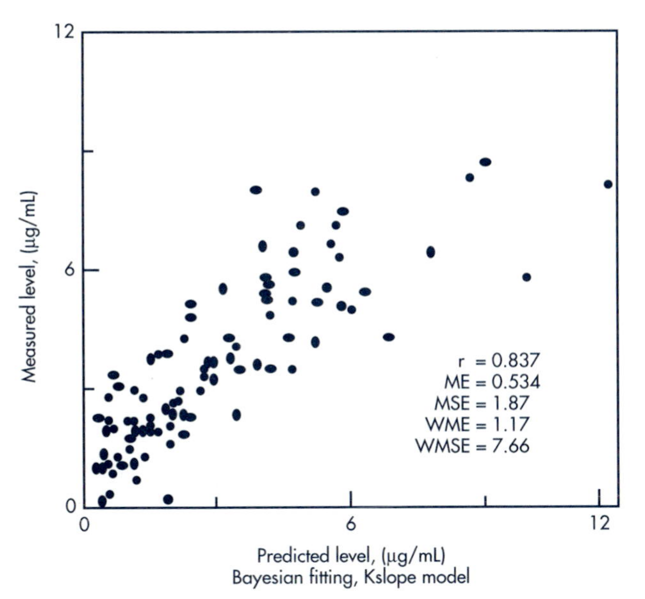

FIGURE B-1. An example of Gentamicin dosing prediction in patients using MAP Bayesian fitting and K slope method (one compartment): Predicted versus measured serum gentamicin. (r = correlation coefficient, ME = mean error, MSE = mean squared error, WME = mean weighted error. WMSE = weighted mean squared error.) (From Jelliffe et al, 1995, with permission.)

vidual patients are entered into files along with parameter and dose-prediction programs for various drugs (eg, aminoglycosides, other antibiotics, and drugs of special interest). Bayesian-fitting procedures are included to fit a selected drug population model to a patient's data of doses and serum concentrations and to adaptive control of the individual dose regimen. Some program selections include:

a. Amikacin (Amik)
b. Gentamicin (Gent)
c. Netilmicin (Net)
d. Tobramycin (Tob)
e. Bayesian General Modeling (MB)
f. Least-Squares General Modeling (MLS)

Many patient-oriented programs for adaptive dosing based on pharmacokinetics and pharmacodynamic are featured in the package. Maximum Aposteriori Probability (MAP) Bayesian Fitting is useful in individual dosing; an example is shown in Figure B-1 for gentamicin dose prediction. This method yields better prediction than conventional clinical methods even in patients with unstable renal function.

PHARMACOKINETIC PROGRAMS ON THE INTERNET

Various pharmacokinetic programs are available on the Internet. These programs may not have been validated by the programmer. Thus, the user is responsible for validating the program. Dr. David Bourne of the University of Oklahoma has compiled a listing of pharmacokinetic programs, general references in pharmacokinetics and pharmacokinetics and other information. The Website http://www.cpb.uokhsc.edu/pkin/soft.html lists numerous pharmacokinetic software packages with user comments. Students should consult the site for updated information.

OTHER PHARMACOKINETIC PROGRAMS

Other pharmacokinetic programs include:

- FUNFIT A parameter estimation regression program.
- LAGRAN A parameter estimation regression program.
- MATLAB A powerful program that handles complex models, mostly in chemical engineering but found useful in pharmacokinetics.
- SAAM A program for pharmacokinetics and other biological models that was developed at NIH.
- TOPFIT A pharmacokinetic program with both data fitting and clinical application.
- BIOPAK A pharmacokinetic program available from SCI Software, for bioavailability / bioequivalence studies.
- BOOMER/MULTI-FORTE A simulation program by D.W.A. Bourne, College of Pharmacy, University of Oklahoma.

GENERAL COMPUTATION SOFTWARE

For general computation, many programs, such as the electronic spreadsheets are very adaptable to calculation and pharmacokinetic curve plotting. Spreadsheet software programs such as Lotus 1-2-3, Quattro, VisiCalc, SuperCalc, and Microsoft Excel are easy to use.

Data are entered in columns (referred to alphabetically as A, B, C . . .) and rows (numerically referred to as 1, 2, 3, . . .). Manuals are generally displayed on screen and can be selected by moving the arrow keys followed by pressing the "return" or "enter" key. An example of a Microsoft Excel worksheet used to generate time versus concentration data after *n* doses of a drug given orally according to a one-compartment model is given in Figure B-2. The parameter inputs are in column B, time is in column D, and concentration is in column E.

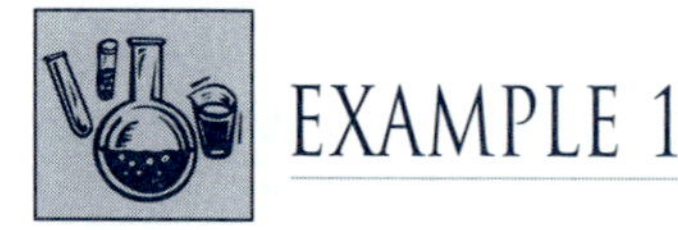

EXAMPLE 1

From a series of time–concentration data (Figure B-3, rows A and B), determine the elimination rate constant using the regression feature of Lotus 1-2-3.

Solution

a. Type in the time and concentration data shown in columns A and B (Fig. B-3).

b. Convert in column C all concentration data to ln concentration. Data point #1 may be omitted because ln of zero cannot be determined.

c. From the main menu, select stepwise:
Data
Regression
X-data range
Output range

	A	B	C	D	E	F
1	D	100000		0	0.00	
2	KA	2		0.1	1.78	
3	K	0.4		0.2	3.16	
4	V	10000		0.3	4.23	
5	TAU	4		0.4	5.04	
6	F	1		0.5	5.64	
7	N	1		0.6	6.07	
8	EXP(-KA*TAU	0.00033546		0.7	6.36	
9	EXP(-K*TAU)	0.20189652		0.8	6.55	
10	FKAD	200000		0.9	6.65	
11	V(K-KA)	-16000		1	6.69	
12	AA	1		1.1	6.67	
13	BB	1		1.2	6.60	
14				1.3	6.50	
15	FD/VK	25	AUC	1.4	6.38	
16				1.5	6.24	
17	FD/V...	8.86435343	Cmax-ss	1.6	6.08	
18				1.7	5.92	
19				1.8	5.74	
20	TMAX	1.0058987	tmax-1	1.9	5.57	
21				2	5.39	
22				2.1	5.21	
23	TMAX-SS	0.86516026	tmax-ss	2.2	5.03	
24				2.3	4.86	
25				2.4	4.68	
26				2.5	4.51	
27				2.6	4.35	
28				2.7	4.19	
29				2.8	4.03	
30				2.9	3.88	
31				3	3.73	
32				3.1	3.59	
33				3.2	3.45	
34				3.3	3.32	
35				3.4	3.19	
36				3.5	3.07	
37				3.6	2.95	
38				3.7	2.84	
39				3.8	2.73	
40				3.9	2.62	
41			tmin	4	2.52	Cmin
42						
43						
44						
45						
46						
47	PARAMETER	PARAM. VAL	PHARM-TERM	TIME (HRS)	CONC (MCG/ML)	

FIGURE B-2. Example of a Microsoft Excel spreadsheet used to calculate time–concentration data according to an oral one-compartment model after N doses.

Go
Use the arrow key to indicate the data range (only 4 points used in the terminal phase of the curve).

d. The slope, given in cell F-19, is −0.09985 (referred to as the x coefficient) in Lotus. Because the ln concentration is plotted versus time, the slope is simply the elimination rate constant. The y intercept is referred to as constant, 9.34. The R squared is the linear regression coefficient squared for this analysis.

Note: To check this result, students may be interested in simulating the data with dose = 10000 μg/kg, VD = 1000 mL/kg, $k_a = 0.8$ hr^{-1}, and $k = 0.1$ hr^{-1}.

```
              A          B          C          D          E          F          G          H
1
2         10000       1000       0.08        0.1
3       hour        conc     LN(CONC)
4             0       0.00
5             2    7049.53       8.86
6             4    7194.95       8.88
7             6    6178.08       8.73
8             8    5116.20       8.54
9            10    4200.50       8.34
10           12    3441.45       8.14
11           14    2818.09       7.94
12           16    2307.36       7.74         Regression Ouput:
13                                   Constant                        9.34 ← Intercept
14                                   Std Err of Y Est                0.00
15                                   R Squared                       1.00
16                                   No. of Observations             4.00
17                                   Degrees of Freedom              2.00
18
19                                   X Coefficient(s) -0.09985 ← Slope
20                                   Std Err of Coef. 0.000052
23-May-90      12:26 PM
```

FIGURE B-3. *A sample Lotus 1-2-3 (version 2.1) spreadsheet showing a set of time-concentration data (column A and B) being analyzed to obtain the slope or elimination constant.*

Copyright (c) 1988 by MathSoft, Inc.

SOLVING A SYSTEM OF DIFFERENTIAL EQUATIONS $k_1 = 0.2 \quad k_2 = 1 \quad k_3 = 3$

x and y are functions of the time variable t, and F and G are the derivatives dx/dt and dy/dt.

$F(t,x,y) = k_2 \cdot y - [k_3 + k_1] \cdot x$

$G(t,x,y) = k_1 \cdot x - k_2 \cdot y$

startt = 0 endt = 4 n = 100 intervals initx = 1 inity = 0

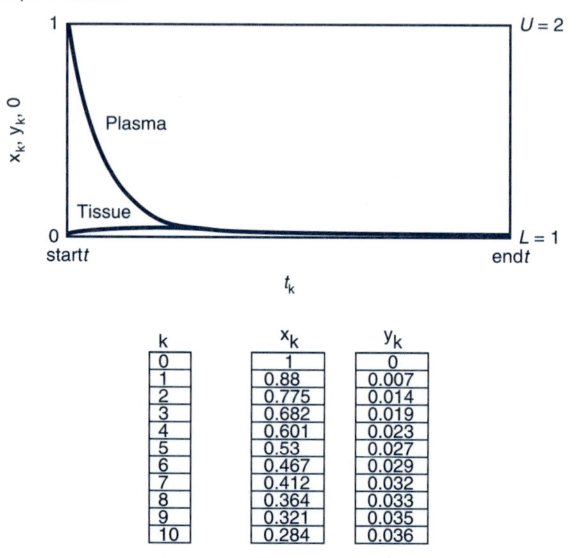

k	x_k	y_k
0	1	0
1	0.88	0.007
2	0.775	0.014
3	0.682	0.019
4	0.601	0.023
5	0.53	0.027
6	0.467	0.029
7	0.412	0.032
8	0.364	0.033
9	0.321	0.035
10	0.284	0.036

FIGURE B-4. *A sample of the MCAD application program used to solve the two-differential equation for a two-compartment model after IV bolus dose. (The first 10 data points are shown.)*

```
                    Summary of Least Squares for dataset oral absorption

          computation time:      1.04 secs   A[1]=  12.801        k[1]=  0.40724
       calculated lag time:     0.00000      k[2]= -12.800        k[2]=  1.9428
     sum of squared residuals:  0.0048572
   Model Selection Criterion:   8.1157
          Weighting Factor:     0.00000
```

time	y-obs	y-calc	resid	wt*res-sq
0.00000	0.00000	0.00051906	-0.00051906	2.694E-007
0.40000	5.0000	4.9919	0.0080675	6.509E-005
0.80000	6.5000	6.5363	-0.036276	0.0013160
1.2000	6.6600	6.6087	0.051306	0.0026323
2.0000	5.3900	5.4062	-0.016228	0.00026334
2.4000	4.6800	4.6961	-0.016060	0.00025791
2.8000	4.0300	4.0373	-0.0072648	5.278E-005
3.2000	3.4500	3.4520	-0.0020411	4.166E-006
3.6000	2.9500	2.9431	0.0069157	4.783E-005
4.0000	2.5200	2.5053	0.014746	0.00021745

press any key to continue

FIGURE B-5. Sample output from RSTRIP pharmacokinetic software showing a good fit of the theoretical data to actual data (columns 2 and 3). The parameters estimated are given in the top right-hand corner.

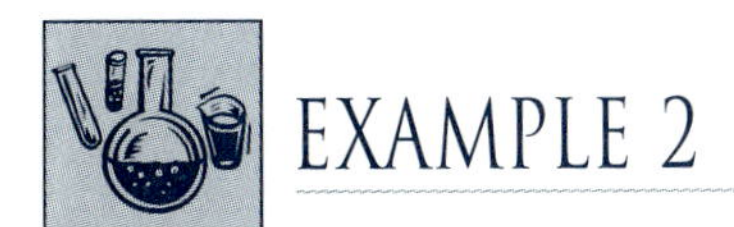

EXAMPLE 2

Generate some data for a two-compartment model using two differential equations. Initial conditions are dose = 1, $V = 1$, and $k_{12} = 0$, $k_{21} = 1$, and $k = 3$:

Solution

The data may be generated with MathCAD (Fig. B-4). Note that k_{12} is abbreviated as k_1, k_{21} is abbreviated as k_2, and k is abbreviated at k_3 in the program for simplicity. Also, $dCp/dt = F(t, x, y)$; $x = C_p$; $y = C_t$; $t =$ time; and $dCt/dt = G(t, x, y)$.

Model Fitting

An example of a set of oral plasma data was fit to a one-compartment model by RSTRIP (Fig. B-5). The software makes an initial estimate as well as a final parameter after several iterations. An example of some oral plasma data was generated with PCNonlin (Figs. B-6A, B, C).

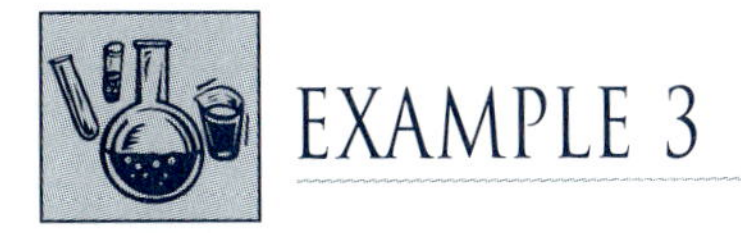

EXAMPLE 3

After a drug is administered orally, a series of plasma drug concentration versus time data may be fitted to a one-compartment model, to estimate the absorption rate constant, elimination rate constant, and volume of distribution. Other phar-

```
LISTING OF INPUT COMMANDS

MODEL 3, 'ONE'
MODEL 3
REMARK   ONE COMPARTMENT MODEL - FIRST ORDER INPUT AND OUTPUT
REMA
REMA    NO.     PARAMETER        CONSTANT         SECONDARY PARM.
REMA    ---     ---------        --------         ---------------
REMA    1        VOLUME            DOSE                AUC
REMA    2         K01                              K01 HALF LIFE
REMA    3         K10                              K10 HALF LIFE
REMA    4                                             TMAX
REMA    5                                             CMAX
REMA*****************************************************************
REMA              I----------------------I
REMA              I                      I
REMA   K01    --> I    COMPARTMENT 1     I   ---> K10
REMA              I                      I
REMA              I----------------------I
REMA*****************************************************************
COMM
NPARM 3
NCON 1
MSEC 5
PNAMES 'VOLUME', 'K01', 'K10'
SNAMES 'AUC', 'K01-HL', K10-HL', 'TMAX', 'CMAX'
END
TEMP
D=CON(1)
V=P(1)
K01=P(2)
K10=P(3)
T=X
END
FUNC1
COEF=D*K01/(V*(K01-K10))
F=COEF*(DEXP(-K10*T)-DEXP(-K01*T))
END
SECO
S(1)=D/V/K10
S(2)=-DLOG(.5)/K01
S(3)=-DLOG(.5)/K10
TMAX=(DLOG(K01/K10)/(K01-K10))
S(4)=TMAX
S(5)=(D/V)*DEXP(-K10*TMAX)
END
EOM
CONS 250
INIT 100.7, 1.03, .13
NOBS 9
DATA
BEGIN

PCNONLIN NONLINEAR ESTIMATION PROGRAM

ITERATION WEIGHTED SS       VOLUME        K01           K10
   0       1.34180          100.7         1.030          .1300
                   TAU  = .1583E-04   RANK = 3   COND = 1049.
   1       .136818          100.7          .5689         .1706
                   TAU  = .1108E-04   RANK = 3   COND = 1701.
   2       .358976E-01      100.7          .4396         .1788
                   TAU  = .1008E-04   RANK = 3   COND = 2489.
   3       .357194E-01      100.7          .4439         .1795
                   TAU  = .1005E-04   RANK = 3   COND = 2451.
   4       .357049E-01      100.7          .4442         .1791
                   TAU  = .1008E-04   RANK = 3   COND = 2447.
   5       .356635E-01      99.63          .4392         .1816
                   TAU  = .9998E-05   RANK = 3   COND = 2473.
   6       .356553E-01      99.63          .4383         .1815
                   TAU  = .1000E-04   RANK = 3   COND = 2481.

CONVERGENCE ACHIEVED
RELATIVE CHANGE IN WEIGHTED SUM OF SQUARES LESS THAN        .000100
    6      .356533E-01      99.57          .4377         .1817
```

FIGURE B-6A. Sample output from PCNONLIN showing data fitted to Model 3, a one-compartment model with first-order absorption and first-order elimination.

PARAMETER	ESTIMATE	STANDARD ERROR	95% CONFIDENCE LIMITS		
VOLUME	99.568030	19.182331	52.630524	146.505537	UNIVARIATE
			24.795837	174.340224	PLANAR
K01	.437738	.117793	.149508	.725969	UNIVARIATE
			-.021417	.896894	PLANAR
K10	.181749	.043746	.074706	.288792	UNIVARIATE
			.011228	.352271	PLANAR

*** SUMMARY OF NONLINEAR ESTIMATION ***

FUNCTION 1

X	OBSERVED Y	CALCULATED Y	RESIDUAL	WEIGHT	SD-YHAT	STANDARDIZED RESIDUAL
1.000	.7000	.8085	-.1085	1.000	.4987E-01	-1.847
2.000	1.200	1.196	.3927E-02	1.000	.4740E-01	.6460E-01
3.000	1.400	1.334	.6581E-01	1.000	.4034E-01	1.002
4.000	1.400	1.330	.7008E-01	1.000	.4253E-01	1.090
6.000	1.100	1.132	-.3226E-01	1.000	.4620E-01	-.5228
8.000	.8000	.8737	-.7371E-01	1.000	.4000E-01	-1.119
10.00	.6000	.6435	-.4349E-01	1.000	.3919E-01	-.6552
12.00	.5000	.4624	.3760E-01	1.000	.4469E-01	.5986
16.00	.3000	.2305	.6954E-01	1.000	.4888E-01	1.167

CORRECTED SUM OF SQUARED OBSERVATIONS = 1.28889
WEIGHTED CORRECTED SUM OF SQUARED OBSERVATIONS = 1.28889
SUM OF SQUARED RESIDUALS = .356533E-01
SUM OF WEIGHTED SQUARED RESIDUALS = .356533E-01
S = .770857E-01 WITH 6 DEGREES OF FREEDOM

SUMMARY OF ESTIMATED SECONDARY PARAMETERS

PARAMETER	ESTIMATE	STANDARD ERROR
AUC	13.814898	.847009
KO1-HL	1.583474	.425680
K10-HL	3.813757	.917038
TMAX	3.433715	.217994
CMAX	1.345203	.040455

FIGURE B-6B. Sample output from PCNONLIN.

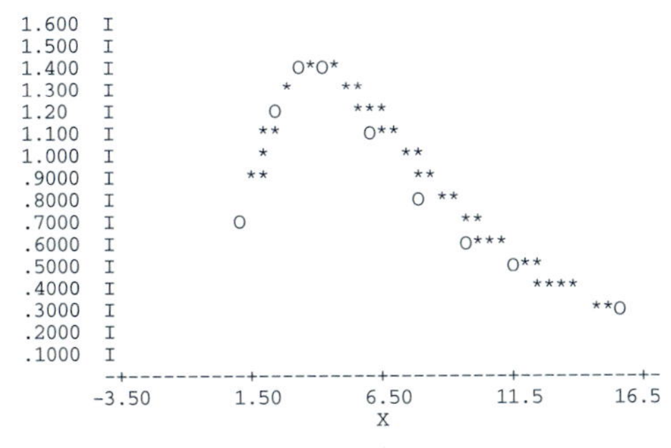

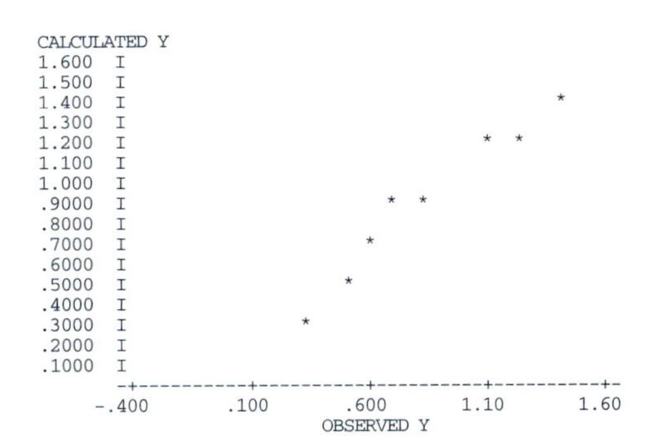

FIGURE B-6C. Sample output from PCNONLIN.

macokinetic parameters of interest may also be calculated using the NONLIN program, as shown in Figure B-6. Three parameters were estimated: V, k_{01}, and k_{10}, representing volume of distribution; k_a; and k (see model). Initial estimates were derived from either curve stripping or feathering. Dose is CON (1). In this case, NOBS = 9, showing that there are 9 data points. There is only one function that describes the model FUNC 1. S (1) represents the calculation of AUC, S (2) the calculation of absorption, and S (3) the elimination half-life.

REFERENCES

Gabrielsson J, Wiener D: *Pharmacokinetics and pharmacodynamic data analysis: Concepts and applications,* Swedish Pharmaceutical Press, 2nd ed., 1998

Heatherington AC, Vicini P, Golde H: A pharmacokinetic/pharmacodynamic comparison of SAAM II and PC/WIN Nonlin Modeling software. *J Pharm Sci 87*:1255–1263, 1998

Jelliffe RW, Schumitzky A, Van Guilder M, Jiang F: User manual for version 10.7 USC*PACK collection of PC programs. USC Laboratory of Applied Pharmacokinetics, University of Southern California, 1995

Maronda R (ed): Selected Topics in Clinical Pharmacology. Clinical applications of pharmacokinetics and control theory: Planning, monitoring, and adjusting dosage regiments of aminoglycosides, lidocaine, digoxitin, and digoxin. In Jelliffe RW: New York, Springer-Verlag, 1986, chap 3

NONMEM User Manuals I–VI. The NONMEM Project Group. San Francisco, University of California, San Francisco, 1995

APPENDIX C

SOLUTIONS TO FREQUENTLY ASKED QUESTIONS (FAQ) AND LEARNING QUESTIONS

CHAPTER 1

FREQUENTLY ASKED QUESTIONS

1. A semilog plot spaces the data at logarithmic intervals on the y-axis and rectangular (evenly spaced) intervals on the x-axis. The paper comes in one or more cycles. A two cycle semilog paper covers two logarithmic intervals (eg, 1 to 100). The semilog scale does not start with zero.
2. A common error in using logs is failing to remember that $\ln x = 2.3 \log x$. For the slope formula using a semilog plot:

$$\text{slope} = \frac{\log y_2 - \log y_1}{x_2 - x_1} = \frac{-k}{2.3}$$

$k = -\text{slope} \times 2.3$ (Did you forget the 2.3 factor?)

Alternatively, if you determine the slope with natural log:

$$\text{slope} = \frac{\ln y_2 - \ln y_1}{x_2 - x_1} = -k$$

$k = \text{slope} -$ (You should not use the 2.3 factor in this case)

3. Use the natural antilog of the intercept, or the inverse of ln.

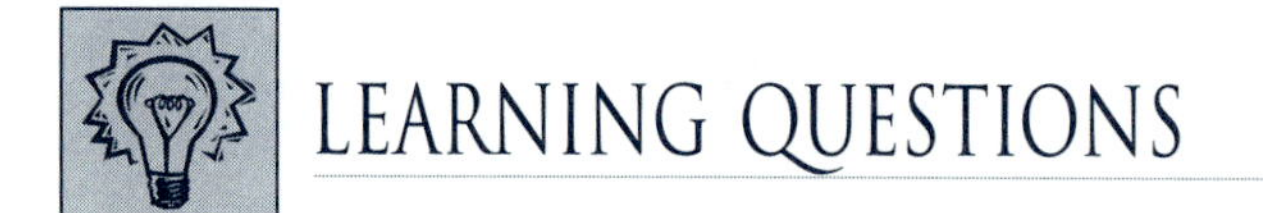

LEARNING QUESTIONS

1. **a.** Zero-order process (Fig. C-1).
   b. Rate constant, k_0:

Method 1

Values obtained from the graph (Fig. C-1):

t(min)	A(mg)
40	71
80	41

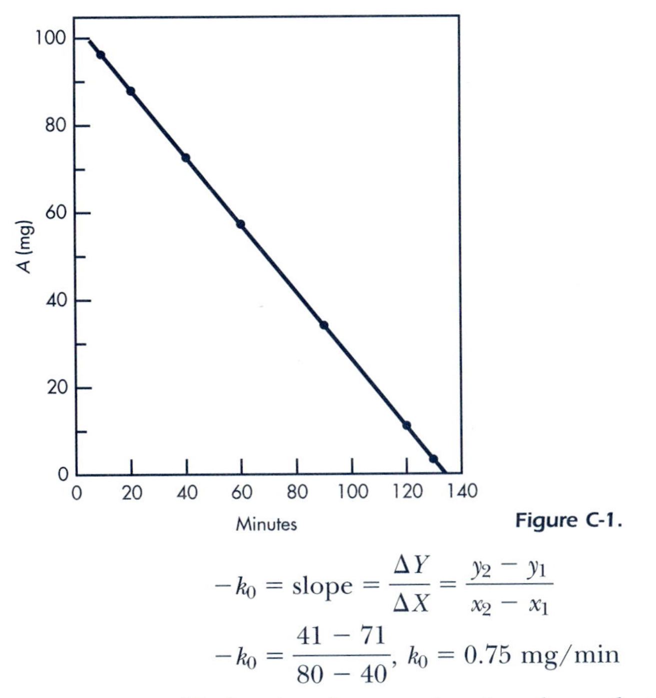

Figure C-1.

$$-k_0 = \text{slope} = \frac{\Delta Y}{\Delta X} = \frac{y_2 - y_1}{x_2 - x_1}$$

$$-k_0 = \frac{41 - 71}{80 - 40}, \; k_0 = 0.75 \text{ mg/min}$$

Notice that the negative sign shows that the slope is declining.

Method 2

By extrapolation:

$A_0 = 103.5$ at $t = 0$; $A = 71$ at $t = 40$ min.

$A = k_0 t + A_0$

$71 = -40k_0 + 103.5$

$k_0 = 0.81$ mg/min

Notice that the answer differs in accordance with the method used.

c. $t_{1/2}$

For zero-order kinetics, the larger the initial amount of drug A_0, the longer the $t_{1/2}$.

Method 1

$$t_{1/2} = \frac{0.5\ A_0}{k_0}$$

$$= \frac{0.5(103.5)}{0.78} = 66 \text{ min}$$

Method 2

The zero-order $t_{1/2}$ may be read directly from the graph (Fig. C-1):

At $t = 0$, $A_0 = 103.5$ mg

At $t_{1/2}$, $A = 51.8$ mg

Therefore, $t_{1/2} = 66$ min

d. The amount of drug A does extrapolate to zero on the x-axis.

e. The equation of the line is:

$$A = -k_0 t + A_0$$
$$= -0.78t + 103.5$$

2. a. First-order process (Fig. C-2).

b. Rate constant, k:

Method 1

Obtain the first-order $t_{1/2}$ from the semilog graph (Fig. C-2):

t(min)	A(mg)
30	30
53	15

$$t_{1/2} = 23 \text{ min}$$
$$k = \frac{0.693}{t_{1/2}} = \frac{0.693}{23} = 0.03 \text{ min}^{-1}$$

Method 2

$$\text{Slope} = \frac{-k}{2.3} = \frac{\log Y_2 - \log Y_1}{X_2 - X_1}$$
$$k = \frac{-2.3(\log 15 - \log 30)}{53 - 30} = 0.03 \text{ min}^{-1}$$

c. $t_{1/2} = 23$ min (see Method 1 above).

d. The amount of drug A does not extrapolate to zero on the x-axis.

e. The equation of the line is

$$\log A = -\frac{kt}{2.3} + \log A_0$$
$$= -\frac{0.03t}{2.3} + \log 78$$
$$A = 78e^{-0.03t}$$

on regular plot, the same data shows a curve (not plotted).

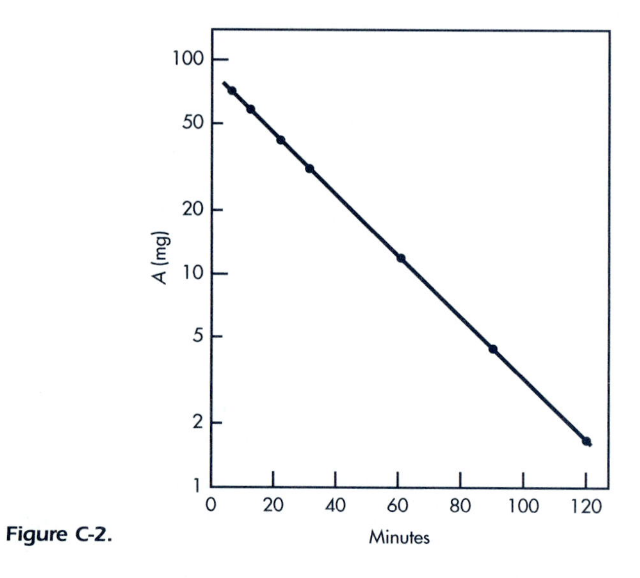

Figure C-2.

3. a. Zero-order process (Fig. C-3).

b. $k_0 = \text{Slope} = \dfrac{\Delta Y}{\Delta X}$

Values obtained from the graph (Fig. C-3).

t(hr)	C(μg/mL)
1.2	80
4.2	60

It is always best to plot the data. Obtain a regression line (ie, the line of best fit), then use points C and t from that line.

$$-k_0 = \frac{60 - 80}{4.2 - 1.2}$$

$$k_0 = 6.67\ \mu\text{g/mL hr}$$

c. By extrapolation:

At t_0, $C_0 = 87.5\ \mu\text{g/mL}$

d. The equation (using ruler only) is:

$$A = -k_0 t + A_0 = -6.67t + 87.5$$

4. Given:

C(mg/mL)	*t*(days)
300	0
75	30

a. $\log C = \dfrac{-kt}{2.3} + \log C_0$

$$\log 75 = \frac{-30k}{2.3} + \log 300$$

$$k = 0.046\ \text{days}^{-1}$$

$$t_{1/2} = \frac{0.693}{k} = \frac{0.693}{0.046} = 15\ \text{days}$$

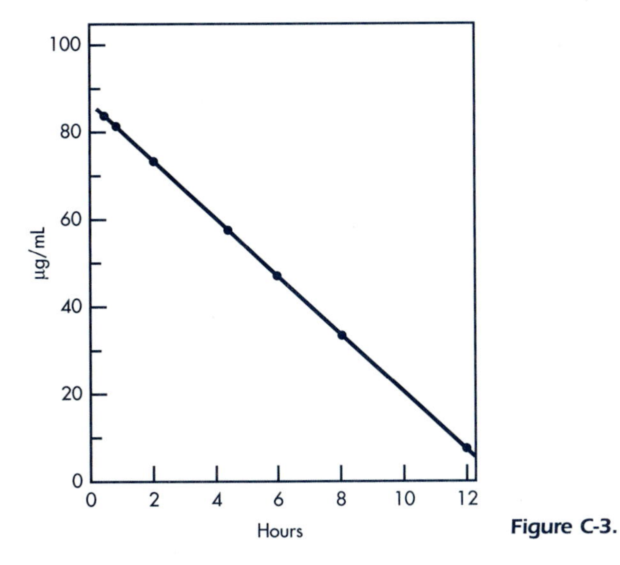

Figure C-3.

b. Method 1

300 mg/mL = C_0 at $t = 0$
75 mg/mL = C at $t = 30$ days
225 mg/mL = difference between initial and final drug concentration

$$k_0 = \frac{225 \text{ mg/mL}}{30 \text{ days}} = 7.5 \text{ mg/mL day}$$

The time, $t_{1/2}$, for the drug to decompose to 1/2 C_0 (from 300 to 150 mg/mL) is calculated by (assuming zero order)

$$t_{1/2} = \frac{150 \text{ mg/mL}}{7.5 \text{ mg/mL day}} = 20 \text{ days}$$

Method 2

$$C = -k_0 t + C_0$$
$$75 = -30k_0 + 300$$
$$k_0 = 7.5 \text{ mg/mL day}$$
$$\text{At } t_{1/2},\ C = 150 \text{ mg/mL}$$
$$150 = -7.5t_{1/2} + 300$$
$$t_{1/2} = 20 \text{ days}$$

Method 3

A $t_{1/2}$ value of 20 days may be obtained directly from the graph by plotting C against t on rectangular coordinates.

5. Assume an original concentration of drug to be 1000 mg/mL.

Method 1

mg/mL	No. of Half-lives	mg/mL	No. of Half-lives
1000	0	15.6	6
500	1	7.81	7
250	2	3.91	8
125	3	1.95	9
62.5	4	0.98	10
31.3	5		

99.9% of 1000 = 999

Concentration of drug remaining = 0.1% of 1000

1000 − 999 = 1 mg/mL

It takes approximately 10 half-lives to eliminate all but 0.1% of the original concentration of drug.

Method 2

Assume any $t_{1/2}$ value:

$$t_{1/2} = \frac{0.693}{k}$$

Then

$$k = \frac{0.693}{t_{1/2}}$$

$$\log C = \frac{-kt}{2.3} + \log C_0$$

$$\log 1.0 = \frac{-kt}{2.3} + \log 1000$$

$$t = 9.9t_{1/2}$$

Substituting $0.693/t_{1/2}$ for k

$$\log 1.0 = \frac{-0.693t}{2.3 \times t_{1/2}} + \log 1000, \qquad 3 \times 2.3t_{1/2} = 0.693t$$

$$t = 9.96\ t_{1/2}$$

6. $t_{1/2} = 12$ hr

$$k = \frac{0.693}{t_{1/2}} = \frac{0.693}{12} = 0.058\ \text{hr}^{-1}$$

If 30% of the drug decomposes, 70% is left.

70% of 125 mg = (0.70)(125) = 87.5 mg

$$A_0 = 125\ \text{mg}$$

$$A = 87.5\ \text{mg}$$

$$k = 0.058\ \text{hr}^{-1}$$

$$\log A = -\frac{kt}{2.3} + \log A_0$$

$$\log 87.5 = -\frac{0.058t}{2.3} + \log 125$$

$$t = 6.1\ \text{hr}$$

7. Immediately after the drug dissolves, the drug degrades at a constant, or zero-order, rate. Since concentration is equal to mass divided by volume, it is necessary to calculate the initial drug concentration (at $t = 0$) to determine the original volume in which the drug was dissolved. From the data, calculate the zero-order rate constant, k_0:

$$-k_0 = \text{slope} = \frac{\Delta Y}{\Delta X} = \frac{0.45 - 0.3}{2.0 - 0.5} \qquad k_0 = 0.1\ \text{mg/mL hr}$$

Then calculate the initial drug concentration, C_0, using the following equation:

$$C = -k_0 t + C_0$$

at $t = 2$ hrs

$$0.3 = -0.1(2) + C_0$$

$$C_0 = 0.5\ \text{mg/mL}$$

Alternatively, at $t = 0.5$ hr

$$0.45 = -0.1(0.5) - C_0$$

$$C_0 = 0.5\ \text{mg/mL}$$

Since the initial mass of drug D_0 dissolved is 300 mg and the initial drug concentration C_0 is 0.5 mg/mL, the original volume may be calculated from the following relationship:

$$C_0 = \frac{D_0}{V}$$

$$0.5\ \text{mg/mL} = \frac{300\ \text{mg}}{V(\text{mL})}$$

$$V = 600\ \text{mL}$$

8. First order.

9. The volume of the culture tube is not important. In 8 hours (480 minutes), the culture tube is completely full. Because the doubling time for the cells is 2 minutes (ie, one $t_{1/2}$), then in 480 minutes less 2 minutes (478 minutes) the culture tube is half full of cells.

10. Data is often reported as the mean ± standard deviation or SD (see Appendix A). One SD above and below the mean represents 95% of the population, assuming a normal distribution of the data. In this example:

    mean + SD = 9.8 L + 4.2 L = 14 L
    mean − SD = 9.8 L − 4.2 L = 5.6 L

    Thus, 95% of the population would have a volume of distribution approximately ranging from 5.6 L to 14 L.

11. The answer is **A.** Each of the equations are in the form of $y = A\,e^{kt}$, where k is the slope of the line connecting the data points. A positive slope indicates that the direction of the line is slanted upward from left to right, whereas a negative slope indicates the line slants downward (declining) from left to right. Answer **C** would have a rising slope.

12. The answer is **C.** Recall that $e^{-kt} = 1/e^{kt}$, and that, as k or t gets larger, the fraction, $1/e^{kt}$ gets smaller. (Note: You may check the values using your calculator.)

13. The answer is **D.** You cannot obtain a log from a negative number.

14. The answer is **B.** Substitute the same value for t in each example and notice your answers.

CHAPTER 2

FREQUENTLY ASKED QUESTIONS

1. Blood is composed of plasma and red blood cells (RBC). Serum is the fluid obtained from blood after it is allowed to clot. Serum and plasma do not contain identical proteins. The RBC may be considered a cellular component of the body in which the drug concentration in the serum or plasma is in equilibrium, in the same way as with the other tissues in the body. Blood samples are generally harder to process and assay than serum or plasma samples.

2. Physiologic models are complex, and require more information for accurate prediction compared to compartment models. Missing information in the physiologic model will lead to bias or error in the model. Compartment models are

more simplistic in that they assume that both arterial and venous drug concentrations are similar. The compartment model accounts for a rapid distribution phase and a slower elimination phase. Physiologic clearance models postulate that arterial blood drug levels are considerably higher than venous blood drug levels. In practice, only venous blood samples are usually sampled. Organ drug clearance is useful in the treatment of cancers and in diagnosis of certain diseases involving arterial perfusion. Physiologic models are difficult to use for general application.

3. The exact site of drug action is generally unknown for most drugs. The time needed for the drug to reach the site of action, produce a pharmacodynamic effect, and reach equilibrium are deduced from studies on the relationship of the time course for the drug concentration and the pharmacodynamic effect. Often, the drug concentration is sampled during the elimination phase after the drug has been distributed and reached equilibrium. For multiple dose studies, both the peak and trough drug concentrations are frequently taken.

LEARNING QUESTIONS

1. The plasma drug level versus time curve describes the pharmacokinetics of the systemically absorbed drug. Once a suitable pharmacokinetic model is obtained, plasma drug concentrations may be predicted following various dosage regimens such as single oral and IV bolus doses, multiple dose regimens, IV infusion, etc. If the pharmacokinetics of the drug relate to its pharmacodynamic activity (or any adverse drug response or toxicity), then a drug regimen based on the drug's pharmacokinetics may be designed to provide optimum drug efficacy. In lieu of a direct pharmacokinetic–pharmacodynamic relationship, the drug's pharmacokinetics describe the bioavailability of the drug including inter- and intrasubject variability; this information allows for the development of drug products that consistently deliver the drug in a predictable manner.
2. The purpose of pharmacokinetic models is to relate the time course of the drug in the body to its pharmacodynamic and/or toxic effects. The pharmacokinetic model also provides a basis for drug product design, the design of dosage regimens, and a better understanding of the action of the body on the drug.
3. (Figure C-4)

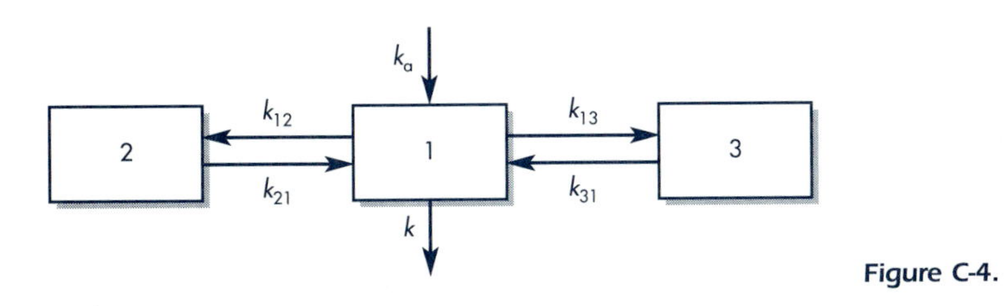

Figure C-4.

4. a. Nine parameters: V_1, V_2, V_3, k_{12}, k_{21}, k_e, k_b, k_m, k_u

b. Compartment 1 and compartment 3 may be sampled.

c. $k = k_b + k_m + k_e$

d. $\dfrac{dC_1}{dt} = k_{21}C_2 - (k_{12} + k_m + k_e + k_b)C_1$

6.

Compartment 1	Compartment 2
C_1	C_2

a. $C_1 > C_2$ are assumed to be the *total* drug concentration in each compartment. $C_1 > C_2$ may occur if the drug concentrates into compartment 1 due to protein binding, (where compartment 1 contains a high amount of protein or special protein binding), due to partitioning, (where compartment 1 has a high lipid content and the drug is poorly water soluble), or if the pH is different in each compartment and the drug is a weak electrolyte (the drug may be more ionized in compartment 1), or if there is an active transport mechanism for the drug to be taken up into the cell (eg, purine drug). Other explanations for $C_1 > C_2$ may be possible.

b. Several different experimental conditions are needed to prove which of the above hypotheses is the most likely cause for $C_1 > C_2$. These experiments may use *in vivo* or *in vitro* methods, including intracellular electrodes to measure pH *in vivo,* protein binding studies *in vitro,* partitioning of drug in chloroform/water *in vitro,* among others.

c. In the case of protein binding, the total concentration of drug in each compartment may be different (eg, $C_1 > C_2$) and, at the same time, the free (nonprotein bound) drug concentration may be equal in each compartment—assuming that the free unbound drug is easily diffusable. Similarly, if $C_1 > C_2$ is due to differences in pH and the nonionized drug is easily diffusable, then the nonionized drug concentration may be the same in each compartment. The total drug concentrations will be $C_1 = C_2$ when there is similar affinity for the drug and similar conditions in each compartment.

d. The total amount of drug, A, in each compartment depends upon the volume, V, of the compartment and the concentration, C, of the drug in the compartment. Since the amount of drug (A) = concentration (C) times volume (V), any condition that causes the product, $C_1V_1 \neq C_2V_2$, will result in $A_1 \neq A_2$. Thus, if $C_1 = C_2$ and $V_1 \neq V_2$, then $A_1 \neq A_2$.

CHAPTER 3

? FREQUENTLY ASKED QUESTIONS

1. A rate represents the change in amount or concentration of drug in the body per time unit. For example, a rate equal to -5 mg/hr means the amount of drug is decreasing at 5 mg per hour. A *positive* or *negative* sign indicates that the rate is increasing or decreasing, respectively. Rates may be zero order, first order, or higher orders. For a first-order rate, the rate of change of drug in the body is determined by the *product of the elimination rate constant, k,* and by the *amount of drug* remaining in the body, ie, rate $= -k\ D_B$, where k represents "the fraction" of the amount of drug in the body that is eliminated per hour. If $k = 0.1\ \text{hr}^{-1}$, and $D_B = 10$ mg, then the rate $= 0.1\ \text{hr}^{-1} \times 10\ \text{mg} = 1\text{mg/hr}$. The rate constant in this example shows that 1/10 of the drug is eliminated, whatever amount of drug is present in the body. For a first-order rate, the rate states the absolute amount eliminated per unit time (which changes with the amount of drug in the body), whereas the first-order rate constant, k, gives the fraction of drug that is eliminated (which is a constant).

2. The first-order rate constant k has no concentration or mass units. In the calculation of the slope, k, the unit for mass or concentration is canceled when taking the log of the number:

$$\text{slope} = \frac{\ln y_2 - \ln y_1}{x_2 - x_1} = \frac{\ln\ [y_2/y_1]}{x_2 - x_1}$$

3. The one-compartment model uses a single homogeneous compartment to represent the fluid and the vascular tissues. This model ignores the heterogeneity of the tissues in the body, so there is no merit in predicting precise tissue–drug levels. However, the model provides useful insight into the mass balance of drug distribution in and out of the plasma fluid in the body. If V_D is larger than the physiologic vascular volume, the conclusion is that there is some drug outside the vascular pool, ie, in the tissues. If V_D is small, then there is little extravascular tissue drug storage, except perhaps in the lung, liver, kidney, and heart. With some knowledge about the lipophilicity of the drug and an understanding of blood flow and perfusion within the body, a postulation may be made as to which organs are involved in storing the extravascular drug. The concentration of a biopsy sample may not support or refute the postulation.

4. Clearance is the volume of plasma fluid that is cleared of drug per unit time. Clearance may also be derived for the physiologic model as the fraction of drug that is eliminated by an organ as blood flows through it. The former definition is equivalent to $Cl = kV_D$ and is readily adapted to dosing since V_D is the volume of distribution. If the drug is solely eliminated by metabolism in the liver, then

$Cl_H = Cl$. However, if Cl_H is estimated directly from blood flow and extraction. Cl_H is not readily used in dosing because Cl_H is computed from organ blood flow and a realistic blood volume instead of the volume of distribution.

5. Since mass balance (ie, relating dose to plasma drug concentration) is based on volume of distribution rather than blood volume, the compartment model is used in determining dose. Generally, the total blood concentrations of most drugs are not known, since only the plasma or serum concentration is assayed. Some drugs have a RBC/plasma drug ratio much greater than 1, making the application of the physiologic model difficult without knowing the apparent volume of distribution.

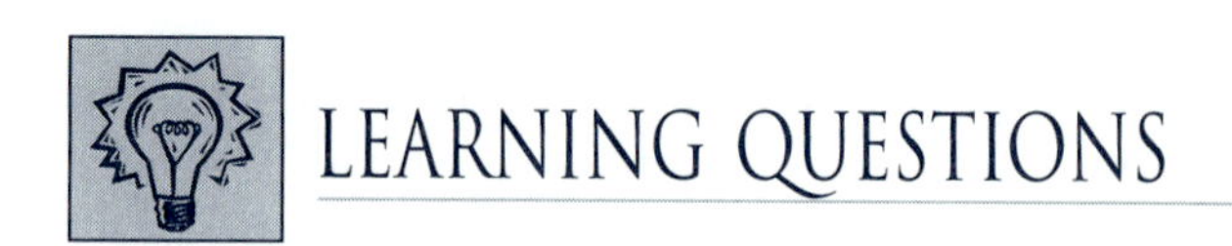

LEARNING QUESTIONS

1. The C_p decreased from 1.2 to 0.3 μg/mL in 3 hours.

t(hr)	**C_p(μg/mL)**
2	1.2
5	0.3

$$\log C_p = -\frac{kt}{2.3} + \log C_p^0$$

$$\log 0.3 = -\frac{k(3)}{2.3} + \log 1.2$$

$$k = 0.462\ \text{hr}^{-1}$$

$$t_{1/2} = \frac{0.693}{k} = \frac{0.693}{0.462}$$

$$t_{1/2} = 1.5\ \text{hrs}$$

This data may also be plotted on a semilog graph and the $t_{1/2}$ obtained from the graph.

2. Dose (IV bolus) = 6 mg/kg × 50 kg = 300 mg

a. $V_D = \dfrac{\text{dose}}{C_p^0} = \dfrac{300\ \text{mg}}{8.4\ \mu\text{g/mL}} = \dfrac{300\ \text{mg}}{8.4\ \text{mg/L}} = 35.7\ \text{L}$

(1) Plot the data on semi-log graph paper and use two points from the line of best fit.

t(hr)	**C_p(μg/mL)**
2	6
6	3

(2) $t_{1/2}$ (from graph) = 4 hrs $\qquad k = \dfrac{0.693}{4} = 0.173\ \text{hr}^{-1}$

b. $C_p^0 = 8.4\ \mu\text{g/mL}, \quad C_p = 2\ \mu\text{g/mL}, \quad k = 0.173\ \text{hr}^{-1}$

$$\log C_p = -\frac{kt}{2.3} + \log C_p^0$$

$$\log 2 = -\frac{0.173t}{2.3} + \log 8.4$$

$$t = 8.29\ \text{hr}$$

Alternatively, time t may be found from a graph of C_p versus t.

c. Time required for 99.9% of the drug to be eliminated:

(1) Approximately $10t_{1/2}$

$$t = 10(4) = 40 \text{ hrs}$$

(2) $C_p^0 = 8.4\ \mu\text{g/mL}$

With 0.1% of drug remaining,

$$C_p = 0.001(8.4\ \mu\text{g/mL}) = 0.0084\ \mu\text{g/mL}$$
$$k = 0.173\ \text{hr}^{-1}$$
$$\log 0.0084 = \frac{-0.173t}{2.3} + \log 8.4$$
$$t = 39.9 \text{ hrs}$$

d. If the dose doubled, then C_p^0 will also double. However, the elimination half-life or first-order rate constant will remain the same. Therefore:

$$C_p^0 = 16.8\ \mu\text{g/mL}, \qquad C_p = 2\ \mu\text{g/mL},\ k = 0.173\ \text{hr}^{-1}$$
$$\log 2 = \frac{0.173t}{2.3} + \log 16.8$$
$$t = 12.3 \text{ hr}$$

Notice that doubling the dose does not double the duration of activity.

3. $D_0 = 200$ mg

$V_D = 10\%$ of body weight $= 0.1(80\ \text{kg}) = 8000\ \text{mL} = 8\text{L}$

At 6 hours:

$$C_p = 1.5\ \text{mg}/100\ \text{mL}$$
$$V_D = \frac{\text{drug in body } (D_B)}{C_p}$$
$$D_B = C_p V_D = \frac{1.5\ \text{mg}}{100\ \text{mL}}(8000\ \text{mL})$$
$$\log D_B = -\frac{kt}{2.3} + \log D_B^0$$
$$\log 120 = -\frac{k(6)}{2.3} + \log 200$$
$$k = 0.085\ \text{hr}^{-1}$$
$$t_{1/2} = \frac{0.693}{k} = \frac{0.693}{0.085} = 8.1 \text{ hr}$$

4. $C_p = 78e^{-0.46t}$ [equation is in the form of $C_p = C_p^0 e^{-kt}$]

$$\ln C_p = \ln 78 - 0.46t$$
$$\ln C_p = -\frac{0.46t}{2.3} + \log 78$$

Thus, $k = 0.46\ \text{hr}^{-1}$, $C_p^0 = 78\ \mu\text{g/mL}$.

a. $$t_{1/2} = \frac{0.693}{k} = \frac{0.693}{0.46} = 1.5 \text{ hr}$$

b. $$V_D = \frac{\text{dose}}{C_p^0} = \frac{300{,}000\ \mu\text{g}}{78\ \mu\text{g/mL}} = 3846\ \text{mL}$$

Dose $= 4\ \text{mg/kg} \times 75\ \text{kg} = 300$ mg

c. (1) $$\log C_p = -\frac{0.46(4)}{2.3} + \log 78 = 1.092$$
$$C_p = 12.4\ \mu\text{g/mL}$$

(2) $C_p = 78e^{-0.46(4)} = 78e^{-1.84} = 78(0.165)$
$C_p = 12.9\ \mu g/mL$

d. At 4 hours:

$$D_B = C_p V_D = 12.4\ \mu g/mL \times 3846\ mL = 47.69\ mg$$

e.

$$V_D = 3846\ mL$$
$$\text{Average weight} = 75\ kg$$
$$\text{Percent body wt} = (3.846\ kg/75\ kg) \times 100 = 5.1\%$$

The apparent V_D approximates the plasma volume.

f. $C_p = 2\ \mu g/mL$
Find t.

$$\log 2 = -\frac{0.46t}{2.3} + \log 78$$
$$t = -\frac{2.3(\log 2 - \log 78)}{0.46}$$
$$= 7.96\ hr \approx 8\ hr$$

Alternate method

$$2 = 78e^{-0.46t}$$
$$\frac{2}{78} = 0.0256 = e^{-0.46t}$$
$$-3.7 = -0.46t$$
$$t = \frac{3.7}{0.46} = 8\ hr$$

6. For first-order elimination kinetics, one-half of the initial quantity is lost each $t_{1/2}$. The following table may be developed:

Time (hr)	Number of $t_{1/2}$	Amount of Drug in Body (mg)	Percent of Drug in Body	Percent of Drug Lost
0	0	200	100	0
6	1	100	50	50
12	2	50	25	75
18	3	25	12.5	87.5
24	4	12.5	6.25	93.75

Method 1

From the above table the percent of drug remaining in the body after each $t_{1/2}$ is equal to 100% times $(1/2)^n$, where n is the number of half-lives, as shown below:

Number of $t_{1/2}$	Percent of Drug in Body	Percent of Drug Remaining in Body after n $t_{1/2}$
0	100	
1	50	$100 \times 1/2$
2	25	$100 \times 1/2 \times 1/2$
3	12.5	$100 \times 1/2 \times 1/2 \times 1/2$
n		$100 \times (1/2)^n$

$$\text{Percent of drug remaining} = \frac{100}{2^n}, \text{ where } n = \text{number of } t_{1/2}$$

$$\text{Percent of drug excreted} = 100 - \frac{100}{2^n}$$

At 24 hours, $n = 4$, since $t_{1/2} = 6$ hours.

$$\text{Percent of drug lost} = 100 - \frac{100}{16} = 93.75\%$$

Method 2

The equation for a first-order elimination after IV bolus injection is

$$\log D_B = \frac{-kt}{2.3} + \log D_0$$

where

D_B = amount of drug remaining in the body
D_0 = dose = 200 mg
k = elimination rate constant = $0.693/t_{1/2} = 0.1155\ \text{hr}^{-1}$
t = 24 hrs

$$\log D_B = \frac{-0.1155(24)}{2.3} + \log 200$$

$$D_B = 12.47\ \text{mg} \simeq 12.5\ \text{mg}$$

$$\%\ \text{of drug lost} = \frac{200 - 12.5}{12.5} \times 100 = 93.75\%$$

7. The zero-order rate constant for alcohol is 10 mL/hr. Since the specific gravity for alcohol is 0.8, then

$0.8\ \text{g/mL} = x(\text{g})/10\ \text{mL} \quad x = 8\ \text{g}$

Therefore, the zero-order rate constant, k_0, is 8 g/hr.

Drug in body at $t = 0$:
$D_B^0 = C_p V_D = 210\ \text{mg}/0.100\ \text{L} \times (0.60)(75\ \text{L}) = 94.5\ \text{g}$

Drug in body at time t:

$D_B = C_p V_D = 100\ \text{mg}/0.100\ \text{L} \times (0.60)(75\ \text{L}) = 45.0\ \text{g}$

For a zero-order reaction:

$D_B = -k_0 t + D_B^0$
$45 = -8t + 94.5$
$t = 6.19$ hr

8. a. $C_p^0 = \dfrac{\text{dose}}{V_D} = \dfrac{500\ \text{mg}}{(0.1\ \text{L/kg})(55\ \text{kg})} = 90.9\ \text{mg/L}$

b. $\log D_B = \dfrac{-kt}{2.3} + \log D_B^0$

$$= \frac{(0.693/0.75)(4)}{2.3} + \log 500$$

$D_B = 12.3$ mg

c. $\log 0.5 = \dfrac{-(0.693/0.75)t}{2.3} + \log 90.0$

$t = 5.62$ hr

9. $\log D_B = \dfrac{-kt}{2.3} + \log D_B^0$

$$\log 25 = \frac{-k(8)}{2.3} + \log 100$$

$k = 0.173\ \text{hr}^{-1}$

$$t_{1/2} = \frac{0.693}{0.173} = 4\ \text{hr}$$

10.

$$\log D_B = \frac{-kt}{2.3} + \log D_B^0$$
$$= \frac{(-0.693/8)(24)}{2.3} + \log 600$$
$$D_B = 74.9 \text{ mg}$$
$$\text{Percent drug lost} = \frac{600 - 74.9}{600} \times 100 = 87.5\%$$

C_p at $t = 24$ hr:

$$C_p = \frac{74.9 \text{ mg}}{(0.4 \text{ L/kg})(62 \text{ kg})} = 3.02 \text{ mg/L}$$

11. The total drug concentration in the plasma is not usually equal to the total drug concentration in the tissues. A one-compartment model implies that the drug is rapidly equilibrated in the body (in plasma and tissues). At equilibrium, the drug concentration in the tissues may differ from the drug concentration in the body due to drug protein binding, partitioning of drug into fat, differences in pH in different regions of the body causing a different degree on ionization for a weak electrolyte drug, an active tissue uptake process, etc.

12. Set up the following table:

Time (hr)	D_u (mg)	D_u/t	mg/hr	t^*
0	0			
4	100	100/4	25	2
8	26	26/4	6.5	6

The elimination half-life may be obtained graphically after plotting mg/hr versus t^*. The $t_{1/2}$ obtained graphically is approximately 2 hours.

$$\log \frac{dD_u}{dt} = \frac{-kt}{2.3} + \log k_e D_B^0$$
$$\text{Slope} = \frac{-k}{2.3} = \frac{\log Y_2 - \log Y_1}{X_2 - X_1} = \frac{\log 6.5 - \log 25}{6 - 2}$$
$$k = 0.336 \text{ hr}^{-1}$$
$$t_{1/2} = \frac{0.693}{k} = \frac{0.693}{0.336} = 2.06 \text{ hr}$$

CHAPTER 4

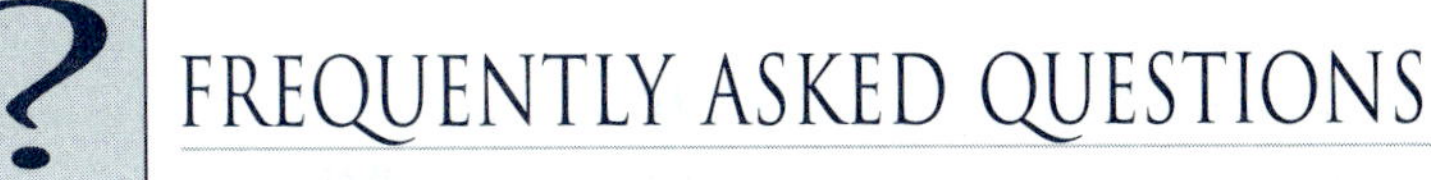

FREQUENTLY ASKED QUESTIONS

1. "Mathematical" or "hypothetical" are indeed vague and noninformative terms. Mathematical equations are developed to calculate how much drug is in the vascular fluid, as well as outside of the vascular fluid (ie, extravascular or in the tissue pool). Hypothetical refers to an unproven model. The assumptions in the compartmental models simply imply that the model simulates the mass transfer of drug between the circulatory system and the tissue pool. The mass balance of drug moving out of the plasma fluid is described even though we know the tissue pool is not real (the tissue pool represents the virtual tissue mass that receives drug from the blood). While the model is a less than a perfect representation, we can interpret it, knowing its limitations. All pharmacokinetic models need interpretation. We use a model when there are no simple ways to obtain needed information. As long as we know the model limitations (ie, that the tissue compartment is not the brain, nor the muscle!) and stay within the bounds of the model, we can extract useful information from it. For example, we may determine that the amount of drug is stored outside the plasma compartment at any desired time point. After an IV bolus drug injection, the drug distributes rapidly throughout the plasma fluid and more slowly into the fluid-filled tissue spaces. Drug distribution is initially rapid and confines to a fixed fluid volume known as the V_p or the initial volume. As drug distribution expands into other tissue regions, the volume of the penetrated spaces increases, until a critical point (steady state) is obtained when all penetrable tissue regions are equilibrated with the drug. Knowing that there is heterogenous drug distribution within and between tissues, the tissues are grouped into compartments to determine the amount of drugs in them. Mass balance, including drug inside and outside the vascular pool accounts for all body drug storage ($D_B = D_t + D_p$). Assuming steady state, the tissue drug concentration equal to the plasma drug concentration $C_{p_{ss}}$, one may determine size of the tissue volume using $D_t/C_{p_{ss}}$. This volume is really a "numerical factor" that is used to describe the relationship of the tissue storage drug relative to the drug in the blood pool. The sum of the two volumes is the steady state volume of distribution. The product of the steady-state concentration $C_{p_{ss}}$ and the (V_D)ss yields the amount of drug in the body at steady state. The amount of drug in the body at steady state is considered vital information in dosing drugs clinically. Students should realize that tissue drug concentrations are not predicted by the model. However, plasma drug concentration is fully predictable after any given dose once the parameters become known. Initial pharmacokinetic parameter estimation may be obtained from the literature using comparable age and weight for a specific individual.

2. Apparent volumes of distribution are not real tissue volumes, but rather reflect the volume in which the drug is contained. For example:

V_p = initial or plasma volume
V_t = tissue volume

$(V_D)_{ss}$ = steady state volume of distribution (most often listed in the literature). The steady state drug concentration multiplied by $(V_D)_{ss}$ yields the amount of drug in the body. $(V_D)_\beta$ is a volume usually determined from area under curve and differs from $(V_D)_{ss}$ somewhat in magnitude. $(V_D)_\beta$ multiplied by b gives clearance of the drug.

3. A physiologic model is a detailed representation of drug disposition in the body. The model requires blood flow, extraction ratio, and specific tissue and organ size. This information is not often available for the individual. Thus, the less sophisticated compartment models are used more often.

4. Clearance is used to calculate the steady-state drug concentration and to calculate the maintenance dose. However, clearance alone is not useful in determining the maximum and minimum drug concentration in a multiple dosing regimen.

5. If the two-compartment model is ignored and the data is treated as a one-compartment model, the estimated values for the pharmacokinetic parameters are distorted. For example, during the distributive phase, the drug declines rapidly according to distribution alpha half-life while in the elimination (terminal) part of the curve, the drug declines according to a beta elimination half-life.

6. Compartment models have been used to develop dosage regimens and for the development of pharmacodynamic models. Compartment models have improved the dosing of drugs such as digoxin, gentamicin, lidocaine, and many others. The principle use of compartment models in dosing is to simulate a plasma drug concentration profile based on pharmacokinetic (PK) parameters. This information allows comparison of PK parameters in patients with only 2 or 3 points to a patient with full profiles using generated PK parameters.

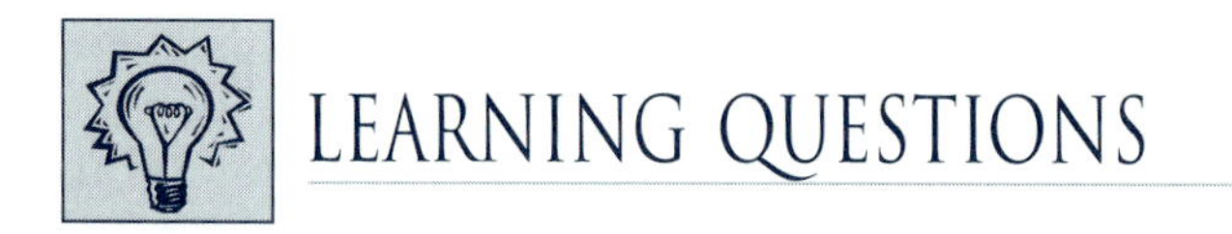

LEARNING QUESTIONS

1. Equation for the curve:

$$C_p = 52e^{-1.39t} + 18e^{-0.135t}$$

$k = 0.41\ \text{hr}^{-1}$ $\quad k_{12} = 0.657\ \text{hr}^{-1}$ $\quad k_{21} = 0.458\ \text{hr}^{-1}$

2. Equation for the curve:

$$C_p = 28e^{-0.63t} + 10.5e^{-0.46t} + 14e^{-0.077t}$$

Note: When feathering curves by hand, a minimum of three points should be used to determine the line. Moreover, the rate constants and y intercepts may vary according to the individual's skill. Therefore, values for C_p should be checked by substitution of various times for t, using the derived equation. The theoretical curve should fit the observed data.

3. $C_p = 11.14\ \mu g/mL$

4. The initial decline in the plasma drug concentration is mainly due to uptake of drug into tissues. During the initial distribution of drug, some drug elimination also takes place. After the drug has equilibrated with the tissues, the drug declines at a slower rate due to drug elimination.

5. A third compartment may indicate that the drug has a slow elimination component. If the drug is eliminated by a very slow elimination component, then drug accumulation may occur with multiple drug doses or long IV drug infusions. Depending upon the blood sampling, a third compartment may be missed. However, some data may fit both a two- or three-compartment model. In this case, if the fit for each compartment model is very close statistically, the more simple compartment model should be used.

6. Due to heterogeneity of the tissues, drug equilibrates into the tissues at different rates and the different drug concentrations are usually observed in the different tissues. The drug concentration in the "tissue" compartment represents an "average" drug concentration and does not represent the drug concentration in any specific tissue.

7.

$$C_p = Ae^{-at} + Be^{-bt}$$

After substitution:

$$C_p = 4.62e^{-8.94t} + 0.64e^{-0.19t}$$

a. $V_p = \dfrac{D_0}{A + B} = \dfrac{75000}{4.62 + 0.64} = 14259 \text{ mL}$

b. $V_t = \dfrac{V_p k_{12}}{k_{21}} = \dfrac{(14259)(6.52)}{(1.25)} = 74375 \text{ mL}$

c. $k_{12} = \dfrac{AB(b-a)^2}{(A + B)(Ab + Ba)}$

$$= \frac{(4.62)(0.64)(0.19 - 8.94)^2}{(4.62 + 0.64)[(4.62)(0.19) + (0.64)(8.94)]}$$

$$= 6.52 \text{ hr}^{-1}$$

$$k_{21} = \frac{Ab + Ba}{A + B} = \frac{(4.62)(0.19) + (0.64)(8.94)}{4.62 + 0.64}$$

$$= 1.25 \text{ hr}^{-1}$$

d. $k = \dfrac{ab(A + B)}{Ab - Ba} = \dfrac{(8.94)(0.19)(4.62 + 0.64)}{(4.62)(0.19) + (0.64)(8.94)}$

$$= 1.35 \text{ hr}^{-1}$$

8. The tissue compartments may not be sampled directly to obtain the drug concentration. Theoretical concentration, C_t, represents the average concentration in all the tissues outside of the central compartment. The amount of drug in the tissue, D_t, represents the total amount of drug outside of the central or plasma compartment. Occasionally C_t may be equal to a particular tissue drug concentration in an organ. However, this C_t may be equivalent by chance only.

9. The data were analyzed by the computer software, RSTRIP, and found to fit a two-compartment model:

$A(1) = 2.0049$, $A(2) = 6.0057$ (two preexponential values)
$k(1) = 0.15053$, $k(2) = 7.0217$ (two exponential values)

The equation that describes the data is:

$C_p = 2.0049\, e^{-0.15053t} + 6.0057 e^{-7.0217t}$

Coefficient of correlation = 0.999 (very good fit)
Model selection criteria = 11.27 (good model)
Sum of squared deviations = 9.3×10^{-5} (There is little deviation between the observed data and the theoretical value.)
Alpha = 7.0217 hr^{-1}, beta = 0.15053 hr^{-1}

10. **a.** Late-time samples were taken in some patients yielding data that resulted in a monoexponential elimination profile. It is also possible that a patient's illness contributes to an impaired drug distribution.
b. The range of distribution half lives is 30–45 minutes.
c. None. Tissue concentrations are not generally well predicted from the two-compartment model. Only the amount of drug in the tissue compartment may be predicted.
d. No. At steady state, the rate in and the rate out of the tissues are the same, but the drug concentrations are not necessarily the same. The plasma and each tissue may have different drug binding.
e. None. Only the pooled tissue is simulated by the tissue compartment.

CHAPTER 5

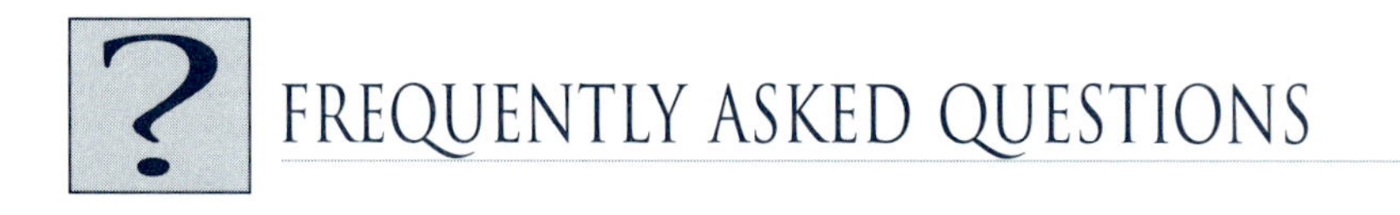

FREQUENTLY ASKED QUESTIONS

1. An *absorption window* refers to the segment of the gastrointestinal tract from which the drug is well absorbed and beyond which the drug is either poorly absorbed or not absorbed at all. After oral administration, most drugs are well absorbed in the duodenum and to a lesser extent in the jejunum. A small amount of drug absorption may occur from the ileum.
2. Food, particularly foods with a high fat content, stimulates the production of bile, which is released into the duodenum. The bile helps to solubilize a lipid soluble drug, thereby increasing drug absorption. Fatty food also slows gastrointestinal motility, resulting in a longer "*residence time*" for the drug to be absorbed from the small intestine.
3. After oral administration, the drug in solution may precipitate in the gastrointestinal

tract. The precipitated drug needs to redissolve prior to absorption. Some drug solutions are prepared with a cosolvent, such as alcohol or glycerin, and form coarse crystals on precipitation that dissolve slowly, whereas other drugs precipitate into fine crystals that redissolve rapidly. The type of precipitate is influenced by the solvent, by the degree of agitation, and by the physical environment. *In vitro* mixing and dilution of the drug solution in artificial gastric juice, artificial intestinal juice, or in other pH buffers may predict the type of drug precipitate that is formed.

In addition, drugs dissolved in a highly viscous solution (eg, simple syrup) may have slower absorption due to the viscosity of the solution. Furthermore, drugs that are readily absorbed across the gastrointestinal membrane may not be completely bioavailable (ie, 100% systemic absorption) due to *first-pass effects* (discussed in Chapter 13).

4. The major biological factor that delays gastrointestinal drug absorption is a delay in gastric emptying time. As discussed in Chapter 5, any factor that delays stomach emptying time, such as fatty food, will delay the drug from entering into the duodenum from the stomach and, thereby, delay drug absorption.

LEARNING QUESTIONS

1. In the presence of food, undissolved aspirin granules larger than 1 mm are retained longer in the stomach, up to several hours longer. In the absence of food, aspirin granules are emptied from the stomach within 1 to 2 hours. When the aspirin granules are emptied slowly into the duodenum, the drug absorption will be as slow-acting as a sustained-release drug product. Enteric-coated aspirin granules taken with an evening meal may provide relief of pain for arthritic patients late into the night.
2. The answer is **b.** A basic drug formulated as a suspension will be dependent on stomach acid for dissolution as the basic drug forms a hydrochloric acid (HCl) salt. If the drug is poorly soluble, adding milk may neutralize some acid so that the drug may not be completely dissolved. Making a HCl salt rather than a suspension of the base ensures that the drug is soluble without dependency on stomach HCl for dissolution.
3. Protein drugs are generally digested by proteolytic enzymes present in the GI tract and therefore are not adequately absorbed by the oral route. Protein drugs are most commonly given parenterally. Other routes of administration, such as intranasal and rectal administration, have had some success or are under current investigation for the system absorption of protein drugs.
4. The answer is **c.** Raising the pH of an acid drug above its pKa will increase the dissociation of the drug, thereby increasing its aqueous solubility.
5. The large intestine is most heavily populated by bacteria, yeasts, and other microflora. Some drugs which are not well absorbed in the small intestine are metabolized by the microflora to products that are absorbed in the large bowel. For example, drugs with an azo link (eg, sulfasalazine) are cleaved by bacteria in the bowel and the cleaved products (eg, 5-aminosalicylic acid and sulfapyridine) are

absorbed. Other drugs, such as antibiotics (eg, tetracyclines), may destroy the bacteria in the large intestine resulting in an overgrowth of yeast (eg, *Candida albicans*) leading to a yeast infection. Destruction of the microflora in the lower bowel can also lead to cramps and diarrhea.

6. First-pass effects are discussed more fully in Chapter 13. Alternative routes of drug administration such as buccal, inhalation, sublingual, intranasal, and parenteral will bypass the first-pass effects observed after oral drug administration.

7. Although antacid statistically decreased the extent of systemic drug absorption ($P < 0.05$) as shown by an $AUC_{0-4\ hr}$ of 349 ± 108 pg hr/mL, compared to the control (fasting) $AUC_{0-4\ hr}$ value of 417 ± 135 pg hr/mL, the effect of antacid is not clinically significant. A high-fat diet decreased the rate of systemic drug absorption, as shown by a longer t_{max} value (64 min) and lower C_{max} value (303 pg/mL).

CHAPTER 6

? FREQUENTLY ASKED QUESTIONS

1. a. For optimal drug absorption after oral administration, the drug should be water soluble and highly permeable to be absorbed throughout the gastrointestinal tract. Ideally, the drug should not change into a polymorphic form that could affect its solubility. The drug should be stable in both gastric and intestinal pH and preferably should not be hygroscopic.

b. For parenteral administration, the drug should be water soluble and stable in solution, preferably at autoclave temperature. The drug should be nonhydroscopic and preferably should not change into another polymorphic form.

2. A lipid-soluble drug may be prepared in an oil-in-water (o/w) emulsion or dissolved in a nonaqueous solution in a soft gelatin capsule. A cosolvent may improve the solubility and dissolution of the drug.

3. The rate of hydrolysis (decomposition) of the ester drug may be reduced by formulating the drug in a cosolvent solution. A reduction in the percent of the aqueous vehicle will decrease the rate of hydrolysis. In addition, the drug should be formulated at the pH in which the drug is most stable.

4. Excipients are needed in a formulation to solubilize the drug, increase the dissolution rate, decrease gastrointestinal transit time, or improve oral absorption by complexation. Excipients can also decrease the rate of oral absorption in the gastrointestinal tract by reducing drug solubility, decreasing the dissolution rate, or forming an insoluble complex.

LEARNING QUESTIONS

1. The rate-limiting steps in the oral absorption of a solid drug product are the rate of drug dissolution within the gastrointestinal tract and the rate of permeation of the drug molecules across the intestinal mucosal cells. Generally, disintegration of the drug product is rapid and not rate limiting. Water-soluble drugs rapidly dissolve in the aqueous environment of the gastrointestinal tract, so that the permeation of the intestinal mucosal cells may be the rate-limiting step. The drug absorption rate may be altered by a variety of methods, all of which depend on knowledge of the biopharmaceutic properties of the drug and the drug product and on the physiology of the gastrointestinal tract. Drug examples are described in detail in this chapter and in the previous chapter.
2. Most drugs are absorbed by passive diffusion. The duodenum area provides a large surface area and blood supply that maintains a large drug concentration gradient favorable for drug absorption from the duodenum into the systemic circulation.
3. If the initial drug absorption rate, dD_A/dt were slower than the drug elimination rate, dD_E/dt, then therapeutic drug concentrations in the body would not be achieved. It should be noted that the rate of absorption is generally first order, $dD_A/dt = D_0k_a$, where, D_0 is the drug dose which is great initially. Even if $k_a < k$, the initial drug absorption rate may be greater than the drug elimination rate. After the drug is absorbed from the absorption site, $dD_A/dt \leq dD_E/dt$.
4. A drug prepared as an oral aqueous drug solution is generally the most bioavailable. However, the same drug prepared as a well-designed immediate-release tablet or capsule may have similar bioavailability. In the case of an oral drug solution, there is no dissolution step; the drug molecules come into contact with intestinal membrane, and the drug is rapidly absorbed. Due to first-pass effects (discussed in Chapter 13), a drug given in an oral drug solution may not be 100% bioavailable. If the drug solution is formulated with a high solute concentration, such as sorbitol solution that yields a high osmotic pressure, gastric motility may be slowed, thus slowing the rate of drug absorption.
5. Anticholinergic drugs prolong gastric emptying which would delay the absorption of an enteric-coated drug product.
6. Erythromycin may be formulated as enteric-coated granules to protect the drug from degradation in the stomach pH. Enteric-coated granules are less affected by gastric emptying and food (which delays gastric emptying) compared to enteric-coated tablets.

CHAPTER 7

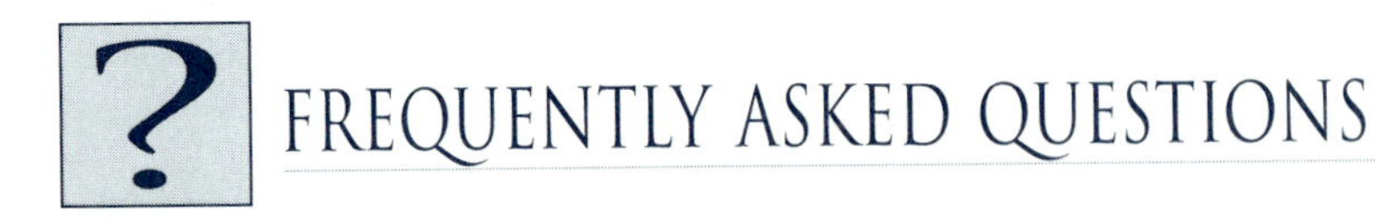

FREQUENTLY ASKED QUESTIONS

1. Controlled-release drug products have many advantages compared to immediate-release drug products as discussed in Chapter 7. However, a controlled-release drug product of a drug that has a long elimination half-life (eg, chlorpheniramine maleate, digoxin, levothyroxine) has no advantage over the same drug given in an immediate-release (conventional) drug product. For some drugs, the clinical rationale for a controlled-release drug product that provides a long sustained drug level is not established. Nitroglycerin, for example, is less likely to produce tolerance with intermittent dosing compared with dosing by a continuous-release product. For some antibiotics, there is also a specific duration of post-antibiotic effect during which bactericidal activity continues even when plasma drug level is depleted. Some drugs are better tolerated with a "pulse" type of drug input into the body.
2. A zero-order rate for drug absorption will give more constant plasma drug concentrations with minimal fluctuations between peak and trough levels compared to first-order drug absorption. Depending upon the therapeutic window for the drug and the relationship between the pharmacokinetics and pharmacodynamics of the drug, zero-order drug absorption may not always be more efficacious than first-order absorption.

LEARNING QUESTIONS

1. **a.** For many drugs, the plasma drug concentration is proportional to the drug concentration at the receptor site and the pharmacodynamic effect. By maintaining a prolonged, constant plasma drug concentration, the pharmacodynamic effect is also maintained.

   b. A drug that releases at a zero-order rate and is absorbed at a zero-order rate provides a more constant plasma drug concentration compared to a first-order drug release.

2. **a.** Both A and B release drug at a zero-order rate (straight line). Curve B shows 100% of drug is released in 12 hours, or about 8.3% per hour.
   b. Product C.
   c. Product C initially releases drug at a zero-order rate (first 3 hours).
   d. Drug release usually slows down toward the end of dissolution because most tablets get smaller as dissolution proceeds, resulting in a smaller surface for water penetration inward and drug diffusion outward. Also, as drug dissolution occurs, the concentration gradient (Fick's law) gets progressively smaller due to the build-up of drug in the bulk solution.
   e. As the surface drug of a sustained-release product is dissolved, the interior drug has to traverse a longer or a more tortuous path to reach the outside, resulting in the slowing rate of dissolution.
3. **a.** A drug given 10 mg 4 times daily would be equivalent to 40 mg/day or 20 mg/12 hr at the rate of 1.67 mg/hr.
   b. 0.5 mL/hr should deliver 1.67 mg of drug. Therefore, the concentration should be

$$1.67/0.5 = 3.34 \text{ mg/mL}$$

4. Using the infusion equation:

$$k = \frac{0.693}{3.5} = 0.198 \text{ hr}^{-1}$$

$$V_D = 10 \text{ L} \qquad C_p = 20 \text{ mg/L}$$

$$R = C_p V_D k = (20)(10)(0.198) = 39.6 \text{ mg/hr}$$

Total drug needed $= R \times 12 \text{ hr} = (39.6)(12) = 475.2$ mg

CHAPTER 8

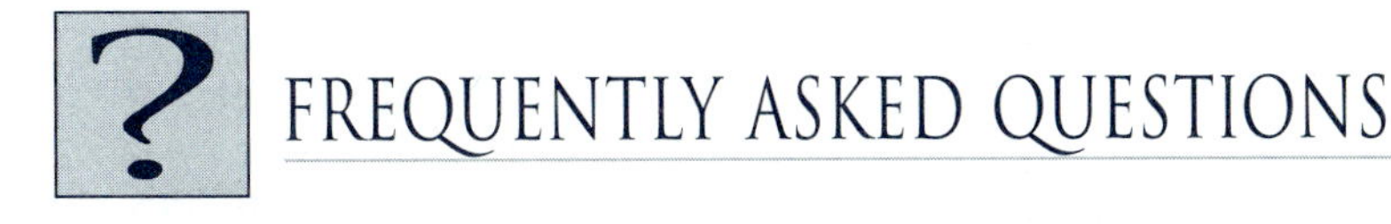

FREQUENTLY ASKED QUESTIONS

1. The most frequent route of administration for biological compounds is parenteral (eg, IM or IV). For example, beta interferon for multiple sclerosis is given IM to allow gradual drug release into the systemic circulation.
2. Glycosylation is the addition of a carbohydrate group to the molecule. For example, Betaseron (interferon beta-1A) is not glycosylated, whereas Avonex (interferon beta-1B) is glycosylated. Glycosylation will increase the water solubility and

the molecular weight of the drug. Although both drugs are beta interferons, glycosylation affects the pharmacokinetics, the stability, and the efficacy of these drugs.

3. The distribution of a biotechnology compound depends upon its physicochemical characteristics. Many peptides, proteins, and nucleotides have polar chains so that a major portion of the drug is distributed in the extracellular fluid with a volume of 7 to 15 liters. Drugs that easily penetrate into the cell have higher volumes of distribution, about 15 to 45 liters due to the larger volume of intracellular fluid.

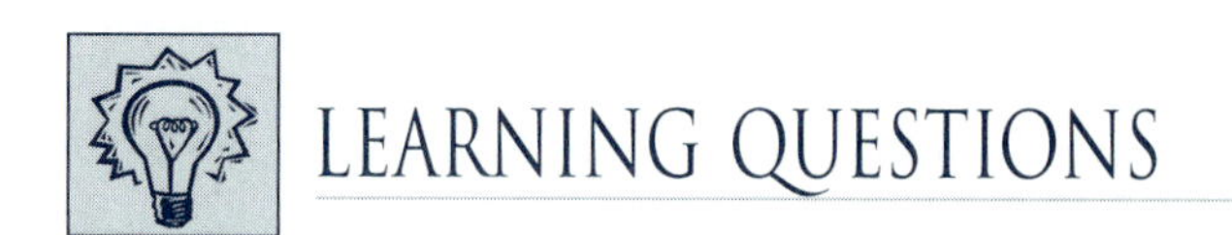

LEARNING QUESTIONS

None

CHAPTER 9

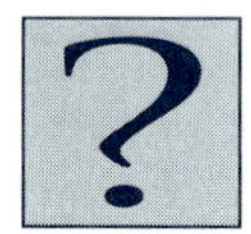

FREQUENTLY ASKED QUESTIONS

1. For drugs absorbed by a first-order process, the absorption half-life is $0.694/k_a$. Although drug absorption involves many stochastic (random) steps, the overall rate process is often approximated by a first-order process, especially with oral solutions and immediate-release drug products such as compressed tablets or capsules. The determination of the absorption rate constant, k_a is most often calculated by the Wagner-Nelson method for drugs that follow a one-compartment model with first-order absorption and first-order elimination.

2. The fraction of drug absorbed, F, and the absorption rate constant, k_a, are independent parameters. A drug in an oral solution may have a more rapid rate of absorption compared to a solid drug product. If the drug is slowly released from the drug product or is formulated so that the drug is slowly absorbed, then the drug may be subjected to first-pass effects, degraded in the gastrointestinal tract, or eliminated in the feces so that less drug (smaller F) may be absorbed systemically compared to the same drug formulated to be more rapidly absorbed from the drug product.

3. A drug with a rate of absorption slower than its rate of elimination would not be able to obtain optimal systemic drug concentrations to achieve efficacy. Such drugs are generally not developed into products.
4. Drug clearance is generally not affected by drug absorption from most absorption sites. In the gastrointestinal tract, a drug is absorbed via the hepatic portal vein to the liver and may be subject to hepatic clearance.
5. The fraction of drug absorbed may be less than 1 (ie, 100% bioavailable) after oral administration.

LEARNING QUESTIONS

1. **a.** The elimination rate constant is 0.1 hr^{-1} ($t_{1/2} = 6.93$ hr).
   b. The absorption rate constant, k_a, is 0.3 hr^{-1} (absorption half life = 2.31 hr).
   The calculated $t_{max} = \dfrac{\mathrm{lm}(k_a/k)}{k_a - k} = 5.49$ hr.
   c. The y intercept was observed as 60 ng/mL. Therefore, the equation that fits the observed data is:
   $$C_p = 60\ [e^{-0.1t} - e^{-0.3t}]$$
   Note: Answers obtained by "hand" feathering the data on semilog graph paper may vary somewhat depending on graphing skills and skill in reading data from a graph.
2. By direct observation of the data, the t_{max} is 6 hours and the C_{max} is 23.01 ng/mL. The apparent volume of distribution, V_D, is obtained from the intercept, I, of the terminal elimination phase, and substituting $F = 0.8$, $D = 10{,}000{,}000$ ng, $k_a = 0.3$ hr^{-1}, $k = 0.1$ hr^{-1}:
   $$I = \frac{Fk_aD_0}{V_D\ (k_a - k)} \qquad 60 = \frac{(0.8)(0.3)(10000000)}{V_D\ (0.3 - 0.1)}$$
   $$V_D = 200\ \mathrm{L}$$
3. The percent of drug unabsorbed method is applicable to any model with first-order elimination regardless of the process of drug input. If the drug is given by IV injection, the elimination rate constant, k, may be accurately determined. If the drug is orally administered, k and k_a may *flip flop* resulting in an error unless IV data is available to determine k. For a drug that follows a two-compartment model, an IV bolus injection is used to determine the rate constants for distribution and elimination.
4. After an IV bolus injection, a drug such as theophylline follows a two-compartment model with a rapid distribution phase. During oral absorption, the drug is distributed during the absorption phase, and no distribution phase is observed. Pharmacokinetic analysis of the plasma drug concentration data obtained after oral drug administration will show that the drug follows a one-compartment model.

5. The equations for a drug that follows the kinetics of a one-compartment model with first-order absorption and elimination is:

$$C_p = \frac{FD_0}{V_D(k_a - k)}(e^{kt} - e^{-k_a t}) \qquad t_{max} = \frac{\ln(k_a/k)}{k_a - k}$$

As shown by these equations:

a. t_{max} is influenced by k_a and k and not by F, D_0, or V_D.

b. C_p is influenced by F, D_0, V_D, k_a, and k.

6. Drug products that might provide a zero-order input is an oral controlled release tablet or a transdermal drug delivery system (patch). An IV drug infusion will also provide a zero-order drug input.

7. The general equation for a one-compartment open model with oral absorption is the following:

$$C_p = \frac{FD_0}{V_D(k_a - k)}(e^{kt} - e^{-k_a t})$$

From

$$C_p = 45(e^{-0.17t} - e^{-1.5t})$$

$$\frac{FD_0 k_a}{V_D(k_a - k)} = 45$$

$$k = 0.17 \text{ hr}^{-1}$$

$$k_a = 1.5 \text{ hr}^{-1}$$

a. $t_{max} = \frac{\ln(k_a/k)}{k_a - k} = \frac{\ln(1.5/0.17)}{1.5 - 0.17} = 1.64 \text{ hr}$

b. $C_{max} = 45(e^{-(0.17)(1.64)} - e^{-(1.5)(1.64)})$

$= 30.2\ \mu\text{g/mL}$

c. $t_{1/2} = \frac{0.693}{k} = \frac{0.693}{0.17} = 4.08 \text{ hr}$

8. a. *Drug A* $\quad t_{max} = \frac{\ln(1.0/0.2)}{1.0 - 0.2} = 2.01 \text{ hr}$

Drug B $\quad t_{max} = \frac{\ln(0.2/1.0)}{0.2 - 1.0} = 2.01 \text{ hr}$

b. $\quad C_{max} = \frac{FD_0 k_a}{V_D(k_a - k)}(e^{-kt_{max}} - e^{-k_a t_{max}})$

Drug A $\quad C_{max} = \frac{(1)(500)(1)}{(10)(1 - 0.2)}(e^{-(0.2)(2)} - e^{-(1)(2)})$

$C_{max} = 33.4\ \mu\text{g/mL}$

Drug B $\quad C_{max} = \frac{(1)(500)(0.2)}{(20)(0.2 - 1.0)}(e^{-1(2)} - e^{-(0.2)(2)})$

$C_{max} = 3.34\ \mu\text{g/mL}$

9. a. The method of residuals using manual graphing methods may give somewhat different answers depending upon personal skill and the quality of the graph paper. Values obtained by the computer program ESTRIP gave the following estimates:

$$k_a = 2.84 \text{ hr}^{-1}, \qquad k = 0.186 \text{ hr}^{-1}, \qquad t_{1/2} = 3.73 \text{ hr}$$

b. A drug in an aqueous solution is in the most absorbable form compared to other oral dosage forms. The assumption that $k_a > k$ is generally true for drug solutions and immediate-release oral dosage forms such as compressed tablets and capsules. Drug absorption from extended-release dosage forms may have $k_a < k$. To unequivocally demonstrate which slope represents the true k, the drug must be given by IV bolus or IV infusion, and the slope of the elimination curve is obtained.

c. The Loo–Riegelman method requires IV data. Therefore, only the method of Wagner–Nelson may be used on these data.

d. Observed t_{max} and C_{max} values are taken directly from the experimental data. In this example, C_{max} is 85.11 ng/mL which occurred at a t_{max} of 1.0 hr. The theoretical t_{max} and C_{max} are obtained as follows:

$$t_{max} = \frac{2.3 \log k_a/k}{k_a - k} = \frac{2.3 \log(2.84/0.186)}{2.84 - 0.186} = 1.03 \text{ hr}$$

$$C_{max} = \frac{FD_0 k_a}{V_D(k_a - k)} [e^{-kt_{max}} - e^{-k_a t_{max}}].$$

Where, $FD_0k_a/V_D(k_a - k)$ is the y-intercept equal to 110 ng/mL and t_{max} = 1.03 hours.

$$C_{max} = (110)(e^{-(0.186)(1.0)} - e^{-(2.84)(1.03)})$$
$$C_{max} = 85 \text{ ng/mL}.$$

e. A more complete model-fitting program, such as PCNONLIN, is needed to statistically fit the data to a one-compartment model.

CHAPTER 10

? FREQUENTLY ASKED QUESTIONS

1. Preclinical animal toxicology and clinical efficacy studies were performed on the marketed *brand* drug product as part of the New Drug Application (NDA) prior to FDA approval. These studies do not have to be repeated for the *generic* bioequivalent drug product. The manufacturer of the generic drug product must submit an Abbreviated New Drug Application (ANDA) to the FDA demonstrating that the generic drug product is a therapeutic equivalent (see definitions in Chapter 10) to the brand drug product.
2. The *sequence* is the order in which the drug products (ie, treatments) are given (eg, brand product followed by generic product or vice versa). Sequence is im-

portant to prevent any bias due to the order of the treatments in the study. The term *washout* refers to the time for total elimination of the dose. The time for the washout is determined by the elimination half-life of the drug. *Period* refers to the drug-dosing day on which the drug is given to the subjects. For example, for Period One, half the subjects receive treatment A, brand product and the other half of the subjects receive treatment B, generic product.

3. Manufacturers are required to perform a food intervention bioavailability study on all drugs whose bioavailability is known to be affected by food. In addition, a food intervention bioavailability study is required on all modified-release products since (1) the modified-release formulation (eg, enteric coating, sustained-release coating) may be affected by the presence of food and (2) modified-release products have a greater potential to be affected by food due to the longer time in the gastrointestinal tract.

4. If the drug is not systemically absorbed from the drug product, then a *surrogate marker* must be used as a measure of bioequivalence. This surrogate marker may be a pharmacodynamic effect or, as in the case of cholestyramine resin, the binding capacity for bile acids *in vitro*.

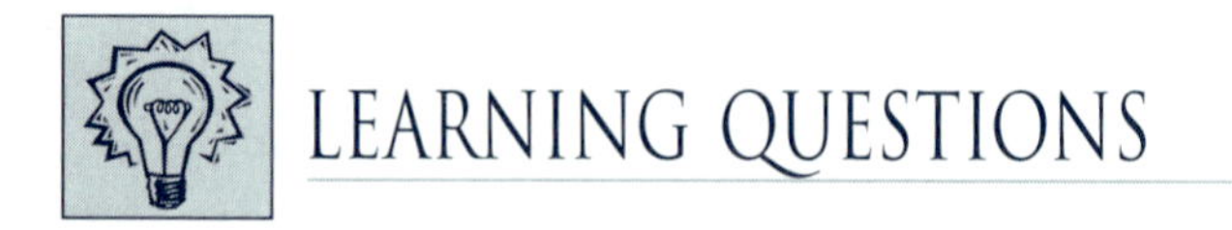

LEARNING QUESTIONS

3. a. Oral solution. The drug is in the most bioavailable form.

b. Oral solution. Same reason as above.

c. $$\text{Absolute bioavailability} = \frac{[\text{AUC}]\text{oral solution/dose}}{[\text{AUC}]_{\text{IV}}/\text{dose}} = \frac{145/10}{29/2} = 1.0$$

d. $$\text{Relative bioavailability} = \frac{[\text{AUC}]\text{tablet/dose}}{[\text{AUC}]\text{solution/dose}} = \frac{116/10}{145/10} = 0.80$$

e. (1) $C_{\text{P}}^0 = 6.67\ \mu\text{g/mL}$ [by extrapolation of IV curve]

$$V_{\text{D}} = \frac{2000\ \mu\text{g/kg}}{6.67\ \mu\text{g/mL}} = 300\ \text{mL/kg}$$

(2) $t_{1/2} = 3.01$ hr

(3) $k = 0.23\ \text{hr}^{-1}$

(4) $Cl_{\text{T}} = kV_{\text{D}} = 69$ mL/kg hr

4. Plot the data on both rectangular and semilog graph paper. The following answers were obtained from estimates from the plotted plasma level–time curves. More exact answers may be obtained mathematically by substitution into the proper formulas.

a. 1.37 hr

b. 13.6 hr

c. 8.75 hr

d. 5 hr

e. 4.21 μg/mL

f. 77.98 μg hr/mL

5.

Subject	Drug Product Period 1	Period 2	Week 3
1	A	B	C
2	B	C	A
3	C	A	B
4	A	C	B
5	C	B	A
6	B	A	C

6. **a.** Absolute bioavailability $= \dfrac{D_{u,PO}^{\infty}/\text{dose}_{PO}}{D_{u,IV}^{\infty}/\text{dose}_{IV}}$

$$= \frac{340/4}{20/0.2} = 0.85 \text{ or } 85\%$$

b. Relative bioavailability $= \dfrac{D_u^{\infty}\ \text{cap}/\text{dose cap}}{D_u^{\infty}\ \text{sol}/\text{dose sol}}$

$$= \frac{360/4}{380/4} = 0.947 \text{ or } 94.7\%$$

7. The fraction of drug absorbed systemically is the absolute bioavailability.

$$\text{Fraction of drug absorbed} = \frac{\%\text{ of dose excreted after PO}}{\%\text{ of dose excreted after IV}}$$

$$= \frac{48\%}{75\%} = 0.64$$

CHAPTER 11

? FREQUENTLY ASKED QUESTIONS

1. No. For some drugs, protein binding does not affect the overall distribution of other drugs. Typically, if a drug is highly bound, there is an increased chance of a significant change in the fraction of free drug when binding is altered.
2. Albumin, α_1-acid glycoprotein, and lipoprotein. For some drugs and hormones, there may be a specific binding protein.
3. Most drugs are assumed to be *restrictively bound*, and binding reduces drug clearance and elimination. However, some *nonrestrictively bound* drugs may be cleared easily. Changes in binding do not affect the rate of elimination of these drugs.

Some drugs, such as some semi-synthetic penicillins, that are bound to plasma protein, they may be actively secreted in the kidney. The elimination rates of these drugs are not affected by protein binding.

4. *Partitioning* refers to the relative distribution of a drug in the lipid and aqueous phases. Generally, a high partition coefficient ($P_{\text{oil/water}}$) favors tissue distribution and leads to a larger volume of distribution. Partitioning is a major factor that determines drug distribution along with protein binding of a drug.

5. It is important to examine why albumin level is reduced in the patient. For example is the reduced albumin level due to uremia or hepatic dysfunction? In general, reduced protein binding will increase free drug concentration. Any change in drug clearance should be considered before reducing the dose since the volume of distribution may be increased partially offsetting the increase in free drug concentration.

6. In general, the early phase after an IV bolus dose is the distributive phase. The elimination phase occurs in the later phase, although distribution may continue for some drugs, especially for a drug with a long elimination half-life. The elimination phase is generally more gradual, since some drug may be returned to the blood from the tissues as drug is eliminated from the body.

7. Generally, the long distribution half-life is caused by a tissue/organ that has a high drug concentration either due to intracellular drug binding or high affinity for tissue distribution. Alternatively, the drug may be metabolized slowly within the tissue.

8. The distribution half-life determines the time it takes for a tissue organ to be equilibrated. It takes 4.32 distribution half-lives for the tissue organ to be 95% equilibrated and one distribution half-life for the drug to be 50% equilibrated. The concept is analogous the dynamics of drug infusion (see Chapter 14).

9. The answer is **False.** The free drug concentration in the tissue and plasma is the same after equilibration, but the total drug concentration in tissue is not the same as the total drug concentration in the plasma. The bound drug concentration may vary depending on local tissue binding or lipid solubility of the drug. Many drugs have a long distributive phase due to tissue drug binding or lipid solubility. Drugs may equilibrate slowly into these tissues and then be slowly eliminated. Drugs with limited tissue affinity are easily equilibrated. Some examples of drugs with a long distributive phase are discussed in the two-compartment model (Chapter 4).

10. The ratio, r, is defined as the ratio of the number of moles of drug bound to the number of moles of protein in the system. For a simple case of one binding site, r reflects the proportion of binding sites occupied; r is affected by (1) the association binding constant, (2) the free drug concentration, and (3) the number of binding sites per mole of protein. When $[D]$, or free drug concentration, is equal to 1 (or the dissociation constant K), the protein is 50% occupied for a drug with 1:1 binding according to Equation 11.14. (This can be verified easily by substituting for $[D]$ into the right side the equation and determining r.) For a drug with n binding sites, 50% of the binding sites are occupied when $[D] = 1/[K_a(n-1)]$. This equation, however, reflects binding *in vitro* when drug concentration is not changing; therefore, its conclusions are somewhat limited.

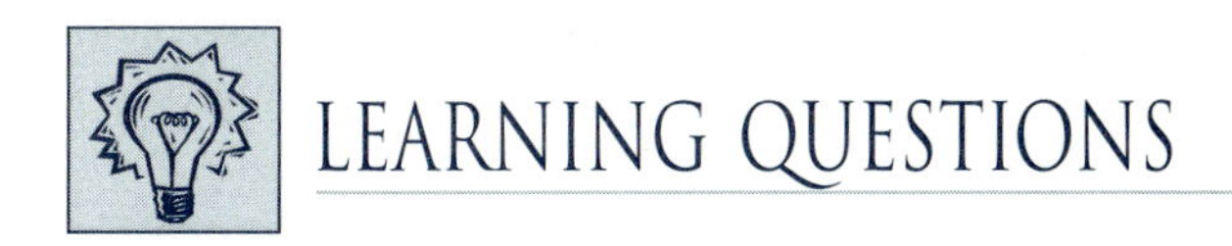

LEARNING QUESTIONS

1. The zone of inhibition for the antibiotic in serum is smaller due to drug–protein binding.

2. Calculate $r/(D)$ versus r; then graph the results on rectangular coordinates.

r	$r/(D \times 10^4)$
0.4	1.21
0.8	0.90
1.2	0.60
1.6	0.30

The y-intercept $= nK_a = 1.5 \times 10^4$
The x-intercept $= n = 2$

Therefore,

$K_a = 1.5 \times 10^4/2 = 0.75 \times 10^4$

K_a may also be found from the slope.

8. The liver is important for the synthesis of plasma proteins. In chronic alcoholic liver disease or cirrhosis, fewer plasma proteins are synthesized in the liver, resulting in a lower plasma protein concentration. Thus, for a given dose of naproxen, less drug is bound to the plasma proteins, and the total plasma drug concentration is smaller.

10. Protein binding may become saturated at any drug concentration in patients with defective proteins or when binding sites are occupied by metabolic wastes generated during disease states (eg, renal disease). Diazoxide is an example of nonlinear binding at therapeutic dose.

11. The answer is **False.** The percent bound refers to the percent of total drug that is bound. The percent bound may be ≥99% bound for some drugs. Saturation may be better estimated using the Scatchard plot approach and by examining "r", which is the number of moles of drug bound divided by the number of males of protein. When r is 0.99, most of the binding sites are occupied. The f_b, or fraction of bound drug, is useful for determining f_u, $f_u = 1 - f_b$.

12. Adenosine is extensively taken up by cells including the blood elements and the vascular endothelium. Adenosine is rapidly metabolised by deamination and/or is used as AMP in phosphorylation. Consequently, adenosine has a short elimination half-life.

CHAPTER 12

? FREQUENTLY ASKED QUESTIONS

1. Elimination half-life, $t_{1/2}$, is a concise and informative term that describes the time needed for half the dose to be removed from the body. Alternatively, the elimination half-life indicates the time for the plasma drug concentration to decline to one-half from whatever concentration it started. Classical pharmacokinetic models are based on $t_{1/2}$ (or k) and V_D. Some pharmacokineticists prefer Cl and V_D, and regard $t_{1/2}$ as a derived parameter.

2. A *parameter* is a model-based numerical constant estimated statistically from the data. Model parameters are used generally to make predictions about the behavior of the real process. A parameter is termed independent if the parameter is not dependent on other parameters of the model. In the classical one-compartment model, k and V_D are independent model parameters, and $t_{1/2}$ and Cl are regarded as derived parameters. In the physiologic model, Cl and V_D are regarded as independent model parameters, while k is a dependent parameter since k depends on Cl/V_D. In practice, both Cl and k are dependent on various physiologic factors, such as blood flow, drug metabolism, renal secretion, and drug reabsorption. Most biological events are the result of many events that are described more aptly as mutually interacting rather than acting independently. Thus, the underlying elimination process may be adequately described as fraction of drug removed per minute (k) or as volume of fluid removed per minute (Cl).

3. With most drugs, total body clearance (often termed "clearance") is the sum of renal and nonrenal clearances. Creatinine is an endogenous marker that accumulates in the blood when renal function is impaired. Creatinine is excreted by glomerular filtration and not reabsorbed. Creatinine clearance is a measure of glomerular filtration rate. Renal clearance is, therefore, proportional to creatinine clearance but not equal, since most drugs are reabsorbed to some extent, and some drugs are actively secreted.

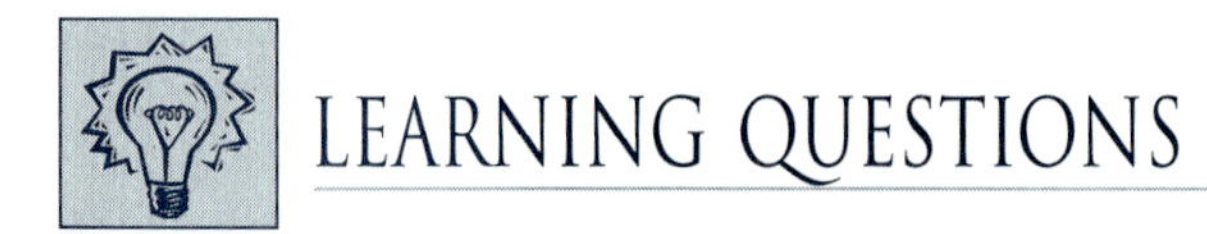

LEARNING QUESTIONS

3. a.

$$Cl_T = V_D k = V_D \frac{0.693}{t_{1/2}}$$

$$\text{Average } Cl_T = \frac{(30)(0.693)}{3.4} = 6.11 \text{ L/hr}$$

$$\text{Upper } Cl_T \text{ limit} = \frac{(30)(0.693)}{1.8} = 11.55 \text{ L/hr}$$

$$\text{Lower } Cl_T \text{ limit} = \frac{(30)(0.693)}{6.8} = 3.06 \text{ L/hr}$$

b. $Cl_R = k_e V_D = 0.36$ L/hr

$$k_e = \frac{0.36}{30} = 0.012 \text{ hr}^{-1}$$

$$Cl_{nr} = Cl_T - Cl_r$$

$$Cl_{nr} = 6.11 - 0.36 = 5.75 \text{ L/hr}$$

$$Cl_{nr} = k_m V_D$$

$$k_m = \frac{5.75}{30} = 0.192 \text{ hr}^{-1}$$

4. a. Apparent $V_D = (0.21)(78{,}000 \text{ mL})$

$$= 16{,}380 \text{ mL}$$

$$Cl_T = kV_D$$

$$= \left(\frac{0.693}{2}\right)(16{,}380)$$

$$= 5676 \text{ mL/hr} = 94.6 \text{ mL/min}$$

b. k_e = 70% of the elimination constant

$$k_e = (0.7)\left(\frac{0.693}{2}\right) = 0.243 \text{ hr}^{-1}$$

$$Cl_R = k_e V_D$$

$$Cl_R = (0.243)(16{,}380) = 3980 \text{ mL/hr} = 66.3 \text{ mL/min}$$

c. Normal GFR = creatinine clearance = 122 mL/min

Cl_R of drug = 66.3 mL

Because the Cl_R of the drug is less than the creatinine clearance, the drug is filtered at the glomerulus and is partially reabsorbed.

5. a. During intravenous infusion, the drug levels will reach more than 99% of the plasma steady-state concentration after seven half-lives of the drug.

$$Cl_T = \frac{\text{R}}{C_{ss}}$$

$$= \frac{300{,}000 \ \mu\text{g/hr}}{11 \ \mu\text{g/mL}} = 27{,}272 \text{ mL/hr}$$

b. $Cl_T = kV_D$

$$V_D = \frac{27{,}272}{0.693} = 39{,}354 \text{ mL}$$

c. Since $k_m = 0$, $\quad k_e \cong k$

$$Cl_T = Cl_R = 27{,}272 \text{ mL/hr}$$

d. $Cl_R = 27{,}272 \text{ mL/hr} = 454 \text{ mL/min}$

Normal GFR is 100 to 130 mL/min. The drug is probably filtered and actively secreted in the kidney.

6. $$Cl_R = \frac{\text{excretion rate}}{C_p} = \frac{200 \text{ mg/2 hr}}{2.5 \text{ mg/100 mL}}$$

$$= 4000 \text{ mL/hr}$$

7. $$Cl_T = \frac{R}{C_{ss}}$$

$$= \frac{5.3 \text{ mg/kg hr}}{17 \text{ mg/L}} = 0.312 \text{ L/kg hr}$$

For 71.7-kg adults

$$Cl_T = (0.312 \text{ L/kg hr})(71.7 \text{ kg}) = 22.4 \text{ L/hr}$$

11. From the data, determine urinary rate of drug excretion per time period by multiplying urinary volume with the urinary concentration for each points. Average C_p for each period by taking the mean of two consecutive points. Plot dD_u/dt versus C_p to determine renal clearance from slope. The renal clearance from slope is 1493.4 mL/hr (Fig. C-5).

Time (hr)	Plasma Concentration, (μg/mL)	Urinary Volume (mL)	Urinary Concentration (μg/mL)	Urinary Rate dD_u/dt (μg/hr)	Average C_p
0	250.00	100.00	0.00	0.00	
1	198.63	125.00	2680.00	334999.56	224.32
2	157.82	140.00	1901.20	266168.41	178.23
3	125.39	100.00	2114.80	211479.74	141.61
4	99.63	80.00	2100.35	168027.76	112.51
5	79.16	250.00	534.01	133503.70	89.39
6	62.89	170.00	623.96	106073.18	71.03
7	49.97	160.00	526.74	84278.70	56.43
8	39.70	90.00	744.03	66962.26	44.84
9	31.55	400.00	133.01	53203.77	35.63

To determine the total body clearance by the area method, the area under the plasma concentration curve [AUC] must be calculated and summed. The tailpiece was extrapolated because the data are not taken to the end. A plot of log C_p versus t (Fig. C-6) yields a slope of $k = 0.23 \text{ hr}^{-1}$. The tailpiece of area was extrapolated using the last data point divided by k or $31.55/0.23 = 137.17$ μg/mL per hour.

Subtotal area	(0–9 hr)	953.97
Tailpiece	(9–∞ hr)	137.17
Total area	(0–∞)	1091.14

$$\text{Total clearance} = Cl_T = \frac{FD_0}{[AUC]_0^\infty} = \frac{2{,}500{,}000}{1091.14} = 2291.2 \text{ mL/hr}$$

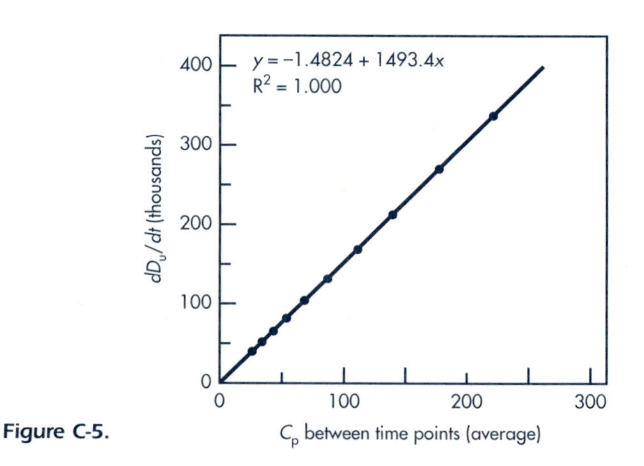

Figure C-5.

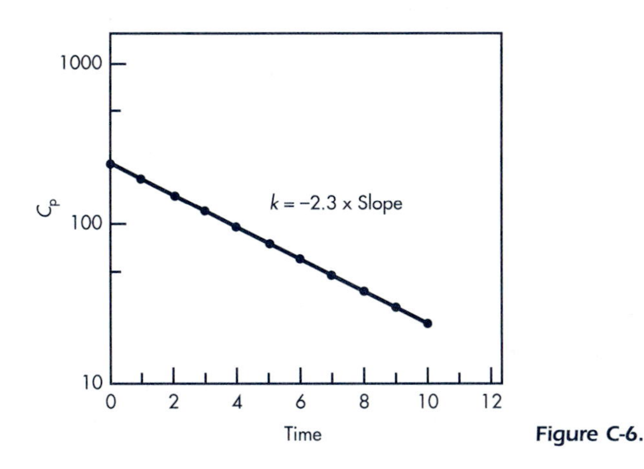

Figure C-6.

Because total body clearance is much larger than renal clearance, the drug is probably also excreted by a nonrenal route.

Nonrenal clearance = 2291.2 − 1493.4 = 797.8 mL/hr

The easiest way to determine clearance by compartmental approach is to estimate k and V_D from the graph. V_D is 10 L and k is 0.23 hr^{-1}. Total clearance is 2300 mL/min (slightly different value when compared with the area method).

CHAPTER 13

FREQUENTLY ASKED QUESTIONS

1. Hepatic drug clearance describes drug metabolism in the liver and accounts for both the effect of blood flow and the intrinsic ability of the liver to metabolize a drug. Hepatic drug clearance is added to renal clearance and other clearances to obtain total (body) clearance, which is important in determining the maintenance dose of a drug. Hepatic drug clearance is often considered nonrenal clearance when measured as the difference between total clearance and renal clearance.
2. Most orally administered drugs pass through the liver prior to systemic absorption. The rate of blood flow can greatly affect the extent of drug that reaches the systemic circulation. Also, intrinsic metabolism may differ among individu-

als and may be genetically determined. These factors may cause drug levels to be more erratic for drugs that undergo extensive metabolism compared to drugs that are excreted renally.

3. Protein synthesis may be altered by liver dysfunction. In general, when drug protein binding is reduced, the free drug may be metabolized more easily. However, some drugs may be metabolized regardless of whether the drug is bound or free (for discussion of nonrestrictive binding, see Chapter 11). In such cases, there is little change in pharmacodynamic activity due to changes in drug protein binding.

4. Erythromycin, morphine, propranolol, various steroids, and other drugs have a large metabolic clearance. Highly potent drugs that have a narrow therapeutic index should be carefully monitored in hepatic disease. Troglitazone (Rezulin), for example, is a drug that can cause severe side effects in patients with liver dysfunction; liver transaminase should be monitored in diabetic patients.

LEARNING QUESTIONS

1. a. $k = k_m + k_e + k_b = 0.20 + 0.25 + 0.15 = 0.60 \text{ hr}^{-1}$

$$t_{1/2} = \frac{0.693}{k} = \frac{0.693}{0.60} = 1.16 \text{ hr}$$

b. $k = k_m + k_e = 0.45 \text{ hr}^{-1}$

$t_{1/2} = 1.54$ hr

c. $k = 0.35 \text{ hr}^{-1}$

$t_{1/2} = 1.98$ hr

d. $k = 0.80 \text{ hr}^{-1}$

$t_{1/2} = 0.87$ hr

2. $k = 0.347 \text{ hr}^{-1}$

$k_e = (0.9)(0.347) = 0.312 \text{ hr}^{-1}$

b. Renal excretion, 90% of the drug is excreted unchanged.

5. Normal hepatic clearance, Cl_H:

$$Cl_H = Q\left(\frac{Cl_{int}}{Q + \text{Cl}_{int}}\right) \qquad Q = 1.5 \text{ L/min}, \qquad Cl_{int} = 0.040 \text{ L/min}$$

$$= 1.5\left(\frac{0.040}{1.5 + 0.040}\right) = 0.039 \text{ L/min}$$

a. Congestive heart failure:

$$Cl_H = 1.0\left(\frac{0.040}{1.0 + 0.040}\right) = 0.038 \text{ L/min}$$

b. Enzyme induction:

$$Cl_H = 1.5\left(\frac{0.090}{1.5 + 0.090}\right) = 0.085 \text{ L/min}$$

Note: A change in blood flow Q did not markedly affect Cl_H for a drug with low Cl_{int}.

6. Normal hepatic clearance:

$$Cl_H = 1.5\left(\frac{12}{1.5 + 12}\right) = 1.33 \text{ L/min}$$

Congestive heart failure (CHF):

$$Cl_H = 1.0\left(\frac{12}{1.0 + 12}\right) = 0.923 \text{ L/min}$$

a.

$$Cl_H = Q(\text{ER}) = Q\left(\frac{Cl_{int}}{Q + Cl_{int}}\right)$$

$$\text{ER} = \frac{Cl_{int}}{Q + Cl_{int}}$$

$$\text{Normal ER} = \frac{12}{1.5 + 12} = 0.89 \text{ L/min}$$

$$\text{CHF ER} = \frac{12}{1.0 + 12} = 0.92 \text{ L/min}$$

b. $F = 1 - \text{ER} = 1 - 0.89$

$F = 0.11$ *or* 11%

10. a. Because <0.5% of the unchanged drug is excreted in the urine, hepatic clearance nearly approximates total body clearance.

$$Cl_H \approx Cl_T = kV_D = (0.693/3.9)(4.3)(80) = 61.1 \text{ L/hr}$$

b. $Cl_H = Q\,\text{ER} \qquad Q = (1.5 \text{ L/min})(60 \text{ min}) = 90 \text{ L/hr}$

$\text{ER} = 61.1/90 = 0.68.$

11. a. $Cl_T = kV_D = (0.693/1.6)(0.78)(81) = 27.4 \text{ L/hr}$

b. $Cl_R = k_e V_D$

$$k_e = 0.12k = (0.12)(0.693/1.6) = 0.052 \text{ hr}^{-1}$$

$$Cl_R = (0.052)(0.78)(81) = 3.29 \text{ L/hr}$$

Alternatively,

$$Cl_R = f_e Cl_T$$

$$Cl_R = 0.12\ Cl_T = (0.12)(27.4) = 3.29 \text{ L/hr}$$

c. $Cl_H = Cl_T - Cl_R = 27.4 - 3.29 = 24.11 \text{ L/hr}$

CHAPTER 14

? FREQUENTLY ASKED QUESTIONS

1. Slow IV infusion may be used to avoid side effects due to rapid drug administration. For example, immune globulin intravenous (human), may cause a rapid fall in blood pressure and possible anaphylactic shock in some patients when rapidly infused intravenously. Some antisense drugs cause a rapid fall in blood pressure also when injected rapidly IV into the body. The rate of infusion is particularly important in administering anti-arrythmic agents in patients. The rapid IV bolus injection of many drugs (eg, lidocaine) that follow the pharmacokinetics of multiple compartment models may cause an adverse response due to the initial high drug concentration in the central (plasma) compartment before slow equilibration with the tissues.
2. The loading drug dose is used to rapidly attain the target drug concentration, which is approximately the steady-state drug concentration. However, the loading dose will not maintain the steady-state level unless an appropriate IV drug infusion rate or maintenance dose is also given. If a larger IV drug infusion rate or maintenance dose is given, the resulting steady-state drug concentration will be much higher and remain sustained at the higher level. A higher infusion rate may be taken if the initial steady-state drug level is inadequate for the patient.
3. The common complications associated with intravenous infusion include phlebitis and infections at the infusion site caused by poor intravenous techniques or indwelling catheters.

LEARNING QUESTIONS

1. **a.** To reach 95% of C_{ss}:

   $$4.32t_{1/2} = (4.32)(7) = 30.2 \text{ hr}$$

   b. $D_L = C_{ss}V_D = (10)(0.231)(65000) = 150 \text{ mg}$

   c. $R = C_{ss}V_Dk = (10)(15000)(0.099) = 14.85 \text{ mg/hr}$

d. $Cl_T = V_D k = (15000)(0.099) = 1485$ mL/hr

e. To establish a new C_{ss} would still take $4.32t_{1/2}$. However, the $t_{1/2}$ would be longer in renal failure.

f. If Cl_T is decreased by 50%, then the infusion rate R should be decreased proportionately:

$$R = 10(0.50)(1485) = 7.425 \text{ mg/hr}$$

2. a. The steady-state level can be found by plotting the IV infusion data. The plasma–drug time curves plateau at 10 μg/mL. Alternatively, V_D and k can be found from the single IV dose data:

$$V_D = 100 \text{ mL/kg} \qquad k = 0.2 \text{ hr}^{-1}$$

b. Using equations developed in Example 2 in the first set of examples in Chapter 14:

$$0.95\frac{R}{V_D k} = \frac{R}{V_D k}(1 - e^{-kt})$$
$$0.95 = 1 - e^{-0.2t}$$
$$0.05 = e^{-0.2t}$$
$$t_{95\%ss} = \frac{\ln 0.05}{-0.2} = 15 \text{ hr}$$

c.

$$Cl_T = V_d k = 100 \times 0.2 = 20 \text{ mL/kg hr}$$

$$V_D = D_0/C_p^0 = 1000/10 = 100 \text{ mL/kg}$$

d. The drug level 4 hours after stopping the IV infusion can be found by considering the drug concentration at the termination of infusion as C_p^0. At the termination of the infusion, the drug level will decline by a first-order process.

$$C_p = C_p^0 e^{-kt}$$
$$= 9.9e^{-(0.2)(4)}$$
$$= 4.5 \ \mu\text{g/mL}$$

e. The infusion rate producing a C_{ss} of 10 μg/mL is 0.2 mg/kg per hour. Therefore, the infusion rate needed for this patient is as follows:

$$0.2 \text{ mg/kg hr} \times 75 \text{ kg} = 15 \text{ mg/hr}$$

f. From the data shown, at 4 hours after the start of the IV infusion, the drug concentration is 5.5 μg/mL; the drug concentration after an IV bolus of 1 mg/kg is 4.5 μg/mL. Therefore, if a 1-mg dose was given and the drug is then infused at 0.2 mg/kg per hr, the plasma drug concentration would be $4.5 + 5.5 = 10$ μg/mL.

3. Infusion rate R for a 75-kg patient:

$$R = (1 \text{ mg/kg hr})(75 \text{ kg}) = 75 \text{ mg/hr}$$

Sterile drug solution contains 25 mg/mL. Therefore, 3 mL contains (3 mL) × (25 mg/mL), or 75 mg. The patient should receive 3 mL (75 mg)/hr by IV infusion.

4. $C_{ss} = \dfrac{R}{V_D k} \qquad R = C_{ss} V_D k$

$$R = (20 \text{ mg/L})(0.5 \text{ L/kg})(75 \text{ kg})\left(\frac{0.693}{3 \text{ hr}}\right) = 173.25 \text{ mg/hr}$$

Drug is supplied as 125 mg/mL. Therefore,

$$125 \text{ mg/mL} = \frac{173.25 \text{ mg}}{X} \qquad X = 1.386 \text{ mL}$$

$$R = 1.386 \text{ mL/hr}$$

$$D_L = C_{ss}V_D = (20 \text{ mg/L})(0.5 \text{ L/kg})(75 \text{ kg}) = 750 \text{ mg}$$

5. $C_{ss} = \dfrac{R}{kV_D} = \dfrac{R}{Cl_T}$

a. $Cl_T = \dfrac{R}{C_{ss}} = \dfrac{5.3 \text{ mg/kg hr} \times 71.71 \text{ kg}}{17 \text{ mg/L}} = 22.4 \text{ L/hr}$

b. At end of IV infusion, $C_p = 17\ \mu\text{g/mL}$. Assuming first-order elimination kinetics:

$$C_p = C_p^0 e^{-kt}$$
$$1.5 = 17e^{-k(2.5)}$$
$$0.0882 = e^{-2.5k}$$
$$\ln 0.0882 = -2.5k$$
$$-2.43 = -2.5k$$
$$k = 0.971 \text{ hr}^{-1}$$
$$t_{1/2} = \frac{0.693}{0.971} = 0.714 \text{ hr}$$

c. $Cl_T = kV_D \qquad V_D = Cl_T/k$

$$V_D = \frac{22.4}{0.971} = 23.1 \text{ L}$$

d. Probenecid blocks active tubular secretion of cephradine.

6. At steady-state, the rate of elimination should equal the rate of absorption. Therefore, the rate of elimination would be 30 mg/hr. The C_{ss} is directly proportional to the rate of infusion R, as shown by:

$$C_{ss} = \frac{R}{kV_D} \qquad kV_D = \frac{R}{C_{ss}}$$

$$\frac{R_{old}}{C_{ss,old}} = \frac{R_{new}}{C_{ss,new}}$$

$$\frac{30 \text{ mg/hr}}{20\ \mu\text{g/mL}} = \frac{40 \text{ mg/hr}}{C_{ss,new}}$$

$$C_{ss,new} = 26.7\ \mu\text{g/mL}$$

The new elimination rate would be 40 mg/hr.

7. a. $R = C_{ss}kV_D$

$R = (20 \text{ mg/L})(0.693/8 \text{ hr})(1.5 \text{ L/kg})(75 \text{ kg}) = 194.9 \text{ mg/hr}$

$R \approx 195 \text{ mg/hr}$

b. $D_L = C_{ss}V_D = (20)(1.5)(75) = 2250$ mg given by IV bolus injection

c. The loading dose is given to obtain steady-state drug concentrations as rapidly as possible.

d. 15 mL of the antibiotic solution contains 225 mg of drug. Thus, an IV infusion rate of 15 mL/hr is equivalent to 225 mg/hr. The C_{ss} achieved by the manufacturer's recommendation is the following:

$$C_{ss} = \frac{R}{kV_D} = \frac{225}{(0.0866)(112.5)} = 23.1 \text{ mg/L}$$

The theoretical C_{ss} of 23.1 mg/L is close to the desired C_{ss} of 20 mg/L. Assuming a reasonable therapeutic window, the manufacturer's suggested starting infusion rate is satisfactory.

CHAPTER 15

? FREQUENTLY ASKED QUESTIONS

1. Some of the advantages for administering a drug by constant IV infusion include: (1) A drug may be infused continuously for many hours without disturbing the patient. (2) Constant infusion provides a stable blood drug level for drugs that have a narrow therapeutic index. (3) Some drugs are better tolerated when infused slowly. (4) Some drugs may be infused simultaneously with electrolytes or other infusion media in an acute-care setting. Disadvantages for administering a drug by constant IV infusion include: (1) Some drugs are more suitable to be administered as a bolus IV injection. For example, some reports show that an aminoglycoside given once daily resulted in fewer side effects compared with dividing the dose into 2 to 3 doses daily. Due to drug accumulation in the kidney and adverse toxicity, aminoglycosides are generally not given by prolonged IV infusions. In contrast, a prolonged period of low drug level for penicillins and tetracyclines may not be as efficacious and may result in a longer cure time for an infection. The pharmacodynamics of the individual drug must be studied to determine the best course of action. (2) Drugs such as nitroglycerin are less likely to produce tolerance when administered intermittently versus continuously.

2. A loading or priming dose is used to rapidly raise the plasma drug concentration to therapeutic drug levels to obtain a more rapid pharmacodynamic response. In addition, the loading dose along with the maintenance dose allows the drug to reach steady state quickly, particularly for drugs with long elimination half-lives.

An alternative way of explaining the loading dose is based on clearance. After multiple IV dosing, the maintenance dose required is based on Cl, C_{ss}, and τ:

$C_{ss} = \text{Dose}/(\tau\ Cl)$,
$\text{Dose} = C_{ss}\ \tau\ Cl$

If C_{ss} and τ are fixed, a drug with a smaller clearance requires a smaller maintenance dose. In practice, the dosing interval is adjustable and may be longer for drugs with a, small Cl if the drug does not need to be dosed frequently. The steady-state drug level is generally determined by the desired therapeutic drug.

3. *Accumulation index* (R) is a ratio that indicates steady-state drug concentration to the drug concentration after the first dose. The accumulation index does not measure the absolute size of overdosing, but measures the amount of drug cumulation that can occur due to frequent drug administration. Factors that affect R are the elimination rate constant, k, and the dosing interval, τ. If the first dose is not chosen appropriately, the steady state level may still be incorrect. Therefore, the first dose and the dosing interval must be determined correctly to avoid any significant drug accumulation. The accumulation index is a good indication of accumulation due to frequent drug dosing, applicable to any drug, regardless of whether the drug is bound to tissues.

4. The loading dose will only affect the initial drug concentrations in the body. Steady-state drug levels are obtained after several elimination half lives (eg, 4.32 $t_{1/2}$ for 95% steady-state level). Only 5% of the drug contributed by the loading dose will remain at 95% steady state. At 99% steady state level, only 1% of the loading dose will remain.

5. Two possible examples are digoxin and amitriptyline.

6. After an IV bolus drug injection, the drug is well distributed within a few minutes. In practice, however, an IV bolus dose may be administered slowly over several minutes or the drug may have a slow distribution phase. Therefore, clinicians often prefer to take a blood sample 15 minutes or 30 minutes after IV bolus injection and refer to that drug concentration as the peak concentration. In some cases, a blood sample is taken an hour later to avoid the fluctuating concentration in the distributive phase. The error due to changing sampling time can be large for a drug with a short elimination half-life.

LEARNING QUESTIONS

1. $V_D = 0.20(50 \text{ kg}) = 10{,}000 \text{ mL}$

a. $$D_{max} = \frac{D_0}{1-f} = \frac{50 \text{ mg}}{1 - e^{-(0.693/2)(8)}} = 53.3 \text{ mg}$$

$$C_{max} = \frac{D_{max}}{V_D} = \frac{53.3 \text{ mg}}{10{,}000 \text{ ml}} = 5.33\ \mu\text{g/mL}$$

b. $$D_{min} = 53.3 - 50 = 3.3 \text{ mg}$$

$$C_{min} = \frac{3.3 \text{ mg}}{10{,}000 \text{ mL}} = 0.33\ \mu\text{g/mL}$$

c. $$C_{av}^{\infty} = \frac{FD_0 1.44 t_{1/2}}{V_D \tau} = \frac{(50)(1.44)(2)}{(10{,}000)(8)} = 1.8\ \mu\text{g/mL}$$

2. a. $$D_0 = \frac{C_{av}^{\infty} V_D \tau}{1.44 t_{1/2}}$$

$$= \frac{(10)(40{,}000)(6)}{(1.44)(5)} = 333 \text{ mg every 6 hr}$$

b. $\tau = \dfrac{FD_0 1.44 t_{1/2}}{V_D C_{av}^{\infty}}$

$= \dfrac{(225{,}000)(1.44)(5)}{(40{,}000)(10)} = 4.05 \text{ hr}$

6. Dose the patient with 200 mg every 3 hours.

$$D_L = \frac{D_0}{1 - e^{-k\tau}} = \frac{200}{1 - e^{-(0.23)(3)}} = 400 \text{ mg}$$

Notice that D_L is twice the maintenance dose, because the drug is given at a dosage interval equal approximately to the $t_{1/2}$ of 3 hours.

8. The plasma drug concentration C_p may be calculated at any time after n doses by Equation 15.21 and proper substitution.

$$C_p = \frac{D_0}{V_D}\left(\frac{1 - e^{-nk\tau}}{1 - e^{-k\tau}}\right) e^{-k\tau}$$

$$C_p = \frac{200}{40}\left(\frac{1 - e^{-(3)(0.347)(4)}}{1 - e^{-(0.347)(4)}}\right) e^{-(0.347)(1)} = 4.63 \text{ mg/L}$$

Alternatively, one may conclude that for a drug whose elimination $t_{1/2}$ is 2 hours, the predicted plasma drug concentration is approximately at steady state after 3 doses or 12 hours. Therefore, the above calculation may be simplified to the following:

$$C_p = \frac{D_0}{V_D} = \left(\frac{1}{1 - e^{-k\tau}}\right) e^{-k\tau}$$

$$C_p = \left(\frac{200}{40}\right)\left(\frac{1}{1 - e^{-(0.347)(4)}}\right) e^{-(0.347)(1)} = 4.71 \text{ mg/L}$$

9. $C_{max}^{\infty} = \dfrac{D_0/V_D}{1 - e^{-k\tau}}$

where

$$V_D = 20\% \text{ of } 82 \text{ kg} = (0.2)(82) = 16.4 \text{ L}$$
$$k = (0.693/3) = 0.231 \text{ hr}^{-1}$$
$$D_0 = V_D C_{max}^{\infty}(1 - e^{-k\tau}) = (16.4)(10)(1 - e^{-(0.231)(8)})$$

a. $D_0 = 138.16$ mg to be given every 8 hours

b. $C_{min}^{\infty} = C_{max}^{\infty}(e^{-k\tau}) = (10)(e^{-(0.231)(8)}) = 1.58 \text{ mg/L}$

c. $C_{av}^{\infty} = \dfrac{D_0}{kV_D\tau} = \dfrac{138.16}{(0.231)(16.4)(8)} = 4.56 \text{ mg/L}$

d. In the above dosage regimen, the C_{min}^{∞} of 1.59 mg/L is below the desired C_{min}^{∞} of 2 mg/L. Alternatively, the dosage interval, τ, could be changed to 6 hours.

$$D_0 = V_D C_{max}^{\infty}(1 - e^{-k\tau}) = (16.4)(10)(1 - e^{-(0.231)(6)})$$
$$D_0 = 123 \text{ mg to be given every 6 hrs}$$
$$C_{min}^{\infty} = C_{max}^{\infty}(e^{-k\tau}) = (10)(e^{-(0.231)(6)}) = 2.5 \text{ mg/L}$$
$$C_{av}^{\infty} = \frac{D_0}{kV_D\tau} = \frac{123}{(0.231)(16.4)(6)} = 5.41 \text{ mg/L}$$

10. a. $C_{av}^{\infty} = \dfrac{FD_0}{kV_D\tau}$

Let $C_{av}^{\infty} = 27.5$ mg/L

$$D_0 = \frac{C_{av}^{\infty} k V_D \tau}{F} = \frac{(27.5)(0.693/10.6)(0.5)(78)(6)}{0.77} = 546.3 \text{ mg}$$

$D_0 = 546.3$ mg every 6 hrs

b. If a 500-mg capsule is given every 6 hours:

$$C_{av}^{\infty} = \frac{FD_0}{kV_D\tau} = \frac{(0.77)(500)}{(0.693/10.6)(0.5)(78)(6)} = 25.2 \text{ mg/L}$$

c. $$D_L = \frac{D_M}{1 - e^{-k\tau}} = \frac{500}{1 - e^{-(0.654)(6)}} = 1543 \text{ mg}$$

$D_L = 3 \times 500$ mg capsules $= 1500$ mg

CHAPTER 16

? FREQUENTLY ASKED QUESTIONS

1. A patient with concomitant hepatic disease may have decreased biotransformation enzyme activity. Infants and young subjects may have immature hepatic enzyme systems. Alcoholics may have liver cirrhosis and lack certain coenzymes. Other patients may experience enzyme saturation at normal doses due to genetic polymorphism. Pharmacokinetics provides a simple way to identify nonlinear kinetics in these patients and to estimate an appropriate dose. Finally, concomitant use of other drugs may cause nonlinear pharmacokinetics at lower drug doses due to enzyme inhibition.
2. A drug following linear pharmacokinetics generally has a constant elimination half-life and a constant clearance with an increase in the dose. The steady-state drug concentrations and AUC are proportional to the size of the dose. Nonlinear pharmacokinetics results in a dose dependent Cl, $t_{1/2}$, and AUC. Nonlinear pharmacokinetics are often described in terms of V_{max} and K_M.
3. The physiologic model based on organ drug clearance describes nonlinear drug metabolism in terms of blood flow and intrinsic hepatic clearance (Chapter 13). Drugs are extracted by the liver as they are presented by blood flow. The physiologic model accounts for the sigmoid profile with changing blood flow and ex-

traction, whereas the Michaelis–Menten model simulates the metabolic profile based on V_{max} and K_M. The Michaelis–Menten model was applied mostly to describe *in vitro* enzymatic reactions. When V_{max} and K_M are estimated in patients, blood flow is not explicitly considered. This semiempirical method was found by many clinicians to be useful in dosing phenytoin. The organ clearance model was more useful in explaining clearance change due to impaired blood flow. In practice, the physiologic model has limited use in dosing patients because blood flow data for patients are not available.

4. *Chronopharmacokinetics* is the main cause of nonlinear pharmacokinetics that is not dose related. The time-dependent or temporal process of drug elimination can be the result of rhythmic changes in the body. For example, nortriptyline and theophylline levels are higher when administered between 7 AM and 9 AM compared to 7 PM to 9 PM after the same dose. Biological rhythmic differences in clearance cause a lower elimination rate in the morning compared to that in the evening. Other factors causing nonlinear pharmacokinetics may result from enzyme induction (eg, carbamazepine) or enzyme inhibition after multiple doses of the drug. Furthermore, the drug or a metabolite may accumulate following multiple dosing and affect the metabolism or renal elimination of the drug.

LEARNING QUESTIONS

2. Capacity-limited processes for drugs include:
- Absorption
  - Active transport
  - Intestinal metabolism by microflora
- Distribution
  - Protein binding
- Elimination
  - Hepatic elimination
  - Biotransformation
  - Active biliary secretion
- Renal excretion
  - Active tubular secretion
  - Active tubular reabsorption

4. $C_p^0 = \frac{\text{dose}}{V_D} = \frac{10{,}000\ \mu\text{g}}{20{,}000\ \text{mL}} = 0.5\ \mu\text{g/mL}$

From Equation 16.1,

$$\text{Elimination rate} = -\frac{dC_p}{dt} = \frac{V_{max} C_p}{k_M + C_p}$$

Because $K_M = 50\ \mu g/mL$, $C_p \ll K_M$ and the reaction rate is first order. Thus, the above equation reduces to Equation 16.3.

$$-\frac{dC_p}{dt} = \frac{V_{max} C_p}{K_M} = k' C_p$$

$$k' = \frac{V_{max}}{K_M} = \frac{20\ \mu g/hr}{50\ \mu g} = 0.4\ hr^{-1}$$

For first-order reactions,

$$t_{1/2} = \frac{0.693}{k'} = \frac{0.693}{0.4} = 1.73\ hr$$

The drug will be 50% metabolized in 1.73 hours.

7. When INH coadminstered, plasma phenytoin concentration is increased due to a reduction in metabolic rate v. Equation 16.1 shows that v and K_M are inversely related (K_M in denominator). An increase in K_M would be accompanied by an increase in plasma drug concentration. Figure 16-4 shows that an increase in K_M is accompanied by an increase in amount of drug in the body at any time t. Equation 16.4 relates drug concentration to K_M, and it can be seen that the two are proportionally related, although they are not linearly proportional to each other due to the complexity of the equation. An actual study in the literature shows that k is increased several-fold in the presence of INH in the body.

8. The K_M has the unit of concentration. In laboratory studies, K_M is expressed in moles per liter, or micromoles per milliliter, because reactions are expressed in moles and not milligrams. In dosing, drugs are given in milligram and plasma drug concentrations are expressed as milligrams per liter or micrograms per milliliter. The units of K_M for pharmacokinetic models are estimated from *in vivo* data. They are, therefore, commonly expressed accordingly as milligrams per liter, which is preferred over micrograms per milliliter because dose is usually expressed in milligrams. The two terms may be shown to be equivalent. Occasionally, when simulating amount of drug metabolized in the body as a function of time, the amount of drug in the body has been assumed to follow Michaelis–Menten kinetics, and K_M would assume the unit of D_0 (eg, mg). In this case, K_M would take on a very different meaning.

CHAPTER 17

FREQUENTLY ASKED QUESTIONS

1. Therapeutic drug monitoring (TDM) may be performed by sampling other biologic fluids, such as saliva or, when available, tissue or ear fluids. However, the sample must be correlated to blood or special tissue level. Urinary drug concentrations generally are not reliable. Saliva is considered an ultrafiltrate of plasma and does not contain significant albumin. Saliva drug concentrations represent free plasma drug levels and have been used with limited success for monitoring some drugs.

   Pharmacodynamic end points such as prothrombin clotting time for warfarin, blood glucose concentrations for antidiabetic drugs, blood pressure for antihypertensive drugs, and other clinical observations are useful indications that the drug is dosed correctly.

2. Most pharmacokinetic models require well-controlled studies in which many blood samples are taken from each subject and the pharmacokinetic parameters estimated. In patient care situations, only a limited number of blood samples is collected, which does not allow for the complete determination of the drug's pharmacokinetic profile in the individual patient. However, the data from blood samples taken from a large demographic sector are more reflective of the diseased states of the patients treated. Population pharmacokinetics allow data from previous patients to be used in addition to the limited blood sample from the individual patient. The type of information obtained is less constrained and sometimes dependent on the model and algorithm used for analysis. However, many successful examples have been reported in the literature.

3. The major considerations in TDM include the pathophysiology of the patient, the blood sample collection, and the data analysis. Clinical assessment of patient history, drug interaction, and demographic factors are all part of a successful program for therapeutic drug monitoring.

4. With the Bayesian approach, the estimate of the patient parameters are constrained more narrowly to allow easier parameter estimation due to information provided from the population. The information is then combined with one or more serum concentrations from the patient to obtain a set of final patient parameters (generally Cl and V_D). When no serum sample is taken, the Bayesian approach is reduced to an *a priori* model using only population parameters.

5. Pharmacokinetics provides a means of studying whether an unusual drug action is related to pharmacokinetic factors, such as drug disposition, distribu-

tion, or binding or is related to pharmacodynamic interaction, such as a difference in receptor sensitivity, drug tolerance, or some other reason. Many drug interactions involving enzyme inhibition, stimulation, and protein binding were discovered as a result of pharmacokinetic and pharmacodynamic investigations.

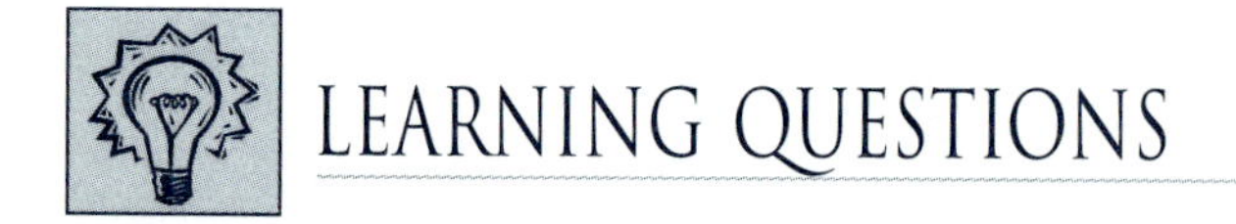

LEARNING QUESTIONS

1. Steady-state drug concentrations are achieved in approximately 5 half-lives. For a drug with a half-life of 36 hours, steady-state drug concentrations are achieved in approximately 180 hours (or 7.5 days). Thus, dose adjustment in patients is difficult for drugs with very long half-lives. In contrast, steady-state drug concentrations are achieved in approximately 20 to 30 hours (or 1 day) for drugs whose half-lives are 4 to 6 hours.

2.
$$C_{\max}^{\infty} = \frac{D_0}{V_D}\left(\frac{1}{1 - e^{-k\tau}}\right) = \frac{250{,}000}{42{,}000}\left(\frac{1}{1 - e^{-(6)(1.034)}}\right) = \frac{250{,}000}{42{,}000}\left(\frac{1}{0.998}\right) = 5.96\ \mu\text{g/mL}$$

At steady state, the peak concentration of penicillin G would be 5.96 μg/mL.

3.
$$C_{\text{av}}^{\infty} = \frac{D}{kV_D\tau} = \frac{250{,}000}{(0.99)(20{,}000)(6)} = 2.10\ \mu\text{g/mL}$$

Free drug concentration at steady state $= 2.10(1 - 0.97) = 0.063\ \mu$g/mL.

4.
$$C_{\text{av}}^{\infty} = \frac{1.44 D_0 F t_{1/2}}{V_D \tau}$$

For the Normal Patient:

$$V_D = (0.392)(1)(1000) = 392\ \text{mL/kg}$$

$$C_{\text{av}}^{\infty} = \frac{(1.44)(D_0)(1)(1.49)}{(392)(6)} = 2\ \mu\text{g/mL}$$

$$D_0 = \frac{(392)(6)(2)}{(1.44)(1.49)} = 2192\ \mu\text{g/kg} = 2.2\ \text{mg/kg}$$

For the Uremic Patient:

$$V_D = (23.75)(1)(1000) = 237.5\ \text{mL/kg}$$

$$C_{\text{av}}^{\infty} = \frac{(1.44)(D_0)(1)(6.03)}{(237.5)(6)} = 2\ \mu\text{g/mL}$$

$$D_0 = \frac{(2)(237.5)(6)}{(1.44)(6.03)} = 328.2\ \mu\text{g/kg} = 0.3\ \text{mg/kg}$$

5. a. $V_D = 306{,}000$ ml Dose $= 0.5 \times 10^6$ ng

$$C_{av}^{\infty} = \frac{(1.44)(DFt_{1/2})}{V_D\tau} = \frac{(1.44)(0.5 \times 10^6)(0.56)(0.95)}{(306{,}000)(1)} = 1.25\ \text{ng/mL}$$

b. The patient is adequately dosed.

c. $F = 1$; using the above equation, the C_{av}^{∞} would be 2.2 ng/mL; although still effective, the C_{av}^{∞} will be closer to the toxic serum concentration of 3 ng/mL.

6. The Cl_{Cr} for this patient shows normal kidney function.

$t_{1/2} = 2$ hr, $\quad k = 0.693/2 = 0.3465\ \text{hr}^{-1}$
$V_D = 0.2\ \text{L/kg} \times 80\ \text{kg} = 16\ \text{L}$

a. $$C_{max}^{\infty} = \frac{D_0/V_D}{1 - e^{-k\tau}} = \frac{250/16}{1 - e^{-(0.3465)(8)}} = 16.68\ \text{mg/L}$$

$$C_{min}^{\infty} = C_{max}^{\infty} e^{-k\tau} = 16.68 e^{-(0.3465)(8)} = 1.04\ \text{mg/L}$$

The dosage regimen of 250 mg every 8 hours gives a C_{max}^{∞} above 16 mg/L and a C_{min}^{∞} below 2 mg/L. Therefore, this dosage regimen is not correct.

b. Several trials might be necessary to obtain a more optimal dosing regimen. One approach is to change the dosage interval, τ, to 6 hours and to calculate the dose, D_0:

$$D_0 = C_{max}^{\infty}\ V_D(1 - e^{-k\tau}) = (16)(14)(1 - e^{-(0.3465)(6)}) = 196\ \text{mg}$$
$$C_{min}^{\infty} = C_{max}^{\infty} e^{-k\tau} = 16 e^{-(0.3465)(6)} = 2\ \text{mg/L}$$

A dose of 196 mg (approximately 200 mg) given every 6 hours should achieve the desired drug concentrations.

10. Assume desired $C_{av}^{\infty} = 0.0015\ \mu\text{g/mL}$ and $\tau = 24$ hours.

$$C_{av}^{\infty} = \frac{FD_0\ 1.44t_{1/2}}{V_D\tau}$$

$$D_0 = \frac{C_{av}^{\infty}\ V_D\tau}{F\,1.44t_{1/2}}$$

$$= \frac{(0.0015)(4)(68)(24)}{(0.80)(1.44)(30)} = 0.283\ \text{mg}$$

Give 0.283 mg every 24 hours.

a. For a dosage regimen of one 0.30-mg tablet daily,

$$C_{av}^{\infty} = \frac{(0.80)(0.3)(1.44)(30)}{(4)(68)(24)} = 0.0016\ \mu\text{g/mL}$$

which is within the therapeutic window.

b. A dosage regimen of 0.15 mg/12 hr would provide smaller fluctuations between C_{max}^{∞} and C_{min}^{∞} compared to a dosage regimen of 0.30 mg/24 hr.

c. Since the elimination half-life is long (30 hours), a loading dose is advisable.

$$D_L = D_m \left(\frac{1}{1 - e^{-k\tau}}\right)$$

$$= 0.30 \left(\frac{1}{1 - e^{-(0.693/30)(24)}}\right) = 0.70\ \text{mg}$$

For cardiotonic drugs related to the digitalis glycosides, it is recommended that the loading dose be administered in several portions with approximately half the total as the first dose. Additional fractions may be given at 6- to 8-hour intervals, with careful assessment of the clinical response before each additional dose.

d. There is no rationale for a controlled-release drug product due to the long elimination half-life of 30 hours inherent in the drug.

11. a. $C_{av}^{\infty} = \dfrac{FD_0\ 1.44t_{1/2}}{V_D\tau}$

$$= \frac{(1500)(1.44)(6)}{(1.3)(63)(4)} = 39.6\ \mu g/mL$$

b. $D_L = D_M \left(\dfrac{1}{1 - e^{-k\tau}}\right)$

c. A D_L of 4.05 g is needed that is equivalent to 8 tablets containing 0.5 g each.

d. The time to achieve 95 to 99% of steady state is, approximately, $5t_{1/2}$ without a loading dose. Therefore,

$$5 \times 6 = 30\ \text{hr}$$

12. a. $C_{ss} = \dfrac{R}{kV_D} \qquad R = C_{ss}kV_D$

$$R = (5)\left(\frac{0.693}{2}\right)(0.173)(75) = 22.479\ \text{mg/hr}$$

$$D_L = C_{ss}V_D = (5)(0.173)(75) = 64.875\ \text{mg}$$

b. $\dfrac{R_{old}}{C_{ss,old}} = \dfrac{R_{new}}{C_{ss,new}}$

$$\frac{22.479}{2} = \frac{R_{new}}{5} \qquad R_{new} = 56.2\ \text{mg/hr}$$

c. $4.32t_{1/2} = 4.32(2) = 8.64\ \text{hr}$

13. $t_{1/2} = 8\ \text{hr} \qquad k = 0.693/8 = 0.0866\ \text{hr}^{-1}$

$V_D = (1.5\ \text{L/kg})(75\ \text{kg}) = 112.5\ \text{L} \qquad C_{ss} = 20\ \mu g/mL$

a. $R = C_{ss}kV_D = (20)(0.0866)(112.5) = 194.85\ \text{mg/hr}$

b. $D_L = C_{ss}V_D = (20)(112.5) = 2250\ \text{mg}$

Alternatively, $D_L = R/k = 194.85/0/0866 = 2250\ \text{mg}$

c. 0.2 mL of a 15 mg/mL solution contains 3 mg.

$$R = 3\ \text{mg/hr/kg} \times 75\ \text{kg} = 225\ \text{mg/hr}$$

$$C_{ss} = \frac{R}{kV_D} = \frac{225}{(0.0866)(112.5)} = 23.1\ \text{mg/L}$$

The proposed starting infusion rate given by the manufacturer should provide adequate drug concentrations.

CHAPTER 18

FREQUENTLY ASKED QUESTIONS

1. Renal disease can cause profound changes in the body that must be evaluated by assessing the patient's condition and medical history. Renal dysfunction is often accompanied by reduced protein drug binding and by reduced glomerular filtration rate in the kidney. Some changes in hepatic clearance may also occur. While there is no accurate method for predicting the resulting *in vivo* changes, a decrease in albumin may increase f_u, or the fraction of free plasma drug concentration in the body. The f_u is estimated from the following: $f_u = 1 - f_b$, where f_b is the fraction of bound plasma drug. For the uremic patient, the fraction of drug bound f_b' is affected by a change in plasma protein: $f_b'/f_b = p'/4.4$, where p is the normal plasma protein concentration (4.4 g/dL assuming albumin is the protein involved) and p' is the uremic plasma protein concentration; f_b' is the fraction of drug bound in the uremic patient. Since f_u', or fraction of unbound drug, is increased in the uremic patient, the free drug concentration may be increased and sometimes lead to more frequent side effects. On the other hand, an increase in plasma free drug in the uremic patient is offset somewhat by a corresponding increase in the volume of distribution as plasma protein drug binding is reduced. Reduction in GFR is more definite; it is invariably accompanied by a reduction in drug clearance and by an increase in the elimination half-life of the drug.
2. Two approaches to dose adjustment in renal disease are the clearance method and the elimination rate constant method. The methods are based on estimating either the uremic Cl_R or uremic k_R after the creatinine clearance is obtained in the uremic patient.
3. Aminoglycosides are given as a larger dose spaced farther apart (once daily). Keeping the same total daily dose of the aminoglycoside improves the response (efficacy) and possibly lessens side effects in many patients. Model simulation shows reduced exposure (AUC) to the effect compartment (toxicity), while the activity is not altered. The higher drug dose produces a higher peak drug concentration. In the case of gentamicin, the marketed drug is chemically composed of three related, but distinctly different, chemical components which may distribute differently in the body.
4. Hepatic disease may reduce albumin and α_1-acid glycoprotein (AAG) concentrations resulting in decreased drug protein binding. Blood flow to the liver may also be affected. Generally, for a drug with linear binding, f_u may be increased as discussed in FAQ #1. Consult Chapter 11 also for a discussion of restrictive

clearance of drugs. Examples of binding to AAG are the protease inhibitors for AIDS.

5. Congestive heart failure (CHF) can reduce renal or hepatic blood flow and decrease hepatic and renal drug clearance. In CHF, less blood flow is available in the splanchnic circulation to the small intestine and may result to less systemic drug bioavailability after oral drug administration. Severe disturbances to blood flow will affect the pharmacokinetics of many drugs. Myocardiac infarction (MI) is a clinical example which often causes drug clearance to be greatly reduced, especially for drugs with large hepatic extraction.

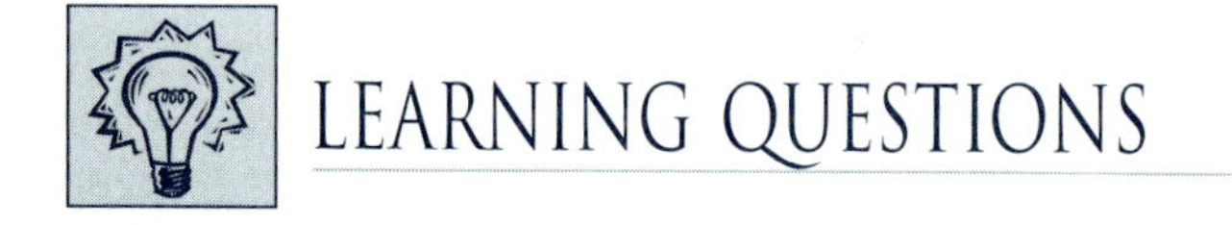

LEARNING QUESTIONS

1. The normal dose of tetracycline is 250 mg PO every 6 hours. The dose of tetracycline for the uremic patient is determined by the k_u/k_N ratio, which is determined by the kidney function, as in Figure 18-5. From line H in the figure, at Cl_{Cr} of 20 mL, $k_u/k_N = 40\%$. In order to maintain the average concentration of tetracycline at the same level as in normal patients, the dose of tetracycline must be reduced.

$$\frac{D_u}{D_N} = \frac{k_u}{k_N} = 40\%$$

$$D_u = (250)(0.40) = 100 \text{ mg}$$

Therefore, 100 mg of tetracycline should be given PO every 6 hours.

2. The drug in this patient is eliminated by the kidneys and the dialysis machine. Therefore,

$$\text{Total drug clearance} = Cl_T + Cl_D$$

Using Equation 18.33,

$$Cl_D = \frac{Q(C_a - C_v)}{C_a}$$

$$= \frac{50(5 - 2.4)}{5} = 26 \text{ mL/min}$$

Total drug clearance = 10 + 26 = 36 mL/min

Since the drug clearance is increased from 10 to 36 mL/min, the dose should be increased if dialysis is going to continue. Since dose is directly proportional to clearance,

$$\frac{D_u}{D_N} = \frac{36}{10} = 3.6$$

The new dose should be 3.6 times the dose given before dialysis if the same level of antibiotics is to be maintained.

4. The creatinine clearance of a patient is determined experimentally by using Equation 18.11,

$$Cl_{Cr} = \frac{C_u V 100}{C_{Cr} 1440}$$

$$= \frac{(0.1)(1800)(100)}{(2.2)(1440)} = 5.68 \text{ mL/min}$$

Assuming the normal Cl_{Cr} in this patient is 100 mL/min, the uremic dose should be 5.7% of the normal dose, since kidney function is drastically reduced:

$$(0.057)(20 \text{ mg/kg}) = 1.14 \text{ mg/kg given every 6 hours}$$

5. From Figure 18-5, line F, at a Cl_{Cr} of 5 mL/min,

$$\frac{k_u}{k_N} = 45\%$$

a. The dose given should be as follows:

$$(0.45)(600 \text{ mg}) = 270 \text{ mg every 12 hours}$$

b. Alternatively, the dose of 600 mg should be given every

$$12 \times \frac{100}{45} = 26.7 \text{ hr}$$

c. Since it may be desirable to give the drug once every 24 hours, both dose and dosing interval may be adjusted so that the patient will still maintain an average therapeutic blood level of the drug, which can then be given at a convenient time. Using the equation for C_{av}^{∞},

$$C_{av}^{\infty} = \frac{D_0}{kV_D\tau}$$

$$D_0 = 600 \text{ mg}$$

$$\tau = 26.7 \text{ hr}$$

$$C_{av}^{\infty} = \frac{600}{kV_D \times 26.7}$$

To maintain C_{av}^{∞} the same, calculate a new dose, D_N, with a new dosing interval, τ_N, of 24 hours.

$$C_{av}^{\infty} = \frac{D_N}{kV_D 24}$$

Thus,

$$\frac{600}{26.7} = \frac{D_N}{24}$$

Therefore,

$$D_N = \frac{24}{26.7} \times 600 = 539 \text{ mg}$$

The drug can also be given at 540 mg daily.

6. For females, use 85% of the Cl_{Cr} value obtained in males.

$$Cl_{Cr} = \frac{0.85[140 - \text{age (yr)}] \text{ body weight (kg)}}{72\ (Cl_{Cr})}$$

$$= \frac{0.85[140 - 38]62}{(72)(1.8)} = 41.5 \text{ mL/min}$$

9. Gentamycin is listed in group K (Table 18-2). From the nomogram in Figure 18-5,

$$Cl_{Cr} = 20 \text{ mL/min} \qquad \frac{k_u}{k_n} = 25\%$$

Uremic dose = 25% of normal dose = (0.25) (1 mg/kg) = 0.25 mg/kg

For a 72-kg Patient:

Uremic dose = (0.25) (75) = 18.8 mg

The patient should receive 18.8 mg every 8 hours by multiple IV bolus injections.

10. **a.** During the first 48 hours postdose, $t_{1/2} = 16$ hours. For IV bolus injection, assuming first-order elimination:

$$D_B = D_0 e^{-kt}$$
$$= 1000e^{-(0.693/16)(48)}$$
$$= 125 \text{ mg remaining in body just prior to dialysis}$$

During dialysis, $t_{1/2} = 4$ hours, and

$$D_B = 125e^{-(0.693/4)(8)} = 31.3 \text{ mg after dialysis}$$

b. $V_D = (0.5 \text{ L/kg})(75 \text{ kg}) = 37.5 \text{ L}$

Drug concentration just prior to dialysis:

$$C_p = 125 \text{ mg}/37.5 \text{ L} = 3.33 \text{ mg/L}$$

Drug concentration just after dialysis:

$$C_p = 31.3 \text{ mg}/3.75 \text{ L} = 0.83 \text{ mg/L}$$

CHAPTER 19

FREQUENTLY ASKED QUESTIONS

1. Doubling a dose does not double the drug response (or the pharmacodynamic effect). The pharmacodynamic effect of a drug is proportional to the log of the plasma drug concentration—usually within 20 to 80% of the maximal response. Near the maximal pharmacodynamic effect, doubling the dose may only cause a very small increase in effect. No further increase in pharmacodynamic effect is achieved by an increase in dose once the maximum pharmacodynamic effect, E_{max}, is obtained.

2. For many drugs, the drug responses over time plotted versus plasma drug concentrations produces a loop-shaped (*hysteresis loop*) profile. The hysteresis loop shows that the plasma drug concentration is not always a good indicator of drug response. A *clockwise* hysteresis loop shows that response decreases with time and may be the result of drug tolerance or formation of an antagonistic metabolite. A *counterclockwise* hysteresis loop may be due to slower equilibration of the drug at the receptor site or to the formation of an agonist metabolite.

3. The *effect compartment* is postulated to describe the pharmacodynamics of drugs that are not well described by drug concentration in the plasma compartment. The effect compartment is assumed to be the receptor site in the body for drug response. Drug concentration in this site is referred to as drug concentration in the effect compartment. The amount of drug in the effect compartment is relatively small and is insignificant compared to the amount of drug in other tissues. Drug elimination from the effect compartment is governed by k_{eo}, a first-order rate constant that is estimated from the pharmacodynamic data. Drug concentration in the effect compartment may be equilibrated with the central compartment when a steady-state plasma drug concentration is reached.

LEARNING QUESTIONS

1. **a.** *True.* Drug concentration is more precise because an identical dose may result in different plasma drug concentration in different subjects due to individual differences in pharmacokinetics.
   b. *True.* The kinetic relationship between drug response and drug concentration is such that the response is proportional to log concentration of the drug.
   c. *True.* The data show that after IV bolus dose, the response begins at the same point indicating that the initial plasma drug concentration is the same. In uremic patients, the volume of distribution may be affected by changes in protein binding and electrolyte levels, which may range from little or no effect to strongly affecting the V_D.
   d. *False.* The drug is likely to be excreted through the kidney since the slope (elimination) is reduced in uremic patients.
   e. *True.* Assuming the volume of distribution is unchanged, the starting pharmacologic response should be the same if the receptor sensitivity is unchanged. In a few cases, receptor sensitivity to the drug can be altered in uremic patients. For example, the effect of digoxin will be more intense if the serum potassium level is depleted.

2. These antibiotics inhibit beta-lactamase by irreversible binding to the enzyme protein via an acylation reaction, similar to antibiotic-binding to the protein in the cell wall. Beta-lactamase breaks the cyclic amide bond of the antibiotics.

3. Several answers are possible:
   a. Pharmacokinetic considerations: Subsequent doses induce the hepatic drug metabolizing enzymes (auto-induction), thereby decreasing the elimination half-life resulting in lower steady-state drug concentrations.

b. Pharmacodynamic considerations: The patient develops tolerance to the drug resulting in the need for a higher dose to produce the same effect.

5. CNS drugs.

6. An allergic response to a drug may be unpredictable and does not generally follow a dose response relationship.

7. PAT (Postantibiotic Time) is the time for continued antibacterial activity even though the plasma antibiotic concentration has fallen below MEC, or minimum effective concentration.

8. AUC/MIC or AUIC is a pharmacokinetic parameter incorporating MIC together in order to provide better prediction of antibiotic response (cure percent). An example is ciprofloxacin. AUIC is a good predictor of percent cure in infection treated at various dose regimens.

CHAPTER 20

? FREQUENTLY ASKED QUESTIONS

1. Differential equations are used to describe the rate of drug transfer between different tissues and the blood. Differential equations have the advantage of being very adaptable to computer simulation without a lot of mathematical manipulations.

2. After an IV bolus drug injection, a drug is diluted rapidly in the venous pool. The venous blood is oxygenated in the lung and becomes arterial blood. The arterial blood containing the diluted drug then perfuses all the body organs through the systemic circulation. Some drug diffuses into the tissue and others are eliminated. In cycling through the body, the blood leaving a tissue (venous) generally has a lower drug concentration than the perfusing blood (arterial). In practice, only venous blood is sampled and assayed. Drug concentration in the venous blood rapidly equilibrates with the tissue and will become the arterial blood in the next perfusion cycle (seconds later) through the body. In pharmacokinetics, the drug concentration is assumed to decline smoothly and continuously. The difference in drug concentration between arterial and venous blood would reflect drug uptake by the tissue, and this difference may have important consequences in drug therapy, such as tumor treatment.

3. Statistical moment is adaptable to being used in mean residence time calculation and is widely used in pharmacokinetics.

4. *Mean residence time* (MRT) represents the average staying time of the drug in a body organ or compartment as the molecules diffuse in and out. MRT is an alternative concept used to describe how long a drug stays in the body. The main advantage of MRT is that it is based on probability and is consistent with how drug molecules behave in the physical world.

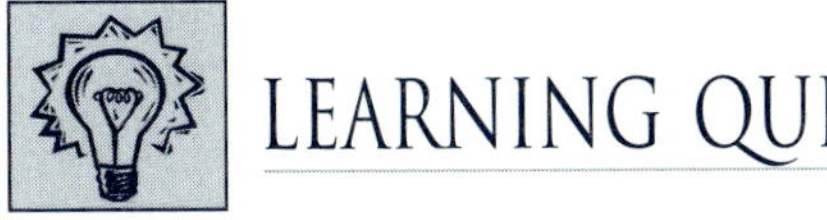

LEARNING QUESTIONS

1. **a.** $\text{MRT} = \dfrac{[\text{AUMC}]_0^\infty}{[\text{AUC}]_0^\infty} = \dfrac{100\ (\text{mg/L})\ \text{hr}^2}{25\ (\text{mg/L})\ \text{hr}} = 4\ \text{hr}$

   b. $Cl_T = \dfrac{D_0}{[\text{AUC}]_0^\infty} = \dfrac{500\ \text{mg}}{20\ (\text{mg/L})\ \text{hr}} = 25\ \text{L/hr}$

   c. V_{ss} may be calculated using Equation 20.49

   $\text{MRT} = Cl_T / V_{ss}$

   Therefore,

   $V_{ss} = Cl_T/\text{MRT} = 25/4 = 6.25\ \text{L}$

2. MRT is not directly calculated based on its definition (AUC/C_0) because it is not possible to determine C_0 except with simple data involving a one-compartment model. Based on rigorous derivation, C_0 is not C_p^0 except in a one-compartment IV bolus dose; rather, it is the concentration D_0/V_D which is equal to $C_p = C_p^0$ in the simple IV bolus dose. With oral absorption data, it is not possible to determine D_0/V_D without using a model.

3. If the data in problem 1 are fitted to obtain k, and $k = 0.25\ \text{hr}^{-1}$,

   $\text{MRT} = 1/\text{k} = 1/0.25 = 4\ \text{hrs}$

   Although the answer agrees with the result calculated above using a noncompartmental approach, the calculation now uses an equation with assumptions of the one-compartment model for IV bolus.

4. The principle considerations in interspecies scaling are size, protein–drug binding, and maximum lifespan potential (MLP) of the species.

5. The model assumptions should be consistent with known information about the system. The number of model parameters should not exceed the available data, and an adequate degree of freedom should be present to test for lack of fit. The law of parsimony should apply at all times.

APPENDIX D

GUIDING PRINCIPLES FOR HUMAN AND ANIMAL RESEARCH

WORLD MEDICAL ASSOCIATION DECLARATION OF HELSINKI

Recommendations guiding physicians
in biomedical research involving human subjects

Adopted by the 18th World Medical Assembly
Helsinki, Finland, June 1964

and amended by the
29th World Medical Assembly
Tokyo, Japan, October 1975
35th World Medical Assembly
Venice, Italy, October 1983
and the
41st World Medical Assembly
Hong Kong, September 1989

INTRODUCTION

It is the mission of the physician to safeguard the health of the people. His or her knowledge and conscience are dedicated to the fullfillment of this mission.

The Declaration of Geneva of the World Medical Association binds the physician with the words, "The health of my patient will be my first consideration," and the International Code of Medical Ethics declares that, "A physician shall act only in the patient's interest when providing medical care which might have the effect of weakening the physical and mental condition of the patient."

The purpose of biomedical research involving human subjects must be to improve diagnostic, therapeutic and prophylactic procedures and the understanding of the aetiology and pathogenesis of disease.

In current medical practice most diagnostic, therapeutic or prophylactic procedures involve hazards. This applies especially to biomedical research.

Medical progress is based on research which ultimately must rest in part on experimentation involving human subjects.

In the field of biomedical research a fundamental distinction must be recognized between medical research in which the aim is essentially diagnostic or therapeutic for a patient, and medical research, the essential object of which is purely scientific and without implying direct diagnostic or therapeutic value to the person subjected to the research.

Special caution must be exercised in the conduct of research which may affect the environment, and the welfare of animals used for research must be respected.

Because it is essential that the results of laboratory experiments be applied to human beings to further scientific knowledge and to help suffering humanity, the World Medical Association has prepared the following recommendations as a guide to every physician in biomedical research involving human subjects. They should be kept under review in the future. It must be stressed that the standards as drafted are only a guide to physicians all over the world. Physicians are not relieved from criminal, civil and ethical responsibilities under the laws of their own countries.

I. BASIC PRINCIPLES

1. Biomedical research involving human subjects must conform to generally accepted scientific principles and should be based on adequately performed laboratory and animal experimentation and a thorough knowledge of the scientific literature.
2. The design and performance of each experimental procedure involving human subjects should be clearly formulated in an experimental protocol which should be transmitted for consideration, comment and guidance to a specially appointed committee independent of the investigator and the sponsor, provided that this independent committee is in conformity with the laws and regulations of the country in which the research experiment is performed.
3. Biomedical research involving human subjects should be conducted only by scientifically qualified persons and under the supervision of a clinically competent medical person. The responsibility for the human subject must always rest with a medically qualified person and never rest on the subject of the research, even though the subject has given his or her consent.
4. Biomedical research involving human subjects cannot legitimately be carried out unless the importance of the objective is in proportion to the inherent risk to the subject.
5. Every biomedical research project involving human subjects should be preceded by careful assessment of predictable risks in comparison with foreseeable benefits to the subject or to others. Concern for the interests of the subject must always prevail over the interests of science and society.
6. The right of the research subject to safeguard his or her integrity must always be respected. Every precaution should be taken to respect the privacy of the subject and to minimize the impact of the study on the subject's physical and mental integrity and on the personality of the subject.
7. Physicians should abstain from engaging in research projects involving human subjects unless they are satisfied that the hazards involved are believed to be

predictable. Physicians should cease any investigation if the hazards are found to outweigh the potential benefits.

8. In publication of the results of his or her research, the physician is obliged to preserve the accuracy of the results. Reports of experimentation not in accordance with the principles laid down in this Declaration should not be accepted for publication.
9. In any research on human beings, each potential subject must be adequately informed of the aims, methods, anticipated benefits and potential hazards of the study and the discomfort it may entail. He or she should be informed that he or she is at liberty to abstain from participation in the study and that he or she is free to withdraw his or her consent to participation at any time. The physician should then obtain the subject's freely-given informed consent, preferably in writing.
10. When obtaining informed consent for the research project the physician should be particularly cautious if the subject is in a dependent relationship to him or her or may consent under duress. In that case the informed consent should be obtained by a physician who is not engaged in the investigation and who is completely independent of this official relationship.
11. In case of legal incompetence, informed consent should be obtained from the legal guardian in accordance with national legislation. Where physical or mental incapacity makes it impossible to obtain informed consent, or when the subject is a minor, permission from the responsible relative replaces that of the subject in accordance with national legislation.

    Whenever the minor child is in fact able to give a consent, the minor's consent must be obtained in addition to the consent of the minor's legal guardian.
12. The research protocol should always contain a statement of the ethical considerations involved and should indicate that the principles enunciated in the present Declaration are compiled with.

II. MEDICAL RESEARCH COMBINED WITH PROFESSIONAL CARE

(Clinical Research)

1. In the treatment of the sick person, the physician must be free to use a new diagnostic and therapeutic measure, if in his or her judgement it offers hope of saving life, reestablishing health or alleviating suffering.
2. The potential benefits, hazards and discomfort of a new method should be weighed against the advantages of the best current diagnostic and therapeutic methods.
3. In any medical study, every patient—including those of a control group, if any—should be assured of the best proven diagnostic and therapeutic method.
4. The refusal of the patient to participate in a study must never interfere with the physician-patient relationship.
5. If the physician considers it essential not to obtain informed consent, the specific reasons for this proposal should be stated in the experimental protocol for transmission to the independent committee (I, 2).
6. The physician can combine medical research with professional care, the objective being the acquisition of new medical knowledge, only to the extent that

medical research is justified by its potential diagnostic or therapeutic value for the patient.

III. NON-THERAPEUTIC BIOMEDICAL RESEARCH INVOLVING HUMAN SUBJECTS

(Non-clinical Biomedical Research)

1. In the purely scientific application of medical research carried out on a human being, it is the duty of the physician to remain the protector of the life and health of that person on whom biomedical research is being carried out.
2. The subjects should be volunteers—either healthy persons or patients for whom the experimental design is not related to the patient's illness.
3. The investigator or the investigating team should discontinue the research if in his/her or their judgement it may, if continued, be harmful to the individual.
4. In research on man, the interest of science and society should never take precedence over considerations related to the wellbeing of the subject.

GUIDING PRINCIPLES IN THE CARE AND USE OF ANIMALS

Animal experiments are to be undertaken only with the purpose of advancing knowledge. Consideration should be given to the appropriateness of experimental procedures, species of animals used, and number of animals required.

Only animals that are lawfully acquired shall be used in the laboratory, and their retention and use shall be in every case in compliance with federal, state, and local laws and regulations and in accordance with the NIH Guide.

Animals in the laboratory must receive every consideration for their comfort; they must be properly housed, fed, and their surroundings kept in a sanitary condition.

Appropriate anesthetics must be used to eliminate sensibility to pain during all surgical procedures. Where recovery from anesthesia is necessary during the study, acceptable technique to minimize pain must be followed. Muscle relaxants or paralytics are not anesthetics and they should not be used alone for surgical restraint. They may be used for surgery in conjunction with drugs known to produce adequate analgesia. Where use of anesthetics would negate the results of the experiment, such procedures should be carried out in strict accordance with the NIH Guide. If the study requires the death of the animal, the animal must be killed in a humane manner at the conclusion of the observations.

The postoperative care of animals shall be such as to minimize discomfort and pain, and in any case shall be equivalent to accepted practices in schools of veterinary medicine.

When animals are used by students for their education or the advancement of science, such work shall be under the direct supervision of an experienced teacher or investigator. The rules for the care of such animals must be the same as for animals used for research.

From Guide for the Care and Use of Laboratory Animals. DHEW publ. no. (NIH) 80-23, revised 1978, reprinted 1980. Bethesda, Office of Science and Health Reports, DDR/NIH.

APPENDIX E

POPULAR DRUGS AND PHARMACOKINETIC PARAMETERS

TABLE E.1 Pharmacokinetic and Pharmacodynamic Parameters for Selected Drugs[1]

DRUG	ORAL AVAILABILITY (%)	URINARY EXCRETION (%)	BOUND IN PLASMA (%)	CLEARANCE[2] (mL/min)	VOLUME OF DISTRIBUTION (L)	HALF-LIFE (hr)	EFFECTIVE[3] CONCENTRATIONS	TOXIC[3] CONCENTRATIONS
Acetaminophen	88 ± 15	3 ± 1	0	350 ± 100	67 ± 8	2.0 ± 0.4	10–20 μg/mL	>300 μg/mL
Acyclovir	15–30	75 ± 10	15 ± 4	330 ± 80	48 ± 13	2.4 ± 0.7		
Alendrenate	0.59 (0.58–0.98)					very long (related to bone turnover)		
Alprazolam	88 ± 16	20	71 ± 3	0.74 ± 0.14 ml/min/kg	0.72 ± 0.12 L/Kg	12 ± 2 hr	20–40 ng/mL	
Alteplase (TPA)	—	LOW	—	10 ± 4 ml/min/kg	0.1 ± 0.01 L/Kg	0.08 ± 0.04 hr		
Amikacin		98	4	91 ± 42	19 ± 4	2.3 ± 0.4		
Amoxicillin	93 ± 10	86 ± 8	18	180 ± 28	15 ± 2	1.7 ± 0.3		
Amphotericin B		2–5	>90	32 ± 14	53 ± 36	18 ± 7		
Ampicillin	62 ± 17	82 ± 10	18 ± 2	270 ± 50	20 ± 5	1.3 ± 0.2		
Aspirin[4]	68 ± 3	1.4 ± 1.2	49	650 ± 80	11 ± 2	0.25 ± 0.3	See Salicyclic acid	
Atenolol	56 ± 30	94 ± 8	<5	170 ± 14	67 ± 11	6.1 ± 2.0	1 μg/mL	
Atropine	50	57 ± 8	14–22	410 ± 250	120 ± 49	4.3 ± 1.7		
Captopril	65	38 ± 11	30 ± 6	840 ± 100	57 ± 13	2.2 ± 0.5	50 ng/mL	
Carbamazepine[4]	>70	<1	74 ± 3	89 ± 37	98 ± 26	15 ± 5	6.5 ± 3 μg/mL	>9 μg/mL
Cephalexin	90 ± 9	91 ± 18	14 ± 3	300 ± 80	18 ± 2	0.90 ± 0.18		
Cephalothin		52	71 ± 3	470 ± 120	18 ± 8	0.57 ± 0.32		
Chloramphenicol	75–90	25 ± 15	53 ± 5	170 ± 14	66 ± 4	2.7 ± 0.8		
Chlordiazepoxide[4]	100	<1	96.5 ± 1.8	38 ± 34	21 ± 2	10 ± 3	>0.7 μg/mL	
Chloroquine[4]	89 ± 16	61 ± 4	61 ± 9	750 ± 120	13,000 ± 4600	8.9 ± 3.1 days	15–30 ng/mL	0.25 μg/mL
Chlorpropamide	>90	20 ± 18	96 ± 1	2.1 ± 0.4	6.8 ± 0.8	33 ± 6		
Cimetidine	62 ± 6	62 ± 20	19	540 ± 130	70 ± 14	1.9 ± 0.3	0.8 μg/mL	
Ciprofloxacin	60 ± 12	65 ± 12	40	420 ± 84	130 ± 28	4.1 ± 0.9		
Clonidine	95	62 ± 11	20	210 ± 84	150 ± 30	12 ± 7	0.2–2 ng/mL	
Cyclosporine	23.7	<1	93 ± 2	410 ± 70	85 ± 15	5.6 ± 2	100–400 ng/mL	>400 ng/mL
Cylosporine	27 ± 9	<1	93 ± 2	5.3 ± 1.5 mL/min/kg	1.3 ± 0.3 L/kg	5.6 ± 0.2 hr		

DRUG	ORAL AVAILABILITY (%)	URINARY EXCRETION (%)	BOUND IN PLASMA (%)	CLEARANCE[2] (mL/min)	VOLUME OF DISTRIBUTION (L)	HALF-LIFE (hr)	EFFECTIVE[3] CONCENTRATIONS	TOXIC[3] CONCENTRATIONS
Diazepam[4]	100	<1	98.7 ± 0.2	27 ± 4	77 ± 20	43 ± 13	300–400 ng/mL	
Digitoxin	>90	32 ± 15	97 ± 1	3.9 ± 1.3	38 ± 10	6.7 ± 1.7 days	>10 ng/mL	>35 ng/mL
Digoxin	70 ± 13	60 ± 11	25 ± 5	130 ± 67	440 ± 150	39 ± 13	>0.8 ng/mL	>2 ng/mL
Diltiazem[4]	44 ± 10	<4	78 ± 3	840 ± 280	220 ± 85	3.7 ± 1.2		
Diflunisal	90	6 ± 3	99.9 ± 0.01	0.1 ± 0.02 mL/min/kg	0.1 ± 0.02 L/kg	11 ± 2 hr		
Dirithromycin	10% (6–14) abs bio (urinary data)	17–25	10–30	226–1040 mL/min	800 L (504–1041)	44 hr (16–65)		
Disopyramide	83 ± 11	55 ± 6	Dose-dependent	84 ± 28	41 ± 11	6.0 ± 1.0	3 ± 1 μg/mL	>8 μg/mL
Erythromycin	35 ± 25	12 ± 7	84 ± 3	640 ± 290	55 ± 31	1.6 ± 0.7		
Erythropoietin				7.88 mL/min	3.70 L per 1.73 m^2	4.92 hr		
Ethambutol	77 ± 8	79 ± 3	<5	600 ± 60	110 ± 14	3.1 ± 0.4		>10 μg/mL
Ethosuximide	—	25 ± 15	0	0.19 ± 0.04 mL/min/kg	0.72 ± 0.16 L/kg	45 ± 8 hr	40–100 μg/mL	
Famciclovir	77 ± 8	74 ± 9	<20	8.0 ± 1.5 mL/min/kg	0.98 ± 0.13 L/kg	2.3 ± 0.4 hr		
Famotidine	45 ± 14	67 ± 15	17 ± 7	7.1 ± 1.7 mL/min/kg	1.3 ± 0.2 L/kg	2.6 ± 1.0 hr	13 ng/ml	
Fluoxetine	>60	<2.5	94	9.6 ± 6.9 mL/min/kg	35 ± 21 L/kg	53 ± 41 hr	<500 ng/mL	
Furosemide	61 ± 17	66 ± 7	98.8 ± 0.2	140 ± 30	7.7 ± 1.4	1.5 ± 0.1		25 μg/mL
Ganciclovir	3	73 ± 31	1–2	4.6 ± 1.8 mL/min/kg	1.1 ± 0.3 L/kg	4.3 ± 1.6 hr		
Gentamicin		>90	<10	90 ± 25	18 ± 6	2–3		
Hydralazine	20–60	1–15	87	3900 ± 900	105 ± 70	1.0 ± 0.3	100 ng/mL	
Imipramine[4]	40 ± 12	<2	90.1 ± 1.4	1050 ± 280	1600 ± 600	18 ± 7	100–300 ng/mL	>1 μg/mL
Indinavir						~3 hr		
Indomethacin	98	15 ± 8	90	140 ± 30	18 ± 5	2.4 ± 0.4	0.3–3 μg/mL	>5 μg/mL
Labetalol	18 ± 5	<5	50	1750 ± 700	660 ± 240	4.9 ± 2.0	0.13 μg/mL	

(Continued)

TABLE E.1 Pharmacokinetic and Pharmacodynamic Parameters for Selected Drugs[1] *(Continued)*

DRUG	ORAL AVAILABILITY (%)	URINARY EXCRETION (%)	BOUND IN PLASMA (%)	CLEARANCE[2] (mL/min)	VOLUME OF DISTRIBUTION (L)	HALF-LIFE (hr)	EFFECTIVE[3] CONCENTRATIONS	TOXIC[3] CONCENTRATIONS
Lidocaine	35 ± 11	2 ± 1	70 ± 5	640 ± 170	77 ± 28	1.8 ± 0.4	1.5–6 μg/mL	>6 μg/mL
Lithium	100	95 ± 15	0	25 ± 8	55 ± 24	22 ± 8	0.5–1.25 meq/L	>2 meq/L
Lomefloxacin	97 ± 2	65 ± 9	10	3.3 ± 0.5 mL/min/kg	2.3 ± 0.3 L/kg	8.0 ± 1.4 hr		
Lovastatin	<5	negligible	95	4–18 mL/min/kg	—	1.1–1.7 hr	—	
Meperidine	52 ± 3	1–25	58 ± 9	1200 ± 350	310 ± 60	3.2 ± 0.8	0.4–0.7 μg/mL	
Methotrexate	70 ± 27	48 ± 18	34 ± 8	150 ± 60	39 ± 13	7.2 ± 2.1		10 μM
Metoprolol	38 ± 14	10 ± 3	11 ± 1	1050 ± 210	290 ± 50	3.2 ± 0.2	25 ng/mL	
Metronidazole[4]	99 ± 8	10 ± 2	10	90 ± 20	52 ± 7	8.5 ± 2.9	3–6 μg/mL	
Mexiletine	87 ± 13	4–15	63 ± 3	6.3 ± 2.7 ml/min/kg	4.9 ± 0.5 L/kg	9.2 ± 2.1 hr	0.5–2.0 μg/mL	>2.0 μg/mL
Midazolam	44 ± 17	56 ± 26	95 ± 2	460 ± 130	77 ± 42	1.9 ± 0.6		
Morphine	24 ± 12	6–10	35 ± 2	1600 ± 700	230 ± 60	1.9 ± 0.5	65 ng/mL	
Moxalactam		76 ± 12	50	120 ± 30	19 ± 6	2.1 ± 0.7		
Notilmicin	—	80–90	<10	1.3 ± 0.2 ml/min/kg	0.2 ± 0.02 L/kg	2.3 ± 0.7 hr		
Nifedipine	50 ± 13	0	96 ± 1	490 ± 130	55 ± 15	1.8 ± 0.4	47 ± 20 ng/mL	
Nortriptyline[4]	51 ± 5	2 ± 1	92 ± 2	500 ± 130	1300 ± 300	31 ± 13	50–140 ng/mL	>500 ng/mL
Phenobarbital	100 ± 11	24 ± 5	51 ± 3	4.3 ± 0.9	38 ± 2	4.1 ± 0.8 days	10–25 μg/mL	>30 μg/mL
Phenytoin	90 ± 3	2	89 ± 23	Dose-dependent	45 ± 3	Dose-dependent	>10 μg/mL	>20 μg/mL
Pravastatin	18 ± 8	47 ± 7	43–48	3.5 ± 2.4 ml/min/kg	0.46 ± 0.04 L/kg	1.8 ± 0.8 hr		
Prazosin	68 ± 17	<1	95 ± 1	210 ± 20	42 ± 9	2.9 ± 0.8		
Procainamide[4]	83 ± 16	67 ± 8	16 ± 5	350–840	130 ± 20	3.0 ± 0.6	3–14 μg/mL	>14 μg/mL
Propranolol[4]	26 ± 10	<0.5	87 ± 6	840 ± 210	270 ± 40	3.9 ± 0.4	20 ng/mL	
Pyridostigmine	14 ± 3	80–90		600 ± 120	77 ± 21	1.9 ± 0.2	50–100 ng/mL	
Quinidine[4]	80 ± 15	18 ± 5	87 ± 3	330 ± 130	190 ± 80	6.2 ± 1.8	2–6 μg/mL	>8 μg/mL
Ranitidine	52 ± 11	69 ± 6	15 ± 3	730 ± 80	91 ± 28	2.1 ± 0.2	100 ng/mL	

DRUG	ORAL AVAILABILITY (%)	URINARY EXCRETION (%)	BOUND IN PLASMA (%)	CLEARANCE[2] (mL/min)	VOLUME OF DISTRIBUTION (L)	HALF-LIFE (hr)	EFFECTIVE[3] CONCENTRATIONS	TOXIC[3] CONCENTRATIONS
Ribavirin	45 ± 5	35 ± 8	0	5 ± 1.0 ml/min/kg	9.3 ± 1.5 L/kg	28 ± 7 hr		
Rifampin[4]		7 ± 3	89 ± 1	240 ± 110	68 ± 25	3.5 ± 0.8		
Ritonavir	<5	high (AAG)				~3 hr		
Saquinavir	<5	high (AAG)		*<989 L/hr	*<1503 L	7–12 hr (beta) (1.38 hr)		
Salicylic acid	100	2–30	80–90[5]	14[5]	12 ± 2	10–15[5]	150–300 µg/mL	>200 µg/mL
Simvastatin	<5	negligible	94	7.6 ml/min/kg	—	1.9 hr	—	—
Sotalol	90–100	>75	0	2.6 ± 0.5 ml/min/kg	2.0 ± 0.4 L/kg	12 ± 3 hr		
Sulfamethoxazole	100	14 ± 2	62 ± 5	22 ± 3	15 ± 1.4	10 ± 5		
Sulfisoxazole	96 ± 14	49 ± 8	91 ± 1	23 ± 3.5	10.5 ± 1.4	6.6 ± 0.7		
Sumatriptan	14 ± 5 (oral) 97 ± 16 (SQ)	22 ± 4	14–21	16 ± 2 ml/min/kg	0.65 ± 0.1 L/kg	1.9 ± 0.3 hr		
Tamoxifen	—	<1	>98	1.4 ml/min/kg	50–60 L/kg	4–11 days		
Terbutaline	14 ± 2	56 ± 4	20	240 ± 40	125 ± 15	14 ± 2	2.3 ± 1.8 ng/mL	
Tetracycline	77	58 ± 8	65 ± 3	120 ± 20	105 ± 6	11 ± 1.5		
Theophylline	96 ± 8	18 ± 3	56 ± 4	48 ± 21	35 ± 11	8.1 ± 2.4	10–20 µg/mL	>20 µg/mL
Tobramycin		90	<10	77	18 ± 6	2.2 ± 0.1		
Tocainide	89 ± 5	38 ± 7	10 ± 15	180 ± 35	210 ± 15	14 ± 2	6–15 µg/mL	
Tolbutamide	93 ± 10	0	96 ± 1	17 ± 3	7 ± 1	5.9 ± 1.4	80–240 µg/mL	
Trimethoprim	100	69 ± 17	44	150 ± 40	130 ± 15	11 ± 1.4		
Tubocurarine		63 ± 35	50 ± 8	135 ± 42	27 ± 8	2.0 ± 1.1	0.6 ± 0.2 µg/mL	
Valproic acid	100 ± 10	1.8 ± 2.4	93 ± 1	7.7 ± 1.4	9.1 ± 2.8	14 ± 3	30–100 µg/mL	>150 µg/mL
Vancomycin		79 ± 11	30 ± 10	98 ± 7	27 ± 4	5.6 ± 1.8		
Verapamil	22 ± 8 (oral) 35 ± 13 (Sublingual)	<3	90 ± 2	15 ± 6 ml/min/kg	5.0 ± 2.1 L/kg	4.0 ± 1.5 hr	120 ± 20 ng/mL	
Warfarin	93 ± 8	<2	99 ± 1	3.2 ± 1.7	9.8 ± 4.2	37 ± 15	2.2 ± 0.4 µg/mL	

(Continued)

TABLE E.1 Pharmacokinetic and Pharmacodynamic Parameters for Selected Drugs[1] *(Continued)*

DRUG	ORAL AVAILABILITY (%)	URINARY EXCRETION (%)	BOUND IN PLASMA (%)	CLEARANCE[2] (mL/min)	VOLUME OF DISTRIBUTION (L)	HALF-LIFE (hr)	EFFECTIVE[3] CONCENTRATIONS	TOXIC[3] CONCENTRATIONS
Zidovudine	63 ± 13	18 ± 5	<25	26 ± 6 ml/min/kg	1.4 ± 0.4 L/kg	1.1 ± 0.2 hr		
Zalcitabine	88 ± 17	65 ± 17	<4	4.1 ± 1.2 ml/min/kg	0.53 ± 0.13 L/kg	2.0 ± 0.8 hr		

[1]The values in this table represent the parameters determined when the drug is administered to healthy normal volunteers or to patients who are generally free from disease except for the condition for which the drug is being prescribed. The values presented here are adapted, with permission, from Hardman JG: Design and optimization of dosage regimens: Pharmacokinetic data. In: *Goodman and Gilman's The Pharmacological Basis of Therapeutics*. 9th ed. Gilman AG et al (editors). McGraw-Hill, 1995. This source must be consulted for the effects of disease states on the pertinent pharmacokinetic parameters.
[2]For a standard 70-kg person.
[3]No pharmacodynamic values are given for antibiotics since these vary depending upon the infecting organism.
[4]One or more metabolites are active. Clearance given for aspirin is for conversion to the active metabolite, salicylic acid; see that compound for further clearance data.
[5]The values are within the therapeutic range for drugs exhibiting dose-dependent pharmacokinetics.
[6]Volume of distribution and clearance determined orally (when F is unknown, *Cl/F*, or V_D/F) are listed as less than actual since F may be less than 1.
[7]Effective levels for antibiotics are variable depending on the susceptibility of the microorganisms.
[8]Generally, the beta half-life is listed, but it may be essential to consult the alpha half-life if the effective concentration is high or the distributive phase is long.
[9]The percent of urinary drug excretion is 100 fe, fe is the fraction of drug excreted unchanged."100–100 fe" yields the percent of drug eliminated by other routes, often assumed to be metabolism. It is worth noting that in some cases the mass balance may be off, and sometimes biliary excretion is significant.
[10]For simplicity, most PK parameters are listed without consideration of the curvilinear phase which is present for most drugs.
[11]Some parameters are listed on a per kilogram basis, whereas others are parameters based on average BW or body surface reported in the study.
From Katzung BG: Basic & Clinical Pharmacology. 7th ed. Norwalk, CT, Appleton & Lange, 1998.

Physician's Desk Reference, 1997

Dirithromycin:
Sides GD et al, Anti Micr. Chem. 31; Supp C: P65–75, 1993

Erythropoetin:
Jensen-JD et al: J-Am-Soc-Nephrol. 1994 Aug; 5(2):177–85

Indinavir:
Lin JH et al: Drug Metab Dispos 1996 Oct;24(10):1111–1120

Alendronate:
Gertz BJ, Holland SD, Kline WF, Matuszewski BK, Freeman A, Quan H, Lasseter KC, Mucklow JC, Porras: Clin Pharmacol Ther, 1995 Sep (3):288–298

Protease inhibitors:
Barry M, Gibbons S, Back D, Mulcahy F: Clin Pharmacokinet 1997 Mar;32(3):194–209

Zidovudine, zalcitabine, and saquinavir:
Vanhove GF, Kastrissios H, Gries JM, Verotta D, Park K, Collier AC, Squires K, Sheiner LB, Blaschke: Antimicrob Agents Chemother 1997 Nov;2428–2432

APPENDIX F

GLOSSARY

Ab	Amount of drug in the body of time t
Ab^{∞}	Total amount of drug in the body
A, B, C	Preexponential constants for three-compartment model equation
a, b, c	Exponents for three-compartment model equation
AUC	Area under the plasma level–time curve
$[AUC]_0^{\infty}$	Area under the plasma level–time curve extrapolated to infinite time
AUMC	Area under the (first) moment versus time curve
C_{av}^{∞}	Average steady-state plasma drug concentration
C_C or C_p	Concentration of drug in the central compartment
C_{Cr}	Serum creatinine concentration, usually expressed as mg%
C_d	Concentration of drug
C_{eff}	Minimum effective drug concentration
C_{GI}	Concentration of drug in gastrointestinal tract
C_m	Metabolite plasma concentration
C_{max}	Maximum concentration of drug
C_{max}^{∞}	Maximum steady-state drug concentration
C_{min}	Minimum concentration of drug
C_{min}^{∞}	Minimum steady-state drug concentration
C_p	Concentration of drug in plasma
C_p^0	Concentration of drug in plasma at zero time ($t = 0$)
C_p^{∞}	Steady-state plasma drug concentration (equivalent to C_{ss})
C_{p_t}	Last measured plasma drug concentration
C_{ss}	Concentration of drug at steady state
C_t	Concentration of drug in tissue
Cl_{Cr}	Creatinine clearance
Cl_D	Dialysis clearance
Cl_h	Hepatic clearance
Cl_{int}	Intrinsic clearance
Cl_{int}	Intrinsic clearance (unbound drug)
Cl_{nr}	Nonrenal clearance
Cl_R	Renal clearance
Cl_T	Total body clearance
D	Amount of drug
D_A	Amount of drug absorbed
D_B	Amunt of drug in body
D_e	Drug eliminated
D_{GI}	Amount of drug in gastrointestinal tract
D_L	Loading (initial) dose
D_m	Maintenance dose
D_0	Dose of drug (same as D^0)
D^0	Amount of drug at zero time ($t = 0$)
D_t	Amount of drug in tissue
D_u	Amount of drug in urine
D_{μ}^{∞}	Total amount of drug excreted in the urine
E	Pharmacologic effect

e	Intercept on y axis of graph relating pharmacologic response against log drug concentration
E_0	Pharmacologic effect at zero drug concentration
E_{max}	Maximum pharmacologic effect
EC_{50}	Drug concentration that produces 50% maximum pharmacologic effect
ELS	Extended least square
ER	Extraction constant
F	Fraction of dose absorbed (bioavailability factor)
f	Fraction of dose remaining in body
f_e	Fraction of drug excreted unchanged in urine
$f(t)$	Function representing drug elimination over time (time is the independent variable)
GFR	Glomerular filtration rate
GI	Gastrointestinal tract
$f'(t)$	Derivative of $f(t)$
k	Overall drug elimination rate constant (first order)
K_a	Association binding constant
k_a	First-order absorption rate constant
k_e	Excretion rate constant (first order)
k_{1e}	Transfer rate constant from the central to the effect compartment
k_{e0}	Transfer rate constant out of the effect compartment
K_M	Michaelis–Menten constant
k_m	Metabolism rate constant (first order)
k_N	Normal elimination rate constant (first order)
k_0	Zero-order absorption rate constant
k_u	Uremic elimination rate constant (first order)
k_{12}	Transfer rate constant (from the central to the tissue compartment)
k_{21}	Transfer rate constant (from the tissue to the central compartment)
LBW	Lean body weight
m	Slope
m	Slope of E versus log C
MAT	Mean absorption time
MDT	Mean dissolution time
MEC	Minimum effective concentration
MLP	Maximum lifespan potential
MRT	Mean residence time
$\mathbf{MRT_c}$	Mean residence time from the central compartment
$\mathbf{MRT_p}$	Mean residence time from the peripheral compartment
$\mathbf{MRT_t}$	Mean residence time from the tissue compartment (same as MRT_p)
MTC	Minimum toxic concentration
$\mathbf{M_u}$	Amount of metabolite excreted in urine
μ_0	Area under the zero moment curve (same as AUC)
μ_1	Area under the first moment curve (same as AUMC)
NON MEN	Nonlinear mixed effect model
P	Amount of protein
Q	Blood flow
R	Pharmacologic response, infusion rate
r	Ratio of mole of drug bound to total moles of protein
R_{max}	Maximum pharmacologic response
τ	Time interval between doses
t	Time
t_{eff}	Duration of pharmacologic response to drug
t_{inf}	Infusion period
t_{max}	Time of occurrence for maximum (peak) drug concentration
t_{lag}	Lag time
t_0	Initial or zero time
$t_{1/2}$	Half-life
v	Velocity
V_C	Volume of central compartment (same as V_p)
V_D	Volume of distribution
$(V_D)_{exp}$	Extrapolated volume of distribution
$(V_D)_{ss}$	Steady-state volume of distribution
V_e	Volume of the effect compartment
V_{max}	Maximum metabolic rate
V_p	Volume of plasma (central compartment)
V_t	Volume of tissue compartment

INDEX

Page numbers in *italics* denote figures; those followed by "t" denote tables.

D

F

G

H

S